Handbook of
Research on Student Engag

Sandra L. Christenson • Amy L. Reschly
Cathy Wylie
Editors

Handbook of Research on Student Engagement

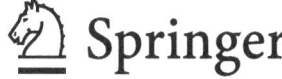

Editors
Sandra L. Christenson
Department of Educational Psychology
University of Minnesota
Minneapolis, MN, USA

Amy L. Reschly
Department of Educational Psychology
and Instructional Technology
University of Georgia
Athens, GA, USA

Cathy Wylie
New Zealand Council
for Educational Research
Wellington, New Zealand

ISBN 978-1-4614-2017-0 (hardcover)   ISBN 978-1-4614-2018-7 (eBook)
ISBN 978-1-4614-6791-5 (softcover)
DOI 10.1007/978-1-4614-2018-7
Springer New York Heidelberg Dordrecht London

Library of Congress Control Number: 2011944509

© Springer Science+Business Media New York 2012, First softcover printing 2013
This work is subject to copyright. All rights are reserved by the Publisher, whether the whole or part of the material is concerned, specifically the rights of translation, reprinting, reuse of illustrations, recitation, broadcasting, reproduction on microfilms or in any other physical way, and transmission or information storage and retrieval, electronic adaptation, computer software, or by similar or dissimilar methodology now known or hereafter developed. Exempted from this legal reservation are brief excerpts in connection with reviews or scholarly analysis or material supplied specifically for the purpose of being entered and executed on a computer system, for exclusive use by the purchaser of the work. Duplication of this publication or parts thereof is permitted only under the provisions of the Copyright Law of the Publisher's location, in its current version, and permission for use must always be obtained from Springer. Permissions for use may be obtained through RightsLink at the Copyright Clearance Center. Violations are liable to prosecution under the respective Copyright Law.
The use of general descriptive names, registered names, trademarks, service marks, etc. in this publication does not imply, even in the absence of a specific statement, that such names are exempt from the relevant protective laws and regulations and therefore free for general use.
While the advice and information in this book are believed to be true and accurate at the date of publication, neither the authors nor the editors nor the publisher can accept any legal responsibility for any errors or omissions that may be made. The publisher makes no warranty, express or implied, with respect to the material contained herein.

Printed on acid-free paper

Springer is part of Springer Science+Business Media (www.springer.com)

Preface

Who are engaged students? And why are students engaged? What are the antecedents and outcomes of engaged students and engaging contexts? How do engaging contexts (schools, families, peers) affect students and, in turn, student outcomes? What is the relationship between engagement, learning, achievement, and other long-term outcomes, such as high school completion and college attendance? What conditions foster reengagement of students who are no longer invested in learning or school? Questions such as these have captured the interest and curiosity of international researchers from a range of disciplines, including educational psychology, developmental psychology, public health, and teacher education for the past two decades.

Active research on student engagement has occurred primarily in the past 25 years, advancing with an article in 1985 by Mosher and McGowan. There are questions and unresolved issues related to engagement, which this volume explores; however, there is also general consensus regarding a number of facets of engagement theory and research, such as:

- Student engagement is considered the primary theoretical model for understanding dropout and promoting school completion, defined as graduation from high school with sufficient academic and social skills to partake in postsecondary educational options and/or the world of work (Christenson et al., 2008; Finn, 2006; Reschly & Christenson, 2006b).
- Engaged students do more than attend or perform academically; they also put forth effort, persist, self-regulate their behavior toward goals, challenge themselves to exceed, and enjoy challenges and learning (Klem & Connell, 2004; National Research Council and the Institute of Medicine [NRC and IoM], 2004).
- Student engagement, irrespective of the specificity of its definition, is generally associated positively with desired academic, social, and emotional learning outcomes (Klem & Connell, 2004).
- Engagement is a multidimensional construct – one that requires an understanding of affective connections within the academic environment (e.g., positive adult-student and peer relationships) and active student behavior (e.g., attendance, participation, effort, prosocial behavior) (Appleton, Christenson, & Furlong, 2008; Newmann, Wehlage, & Lamborn, 1992).
- The role of context cannot be ignored. Engagement is not conceptualized as an attribute of the student but rather as an alterable state of being that is highly influenced by the capacity of school, family, and peers to provide

consistent expectations and supports for learning (Reschly & Christenson, 2006a, 2006b). Engagement is an active image (Wylie, 2009) depicting effortful learning through interaction with the teacher and the classroom learning opportunities. In short, both the individual and context matter.
- Student engagement reinforces the notion that effective instruction explicitly considers and programs for the role of student motivation on learning outcomes (NRC and IoM, 2004; Russell, Ainley, & Frydenberg, 2005).
- The increase in student engagement measures with adequate psychometric properties has cemented the power and value of student engagement as a useful variable for data-driven decision-making efforts in schools (Appleton, Christenson, Kim, & Reschly, 2006; Betts, Appleton, Reschly, Christenson, & Huebner, 2010; Darr, 2009; Fredricks et al., 2011).
- There is an emerging intervention database that suggests evidence-based or promising strategies for educators to employ to enhance student engagement (Christenson et al., 2008).

This volume seeks to address a number of the "unknowns" that characterize theory and research on student engagement. These unknowns, or in some cases controversies in the field, affect the advancement of research on student engagement and, consequently, our knowledge base for improving student learning outcomes. We offer the following:

- Some researchers consider student engagement a "metaconstruct" or an organizing framework – one that integrates such areas as belonging, behavioral participation, motivation, self-efficacy, school connectedness, and so forth (Fredricks, Blumenfeld, & Paris, 2004), while others disagree, believing that engagement must have clearly defined boundaries (Finn & Kasza, 2009).
- Although researchers have reached consensus that student engagement is multidimensional, agreement on the multidimensionality differs from agreement on the number and types of engagement dimensions, which ranges from two to four. It may be that consensus only will be achieved with respect that student engagement is multidimensional, and, if so, researchers will need to define clearly their conceptualization in each study.
- Other methodological considerations (e.g., selection of informants, validity of self-report, common agreement of items within dimensions, development of instruments with strong psychometric properties) must be addressed if the construct and application of student engagement to practice will be advanced.
- The relationship between and/or differentiation of engagement and motivation is subject to debate (Appleton et al., 2006, 2008). What is the relationship between these two constructs? Are motivation and engagement separate? Can one be motivated but not actively engaged in a task or goal accomplishment?

Recently, there has been a proliferation of definitions of student engagement. Definitions of the terms of engagement, student engagement, school engagement, engagement in schoolwork, and academic engagement have been offered. These conceptualizations vary further along a number of other dimensions, such as participation, behavior, action, emotion, investment, motivation, and so on (see Appleton et al., 2008). Some studies have considered engagement as a process, while others conceptualize it as an outcome (Appleton et al., 2008; Skinner, Furrer, Marchand, & Kinderman, 2008). We contend that establishing construct validity for student engagement requires common agreement regarding what comprises the engagement construct – or what engagement is and what it is not. It demands an understanding of whether engagement is the outcome, a process to other desired outcomes, or plays a dual role. The constancy of the construct across researchers – in conceptualization and measurement – is a worthy endeavor, one with practical, scientific, and policy implications.

To date, conceptual clarity and methodological rigor (e.g., use of psychometrically sound measures) have not been achieved; they are considered a prerequisite to advance the emerging construct of student engagement and its usefulness in interventions and school programs. A particular concern addressed in this volume is the apparent overlap and confusion of engagement with motivation-to-learn variables. We designed this handbook as a way to create a dialogue among engagement and motivational researchers. To do so, we invited authors to cover their research topic and to respond to the following questions:

- What is your definition of engagement and motivation? How do you differentiate the two?
- What overarching framework or theory do you use to study/explain engagement or motivation?
- What is the role of context in explaining engagement or motivation?
- Focusing on the emerging construct of student engagement, what are necessary advances in theory, research, and practice to propel this construct forward?

The 34 chapters were placed into one of these 5 parts: (1) What Is Student Engagement? (2) Engagement as Linked to Motivational Variables, (3) Engagement and Contextual Influences, (4) Student Engagement: Determinants and Student Outcomes, and (5) Measurement Issues, Instruments, and Approaches. We also solicited an expert commentary for each of the above parts, for a total of 39 chapters. As coeditors, we are grateful to both the chapter and commentary authors.

Engagement is thought to be especially important for apathetic and discouraged learners (Brophy, 2004) and those at high risk for dropping out, but the primary appeal of the engagement construct is that it is relevant for *all* students. The universal appeal of engagement is underscored by high school reform efforts that explicitly address students' motivation to learn and engagement with school (NRC and IoM, 2004). Thus, student engagement underlies school reform – or what we seek to engender for all students through the school environment, teaching, and coursework. In addition, indicators of engagement may be used for screening and early detection of disengagement; these indicators provide links to intervention targets to reengage students at school and with learning.

Establishing construct validity for student engagement is integral to its utility in classrooms and the value of future scientific studies. The authors in this volume provided definitions for student engagement, offered their perspective on engagement and motivation, underscored the role of contextual influences, and proposed a range of future research directions. It is our hope, as coeditors, that this comprehensive volume stimulates the quality of student engagement research and advances the field. Let the dialogue begin.

Minneapolis, MN, USA	Sandra L. Christenson
Athens, GA, USA	Amy L. Reschly
Wellington, New Zealand	Cathy Wylie

References

Appleton, J., Christenson, S. L., Kim, D., & Reschly, A. (2006). Measuring cognitive and psychological engagement: Validation of the Student Engagement Instrument. *Journal of School Psychology, 44*, 427–445.

Appleton, J. J., Christenson, S. L., & Furlong, M. J. (2008). Student engagement with school: Critical conceptual and methodological issues of the construct. *Psychology in the Schools, 45*, 369–386.

Betts, J., Appleton, J. J., Reschly, A. L., Christenson, S. L., & Huebner, E. S. (2010). A study of the reliability and construct validity of the Student Engagement Instrument across multiple grades. *School Psychology Quarterly, 25*, 84–93.

Brophy, J. (2004). *Motivating students to learn* (2nd ed.). Mahwah, NJ: Lawrence Erlbaum.

Christenson, S. L., Reschly, A. L., Appleton, J. J., Berman, S., Spanjers, D., & Varro, P. (2008). Best practices in fostering student engagement. In A. Thomas, & J. Grimes (Eds.), *Best practices in school psychology* (5th ed.). Bethesda, MD: National Association of School Psychologists.

Darr, C. (2009). The me and my school survey. In J. Morton (Ed.), *Engaging young people in learning: Why does it matter and what can we do?: Conference proceedings* (pp. 85–100). Wellington, New Zealand: New Zealand Council for Educational Research.

Finn, J. D. (2006). *The adult lives of at-risk students: The roles of attainment and engagement in high school* (NCES 2006–328). Washington, DC: U.S. Department of Education, National Center for Education Statistics.

Finn, J. D., & Kasza, K. A. (2009). Disengagement from School. In *Engaging young people in learning: Why does it matter and what can we do?* (pp. 4–35). Wellington, New Zealand: New Zealand Council for Educational Research.

Fredricks, J., McColskey, W., Meli, J., Mordica, J., Montrosse, B., & Mooney, K. (2011). *Measuring student engagement in upper elementary through high school: A description of 21 instruments* (Issues & Answers Report, REL 2011–No. 098). Washington, DC: U.S. Department of Education, Institute of Education Sciences, National Center for Education Evaluation and Regional Assistance, Regional Educational Laboratory Southeast. Retrieved from http://ies.ed.gov/ncee/edlabs

Fredricks, J. A., Blumenfeld, P. C., & Paris, A. H. (2004). School engagement: Potential of the concept, state of the evidence. *Review of Educational Research, 74*, 59–109.

Klem, A. M., & Connell, J. P. (2004). Relationships matter: Linking teacher support to student engagement and achievement. *Journal of School Health, 74*(7), 262–273.

Mosher, R., & McGowan, B. (1985). Assessing student engagement in secondary schools: Alternative conceptions, strategies of assessing, and instruments. University of Wisconsin, Research and Development Center (ERIC Document Reproduction Service No. ED 272812).

National Research Council and the Institute of Medicine [NRC and IoM] (2004). *Engaging schools: Fostering high school students' motivation to learn*. Washington, DC: The National Academies Press.

Newmann, F. M., Wehlage, G. G., & Lamborn, S. D. (1992). The significance and sources of student engagement. In F. M. Newmann (Ed.), *Student engagement and achievement in American secondary schools* (pp. 11–39). New York: Teachers College Press.

Reschly, A., & Christenson, S. L. (2006a). Prediction of dropout among students with mild disabilities: A case for the inclusion of student engagement variables. *Remedial and Special Education, 27*, 276–292.

Reschly, A., & Christenson, S. L. (2006b). Promoting school completion. In G. Bear, & K. Minke (Eds.), *Children's needs III: Understanding and addressing the developmental needs of children*. Bethesda, MD: National Association of School Psychologists.

Russell, V. J., Ainley, M., & Frydenberg, E. (2005). Schooling issues digest: Student motivation and engagement. Retrieved November 9, 2005, from http://www.dest.gov.au/sectors/school education/publications resources/schooling issues digest/schooling issues digest motivation engagement.htm

Skinner, E., Furrer, C., Marchand, G., & Kinderman, T. (2008). Engagement and disaffection in the classroom: Part of a larger motivational dynamic? *Journal of Educational Psychology, 100*, 765–781.

Wylie, C. (2009). Introduction. J. Morton (Ed.), *Engaging young people in learning: Why does it matter and what can we do?: Conference proceedings* (pp. 1–3). Wellington, New Zealand: New Zealand Council for Educational Research.

About the Editors

Sandra L. Christenson is the Birkmaier professor of Educational Leadership, professor of Educational Psychology, and faculty member in the School Psychology Program at the University of Minnesota. Her research focuses on interventions that enhance engagement at school and with learning for marginalized students with and without disabilities. She is particularly interested in the identification of contextual factors that facilitate student engagement and increase the probability for student success in school and the identification of the effect of family-school partnership variables.

Amy L. Reschly is an associate professor and training director in the School Psychology Program, Department of Educational Psychology & Instructional Technology, at the University of Georgia. Her areas of expertise include engagement and dropout prevention, working with families and schools to promote student success, and curriculum-based measurement (CBM) and problem solving.

Cathy Wylie is a chief researcher with the New Zealand Council for Educational Research. She has led the longitudinal Competent Learners project since 1993. Her research interests include the interaction between experiences and student development and identifying policies that best support school capability to provide engaging and productive learning. Her research into policy includes the impact on schools and students of New Zealand national policies, including the shift to self-managed schools since 1989.

Contents

Part I What Is Student Engagement?

1. **Jingle, Jangle, and Conceptual Haziness: Evolution and Future Directions of the Engagement Construct** 3
   Amy L. Reschly and Sandra L. Christenson

2. **Developmental Dynamics of Student Engagement, Coping, and Everyday Resilience** 21
   Ellen A. Skinner and Jennifer R. Pitzer

3. **Engagement Across Developmental Periods** 45
   Duhita Mahatmya, Brenda J. Lohman, Jennifer L. Matjasko, and Amy Feldman Farb

4. **Ethnicity and Student Engagement** 65
   Gary E. Bingham and Lynn Okagaki

5. **Student Engagement: What Is It? Why Does It Matter?** 97
   Jeremy D. Finn and Kayla S. Zimmer

6. **Part I Commentary: So What Is Student Engagement Anyway?** 133
   Jacquelynne Eccles and Ming-Te Wang

Part II Engagement as Linked to Motivational Variables

7. **A Self-determination Theory Perspective on Student Engagement** 149
   Johnmarshall Reeve

8. **Achievement Goal Theory, Conceptualization of Ability/Intelligence, and Classroom Climate** 173
   Eric M. Anderman and Helen Patrick

9. **School Identification** 193
   Kristin E. Voelkl

10	Self-Efficacy as an Engaged Learner	219
	Dale H. Schunk and Carol A. Mullen	
11	A Cyclical Self-Regulatory Account of Student Engagement: Theoretical Foundations and Applications	237
	Timothy J. Cleary and Barry J. Zimmerman	
12	Academic Emotions and Student Engagement	259
	Reinhard Pekrun and Lisa Linnenbrink-Garcia	
13	Students' Interest and Engagement in Classroom Activities	283
	Mary Ainley	
14	Part II Commentary: Motivation and Engagement: Conceptual, Operational, and Empirical Clarity	303
	Andrew J. Martin	

Part III Engagement and Contextual Influences

15	Parental Influences on Achievement Motivation and Student Engagement	315
	Janine Bempechat and David J. Shernoff	
16	Families as Facilitators of Student Engagement: Toward a Home-School Partnership Model	343
	Jacquelyn N. Raftery, Wendy S. Grolnick, and Elizabeth S. Flamm	
17	Teacher-Student Relationships and Engagement: Conceptualizing, Measuring, and Improving the Capacity of Classroom Interactions	365
	Robert C. Pianta, Bridget K. Hamre, and Joseph P. Allen	
18	The Role of Peer Relationships in Student Academic and Extracurricular Engagement	387
	Jaana Juvonen, Guadalupe Espinoza, and Casey Knifsend	
19	Understanding Student Engagement with a Contextual Model	403
	Shui-fong Lam, Bernard P.H. Wong, Hongfei Yang, and Yi Liu	
20	Allowing Choice and Nurturing an Inner Compass: Educational Practices Supporting Students' Need for Autonomy	421
	Avi Assor	
21	The Engaging Nature of Teaching for Competency Development	441
	Rosemary Hipkins	
22	Assessment as a Context for Student Engagement	457
	Sharon L. Nichols and Heather S. Dawson	

23 Part III Commentary: Socio-Cultural Contexts,
    Social Competence, and Engagement at School 479
    Kathryn Wentzel

Part IV Student Engagement: Determinants and Student Outcomes

24 The Relationship Between Engagement
    and High School Dropout 491
    Russell W. Rumberger and Susan Rotermund

25 High School Reform and Student Engagement 515
    Marcia H. Davis and James M. McPartland

26 The Power of Mindsets: Nurturing Engagement,
    Motivation, and Resilience in Students 541
    Robert Brooks, Suzanne Brooks, and Sam Goldstein

27 The Relations of Adolescent Student Engagement
    with Troubling and High-Risk Behaviors 563
    Amy-Jane Griffiths, Elena Lilles, Michael J. Furlong,
    and Jennifer Sidhwa

28 Trajectories and Patterns of Student Engagement:
    Evidence from a Longitudinal Study 585
    Cathy Wylie and Edith Hodgen

29 Instructional Contexts for Engagement
    and Achievement in Reading 601
    John T. Guthrie, Allan Wigfield, and Wei You

30 A Self-regulated Learning Perspective
    on Student Engagement 635
    Christopher A. Wolters and Daniel J. Taylor

31 Classroom Strategies to Enhance Academic
    Engaged Time 653
    Maribeth Gettinger and Martha J. Walter

32 Deep Engagement as a Complex System:
    Identity, Learning Power and Authentic Enquiry 675
    Ruth Deakin Crick

33 Part IV Commentary: Outcomes of Engagement
    and Engagement as an Outcome: Some Consensus,
    Divergences, and Unanswered Questions 695
    Michel Janosz

Part V Measurement Issues, Instruments, and Approaches

34 Measuring Student Engagement: The Development
    of a Scale for Formative Use 707
    Charles W. Darr

35 Systems Consultation: Developing the Assessment-to-Intervention Link with the Student Engagement Instrument 725
James J. Appleton

36 Finding the Humanity in the Data: Understanding, Measuring, and Strengthening Student Engagement 743
Ethan Yazzie-Mintz and Kim McCormick

37 The Measurement of Student Engagement: A Comparative Analysis of Various Methods and Student Self-report Instruments 763
Jennifer A. Fredricks and Wendy McColskey

38 Issues and Methods in the Measurement of Student Engagement: Advancing the Construct Through Statistical Modeling 783
Joseph Betts

39 Part V Commentary: Possible New Directions in the Measurement of Student Engagement 805
Karen M. Samuelsen

Epilogue 813

Index 819

Contributors

Mary Ainley is an associate professor in Psychological Sciences at the University of Melbourne, Australia. Her experience and research interests are in developmental and educational psychology. Most recently, these interests have been applied to investigating the experience of interest and exploring the psychological processes that are involved when students engage with (and disengage from) achievement tasks. This has resulted in the development of software for tracking students' choices and affective responses as they are tackling specific reading and problem-solving tasks. The goal of this research is to understand how to support positive educational experiences for students of all ages.

Joseph P. Allen is professor of psychology at the University of Virginia and director of the clinical psychology doctoral program in the Department of Psychology. His interests include adolescent and young adult social development and interventions to enhance behavioral and academic outcomes for adolescents.

Eric M. Anderman is a professor in the School of Educational Policy and Leadership at the Ohio State University. His research examines academic motivation. His studies have focused specifically on school transitions, prevention of risky behaviors, and academic cheating.

James J. Appleton is employed within the Research and Evaluation Office of Gwinnett County Public Schools, GA (a district of around 160,000 students). His publications include the area of student engagement with school, a pathway for dropping out, and he presents and consults nationally on this topic. Dr. Appleton has research and evaluation experience in district advisement and graduation coach programs, school initiatives, accountability metrics, and nested data. He has work experience in research and consultation within large urban and small rural school districts. Dr. Appleton has also served as mentor and researcher within the Check & Connect school completion intervention. He has codeveloped the Student Engagement Instrument (SEI).

Avi Assor is professor and former head of the Educational and School Psychology Program in Ben Gurion University, Israel. His research focuses on processes affecting children's autonomous internalization of values and practices that affect students' and teachers' motivation. In addition, he is involved in the development and assessment of school reforms aimed at enhancing students' and teachers' basic psychological needs, intrinsic motivation, and caring for others. He has published in the *Journal of Personality and Social Psychology, Child Development,* the *Journal of Educational Psychology,* the *Journal of Personality,* the *Journal of Educational Administration*, and *Learning and Instruction*.

Janine Bempechat is an associate professor in the Department of Human Development at Wheelock College. Her research interests include the achievement motivation of low-income students, school and family influences in achievement motivation, and ethnic and cultural influences in the development of achievement beliefs.

Joseph Betts is the director of research and principal research scientist at Riverside Publishing. He also serves as the senior research consultant for the Center for Cultural Diversity & Minority Education. Joe has participated in the development of computerized adaptive tests and worked as a practicing psychologist. In addition to student engagement, his research interests involve the applications of latent variable models to various educational research and assessment issues. The study of children's early literacy and mathematics developmental trajectories has been an area of research for a number of years, and he has recently developed growth norms for use in progress monitoring in the areas of reading, mathematics, and early literacy.

Gary E. Bingham is an assistant professor in the Department of Early Childhood Education in the College of Education at Georgia State University. He received his Ph.D. from Purdue University with an emphasis in early childhood education and child development. His research examines how children's early experiences within multiple contexts (i.e., home environment and early childhood educational settings) impact their language, literacy, and social development. As a result of this focus, much of his research seeks to understand the connection of culture to family and educational processes, particularly in relation to the engagement and achievement patterns of ethnically and economically diverse children and youth.

Robert Brooks is an assistant clinical professor of psychology at Harvard Medical School and former director of the Department of Psychology at McLean Hospital. He is the author or coauthor of 14 books and dozens of chapters and peer-reviewed articles. His interests pertain to topics of resilience, motivation, school climate, and the mindset and strategies of effective students, educators, and other professionals.

Suzanne Brooks is a clinical and school psychologist. In addition to working as a school psychologist in the Weston, MA Public Schools, she also has a part-time private practice in which she sees children, adolescents, and families. She has a special interest in assessing and treating students with learning and behavior problems and collaborating with teachers to develop effective classroom interventions for these youngsters.

Timothy J. Cleary is an associate professor in the Department of Educational Psychology and the training director of the School Psychology Program at the University of Wisconsin, Milwaukee. His research interests include developing alternative assessment tools targeting student motivation and self-regulation, developing and evaluating efficacy of self-regulation interventions in math and science, and examining trends in school psychology and education.

Ruth Deakin Crick is a reader in education at the Graduate School of Education in the University of Bristol and conjoint professor of education at the University of Newcastle in Australia. Her research interests include the theory and practice of learning power, pedagogies for deep engagement, systems learning and leadership, and approaches to engagement and social enterprise which integrate research, policy, practice, and enterprise.

Charles W. Darr is a senior researcher at the New Zealand Council for Educational Research and manager of the Assessment Design and Reporting Team. Charles' research interests include the measurement of student engagement, the development of assessment tools across the curriculum, and the application of computer technologies to administer assessments, and report and analyze assessment data.

Marcia H. Davis is an associate research scientist at the Center for Social Organization of Schools, Johns Hopkins University. She holds a doctorate in educational psychology from the University of Maryland and a master's degree in educational statistics. Her research interests include reading comprehension measurement, reading motivation, and school engagement as it relates to dropout prevention.

Heather S. Dawson is a Ph.D. candidate in the Department of Educational Policy and Leadership at the Ohio State University. Her research interests include examining the relationship between education policy and teacher and student motivation.

Dr. Jacquelynne Eccles (McKeachie/Pintrich Distinguished University professor of psychology at the University of Michigan) received her Ph.D. from UCLA in 1973. She was chair of the MacArthur Foundation Network on Successful Pathways through Middle Childhood, chair of the NAS Committee on After School Programs for Youth, and president of both the Society for Research on Adolescence and Division 35 of APA. She is currently editor of *Developmental Psychology* and is past editor of the *Journal of Research on Adolescence*. Her awards include the Spencer Foundation Fellowship for Outstanding Young Scholar in Educational Research, the Sarah Goddard Power Award for Outstanding Service from the University of Michigan, the APS Cattell Fellows Award for Outstanding Applied Work in Psychology, SPSSI's Kurt Lewin Award for outstanding research, the Distinguished Career Awards from SRA and Division 15 APA, and the University of Michigan Faculty Recognition Award for Outstanding Scholarship. Her research ranges from gender-role socialization, teacher expectancies, and classroom influences on student motivation to social development in the family and school context.

Guadalupe Espinoza is doctoral student in developmental psychology at the University of California, Los Angeles. Her research interests include examining how social contexts impact school functioning and peer relationships (e.g., bullying) within the school and online context, particularly among Latino adolescents.

Amy Feldman Farb is an evaluation specialist with the Office of Adolescent Health in the US Department of Health and Human Services. She manages federal evaluations of teen pregnancy prevention programs and development of performance measures and participates in an ongoing evidence review. Prior to this position, Dr. Farb was a research scientist with the US Department of Education, where she managed a contract conducting methodological investigations to advance the field of education research and a technical peer review process for the Regional Educational Laboratory program.

Jeremy D. Finn is professor of education (quantitative methods) at the State University of New York at Buffalo. His research interests include issues of educational equity that are affected by school policies and practices: class size reduction, educational risk and resilience, gender differences in behavior and performance, and student disengagement and dropping out. He has conducted a number of long-term studies of student attitudes and performance.

Elizabeth S. Flamm is a doctoral student in the Clark University Clinical Psychology Program. Her research explores the social and environmental contexts that facilitate motivation, achievement, and well-being in children and adolescents.

Jennifer A. Fredricks is an associate professor of Human Development at Connecticut College where she teaches courses in adolescence and child and family policy. Her research interests include school engagement, motivation, organized activity participation, youth sports, and adolescent development.

Michael J. Furlong is a professor in the Counseling, Clinical, and School Psychology Department at the University of California, Santa Barbara. He is the director of the Center for School-Based Youth Development and the editor of the *Journal of School Violence*.

Maribeth Gettinger is a professor in the School Psychology Program, Department of Educational Psychology, at the University of Wisconsin, Madison. Her research focuses on classroom environments that support academic success and evidence-based practices to promote skill development among high-risk children.

Sam Goldstein is an assistant clinical professor at the University of Utah School of Medicine. He is the clinical director of the Neurology, Learning and Behavior Center in Salt Lake City, Utah. Dr. Goldstein has authored 32 books and dozens of chapters and peer-reviewed research articles. He also serves as editor in chief of the *Journal of Attention Disorders* and coeditor in chief of *Encyclopedia of Child Development*.

Amy-Jane Griffiths is the assistant director at The Help Group's residential treatment center for adolescents with social, emotional, and behavioral challenges. Her research interests include empirically supported interventions for children engaging in high-risk behaviors, system level change, and positive school adaptation.

Wendy S. Grolnick is a professor of psychology in the Frances L. Hiatt School of Psychology at Clark University. Her research, which has been supported by NIMH, The William T. Grant Foundation, and the Spencer Foundation, has focused on the effects of home and school environments on children's motivation as well as factors affecting the environments that parents and teachers create for their children.

John T. Guthrie is the Jean Mullan Professor of Literacy Emeritus in the Department of Human Development at the University of Maryland. He currently directs an NICHD grant on adolescent motivation and achievement in reading, with an emphasis on ethnic variations. The project includes a reading intervention for all seventh-grade students in one school district.

Bridget K. Hamre is associate director of the Center for Advanced Study of Teaching and Learning at the University of Virginia. Her areas of expertise include large-scale assessment of teacher-student relationships and classroom processes that promote positive academic and social development for children and adolescents.

Rosemary Hipkins is a chief researcher at the New Zealand Council for Educational Research. She is interested in educating for competencies and the challenges of transforming curriculum, teaching, and assessment practices to meet "twenty-first century" learning needs. Her expertise is in high school education and science education.

Edith Hodgen is the chief statistician at the New Zealand Council for Educational Research, undertaking the analysis for the longitudinal Competent Learners project and for a range of research and evaluation studies, with a focus on analyzing changes over time.

Michel Janosz is director of the School Environment Research Group and professor at the School of Psychoeducation, University of Montreal. His research interests concern the etiologies and prevention of school dropout and violence and the specific role of school environments. His current work focuses upon (1) the efficacy of school-level interventions and the effectiveness of large-scale government initiatives to improve school success in disadvantaged populations, (2) the relationship between school climate and practices and student adjustment, and (3) the bidirectional links between internalizing/externalizing problems and school adjustment.

Jaana Juvonen is a professor in the Department of Psychology at the University of California, Los Angeles. She conducts research on school-based peer relationships and school adjustment. Much of her work focuses on bullying in middle schools.

Casey Knifsend is a doctoral student in Developmental Psychology at the University of California, Los Angeles. Her research interests include examining social identity development through ascribed (e.g., ethnicity) and achieved (e.g., extracurricular activities) group memberships and, specifically, how multiple social identities contribute to adolescent adjustment and intergroup attitudes.

Shui-fong Lam is an associate professor in the Department of Psychology at the University of Hong Kong. She is the director of a professional training program for educational psychologists. Her research interests include achievement motivation, parenting, school engagement, instructional strategies, and school-based prevention programs.

Elena Lilles is a doctoral candidate student at the University of California, Santa Barbara. Her research interests include early intervention with children ages 0–5 to promote academic readiness, social-emotional well-being, and school success.

Lisa Linnenbrink-Garcia is an assistant professor of Developmental Psychology in the Department of Psychology and Neuroscience, with a secondary appointment in Education, at Duke University. Her research focuses on the development of achievement motivation in school settings and the interplay among achievement motivation, emotions, and learning, especially in the domains of science and mathematics.

Yi Liu is an associate researcher in the Urban Community and Mental Health Education Office at the Yunnan Health Education Institute. She is also a social worker providing services to students and patients. Her research interests include student mental health education in impoverished minority areas, tobacco control, and quitting smoking.

Brenda J. Lohman is the director of Graduate Education and an associate professor in the Department of Human Development and Family Studies at Iowa State University. Utilizing a multidisciplinary framework, her research interests focus on the successful academic, psychological, social, and sexual adjustment of adolescents, especially those from economically disadvantaged minority families and communities.

Duhita Mahatmya is an assistant professor in the New Century College at George Mason University. Anchored in the ecological theory of human development and a positive youth development framework, her research emphasizes the multicontextual effects of the family, school, and neighborhood on adolescent engagement and well-being.

Andrew J. Martin is a professorial research fellow in the Faculty of Education and Social Work at the University of Sydney. His research interests include motivation, engagement, achievement, and quantitative research methods.

Jennifer L. Matjasko is a an adjunct assistant professor at the University of Texas at Austin and a behavioral scientist in the Division of Violence Prevention at the National Center for Injury Prevention and Control located at the Centers for Disease Control and Prevention. She received her Ph.D. in Public Policy from the University of Chicago. Her research interests focus on the development of at-risk adolescents and the factors that promote their health and well-being. Her research emphasizes the use of ecological, life-course, and person-centered approaches in understanding the relationship between individual, family, school, and community factors and adolescent functioning in order to inform prevention, intervention, and policy efforts targeted toward at-risk youth.

Wendy McColskey is a program director with the SERVE Center at the University of North Carolina at Greensboro. Her research interests include student engagement and motivation, formative and classroom assessment processes, and use of research and evaluation by educators.

Kim McCormick is a doctoral student in the Department of Counseling and Educational Psychology at the Indiana University School of Education in Bloomington, Indiana. Her research interests include student engagement and gifted and talented education.

James M. McPartland is research professor of sociology and codirector of the Center for Social Organization of Schools, Johns Hopkins University. His research specialties include high school reform and scale-up processes, effects of school formal and informal organization on student outcomes, and adolescent literacy innovations and impacts.

Carol A. Mullen is professor and chair of the Department of Educational Leadership and Cultural Foundations at the University of North Carolina at Greensboro. Her research interests include mentoring, leadership, and social justice in higher education and K–12 settings.

Sharon L. Nichols is an associate professor in the Department of Educational Psychology at the University of Texas at San Antonio. Her research interests include the intended and unintended consequences of high-stakes testing accountability on teachers and teaching and the ways in which test-related practices connect to students' motivational development.

Lynn Okagaki is Dean of the College of Education and Human Development at the University of Delaware. Her research focuses on academic achievement as influenced by culture and family values. From 2002–2005, she served as the first Deputy Director for Science in the U.S. Department of Education's Institute of Education Sciences. In December 2005, she was appointed for a six-year term as Commissioner for Education Research at the Institute of Education Sciences. Prior to 2002, she held appointments at Purdue University, Yale University, and the University of Houston. Dr. Okagaki received her bachelor of science degree in applied behavioral sciences from the University of California Davis and her doctoral degree in developmental psychology from Cornell University.

Helen Patrick is a professor in the Department of Educational Studies at Purdue University. Her research interests involve student motivation, including classroom processes and contexts that support motivation and engagement.

Reinhard Pekrun holds the chair for Personality and Educational Psychology in the Department of Psychology at the University of Munich. His research interests pertain to achievement emotion and motivation, students' personality development, and educational assessment and evaluation, including international large-scale assessments of student achievement.

Robert C. Pianta is Novartis US Foundation professor of education and dean of the Curry School of Education at the University of Virginia. His interests include theory, assessment, and intervention focused on teacher-student interactions and relationships, as well as policies that support increased attention to interactions in the classroom.

Jennifer R. Pitzer is a graduate student in the Department of Psychology at Portland State University. Her research interests include the influence of teacher support (e.g., warmth, structure, and autonomy support) on student reengagement, everyday resilience, and coping.

Jacquelyn N. Raftery is a graduate student in the Department of Psychology at Clark University. Her research interests include the development of coping with a special focus on how social contexts facilitate more adaptive coping.

Johnmarshall Reeve is a WCU (World Class University) professor in the Department of Education at Korea University in Seoul, Korea. Professor Reeve's research interests center on the empirical study of all aspects of human motivation and emotion, though he particularly emphasizes student motivation, student engagement, and teachers' motivating styles toward students.

Susan Rotermund is a research associate at MPR Associates in Berkeley, CA. Her research interests include student engagement, school climate, and how these factors can be altered to reduce dropouts. She uses a variety of quantitative methodologies for her research, including factor analysis, structural equation modeling, and latent class analysis.

Russell W. Rumberger is the vice provost for Education Partnerships, University of California Office of the President, and professor of Education in the Gevirtz Graduate School of Education at UC Santa Barbara. His research interests include education and work; the schooling of disadvantaged students, particularly school dropouts and linguistic minority students; school effectiveness; and education policy. He recently completed a book on high school dropouts published by Harvard University Press in 2011.

Karen M. Samuelsen is an assistant professor in the Department of Educational Psychology and Instructional Technology at the University of Georgia. She holds a doctorate in measurement, statistics, and evaluation from the University of Maryland. Dr. Samuelsen currently teaches graduate courses in measurement and statistics and serves as the director on a federally funded research project examining the efficacy of a conversational pedagogy for English language learners. Her research interests are in the fields of differential item functioning, latent mixture models, and validity. Before getting her Ph.D., Dr. Samuelsen was a high school science teacher with a certification in physics.

Dale H. Schunk is dean in the School of Education and professor of Teacher Education and Higher Education at the University of North Carolina at Greensboro. His research interests include social cognitive learning, motivation, and self-regulation.

David J. Shernoff is an associate professor in the Department of Leadership, Educational Psychology, and Foundations at Northern Illinois University. His research interests include the motivation and engagement of adolescents in school and after-school contexts, mentoring, early career development, and positive psychology.

Jennifer Sidhwa is a graduate student in the Educational Leadership and Organizations program at the Gevirtz Graduate School of Education, University of California, Santa Barbara. Her research interests focus on factors that promote positive organizational climate.

Ellen A. Skinner is a professor of developmental science and education in the Department of Psychology at Portland State University. Her research focuses on the dynamics of motivational development and resilience during childhood and adolescence and examines how school contexts and students' self-system processes shape the development of constructive engagement, coping, and (eventually) the emergence of a sense of purpose and ownership for one's own progress in school and beyond. In the last several years, she has become very interested in the development of teacher engagement and coping.

Daniel J. Taylor is a doctoral student in the Department of Educational Psychology at the University of Houston. His research interests include student motivation and academic achievement. His most recent empirical work examines motivational factors involved in the effects of stereotype threat in college populations.

Kristin E. Voelkl is an associate professor in the Department of Adolescence Education at Canisius College in Buffalo, New York. Her research interests include students' attitudes toward school and adolescent misbehavior including school-related substance use, academic dishonesty, and aggression in school. She continues to research engagement in school as it relates to other forms of risky and health-related behavior.

Martha J. Walter is a graduate student in the Department of Educational Psychology at the University of Wisconsin, Madison. Her current research interests include response to intervention, universal screening, and the social and emotional development of preschool children.

Ming-Te Wang is a research scientist in the Institute for Social Research at the University of Michigan and assistant professor of Applied Developmental Psychology at the University of Pittsburgh. He received his doctoral degree in Human Development and Psychology from Harvard University. His research has focused on the impact of school/classroom climate on adolescents' motivational beliefs and engagement and the effects of multiple ecological systems on the behavioral, social, and emotional development of youth from diverse socioeconomic and cultural backgrounds. His work emphasizes the interplay of developmental processes across both academic and social domains in adolescence and situates these processes within family, school, and community contexts.

Kathryn Wentzel is a professor in the Department of Human Development at the University of Maryland, College Park. Her research interests focus on parents, peers, and teachers as motivators of adolescents' classroom behavior and academic accomplishments. She has published over 100 articles and book chapters based on this work and has coedited books on achievement motivation. She is currently coeditor of the *Journal of Applied Developmental Psychology*. Dr. Wentzel is past vice president of Division E (Counseling and Human Development, AERA) and a fellow of the American Psychological Association, Division 15, and of the American Educational Research Association.

Allan Wigfield is professor and chair of the Department of Human Development at the University of Maryland. His research interests include the development and socialization of children's achievement motivation in different areas, and the effects of different kinds of reading comprehension instructional practice on children's reading motivation and achievement.

Christopher A. Wolters received his Ph.D. in Education and Psychology (1996) from the University of Michigan in Ann Arbor. He is now a professor in the Department of Educational Psychology at the University of Houston. He teaches master's- and doctoral-level courses that focus on theories of learning, motivation, and self-regulated learning. His research interests focus on the interface of motivational, cognitive, and metacognitive processes and their relation to students' learning and achievement, especially during adolescence.

Bernard P.H. Wong is a Ph.D. candidate in the Department of Psychology at the University of Hong Kong. His research interests include student engagement and disengagement in school, social-cognitive and identity development during adolescence, school-based intervention, and program evaluation.

Hongfei Yang is an associate professor in the Department of Psychology and Behavioral Sciences at the University of Zhejiang. He is a graduate advisor of counseling psychology. His research interests include counseling outcome assessment, perfectionism, mental health education, Chinese culture, and mental health.

Ethan Yazzie-Mintz was director of the High School Survey of Student Engagement and assistant research scientist at Indiana University from 2005 through 2011. Prior to coming to Indiana University, he worked in a number of large urban school districts – including Boston and New York – as a leadership trainer, data analysis consultant, and curriculum consultant. His research centers on student engagement, educational leadership and policy, and arts (specifically drama) and education. Dr. Yazzie-Mintz is coeditor of *The Complex World of Teaching: Perspectives from Theory and Practice* and is currently director of the First Light Education Project and an independent consultant based in Denver, Colorado.

Wei You is a doctoral student in the Department of Curriculum & Instruction at the University of Maryland. Her research interests include reading motivation and achievement, the interplay between reading engagement and reading comprehension, and measurement issues in reading research.

Kayla S. Zimmer is a lecturer in Elementary Education at St. Bonaventure University and a doctoral candidate at the State University of New York at

Buffalo. Her research interests include student-generated questions and how preservice teachers can be prepared to create the supportive environment that facilitates question generation and engagement.

Barry J. Zimmerman is a distinguished professor of Educational Psychology and head of Learning, Development, and Instruction area at the Graduate School and University Center of the City University of New York. He has devoted his career to investigating social cognitive and self-regulatory processes of children and youth in diverse areas of academic functioning, such as mathematics, writing, and science, as well as in sport and health functioning.

Part I

What Is Student Engagement?

Jingle, Jangle,[1] and Conceptual Haziness[2]: Evolution and Future Directions of the Engagement Construct

Amy L. Reschly and Sandra L. Christenson

Abstract

This chapter serves as an introduction to the history and study of student engagement. We describe the evolution of the construct of engagement and disciplinary differences in theories and use of the engagement construct. We highlight how our work on engagement, arising out of dropout intervention, has changed over the last decade. In addition, we delineate current issues in the study of engagement. The chapter ends with a discussion of future directions to advance the theoretical and applied use of student engagement to enhance outcomes for youth.

Introduction

The roots of interest in engagement are, at least in part, driven by the desire to enhance student learning. There is a long history of research on the relevance of academic engaged time for improving student achievement (Fisher & Berliner, 1985). Indeed, many current definitions of student engagement (see Epilogue, this volume) are explicitly linked to academic tasks and activities.

However, engagement has long been viewed as more than academic engaged time. From the earliest review to include the term engagement (Mosher & McGowan, 1985), to the publication of seminal theory about the underpinnings of school dropout and completion (Finn, 1989), to more recent conceptualizations (see Epilogue, this volume), engagement is viewed as multidimensional, involving aspects of students' emotion, behavior (participation, academic learning time), and cognition (Fredricks, Blumenfeld, & Paris, 2004). In other words, academic engaged time is important but not enough to accomplish the goals of schooling—student learning across academic, social-emotional, and behavioral domains. Student engagement is the glue, or mediator, that links important contexts—home, school, peers, and community—to students and, in turn, to outcomes of interest.

A.L. Reschly (✉)
Department of Educational Psychology
& Instructional Technology, University of Georgia,
325N Aderhold Hall, Athens, GA 30602, USA
e-mail: Reschly@uga.edu

S.L. Christenson
Department of Educational Psychology,
University of Minnesota, 250 Educational Sciences
Building 56 East River Road, Minneapolis,
MN 55455, USA
e-mail: Chris002@umn.edu

Our work in engagement began with direct intervention provided to students at elevated risk for dropping out of high school. Through this work, the importance of the social context of schooling (e.g., relationships with teachers and peers, belonging) and the need to foster students' personal investment became apparent. Our goal shifted from dropout prevention to school completion. The successful completion of high school is much more than simply staying in school, and thus, much more than the dropout problem—it involves meeting the defined academic, social, and behavioral standards of schooling to succeed in school and ensure access to and success in postsecondary enrollment options (Christenson, Sinclair, Lehr, & Godber, 2001; Reschly & Christenson, 2006b). When the goal is promoting school completion, the major foci of interventions are strategies that help students acquire skills to meet the demands and expectations of the school environment, create relationships with adults and students to facilitate their active participation in learning and school, and engage in future-oriented thinking that links skill acquisition to postsecondary enrollment success. As will be illustrated in this chapter and volume, engagement not only drives learning but also predicts school success.

The purpose of this chapter is to describe the evolution of the construct of engagement, with roots in the dropout prevention literature, to more recent conceptualizations of engagement as the basis of high school reform and school-based interventions to enhance student outcomes across academic, social, behavioral, and emotional domains. In this endeavor, we first detail how our own theorizing and measurement of student engagement has changed with time and our experiences with implementing a dropout prevention program. Next, we delineate several issues that have arisen in the study of engagement, including the number of types and definitions of engagement; the differentiation of indicators from facilitators of engagement; whether engagement is understood as a process or outcome and conceptualized on a single continuum or two continua of engagement and disengagement/disaffection; the differentiation of the constructs of motivation and engagement; and technical and related conceptual issues in the measurement of student engagement. Finally, we proposed directions for research to advance the theoretical and applied use of student engagement to enhance outcomes for youth.

Student Engagement and High School Completion

The Participation–Identification Model, postulated by Finn (1989), was a seminal theory addressing critical variables of student engagement and the process of both dropout and completion. According to the theory, dropout and completion are conceptualized, respectively, as ongoing processes of *participation* → *school success* → *identification* (completion) or of *non-participation* → *poor school performance* → *emotional withdrawal* (dropout). In other words, dropout and completion are not events but long-term processes of disengagement or engagement with school. In this view, engagement is comprised of behavior (participation) and affect, in the form of belonging and valuing school. Further, this theory highlighted the importance of student development prior to school entry in that there are differences in students' skills, attitudes, and behaviors (preparation) at the time of the commencement of formal schooling that affect the likelihood of successful participation, success, and identification with school.

There is a great deal of research that supports the importance of the main components of this theory. For example, developmental pathways to dropout and completion have been delineated from early childhood (Evans & DiBenedetto, 1990; Garnier, Stein, & Jacobs, 1997; Jimerson, Egeland, Sroufe, & Carlson, 2000). In addition, several studies have reported long-term positive effects of intensive early childhood programs on academic achievement and high school graduation (Reynolds, 2001; Schweinhart & Weikart, 1999), which presumably affect long-term engagement by increasing students' readiness in terms of academic skills and behavior, thereby facilitating the participation–success–identification cycle. Other research has shown dropout and completion may be predicted fairly accurately from data such as attendance, behavior, academic performance, and attachment to school in grades 1–3 (e.g., Alexander, Entwisle, & Horsey, 1997; Barrington & Hendricks, 1989; Ensminger & Slusarcick, 1992) and later elementary school. For example, Balfanz, Herzog, and Mac Iver (2007) were able to identify 60% of high school dropouts from sixth-grade attendance, misbehavior, and course failures. Similarly, robust conclusions can be drawn from the literature on classroom (e.g., Finn & Cox, 1992) and extracurricular participation (Feldman & Matjasko, 2005) and with respect to the importance of belonging and identification (see Voelkl, 2012). Finally, student engagement in high school has also been found to be related to postsecondary outcomes (Finn, 2006).

Among the most compelling evidence are those studies that differentiate student outcomes, within groups of students considered to be at risk given certain demographics, based on their engagement (attendance, participation, belonging) with school. Using a national, longitudinal dataset, Finn and Rock (1997) identified minority students from low-income backgrounds, two powerful demographic risk factors for poor outcomes in the USA, and classified them into three groups: resilient completers (higher achieving students, on track to graduate), nonresilient completers (likely to graduate but with poorer academic performance), and noncompleters (dropouts). The groups differed in expected ways according to a number of other demographic and social variables (e.g., percent of students living with both parents, family income, amount of schooling parents expected students to complete). After controlling for socioeconomic status and family structure, the three groups of students differed significantly in terms of teacher-rated and student self-reported engagement (e.g., attendance, working hard, paying attention in class, preparing for class/school, behavior problems). In other words, within a group of students who were demographically at risk for poor school outcomes, engagement variables significantly differentiated those who were academically successful from lower achieving school completers and high school dropouts. In a similar vein, Reschly and Christenson (2006a) found that student engagement variables, as measured in the eighth grade, were predictive of high school dropout and completion after achievement, grade retention, and socioeconomic status were statistically controlled, for another population of students with high rates of dropout (i.e., those with high-incidence disabilities).

Engagement and Dropout Prevention

The number of students who leave US high schools prematurely as dropouts has been of concern for several decades. Interestingly, despite publicity and great interest in preventing dropout, many commonly used interventions have been found to have negligible effects (Christenson et al., 2001; Dynarski & Gleason, 2002; c.f., What Works Clearinghouse, ND). Of those interventions that appear to be most promising, many of these may be characterized as addressing students' engagement at school and with learning. Thus, in addition to the prominent role ascribed student engagement in theory underlying student completion and dropout, student engagement is the cornerstone of our most promising dropout prevention and intervention efforts (Christenson et al., 2008).

One important difference, however, between theory (Finn, 1989) and direct intervention is the importance of contexts—families, schools, peers, and communities—as targets of intervention to engender or enhance students' engagement (Christenson et al., 2008; Reschly & Christenson, 2006b). Dozens of predictors of dropout and completion have been identified (Hammond, Linton, Smink, & Drew, 2007; Reschly & Christenson, 2006b; Rosenthal, 1998; Rumberger & Lim, 2008). Some predictors are inherent to the individual students and families (e.g., race/ethnicity) or are impractical or too difficult to address in even the most comprehensive dropout prevention program (e.g., socioeconomic status, single parents). However, a number of variables are alterable, represent behaviors or indicators that directly impact student behavior, preparation, and success in school, and may be found in external contexts, such as families and schools. Categorizations of variables (e.g., nonschool correlates, status and alterable, proximal and distal) predictive of dropout and completion may be found in Table 1.1.

Table 1.1 Categorizations of variables predictive of high school dropout and completion

Nonschool correlates (Rosenthal, 1998)		Status variables (Reschly & Christenson, 2006b)
SES	*Family process*	*Dropout*
Minority group status	Those with parental involvement and monitoring less likely to drop out	Low SES
Gender		Reside in southeastern and western regions of the USA
Males slightly more likely to drop out	*Student involvement with education*	Students with disabilities
Community characteristics	Dropouts have lower aspirations and achievement, less participation, etc.	English language learners
Dropout more likely in urban areas, Southeastern and Western USA, poorer communities, single-parent families, nonwhite communities, communities with high rates of foreign-born individuals	*Social conformity vs. autonomy* Dropouts have a higher need for autonomy, less conformity and less accepting of authority, lower church involvement, etc.	From Native American, Hispanic, or Black racial/ethnic backgrounds
Household stress	*Social deviance*	
Several stress variables related to dropout (e.g., single parenting, substance abuse, mobility, neighborhood violence)	Dropouts more likely to be deviant (e.g., substance abuse, conduct disorder, runaway)	
Taking adult roles	*Personality*	
Teen pregnancy, employment, other adult responsibilities	Dropouts have lower self-esteem and confidence, more impulsive, difficulty communicating, etc.	
Social support for staying in school		
Valuing education by parents and peers reduces likelihood of dropout (e.g., parental expectations and achievement)		

Alterable variables (Reschly & Christenson, 2006b)
By context

	Protective	Risk
Student	Complete homework Come to class prepared High locus of control Good self-concept Expectations for school completion	High rates of absences Behavior problems Poor academic performance Grade retention Working
Family	Academic support (e.g., help with homework) and motivational support (e.g., high expectations, talk to children about school) for learning Parental monitoring	Low educational expectations Mobility Permissive parenting styles
School	Orderly school environments Committed, caring teachers Fair discipline policies	Weak adult authority Large school size (>1,000 students) High pupil–teacher ratios Few caring relationships between staff and students Poor or uninteresting curricula Low expectations and high rates of truancy

Push	*Pull* (Jordan, McPartland, & Lara, 1999)	*Proximal*	*Distal* (Rumberger, 1995)
Conditions or events in the school environment that push kids out (e.g., disciplinary policies, grade retention)	Events or conditions outside of school that pull kids away (e.g., caring for a family member, having to get a job).	e.g., school attendance and behavior	e.g., family background, early school experiences

	Demographic risk variables	*Functional risk* (Christenson, 2008)
	SES, disability or English learner, status, race/ethnicity, etc.	Attendance, behavior, academic performance, credits earned, low levels of participation, etc.

Sources: Rosenthal (1998); Reschly and Christenson (2006b); Jordan et al. (1999); Rumberger (1995); Christenson (2008)

These various categorizations of variables predictive of dropout and completion clearly indicate the importance of contexts. Some variables are more useful than others for determining which students are at greatest risk for disengagement and dropout and monitoring the effects of intervention. Christenson's (2008) distinction between demographic and functional risk builds on student engagement research that showed within demographically high-risk groups of students engagement variables differentiate those who graduate from those who do not (e.g., Finn & Rock, 1997; Reschly & Christenson, 2006a) and further identifies those variables that are sensitive to small changes in student performance and may be used to monitor the effects of intervention. From a practical standpoint, it is not feasible to implement individually focused intervention to all students within a demographically higher risk category, for example, in the USA, to all Hispanic students, or all students identified as receiving free or reduced lunch (a broad, widely used indicator of low socioeconomic status), and more importantly, not every student within one of these demographically high-risk groups needs intervention. Thus, functional risk—attendance, behavior, low levels of involvement, and few relationships at schools—differentiates those who would benefit from interventions from those who do not need additional support or services. Developmental changes and progression across levels of schooling necessitate that indicators of functional risk are further differentiated by elementary and middle/high school levels (Christenson & Reschly, 2010).

Interest in both dropout prevention and student engagement has grown steadily from the publication of Finn's seminal theory in the late 1980s. The applied nature of engagement as a basis of dropout prevention and the importance of contexts as targets of intervention have led to expansion from the two-factor Participation–Identification Model. Indeed, our own theorizing about the nature of engagement and our attempts to measure this construct have been heavily influenced by our dropout prevention work with Check & Connect.

Check & Connect

The notion of alterable variables drawn from Finn's (1989) Participation–Identification Model was applied to the development of Check & Connect (Christenson & Reschly, 2010). Check & Connect is a structured mentoring intervention to promote student success and engagement at school and with learning, through relationship building and systematic use of data to design personalized "connect" interventions. A targeted intervention intended to complement universal intervention initiatives of schools and districts, Check & Connect is designed to promote student engagement through relationship building, problem solving, and persistence for marginalized students. The intervention has four components: (1) a *mentor* who works with students and families for a minimum of 2 years; (2) regular *checks*, utilizing data schools collect, on school adjustment, behavior, and educational progress of the student; (3) timely interventions, driven by data, to reestablish and maintain the student's *connection* to school and learning and to enhance the student's social and academic competencies; and (4) a *partnership with families*.

Since its inception in 1995, a seminal assumption of the Check & Connect student engagement intervention is that students are placed at risk when the learning environment does not respond to their needs (we differentiate this from the common phrase of "at-risk" students). Four theoretical perspectives undergird Check & Connect: systems-ecological, resilience, cognitive–behavioral, and autonomous motivation (Connell & Wellborn, 1991; Ryan & Deci, 2002). With respect to systems theory, it is assumed that students benefit from congruent and consistent messages about expectations and goals across home and school and within the school setting and that to promote student success, the needs of students must be considered in the context of their family, classroom, peers, and community.

Drawing on resilience theory, the mentor is the significant person with a long-term relationship with youth. However, mentors recognize that context matters—what parents and teachers do to support the student toward school completion makes a difference. They draw upon community resources as much as feasible, avoiding "reinventing the wheel." Finally, irrespective of family circumstances (e.g., status variables), mentors believe in students' capability to change their trajectory when standards for performance are paired with persistent support. Mentors consider student perspectives and personal goals, and they use problem solving to maintain a focus on developing self-determined, self-directed, and self-regulated learners, avoiding dependence on the mentor. We have always said that mentors "fuel the academic motivation" of students by underscoring autonomous motivation and providing instrumental support—facilitating problem solving toward students' personal goals; giving regular, systematic, informed feedback in a nonjudgmental way; encouraging the student to self-observe, self-evaluate, and self-reflect on progress toward goals; emphasizing the importance of effort, persistence, and trying again to help the student self-regulate their motivation; and making a long-term commitment, at least 2 years, to be a persistent source of support for the student and family.

Research Findings

Check & Connect has met the evidence-based standards of the US Department of Education's What Works Clearinghouse (2006) for students with disabilities who were at risk of disengagement and dropout. Specifically, two experimental studies with secondary students with disabilities (Ns of 94 and 144) revealed that Check & Connect youth were more likely to be enrolled in school (i.e., attendance), never interrupted their schooling, have persisted in school with no periods of 15 days or more absences, were less likely to have dropped out, and were more likely be on track to graduate within 5 years, be enrolled in an educational program (alternative, GED), or to have completed high school in 2 years than students in the control group (Sinclair, Christenson, Evelo, & Hurley, 1998; Sinclair, Christenson, & Thurlow, 2005). The effect size for treatment and control student differences for a 5-year graduation rate was significant and moderate ($ES=.53$). Christenson (2009) concluded that Check & Connect improves indicators of students' academic (e.g., credits earned, homework completion) and behavioral engagement (attendance, ratings of social skills) and demonstrates the necessity of sustained intervention for students who are disengaged from learning.

Consistent with the experimental studies, two other longitudinal studies using a pre-post measurement design revealed similar positive results (reduced rates of truancy, out-of-school suspensions, and course failures and increased rates of attendance) for students both with and without disabilities who attended elementary and secondary schools in suburban settings (Lehr, Sinclair, & Christenson, 2004; Sinclair & Kaibel, 2002). Also, closer relationships between Check & Connect intervention staff and students were associated with improved engagement (Anderson, Christenson, Sinclair, & Lehr, 2004). Specifically, the mentor perspective of the relationship predicted teacher-rated academic engagement, while the student perspective of the relationship approached significance as a predictor of teacher-rated academic engagement. Lastly, our findings suggest that Check & Connect is working to actively engage students and their families with school and with learning (Lehr et al., 2004). For example, 87% of parents of students in grades K–8 ($N=147$) who took part in Check & Connect for 2 years were rated by different teachers as more supportive of their children's education (defined as parental follow-through, communication with school, and homework completion). Furthermore, teachers' perceptions ($N=123$) of student behavior were positive—90% indicated students in grades K–8 were showing improvement in homework completion, interest in school, and attendance. Teachers' observations of students who received 2 years of sustained intervention were very positive. Teachers rated these students significantly more likely to be eager to learn, follow school rules, think ahead about consequences, get along with others, show respect for others' rights and feelings, and persist when challenged by difficult tasks, all critical competencies and habits of learning success.

In sum, analysis of Check & Connect program impact data consistently yields positive results: reduced rates of truancy, tardiness, suspensions, course failures, and dropout and increased rates of attendance. In particular, treatment–control differences in critical student engagement variables such as participation (attendance), behavior (social skills ratings), academics (credits earned), and, ultimately, graduation rates have been demonstrated for middle and high school students with learning and behavioral disabilities (Sinclair et al., 1998, 2005). Our current research projects are focused on (a) assessing the efficacy of Check & Connect with a general education population in three large urban school districts and (b) modifying Check & Connect for use in community college settings or assisting secondary school students with college readiness information and support. Beginning with the 2010 school year, Check & Connect has been supported by the core budget of the Minneapolis Public Schools (MPS); hence, sustainability of an intervention that was developed with MPS during 1990–1995 has been achieved.

Measuring Student Engagement

Important to the ability to examine outcomes of Check & Connect with different populations and under different conditions in our engagement research has been the development of the Student Engagement Instrument (SEI) (Appleton, Christenson, Kim, & Reschly, 2006; Betts, Appleton, Reschly, Christenson, & Huebner, 2010). As noted previously, the dependent variables for the research on Check & Connect implementations have been indicators of academic or behavioral engagement (e.g., credits earned, extracurricular participation, homework completion, attendance). Ongoing comments from the Check & Connect high school students with emotional disabilities (Sinclair et al., 2005) assisted us in broadening our indicators and theory of student engagement. These students quite regularly and persistently reported in various ways to their mentors that they "can't do the schoolwork," "won't try anymore," and that "no one likes them anyway." In response to our students' questioning of their personal competence and control (I can), values and goals (I want to), and social connectedness (I belong) around schooling and learning, we created the SEI to measure affective (perceived connection to others) and cognitive engagement (perceived relevance and motivation to learn). Coincidently, our Check & Connect intervention—within the dropout arena—drew upon similar theoretical underpinnings (intrinsic motivation, expectations, and supports) as the Committee on Increasing High School Students' Engagement and Motivation to Learn (National Research Council, 2004).

At this point, we posit that the theory of student engagement that undergirds Check & Connect is multidimensional; the four subtypes (academic, behavioral, cognitive, affective) serve as a heuristic for designing interventions that maximize the person–environment fit for students who are disengaged, alienated, or marginalized from learning. Inherent in our theorizing on student engagement is the belief that students are able to accurately report on their own engagement and environments and, further, that their perspectives are integral to the selection, implementation, and monitoring of interventions. In our view, engagement can be considered an outcome and a process. In Check & Connect, we want students to improve on all subtypes of engagement (outcomes). However, we recognize that student engagement is also a mediator between the contextual influences (facilitators) and our desired learning outcomes across academic, social, and emotional domains. We speculate that cognitive and affective engagement are potentially mediators of academic and behavioral engagement (Reschly & Christenson, 2006a), or in other words, engaging or disengaging students cognitively and affectively precedes changes in students' behavior and academic engagement. As others have posited (Furrer, Skinner, Marchand, & Kindermann, 2006), we hypothesize that there are Matthew Effects (Ceci & Papierno, 2005) between contexts and engagement wherein as students are engaged, contexts provide feedback and support that promote ever greater engagement (Reschly, 2010). A representation of this model may be found in Fig. 1.1. Inherent in our model is the belief that the student perspective is essential for change in student learning and behavior.

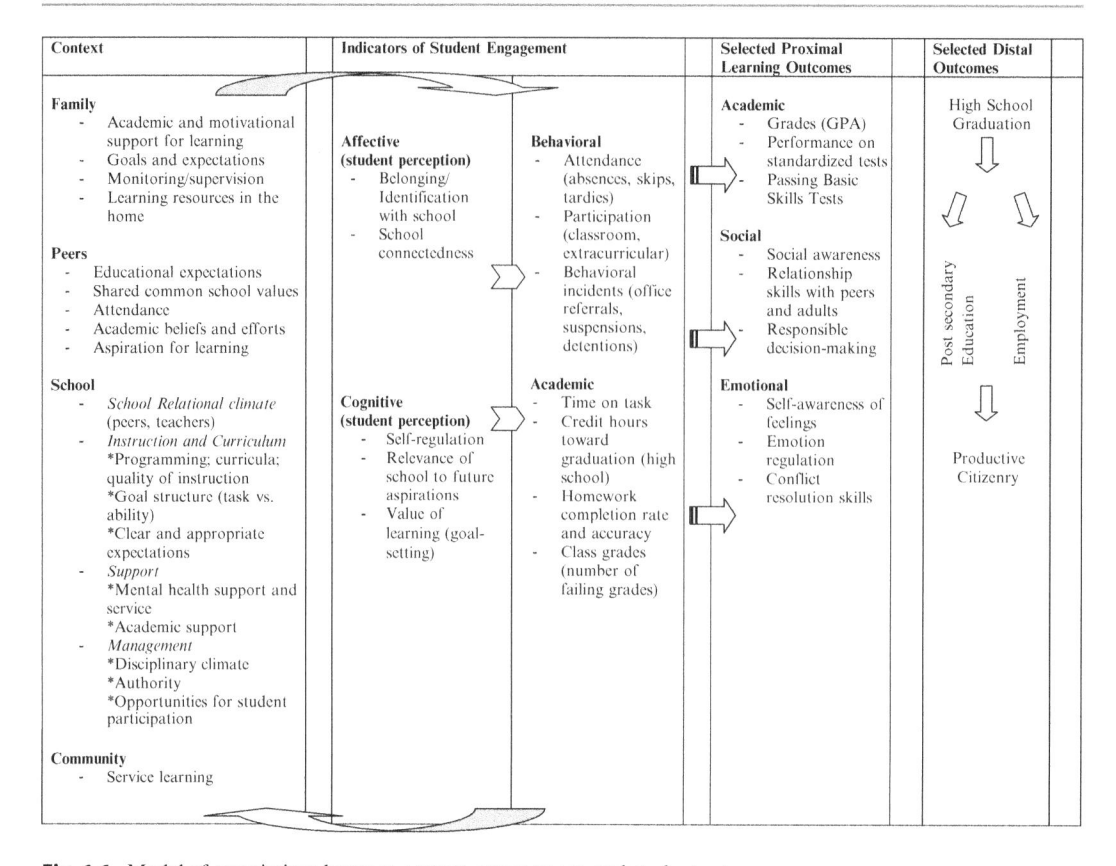

Context	Indicators of Student Engagement		Selected Proximal Learning Outcomes	Selected Distal Outcomes

Family
- Academic and motivational support for learning
- Goals and expectations
- Monitoring/supervision
- Learning resources in the home
 	
Peers
- Educational expectations
- Shared common school values
- Attendance
- Academic beliefs and efforts
- Aspiration for learning
 	
School
- *School Relational climate* (peers, teachers)
- *Instruction and Curriculum*
  *Programming; curricula; quality of instruction
  *Goal structure (task vs. ability)
  *Clear and appropriate expectations
- *Support*
  *Mental health support and service
  *Academic support
- *Management*
  *Disciplinary climate
  *Authority
  *Opportunities for student participation
 	
Community
- Service learning
	Affective
	(student perception)
	- Belonging/ Identification with school
	- School connectedness
	
	Cognitive
	(student perception)
	- Self-regulation
	- Relevance of school to future aspirations
	- Value of learning (goal-setting)
		Behavioral
		- Attendance (absences, skips, tardies)
		- Participation (classroom, extracurricular)
		- Behavioral incidents (office referrals, suspensions, detentions)
		
		Academic
		- Time on task
		- Credit hours toward graduation (high school)
		- Homework completion rate and accuracy
		- Class grades (number of failing grades)
			Academic
			- Grades (GPA)
			- Performance on standardized tests
			- Passing Basic Skills Tests
			
			Social
			- Social awareness
			- Relationship skills with peers and adults
			- Responsible decision-making
			
			Emotional
			- Self-awareness of feelings
			- Emotion regulation
			- Conflict resolution skills
				High School Graduation
				
				⇩
				
				Post secondary Education / Employment
				
				⇩
				
				Productive Citizenry

Fig. 1.1 Model of associations between context, engagement, and student outcomes

The academic lens maintained for Check & Connect students by mentors is paramount. They employ a problem-solving orientation with the student, teacher, and family to foster a person–environment fit for the student at school and with learning; provide persistent, ongoing support to enhance the student's capacity to meet the academic, social, and behavioral standards of the school environment; and aim to improve students' academic, social, and emotional learning outcomes by fostering the academic, behavioral, cognitive, and affective engagement of students.

Expansion of Engagement: Metaconstruct and School Reform

While engagement theory and intervention were expanding within the dropout prevention literature, a more general interest in engagement was burgeoning as a central construct to understanding student achievement and behavior for all students (Fredricks et al., 2004). Engagement was also given a central role in high school reform efforts (National Research Council, 2004).

Underscoring the predominant view in the dropout prevention arena, Fredricks et al. (2004) also conceptualized engagement as a multidimensional construct that is amenable to the effects of intervention and highly affected by contexts—teachers, families, etc. The authors' extensive review of the literature was organized around three types of engagement: behavioral, cognitive, and emotional. Behavioral engagement is defined by participation in academic, social, or extracurricular activities. Emotional engagement is comprised of affect (positive and negative) in interactions with teachers, peers, schoolwork, and the school. The definition of cognitive engagement was rooted in personal investment, self-regulation, and striving for mastery (Fredricks et al., 2004). Unique to the

Fredricks et al. conceptualization of engagement, however, was the elevation of engagement to the level of a metaconstruct that brings together many previously separate lines of research and may subsume the construct of motivation as a form of engagement.

There are essentially three schools of thought on student engagement: one arising from the dropout prevention theory and intervention area, another from a more general school reform perspective (i.e., National Research Council, 2004), and the third arising out of the motivational literature (e.g., Skinner, Furrer, Marchand, & Kinderman, 2008; Skinner, Kinderman, & Furrer, 2009). Overlapping with these schools of thought are subdisciplines within the academic field of psychology. Some scholars, ourselves included, are educational psychologists whose interests are more educationally focused and applied in orientation, while others are developmental psychologists with more theoretical interests in motivation and basic (i.e., theory-testing) research. It is perhaps not surprising that given the relatively recent ascendance of the engagement construct and somewhat varying origins of interest in engagement, there are a number of issues that have yet to be resolved, including those related to theory, definitions, and measurement. These issues are explicated in the paragraphs that follow.

Types and Definitions

The study of engagement is hindered by lack of consensus in both the number of subtypes and definitions of student engagement. Two-, three-, and four-subtype models are prevalent in the literature. There is agreement that at a minimum, engagement is comprised of participatory behavior and some affective component. Other scholars add cognitive engagement (Appleton et al., 2006; Christenson & Anderson, 2002; Fredricks et al., 2004) and/or bifurcate behavioral engagement into two subtypes: academic (e.g., time on task) and behavioral (participation) (Appleton et al., 2006; Christenson et al., 2008).

Although a number of authors, many in this volume included, ascribe to the three-part typology, there is little agreement about the definition of each subtype of engagement. Block (2000) applied traditional psychology terms of jingle (Thorndike, 1904) and jangle (Kelly, 1927) to describe the confusing way terms and concepts were used in personality psychology. Engagement currently suffers from a similar problem wherein the same term is used to refer to different things (jingle) and different terms are used for the same construct (jangle). For example, Finn (2006) classified perceived relevance, or utility, of school as affective engagement, whereas we would characterize it as cognitive engagement (Appleton et al., 2006; Christenson et al., 2008) and others as motivation (Wylie & Hodgen, 2012). Or, we described student-perceived relationships with teachers and peers and feelings of belonging as affective engagement (Appleton et al., 2006), while Yazzie-Mintz and colleagues from the High School Survey of Student Engagement include interaction with others and connection to community in the scale Social/Behavioral/Participatory Engagement and feelings of connection to others as emotional engagement (Yazzie-Mintz & McCormick, 2012). Selected engagement theories and respective indicators may be found in Table 1.2.

Process or Outcome

In Connell and Wellborn's (1991) influential model of self-system processes, engagement was viewed as a mediator between context, individuals' needs for autonomy, competence, and relatedness, and outcomes (context–self-action [engagement/disaffection]–outcomes). The notion that engagement connects contexts and student outcomes is prevalent in other engagement theories (Appleton et al., 2006; Skinner et al., 2008). When one considers developmental changes and the passage of time in addition to this mediating role, questions about engagement as process or outcome arise. Phrased differently, how can engagement be both a mediator and an outcome? The answer lies in how long range one's view is: a semester? A year? Over several years? Given the conclusion that dropout and completion are

Table 1.2 Comparisons of prominent engagement models on key dimensions

	Number of types	Definitions/indicators	Continuum/continua[a]
Finn (1989)	2	*Participation* Respond to requirements Class-related initiative Extracurricular activities Decision-making	Measured as continuum
		Identification Belonging Valuing	
Appleton, Christenson, and colleagues[b]	4	*Academic* Time on task, credit accrual, homework completion	Continuum
		Behavioral Attendance, participation, preparation for class/school	
		Cognitive Value/relevance, self-regulation, goal setting	
		Affective Belonging, identification with school	
Skinner and colleagues[c]	4 (2 Engagement, 2 Disaffection)	*Behavioral engagement* Action initiation, effort, persistence, intensity, attention, absorption, involvement	Continua
		Behavioral disaffection Passivity, giving up, withdrawal, inattentive, unprepared, distracted, mentally disengaged	
		Emotional engagement Enthusiasm, interest, enjoyment, satisfaction, pride, vitality, zest	
		Emotional disaffection Boredom, disinterest, frustration, sadness, worry/anxiety, shame, self-blame	
Martin (2007)	4 Higher order factors, 11 total	*Adaptive cognition* Valuing, mastery orientation, self-efficacy	Continua
		Adaptive behavior Persistence, planning, task management	
		Maladaptive behavior Disengagement, self-handicapping	
		Impeding/maladaptive cognition Uncertain control, failure avoidance	

[a] Continuum refers to a single dimension of engagement (ranging from high to low); continua refers to the separation of engagement and disengagement/disaffection into two dimensions (each ranging from high to low)
[b] Appleton et al. (2006) and Christenson et al. (2008)
[c] Skinner et al. (2008, 2009)

long-term processes of engagement and disengagement from school over several years, it is appropriate that engagement is both process (mediator) and outcome. For example, an outcome at one-time point, such as attendance or skipping classes, may be considered important process variables (i.e., indicators of engagement) for another later outcome, such as grades or credits earned, which in turn are process variables for even longer range outcomes, such as high school graduation and postsecondary enrollment.

Continuum or Continua

Another difference among various scholars' conceptualizations and measures of engagement is whether engagement is viewed and measured on a single continuum or whether engagement and disengagement, often referred to as disaffection, are separate continua. A parallel may be found in the field of positive psychology where it is argued that mental health and happiness are distinct from mental illness (Seligman & Csikszentmihalyi, 2000). Thus, health and happiness are more than the absence of psychopathology. The parallel for engagement may be that having low engagement is different from being disengaged/disaffected. In our own work, we have measured engagement on a single continuum ranging from low to high whereas other scholars measure both engagement and disaffection (Martin, 2007; Skinner et al., 2008).

Another parallel may be drawn from the research within positive psychology. There is some question as to whether there is a threshold on the benefits of happiness. Research generally finds that most people report being above the neutral point in happiness (Oishi, Diener, & Lucas, 2007); we find similar results in our survey work on student engagement (Appleton, Reschly, & Martin, 2012). Research finds that those who are happiest are most successful in terms of relationships and volunteer work, while those with somewhat lower levels of happiness are most successful in other domains, such as income and education (Oishi et al., 2007). Questions that may be raised for engagement include: Is there a point at which greater engagement no longer confers additional benefits? Or at which one is so highly engaged it is no longer adaptive but maladaptive? Continuing in this vein, how much engagement is needed to produce corresponding changes in desired outcomes—academic, social, and behavioral?

Indicators and Facilitators

Scholarly debate has also touched on whether it is important to distinguish facilitators of engagement from true indicators of the engagement construct (Skinner et al., 2008). Based on our dropout intervention work, we originally proposed the distinction between indicators and facilitators to guide screening and monitoring practices for targeted students (indicators) and direct attention to contexts that are logical foci of intervention efforts (facilitators; Christenson et al., 2008; Sinclair, Christenson, Lehr & Anderson, 2003). From an intervention perspective, we posited that it is important to assess both indicators and facilitators of this construct. Theoretically, it is our contention that cognitive and affective engagement are inherently individual internal processes and, thus, students are the most accurate source of information about these forms of engagement.

Skinner and colleagues, however, have argued for the separation of indicators and facilitators, a position echoed by other scholars (Lam, Wong, Yang, & Liu, 2012), in order to more fully examine the effects of context on engagement (Skinner et al., 2008). We value different explications and believe productive scholarly debate is necessary to propel the field forward. These different viewpoints may align with the aforementioned disciplinary differences between educational and developmental psychology and purpose of measurement (theory testing vs. prevention/intervention). Or, these dissimilar viewpoints represent differences in views on how context affects engagement and outcomes. For example, in the self-system process model (Connell & Wellborn, 1991), engagement is a bridge between context and outcomes (context–self-action–outcome). How does one separate objective measures of context, such as mastery goal orientation or school climate, from students' internal processes of these?

A final, related point concerns the source of engagement data. It is our belief that students can accurately report on their school experiences, and in fact, their reports are likely more accurate, or at a minimum an important addition to, the information obtained from other sources (peers, adults, etc.). Do parents and teachers know if students feel like they belong at school? Or whether a student thinks a class is relevant to his/her future? Perhaps it is necessary to separate parent or teacher reports regarding contextual facilitators of engagement from those collected from students. We believe the student perspective is critical to understanding the person–environment fit and to efforts to enhance student engagement. In fact, the seminal nature of the student perspective is reflected in our framework of engagement (see Fig. 1.1). Teacher–student relationships as perceived and reported by the student (an indicator of affective engagement) are conceptually distinct from teacher–student relationships as reported by the teacher or others (facilitators of students' engagement). Hence, we posit that the source of the informant must be considered and is critical for understanding the distinction between facilitators and indicators. Considering the source of the informant maintains the independence between facilitators and indicators that is deemed essential in measurement (Skinner et al., 2008). Differences in the perspectives of the informants, we would surmise, influence the teacher–student interaction that often shapes student engagement.

Engagement and Motivation

A prominent, lingering issue in the study of engagement is the relationship between engagement and motivation. Some scholars use the terms engagement and motivation interchangeably (e.g., Martin, 2007; National Research Council, 2004); others have proposed that the metaconstruct of student engagement subsumes motivation (Fredricks et al., 2004), while others ascribe to the position that engagement and motivation are distinct, related constructs wherein motivation represents intention and engagement is action (see Epilogue, this volume).

For intervention work, it may be unimportant to differentiate these constructs. Indeed, Martin's work with the Motivation–Engagement Scale and affiliated workbook intervention (Martin, 2006, 2008) follow this course. To this end, it is generally accepted that both motivation and engagement are influenced by context, that there are individual differences in how students respond to the environment, and that these constructs are linked to important student outcomes. However, theoretical advancement of the constructs of engagement and motivation requires that the association between the two be clearly specified and tested.

One issue in the theoretical differentiation of motivation and engagement is the time of existence and extensiveness of the scholarly literature. Fredricks et al. (2004) noted that motivation has more elaborate and differentiated definitions than currently exist for student engagement. Indeed, motivation has a long, rich history and extensive literature. Conversely, engagement is the proverbial new kid on the block, with the first appearance of the term engagement occurring in the 1980s (Appleton, Christenson, & Furlong, 2008).

A number of authors in this volume endorsed the three-type model of engagement: emotional/affective, cognitive, and behavioral (see Epilogue, this volume). Although there are jingle/jangle problems among each of these types, the greatest confusion arises over what we have classified as more internal forms: cognitive engagement and affective engagement and between each of these and motivation. In congruence with the engagement as a metaconstruct idea (Fredricks et al., 2004), it is possible that cognitive engagement and motivation are in fact very similar or even that same subconstruct, as evidenced by the use of traditional motivational concepts like self-regulation in definitions of cognitive engagement (Wolters & Taylor, 2012). The distinction between cognitive engagement and motivation is even murkier when one considers the differentiation of motivation and engagement that is espoused by many scholars (see Epilogue, this volume). In this view, motivation is considered to be intent and engagement as action. Thus, engagement is defined by an observable, action-oriented subtype (behavioral) and two internal ones (cognitive and affective engagement) but then is differentiated from motivation as engagement being action (observable behavior), motivation as intent (internal).

In our writings on engagement, we have frequently acknowledged that there are both theoretical and measurement issues relative to motivation and engagement (e.g., Appleton et al., 2006, 2008; Reschly, 2010). And, as described earlier in this chapter, Check & Connect has motivational underpinnings. We have argued that engagement and motivation are separate, but related constructs, wherein motivation is necessary but not sufficient for engagement (Appleton et al.). In one of our first studies of engagement, we used items representing boredom and perceived utility of education to one's future from the NELS:88 longitudinal dataset as indicators of cognitive engagement (Reschly & Christenson,

2006a). In the SEI, cognitive engagement is measured by the scales: control and relevance of school work, future aspirations and goals, and extrinsic motivation (Appleton et al.). Clearly, there is overlap between our operationalization of cognitive engagement and some motivational concepts (e.g., intrinsic/extrinsic motivation, goal-setting). Our model conceives of engagement as a multidimensional construct. Our operationalization of cognitive engagement may be characterized as motivation to learn as evidenced by the internal processes such as perceived relevance to future, goal setting, and so on. This internal motivation to learn is inherently individual and influenced by the motivational contexts (e.g., classroom goal structures, school climate and messages regarding effort and ability, peer group norms relative to academic behavior). A goal of this volume was to elucidate scholars' thinking on motivation and engagement (see Prologue/Epilogue, this volume). It is clear that the theoretical differentiation of the constructs of engagement and motivation continues to be an important area to be addressed in future scholarly work.

Measurement

Advances in theory require concomitant advances in measurement technology. At the time we began the development of our instrument, the SEI, there were few comprehensive measures of engagement based in any theoretical model. Of those available, some were created from larger, existing surveys to represent aspects of certain types of engagement, and jangling (i.e., items jumping from subtype to subtype, depending on author) was common. A recent review of instruments (Fredricks et al., 2011) provides evidence that the number of instruments intended to measure, in the scale's entirety or via subscales, student engagement has grown dramatically. The available measures differ in terms of the source of data (student self-report; teacher-report; observation instruments), how many types of engagement are measured, and whether designed to measure engagement generally or with reference to a specific subject area (Fredricks et al.). Research with engagement measures has also differed according to whether data were collected via active or passive parental consent. Elsewhere, we have speculated that studies requiring active parental consent may be subject to a positive engagement bias because those children whose parents are less likely to return forms may also be students at risk for disengaging and dropping out of school (Reschly et al., 2008). Methodologies also differ as to whether students complete surveys anonymously or whether the data are confidential from teachers but maintained with identifying student information and linked over time.

In summary, efforts to measure student engagement are in the earliest stages. Advances in measurement are needed to clarify the theoretical issues in the engagement construct, from differentiating engagement and motivation to the utility of conceptualizing engagement on a single continuum or as continua of engagement and disengagement/disaffection. These and other directions for future research are addressed in the next section.

Future Directions

The issues described in this chapter, and throughout this volume (Epilogue), indicate that excitement about the engagement construct should be tempered with knowledge of these issues and the limitations of our current knowledge base. However, enthusiasm about engagement as a basis of theory for conceptualizing important processes and outcomes and interventions to enhance these outcomes support the need for continued scholarship and research. Issues, such as the number of types of engagement, lack of consensus regarding definitions, and differentiating constructs of motivation and engagement, are clear targets of future research efforts. These, and other directions, are described in the following paragraphs.

Block (2000) delineated how jingle/jangle problems limit the conclusions that can be reached through research. Thus, addressing jingle/jangle problems in theory and measurement is a logical step for moving forward. In addition, differentiating the purpose of measurement (e.g., theory testing vs. linking to intervention) may facilitate greater conceptual clarity with the engagement construct. Indeed, measurement technologies are needed to answer important questions about engagement. Of currently available measures, a number of authors have provided correlational evidence of associations between engagement and achievement (Fredricks et al., 2011); however, there are few studies of convergent and divergent validity among measures of engagement and between measures of engagement and motivation.

Currently, there are few longitudinal studies that utilize a comprehensive, theory-based measure of student engagement. This type of research is needed to investigate developmental changes in the engagement construct. Currently, the Motivation–Engagement Scale (MES) has been examined cross-sectionally with students from elementary through college age (Martin, 2009). Similarly, we have recently piloted elementary- and college-age versions of the SEI (Carter, Reschly, Lovelace, Appleton, & Thompson, 2012; Waldrop & Reschly, 2011, respectively). Longitudinal engagement research will also facilitate the examination of (a) trajectories of engagement and the relationship between engagement and student outcomes over time, as well as (b) the importance of different subtypes of engagement to these outcomes. We have proposed that there is a hierarchy of types of engagement (Reschly & Christenson, 2006a) such that affective and cognitive changes (greater belonging, better relationships with teachers and peers) precede the observable, behavioral changes in important variables such as attendance and behavior. Initial research appears to support this contention (Lam et al., 2012; Skinner et al., 2008; Wylie & Hodgen, 2012).

Future research is also needed to address whether engagement is best conceptualized on a single continuum or as two continua of engagement and disengagement/disaffection. In the examination of their measure of engagement, Skinner et al. (2009) found engagement and disaffection to be distinct subscales. Our research suggests that there may be some additive benefits of measuring disengagement as well as engagement (Reschly et al., 2012), something we will consider in our ongoing examinations and potential revision of the SEI (Appleton et al., 2006; Betts et al., 2010). Research is needed to explore the combination of engagement and disengagement/disaffection that yields the most psychometrically sound measure of the construct.

Another direction for research is to examine whether there are cultural differences in the construct of student engagement. Differences may be found in the relative importance of contextual variables (e.g., influence of peers, classroom/school structures, family involvement or support) or the construct may be different across youth in different countries. A small study we conducted using the SEI and Martin's MES (previously only examined with Australian students) indicated that there may be differences in how US and Australian students respond to these measures (Reschly et al., 2012).

Our knowledge base regarding the outcomes of engagement interventions is limited. Some interventions focus on changing students to function more effectively in the environment, others on curriculum and pedagogy, and still others on the school environment with the goal of personalizing education and enhancing relationships among students and between students and staff. As engagement is increasingly conceptualized as an organizing heuristic for interventions delivered at universal-level, for all students, as well as those who are at elevated risk for poor outcomes (targeted or intensive; Christenson et al., 2008), more work is needed to evaluate interventions to determine what works, for whom, and under what conditions. Particularly concerning is the notion of sustained intervention for students disengaged from learning or on the trajectory for school dropout. Specifically, for how long and with what intensity must intervention support be provided to achieve positive learning outcomes? In addition, improved measurement methodology is needed to link assessment to intervention. Our work with Check & Connect underscored the importance of systematic monitoring of student data so that interventions could be delivered at the first sign of disengagement.

In summary, student engagement is a burgeoning construct. It is viewed as a basis of theory and interventions related to high school dropout, high school reform, and as a necessary element for improving student outcomes. The construct of engagement has evolved rapidly in the last 10 years. Although there are numerous conceptual and measurement issues, scholarship around engagement is robust. It continues to be a fruitful and important area of research.

Authors' Notes

1. The jingle/jangle distinction was used to describe personality psychology by Block (2000).
2. Conceptual haziness used to characterize the construct of engagement by Appleton et al. (2008).

References

Alexander, K. L., Entwisle, D. R., & Horsey, C. S. (1997). From first grade forward: Early foundations of high school dropouts. *Sociology of Education, 70*, 87–107.

Anderson, A. R., Christenson, S. L., Sinclair, M. F., & Lehr, C. (2004). Check & Connect: The importance of relationships for promoting engagement with school. *Journal of School Psychology, 42*(2), 95–113.

Appleton, J. J., Christenson, S. L., & Furlong, M. J. (2008). Student engagement with school: Critical conceptual and methodological issues of the construct. *Psychology in the Schools, 45*, 369–386.

Appleton, J. J., Christenson, S. L., Kim, D., & Reschly, A. L. (2006). Measuring cognitive and psychological engagement: Validation of the Student Engagement Instrument. *Journal of School Psychology, 44*, 427–445.

Appleton, J. J., Reschly, A. L., & Martin, C. (2012). Research to practice: Measuring and reporting student engagement. Manuscript under review.

Balfanz, R., Herzog, L., & Mac Iver, D. J. (2007). Preventing student disengagement and keeping students on the graduation path in urban middle-grades schools: Early identification and effective interventions. *Educational Psychologist, 42*, 223–235.

Barrington, B. L., & Hendricks, B. (1989). Differentiating characteristics of high school graduates, dropouts, and nongraduates. *The Journal of Educational Research, 89*, 309–319.

Betts, J., Appleton, J. J., Reschly, A. L., Christenson, S. L., & Huebner, E. S. (2010). A study of the reliability and construct validity of the School Engagement Instrument across multiple grades. *School Psychology Quarterly, 25*, 84–93.

Block, J. (2000). Three tasks for personality psychology. In L. R. Bergman, R. B. Cairns, L.-G. Nilsson, & L. Nystedt (Eds.), *Developmental science and the holistic approach* (pp. 155–164). Mahwah, NJ: Erlbaum.

Carter, C., Reschly, A. L., Lovelace, M. D., Appleton, J. J., & Thompson, D. (2012). Measuring student engagement among elementary students: Pilot of the Elementary Student Engagement Instrument. Manuscript under review.

Ceci, S. J., & Papierno, P. B. (2005). The rhetoric and reality of gap closing: When the "have-nots" gain but the "haves" gain even more. *American Psychologist, 60*, 149–160.

Christenson, S. L. (2008, January 22). *Engaging students with school: The essential dimension of dropout prevention programs*. [Webinar]. National Dropout Prevention Center for Students with Disabilities.

Christenson, S. L. (2009). The relevance of engagement for students at-risk of educational failure: Findings and lessons from Check & Connect research. In J. Morton (Ed.), *Engaging young people in learning: Why does it matter and what can we do?: Conference proceedings* (pp. 36–84). Wellington, New Zealand: NZCER Press.

Christenson, S. L., & Anderson, A. R. (2002). Commentary: The centrality of the learning context for students' academic enabler skills. *School Psychology Review, 31*, 378–393.

Christenson, S. L., & Reschly, A. L. (2010). Check & Connect: Enhancing school completion through student engagement. In E. Doll & J. Charvat (Eds.), *Handbook of prevention science*. Mahwah, NJ: Lawrence Erlbaum Associates, Inc.

Christenson, S. L., Reschly, A. L., Appleton, J. J., Berman, S., Spanjers, D., & Varro, P. (2008). Best practices in fostering student engagement. In A. Thomas & J. Grimes (Eds.), *Best practices in school psychology* (5th ed.). Bethesda, MD: National Association of School Psychologists.

Christenson, S. L., Sinclair, M. F., Lehr, C. A., & Godber, Y. (2001). Promoting successful school completion: Critical conceptual and methodological guidelines. *School Psychology Quarterly, 16*, 468–484.

Connell, J. P., & Wellborn, J. G. (1991). Competence, autonomy, and relatedness: A motivational analysis of self system processes. In M. R. Gunnar & L. A. Sroufe (Eds.), *Self processes and development: The Minnesota symposia on child psychology* (Vol. 23, pp. 43–77). Hillsdale, NJ: L. Erlbaum Associates.

Dynarski, M., & Gleason, P. (2002). How can we help? What we have learned from recent federal dropout prevention evaluations. *Journal of Education for Students Placed At-Risk, 7*, 43–69.

Ensminger, M. E., & Slusarcick, A. L. (1992). Paths to high school graduation or dropout: A longitudinal study of a first-grade cohort. *Sociology of Education, 65*, 95–113.

Evans, I., & DiBenedetto, A. (1990). Pathways to school dropout: A conceptual model for early prevention. *Special Services in School, 6*, 63–80.

Feldman, A. F., & Matjasko, J. L. (2005). The role of school-based extracurricular activities in adolescent development: A comprehensive review and future directions. *Review of Educational Research, 75*(2), 159–210.

Finn, J. D. (1989). Withdrawing from school. *Review of Educational Research, 59*, 117–142.

Finn, J. D. (2006). *The adult lives of at-risk students: The roles of attainment and engagement in high school* (NCES 2006–328). Washington, DC: National Center for Education Statistics, U.S. Department of Education.

Finn, J. D., & Cox, D. (1992). Participation and withdrawal among fourth-grade pupils. *American Educational Research Journal, 29*, 141–162.

Finn, J. D., & Rock, D. A. (1997). Academic success among students at risk for school failure. *Journal of Applied Psychology, 82*(2), 221–234.

Fisher, C. W., & Berliner, D. C. (1985). *Perspectives on instructional time.* New York: Longman.

Fredricks, J., McColskey, W., Meli, J., Mordica, J., Montrosse, B., & Mooney, K. (2011). *Measuring student engagement in upper elementary through high school: A description of 21 instruments* (Issues & Answers Report, REL 2011–No. 098). Washington, DC: U.S. Department of Education, Institute of Education Sciences, National Center for Education Evaluation and Regional Assistance, Regional Educational Laboratory Southeast. Retrieved from http://ies.ed.gov/ncee/edlabs.

Fredricks, J. A., Blumenfeld, P. C., & Paris, A. H. (2004). School engagement: Potential of the concept, state of the evidence. *Review of Educational Research, 74*, 59–109.

Furrer, C. J., Skinner, E., Marchand, G., & Kindermann, T. A. (2006, March). *Engagement vs. disaffection as central constructs in the dynamics of motivational development.* Paper presented at the annual meeting of the Society for Research on Adolescence, San Francisco, CA.

Garnier, H., Stein, J., & Jacobs, J. (1997). The process of dropping out of high school: A 19-year perspective. *American Educational Research Journal, 34*(2), 395–419.

Hammond, C., Linton, D., Smink, J., & Drew, S. (2007). *Dropout risk factors and exemplary programs: A technical report.* Clemson, SC: National Dropout Prevention Center, Communities in Schools, Inc.

Jimerson, S. R., Egeland, B., Sroufe, L. A., & Carlson, E. (2000). A prospective longitudinal study of high school dropouts: Examining multiple predictors across development. *Journal of School Psychology, 38*(6), 525–549.

Jordan, W. J., McPartland, J. M., & Lara, J. (1999). Rethinking the causes of high school dropout. *The Prevention Researcher, 6*, 1–4.

Kelley, T. L. (1927). *Interpretation of educational measurements.* Yonkers, NY: World Book.

Lam, S., Wong, B. P. H., Yang, H., & Liu, Y. (2012). Understanding student engagement with a contextual model. In S. L. Christenson, A. L. Reschly & C. Wylie (Eds.), *Handbook of research on student engagement* (pp. 403–419). New York: Springer.

Lehr, C. A., Sinclair, M. F., & Christenson, S. L. (2004). Addressing student engagement and truancy prevention during the elementary years: A replication study of the Check & Connect model. *Journal of Education for Students Placed At-Risk, 9*(3), 279–301.

Martin, A. J. (2006). Enhancing student motivation and engagement: The effects of a multidimensional intervention. *Contemporary Educational Psychology, 33*, 239–269.

Martin, A. J. (2007). Examining a multidimensional model of student motivation and engagement using a construct validation approach. *British Journal of Educational Psychology, 77*, 413–440.

Martin, A. J. (2008). *Motivation and engagement scale and workbook: Testing and administration guidelines.* Lifelong Achievement Group, New South Wales, Australia.

Martin, A. J. (2009). Motivation and engagement across the academic life span: A developmental construct validity study of elementary school, high school, and university/college students. *Educational and Psychological Measurement, 69*, 794–824.

Mosher, R., & McGowan, B. (1985). *Assessing student engagement in secondary schools: Alternative conceptions, strategies of assessing, and instruments.* University of Wisconsin, Research and Development Center. (ERIC Document Reproduction Service No. ED 272812).

National Research Council and the Institute of Medicine. (2004). *Engaging schools: Fostering high school students' motivation to learn.* Washington, DC: The National Academies Press.

Oishi, S., Diener, E., & Lucas, R. E. (2007). The optimum level of well-being: Can people be too happy? *Perspectives on Psychological Science, 2*(4), 346–360.

Reschly, A. L., Betts, J., & Appleton, J. J. (2012). *Student Engagement Instrument: Evidence of convergent and divergent validity across measures of engagement and motivation.* Manuscript under review.

Reschly, A. (2010). Reading and school completion: Critical connections and Matthew effects. *Reading and Writing Quarterly, 26*, 1–23.

Reschly, A. L., Huebner, E. S., Appleton, J. J., & Antaramian, S. (2008). Engagement as flourishing: The role of positive emotions and coping in student engagement at school and with learning. *Psychology in the Schools, 45*(5), 419–431.

Reschly, A., & Christenson, S. L. (2006a). Prediction of dropout among students with mild disabilities: A case for the inclusion of student engagement variables. *Remedial and Special Education, 27*, 276–292.

Reschly, A., & Christenson, S. L. (2006b). Promoting school completion. In G. Bear & K. Minke (Eds.), *Children's needs III: Understanding and addressing the developmental needs of children.* Bethesda, MD: National Association of School Psychologists.

Reynolds, A. J. (2001). Press release: *Long-term effects of CPC program.* Retrieved October 3, 2006, from http://www.waisman.wisc.edu/cls/PRESS01.PDF.

Rosenthal, B. S. (1998). Non-school correlates of dropout: An integrative review of the literature. *Children and Youth Services Review, 20,* 413–433.

Rumberger, R. W. (1995). Dropping out of middle school: A multilevel analysis of students and schools. *American Educational Research Journal, 32,* 583–625.

Rumberger, R. W., & Lim, S. A. (2008). *Why students drop out of school: A review of 25 years of research* (California Dropout Research Project Report #15). University of California Santa Barbara.

Ryan, R. M., & Deci, E. L. (2002). An overview of self-determination theory: An organismic-dialectical perspective. In E. L. Deci & R. M. Ryan (Eds.), *Handbook of self-determination research* (pp. 3–33). Rochester, NY: University of Rochester Press.

Schweinhart, L. J., & Weikart, D. P. (1999, September). The advantages of High/Scope: Helping children lead successful lives. *Educational Leadership, 57*(1), 77–78.

Seligman, M. E. P., & Csikszentmihalyi, M. (2000). Positive psychology: An introduction. *American Psychologist, 55,* 5–14.

Sinclair, M. F., Christenson, S. L., Evelo, D., & Hurley, C. (1998). Dropout prevention for high-risk youth with disabilities: Efficacy of a sustained school engagement procedure. *Exceptional Children, 65,* 7–21.

Sinclair, M. F., Christenson, S. L., Lehr, C. A., & Anderson, A. R. (2003). Facilitating 890 student engagement: Lessons learned from check & connect longitudinal studies. *The California School Psychologist, 8,* 29–42.

Sinclair, M. F., Christenson, S. L., & Thurlow, M. L. (2005). Promoting school completion of urban secondary youth with emotional or behavioral disabilities. *Exceptional Children, 71,* 465–482.

Sinclair, M. F., & Kaibel, C. (2002). *2002 Dakota county: Secondary Check & Connect program. Program evaluation 2002 final summary report.* Minneapolis, MN: University of Minnesota, Institute on Community Integration.

Skinner, E., Furrer, C., Marchand, G., & Kinderman, T. (2008). Engagement and disaffection in the classroom: Part of a larger motivational dynamic? *Journal of Educational Psychology, 100,* 765–781.

Skinner, E. A., Kinderman, T. A., & Furrer, C. J. (2009). A motivational perspective on engagement and disaffection: Conceptualization and assessment of children's behavioral and emotional participation in academic activities in the classroom. *Educational and Psychological Measurement, 69,* 493–525.

Thorndike, E. L. (1904). An introduction to the theory of mental and social measurements. New York: Teachers College, Columbia University.

Voelkl, K. E. (2012). School identification. In S. L. Christenson, A. L. Reschly & C. Wylie (Eds.), *Handbook of research on student engagement* (pp. 193–218). New York: Springer.

Waldrop, D., & Reschly, A. L. (2011, February). *Examining student engagement and motivation among college students.* Accepted presentation at the annual meeting of the National Association of School Psychologists. San Francisco, CA.

What Works Clearinghouse. (2006). *Dropout prevention: Check & Connect.* Institute of Education Sciences, Department of Education. Downloaded August 8, 2011, from http://ies.ed.gov/ncee/wwc/pdf/WWC_Check_Connect_092106.pdf.

What Works Clearinghouse, Institute of Education Sciences, Department of Education. http://ies.ed.gov/ncee/wwc/reports/advancedss.aspx.

Wolters, C. A., & Taylor, D. J. (2012). A self-regulated learning perspective on student engagement. In S. L. Christenson, A. L. Reschly & C. Wylie (Eds.), *Handbook of research on student engagement* (pp. 635–651). New York: Springer.

Wylie, C., & Hodgen, E. (2012). Trajectories and patterns of student engagement: Evidence from a longitudinal study. In S. L. Christenson, A. L. Reschly & C. Wylie (Eds.), *Handbook of research on student engagement* (pp. 585–599). New York: Springer.

Yazzie-Mintz, E., & McCormick, K. (2012). Finding the humanity in the data: Understanding, measuring and strengthening student engagement. In S. L. Christenson, A. L. Reschly & C. Wylie (Eds.), *Handbook of research on student engagement* (pp. 743–761). New York: Springer.

Developmental Dynamics of Student Engagement, Coping, and Everyday Resilience

Ellen A. Skinner and Jennifer R. Pitzer

Abstract

The goal of this chapter is to present a perspective on student engagement with academic work that emphasizes its role in organizing the daily school experiences of children and youth as well as their cumulative learning, long-term achievement, and eventual academic success. A model grounded in self-determination theory, and organized around student engagement and disaffection with learning activities, seems to offer promise to the study of academic development by specifying the dynamic cycles of context, self, action, and outcomes that are self-stablizing or self-amplifying, and may underlie trajectories of motivation across many school years. The study of ongoing engagement can be enriched by the incorporation of concepts of everyday resilience, focusing on what happens when students make mistakes and encounter difficulties and failures in school. The same personal and interpersonal resources that promote engagement may shape students' reactions to challenges and obstacles, with academic coping an especially important bridge back to reengagement. Future research can examine how these motivational dynamics contribute to the development of durable academic assets, such as self-regulated learning and proactive coping, and an academic identity that allows students eventually to take ownership for their own learning and success in school.

The last two decades have witnessed an explosion of interest in the construct of *academic engagement*, based on evidence that engagement is both a malleable state that can be shaped by schools *and* a robust predictor of students' learning, grades, achievement test scores, retention, and graduation (Appleton, Christenson & Furlong, 2008; Finn, 1993; Fredricks, Blumenfeld, & Paris, 2004; Furlong & Christenson, 2008; Jimerson, Campos, & Grief, 2003; Klem & Connell, 2004; Newmann, Wehlage, & Lamborn,

E.A. Skinner, Ph.D. (✉) • J.R. Pitzer, MS
Department of Psychology, Portland State University,
Portland, OR, USA
e-mail: ellen.skinner@pdx.edu; jenniferpitzer@gmail.com

1992; National Research Council [NRC], 2004; Sinclair, Christenson, Lehr, & Anderson, 2003). As enthusiasm for the notion of engagement has grown, however, so too has an appreciation for the complexity of the construct (Appleton et al., 2008; Fredricks et al., 2004). Engagement not only has an intuitively appealing holistic meaning that focuses on the quality of a student's involvement with school, but it also incorporates multiple distinguishable features, such as behavioral, emotional, cognitive, and psychological engagement. Definitions differ about whether to include the opposite of engagement; some do, using labels such as disengagement, disaffection, alienation, or burnout (Miceli & Castelfranchi, 2000; Salmela-Aro, Kiuru, Leskinen, & Nurmi, 2009; Vallerand et al., 1993). Conceptualizations disagree about the components that should be incorporated into the construct proper—some include academic outcomes such as grades and performance, whereas others include a student's feelings of bonding, academic identity, or positive relationships with teachers and classmates.

As the popularity of engagement grows, it has become increasingly important for researchers to clarify their conceptualizations, both the definition of engagement itself and the larger assumptions and models explaining how it operates. In our work, we view engagement as the outward manifestation of motivation (Skinner, Kindermann, Connell, & Wellborn, 2009a). At their heart, theories of motivation are most fundamentally concerned with the psychological processes that underlie *energy, purpose,* and *durability* of human action (Deci, 1992a). Engagement's characteristic effort, exertion, vigor, intensity, vitality, zest, and enthusiasm are markers of *energy*; its interest, focus, and concentration are outward expressions of *purpose* or *direction*; and its absorption, determination, and persistence are signs of *durability*. Motivation refers to the underlying sources of energy, purpose, and durability, whereas engagement refers to their visible manifestation. That is why constructs of engagement and disaffection have always been central to theories of motivation. In fact, every model of motivation in the field today includes an action component that shares core features with engagement (Skinner et al., 2009a; Wigfield, Eccles, Schiefele, Roeser, & Davis-Kean, 2006).

Our motivational conceptualization is located within a multilevel model of positive youth development and resilience, which recognizes engagement with school and other prosocial institutions as a protective factor and a positive force in the lives of children and youth, especially those who are at risk for underachievement and dropout. Engagement has been studied on at least four nested levels, as shown in Fig. 2.1. At the most general level, engagement refers to the involvement of children and youth in school as a prosocial institution, along with other institutions, such as church, youth groups, and community organizations. This kind of engagement promotes positive youth development and protects children from risks that emerge during early adolescence, such as delinquency, gang involvement, substance use, and unsafe sexual activity (e.g., Morrison, Robertson, Laurie & Kelly, 2002). At the second level, engagement with school refers to the involvement of children and youth in school activities, including academics, sports, band, student government, and extracurricular pursuits. This kind of engagement promotes students' completion and graduation from high school, and protects against absenteeism and dropout.

Nested within the classroom is the kind of engagement we are most interested in: student engagement with academic work, which we define as constructive, enthusiastic, willing, emotionally positive, and cognitively focused participation with learning activities in school (Connell & Wellborn, 1991; Skinner, Kindermann, Connell, et al., 2009a; Skinner, Kindermann, & Furrer, 2009b). This kind of engagement is critical for three reasons. First, it is a necessary condition for students to learn. Only if students participate in academic activities with both "hands-on" and "heads-on" will the time they spend in classrooms result in the acquisition of knowledge and skills. No matter how many extracurriculars students undertake or how attached they are to school, they will not learn or achieve

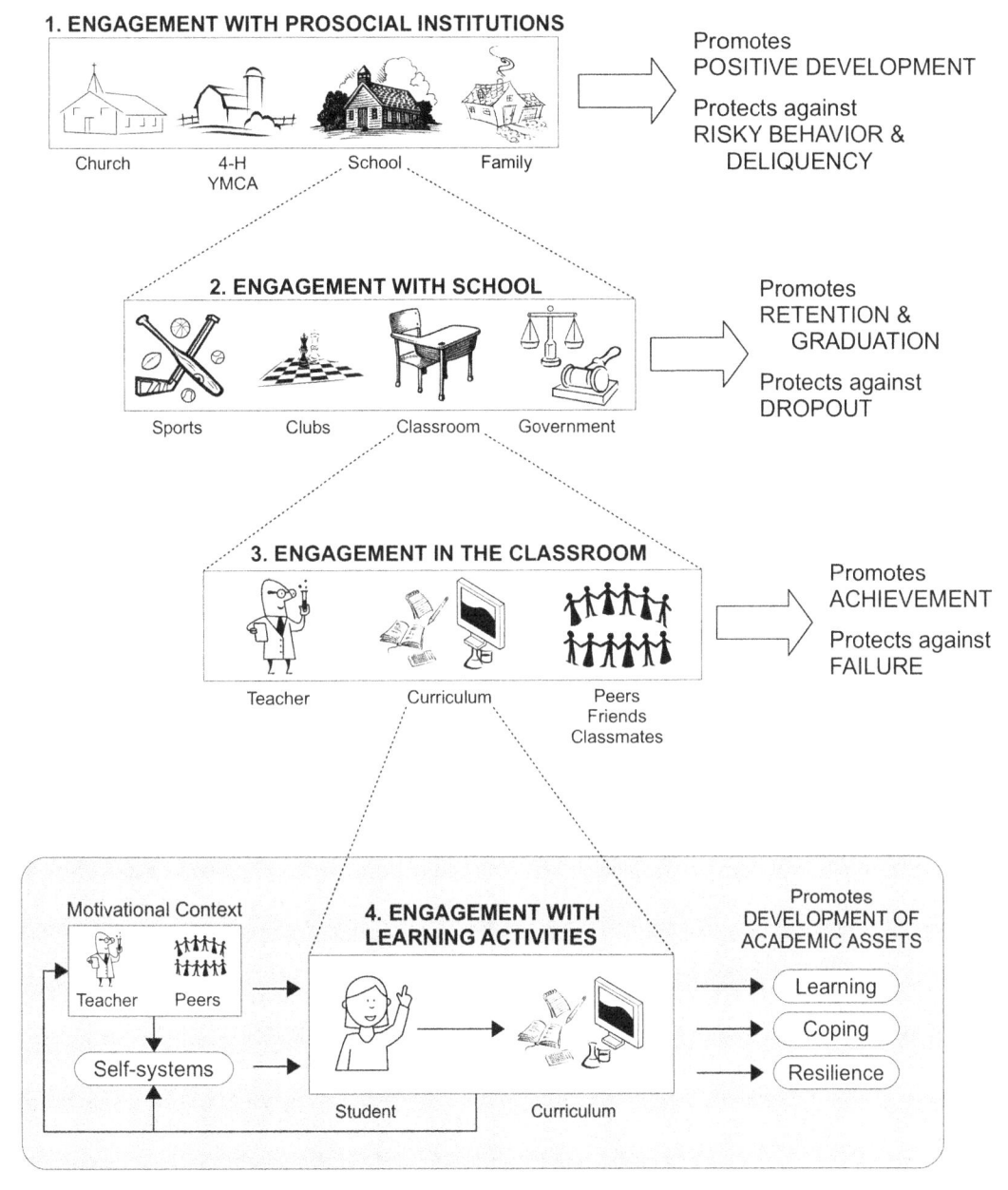

Model of Motivational Dynamics

Fig. 2.1 A multilevel perspective on engagement with school that highlights student engagement with learning activities as central to an understanding of the development of motivational dynamics

unless they are constructively engaged with the academic work of the classroom. Engagement is the active verb between the curriculum and actual learning. Engagement depicts the "proximal processes" that ecological models (e.g., Bronfenbrenner & Morris, 1998) posit are the primary engines of development. As a result, engagement is the direct (and only) pathway to cumulative learning, long-term achievement, and eventual academic success.

Second, engagement shapes students' everyday experiences in school, both psychologically and socially. High-quality engagement and its resultant learning and scholastic success lead students to feel more academically competent and connected, and elicit more positive interactions and support from teachers. Moreover, engaged students are allowed entry into friendships and peer groups with more engaged classmates. In contrast, disengaged students tend to perform poorly in school and so feel marginalized, resentful, and ineffective. Teachers respond to such students with less support and more coercion, and disaffected students are more likely to join disengaged peer groups and become friends with other disaffected students. Hence, students' classroom engagement plays an important role in the quality of their daily experiences while they are attending school.

Third, engagement is a critical contributor to students' academic development. Engagement is a part of the process of everyday academic resilience, and an energetic resource that helps students cope more adaptively with daily stressors, challenges, and setbacks in school. From episodes of effective coping may come the development of durable long-term motivational mindsets and skill sets, such as an autonomous learning style or mastery orientation, self-regulated learning, a positive academic identity, and eventually ownership for one's own progress in high school (and beyond). Therefore, engagement can be seen as a key player in the development of academic assets that takes place across the school year and over the arc of a student's entire educational career.

Purpose of the Chapter

This chapter is structured around these themes, which we refer to collectively as the dynamics of motivational development. First, we provide our conceptualization of engagement and explain the larger motivational model that depicts its functioning. We then review evidence that engagement is central to feed-forward and feedback loops that shape educational pathways. Third, we explain how these cycles of engagement may influence the development of everyday academic resilience, and specifically, how children and youth cope with challenges and setbacks in school. We also speculate how these dynamics may cumulatively shape the development of important but elusive personal assets and social resources at multiple points in a student's academic career. In the final section, we explore some important implications for educational practice.

Motivational Model of Context, Self, Action, and Outcomes

Engagement is the *action* component of our model of motivational development (Connell & Wellborn, 1991; Deci & Ryan, 1985, 2000; Skinner & Wellborn, 1994). In this context, "action" refers to goal-directed emotion-infused behaviors, reflecting the idea that actions are the natural unit of analysis for conceptualizing transactions between people and their social and physical contexts (Boesch, 1976; Brandtstädter, 1998; Chapman, 1984). Hence, engagement refers to energized, directed, and sustained action, or the observable qualities of students' actual interactions with academic tasks.

As a result, as depicted in Fig. 2.2, the motivational conceptualization of engagement includes not only behavior but also emotion and cognitive orientation: the behavioral dimension of engagement includes effort, intensity, persistence, determination, and perseverance in the face of obstacles and difficulties; emotional or affective engagement includes enthusiasm, enjoyment, fun, and satisfaction; and cognitive engagement encompasses attention, concentration, focus, absorption, "heads-on" participation, and a willingness to go beyond what is required. This conceptualization also includes the opposite of engagement, referred to as *disaffection* or burnout. Motivational conceptualizations of disaffection comprise the ways in which students withdraw

	Engagement	Disaffection
Behavior Initiation Ongoing participation Re-engagement	Action initiation Effort, Exertion Working hard Attempts Persistence Intensity Focus, Attention Concentration Absorption Involvement	Passivity, Procrastination Giving up Restlessness Half-hearted Unfocused, Inattentive Distracted Mentally withdrawn Burned out, Exhausted Unprepared Absent
Emotion Initiation Ongoing participation Re-engagement	Enthusiasm Interest Enjoyment Satisfaction Pride Vitality Zest	Boredom Disinterest Frustration/anger Sadness Worry/anxiety Shame Self-blame
Cognitive Orientation Initiation Ongoing participation Re-engagement	Purposeful Approach Goal strivings Strategy search Willing participation Preference for challenge Mastery Follow-through, care Thoroughness	Aimless Helpless Resigned Unwilling Opposition Avoidance Apathy Hopeless Pressured

Fig. 2.2 A motivational conceptualization of engagement and disaffection in the classroom

from learning tasks, including physical withdrawal of effort, such as lack of exertion, passivity, merely going through the motions, or exhaustion as well as their mental counterparts, such as lack of concentration, apathy, inattention, or amotivation. Emotional reactions are critical components of disaffection because patterns of action differ depending on whether lack of participation is based on boredom, anxiety, shame, sadness, or frustration.

Indicators Versus Facilitators of Engagement

In order to study how it functions, indicators of engagement must be distinguished from facilitators of engagement (Sinclair et al., 2003). In general, *indicators* are markers or descriptive parts *inside* a target construct, whereas *facilitators* are explanatory causal factors, *outside* the target construct, that have the potential to influence the target. For example, if a target of study is weight loss, then indicators of weight loss include pounds on a scale, dimensions of the body, and the body mass index. Potential facilitators of weight loss include a healthy diet and exercise. It is an empirical question whether a particular pattern of eating and exercise actually produces any weight loss, and even if they are highly correlated, it does not mean that diet is part of weight loss. In fact, it is essential to conceptually distinguish them and to measure them separately, in order to determine whether the potential facilitators can actually influence indicators of the target. Both indicators and facilitators can be distinguished from the *outcomes* of engagement, which refer to the results that engagement itself can produce. In the weight loss example, outcomes or effects of weight loss might include lowered blood pressure or increased energy. It is an empirical question whether weight loss can influence these outcomes, however, and even if weight loss and outcomes are highly correlated, lowered blood pressure is not an indicator of weight loss.

Maintaining the distinctions among indicators, facilitators, and outcomes of engagement can add clarity to conceptualizations and improve studies of engagement. In the motivational model, indicators of engagement must be *action* components, and so in addition to the behavioral, emotional, and cognitive features of action described previously, we would accept as indicators of engagement other observable student interactions with academic activities, such as on-task behavior or homework completion. In contrast, academic performance (grades on tests or homework, semester grades, achievement test scores) would *not* be indicators of engagement. They are potential *outcomes*. Any studies that measure engagement by combining, for example, GPA with on-task behavior, are confusing because they do not allow the examination of whether more on-task behavior (an indicator) produces a higher GPA (an outcome).

In work on engagement, the greatest confusion is between indicators and facilitators of engagement. Many conceptualizations and measures combine them. In the motivational model, we distinguish two kinds of potential facilitators: personal and social. Personal facilitators are students' self-perceptions or *self-system processes* which refer to durable appraisals of multiple features of the self, such as self-efficacy or a sense of belongingness in school. Social facilitators, also referred to as *social contexts*, are interpersonal interactions with important social partners, such as teachers, peers, and parents, and include their quality and nature, such as whether they are warm, dependable, or controlling.

Explanatory research and intervention efforts require a clear demarcation between indicators and facilitators. If, for example, theories hold that supportive interactions with teachers are an indicator of engagement itself, as opposed to a facilitator that potentially contributes to engagement, research that combines these factors into a "meta-construct" can never investigate whether teacher support influences student engagement. In order to empirically explore whether interpersonal factors and self-perceptions shape the development of engagement and disaffection, it is essential to conceptualize and measure facilitators separately from indicators.

Sources of Engagement: Self-determination Theory

Many important facilitators and outcomes of engagement have been integrated into a model of positive motivational development grounded in self-determination theory, called the Self-System Model of Motivational Development (SSMMD; Connell & Wellborn, 1991; Deci, Connell & Ryan, 1985; Deci & Ryan, 1985, 2000; Deci, Vallerand, Pelletier & Ryan, 1991; Reeve, 2002; Ryan, Connell & Deci, 1985; Skinner & Wellborn, 1994). This model is rooted in organismic assumptions about intrinsic motivation, asserting that "people are innately curious, interested creatures who possess a natural love of learning and who desire to internalize the knowledge, customs, and values that surround them" (Niemiec & Ryan, 2009, p. 133). The core idea is that humans come with basic needs, and when these needs are met by social contexts or activities, people will engage constructively with them. When these needs are thwarted, people become disaffected, that is, they withdraw, escape, or act out.

The model posits three fundamental psychological needs that are based in physiology and are evolutionarily adaptive: the needs for relatedness, competence, and autonomy. School contexts influence engagement by supporting (or undermining) students' experiences of themselves as related in school, as competent to succeed, and as autonomous or self-determined learners. From these experiences, children cumulatively construct views of themselves, referred to as *self-system processes* (Connell & Wellborn, 1991). These beliefs are not fleeting self-perceptions; they are durable convictions that shape apparent reality and so guide action. *Relatedness* refers to the need to experience oneself as connected to other people, as belonging; it is hypothesized to underlie processes of attachment (Ainsworth, 1979; Bowlby, 1969/1973; Bretherton, 1985; Crittenden, 1990) and has been studied across the lifespan as the "need to belong" (Baldwin, 1992; Baumeister & Leary, 1995). Although relatedness is a relatively recent addition to research in the academic domain, studies find links between a sense of belonging in school and multiple indicators of motivation, engagement, and adjustment (e.g., Anderman, 1999; Battistich, Solomon, Kim, Watson, & Schnaps, 1995; Booker, 2006; Eccles & Midgley, 1989; Furrer & Skinner, 2003; Goodenow, 1993; Kuperminc, Blatt, Shahar, Henrich, & Leadbetter, 2004; Lynch & Cicchetti, 1992, 1997; Roeser, Midgley, & Urdan, 1996; Ryan, Stiller, & Lynch, 1994; Wentzel, 1997, 1998, 1999).

Competence refers to the need to experience oneself as effective in one's interactions with the social and physical environments (Elliot & Dweck, 2005; Harter, 1978; Koestner & McClelland, 1990; White, 1959) and is hypothesized to underlie processes of control (Bandura, 1997; Peterson, Maier, & Seligman, 1993; Seligman, 1975). For competence, self-system processes have been studied as perceptions of control (Bandura, 1997; Dweck, 1991; Heckhausen & Schultz, 1995; Skinner, 1996; Weisz, 1986); these are perhaps the most frequently studied academic self-perceptions (Wigfield et al., 2006). Perceptions of self-efficacy, ability, academic competence, and control are robust predictors of student engagement and eventual learning, academic performance, and achievement (see Bandura, 1997; Dweck, 1999; Harter, 1982; Skinner, 1995, 1996; Skinner, Zimmer-Gembeck, & Connell, 1998; Stipek, 2002a; Weiner, 2005; Wigfield et al., 2006).

Autonomy refers to the need to express one's authentic self and to experience that self as the source of action, and is hypothesized to underlie processes of self-determination (Deci & Ryan, 1985, 2000, 2002a). For autonomy, self-system processes have been studied as autonomy or goal orientations (Deci & Ryan, 1985, 1991; Dweck, 1991; Kuhl, 1987; Ryan & Connell, 1989) and contain views about the self as motivated for self-determined or intrinsic reasons (or for extrinsic reasons). Students with a greater sense of *autonomy* in school also show higher levels of classroom engagement, enjoyment, persistence, achievement, and learning (e.g., Deci & Ryan, 2002b; Grolnick & Ryan, 1987; Hardre & Reeve, 2003; Miserandino, 1996; Otis, Grouzet, & Pelletier, 2005; Patrick, Skinner, & Connell, 1993; Vallerand, Fortier, & Guay, 1997; Vasalampi, Salmela-Aro, & Nurmi, 2009).

Schools, Teachers, Peers, Parents, and the Social Context

Although all children and youth come with the needs for relatedness, competence, and autonomy, they act on the motivations provided by these needs in social contexts, like schools, that are differentially responsive to them. The motivational model emphasizes the importance of supportive interactions with teachers, peers, and parents, and intrinsically interesting academic work.

Teachers Shape Engagement

According to the model, three important qualities of student-teacher interactions are pedagogical caring (which supports experiences of relatedness), optimal structure (which facilitates competence), and autonomy support (which promotes self-determined motivation). Research validates the notion that all three are important in shaping motivation and engagement in the classroom (Hamre & Pianta, 2001; Murray & Greenberg, 2000; Pianta, 1999, 2006; Ryan & Stiller, 1991; Stipek, 2002b; Wentzel, 1998, 2009; Wigfield et al., 2006). Early work showed that properly structured classrooms promote student motivation (e.g., Ames & Ames, 1985; Rosenholtz & Wilson, 1980). Subsequently, the quality of student-teacher relationships, in the form of caring supportive alliances, was emphasized as a predictor of motivation and achievement (Birch & Ladd, 1997, 1998; Goodenow, 1993; Murray & Murray, 2004; Ryan & Powelson, 1991). Recently, autonomy supportive instruction (giving choices, making learning relevant) has been linked to engagement (Deci & Ryan 2002b Guthrie & Davis, 2003; Reeve, Jang, Carrell, Jeon & Barch, 2004).

The model focuses on all three facets of teacher support: warmth, provision of structure, and autonomy support, all of which have been shown to contribute to students' positive self-perceptions as well as to classroom engagement (e.g., Skinner & Belmont, 1993). Close and caring relationships with teachers and other adults in school have been shown to be an important predictor of student engagement across race, ethnicity, and class (e.g., Brewster & Bowen, 2004; Connell, Halpern-Felsher, Clifford, Crichlow, & Usinger, 1995; Connell, Spencer, & Aber, 1994; Garcia-Reid, Reid & Peterson, 2002; Wooley & Bowen, 2007).

Peers Shape Engagement
In addition to teachers, peers and parents also influence student motivation and engagement (Wentzel, 1998). Although many studies highlight negative developmental influences from friends, in recent years, an increasing number show that children's friendships in school can also exert positive effects on academic development (e.g., Altermatt & Pomeranz, 2003; Hallinan & Williams, 1990; Kandel, 1978; Ladd, 1990; Ladd, Kochenderfer & Coleman, 1997; Ryan, 2001; Wentzel, McNamara-Barry, & Caldwell, 2004; for a review, see Bukowski, Motzoi & Meyer, 2009), especially school motivation and achievement (e.g., Berndt, 2004; Berndt, Hawkins & Jiao, 1999; Berndt & Keefe, 1995; Berndt, Laychak & Park, 1990). Moreover, studies of naturally occurring peer groups also suggest that peers influence students' motivation, behavior, and achievement in school (e.g., Cairns, Neckerman & Cairns, 1989; Chen, Chang & He, 2003; Estell, Farmer, Cairns & Cairns, 2002; Gest, Rulison, Davidson & Welsh, 2008; Kindermann, 1993, 2007; Kindermann, McCollam & Gibson, 1996; Kindermann & Skinner, 2009, in press).

Parents Shape Engagement
Following up on the large body of work demonstrating a connection between parenting practices and school achievement, studies are accumulating which suggest that one pathway through which parenting has an impact on children's school performance is by shaping children's classroom engagement, intrinsic motivation, preference for challenge, valuing and commitment to school, and enthusiasm, enjoyment, and interest in schoolwork (Connell & Wellborn, 1991; Epstein & Sanders, 2002; Ginsberg & Bronstein, 1993; Gottfried, Fleming, & Gottfried, 1994; Grolnick & Ryan, 1989, 1992; Grolnick, Ryan, & Deci, 1991; Grolnick & Slowiaczek, 1994; Jeynes, 2007; Pomerantz, Grolnick, & Price, 2005; Reynolds & Clements, 2005; Steinberg, Elmen, & Mounts, 1989; Wigfield et al., 2006). Longitudinal studies of the motivational mediators between authoritative parenting and children's school performance are especially informative (e.g., Steinberg et al., 1989) as are studies that examine parents' use of specific motivational practices (e.g., Gottfried, Marcoulides, Gottfried, & Oliver, 2009; Grolnick & Slowiaczek, 1994).

The Nature of Academic Work
Especially important determinants of motivation and engagement are the academic tasks students undertake in the classroom (Newmann, King, & Carmichael, 2007; Newmann et al., 1992; Wigfield et al., 2006). Because learning activities are the "interaction partners" with which students engage, their qualities influence the nature of the interaction. Hence, active participation, engagement, and effort are promoted by tasks that are hands-on, heads-on, project-based, relevant,

progressive, and integrated across subject matter, or in other words, intrinsically motivating, inherently interesting, and fun (Deci, 1992b, 1998; Renninger, 2000). *Authentic work* is a term used to characterize "tasks that are considered meaningful, valuable, significant, and worthy of one's effort, in contrast to those considered nonsensical, useless, contrived, trivial, and therefore unworthy of effort" (Newmann et al., 1992, p. 23). By connecting to the "real world" beyond school, such tasks offer students a sense of purpose and ownership (Newmann et al., 2007).

Motivational Dynamics of Engagement and Disaffection

The motivational model is depicted graphically in Fig. 2.3. According to the model, school contexts differentially provide children and youth with opportunities to fulfill their fundamental psychological needs (through provision of warmth/involvement, structure, and autonomy support). Based on these experiences, students construct self-system processes which are organized around relatedness, competence, and autonomy. These self-system processes in turn provide a motivational basis for their patterns of engagement versus disaffection with learning activities. Constructive engagement is considered to be a critical mechanism through which motivational processes contribute to learning and achievement.

Reciprocal Feedback Effects of Engagement

As can be seen in Fig. 2.3, engagement not only contributes to students' subsequent learning and performance, but it has a reciprocal connection to teachers, parents, and peers. The key idea is that students' motivation, as expressed through their engagement, is salient to their social partners and so has an impact on the way that others respond to them. Most of the research that links motivational support (from teachers, parents, or peers) to student engagement is correlational and cross-sectional, and is typically interpreted as reflecting the feed-forward effects of social partners on students' motivation. However, a few experimental and longitudinal studies have been conducted which show that adults respond to children differentially depending on their on-task, engaged, or disruptive behaviors, and that children join or are allowed entry into friendships and peer groups based on their engagement in school.

Effects of Engagement on Teachers
Only a few studies have explicitly investigated whether students' engagement shapes how teachers subsequently respond to them (Furrer &

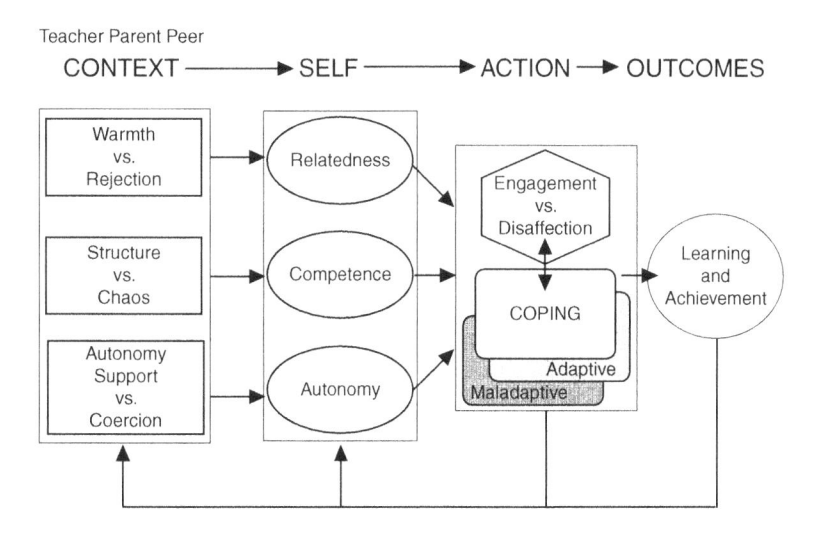

Fig. 2.3 A dynamic model of motivational development organized around student engagement and disaffection

Skinner, 2009; Pelletier & Vallerand, 1996). For example, kindergarteners who were more behaviorally engaged in the classroom tended to develop closer relationships with their teachers over time than did those who were less engaged (Ladd, Birch, & Buhs, 1999). Similarly, elementary school students (in grades 3 through 5) with higher behavioral engagement in the fall experienced increases in teacher support over the school year, and students with higher emotional engagement experienced increases in teacher autonomy granting as the year progressed (Furrer & Skinner, 2009; Skinner & Belmont, 1993). In the same vein, two observational studies, one of middle schoolers (Altermatt, Jovanovic, & Perry, 1998) and one of junior high and high schoolers (Fiedler, 1975), revealed that students who showed more participation in class elicited greater teacher responsiveness.

Effects of Engagement on Parents

A growing body of research also examines children's effects on their parents (Bell, 1968, 1979; Patterson, 1982). A portion of this research looks directly at parental reactions to children who are resistant, unresponsive, uncooperative, or off-task (or who are perceived to be so), and suggests that parents respond to such children by withdrawing their involvement or becoming more controlling (power assertive and coercive; Anderson, Lytton, & Romney, 1996; Grolnick & Apostoleris, 2002; Patterson, 1982). Especially interesting are the few experimental studies in which child behavior was manipulated or assigned. In one study, children ages 9–11 were trained as confederates to be difficult, uncooperative, and disinterested (versus easy, cooperative, and interested); mothers who were trying to teach children anagrams were more controlling with the "difficult" children (Jelsma, 1982). Taken together, these studies suggest that students' academic engagement is likely to shape how adults, both teachers and parents, respond to them.

Effects of Engagement on Peers

In research on the effects of children's friendships and peer groups on their academic performance, a few studies examine what are referred to as *selection* effects, or how children enter and leave friendship and peer relationships. The key idea is that children select and are selected by other children based in part on their engagement in school, with more engaged children and youth joining peer and friendship groups with more engaged peers, and more disaffected children and youth joining groups of more disaffected peers. Evidence comes from cross-sectional studies showing that students' own levels of engagement are correlated with those of their friendship networks and peer groups (Kindermann & Skinner, in press), and longitudinal studies which show that despite high turnover in actual members over a school year, there is relatively high stability in the motivational composition (average levels of engagement) of children's peer groups (Kindermann, 1993, 2007). Taken together, this work suggests that children who are more engaged join peer and friendship networks of other children who are likewise more engaged in school.

Cycles of Engagement and Disaffection

Motivational dynamics involve the feed-forward and feedback causal effects among context, self, action, and outcomes, which result in feedback loops or "cycles" of engagement. Supportive interactions with teachers, parents, and peers contribute to positive self-perceptions, which promote student engagement with interesting and meaningful academic activities—which facilitates learning and the development of competence. High-quality engagement and achievement in turn bolster students' positive self-perceptions, elicit further teacher and parent support, and allow children to join networks of engaged peers and friends. In contrast, unsupportive interpersonal interactions or perceptions of the self as unwelcome, incompetent, or pressured in school lead to disaffection—which undermines learning and achievement. Disaffection and failure in turn undercut students' sense of self, can result in withdrawal of support or increasing coercion from teachers and parents, and lead children to join more disengaged friendship and peer groups.

These feedback loops are self-amplifying, forming *virtuous* or *vicious* cycles that magnify initial individual differences across time, making motivationally "rich" students richer, and motivationally "poor" students poorer. Studies examining engagement at multiple time points have empirically captured some of these dynamics, some involving motivational resources, such as perceived control (e.g., Schmitz & Skinner, 1993), achievement (e.g., Gottfried, Marcoulides, Gottfried, Oliver, & Guerin, 2007), or teacher support (e.g., Altermatt et al., 1998; Fiedler, 1975; Skinner & Belmont, 1993), and some involving multiple components (e.g., Skinner, Furrer, Marchand, & Kindermann, 2008; Skinner et al., 1998). Although other kinds of cycles are theoretically possible, all the dynamics that have been documented so far have turned out to be self-amplifying or self-stabilizing, in that they magnify or verify the pattern of individual differences present in the initial conditions.

Trajectories of Engagement

These dynamics may be responsible for the high stability of engagement and disaffection, and may underlie interindividual differences in trajectories of motivation over a student's school career. Although there is an overall normative decline in engagement across school years (Wigfield et al., 2006), research also documents a high level of interindividual stability. That is, children's levels of engagement at the beginning of the school year are highly correlated with their levels at the end of the school year (e.g., Skinner & Belmont, 1993); engagement during one grade is highly correlated with engagement in neighboring grades (e.g., Gottfried, Fleming, & Gottfried, 2001); and children's engagement in the early elementary school years is highly correlated with their engagement in middle school (e.g., Gottfried et al., 2007; Skinner et al., 1998) and high school (Gottfried et al., 2001; Marks, 2000; Otis et al., 2005). In fact, in the few studies comparing such relations, interindividual stability seems to *increase* as students move through junior high and high school (Gottfried, 1990; Gottfried et al., 2001).

Although it can be tempting to interpret such high cross-time correlations as evidence that engagement is a fixed motivational trait, research on the dynamics of engagement contradict this conclusion. Taken together, studies demonstrate that engagement is a malleable state, open to contextual conditions, that can be shaped by interpersonal and task characteristics. Dynamic stability is continually recreated by the feedback loops between students' engaged and disaffected actions, on the one hand, and their facilitators and outcomes, on the other, including the context created by teachers, parents, peers, and the nature of academic work, students' self-perceptions, and their performance outcomes. It is the thousands of episodes of engaged participation or disaffected withdrawal that organize these feedback loops, which is why engagement is a sensitive indicator of the state of the whole motivational system.

Engagement and the Development of Coping and Everyday Resilience

Cycles of ongoing engagement also create a motivational context that may shape how students deal with everyday difficulties, challenges, and obstacles in school. As studied under the name "everyday resilience" or "academic buoyancy" (Martin & Marsh, 2006, 2008a, 2008b, 2009), these processes refer to resources students can access to help them bounce back from setbacks and failures, and allow them to constructively reengage with challenging academic tasks after running into obstacles or problems. Academic buoyancy refers to "students' ability to successfully deal with academic setbacks and challenges that are typical of the ordinary course of school life (e.g., poor grades, competing deadlines, exam pressure, difficult schoolwork)" (Martin & Marsh, 2008a, p. 72). The motivational model suggests that both interpersonal resources, such as teacher warmth or peer engagement, and personal resources, such as a sense of competence, relatedness, and autonomy, are assets that can support everyday resilience and reengagement.

Academic Coping as a Mechanism of Everyday Resilience

A primary process of resilience in school is *coping*, which describes how students deal with challenges, threats, and failures in their daily experiences with academic tasks (Skinner & Wellborn, 1994, 1997). Work on coping is distinguished by its focus on what children and youth actually do in their real-life encounters with stressful events. These reactions can be classified into *families of coping*, such as problem-solving, support seeking, or escape (Skinner, Edge, Altman, & Sherwood, 2003). Many of these ways of coping have been studied individually, but when considered as a *profile* or *repertoire* of ways of coping, it is possible to examine how they work together cumulatively as a series of adaptive (or maladaptive) responses to problems and difficulties with schoolwork or other stressful events in school.

A developmental model has identified a dozen families of coping (Skinner et al., 2003), some of which promote reengagement (e.g., problem-solving or help seeking) and some of which lead to giving up (e.g., helplessness or social isolation) or getting in trouble (e.g., delegation or opposition). Help seeking seems to be an especially adaptive strategy for dealing with problems (Newman, 1994, 2000). In fact, it is the most common all-purpose strategy used by children (Zimmer-Gembeck & Skinner, 2011) and a common way of coping even for adolescents and adults (Skinner et al., 2003). One reason it is so adaptive is that interactions with competent and supportive social partners (like teachers) can help students reengage with difficult material and eventually develop strategies like problem-solving and self-reliance that they can then employ in dealing with (or preventing) subsequent stressors (Nelson-Le Gall, Gumerman, & Scott-Jones, 1983). Unfortunately, over the same age range that children and adolescents show declines in motivation, they also evince declines in the use of help seeking (Marchand & Skinner, 2007; Newman, 2002; Ryan, Patrick, & Shim, 2005).

Emergence of Academic Resources for Resilience

Over time, ongoing engagement, constructive coping, and reengagement following failures and setbacks may work together to shape children's academic development. The central idea is that these cycles of engagement and coping, over months or years, give rise to the development of qualitatively different mindsets and skill sets at different ages. For example, early research on participation-identification models of engagement argued that positive patterns of engagement lead to a sense of belonging in school and valuing of school-related goals (Finn, 1989). And reviews of coping show that (compared with younger children) older children are able to use more complex cognitive coping strategies and to more flexibly match the demands of the stressor to the family of coping (Zimmer-Gembeck & Skinner, 2011).

Although educators and parents stress how important it is for students to take responsibility or ownership for their own academic progress, very little is known about how and at what ages specific qualitativly new resources emerge during a student's scholastic career. It is clear that some qualitative growth must be taking place, in that kindergarten and first-grade students do not have the means to form a complex academic identity, use sophisticated cognitive strategies, or flexibly regulate their own learning. Researchers have begun to identify some of the cognitive and meta-cognitive abilities students need to become more proactive, self-reliant, and autonomous in their own learning (Otis et al., 2005; Schunk & Zimmerman, 2007) and in their adaptive help seeking (Newman, 2002), but little research examines the effects of these underlying processes on students' development.

Early adolescence seems to be a key developmental period for students to construct an identity as academically capable, socially integrated, and committed to learning (Roeser, Peck, & Nasir, 2006; Wentzel, 1991), but it is possible that qualitative changes in academic resources occur at other points as well, for example, during the five to seven shift (Sameroff & Haith, 1996) or the third-grade shift. One indicator of a transition might be steeper rates of normative decline in engagement, signaling a window of opportunity as well as of vulnerability. A noticeable trend in findings from the study of all such forms of potential academic development is that these desirable attributes are quite rare even in older academically successful students (Miserandino, 1996). Future research can examine how positive motivational dynamics may contribute to the development of self-regulated learning and proactive coping, and an academic identity that allows students to eventually take ownership for their own learning and success in school.

Educational Implications for Promoting Engagement, Coping, and Everyday Resilience

The motivational model of engagement and disaffection inspired by self-determination theory has several important implications for the structuring of learning environments (see also Deci, Connell, & Ryan, 1985; Niemiec & Ryan, 2009; Reeve, 2002) and comprehensive school reform (Connell, Klem, Lacher, Leiderman, & Moore, 2009; Deci, 2009). The most important is the core assumption that all students come with a wellspring of intrinsic motivation that does not have to be acquired and cannot be lost. However, steady declines in students' intrinsic motivation and engagement signal that schools are not nurturing this precious energetic resource (Eccles et al., 1993; Wigfield et al., 2006). We highlight three important antidotes (see Fig. 2.4).

Focus on Engagement and Disaffection

The motivational model encourages schools and teachers, when formulating their target outcomes, to insist on a dual focus on learning *and* engagement. High grades or high achievement test scores cannot be considered a success if they come at the cost of undermining engagement and increasing student disaffection. The good news is that constructive engagement, when combined with a challenging curriculum and authentic learning activities, creates opportunities for increased learning and so is a direct pathway to better performance. It is important to include the entire complex construct of engagement in target outcomes. Teachers and parents can easily focus on only the behavioral component—on-task behavior—and lose track of emotion, cognition, and orientation, as embodied, for example, by enthusiasm, interest, excitement, willingness, preference for challenge, and "heads-on" participation. Although behavioral engagement seems to be the primary driver of actual performance, emotion is likely the fuel for the kind of behavioral and cognitive engagement that leads to high-quality learning (Skinner et al., 2008).

Tracking Engagement

Additional good news is that the action component of student engagement with academic work is directly observable, and so teachers can track it at the classroom level (Reeve et al., 2004) or at the level of individual students (Skinner et al., 2009a, 2009b). The positive and significant correlations between teachers' ratings of engagement and both student ratings and observers' reports indicate that teachers seem to do this spontaneously and accurately, suggesting that student engagement is a source of information available to teachers in designing and delivering their lesson plans. Student engagement with learning activities is a marker of the whole motivational system and so provides teachers a diagnostic window into other important motivational processes that are not directly observable, such as students' self-system processes of belonging, competence, or value (Furrer, Kelly, & Skinner, 2003). Researchers and interventionists who want to support students' motivation and learning can also take advantage of engagement as a key summary marker of the quality of students' school experiences.

Focus on Engagement and Disaffection

1. Adopt as a central goal the *promotion of engagement in academic work*, tracking especially student orientation, emotional, and cognitive engagement, as expressed through student enthusiasm, interest, excitement, willingness, preference for challenge, and "heads-on" participation.

2. Use student disaffection as a *diagnostic tool* signaling that a student needs *more* warmth, involvement, structure, and/or autonomy support. View students' misunderstandings and failures as opportunities for students to learn something new about the subject and about how to cope more constructively.

3. Provide *academic tasks* that are authentic, challenging, relevant to students' experiences and concerns, hands-on, project-based, integrated across subject areas, and that allow students some freedom to choose their own direction and to work closely in cooperative groups over long periods of time.

Focus on the Social Learning Environment

1. Promote students' *intrinsic motivation*, by offering challenging and fun learning activities, allowing and encouraging students to discover and follow their own interests and goals, and providing clear instruction and feedback about how to reach them.

2. *Meet students' needs* for relatedness, competence, and autonomy: Foster caring relationships (warmth and involvement), provide challenging learning activities with high expectations and clear feedback (optimal structure), and explain the relevance and importance of activities and rules while soliciting input from students and respecting their opinions (autonomy support).

3. Promote *classroom goals* that focus on mastery, by creating a climate that emphasizes hard work, sustained effort, self-improvement, deep understanding, and the recognition that "mistakes," "setbacks," and "failures" can be interesting detours and good information about next steps.

Focus on Teachers

1. Model your *own engagement* in teaching, by showing your enthusiasm, hard work, careful thought, and excitement about a subject area. Model *constructive coping* in the classroom. Admit mistakes and tell stories of your own past failures and struggles.

2. View student *amotivation as a fascinating challenge*, a puzzle to be solved, and an opportunity to learn more about teaching and more about coping successfully with challenging students.

3. Remember that *teachers have their own needs* for relatedness, competence, and autonomy, and when they are met, it provides opportunities for more constructive engagement and coping, everyday resilience, vigor, vitality, and the development of teaching expertise.

Fig. 2.4 Educational practices that promote the development of engagement, coping, and everyday resilience

Coping with Student Disaffection and Failure

Just because teachers are accurate monitors of engagement and disaffection does not mean that they always respond to students' motivation in the optimal fashion. In fact, as described previously, the feedback loops from student engagement to teacher support found in several studies suggest that teachers typically react to students' disaffection in the classroom by withdrawing their support or increasing coercion. In other words, teachers typically respond in ways that are likely to further undermine students' engagement, making matters worse. Little research examines the mindsets or contextual conditions that would allow teachers to react to disengaged students with *increased* warmth, involvement, and autonomy support. Perhaps teachers could respond more positively if they could see student disaffection, not as a personal insult to them or a character flaw in the student, but as a handy diagnostic tool signaling times when a student is encountering resistance and need more support. It might be likewise helpful if teachers could see students' misunderstandings and failures, not as shortcomings of teacher or student, but as opportunities for students to learn something new about the subject and about how to deal more constructively with challenging learning tasks.

The Nature of Academic Work

For educators and researchers interested in classroom engagement, it is evident that the primary interaction partners for students, if they are to learn, are the academic tasks that we require them to undertake as part of the curriculum in schools. The nature of these learning activities is a definitive determinant of students' intrinsic interest and can make much easier (or much harder) the job of the teacher in facilitating motivation. Curricula and academic tasks will naturally arouse intrinsic motivation the more they are authentic, challenging, relevant to students' experiences and concerns, hands-on or project-based, integrated across subject areas and into students' real lives, and reflect students' own interests and goals—in other words, are fun and interesting (Deci & Ryan, 1985; Newmann et al., 1992). Complex learning environments, which include project-based curricula, integrated across subject matter, that allow students some freedom to chose their direction and to work closely in cooperative groups over long periods of time, awaken and sustain students' natural curiosity and love of learning.

In general, these are the learning environments provided by high-quality preschools and graduate schools, two levels of schooling at which intrinsic motivation and engagement flourish. Unfortunately, they are not the norm for the grades in between. However, simply ask any adults about their favorite memories of school (as we recently did in our research group) and you will find that they nevertheless do appear as individual unforgettable experiences. We heard enthusiastic tales of an opera written and performed by third graders, the creation of an Egyptian museum in elementary school, a Japanese tea house in sixth grade, a CSI-type investigation of a "dead" body in science and English class during middle school, and a radio program covering the Red Scare of the 1920s performed in high school. Ten, twenty, thirty years later, these experiences evoke smiles and detailed indelible memories of wholehearted engagement. Our research group is currently studying the effects of garden-based science education programs for at-risk middle school students—and finding that the holistic, authentic, cooperative, fun, environmentally friendly activities of gardening promote both students' engagement *and* their achievement (Ratcliffe, Goldberg, Rogers, & Merrigan, 2010; Skinner, Chi, & the LEAG, 2012).

Focus on the Social Learning Environment

Formal classroom curricula are essential, of course, but so too are the informal or tacit curricula—answers to the questions: What are we doing here? What is the purpose of school? Although it seems obvious—we are here to learn—research on goal orientations over the last 25 years eloquently demonstrates that teachers and schools seem to be consistently communicating to students, especially as they grow older, that schools have an agenda that is not fully aligned with learning and mastery (e.g., Ames, 1992; Midgley & Edelin, 1998; Roeser et al., 1996). Although questions remain about the exact meaning of achievement goal constructs (Hulleman, Schrager, Bodman, & Harachiewicz, 2010), it is clear that engagement, joy, high-quality conceptual learning, creativity, and constructive coping are all undermined by the external and internal pressures created by a focus on performance and grades, the evaluation of fixed abilities, and the shame and embarrassment of mistakes and failures (Deci, Koestner, & Ryan, 1999; Dweck, 1991; Hulleman et al., 2010; Pintrich, 2003). A complement to curricula designed to tap intrinsic motivation is the establishment of a classroom climate focused on *mastery*, that is, hard work, sustained effort, self-improvement, deep understanding, the unshakable conviction that everyone can excel, and the recognition that "mistakes," "setbacks," and "failures" can not only be interesting detours but are also informative about next steps in one's own thinking and progress.

Teacher-Student Interactions as Facilitators of Engagement

The nature of the interactions teachers have with their students can shape student engagement in the classroom in at least two ways. The first is by promoting students' intrinsic motivation: by offering challenging and fun learning activities, allowing and encouraging students to discover and follow their own interests and goals, and providing clear instruction and feedback about how to reach them. The second is by creating classroom contexts that support the development of increasingly more self-determined reasons for accomplishing the parts of learning that are not intrinsically fun. All worthwhile tasks involve a mix of inspiration and perspiration, and self-determination theory posits that activities that are extrinsically motivated can nevertheless be completed autonomously if students identify with their value and relevance (Ryan, 1995; Ryan & Connell, 1989). Students are more likely to internalize autonomous reasons for completing extrinsically motivated tasks in school when they learn from teachers who display the three features of motivational support described previously: when teachers foster caring relationships (warmth and involvement), provide challenging learning activities with high expectations and clear feedback (optimal structure), and explain the relevance and importance of activities and rules while soliciting input from students and respecting their opinions (autonomy support) (Connell & Wellborn, 1991; Deci & Ryan, 2000).

Focus on Teacher Motivation, Engagement, Coping, and Resilience

Teachers can facilitate students' engagement and constructive coping directly through their own actions and modeling in the classroom. Teachers' enthusiasm and excitement about a subject can be contagious (Patrick, Hisley, Kempler, & College, 2000). Teachers' hard work and careful thought can communicate the importance and value of knowledge and skills. Perhaps most important are the ways in which teachers model how to deal with roadblocks, confusion, and mistakes. Teachers can demonstrate constructive coping through such simple (and challenging) means as admitting that they do not know something or that their own current understandings can sometimes be contradictory and uncertain, and then taking the time to straighten them out or to find out more, by identifying areas of confusion and consulting resources or experts. Constructive coping can also involve telling stories of one's own past failures and mistakes, as inspiration for students who are currently struggling. Compared to the effects of parents (Bradley, 2007; Power, 2004), much less research examines how teachers can promote the development of constructive coping and everyday resilience in their students, making this a fruitful area for research.

Teacher Motivation and Engagement

The motivational model holds that teachers have the same needs as students and so provides a useful lens through which to hypothesize about the effects of students' motivational problems on teachers. If teachers experience low student motivation as an obstacle to their teaching and lesson plans, then it thwarts teacher autonomy. If it is perceived as a signal that teachers are bad at teaching, then it undercuts teachers' sense of competence. If it is seen as evidence that students don't like the teacher, it can undermine teachers' feelings of relatedness. According to the motivational model, any of these interpretations should lead teachers to become disaffected from the target students, and could produce the withdrawal, hostility, or coercion found in studies of the reciprocal effects of student motivation on teacher behaviors. If, however, in contrast, teachers can see student amotivation as a fascinating challenge, an interesting puzzle which they are confident they can solve, then the boredom, passivity, or disruptive behavior students show in class can be opportunities for teachers to learn more about teaching and more about how to cope successfully with challenging students (Hakanen, Bakker, & Schaufeli, 2006; Martin & Marsh, 2008b).

Teachers Within the Larger School Context

Student engagement is a precious energetic resource, not only for students, but also for teachers' own enjoyment and engagement in teaching. When students are trying hard, taking on challenges, seeking and providing help, and making strides in their learning, teachers remember why they decided to become teachers in the first place. The research on reciprocal effects suggests that teacher and student engagement can create a virtuous circle—one that supports both partners (and by implication the whole classroom) in self-stabilizing cycles of hard work, joy, and learning, as well as increasing feelings of connectedness to each other as a learning community, competence in learning and teaching, and autonomy toward the activities and enterprise of schooling. Comprehensive school reforms based on self-determination theory have the goal of creating such vibrant self-renewing communities, and highlight the larger contextual supports that need to be in place to create and sustain them (Connell et al., 2009; Deci, 2009).

Conclusion

For many schools and teachers, the creation and continual renegotiation of an intrinsically motivating curriculum and a supportive classroom climate may appear to require too much work and coordination among teachers, and to produce too uncertain a path to the achievement test scores upon which evaluations and accountability of teachers and schools are now based (Ryan & Brown, 2005). However, the downward spirals of student and teacher engagement, the draining away of students' intrinsic motivation, and the rates of student dropout and teacher burnout, are all reminders of the costs associated with the current situation. Self-determination theory and the motivational model it inspires offer an alternative vision (Connell et al., 2009; Deci, 2009).

In the current chapter, we have attempted to show how a motivational model grounded in self-determination theory can be used as a framework to both clarify and enrich the study of student engagement. We suggest that, within a multilevel perspective on engagement, student constructive participation in academic work enjoys a privileged status as the focus of research on engagement because it is the only gateway to learning and scholastic development. We have emphasized the importance of distinguishing indicators of engagement from its facilitators, and along with many other researchers, we favor indicators of engagement as an action construct that capture its behavioral, cognitive, and emotional facets. We have suggested sets of important social and personal facilitators that highlight the nature of academic work, and include many of the self-system processes studied in research on motivation today. Facilitators also take into account a range of interpersonal relationships that can satisfy or undermine students' needs for relatedness, competence, and autonomy, including interactions with parents, friends, and peer group members, but emphasizing as fundamental students' relationships with their teachers.

The episodes of students' daily lives in school, which are shaped by their engagement and disaffection, have only recently become the focus of research on the development of motivational dynamics. However, such dynamics hold promise for helping to explain the durability of students' motivation across the school year and for identifying underlying processes that contribute to interindividual trajectories of motivation across multiple years. We have suggested directions for future research that can examine the role that cycles of engagement may play in the emergence of everyday resilience and constructive coping. Taken together, these ideas may provide tools to help researchers explore and educators nurture the long-term development of valuable (but rare) academic assets, such as self-regulated and autonomous learning, and an academic identity and sense of purpose that allow students to take ownership for their own progress in school and beyond.

References

Ainsworth, M. D. S. (1979). Infant–mother attachment. *American Psychologist, 34*, 932–937.
Altermatt, E. R., Jovanovic, J., & Perry, M. (1998). Bias or responsivity? Sex and achievement level effects on teachers' classroom questioning practices. *Journal of Educational Psychology, 90*, 516–527.
Altermatt, E. R., & Pomerantz, E. M. (2003). The development of competence-related and motivational beliefs: An investigation of similarity and influence among friends. *Journal of Educational Psychology, 95*, 111–123.
Ames, C. (1992). Classrooms: Goals, structures, and student motivation. *Journal of Educational Psychology, 84*, 261–271.
Ames, C., & Ames, R. (1985). *Research on motivation in education* (The classroom milieu, Vol. 2). San Diego, CA: Academic.
Anderman, L. H. (1999). Classroom goal orientation, school belonging, and social goals as predictors of students' positive and negative affect following transition to middle school. *Journal of Research and Development in Education, 32*, 89–103.
Anderson, K. E., Lytton, H., & Romney, D. (1996). Mothers' interactions with normal and conduct disordered boys: Who affects whom? *Developmental Psychology, 22*, 604–609.
Appleton, J. J., Christenson, S. L., & Furlong, M. J. (2008). Student engagement with school: Critical conceptual and methodological issues of the construct. *Psychology in the Schools, 45*, 369–386.
Baldwin, M. W. (1992). Relational schemas and the processing of social information. *Psychological Bulletin, 112*, 461–484.
Bandura, A. (1997). *Self-efficacy: The exercise of control*. New York: Freeman.
Battistich, V., Solomon, D., Kim, D., Watson, M., & Schnaps, K. (1995). Schools as communities, poverty levels of student populations, and students' attitudes and performance: A multilevel analysis. *American Educational Research Journal, 32*(3), 627–658.
Baumeister, R. F., & Leary, M. R. (1995). The need to belong: Desire for interpersonal attachments as a fundamental human motivation. *Psychological Bulletin, 117*, 497–529.
Bell, R. Q. (1968). A reinterpretation of the direction of effects in studies of socialization. *Psychological Review, 75*, 81–95.
Bell, R. Q. (1979). Parent, child, and reciprocal influences. *The American Psychologist, 34*, 821–826.
Berndt, T. J. (2004). Children's friendships: Shifts over a half-century in perspectives on their development and effects. *Merill-Palmer Quarterly, 50*, 206–223.
Berndt, T. J., Hawkins, J. A., & Jiao, Z. (1999). Influences of friends and friendships on adjustment to junior high school. *Merrill-Palmer Quarterly, 45*, 13–41.
Berndt, T. J., & Keefe, K. (1995). Friends' influences on adolescents' adjustment to school. *Child Development, 66*, 1312–1329.
Berndt, T. J., Laychak, A. E., & Park, K. (1990). Friends' influence on adolescents' academic achievement motivation: An experimental study. *Journal of Educational Psychology, 82*, 664–670.
Birch, S. H., & Ladd, G. W. (1997). The teacher–child relationship and children's early school. *Journal of School Psychology, 35*, 61–79.
Birch, S. H., & Ladd, G. W. (1998). Children's interpersonal behaviors and the teacher–child relationship. *Developmental Psychology, 34*, 934–946.
Boesch, E. E. (1976). *Psychopathologie des alltags [Everyday psychopathology]*. Bern, Switzerland: Huber.
Booker, K. C. (2006). School belonging and the African-American adolescent: What do we know and where should we go? *The High School Journal, 89*, 1–7.
Bowlby, J. (1969/1973). *Attachment and loss* (Vols. 1 and 2). New York: Basic Books.
Bradley, R. H. (2007). Parenting in the breach: How parents help children cope with developmentally challenging circumstances. *Parenting: Science and Practice, 7*, 99–148.
Brandtstädter, J. (1998). Action perspectives on human development. In W. Damon (Series Ed.) & R. M. Lerner (Vol. Ed.), *Handbook of child psychology: Vol. 1. Theoretical models of human development* (pp. 807–863). New York: Wiley.
Bretherton, I. (1985). Attachment theory: Retrospect and prospect. *Monographs of the Society for Research in Child Development, 50* (1–2, Serial No. 209), 276–297.
Brewster, A. B., & Bowen, G. L. (2004). Teacher support and the school engagement of Latino middle and high school students at risk of school failure. *Child and Adolescent Social Work Journal, 21*, 47–67.
Bronfenbrenner, U., & Morris, P. A. (1998). The ecology of developmental processes. In W. Damon & R. Lerner (Eds.), *Handbook of child psychology: Vol. 1: Theoretical models of human development* (5th ed., pp. 993–1028). Hoboken, NJ: Wiley.
Bukowski, W. M., Motzoi, C., & Meyer, F. (2009). Friendship as process, function, and outcome. In K. H. Rubin, W. M. Bukowski, & B. Laursen (Eds.), *Handbook of peer interactions, relationships, and groups* (pp. 217–231). New York: Guilford.
Cairns, R. B., Neckerman, H. J., & Cairns, B. D. (1989). Social networks and shadows of synchrony. In G. R. Adams, R. Montemayor, & T. P. Gullota (Eds.), *Biology of adolescent behavior and development* (pp. 275–305). Beverly Hills, CA: Sage.
Chapman, M. (1984). Intentional action as a paradigm for developmental psychology: A symposium. *Human Development, 27*, 113–114.
Chen, X., Chang, L., & He, Y. (2003). The peer group as a context: Mediating and moderating effects on relations between academic achievement and social functioning in Chinese children. *Child Development, 74*, 710–727.
Connell, J. P., Halpern-Felsher, B. L., Clifford, E., Crichlow, W., & Usinger, P. (1995). Hanging in there: Behavioral, psychological, and contextual factors

affecting whether African-American adolescents stay in high school. *Journal of Adolescent Research, 10*, 41–63.

Connell, J. P., Klem, A. M., Lacher, T., Leiderman, S., & Moore, w., with Deci, E. L. (2009). First Things First: Theory, research, and practice. Toms River, NJ: Institute for Research and Reform in Education. Available online: http://www.irre.orglpublications.

Connell, J. P., Spencer, M. B., & Aber, J. L. (1994). Educational risk and resilience in African American youth: Context, self, and action outcomes in school. *Child Development, 65*, 493–506.

Connell, J. P., & Wellborn, J. G. (1991). Competence, autonomy and relatedness: A motivational analysis of self-system processes. In M. Gunnar & L. A. Sroufe (Eds.), *Minnesota symposium on child psychology: Vol. 23. Self processes in development* (pp. 43–77). Chicago: University of Chicago Press.

Crittenden, P. M. (1990). Internal representational models of attachment relationships. *Infant Mental Health Journal, 11*, 259–277.

Deci, E. L. (1992a). On the nature and function of motivational theories. *Psychological Science, 3*, 167–171.

Deci, E. L. (1992b). The relation of interest to the motivation of behavior: A self-determination theory perspective. In K. A. Renninger, S. Hidi, & A. Krapp (Eds.), *The role of interest in learning and development* (pp. 43–70). Hillsdale, NJ: Erlbaum.

Deci, E. L. (1998). The relation of interest to motivation and human needs: The self-determination theory viewpoint. In L. Hoffmann, A. Krapp, K. A. Renninger, & J. Baumert (Eds.), *Interest and learning* (pp. 146–162). Kiel, Germany: Institute for Science Education.

Deci, E. L. (2009). Large-scale school reform as viewed from the self-determination theory perspective. *Theory and Research in Education, 7*, 244–253.

Deci, E. L., Connell, J. P., & Ryan, R. M. (1985). A motivational analysis of self-determination and self-regulation in the classroom. In C. Ames & R. Ames (Eds.), *Research on motivation in education: Vol. 2: The classroom milieu* (pp. 13–52). San Diego, CA: Academic.

Deci, E. L., Koestner, R., & Ryan, R. M. (1999). A meta-analytic review of experiments examining the effects of extrinsic motivation on intrinsic rewards. *Psychological Bulletin, 125*, 627–668.

Deci, E. L., & Ryan, R. M. (1985). *Intrinsic motivation and self-determination in human behavior*. New York: Plenum Press.

Deci, E. L., & Ryan, R. M. (1991). A motivational approach to self: Integration in personality. In R. Dienstbier (Ed.), *Nebraska symposium on motivation: Vol. 38. Perspectives on motivation* (pp. 237–288). Lincoln, NE: University of Nebraska Press.

Deci, E. L., & Ryan, R. M. (2000). The "what" and "why" of goal pursuits: Human needs and the self-determination of behavior. *Psychological Inquiry, 11*, 227–268.

Deci, E. L., & Ryan, R. M. (2002a). The paradox of achievement: The harder you push, the worse it gets. In J. Aronson (Ed.), *Improving academic achievement: Impact of psychological factors on education* (pp. 61–87). San Diego, CA: Academic.

Deci, E. L., & Ryan, R. M. (Eds.). (2002b). *The handbook of self-determination research*. Rochester, NY: University of Rochester Press.

Deci, E. L., Vallerand, R. J., Pelletier, L. G., & Ryan, R. M. (1991). Motivation and education: The self-determination perspective. *Educational Psychologist, 26*, 642–650.

Dweck, C. S. (1991). Self-theories and goals: Their role in motivation, personality, and development. In R. A. Dienstbier (Ed.), *Perspectives on motivation: Nebraska symposium on motivation* (Vol. 38). Lincoln, NE: University of Nebraska Press.

Dweck, C. S. (1999). *Self-theories: Their role in motivation, personality, and development*. Philadelphia: Psychology Press.

Eccles, J. S., & Midgley, C. (1989). Stage-environment fit: Developmentally appropriate classrooms for early adolescents. In R. E. Ames & C. Ames (Eds.), *Research on motivation in education: Goals and cognitions* (Vol. 3, pp. 13–44). New York: Academic.

Eccles., J. S., Midgley, C., Wigfield, A., Buchanan, C. M., Reuman, D., Flanagan, C., et al. (1993). Development during adolescence: The impact of stage-environment fit on adolescents' experiences in schools and families. *American Psychologist, 48*, 90–101.

Elliot, A. J., & Dweck, C. S. (Eds.). (2005). *Handbook of competence and motivation*. New York: Guilford.

Epstein, J. L., & Sanders, M. G. (2002). Family, school, and community partnerships. In M. Bornstein (Ed.), *Handbook of parenting* (Practical issues in parenting 2nd ed., Vol. 5, pp. 407–438). Mahwah, NJ: Erlbaum.

Estell, D. B., Farmer, T. W., Cairns, R. B., & Cairns, B. D. (2002). Social relations and academic achievement in inner-city early elementary classrooms. *International Journal of Behavioral Development, 26*, 518–528.

Fiedler, M. L. (1975). Bidirectionality of influence in classroom interactions. *Journal of Educational Psychology, 87*, 735–744.

Finn, J. D. (1989). Withdrawing from school. *Review of Educational Research, 59*, 117–142.

Finn, J. D. (1993). *School engagement and students at risk*. Washington, DC: National Center of Educational Statistics.

Fredricks, J. A., Blumenfeld, P. C., & Paris, A. H. (2004). School engagement: Potential of the concept, state of the evidence. *Review of Educational Research, 74*(1), 59–109.

Furlong, M. J., & Christenson, S. L. (2008). Engaging students at school with learning: A relevant construct for *all* students. *Psychology in the Schools, 45*, 365–368.

Furrer, C., Kelly, G., & Skinner, E. (2003, April). *Can teachers use children's emotions in the classroom to diagnose and treat underlying motivational problems?* Poster presented at the biennial meetings of the Society for Research in Child Development, Tampa, FL.

Furrer, C., & Skinner, E. (2003). Sense of relatedness as a factor in children's academic engagement and performance. *Journal of Educational Psychology, 95*, 148–162.

Furrer, C. J., & Skinner, E. A. (2009, April). *Reciprocal effects of student engagement in the classroom on changes in teacher support over the school year.* Poster at the Society for Research in Child Development, Denver, CO.

Garcia-Reid, P., Reid, R., & Peterson, N. (2002). School engagement among Latino youth in an urban middle school context: Valuing the role of social support. *Education and Urban Society, 37*, 257–275.

Gest, S. D., Rulison, K. L., Davidson, A. J., & Welsh, J. A. (2008). A reputation for success (or failure): The association of peer academic reputations with academic self-concept, effort, and performance across the upper elementary grades. *Developmental Psychology, 44*(3), 625–636.

Ginsberg, G. S., & Bronstein, P. (1993). Family factors related to children's intrinsic/extrinsic motivational orientation and academic performance. *Child Development, 64*, 1461–1474.

Goodenow, C. (1993). Classroom belonging among early adolescent students: Relationships to motivation and achievement. *Journal of Early Adolescence, 13*, 21–43.

Gottfried, A. E. (1990). Academic intrinsic motivation in young elementary school children. *Journal of Educational Psychology, 82*, 525–538.

Gottfried, A. E., Fleming, J. S., & Gottfried, A. W. (1994). Role of parental motivational practices in children's academic intrinsic motivation and achievement. *Journal of Educational Psychology, 86*, 104–113.

Gottfried, A. E., Fleming, J. S., & Gottfried, A. W. (2001). Continuity of academic intrinsic motivation from childhood through late adolescence: A longitudinal study. *Journal of Educational Psychology, 93*, 3–13.

Gottfried, A. E., Marcoulides, G. A., Gottfried, A. W., & Oliver, P. H. (2009). A latent curve model of parental motivational practices and developmental decline in math and science academic intrinsic motivation. *Journal of Educational Psychology, 3*, 729–739.

Gottfried, A. E., Marcoulides, G. A., Gottfried, A. W., Oliver, P. H., & Guerin, D. W. (2007). Multivariate latent change modeling of developmental decline in academic intrinsic math motivation and achievement: Childhood through adolescence. *International Journal of Behavioral Development, 31*, 317–327.

Grolnick, W. S., & Apostoleris, N. H. (2002). What makes parents controlling? In E. L. Deci & R. M. Ryan (Eds.), *Handbook of self-determination research* (pp. 161–181). Rochester, NY: University of Rochester Press.

Grolnick, W. S., & Ryan, R. M. (1987). Autonomy in children's learning: An experimental and individual difference investigation. *Journal of Personality and Social Psychology, 52*, 890–898.

Grolnick, W. S., & Ryan, R. M. (1989). Parent styles associated with children's self-regulation and competence: A social contextual perspective. *Journal of Educational Psychology, 81*, 143–154.

Grolnick, W. S., & Ryan, R. M. (1992). Parental resources and the developing child in school. In M. E. Procidano & C. B. F. Fisher (Eds.), *Contemporary families: A handbook for school professionals* (pp. 275–291). New York: Teachers College Press.

Grolnick, W. S., Ryan, R. M., & Deci, E. L. (1991). Inner resources for school achievement: Motivational mediators of children's perceptions of their parents. *Journal of Educational Psychology, 83*, 508–517.

Grolnick, W. S., & Slowiaczek, J. L. (1994). Parental involvement in children's schooling: A multidimensional conceptualization and motivational model. *Child Development, 65*, 237–252.

Guthrie, J. T., & Davis, M. H. (2003). Motivating struggling readers in middle school through an engagement model of classroom practice. *Reading & Writing Quarterly, 19*, 59–85.

Hakanen, J. J., Bakker, A. B., & Schaufeli, W. B. (2006). Burnout and work engagement among teachers. *Journal of School Psychology, 43*, 495–513.

Hallinan, M. T., & Williams, R. A. (1990). Students' characteristics and the peer-influence process. *Sociology of Education, 63*, 122–132.

Hamre, B. K., & Pianta, R. C. (2001). Early teacher-child relationships and the trajectory of children's school outcomes through eighth grade. *Child Development, 72*, 625–638.

Hardre, P. L., & Reeve, J. (2003). A motivational model of students' intentions to persist in, versus drop out of, high school. *Journal of Educational Psychology, 95*, 347–356.

Harter, S. (1978). Effectance motivation reconsidered: Toward a developmental model. *Human Development, 21*, 36–64.

Harter, S. (1982). The perceived competence scale for children. *Child Development, 53*, 89–97.

Heckhausen, J., & Schulz, R. (1995). A life-span theory of control. *Psychological Review, 102*, 284–304.

Hulleman, C. S., Schrager, S. M., Bodman, S. M., & Harachiewicz, J. M. (2010). A meta-analytic review of achievement goal measures: Different labels for the same constructs or different constructs with similar labels? *Psychological Bulletin, 136*, 422–449.

Jelsma, B. M. (1982). *Adult control behaviors: The interaction between orientation toward control in women and activity level of children.* Unpublished doctoral Dissertation, University of Rochester, Rochester, NY.

Jeynes, W. H. (2007). The relationship between parental involvement and urban secondary school student academic achievement: A meta-analysis. *Urban Education, 42*, 82–110.

Jimerson, S. J., Campos, E., & Greif, J. L. (2003). Towards an understanding of definitions and measures of school engagement and related terms. *The California School Psychologist, 8*, 7–27.

Kandel, D. B. (1978). Homophily, selection, and socialization in adolescent friendships. *The American Journal of Sociology, 84*, 427–436.

Kindermann, T. A. (1993). Natural peer groups as contexts for individual development: The case of children's motivation in school. *Developmental Psychology, 29*, 970–977.

Kindermann, T. A. (2007). Effects of naturally existing peer groups on changes in academic engagement in a cohort of sixth graders. *Child Development, 78*, 1186–1203.

Kindermann, T. A., McCollam, T. L., & Gibson, E. (1996). Peer group influences on children's developing school motivation. In K. Wentzel & J. Juvonen (Eds.), *Social motivation: Understanding children's school adjustment* (pp. 279–312). Newbury Park, CA: Sage.

Kindermann, T. A., & Skinner, E. A. (2009). How do naturally existing peer groups shape children's academic development during sixth grade? *European Journal of Psychological Science, 3*, 31–43.

Kindermann, T. A., & Skinner, E. A. (in press). Will the real peer group please stand up? A "tensegrity" approach to examining the synergistic influences of peer groups and friendship networks on academic development. In F. Pajares & T. Urdan (Series Eds.), *Adolescents and education*, A. Ryan & G. Ladd (Vol. Eds.), *Peer relationships and adjustment at school*. New York: Information Age Publishing.

Klem, A. M., & Connell, J. P. (2004). Relationships matter: Linking teacher support to student engagement and achievement. *The Journal of School Health, 74*, 262–273.

Koestner, R., & McClelland, D. C. (1990). Perspectives on competence motivation. In L. A. Pervin (Ed.), *Handbook of personality: Theory and research* (pp. 527–548). New York: Guilford.

Kuhl, J. (1987). Action control: The maintenance of motivational states. In F. Halisch & J. Kuhl (Eds.), *Motivation, intention, and volition* (pp. 279–291). New York: Springer.

Kuperminc, G. P., Blatt, S. J., Shahar, G., Henrich, C., & Leadbetter, B. J. (2004). Cultural equivalence and cultural variance in longitudinal associations of young adolescent self-definition and interpersonal relatedness to psychological and school adjustment. *Journal of Youth and Adolescence, 33*(1), 13–30.

Ladd, G. W. (1990). Having friends, keeping friends, making friends, and being liked by peers in the classroom: Predictors of children's early school adjustment? *Child Development, 61*, 1081–1100.

Ladd, G. W., Birch, S. H., & Buhs, E. S. (1999). Children's social and scholastic lives in kindergarten: Related spheres of influence? *Child Development, 70*, 1373–1400.

Ladd, G. W., Kochenderfer, B. J., & Coleman, C. C. (1997). Classroom peer acceptance, friendship, and victimization: Distinct relational systems that contribute uniquely to children's school adjustment? *Child Development, 68*, 1181–1197.

Lynch, M., & Cicchetti, D. (1992). Maltreated children's reports of relatedness to their teachers. In R. C. Pianta (Ed.), *New directions for child development: No. 57. Beyond the parent: The role of other adults in children's lives* (pp. 81–107). San Francisco: Jossey-Bass.

Lynch, M., & Cicchetti, D. (1997). Children's relationships with adults and peers: An examination of elementary and junior high school students. *Journal of School Psychology, 35*, 81–99.

Marchand, G., & Skinner, E. A. (2007). Motivational dynamics of children's academic help-seeking and concealment. *Journal of Educational Psychology, 99*(1), 65–82.

Marks, H. M. (2000). Student engagement in instructional activity: Patterns in the elementary, middle, and high school years. *American Educational Research Journal, 37*, 153–184.

Martin, A. J., & Marsh, H. W. (2006). Academic resilience and its psychological and educational correlates: A construct validity approach. *Psychology in the Schools, 43*, 267–282.

Martin, A. J., & Marsh, H. W. (2008a). Academic buoyancy: Towards an understanding of students' everyday academic resilience. *Journal of School Psychology, 46*, 53–83.

Martin, A. J., & Marsh, H. W. (2008b). Workplace and academic buoyancy: Psychometric assessment and construct validity amongst school personnel and students. *Journal of Psychoeducational Assessment, 26*, 168–184.

Martin, A. J., & Marsh, H. W. (2009). Academic resilience and academic buoyancy: Multidimensional and hierarchical conceptual framing of causes, correlates and cognate constructs. *Oxford Review of Education, 35*, 353–370.

Miceli, M., & Castelfranchi, C. (2000). Nature and mechanisms of loss of motivation. *Review of General Psychology, 4*(3), 238–263.

Midgley, C., & Edelin, K. C. (1998). Middle school reform and early adolescent well-being: The good news and the bad. *Educational Psychologist, 33*, 195–206.

Miserandino, M. (1996). Children who do well in school: Individual differences in perceived competence and autonomy in above-average children. *Journal of Educational Psychology, 88*, 203–214.

Morrison, G. M., Robertson, L., Laurie, B., & Kelly, J. (2002). Protective factors related to antisocial behavior trajectories. *Journal of Clinical Psychology, 58*, 277–290.

Murray, C., & Greenberg, M. T. (2000). Children's relationship with teachers and bonds with school. *Journal of School Psychology, 38*, 423–445.

Murray, C., & Murray, K. M. (2004). Child level correlates of teacher-student relationships: An examination of demographic characteristics, academic orientations, and behavioral orientations. *Psychology in the Schools, 41*(7), 751–762.

National Research Council. (2004). *Engaging schools: Fostering high school students' motivation to learn*. Washington, DC: National Academies Press.

Nelson-Le Gall, S., Gumerman, R. A., & Scott-Jones, D. (1983). Instrumental help-seeking and everyday problem-solving: A developmental perspective. In B. DePaulo, A. Nadler, & J. Fisher (Eds.), *New directions* in helping: Help-seeking (Vol. 2, pp. 265–284). New York: Academic.

Newman, R. S. (1994). Adaptive help seeking: A strategy of self-regulated learning. In D. H. Schunk & B. J. Zimmerman (Eds.), *Self-regulation of learning and performance: Issues and educational applications* (pp. 283–301). Hillsdale, NJ: Erlbaum.

Newman, R. S. (2000). Social influences on the development of children's adaptive help seeking: The role of parents, teachers, and peers. *Developmental Review, 20*(3), 350–404.

Newman, R. S. (2002). What do I need to do to succeed… when I don't understand what I am doing!? Developmental influences on students' adaptive help-seeking. In A. Wigfield & J. S. Eccles (Eds.), *Development of achievement motivation* (pp. 285–306). San Diego, CA: Academic.

Newmann, F. M., King, M. B., & Carmichael, D. L. (2007). *Authentic instruction and assessment: Common standards for rigor and relevance in teaching academic subjects*. Des Moines, IA: Iowa Department of Education.

Newmann, F., Wehlage, G. G., & Lamborn, S. D. (1992). The significance and sources of student engagement. In F. Newmann (Ed.), *Student engagement and achievement in American secondary schools* (pp. 11–39). New York: Teachers College Press.

Niemiec, C. P., & Ryan, R. M. (2009). Autonomy, competence, and relatedness in the classroom: Applying self-determination theory to educational practice. *Theory and Research in Education, 7*(2), 133–144.

Otis, N., Grouzet, F. M. E., & Pelletier, L. G. (2005). Latent motivational change in an academic setting: A 3-year longitudinal study. *Journal of Educational Psychology, 97*, 170–183.

Patrick, B. C., Hisley, J., Kempler, T., & College, G. (2000). "What's everybody so excited about?": The effects of teacher enthusiasm on student intrinsic motivation and vitality. *The Journal of Experimental Education, 68*, 217–236.

Patrick, B. C., Skinner, E. A., & Connell, J. P. (1993). What motivates children's behavior and emotion? The joint effects of perceived control and autonomy in the academic domain. *Journal of Personality and Social Psychology, 65*(4), 781–791.

Patterson, G. R. (1982). *Coercive family processes*. Eugene, OR: Castalia Press.

Pelletier, L. G., & Vallerand, R. J. (1996). Supervisors' beliefs and subordinates' intrinsic motivation: A behavioral confirmation analysis. *Journal of Personality and Social Psychology, 71*, 331–340.

Peterson, C., Maier, S. F., & Seligman, M. E. P. (1993). *Learned helplessness: A theory for the age of personal control*. New York: Oxford University Press.

Pianta, R. C. (1999). *Enhancing relationships between children and teachers*. Washington, DC: American Psychologist Association.

Pianta, R. C. (2006). Classroom management and relationships between children and teachers: Implications for research and practice. In C. M. Evertson & C. S. Weinstein (Eds.), *Handbook of classroom management: Research, practice, and contemporary issues* (pp. 85–710). Mahwah, NJ: Erlbaum.

Pintrich, P. R. (2003). A motivational science perspective of the role of student motivation in learning and teaching contexts. *Journal of Educational Psychology, 95*, 667–686.

Pomerantz, E. M., Grolnick, W. S., & Price, C. E. (2005). The role of parents in how children approach achievement: A dynamic process perspective. In A. J. Elliot & C. S. Dweck (Eds.), *Handbook of competence and motivation* (pp. 259–278). New York: Guilford.

Power, T. G. (2004). Stress and coping in childhood: The parents' role. *Parenting: Science and Practice, 4*, 271–317.

Ratcliffe, M. M., Goldberg, J., Rogers, B., & Merrigan, K. (2010). *A model of garden-based education in school settings: Development of a conceptual framework to improve children's academic achievement, ecoliteracy, health and wellness while enhancing schools, communities, and bioregions*. Unpublished manuscript, Friedman School of Nutrition Science and Policy, Tufts University, Medford, MA.

Reeve, J. (2002). Self-determination theory applied to educational settings. In E. L. Deci & R. M. Ryan (Eds.), *The handbook of self-determination research* (pp. 183–203). Rochester, NY: University of Rochester Press.

Reeve, J., Jang, H., Carrell, D., Jeon, S., & Barch, J. (2004). Enhancing students' engagement by increasing teachers' autonomy support. *Motivation and Emotion, 28*, 147–169.

Renninger, K. A. (2000). Individual interest and its implications for understanding intrinsic motivation. In C. Sansone & J. M. Harackiewicz (Eds.), *Intrinsic and extrinsic motivation: The search for optimal motivation and performance* (pp. 373–404). San Diego, CA: Academic.

Reynolds, A. J., & Clements, M. (2005). Parental involvement and children's school success. In E. N. Patrikakou, R. P. Weisberg, S. Redding, & H. J. Walberg (Eds.), *School-family partnerships for children's success*. New York: Teachers College Press.

Roeser, R. W., Midgley, C., & Urdan, T. C. (1996). Perceptions of the school psychological environment and early adolescents' psychological and behavioral functioning in school: The mediating role of goals and belonging. *Journal of Educational Psychology, 88*, 408–422.

Roeser, R. W., Peck, S. C., & Nasir, N. S. (2006). Self and identity processes in school motivation, learning, and achievement. In P. Alexander & P. H. Winne (Eds.), *Handbook of educational psychology* (2nd ed., pp. 391–424). Mahwah, NJ: Lawrence Erlbaum.

Rosenholtz, S. J., & Wilson, B. (1980). The effect of classroom structure on shared perceptions of ability. *American Educational Research Journal, 17*, 75–82.

Ryan, R. M. (1995). Psychological needs and the facilitation of integrative processes. *Journal of Personality, 63*, 397–427.

Ryan, A. M. (2001). The peer group as a context for the development of young adolescents' motivation and achievement. *Child Development, 72*, 1135–1150.

Ryan, R. M., & Brown, K. W. (2005). Legislating competence: High-stakes testing policies and their relations with psychological theories and research. In A. J. Elliot & C. S. Dweck (Eds.), *Handbook of competence and motivation* (pp. 354–372). New York: Guilford.

Ryan, R. M., & Connell, J. P. (1989). Perceived locus of causality and internalization: Examining reasons for acting in two domains. *Journal of Personality and Social Psychology, 57*, 749–761.

Ryan, R. M., Connell, J. P., & Deci, E. L. (1985). A motivational analysis of self-determination and self-regulation in education. In C. Ames & R. E. Ames (Eds.), *Research on motivation in education: The classroom milieu* (pp. 13–51). New York: Academic.

Ryan, A. M., Patrick, H., & Shim, S. (2005). Differential profiles of students identified by their teacher as having avoidant, appropriate, or dependent help-seeking tendencies in the classroom. *Journal of Educational Psychology, 97*(2), 275–285.

Ryan, R. M., & Powelson, C. L. (1991). Autonomy and relatedness as fundamental to motivation and education. *The Journal of Experimental Education, 60*, 49–66.

Ryan, R. M., & Stiller, J. (1991). The social contexts of internalization: Parent and teacher influences on autonomy, motivation, and learning. In M. L. Maehr & P. L. Pintrich (Eds.), *Advances in motivation and achievement* (Vol. 7, pp. 115–149). Greenwich, CT: JAI Press.

Ryan, R. M., Stiller, J. D., & Lynch, J. H. (1994). Representations and relationships to teachers, parents, and friends as predictors of academic motivation and self-esteem. *Journal of Early Adolescence, 14*, 226–249.

Salmela-Aro, K., Kiuru, N., Leskinen, E., & Nurmi, J.-E. (2009). School-Burnout Inventory. *European Journal of Psychological Assessment, 25*, 48–57.

Sameroff, A. J., & Haith, M. M. (Eds.). (1996). *The five to seven year shift: The age of reason and responsibility*. Chicago: University of Chicago Press.

Schmitz, B., & Skinner, E. (1993). Perceived control, effort, and academic performance: Interindividual, intraindividual, and multivariate time-series analyses. *Journal of Personality and Social Psychology, 64*(6), 1010–1028.

Schunk, D. H., & Zimmerman, B. J. (Eds.). (2007). *Motivation and self-regulated learning: Theory, research, and practice*. Hillsdale, NJ: Lawrence Erlbaum Associates.

Seligman, M. E. P. (1975). *Helplessness: On depression, development, and death*. San Francisco: Freeman.

Sinclair, M. F., Christenson, S. L., Lehr, C. A., & Anderson, A. R. (2003). Facilitating student learning and engagement: Lessons learned from Check & Connect longitudinal studies. *The California School Psychologist, 8*, 29–41.

Skinner, E. A. (1995). *Perceived control, motivation, and coping*. Newbury Park, CA: Sage.

Skinner, E. A. (1996). A guide to constructs of control. *Journal of Personality and Social Psychology, 71*, 549–570.

Skinner, E. A., & Belmont, M. J. (1993). Motivation in the classroom: Reciprocal effects of teacher behavior and student engagement across the school year. *Journal of Educational Psychology, 85*, 571–581.

Skinner, E. A., Chi, U., & the Learning-Gardens Educational Assessment Group (2012). Intrinsic motivation and engagement as "active ingredients" in garden-based education: Examining models and measures derived from self-determination theory. *Journal of Environmental Education, 43*(1), 16–36.

Skinner, E., Edge, K., Altman, J., & Sherwood, H. (2003). Searching for the structure of coping: A review and critique of category systems for classifying ways of coping. *Psychological Bulletin, 129*, 216–269.

Skinner, E. A., Furrer, C., Marchand, G., & Kindermann, T. (2008). Engagement and disaffection in the classroom: Part of a larger motivational dynamic? *Journal of Educational Psychology, 100*, 765–781.

Skinner, E. A., Kindermann, T. A., Connell, J. P., & Wellborn, J. G. (2009a). Engagement as an organizational construct in the dynamics of motivational development. In K. Wentzel & A. Wigfield (Eds.), *Handbook of motivation at school* (pp. 223–245). Malwah, NJ: Erlbaum.

Skinner, E. A., Kindermann, T. A., & Furrer, C. (2009b). A motivational perspective on engagement and disaffection: Conceptualization and assessment of children's behavioral and emotional participation in academic activities in the classroom. *Educational and Psychological Measurement, 69*, 493–525.

Skinner, E. A., & Wellborn, J. G. (1994). Coping during childhood and adolescence: A motivational perspective. In D. Featherman, R. Lerner, & M. Perlmutter (Eds.), *Life-span development and behavior* (Vol. 12, pp. 91–133). Hillsdale, NJ: Erlbaum.

Skinner, E. A., & Wellborn, J. G. (1997). Children's coping in the academic domain. In S. A. Wolchik & I. N. Sandler (Eds.), *Handbook of children's coping with common stressors: Linking theory and intervention* (pp. 387–422). New York: Plenum Press.

Skinner, E. A., Zimmer-Gembeck, M. J., & Connell, J. P. (1998). Individual differences and the development of perceived control. *Monographs of the Society for Research in Child Development, 63* (nos. 2 and 3) whole no. 254, pp. 1–220.

Steinberg, L., Elmen, J. D., & Mounts, N. S. (1989). Authoritative parenting, psychosocial maturity, and academic success in adolescents. *Child Development, 60*, 1424–1436.

Stipek, D. J. (2002a). Good instruction is motivating. In A. Wigfield & J. S. Eccles (Eds.), *Development of achievement motivation* (pp. 309–332). San Diego, CA: Academic.

Stipek, D. J. (2002b). *Motivation to learn: From theory to practice* (4th ed.). Needham Heights, MA: Allyn & Bacon.

Vallerand, R. J., Fortier, M. S., & Guay, F. (1997). Self-determination and persistence in a real-life setting: Toward a motivational model of high school dropout.

Journal of Personality and Social Psychology, 72(1161), 1176.

Vallerand, R. J., Pelletier, L. G., Blais, M. R., Brière, N. M., Senécal, C. B., & Vallières, E. F. (1993). On the assessment of intrinsic, extrinsic, and amotivation in education: Evidence on the concurrent and construct validity of the Academic Motivation Scale. *Educational and Psychological Measurement, 53*, 159–172.

Vasalampi, K., Salmela-Aro, K., & Nurmi, J.-E. (2009). Adolescents' self-concordance, school engagement, and burnout predict their educational trajectories. *European Psychologist, 14*, 1–11.

Weiner, B. (2005). Motivation from an attributional perspective and the social psychology of perceived competence. In A. J. Elliot & C. S. Dweck (Eds.), *Handbook of competence and motivation* (pp. 73–84). New York: Guilford.

Weisz, J. R. (1986). Understanding the developing understanding of control. In M. Perlmutter (Ed.), *Minnesota symposium on child psychology: Vol. 18. Social cognition* (pp. 219–278). Hillsdale, NJ: Erlbaum.

Wentzel, K. R. (1991). Social competence at school: Relation between social responsibility and academic achievement. *Review of Educational Research, 61*, 1–24.

Wentzel, K. R. (1997). Student motivation in middle school: The role of perceived pedagogical caring. *Journal of Educational Psychology, 89*(3), 411–419.

Wentzel, K. R. (1998). Social relationships and motivation in middle school: The role of parents, teachers, and peers. *Journal of Educational Psychology, 90*(2), 202–209.

Wentzel, K. R. (1999). Social-motivational processes and interpersonal relationships: Implications for understanding motivation at school. *Journal of Educational Psychology, 91*, 76–97.

Wentzel, K. (2009). Students' relationships with teachers as motivation contexts. In K. Wentzel & A. Wigfield (Eds.), *Handbook of motivation in school* (pp. 301–322). Malwah, NJ: Erlbaum.

Wentzel, K. R., McNamara-Barry, C., & Caldwell, K. A. (2004). Friendships in middle school: Influences on motivation and school adjustment. *Journal of Educational Psychology, 96*, 195–203.

White, R. W. (1959). Motivation reconsidered: The concept of competence. *Psychological Review, 66*, 297–333.

Wigfield, A., Eccles, J. S., Schiefele, U., Roeser, R., & Davis-Kean, P. (2006). Development of achievement motivation. In W. Damon (Series Ed.) & N. Eisenberg (Vol. Ed.), *Handbook of child psychology, 6th Ed. Vol. 3. Social, emotional, and personality development* (pp. 933–1002). New York: John Wiley.

Wooley, M. E., & Bowen, G. L. (2007). In the context of risk: Supportive adults and the school engagement of middle-school students. *Family Relations, 56*, 92–104.

Zimmer-Gembeck, M. J., & Skinner, E. A. (2011). The development of coping across childhood and adolescence: An integrative review and critique of research. *International Journal of Behavioral Development, 35*, 1–17.

Engagement Across Developmental Periods

Duhita Mahatmya, Brenda J. Lohman, Jennifer L. Matjasko, and Amy Feldman Farb

Abstract

The goal of this chapter is to provide a cohesive developmental framework and foundation for which to understand student engagement across early childhood, middle childhood, and adolescence. Guided by the bioecological theory of human development and the person-environment fit perspective, this chapter extends Finn's participation-identification model of engagement by mapping student engagement within a larger developmental sequence. This chapter discusses student engagement within specific developmental periods that are tied to the developmental tasks, opportunities, and challenges unique to early childhood, middle childhood, and adolescence. Student engagement is found to be a nuanced developmental outcome, and the differences may be a result of the maturation of biological, cognitive, and socioemotional developmental tasks and the changing contextual landscape for the children and adolescents. Recommendations for future research as well as policy implications are also discussed.

Chapter Aim and Overview

Research consistently shows that student engagement plays a critical role in the development of positive outcomes in children and adolescents such as increasing academic achievement (Carbonaro, 1998; Eccles, 2004; Manke, McGuire, Reiss, Hetherington, & Plomin, 1995; Portes, 2000) and facilitating the development of new social competencies (Karcher, Kuperminc, Portwood, Sipe, & Taylor, 2006; Parra, Dubois, Neville, Pugh-Lilly, & Povinelli, 2002). While it is important to consider the factors that shape student engagement and its potential consequences, we argue that understanding student engagement within the context of the individual's

D. Mahatmya, Ph.D. (✉)
New Century College, George Mason University,
Fairfax, VA, USA
e-mail: dmahatmy@gmu.edu

B.J. Lohman, Ph.D.
Human Development and Family Studies,
Iowa State University, Ames, IA, USA
e-mail: blohman@iastate.edu

J.L. Matjasko, Ph.D.
University of Texas, Austin, TX, USA
e-mail: jmatjasko@cdc.gov

A.F. Farb, Ph.D.
Office of Adolescent Health,
US Department of Health and Human Services,
Washington, DC, USA
e-mail: amy.farb@hhs.gov

developmental history is also important. The goal of this chapter is to provide a cohesive developmental framework and foundation for which to understand student engagement across early childhood, middle childhood, and adolescence. For the purposes of this chapter, we limit our discussion on engagement to school-related activities. School-related activities comprise both schoolwork (e.g., engagement on academic-specific tasks both within and outside of school) and nonacademic school-related activities (e.g., extracurricular activities).

Moreover, this chapter highlights the importance of accounting for changes in developmental tasks (defined in the following sections) and how they codevelop with student engagement over the childhood and adolescent years. Indeed, while much of the student engagement literature has focused on defining the specific components of student engagement, mainly behavioral, cognitive, and emotional engagement (Appleton, Christenson, & Furlong, 2008; Marks, 2000; Rose-Krasnor, 2009), the research examining the interplay of developmental tasks and the development of student engagement is limited. Echoing Finn's (1989) statement about school dropouts initiated by a "chain of events" (Finn, 1989, p. 119), we conceptualize the interplay of developmental tasks and the development of student engagement as a reciprocal process that also occurs over a period of time. In this way, we adapt Finn's original argument for the participation-identification model of engagement (Finn, 1989; Reschly, 2010) by imparting concepts from the developmental literature to identify the direct and indirect effects of developmental tasks on student engagement and vice versa.

Indeed, childhood and adolescence is a time of rapid growth signified by key developmental tasks that capture overt biological and physiological changes, significant cognitive advancements, emotional maturation, as well as new social relationships. The specific manifestation of the developmental tasks within each developmental period, however, will likely vary across individuals and contexts, and these manifestations can in turn be linked to the developing child or adolescent's student engagement. For instance, the social skills children first gain through participation in peer play, a developmental task of early childhood, and further cultivate during middle childhood and adolescence, may promote his/her student engagement in school-related activities. Children and adolescents who are more engaged may subsequently increase their likelihood of successfully reaching a developmental task. Not only does this suggest that student engagement is more likely to happen if children's and adolescents' school experiences are framed within the developmental tasks fitting the general developmental period, but also student engagement can strengthen the accomplishment of developmental tasks. Based on this, the two main questions that guide this chapter are:

1. How do developmental tasks encourage or discourage the development of student engagement?
2. How can student engagement strengthen the acquisition of developmental tasks?

To further understand the reciprocal processes, we first define student engagement. Second, we briefly describe the prominent developmental tasks of early childhood, middle childhood, and adolescence, and the links between these developmental tasks and student engagement. Next, we detail our overarching theoretical framework that stresses the importance of understanding the emergence of the developmental tasks to enhance our knowledge of the development of student engagement. The bulk of this chapter addresses student engagement across these developmental periods and how the key behavioral, cognitive, and socioemotional developmental tasks in childhood and adolescence are related. It must be noted that the majority of the work assessing student engagement discussed here draws from literature that is nonexperimental in nature. As a result, we cannot make any causal statements about the link between developmental periods and student engagement. Where appropriate, we note findings from experimental research and those that are nationally representative or longitudinal in nature. Throughout these sections, we discuss the importance of understanding growth and development and how it codevelops with student engagement. Finally, we conclude with brief remarks summarizing future research directions in this area and the importance of family, school, and community partnerships for enhancing student engagement across developmental periods.

Defining Student Engagement

In defining student engagement, prior research has identified three distinct dimensions to the construct (e.g., Appleton et al., 2008; Fredricks, Blumenfeld, & Paris, 2004), mainly, behavioral, cognitive, and emotional engagement. According to Fredricks and colleagues (2004) and Blumenfeld and colleagues (2005):

1. *Behavioral engagement* draws on the idea of participation; it includes involvement in academic and social or extracurricular activities. It is usually defined in three ways. The first entails positive conduct, as well as the absence of disruptive behaviors such as skipping school. The second definition concerns involvement in learning and academic tasks and includes behaviors such as effort, persistence, concentration, attention, asking questions, etc. A third definition involves participation in school-related activities such as athletics or school governance.
2. *Cognitive engagement* draws on the idea of investment; it incorporates thoughtfulness and willingness to exert the effort necessary to comprehend complex ideas and master difficult skills.
3. *Emotional engagement* encompasses positive and negative reactions to teachers, classmates, academics, and school, and is presumed to create ties to an institution and influence willingness to do the work. It refers to students' affective reactions in the classroom, including interest, boredom, happiness, sadness, and anxiety.

Appleton and colleagues (2008) build on this characterization by further operationalizing the three engagement constructs. For example, attendance, suspensions, voluntary classroom participation, and extracurricular activity participation are part of behavioral engagement (Appleton et al., 2008). They also claim that both cognitive and emotional engagement are not easily observed and are determined by the extent to which the individual values and identifies with the activities and whether they believe the activities are relevant to their future. We expand the latter statement and argue that the components of student engagement cannot be fully observed without the appropriate developmental foundation via the attainment of developmental tasks, which are described in the next section.

Developmental Tasks of Childhood and Adolescence

Developmental tasks describe the main changes and challenges that occur during a certain developmental period. Generally, they represent any number of things from physical milestones to societal expectations for individuals based on age. Beginning in early childhood (birth to 6 years), children are increasingly faced with new and complex socialization forces that influence their behavioral, cognitive, and emotional development. For instance, as noted above, one main developmental task during early childhood is participation in peer play (Newman & Newman, 2009). Through the process of learning rules and playing cooperatively with others, children begin to form meaningful friendships and mental representations of ways of participating in groups. Entry into the formal school setting also brings new opportunities, new information, and new interactions with teachers and peers that can foster or inhibit the child's maturation.

Moving into middle childhood (6–12 years), there is continued growth in intellectual capacities, mastery, competence, and steady physical development. During this time, children are learning the fundamental skills and values that are associated with their particular environment, which increasingly involves the school environment. As children become adolescents (12–18 years), academic expectations increase in complexity and responsibility; youths are expected to learn and to follow the rules and laws that govern conduct in adult society, and they begin to learn about responsible dating and romantic social conduct in their community and culture. Adolescence is also a period marked by increased exposure to environments outside of the family, and a large developmental task is achieving a psychological sense of autonomy from one's parents (Newman & Newman, 2009). Many parents also consider it important for a child to contribute to the family or community through chores or good deeds, or at least not to destroy and to harm others or community property.

Acceptable performances in these tasks represent important milestones in the eyes of the stakeholders for positive child development, including parents, teachers, other community members, and children themselves. Failing in these domains by not meeting expectations may have consequences for children's current and future opportunities, peer reputation, social support, self-esteem, family relationships, and, of particular relevance of this chapter, student engagement.

Linking Developmental Tasks and Engagement

By acknowledging the larger context of positive development, we can further our understanding of student engagement. For instance, a child or adolescent may be having problems behaviorally engaging in school-related activities if he/she lacks necessary motor or social skills to participate. Social skills may be obtained through participation in peer play, a main developmental task in early childhood (as noted above) that continues to grow in middle childhood. During middle childhood, friendships become based on who plays together, likes the same activities, shares common interests, enjoys each other's company, and counts on each other for help. In addition, children are introduced to the concept of group cooperation through organized activities and team play, which enhances their abilities to analyze and manage social relationships, such as group cooperation. These social skills can in turn influence a child's likelihood to be engaged, and a child that is more engaged may increase his/her likelihood of successfully reaching a developmental task related to friendship formation.

Likewise, a child's or adolescent's ability to become cognitively engaged may be restricted by the development of his/her prefrontal cortex and limbic system, which inform higher order reasoning capabilities. The opposite may be true as well, where cognitive development can be improved by being more engaged. It is not until adolescence that youth begin to have greater self-reflection, become more deliberate and focused, and are able to hypothesize and think about several strategies or outcomes for these hypotheses simultaneously rather than focusing on just one domain or issue at a time (Keating, 2004). Thus, the ability to become cognitively engaged with school is greater during adolescence compared to both early and middle childhood. Increased cognitive student engagement may not only show benefits for academic achievement, but also the continued maturation of cognitive and socioemotional developmental tasks.

With regard to emotional engagement, deficits in the development of the limbic system or social competencies can hinder a child's or adolescent's ability to have affective connections to other people or contexts. As mentioned, peer play begins in early childhood, becomes more purposeful in middle childhood, and then continues to change in composition and importance during adolescence. The continued growth and maturation of these behavioral, cognitive, and socioemotional competencies, paired with the accumulation of learning experiences in and out of the classroom, make it important to understand the links among the developmental tasks and student engagement across developmental periods.

Moreover, it is important to understand the multidimensionality of student engagement because research has shown that engagement helps to mediate the relationship between involvement in school-related activities and healthy developmental outcomes (Bartko, 2005; Weiss, Little, & Blumenfeld, 2005). Indeed, Blumenfeld and colleagues (2005) go so far as to claim that student engagement is necessary to prepare children and adolescents for the transition into adulthood. Furthermore, supporting our argument for the codevelopment of developmental tasks and student engagement, research has found that different behavioral, cognitive, and emotional patterns and psychological states are linked to different developmental outcomes across individuals such as mood, internalizing and externalizing behaviors, and motivation (Blumenfeld et al., 2005; Larson, 2000; Shernoff, 2010).

With regard to motivation in particular, some scholars have emphasized that student motivation and engagement are separate constructs, while others have argued that motivation is a necessary but not a sufficient condition for engagement (Blumenfeld, Kempler, & Krajcik, 2006). Connell's process model of motivation outlines the process through which motivation influences student engagement (Connell, Spencer, & Aber, 1994; Connell & Wellborn, 1991). The model states that the perceived social context influences students' perceived autonomy and relatedness. This perceived autonomy and relatedness then leads to student behavioral, cognitive, and emotional engagement. Similarly, Blumenfeld and colleagues (2006) stated that motivation is a precursor to cognitive engagement and achievement. We assume that motivation is a precursor to all three types of engagement. Therefore, it is an implicit part of our definition of student engagement.

This suggests that in order to adequately capture the multidimensional construct of student engagement, it is necessary to observe the extent to which children and adolescents are involved with their schoolwork and extracurricular activities while also assessing whether one believes that the activities are relevant to their current and future goals. In addition, capacities for and expressions of student engagement will vary by developmental periods. In discussing the developmental-stage-specific forms of student engagement during early childhood, middle childhood, and adolescence, we rely on the bioecological theory of human development and the person-environment fit perspective. A description of both theories follows.

Theoretical Considerations

The bioecological theory of human development (Bronfenbrenner & Morris, 1998) and the person-environment fit perspective (Eccles, 2004; Gutman & Eccles, 2007) put forward a way to integrate the extant literature on child and adolescent development and student engagement. First, Bronfenbrenner's bioecological theory asserts that development is a function of the interaction between the developing person and his/her environments. Bronfenbrenner and Morris (1998) defined those interactions as proximal processes and posited that they are the primary vehicle for development. Couched within those proximal processes are two other considerations: the individual's context and characteristics. An individual's context reflects the idea that development is situated within a set of overlapping and multifaceted environmental systems such as the home, school, neighborhood, and larger sociohistorical context that also interact to shape development. For children and adolescents in particular, the family and the school environments are central developmental contexts and have been shown to be significantly related to student engagement (Lohman, Kaura, & Newman, 2007; Roeser & Eccles, 1998; Steinberg, Bradford, & Dornbusch, 1996).

Second, an individual's characteristics can determine whether these proximal processes occur and how an individual experiences his/her contexts. For example, Finn (1989) discussed how race, socioeconomic status, school ability and performance, and autonomy (an important developmental task realized in adolescence) are often reasons given for a school dropout. In this way, the student's demographic and academic characteristics influenced his/her experience of school and subsequent likelihood of dropping out. Likewise, and of particular interest in this chapter, certain developmental tasks may interact with the individual's motivation for, or experiences in, school-related activities to influence the development of student engagement. Child and adolescent characteristics may interact with the family and school contexts in determining student engagement as well. Student engagement itself can also be seen as a personal characteristic that may contribute to the attainment of developmental tasks.

Integrating concepts from the person-environment fit perspective (Eccles, Midgefield, & Wigfield, 1993), we highlight that one size does not fit all in terms of the optimal organization of developmental tasks and ecologies that promote student engagement and vice versa. According to person-environment fit, processes and characteristics within one context may be coupled with congruent or divergent processes and characteristics in another to shape an individual's development (Catalano, Berglund, Ryan, Lonczak, & Hawkins, 2004; Eccles, 2004; Larson, 2000; Lerner, Brentano, Dowling, & Anderson, 2002; Lerner & Castellino, 2002). With respect to student engagement, this may mean synchrony across the values and practices espoused by families and schools to encourage engagement. Indeed, while Bronfenbrenner originally suggested that contextual levels overlap with each other and tend to be consistent within a society (Epstein, 1983; Miller, 2002), researchers have noted that this is not always the case as contexts may also vary in their degree of embeddedness with one another and are sometimes even at odds with each other (Sternberg & Grigorenko, 2001). Thus, a child's or an adolescent's developmental course may be dependent on whether contexts are in synchrony or in dissynchrony (Bronfenbrenner & Ceci, 1994; Mahoney & Bergman, 2002; Mahoney & Magnusson, 2001). We argue that congruence or synchrony across environments may help foster student engagement, while dissynchrony, incongruence or a mismatch in environments, may hinder student engagement (Goodenow, 1995; Lohman et al., 2007).

Researchers can explore this overlap by taking an ecological approach (i.e., including multiple ecological contexts) in inquiries regarding student engagement during the child and adolescent years. Indeed, a handful of studies have begun to address the individual, family, and contextual factors that are associated with participation and lack of participation in organized activities (Dearing et al., 2009; Mahoney, Vandell, Simpkins, & Zarrett, 2009; Persson, Kerr, & Stattin, 2007). However, most of the work has focused on demographic characteristics that are associated with activity participation (see Anderson, Funk, Elliot, & Smith, 2003; Bohnert, Fredricks, & Randall, 2010; Denault & Poulin, 2009; Fletcher, Elder, & Mekos, 2000, for exceptions); therefore, it is not clear from the extant literature if the factors that are related to who initially participates are the same as the factors that are associated with ongoing activity involvement and different levels of participation across each of the activity dimensions (Eccles, 2005).

To that end, we argue for a more comprehensive and integrative developmental-contextual approach. There is a need for research that explores the individual and contextual factors that are predictive of student engagement and that examines whether these facets of engagement are more or less important depending on the characteristics of the child/adolescent or the ecological context in which they live. In considering the developmental correlates and manifestation of student engagement specifically, longitudinal studies that adjust for some of the individual, family, and neighborhood factors associated with these facets of engagement can help to disentangle the extent to which findings are a function of involvement in organized contexts and how much they reflect self-selection effects (Larson, 2000). From there, researchers, educators, and professionals can determine the optimal developmental correlates to, and of, student engagement.

The Developmental Context of Student Engagement

Guided by Bronfenbrenner's bioecological theory of human development and a person-environment fit framework, what follows is a discussion of student engagement within the specific developmental periods that are tied to the specific developmental tasks, opportunities, and challenges of early childhood, middle childhood, and adolescence.

Early Childhood

Much of the context for student engagement research centers on early childhood education and intervention programs such as Head Start (Barnett, 1995), of which Bronfenbrenner was an early proponent (Bronfenbrenner, 1975). The emphasis is on providing effective learning opportunities to develop the building blocks for cognitive and linguistic development, literacy, and social competencies (Bierman et al., 2008;

McWilliam & Casey, 2008; Ramey & Ramey, 2004), which parallel the important developmental tasks of this period. To that end, the early childhood engagement literature is more concerned with the developmental markers associated with a child's school readiness potential rather than student engagement itself (Blair, 2002; Hair, Halle, & Terry-Human, 2006; Kagan, 1990; McCormick et al., 2006; Ramey & Ramey, 2004). Ramey and Ramey, however, argued that a child's school readiness in early childhood can influence his/her future student engagement.

Indeed, research has found that participation in early childhood education programs such as Head Start promotes cognitive, behavioral, and socioemotional competencies that influence later well-being and academic achievement (Barnett, 1995; Fantuzzo & McWayne, 2002; Hair et al., 2006; Luo, Hughes, Liew, & Kwok, 2009; McCormick et al., 2006). The success of early childhood programs comes from structured curricula that emphasize strategic learning interactions, positive teacher-student relationships, and brain development, with the overall objective of promoting school readiness (Barnett, 1995; Bierman et al., 2008; Currie, 2001; Ramey & Ramey, 2004). The early childhood education literature defines school readiness as the acquisition of basic behavioral, cognitive, and socioemotional skills needed to meet school demands in reading, writing, and math (Kagan, 1990; Ramey & Ramey, 2004). In this way, the main developmental tasks of early childhood are framed within the school context. For example, school readiness is generally measured via the child's behaviors in the classroom, which focuses the discussion of student engagement on the ability to follow classroom rules, perform tasks, or engage in cooperative participation with classmates (Bierman et al., 2008; Luo et al., 2009; McWilliam & Bailey, 1992; McWilliam & Casey, 2008), which reflect the developmental tasks of moral development and peer play. A further discussion of how the developmental tasks of early childhood map onto concepts of student engagement follows; additional early childhood education literature not specific to engagement will be used to supplement the discussion.

Behavioral Engagement

The behavioral component of engagement has been an area of emphasis in the early childhood literature (Coolahan, Fantuzzo, Mendez, & McDermott, 2000; Fantuzzo & McWayne, 2002; McWilliam & Bailey, 1992; McWilliam & Casey, 2008) given that children's behavioral problems in the classroom are often cited as a risk factor for poor school readiness and long-term academic performance (Coolahan et al., 2000; Fantuzzo & McWayne, 2002; Kuperschmidt, Bryant, & Willoughby, 2000; Raver, 2002). This further demonstrates the bioecological idea of how a child's characteristics can influence his/her interaction with the environment, in this case, the classroom. Thus, care should be taken to provide children with the space and resources needed to maintain a level of focused attention and constructive behaviors (McWilliam & Casey, 2008). Staying on task and the ability to follow rules and directions in the classroom become ways to define positive student engagement in early childhood (Bierman et al., 2008; Liew, McTigue, Barrois, & Hughes, 2008; Luo et al., 2009). Moreover, the extent to which a child has a self-theory, a developmental task of early childhood, may influence the degree to which a child can follow rules and directions in the classroom (Wigfield & Karpathian, 1991).

Another behavioral component to student engagement in early childhood, and a developmental task, is peer play as noted above (Coolahan et al., 2000; Fantuzzo & McWayne, 2002). Peer play captures the child's interaction with his/her peer group and carrying out shared activities (Fantuzzo & McWayne, 2002). Research has shown that peer play can be an antecedent to long-term school success (Coolahan et al., 2000; Fantuzzo & McWayne, 2002) as well as self-regulation (Bierman et al., 2008). Specifically, interactive play is associated with active engagement in classroom learning activities, prosocial classroom behavior such as helping and sharing, a motivation to learn, task persistence, and autonomy (Bierman et al., 2008; Coolahan et al., 2000; Fantuzzo & McWayne, 2002).

Cognitive Engagement

A child's ability to follow rules and instructions and otherwise be behaviorally engaged can be influenced by, and also influence, the child's cognitive development. The research on early childhood cognitive development finds that children at this stage begin to transition from externally to internally regulated actions (Kochanska, Coy, & Murray, 2001; Kochanska & Knaack, 2003). This is defined as self-regulation and effortful control whereby the child learns how to control and inhibit his/her own emotions and behaviors (Liew et al., 2008; Kochanska & Knaack, 2003; Kochanska et al., 2001), and may also reflect the child's acquisition of a personal self-theory, which, as previously described, is an important developmental task in early childhood. The extent to which a child has an internal sense of control and can self-regulate his/her behaviors has been shown to influence that child's engagement in a learning environment, specifically the child's ability to participate in classroom activities, control attention, and stay on task (Bierman et al., 2008). Again, student engagement in school during early childhood is often measured by the child's classroom behaviors and is a function of his/her interaction with the school context.

Emotional Engagement

A child's emotional engagement has implications for school readiness and academic achievement (Bierman et al., 2008; Liew et al., 2008; Raver, 2002). Particularly in early childhood, children are beginning to interact with persons other than their parents such as peers and teachers. Having positive interactions with multiple people, such as parents and other caring individuals, can help promote learning and build a warm and responsive social context (Ramey & Ramey, 2004). These interactions in turn can encourage a sense of belonging and liking in school and the development of social-emotional competencies, which has been shown to decrease off-task and aggressive behavior and increase prosocial classroom and task engagement (Bierman et al., 2008; Raver, 2002). Teachers especially can help nurture interest in school and learning activities (Bierman et al., 2008). Likewise, the added influence of interacting with nonfamilial adults can contribute to the child's emotional maturation more generally and shows the importance for synchrony across contexts, or person-environment fit. In other words, the multiple opportunities for positive interactions can have multiplicative effects for encouraging the child's engagement.

Future Research

Research in early childhood education demonstrates that participating in early childhood programs can improve a child's school readiness, which has important implications for a child's future academic success by providing another context that encourages positive development. Indeed, the results from research show children who participate in early childhood programs make gains in vocabulary and math, behavioral, and social skills (Barnett, 1995; Bierman et al., 2008). Beyond those findings, early childhood education research has yet to investigate the relationship between school readiness and student engagement specifically (Blair, 2002). For instance, research is needed to examine how student engagement might vary by school readiness levels, which in turn may be influenced by whether the child possesses certain developmental tasks and the contextual factors associated with engagement. Thus, early childhood researchers should work to integrate the research in early childhood education and other developmental research into a cohesive framework that captures all three components of student engagement. Moreover, engagement research in the early childhood literature should expand its scope to include nonschool/learning environments in understanding the developmental precursors to student engagement in early childhood education. As the theoretical considerations we propose suggest, it is important to take an ecological approach to the study of developmental outcomes, student engagement included. Currently, most of the literature has focused specifically on the preschool, kindergarten, and special education environments (e.g., Mahoney & Wheeden, 1999; Malmskog & McDonnell, 1999; McWilliam & Casey, 2008).

Middle Childhood

During this time, children continue to transition into more formal schooling and learning environments, and there is a concurrent increase in the literature on student engagement, especially as it pertains to academic achievement and school adjustment (Ripke, Huston, & Casey, 2006; Simpkins, Fredricks, Davis-Kean, & Eccles, 2006; Skinner, Furrer, Marchand, & Kinderman, 2008). The increase in literature, however, is limited to research within the school context. Indeed, during middle childhood, the classroom becomes the most salient learning environment, with additional learning experiences provided through after-school activities. The accumulation of these experiences is said to contribute to the development of student engagement in middle childhood (Ripke et al., 2006; Rose-Krasnor, 2009; Simpkins et al., 2006).

As with development in general (according to the bioecological theory), engagement in middle childhood has been defined as a function of individual student characteristics and learning experiences (Marks, 2000), and sustained interactions between the student and activity context (Appleton et al., 2008; Rose-Krasnor, 2009).

Moreover, student engagement during middle childhood increases in importance as the role of parents and teachers in promoting classroom and participation in extracurricular activities begins to wane (Ripke et al., 2006; Simpkins et al., 2006; Skinner et al., 2008). Engagement is also at its peak during middle childhood while children are in elementary school (Marks, 2000), perhaps paralleling the development of children's abilities to manage group cooperation (i.e., team play). In this way, learning to manage group work may foster engagement, and being engaged may facilitate team play. In addition, research on engagement in middle childhood begins to differentiate between behavioral, cognitive, and emotional engagement. The definitions and influences of these three types of engagement are discussed in further detail in the following sections.

Behavioral Engagement

Results taken from teacher's reports of students' behaviors show that behaviorally engaged students are characterized as being attentive in class, responsive to rules and instructions, and initiate action (Finn, 1989; Luo et al., 2009). Indeed, the classroom becomes an important learning environment for youth in middle childhood, and the extent to which children actively participate and are involved in classroom tasks and activities has been argued as a prerequisite for achievement and engagement (Finn, Folger, & Cox, 1991; Ladd, Birch, & Buhs, 1999; Skinner et al., 2008). This demonstrates the bioecological argument that active interactions with a person's environment drive development. Moreover, the continued maturation of developmental tasks during middle childhood may facilitate or hinder engagement; developmental tasks may facilitate the development of student engagement if the child has successfully reached the task, whereas difficulties in coping with new developmental tasks can hinder the development of engagement. As the main propositions of the person-environment fit perspective suggest, the extent to which the child's contexts fit his/her developmental needs can also contribute to the expression of engagement.

Beyond the classroom environment, after-school activities offer another context and opportunity for students to become engaged behaviorally (Simpkins et al., 2006; Vandell, Pierce, & Dadisman, 2005). Behavioral engagement in after-school activities is defined as the child's attendance and involvement in the activities (Morris & Kalil, 2006; Rose-Krasnor, 2009; Vandell et al., 2005). Middle childhood is often when children begin to become involved in activities outside of school; participating in activities such as sports, and arts and music lessons has been shown to promote psychosocial and academic outcomes for children (Dumais, 2006; Ripke et al., 2006). Research has also shown that positive experiences outside of the classroom can supplement and benefit the child's engagement in the classroom (Luo et al., 2009; Rose-Krasnor, 2009). Hence, synchrony among school-related activities can positively influence the development of student engagement. Moreover, the literature suggests that a child's behavioral engagement is a precursor to skill development, positive social interactions, and emotional engagement (Morris & Kalil, 2006; Rose-Krasnor, 2009).

Cognitive Engagement

While behavioral engagement reflects a child's attendance and participation with an activity, cognitive engagement captures the child's knowledge and beliefs about the activity and self (Appleton et al., 2008; Ripke et al., 2006; Rose-Krasnor, 2009; Simpkins et al., 2006). The key developmental tasks in middle childhood include the development of concrete operational reasoning, skill learning, and self-evaluation (Newman & Newman, 2009); thus, children continue to develop their self-regulatory skills that encourage self-perceptions of competence and intrinsic motivation (Appleton et al., 2008; Ripke et al., 2006; Simpkins et al., 2006; Skinner et al., 2008). Having positive self-perceptions and self-efficacy beliefs has been linked to academic achievement as well as future activity participation (Appleton et al., 2008; Simpkins et al., 2006). In middle childhood, students with high cognitive engagement are characterized as having high self-efficacy beliefs and being mastery oriented (Luo et al., 2009). Subsequently, children demonstrating high cognitive engagement are more likely to sustain their engagement in school and activities over time (Ripke et al., 2006; Rose-Krasnor, 2009). In this way, cognitive engagement is an individual characteristic that facilitates interactions within the school context and that encourages engagement.

The child's engagement in activities also becomes more self-directed compared to early childhood; as children develop a greater sense of self-efficacy, the role of parents' and teachers' demands on classroom and activity engagement wane (Hughes, Luo, Kwok, & Loyd, 2008; Skinner et al., 2008). In other words, while parents and teachers may still introduce children to activities and promote activity participation, children can begin to develop their own beliefs and interests toward the activity, which drives their future engagement (Ripke et al., 2006).

Emotional Engagement

A child's emotional engagement is represented by the extent to which the child feels a sense of belonging to his/her school, values learning and shows excitement toward classroom and after-school activities (Finn, 1989; Luo et al., 2009; Rose-Krasnor, 2009). During middle childhood, the student-teacher relationship and the child's relationship with friends contribute to the child's social skill development, which demonstrate how the accumulation of positive interactions across multiple people and contexts can reinforce both positive development and student engagement. Indeed, Ladd et al. (1999) found that stressful teacher and peer relationships negatively influenced classroom engagement, which was defined by participation in classroom activities and academic achievement. A warm and supportive student-teacher relationship has been shown to facilitate gains in achievement (Birch & Ladd, 1997; Hughes et al., 2008; Skinner et al., 2008) with elementary school students reporting greater classroom support than in middle and high school (Marks, 2000). Peer validation has been shown to improve school living and engagement, with engagement defined as classroom involvement and behaviors (Ladd et al., 1999).

Future Research

Extant research has identified middle childhood as the prime developmental period to cultivate student engagement given that children become increasingly involved in relationships outside of the home and move into formal schooling. As such, the literature's focus on the school context is justifiable because it is through these increased school experiences that children gain opportunities to develop their academic engagement. However, we cannot neglect the potential influence that other contexts, such as the home and neighborhood, still have on a child's development and student engagement. Indeed, related research on adolescents has shown that having positive bonds with one's parents, peers, and teachers lays the foundation for supportive learning environments, which in turn increase academic achievement and social skill development (Eccles, 2004; Libbey, 2004). Thus, to expand our understanding of the multidimensionality of student engagement, similar research on the implications of person-environment fit on engagement during the middle childhood and elementary school years is needed; longitudinal research on early and middle childhood can enhance the discussion on student engagement, especially when considering student engagement within a developmental and ecological context.

Adolescence

Given that engagement research started off as a model for understanding dropout (Finn, 1989), there are a multitude of studies that cover the adolescent years—the time when youth have the opportunity to dropout. Moreover, Eccles et al. (1993) showed a decline in student engagement during the transition to junior high school. They documented that these changes in engagement are a function of poor person-environment fit through decreased opportunities for autonomy and relatedness at critical point in development when both aspects are important in explaining healthy developmental outcomes (Eccles et al., 1993). After this period of early adolescence, Janosz, Archambault, Morizot, and Pagani (2008) found that student engagement tends to be stable for many over the course of adolescence and that many display moderate to high levels of behavioral, cognitive, and emotional engagement, albeit lower than in the middle schooling years.

Developmentally, during adolescence, individuals experience rapid physical maturation as well as rapid development of cognitive skills. Youth begin to have greater self-reflection, become more deliberate and focused, and are able to hypothesize and think about several strategies or outcomes for these hypotheses simultaneously rather than focusing on just one domain or issue at a time (Keating, 2004). Thus, the ability to become cognitively engaged with school is greater during adolescence compared to both early and middle childhood. Peers also become even more salient compared to prior developmental periods, and Ryan (2001) demonstrated that peers significantly predicted changes in academic performance over time. Experiences with peers coupled with the family, classroom, and school context are important determinants of student engagement during adolescence (Libbey, 2004; Mullis, Rathge & Mullis, 2003). Overall, compared to the literature on student engagement in early and middle childhood, research on student engagement during adolescence has clearly delineated between behavioral, cognitive, and emotional engagement.

Behavioral Engagement

For adolescents, behavioral engagement is consistently defined as time on task, study behaviors, school and class attendance, and participation in class discussions. Often, teacher reports of student behaviors are used to gauge behavioral engagement. In addition, official school attendance records and adolescent self-reports are also widely used in the literature. Most of the research on adolescent behavioral engagement has focused on student truancy and dropout, which Blumenfeld et al. (2005) argued reflects the disengaged student. Many disengaged students are dissatisfied with school, are disruptive in the classroom, have parents that are more controlling, and have more family conflict (Corville-Smith, Ryan, Adams, & Dalicandro, 1998). With regard to the family's influence, Leone and Richards (1989) found that adolescents who completed their homework with their parents had higher achievement scores. Shumow and Miller (2001) also found that parental assistance with homework was positively associated with measures of school engagement. Beyond the family, peers, teachers, and extracurricular activities can influence the development of student engagement during adolescence. As described in the developmental section, two key developmental tasks during adolescence is the increasing salience and influence of platonic and romantic peer relationships. For instance, several studies suggest that peers are particularly influential on adolescents' day-to-day school activities such as doing homework and the effort put forth during class (Midgely & Urdan, 1995; Steinberg et al., 1996). Klem and Connell (2004) found that middle-school student attendance was higher when their teachers created caring, well-structured classroom environments. Extracurricular and after-school activities provide another way for adolescents to be behaviorally engaged with the school context outside of the classroom environment (Feldman & Matjasko, 2005). This further serves to illustrate the importance of recognizing how individual interactions and characteristics within one context (e.g., school, afterschool) may be coupled with congruent or divergent processes in another (e.g., home) to drive an individual toward engagement.

Cognitive Engagement

Cognitive engagement is defined as attention to task, task mastery, and preference for challenging tasks. During adolescence, youth have developed the self-regulatory skills necessary for the self-perceptions of competence and intrinsic motivation, and abstract thinking. Furthermore, as students move from elementary to middle school, their desire for easy work increases. However, the standards-based educational context in the USA tends to foster extrinsic motivation, which can create dissonance between the adolescent's developmental characteristics and the learning environments in which they participate. Indeed, as students progress from elementary through high school, their self-worth increasingly depends more on their ability to achieve competitively (Harari & Covington, 1981). Extrinsic rewards for learning, such as good grades and performance on standardized tests, are symbols of success that maintain one's self-worth. The increased emphasis on competition and evaluation of student performance from elementary through high school (Gottfried, Fleming, & Gottfried, 2001) may, in part, contribute to the documented decline in students' intrinsic motivation from elementary through middle school (Lepper, Corpus, & Iyengar, 2005) and preference for challenge, curiosity, interest, and mastery from elementary school to high school (Harter & Jackson, 1992).

Despite this decline in intrinsic motivation over the course of childhood and adolescence, certain contextual conditions are related to higher levels of intrinsic motivation. Gottfried, Fleming, and Gottfried (1998) found that a cognitively stimulating home environment (e.g., access to hobbies, books, trips to museums) was significantly related to academic intrinsic motivation over the course of childhood and adolescence.

Steinberg, Lamborn, Dornbusch, and Darling (1992) found a positive relationship between authoritative parenting and cognitive engagement. Ryan and Patrick (2001) found that students' perceptions of teacher support were a significant predictor of cognitive engagement during middle school. Ryan and Patrick (2001) found that peer group characteristics were significantly related to achievement orientation (i.e., intrinsic motivation) and that peers significantly predicted decreases in achievement orientation over time. However, Goodenow and Grady (1993) found that peer academic values were less important than feelings of school belonging in explaining adolescent academic motivation. In an experimental study conducted on a sample of college students, Patrick, Tisley, and Kempler (2000) found that teacher enthusiasm was related to higher intrinsic motivation scores. Thus, echoing the theoretical considerations we described, students' cognitive engagement is situated within a set of overlapping environmental systems that interact to shape development.

Emotional Engagement

Emotions such as fear, anxiety, boredom, or enthusiasm about a school-related task have been considered in investigations of emotional engagement in academic tasks. Along with behavioral and cognitive engagement, emotional engagement also tends to decrease upon the transition to adolescence (Eccles et al., 1993). Caraway, Tucker, Reinke, and Hall (2003) investigated the relationship between fear of failure and academic engagement. They found that fear of failure significantly predicted a decrease in GPA. In addition, test anxiety was negatively related to grades, but it was not significantly related to student engagement or attendance. McNeely, Nonnemaker, and Blum (2002) found that adolescents who report higher levels of school connectedness had higher grades and were less likely to skip school. Furthermore, certain schools were more likely to have students who reported higher levels of school connectedness. Smaller schools and those with less harsh disciplinary policies tended to have students who reported feeling connected to their schools.

In a study using experiential sampling methods, Shernoff (2010) investigated whether the quality of experience in after-school programs mediated the relationship between program participation and academic achievement. He found that feelings of challenge and importance while participating in after-school programs were positively related to academic achievement (Shernoff 2010).

Knollmann and Wild (2007) explored whether the relationship between parental support for autonomy and emotional engagement with homework varied by adolescent cognitive engagement (i.e., intrinsic vs. extrinsic motivation). Even though autonomy is a key developmental task of adolescence, Knollmann and Wild found that extrinsically motivated students reported more negative affect under autonomy-supportive conditions while the opposite was true for intrinsically motivated adolescents. This suggests that cognitive engagement moderates the influence of family factors on emotional engagement. In this, we once again see the interplay between the individual's developmental characteristics and the manifestation of student engagement.

Future Research

While a large amount of research on student engagement during adolescence exists, there are some notable gaps. First, longitudinal work is needed that links all three aspects of student engagement during adolescence with early and middle childhood measures of engagement. Making such links will allow us to understand the important precursors of adolescent student engagement and the potential reciprocal processes that exist between developmental tasks and student engagement. Furthermore, research on the specific forms of behavioral engagement is needed. We know relatively little about time on task, disruptive classroom behavior, and participation in classroom discussions during adolescence. In addition, studies that use experiential sampling methodology will continue to document the links between behaviors, cognitions, and emotions around school-related tasks during adolescence.

Conclusion

At the onset of this chapter, we offered two main guiding questions, essentially how developmental tasks influence student engagement and vice versa. These two questions capture the idea that human development and the development of student engagement can and most likely occur in tandem. All things considered, there are potential connections between research on child and adolescent development and the development of student engagement. The connections, however, are not always transparent, and thus this chapter aimed to present one interpretation of the two streams of theory and research.

As discussed in this chapter, theoretically, a combination of the bioecological theory of human development (Bronfenbrenner & Morris, 1998), person-environment fit perspective (Eccles et al., 1993), and the participation-identification model (Finn, 1989; Reschly, 2010) can create a more comprehensive picture of student engagement, its correlates, and its consequences. Where the participation-identification model excels in outlining the development of student engagement, it does not map out how student engagement itself occurs within a larger developmental sequence. The student engagement literature does point out that engagement changes as students progress through school (Finn, 1989) because of changing opportunities for engagement due to changing contexts. Furthermore, it is important to include a discussion of developmental tasks because children and adolescent may face challenges in successfully reaching those tasks, which may cause some youth to be ill-equipped to reach their full potential for student engagement. The opposite may be true as well, where changes and challenges in student engagement influence successful developmental transitions.

The emphasis on the proximal processes, contexts, and individual characteristics that contribute to human development in the bioecological theory and person-environment fit perspective further help to enhance our understanding of the developmental context of student engagement. First, the bioecological theory recognizes that development is shaped by interactions between people, their characteristics, and their contexts (Bronfenbrenner & Morris, 1998). Applying this to the student engagement research discussed in this chapter, we see that the manifestation of behavioral, cognitive, and emotional engagement at the different developmental periods is often a result of the individual's own capacities and his/her participation in the family, and especially, school contexts. As Finn (1989) mentioned as well, the contexts are themselves important as they provide the opportunities for children and adolescents to be engaged. More generally, the contexts provide the social and structural resources that can mold healthy development. Additionally, it is important to have congruence between the person and their contexts. As espoused by the person-environment fit perspective (Eccles et al., 1993), having synchrony across healthy environments fosters healthy development and in the same vein can facilitate the development of student engagement. As discussed in this chapter, behavioral, cognitive, and emotional engagement are conceptually and methodologically distinct at each developmental period. These differences may be a result of the maturation of developmental tasks and the changing contextual landscape for the children and adolescents. Taken together, student engagement is a nuanced developmental outcome.

Future Research

To further understand the differences in student engagement across developmental periods, developmental and engagement research should focus on growing the empirical evidence for the ecologies and interplay of developmental tasks and the development of student engagement. Indeed, as discussed in this chapter, the research on student engagement in early and middle childhood is especially lacking, and a majority of the research on student engagement has focused on just the school context. While the school context does become increasingly salient in the lives of children and adolescents, it is necessary to understand the developmental processes that occur across multiple contexts such as the school, home, and neighborhood to not only encourage healthy human development, but the development of student engagement as well. According to bioecological theory, it is important to account for multiple contexts in understanding student engagement. Additional research is needed on the family context and how parents support or detract from the development of student engagement. Furthermore, the person-environment fit perspective calls attention to whether specific contexts fit with the developmental needs of children and adolescents, whether these contexts are in synchrony with each other, and the changing nature and consequences of contextual synchrony/dissynchrony across early childhood, middle childhood, and adolescence. Methodologically, we recommend further development of observational (Pittman, Merita, Tolman, Yohalem, & Ferber, 2003) and survey measures (Bohnert et al., 2010; Lippman & Rivers, 2008) of individual-level behavioral, emotional, and cognitive student engagement, and that these measures be integrated into the multifaceted and longitudinal studies of student educational attainment and student activity involvement.

Application and Policy Implications

There is growing recognition among educators and policymakers that student engagement inside and outside (i.e., civic engagement; not discussed in this chapter) of school settings is important for the positive growth and development of America's young children. In addition, a new report finds that student engagement may be particularly important for older adolescents who are preparing for the roles of adult life (Deschenes et al., 2010); yet the extant literature on the developmental precursors of student engagement or how student engagement may manifest across developmental periods is limited, resulting in potentially discontinuous developmental transitions into adult roles (Sherrod & Lauckhard, 2009). Again, there is an important interplay between the development of engagement and human development more generally that needs to be recognized.

To facilitate the many transitions children and adolescents face, family, school, and community initiatives that promote student engagement may be crucial for the growth and development of student engagement. Moreover, we argue for the potential importance of creating integrative multicontextual partnerships that enhance student engagement across developmental periods. Indeed, the bioecological theory and person-environment fit perspective paired with the developmental and engagement research reviewed in this chapter suggest that what might be the most optimal for successful student engagement and human development is consistency through the developmental periods in providing adequate resources to address the developmental and educational challenges in childhood and adolescence. As we began this chapter saying, the development of student engagement must be understood within the context of the individual's developmental history. The two are not separate outcomes, rather they complement each other; both involve a sequence of events, and by recognizing that these sequences occur simultaneously, educators, researchers, policy makers, and other professionals can build environments that promote positive development in multiple domains.

References

Anderson, J. C., Funk, J. B., Elliot, R., & Smith, P. H. (2003). Parental support and pressure and children's extracurricular activities: Relationships with amount of involvement and affective experience of participation. *Journal of Applied Developmental Psychology, 24*, 241–257.

Appleton, J. J., Christenson, S. L., & Furlong, M. J. (2008). Student engagement with school: Critical conceptual and methodological issues of the construct. *Psychology in the Schools, 45*, 369–386.

Barnett, S. (1995). Long-term effects of early childhood programs on cognitive and school outcomes. *The Future of Children, 5*, 25–50.

Bartko, T. W. (2005). The ABCS of engagement in out-of-school programs. *New Directions for Youth Development, 105*, 109–120.

Bierman, K. L., Domitrovich, C. E., Nix, R. L., Gest, S. D., Welsh, J. A., Greenberg, M. T., & Gill, S. (2008). Promoting academic and socioal-emotional school readiness: The head start REDI program. *Child Development, 79*, 1802–1817.

Birch, S. H., & Ladd, G. W. (1997). The teacher-child relationship and children's early school adjustment. *Journal of School Psychology, 35*, 61–79.

Blair, C. (2002). School readiness: Integrating cognition and emotion in a neurobiological conceptualization of children's functioning at school entry. *American Psychologist, 57*, 111–127.

Blumenfeld, P. C., Kempler, T. M., & Krajcik, J. S. (2006). Motivation and cognitive engagement in learning environments. In R. K. Sawyer (Ed.), *The Cambridge handbook of the learning sciences* (pp. 475–488). New York: Cambridge University Press.

Blumenfeld, P. C., Modell, J., Bartko, W. T., Secada, W., Fredricks, J., Friedel, J., & Parks, A. (2005). School engagement of inner city students during middle childhood. In C. R. Cooper, C. Garcia-Coll, W. T. Bartko, H. M. Davis, & C. Chatman (Eds.), *Developmental pathways through middle childhood: Rethinking diversity and contexts as recourses* (pp. 145–170). Mahwah, NJ: Lawrence Erlbaum.

Bohnert, A., Fredricks, J., & Randall, E. (2010). Capturing unique dimensions of youth organized activity involvement: Theoretical and methodological considerations. *Review of Educational Research*, Online First, May 2010.

Bronfenbrenner, U. (1975). Is early intervention effective? In E. Stuening & M. Guttentag (Eds.), *Handbook of evaluation research* (Vol. 2, pp. 519–603). Beverly Hills, CA: Sage.

Bronfenbrenner, U., & Ceci, S. J. (1994). Nature-nurture reconceptualized in developmental perspective: A bio-ecological model. *Psychological Review, 101*, 568–586.

Bronfenbrenner, U., & Morris, P. A. (1998). The ecology of developmental processes. In W. Damon (Series Ed.) & R. Lerner (Vol. Ed.), *Handbook of child psychology: Vol. 1. Theory* (5th ed., pp. 993–1028). New York: John Wiley.

Caraway, K., Tucker, C. M., Reinke, W. M., & Hall, C. (2003). Self-efficacy, goal orientation, and fear of failure as predictors of school engagement with high school students. *Psychology in the Schools, 40*, 417–427.

Carbonaro, W. J. (1998). A little help from my friend's parents: Social closure and educational outcomes. *Sociology of Education, 71*, 295–313.

Catalano, R. F., Berglund, M. L., Ryan, J. A. M., Lonczack, H. S., & Hawkins, J. D. (2004). Positive youth development in the United States: Research findings on evaluations of positive youth development programs. *The Annals of the American Academy of Political and Social Science, 591*, 98–124.

Connell, J. P., Spencer, M. B., & Aber, J. L. (1994). Educational risk and resilience in African-American youth: Context, self, action, and outcomes in school. *Child Development, 65,* 493–506.

Connell, J. P., & Wellborn, J. (1991). Competence, autonomy, and relatedness: A motivational analysis of self-system processes. In M. Gunnar & A. Sroufe (Eds.), *Minnesota symposium on child development* (Vol. 22, pp. 43–77). Hillsdale, NJ: Erlbaum.

Coolahan, K., Fantuzzo, J., Mendez, J., & McDermott, P. (2000). Preschool peer interactions and readiness to learn: Relationships between classroom peer play and learning behaviors and conduct. *Journal of Educational Psychology, 92,* 458–465.

Corville-Smith, J., Ryan, B. A., Adams, G. R., & Dalicandro, T. (1998). Distinguishing absentee students from regular attenders: The combined influence of personal, family, and school factors. *Journal of Youth and Adolescence, 27,* 629–640.

Currie, J. (2001). Early childhood education programs. *Journal of Economic Perspectives, 15,* 213–238.

Dearing, E., Wimer, C., Simpkins, S., Lund, T., Bouffard, W., Caronongan, P., et al. (2009). Do neighborhood and home contexts help explain why low-income children miss opportunities to participate in activities outside of school? *Developmental Psychology, 45,* 1545–1562.

Denault, A. S., & Poulin, F. (2009). Intensity and breadth of participation in organized activities during the adolescent years: Multiple associations with youth outcomes. *Journal of Youth and Adolescence, 9,* 119–1213.

Deschenes, S. N., Arbreton, A., Little, P. M., Herrera, C., Grossman, J. B., Weiss, H. B., et al. (2010). *Engaging older youth: Program and city-level strategies to support sustained participation in out-of-school time.* Harvard Family Research Project. Retrieved from http://www.hfrp.org/out-of-school-time/publications-resources/engaging-older-youth-program-and-city-level-strategies-to-support-sustained-participation-in-out-of-school-time.

Dumais, S. A. (2006). Elementary school students' extracurricular activities: The effects of participation on achievement and teachers' evaluations. *Sociological Spectrum, 26,* 117–147.

Eccles, J. S. (2004). Schools, academic motivation, and stage-environment fit. In R. M. Lerner & L. Steinberg (Eds.), *Handbook of adolescent psychology* (2nd ed., pp. 125–153). Hoboken, NJ: Wiley.

Eccles, J. S. (2005). The present and future of research on activity settings as developmental contexts. In J. Mahoney, R. W. Larson, & J. S. Eccles (Eds.), *Organized activities as contexts of development: Extracurricular activities, after-school and community programs* (pp. 353–374). Mahwah, NJ: Lawrence Erlbaum.

Eccles, J. S., Midgefield, C., & Wigfield, A. (1993). Development during adolescence: The impact of stage-environment fit on young adolescents' experiences in schools and in families. *American Psychologist, 48,* 90–101.

Epstein, J. (1983). Selecting friends in contrasting secondary school environments. In J. Epstein & N. Karweit (Eds.), *Friends in school.* New York: Academic.

Fantuzzo, J., & McWayne, C. (2002). The relationship between peer-play interactions in the family context and dimensions of school readiness for low-income preschool children. *Journal of Educational Psychology, 94,* 79–87.

Feldman, A. F., & Matjasko, J. L. (2005). The role of school-based extracurricular activities in adolescent development: A comprehensive review and future directions. *Review of Educational Research, 75,* 159–210.

Finn, J. D. (1989). Withdrawing from school. *Review of Educational Research, 59,* 117–142.

Finn, J. D., Folger, J., & Cox, D. (1991). Measuring participation among elementary grade students. *Educational and Psychological Measurement, 51,* 393–402.

Fletcher, A. C., Elder, G. H., Jr., & Mekos, D. (2000). Parental influences on adolescent involvement in community activities. *Journal of Research on Adolescence, 10,* 29–48.

Fredricks, J. A., Blumenfeld, P. C., & Paris, A. H. (2004). School engagement: Potential of the concept, state of the evidence. *Review of Educational Research, 74,* 59–109.

Goodenow, C., & Grady, K. E. (1993). The relationship of school belonging and friends' values to academic motivation among urban adolescent students. *The Journal of Experimental Education, 62,* 60–71.

Goodenow, J. (1995). Differentiating among social contexts: By spatial features, forms of participation, and social contracts. In P. Moen, G. H. Elder Jr., & K. Luschner (Eds.), *Examining lives in context: Perspective on the ecology of human development* (pp. 269–302). Washington, DC: American Psychological Association.

Gottfried, A. E., Fleming, J. S., & Gottfried, A. W. (1998). Role of cognitively stimulating home environment in children's academic intrinsic motivation: A longitudinal study. *Child Development, 69,* 1448–1460.

Gottfried, A. E., Fleming, J. S., & Gottfried, A. W. (2001). Continuity of academic intrinsic motivation from childhood through late adolescence: A longitudinal study. *Journal of Educational Psychology, 93,* 3–13.

Gutman, L. M., & Eccles, J. S. (2007). Stage-environment fit during adolescence: Trajectories of family relations and adolescent outcomes. *Developmental Psychology, 43,* 522–537.

Hair, E., Halle, T., & Terry-Humen, E. (2006). Children's school readiness in the ECLS-K: Predictions to academic, health, and social outcomes in first grade. *Early Childhood Research Quarterly, 21,* 431–454.

Harari, O., & Covington, M. V. (1981). Reactions to achievement behavior from a teacher and student perspective: A developmental analysis. *American Educational Research Journal, 18,* 15–28.

Harter, S., & Jackson, B. K. (1992). Trait vs. nontrait conceptualizations of intrinsic/extrinsic motivational orientation. *Motivation and Emotion, 16*, 209–230.

Hughes, J. N., Luo, W., Kwok, O. M., & Loyd, L. K. (2008). Teacher-student support, effortful engagement, and achievement: A 3-year longitudinal study. *Journal of Educational Psychology, 100*, 1–14.

Janosz, M., Archambault, I., Morizot, J., & Pagani, L. S. (2008). School engagement trajectories and their differential predictive relations to dropout. *Journal of Social Issues, 64*, 21–40.

Kagan, S. L. (1990). Readiness 2000: Rethinking rhetoric and responsibility. *The Phi Delta Kappan, 72*, 272–279.

Karcher, M. J., Kuperminc, G. P., Portwood, S. G., Sipe, C. L., & Taylor, A. S. (2006). Mentoring programs: A framework to inform program development, research, and evaluation. *Journal of Community Psychology, 34*, 709–725.

Keating, D. P. (2004). Cognitive and brain development. In R. M. Lerner & L. Steinberg (Eds.), *Handbook of adolescent psychology* (2nd ed., pp. 45–84). New York: Wiley.

Klem, A. M., & Connell, J. P. (2004). Relationships matter: Linking teacher support to student engagement and achievement. *Journal of School Health, 74*, 262–282.

Knollmann, M., & Wild, E. (2007). Quality of parental support and students' emotions during homework: Moderating effects of students' motivational orientations. *European Journal of Psychology of Education, 22*, 63–76.

Kochanska, G., Coy, K. C., & Murray, K. T. (2001). The development of self-regulation in the first four years of life. *Child Development, 72*, 1091–1111.

Kochanska, G., & Knaack, A. (2003). Effortful control as a personality characteristic of young children: Antecedents, correlates, and consequences. *Journal of Personality, 71*, 1087.

Kuperschmidt, J. B., Bryant, D., & Willoughby, M. (2000). Prevalence of aggressive behaviors among preschoolers in Head Start and community child care programs. *Behavioral Disorders, 26*, 42–52.

Ladd, G. W., Birch, S. H., & Buhs, E. S. (1999). Children's social and scholastic lives in kindergarten: Related spheres of influence. *Child Development, 70*, 1373–1400.

Larson, R. W. (2000). Toward a psychology of positive youth development. *American Psychologist, 55*, 170–183.

Leone, C. M., & Richards, M. H. (1989). Classwork and homework in early adolescence: The ecology of achievement. *Journal of Youth and Adolescence, 18*, 531–548.

Lepper, M. R., Corpus, J. H., & Iyengar, S. S. (2005). Intrinsic and extrinsic motivational orientations in the classroom: Age differences and academic correlates. *Journal of Educational Psychology, 97*, 184–196.

Lerner, R. M., Brentano, C., Dowling, E. M., & Anderson, P. M. (2002). Positive youth development: Thriving as the basis of personhood and civil society. *New Directions for Youth Development, 95*, 11–33.

Lerner, R. M., & Castellino, D. R. (2002). Contemporary developmental theory and adolescence: Developmental systems and applied developmental science. *Journal of Adolescent Health, 31*, 122–135.

Libbey, H. P. (2004). Measuring student relationships to school: Attachment, bonding, connectedness, and engagement. *Journal of School Health, 74*, 274–283.

Liew, J., McTigue, E., Barrois, L., & Hughes, J. (2008). Adaptive and effortful control and academic self-efficacy beliefs on achievement: A longitudinal study of 1 through 3 graders. *Early Child Research Quarterly, 23*, 515–526.

Lippman, L., & Rivers, A. (2008). Assessing school engagement: A guide for out-of-school time program practitioners. *Child Trends Research Brief, 39*, 1–5.

Lohman, B. J., Kaura, S. A., & Newman, B. M. (2007). Matched or mismatched environments? The relationship of family and school differentiation to adolescents' psychosocial adjustment. *Youth & Society, 39*, 3–32.

Luo, W., Hughes, J. A., Liew, J., & Kwok, O. (2009). Classifying academically at-risk first graders into engagement types: Association with long-term achievement trajectories. *The Elementary School Journal, 109*, 380.

Mahoney, J., & Bergman, L. (2002). Conceptual and methodological considerations in a developmental approach to the study of positive adaptation. *Applied Developmental Psychology, 23*, 195–217.

Mahoney, J., & Magnusson, D. (2001). Parent participation in community activities and the persistence of criminality. *Development and Psychopathology, 13*, 125–141.

Mahoney, J., Vandell, D. L., Simpkins, S., & Zarrett, N. (2009). Adolescent out-of-school activities. In R. M. Lerner & L. Steinberg (Eds.), *Handbook of adolescent psychology* (3rd ed., pp. 228–269). New York: John Wiley.

Mahoney, J., & Wheeden, C. A. (1999). The effect of teacher style of interactive engagement of preschool-aged children with special learning needs. *Early Childhood Research Quarterly, 14*, 51–68.

Malmskog, S., & McDonnell, A. P. (1999). Teacher-mediated facilitation of engagement of children with developmental delays in inclusive preschools. *Topics in Early Childhood Special Education, 19*, 203–216.

Manke, B., McGuire, S., Reiss, D., Hetherington, E. M., & Plomin, R. (1995). Genetic contributions to adolescents' extrafamilial social interactions: Teachers, best friends, and peers. *Social Development, 4*, 238–256.

Marks, H. M. (2000). Student engagement in instructional activity: Patterns in the elementary, middle, and high school years. *American Educational Research Journal, 37*, 153–184.

McCormick, M. C., Brooks-Gunn, J., Buka, S. L., Goldman, J., Yu, J., Salganik, M., et al. (2006). Early intervention in LBW premature infants: Results at 18 years of age for infant health and development program. *Pediatrics, 117*, 771–780.

McNeely, C. A., Nonnemaker, J. M., & Blum, R. W. (2002). Promoting school connectedness: Evidence from the National Longitudinal Study of Adolescent Health. *Journal of School Health, 72*, 138–146.

McWilliam, R. A., & Bailey, D. B. (1992). Promoting engagement and mastery. In D. B. Bailty & M. Wolery (Eds.), *Teaching infants and preschoolers with disabilities* (2nd ed., pp. 230–255). New York: MacMillian.

McWilliam, R. A., & Casey, A. M. (2008). *Engagement of every child in the preschool classroom*. Baltimore: Paul H. Brooke s Publishing Co.

Midgely, C., & Urdan, T. (1995). Predictors of middle school students' use of self-handicapping strategies. *Journal of Early Adolescence, 15*, 389–411.

Miller, P. H. (2002). *Theories of developmental psychology* (4th ed.). New York: Worth.

Morris, P., & Kalil, A. (2006). Out-of-school time use during middle childhood in a low-income sample: Do combinations of activities affect achievement and behavior? In A. Huston & M. Ripke (Eds.), *Developmental contexts in middle childhood: Bridges to adolescence and adulthood* (pp. 237–259). New York: Cambridge University Press.

Mullis, R. L., Rathge, R., & Mullis, A. K. (2003). Predictors of academic performance during early adolescence: A contextual view. *International Journal of Behavioral Development, 27*, 541–548.

Newman, B. M., & Newman, P. R. (2009). *Development through life: A psychosocial approach* (10th ed.). Belmont, CA: Wadsworth Cenage Learning.

Parra, G. R., Dubois, D. L., Neville, H. A., Pugh-Lilly, A. O., & Povinelli, N. (2002). Mentoring relationships for youth: Investigation of a process-oriented model. *Journal of Community Psychology, 30*, 367–388.

Patrick, B. C., Tinsely, J., & Kempler, T. (2000). "What's everyone so excited about?": The effects of teacher enthusiasm on teacher on student intrinsic motivation and vitality. *The Journal of Experimental Education, 68*, 217–236.

Persson, A., Kerr, M., & Stattin, H. (2007). Staying in or moving away from structured activities: Explanations involving parents and peers. *Developmental Psychology, 43*, 197–207.

Pittman, K. J., Merita, I., Tolman, J., Yohalem, N., & Ferber, T. (2003). *Preventing problems, promoting development, encouraging engagement: Competing priorities or inseparable goals?* Washington, DC: Forum for Youth Investment.

Portes, A. (2000). The two meanings of social capital. *Sociological Forum, 15*, 1–12.

Ramey, C. T., & Ramey, S. L. (2004). Early learning and school readiness: Can early intervention make a difference? *Merrill-Palmer Quarterly, 50*, 471–491.

Raver, C. C. (2002). Emotions matter: Making the case for the role of young children's emotional development for early school readiness. *Social Policy Report, 16*, 3–18.

Reschly, A. L. (2010). Reading and school completion: Critical connections and Matthew effects. *Reading & Writing Quarterly, 26*, 67–90.

Ripke, M. N., Huston, A. C., & Casey, D. M. (2006). Low-income children's activity participation as a predictor of psychosocial and academic outcomes in middle childhood and adolescence. In A. C. Huston & M. N. Ripke (Eds.), *Developmental contexts of middle childhood: Bridges to adolescence and adulthood* (pp. 260–282). New York: Cambridge University Press.

Roeser, R. W., & Eccles, J. S. (1998). Adolescents' perceptions of middle school: Relation to longitudinal changes in academic and psychological adjustment. *Journal of Research on Adolescence, 86*, 123–158.

Rose-Krasnor, L. (2009). Future directions in youth involvement research. *Social Development, 18*, 497–509.

Ryan, A. (2001). The peer group as a context for the development of young adolescent motivation and achievement. *Child Development, 72*, 1135–1150.

Ryan, A. M., & Patrick, H. (2001). The classroom social environment and changes in adolescents' motivation and engagement during middle school. *American Educational Research Journal, 38*, 437–460.

Shernoff, D. J. (2010). Engagement in after-school programs as a predictor of social competence and academic performance. *American Journal of Community Psychology, 45*, 325–337.

Sherrod, L. R., & Lauckhardt, J. (2009). The development of citizenship. In R. M. Lerner & L. Steinberg (Eds.), *Handbook of adolescent psychology* (3rd ed., pp. 372–407). Hoboken, NJ: Wiley.

Shumow, L., & Miller, J. D. (2001). Parents' at-home and at-school academic involvement with young adolescents. *Journal of Early Adolescence, 21*, 68–91.

Simpkins, S. D., Fredricks, J. A., Davis-Kean, P. E., & Eccles, J. S. (2006). Healthy mind, healthy habits: The influence of activity involvement in middle childhood. In A. C. Huston & M. N. Ripke (Eds.), *Developmental contexts of middle childhood: Bridges to adolescence and adulthood* (pp. 283–302). New York: Cambridge University Press.

Skinner, E., Furrer, C., Marchand, G., & Kinderman, T. (2008). Engagement and disaffection in the classroom: Part of a larger motivational dynamic? *Journal of Educational Psychology, 100*, 765–781.

Steinberg, L., Bradford, B., & Dornbusch, S. (1996). *Beyond the classroom: Why school reform has failed and what parents need to do*. New York: Simon & Schuster.

Steinberg, L., Lamborn, S. D., Dornbusch, S. M., & Darling, N. (1992). Impact of parenting practices on adolescent achievement: Authoritative parenting, school involvement, and encouragement to succeed. *Child Development, 63*, 1266–1281.

Sternberg, R. J., & Grigorenko, E. L. (2001). Degree of embeddedness of ecological systems as a measure of ease of adaptation to the environment. In E. L. Grigorenko & R. J. Sternberg (Eds.), *Family environment and intellectual functioning: A lifespan perspective* (pp. 243–262). Mahwah, NJ: Erlbaum.

Vandell, D. L., Pierce, K. M., & Dadisman, K. (2005). Out-of-school settings as a developmental context for children and youth. *Advances in Child Development and Behavior, 33*, 43–77.

Weiss, H. B., Little, P. M. D., & Bouffard, S. M. (2005). More than just being there: Balancing the participation equation. *New Directions for Youth Development, 105*, 15–31.

Wigfield, A., & Karpathia, M. (1991). Who am I and what can I do? Children's self-concepts and motivation in achievement situations. *Educational Psychologist, 26*, 233–261.

Ethnicity and Student Engagement

Gary E. Bingham and Lynn Okagaki

Abstract

The underachievement of African American, Latino, and American Indian students in the United States has been partially attributed to poor engagement in school (e.g., Connell, Spencer & Aber, 1994; Steele, 1997). In this chapter, we consider the role of ethnicity in student engagement. A number of factors have been posited to influence minority students' engagement in school. Okagaki (2001) conceptualized these factors into three broad domains: the roles of the student, the family, and the school. We begin with a discussion of factors within the student, such as students' ethnic identity beliefs, experiences with discrimination, and bicultural efficacy, and the relations of these factors to students' engagement in school. In the second section, we examine the role that parents' beliefs, expectations, and behaviors play in ethnic minority students' engagement in school, paying particular attention to beliefs and values that can be attributed to parents' cultural models of education (Gallimore & Goldenberg, 2001; Lareau, 1996). Third, we consider how factors associated with teachers, peers, and friends relate to ethnic minority students' engagement in school. In particular, we focus on students' access to same ethnic teachers and peers, the quality of relationships with teachers and friends, and pedagogical practices that may facilitate ethnic minority students' engagement in school. Finally, we identify the need for stronger empirical research around the identification and amelioration of the discontinuities between home and school cultures.

G.E. Bingham, Ph.D. (✉)
Department of Early Childhood Education,
College of Education, Georgia State University,
Atlanta, GA, USA
e-mail: gbingham@gsu.edu

L. Okagaki, Ph.D.
College of Education and Human Development,
University of Delaware, Newark, DE 19716, USA

> In a reading class I observed, the teacher said, "We are studying tall tales. This is something that cannot be true. Like Pecos Bill. They said he lived with the coyotes. You see, it can't be true." Two Navajo students look at each other and in unison said, "But us Navajo, we live on the reservation with the coyotes." The teacher replied, "Well, I don't know anything about that. Let's talk about parables now." (Deyhle, 1995)

What does engagement mean for a Navajo student who lives his life traversing two very different worlds—home and school—each day? In this chapter, we consider the role of ethnicity in student engagement. We begin with some caveats. First, in the literature on student engagement, researchers have defined engagement in multiple ways and have often used measures that combine different aspects of engagement or include items representing constructs other than engagement (Fredricks, Blumenfeld, & Paris, 2004; Libbey, 2004). Within the last decade, however, researchers have focused considerable efforts to refine the construct distinguishing among types of engagement (e.g., emotional, behavioral, cognitive) and move the field toward alignment of measurement with type of engagement (e.g., Appleton, Christenson, & Furlong, 2008; Fredricks et al., 2004; Glanville & Wildhagen, 2007; Libbey, 2004).

For this chapter, we draw primarily from Fredericks and colleagues' (2004) definition of engagement and consider the emotional, behavioral, and cognitive aspects as separate, but overlapping, constructs. We consider emotional engagement to include students' attitudes toward and feelings about school and schoolwork and their relationships with teachers and students. In contrast, behavioral engagement has been broadly defined as including activities and behaviors that suggest compliance with school norms, involvement in extracurricular activities at school (e.g., music, sports, student council), and participation in class (e.g., asking questions, being attentive, contributing to class discussions, staying on task). Finally, cognitive engagement encompasses intrinsic motivation for learning and metacognitive strategy use (e.g., planning, monitoring). Utilizing this framework, we situate student motivational processes as an overlapping construct within the dimension of emotional and cognitive engagement. As Skinner and colleagues articulate (Skinner, Kindermann, & Furrer, 2009; Skinner, Marchand, Furrer, & Kindermann, 2008), the relation between student engagement and motivation is cyclical and heavily influenced by contextual variables outside the learner. Given the relatively complex social worlds that many ethnic minority children and youth navigate, considering both engagement and motivational factors may be important to ensuring their academic success.

Second, researchers have defined ethnicity in different ways (e.g., Harwood, Handwerker, Schoelmerich, & Leyendecker, 2001; Phinney, 1996) and identified ethnic groups in various ways. For example, researchers sometimes report on Hispanic or Latino Americans as one ethnic group. However, this broad category masks the variation in cultural heritage within the group, which includes individuals who may identify themselves as being, for example, Mexican, Puerto Rican, Cuban, Dominican, Guatemalan, or Ecuadorian. The histories, customs, economies, and political contexts of each of the countries of origin contribute to the heterogeneity of the Hispanic population (e.g., Carrasquillo, 1991; Torres, 2004). Not only do these ethnic subgroups differ on basic demographic characteristics, such as age (U.S. Department of Commerce, Census Bureau, 2001) and country of origin (U.S. Department of Commerce, Census Bureau, 1993), they also differ on characteristics that may be relevant to children's engagement with school, such as fluency in English (U.S. Department of Education, 2001a). Although there is great diversity within ethnic groups, researchers are often limited by pragmatic constraints (e.g., financial resources) and collapse across subgroups in order to have a reasonable sample size for their study. In secondary data analyses, researchers are limited by the definitions of ethnicity that were obtained for the original study. In this chapter, ethnic groups are identified by the labels used by the authors of the cited studies, and readers should recognize that a sample that is identified by a broad ethnic or racial group category (e.g., African American, Asian, Hispanic, Native American) in one study may be very different from a similarly identified sample in another study.

Third, although ethnic group variation is associated with differential learning outcomes in many countries, the discussion in this chapter is limited to ethnicity and education in the United States. In addition, this chapter focuses on ethnic groups of color, and both racial and ethnic minority groups are included in this discussion. Using the term "ethnic group" in this way is not without its problems (e.g., Gutiérrez & Rogoff, 2003; Helms & Talleyrand, 1997). At minimum, it overlooks the great variation and richness in the ethnic backgrounds of White Americans. In general, however, the majority of research conducted on engagement has focused on majority students and is covered in other chapters in this handbook. Moreover, research on ethnicity, engagement, and student outcomes has grown out of recognition of the differential achievement across ethnic groups and concern for the underachievement of many ethnic groups of color. In 2008, out of approximately 48 million public school students in the United States, 45% were children and adolescents from ethnic groups of color (Aud et al., 2010). Despite improvements in achievement over the last 40 years and a narrowing of the achievement gap, Black and Hispanic students continue to lag behind their White counterparts (Rampey, Dion, & Donahue, 2009). A number of researchers have theorized that student engagement may explain variation in student achievement across ethnic groups (e.g., Connell, Spencer, & Aber, 1994; Finn & Rock, 1997; Steele, 1997).

Fourth, some have argued that the variation observed across racial and ethnic groups may be more attributable to socioeconomic differences within a culture than differences across cultural groups (e.g., Hoff, Laursen, & Tardiff, 2002). Research that teases apart the contributions of racial/ethnic background and socioeconomic backgrounds to cultural models of education is relatively limited. Where possible, we make explicit differences that reflect racial and ethnic cultures versus socioeconomic differences. In the descriptions of individual studies, we use the terminology for describing particular groups (e.g., Latino, Hispanic) that was chosen by the authors of the studies.

This chapter provides a framework for organizing the research on and understanding the role of ethnicity in student engagement. Examples of research on different ethnic groups are used to illustrate points.

Ethnicity and Student Engagement

Why might one expect student engagement in school to vary across ethnic groups? Behavioral scientists have generally taken one of two perspectives to understanding the engagement and achievement of students of color. The *cultural discontinuity* view focuses on specific differences (e.g., language, behavioral norms) between the ethnic culture and the mainstream culture (e.g., Machamer & Gruber, 1998; Tharp, 1989; Trueba, 1987; Tyler et al., 2008; Weisner, Gallimore, & Jordan, 1988) and the extent to which the discontinuity between those beliefs and practices interferes with students' engagement and learning in school. Researchers holding a contextual view of cognition (e.g., Laboratory of Comparative Human Cognition, 1982; Rogoff, 1990) have argued that: (a) cultural context affects the development of social and cognitive processes, (b) there are important differences between ethnic minority cultures and the mainstream culture, and (c) these cultural differences lead to the development of different sets of cognitive and social behavioral repertoires. When children from ethnic minority cultures begin school, for example, they may find it difficult to decode the cues that are presented in the classroom and actively engage in the teaching and learning process. They may experience failure. They may perceive their own cultural practices to be devalued in the school context. Ultimately, the enactment of this process is hypothesized to lead to a lack of engagement in school.

An alternative perspective, the *cultural ecological* or secondary discontinuity model, emphasizes processes of oppression and discrimination toward racial and ethnic minority groups. Ogbu (e.g., Gibson & Ogbu, 1991; Ogbu, 1986) argued that certain minority groups—those who became part of the United States through conquest or slavery—are treated at the institutional and policy levels within our society in ways that limit their ability to succeed economically, professionally, socially, and politically. In such cases, poor school achievement may be a conscious choice, an active response to a system that has failed to work for a particular group of people. For example, Fordham and Ogbu (1986) described African American adolescents as developing identities that were in opposition to the values of the mainstream culture, including intentionally not engaging in school. Ogbu (1992) posited that those who face barriers to their success because of discriminatory practices and policies will find alternative venues in which to achieve and will disengage themselves from trying to achieve in those domains in which discrimination keeps them from succeeding. Psychologists (e.g., Osborne, 1997; Steele, 1997) have suggested that members of groups that have been stigmatized as having low ability in a particular domain will psychologically distance themselves from or "disidentify" with that domain. Disidentification with a domain is hypothesized to protect the individual's self-esteem should the individual do poorly in that domain. Along the same lines, some have proposed that perception of discrimination may lead students to believe that achieving school will not make a difference in their lives, and this belief may result in a lack of engagement in school (e.g., Mickelson, 1990).

Finally, there are models that build on elements of both the cultural discontinuity framework and the cultural ecological model. For example, Deyhle argued that the discontinuity between the Navajo culture and the mainstream culture coupled with discrimination against the Navajo community led Navajo youth to resist assimilation into the behaviors of the mainstream culture. Behaviors that appeared to be lack of engagement in school were not the development of an oppositional identity as theorized by Ogbu but rather the expression of their Navajo culture. Based on work with Navajo youth, Deyhle (1995) has posited that behaviors that are typically interpreted by teachers and school administrators as a student's lack of engagement in school (e.g., dropping out of college to return to the reservation) should be viewed from the perspective of the Navajo culture (e.g., returning to the reservation and one's Navajo community is a positive action). In such cases, the behaviors may be motivated primarily by a desire to express the Navajo culture rather than a reflection of the individual's disinterest in school.

Without a doubt, our education system has historically been differentially successful in educating students across racial and ethnic groups (Farkas, 2003; KewalRamani, Gilbertson, Fox, & Provasnik, 2007; Miller, 1995). Among the theories that have been generated to explain differential achievement across racial and ethnic groups are hypotheses that hinge on variation in student engagement in school. A number of factors have been posited to influence minority students' engagement with school and achievement. Okagaki (2001) conceptualized these factors into three broad domains: the roles of the individual, the family, and the school. These factors are discussed in the following three sections, beginning with a discussion of racial and ethnic minority students' beliefs about their ethnicity. In the next section, we consider how families of color support their child's engagement in school. The last section examines ways in which the nature and structure of the school may support or inhibit the engagement of students of color.

The Role of the Student: Beliefs About Ethnicity and Student Engagement in School

In what ways are students' beliefs about their ethnicity related to their beliefs about, attitudes toward, and behavior in school? In this section, we consider the ways in which ethnic identity, perception of discrimination, and bicultural identity have been linked to students' engagement in school. Ethnic identity is generally viewed as being multidimensional, varying across members of an ethnic group, and changing over time within an individual, and the literature on ethnic identity reflects multiple ways in which ethnic identity has been conceptualized and measured by researchers (Phinney, 1990). Broadly defined, beliefs, feelings, and behaviors contributing to one's ethnic identity include a cognitive component (e.g., knowledge about one's ethnic culture), an emotional component (e.g., attitudes toward one's ethnic culture, feelings of commitment and belonging to one's ethnic group, and attitudes toward the majority culture), and a behavioral component (e.g., participation in traditional cultural activities, interaction with the majority culture). Great diversity exists within any ethnic group in terms of members' ethnic identity (e.g., Chavous et al., 2003; Keefe & Padilla, 1987; Okagaki & Moore, 2000; Witherspoon, Speight, & Thomas, 1997). Diversity comes in part because an individual's ethnic identity develops over time (e.g., Phinney, 1996), because individuals within a group differ in their orientation to their ethnic culture and to the mainstream culture (e.g., Buriel & DeMent, 1997), because within a group, what is important to each group member's ethnic identity varies (Phinney), and because ethnic communities are living entities whose experiences, shared beliefs, and practices evolve over time (Gutiérrez & Rogoff, 2003).

Ogbu (1992; Ogbu & Matute-Bianchi, 1986) argued that to the extent that formal schooling is associated with mainstream culture in the United States and not with a minority culture, doing well in school may be perceived by students from that minority culture as not being compatible with their cultural identity. Further, in response to discrimination, minority students develop an identity that is in opposition to the mainstream culture. In their classic ethnographic study of Black adolescents, Fordham and Ogbu (1986) introduced the concept of "the burden of acting White." They asserted that Black students who do well in school must do so at the cost of maintaining their own racial identity. In their study, Black adolescents said that Black students who were actively engaged in school (e.g., studying, working hard on school work) were in effect trying to act White. High-achieving Black students in their study employed strategies to conceal their engagement in school work. Although the notion of "acting White" has become a popular explanation for the underachievement of minority students (Starkey & Eaton, 2008), subsequent empirical support for the hypothesis has not been strong (e.g., Flores-González, 1999; Spencer, Noll, Stoltzfus, & Harpalani, 2001; Taylor, Casten, Flickinger, Roberts, & Fulmore, 1994).

Based on studies in which ethnic identity and engagement have been measured, it appears that ethnic minority students who have strong ethnic identities are more likely to be engaged in school than those who do not. For example, in a study of 606 African American adolescents, Chavous and colleagues (2003) examined three components of racial identity: (a) centrality, the degree to which a Black identity was important to their personal identity and having relationships with other Black people was important to them; (b) private regard, the positive or negative valence of their feelings about being Black and Black people; and (c) public regard, their perception of other people's views of Black people. Based on this multidimensional approach to racial identity, four clusters of students were identified, and differences across groups on measures of student engagement and academic attainment were observed, with the most distinct differences being for those who exhibited alienation from their Black identity (i.e., low centrality, low private regard, low public regard) and those who had strong positive Black identities (i.e., high centrality, high private regard, low public regard). Relative to other students, those students who exhibited alienation from their Black identity had lower school attachment (degree to which students liked school) and school efficacy (belief in one's ability to do well in school) scores. Moreover, compared to students in the other groups, these adolescents were less likely than other students to be in school at the time of the interviews and less likely to be enrolled in college 2 years after their expected on-time high school graduation (i.e., 6 years after they entered ninth grade). In contrast, compared to other groups, students with a strong, positive racial identity were more likely to be in school at the time of the interview and more likely to be enrolled in college 2 years after their expected on-time high school graduation. Thus, in this study, having a weak racial identity was associated with poor student engagement; a strong racial identity was linked to stronger student engagement.

In a study of 390 African American middle and high school students, Smalls and colleagues (Smalls, White, Chavous, & Sellers, 2007) assessed racial centrality (i.e., the degree to which being Black is important to how the student views himself or herself), perception of discrimination, academic persistence (i.e., the degree to which the student reports persevering when faced with an academic challenge), academic curiosity (i.e., interest in new academic topics), negative school behavior (e.g., cutting classes, cheating on tests), and efforts to conceal engagement in school from their peers. In addition, they measured the degree to which students agreed with four types of racial ideology: assimilation (i.e., the belief that African Americans should be more like European Americans to be successful), humanist (i.e., the belief that people should emphasize how groups are similar rather than different), minority (i.e., the view that African Americans share common experiences with other oppressed minority groups), and nationalist (i.e., the belief that African Americans should embrace their unique African American culture and identity). In a series of hierarchical regressions controlling for gender, grade level, prior school performance, parent education, and racial centrality, they examined whether assimilation, humanism, minority, nationalism, and racial discrimination predicted measures of student engagement in school and efforts to conceal engagement from peers. Assimilation was negatively correlated with academic persistence and academic curiosity (marginally significant), and positively correlated with negative school behaviors and efforts to conceal engagement in school from peers. These findings do not support the notion that African American students who are engaged in school must give up their racial identity. Instead, these results suggest that African American students who are less engaged in school are more likely to believe that they need to be more like their White counterparts in order to succeed in school. However, they also report a negative association between nationalism and academic persistence, but nationalism was not predictive of the other measures. The belief that African Americans share a common experience with other oppressed minority groups was positively associated with academic persistence and negatively associated with efforts to conceal engagement in school from peers. (Findings pertaining to discrimination are discussed below).

In general, the basic thesis that ethnic minority students must give up their ethnic identity to be engaged in school is not supported by current research. In addition to the work by Chavous and colleagues (2003; Smalls et al., 2007), other researchers have also found positive relations between ethnic identity and student engagement with school and achievement for African American youth (e.g., Bennett, 2006; Dotterer, McHale, & Crouter, 2009; Spencer et al., 2001; Taylor et al., 1994). In her work with Navajo adolescents, Deyhle (1995) observed that the Navajo students who were well grounded in their Navajo culture and identity were better able to be engaged in school than were those who did not have a strong ethnic identity.

Similarly, the belief that minority students who do well in school must hide their efforts to be engaged in school from their peers is not well supported (Smalls et al., 2007). Researchers have found that publicly distancing oneself from the appearance of working hard in school is a strategy employed by both Black and White adolescents and that positive attitudes toward doing school work and the importance of doing well in school for one's future were associated with feelings of alienation from peers for both groups (Arroyo & Zigler, 1995). However, there is some evidence that racial and ethnic minority youth from traditionally underachieving groups may not consider academic engagement and achievement to be part of their identity (Oyserman, Kemmelmeier, Fryberg, Brosh, & Hart-Johnson, 2003).

Do students of color identify characteristics of academic engagement with members of their ethnic group? In a study on stereotypes (Hudley & Graham, 2001), African American, Latino, and Anglo middle school students were shown pictures of African American, Latino, and Anglo boys and girls and were given short descriptions of academically engaged students (e.g., someone who works hard on school work, studies, pays attention, and participates in class discussions) and unengaged students (e.g., someone who fools around in class, does not do homework, cuts classes). Based on their "first impressions," students were asked to pick the picture of the student who best fits the description. Across racial and ethnic groups, girls and boys were more likely to identify girls as being academically engaged and boys as being unengaged in school. African American girls were more likely to identify African American and Anglo girls as being academically engaged. African American boys were more likely to select pictures of African American girls as being the best fit for an engaged student. Latino and Anglo girls and boys were more likely to identify pictures of Anglo girls as being academically engaged. All students were more likely to select an African American or Latino boy as fitting the descriptor for a student who is uninterested in school. For our purposes, these data suggest that although African American boys and girls hold an image of African American girls that encompasses being engaged in school, African American boys and Latino boys and girls did not identify someone like themselves as being highly engaged in school. Moreover, all boys and girls were more likely select pictures of African American or Latino boys as fitting the description of someone who is unengaged in school.

Graham (1994; Graham, Taylor, & Hudley, 1998) proposed that underachieving ethnic minority students are not engaged in school because they have aspirations other than to do well in school—that lack of motivation to achieve in school stems from having different goals and values. To examine students' values, Graham and colleagues (1998) asked Black, Hispanic, and White middle school students to identify classmates whom they admired, respected, and wanted to be like. In general, girls were more likely to identify girls of the same race and girls who were high or average achieving over those who were low achieving. The pattern of nominations for White boys paralleled those of the girls—a preference for average- and high-achieving boys of the same race. In contrast, Black and Hispanic boys admired low-achieving boys of their own race. Strambler and Weinstein (2010) extended these results by finding that the degree to which African American and Latino elementary school students identified with nonacademic domains (i.e., being cool, tough, popular, oppositional, liked by girls, liked by boys, or fashionable) was negatively associated with teachers' ratings of students' behavioral engagement (e.g., follows directions, completes homework). Taken together, these studies suggest that Black and Hispanic boys may not view engaging in school as an appropriate component of their identity.

Behavioral scientists have posited that the degree to which students of color perceive or experience discrimination may affect their engagement and achievement in school. On the one hand, if students perceive discrimination against themselves or members of their ethnic group, they may not believe that teachers treat them fairly and may not see any reason to try hard in school or even be in school (e.g., Huffman, 1991; Ogbu, 1992; Wong, Eccles, & Sameroff, 2003). Alternatively, if students perceive discrimination against their ethnic group, they may believe that a good education is the means for overcoming discriminatory barriers that they may encounter in the future (e.g., Sue & Okazaki, 1990). Current research indicates that the relation between discrimination and students' engagement in school is not consistent across or within racial and ethnic groups. Some studies have found a negative correlation between students' perception of discrimination and measures of engagement, particularly students' belief in the importance or value of education (e.g., Dotterer et al., 2009; Okagaki, Frensch, & Dodson, 1996; Smalls et al., 2007; Wong et al., 2003). Others have obtained mixed results (e.g., Taylor et al., 1994) or positive relations between discrimination and aspects of engagement (e.g., Okagaki, Helling, & Bingham, 2009; Sanders, 1997).

Consistent with the hypothesis that racism leads to disengagement from school by ethnic minority students, data from a study of fourth- and fifth-grade Mexican American students indicated that students' perception of general discrimination against members of their ethnic group was negatively correlated with their engagement in school (items included aspects of behavioral and emotional engagement), negatively correlated with intrinsic motivation for learning, and negatively correlated with their belief that school is an appropriate domain in which Mexican American children can and should excel (Okagaki et al., 1996). Among these elementary school students, however, perception of discrimination was not correlated with students' academic performance. Similarly, in their study of African American middle and high school students, Smalls and colleagues (2007) found that students' perceptions of general discrimination within the last year were negatively associated with academic persistence and academic curiosity and positively correlated with negative school behaviors.

In a study of 164 public school and 180 Catholic school African American adolescents from working class families, Taylor and colleagues (1994) assessed students' perceptions of discrimination in employment practices, belief in the importance of education, behavioral engagement in school (e.g., cutting class, spending time on homework, paying attention in class), ethnic identity, self-concept of academic ability, and school performance. Path analyses with the public school data revealed that perception of discrimination was negatively associated with belief in the importance of education, which in turn was positively related to behavioral engagement in school. For Catholic school African American students, path analyses indicated that perception of discrimination was also negatively related to importance of education, but the relation between importance of education and behavioral engagement was not significant. The difference in findings between the public school and Catholic school students highlights within-group differences in the relation between discrimination and importance of education in a study in which the measures and procedures were the same for both groups. The authors speculated that local contextual factors (e.g., differences between Catholic and public schools, parental involvement in education) may moderate the links between perception of discrimination, importance of education, and behavioral engagement for African American students.

Although not directly assessing engagement, Oyserman, Harrison, and Bybee (2001) examined the relation between academic efficacy (e.g., belief that one can do well on school tasks) measured at the end of the school year and three aspects of racial identity measured in the fall (start) of that school year: (a) awareness of racism, (b) feelings of connectedness with one's racial group, and (c) the degree to which students believed that academic achievement was congruent with their racial identity. Among African American middle school boys, perceptions of racism in the fall did not predict school efficacy. However, awareness of racism then was negatively associated with academic efficacy for African American girls. In particular, academic efficacy was negatively associated with awareness of racism among girls who felt more closely connected to the African American community and whose racial identity did not have a strong academic achievement component. Believing that academic achievement is a characteristic of one's racial group may help protect the academic efficacy of African American girls in the context of discrimination.

There is considerable variability across individuals in response to discrimination. For example, Deyhle (1995) conducted an extensive ethnographic study of Navajo youth in a border reservation community, including adolescents who were in high school and those who did not complete high school. Among the 168 Navajo students who did not complete high school, more than half of these youth cited problems of discrimination as contributing to their decision to leave school. However, she asserted that among those students who were most engaged in learning, were persisting in school, and were academically successful were ones who were realistic in recognizing and acknowledging discrimination in their school and community. In a study of 67 American Indian college students, Okagaki et al. (2009) examined the relation between perception of discrimination and students' belief in the pragmatic benefits of education (e.g., a college education is necessary for obtaining a good job). A positive relation between perception of discrimination and students' belief in the value of education was obtained. Scores on the perception of discrimination scale ranged from 1.3 to 5.5 on a 6-point scale, indicating substantial variability among students in their perception of discrimination against American Indians. To explore the finding, the authors split the sample at the median on the discrimination scale. Among those who perceived less discrimination, there was essentially no correlation between discrimination and students' belief in the instrumental importance of education. For students who perceived greater discrimination, the correlation was positive. However, in a similar study with American Indian adolescents, Bingham, Helling, and Okagaki (2001) found no relation between students' perception of discrimination and their motivation in school, expectations for achievement in school, or time spent on homework.

In general, the research to date suggests that there is not a simple and consistent relation between perception of discrimination and student engagement. To explain Asian American students' achievement, Sue and Okazaki (1990) posited that when other avenues to upward mobility are blocked (e.g., business, politics, sports) because of discrimination, then education becomes more important as the means to upward mobility. Several behavioral scientists have suggested that the degree to which racial and ethnic minority students believe that doing well in school will have pragmatic benefits for their lives contributes to students' engagement and achievement in school (e.g., Matute-Bianchi, 1986; Mickelson, 1990; Suarez-Orozco, 1993; Sue & Okazaki, 1990). For example, in a study of Black and White high school seniors, Mickelson found that the belief in the instrumental importance of education, rather than a general belief in the value of education, was related to school achievement. In a study of about 15,000 adolescents, Steinberg, Dornbusch, and Brown (1992) reported that adolescents across ethnic groups believed that getting a good education would be beneficial to them (e.g., help them get a good job). Where the ethnic groups differed is in their response to the consequences of not getting a good education. Compared to other students, Asian American adolescents were more likely to believe that they would not be able to get a good job if they did not do well in school. In contrast, Hispanic and African American youth were more likely to maintain that they would be able to obtain a good job even if they did not get a good education in high school. Steinberg and colleagues described the motivation of the Asian American students as fear of the negative consequences of a poor education.

In addition to belief in the instrumental importance of school, some researchers have posited that minority students must believe that they can be true to their ethnic identity and still participate effectively in the mainstream culture if they are to function well in the mainstream culture and not be alienated from their ethnic community (e.g., Buriel & DeMent, 1997; LaFromboise, Coleman & Gerton, 1993; Miller, 1999; Ogbu, 1992; Okagaki, 2001). For student engagement and achievement, this means that ethnic minority students need to develop a positive academic identity while holding onto positive ethnic identity. In a study of American Indian college students, a measure of academic identity (e.g., "Doing well in school and graduating from college are important to my view of myself") was positively correlated with a measure of bicultural efficacy (e.g., "I believe I can maintain my tribal identity and still participate in activities that are traditionally part of the White culture"; Okagaki et al., 2009). That is, the more strongly students believed that they could be a good member of their tribal community and at the same time, do well in school, the more positive their academic identity was. Among Hispanic high school students, bicultural efficacy has been positively correlated with students' self-reported grades (Okagaki, Izarraraz, & Bojczyk, 2003).

The idea of bicultural efficacy or a bicultural identity is related to research on racial-ethnic self-schemas (Oyserman et al., 2003). Racial-ethnic self-schemas refer to an individual's self-concept that forms through the integration of emotions, attitudes, and beliefs into a coherent cognitive structure about one's membership of an ethnic group (Oyserman et al.). It is hypothesized that individuals who develop racial-ethnic schemas that incorporate both in-group (i.e., identification with one's racial group) and larger society racial-ethnic schemas (i.e., positive identification with the majority culture) will do better in school than individuals who do not. Although not directly measuring student engagement with school, in a series of studies, Oyserman and colleagues obtained support for this hypothesis with respect to school achievement. For example, they found that, after controlling for fall grades, ethnically diverse middle school students with both in-group and larger society racial-ethnic schemas received significantly higher last-quarter grades than students without racial-ethnic schemas or in-group-only racial-ethnic schemas students (Oyserman et al.). In a separate study, students with both in-group and larger society racial-ethnic schemas evidenced more persistence on a math task compared to youth without racial-ethnic schemas (Oyserman, Bybee, Terry, & Hart-Johnson, 2004). These data suggest that students' beliefs about themselves and their ability to function within their own ethnic culture and within the larger society may play a role in their engagement in school.

In a study of 98 American Indian adolescents, the degrees to which students' ethnic identity, bicultural efficacy, belief in the instrumental importance of school, and students' general perceptions of discrimination predicted emotional engagement (as measured by interest in school and educational expectations), behavioral engagement (as measured by time spent studying), and school achievement were examined (Bingham et al., 2001). Ethnic identity was measured by the Multigroup Ethnic Identity Measure (Phinney, 1992; Roberts et al., 1999) and captured the individual's sense of belonging to their ethnic group and their active engagement in learning about their ethnic group. Multivariate analyses of covariance indicated that ethnic identity and belief in the instrumental importance of school predicted students' orientation to school. In particular, stronger identification with and participation in their American Indian community was associated with greater interest in school for American Indian adolescents. Instrumental importance of school was consistently and positively correlated with all aspects of engagement—interest in school, educational expectations, and time spent studying. Although bicultural efficacy did not predict student engagement, bicultural identity, which was measured in the fall of the school year, was positively related to students' grades at the end of the academic year, even after controlling for prior grades. Perception of discrimination was not related to engagement or achievement. In this study, the students had spent most of their lives on a reservation, and most were attending tribal schools or public schools near the reservation at the time of the study. It is possible that discrimination did not play a strong role in these adolescents' daily lives.

Summary According to social identity theorists and researchers, individuals have multiple ways of defining themselves that depend on the social groups to which they belong by birth (e.g., ethnicity, gender), achievement (e.g., prize-winning author or dancer), or choice (e.g., church member, community activist) (e.g., Bernal, Saenz, & Knight, 1991; Harwood et al., 2001; Tajfel, 1981). To the extent that individuals have multiple social identities, having a strong ethnic identity need not be incompatible with a strong academic identity. In general, the research seems to indicate that racial and ethnic minority students can maintain a strong racial and ethnic identity and be engaged in school. Generally, perception of discrimination is negatively associated with engagement. However, when students believe that achieving in school is appropriate for members of their racial or ethnic group or they develop a bicultural identity, it appears that this belief may act as a buffer to the negative effects of discrimination on student engagement.

The Role of Parents: Expectations, Support, and Cultural Socialization

Much of the research on parenting and student engagement and achievement in racial and ethnic minority families has mirrored research among mainstream families. Researchers have found, for instance, that parental involvement is positively related to student engagement among African American youth (e.g., Connell et al., 1994).

In this section, we discuss parental expectations, support, and cultural socialization as they pertain to racial and ethnic minority students' engagement in school.

A meta-analysis of parenting and school achievement indicate that among the various components of parenting (e.g., communication, supervision, school contact and participation, general involvement with child) parents' aspirations and expectations for their children have the strongest relation to children's achievement (Fan & Chen, 2001). In general, parents' expectations for academic achievement differ across racial and ethnic groups (e.g., Alexander, Entwisle, & Bedinger, 1994; Hao & Bonstead-Bruns, 1998; Okagaki & Frensch, 1998), and their expectations are correlated with children's school performance among economically disadvantaged Black families (e.g., Gill & Reynolds, 1999; Halle, Kurtz-Costes, & Mahoney, 1997; Luster & McAdoo, 1996), Asian American families (Hao & Bonstead-Bruns, 1998; Okagaki & Frensch, 1998), and Hispanic families (e.g., Goldenberg, Gallimore, Reese, & Garnier, 2001; Hao & Bonstead-Bruns, 1998). Although most of this literature has focused on the relation between expectations and achievement, rather than on student engagement, researchers have found that parental expectations are associated with student engagement among racial and ethnic minority students (e.g., Murray, 2009; Taylor & Lopez, 2005).

In a study of 104 low-income students in which 91% of the students were Latino, 4% African American, and 5% White, Murray (2009) examined the relations between students' engagement and support from parents and teachers. Because the analyses are not broken apart by ethnic and racial group, we discuss the results as reflecting generally Latino and African American families. Along with aspects of the teacher-student relationship, four aspects of parenting were identified: (a) closeness of the parent–child relationship, (b) parental involvement in the child's life, (c) unclear parental academic expectations, and (d) poor accessibility of parents. Students reported on their behavioral engagement in school (e.g., "Trying hard is the best way for me to do well in school"; "I can work really hard in school") and their competence in school. Utilizing hierarchical regression analyses, Murray examined parent and teacher contributions to explaining the variance in students' engagement after controlling for students' reading and math achievement. Parental variables accounted for about 24% of the variance in engagement; teacher variables explained an additional 25% of the variance. Of the parental variables, unclear parental expectations predicted student engagement such that higher scores on unclear parental expectations were associated with lower student engagement. Parenting also accounted for about 18% of the variance in self-reported school competence. Higher scores on positive involvement with the child were associated with higher school competence scores; higher scores on unclear parental expectations were associated with lower school competence scores.

In a study of 95 low-income African American adolescents and their mothers, Taylor and Lopez (2005) examined whether the degree to which African American families maintained predictable routines and mother's expectations for their child's achievement was related to student engagement with school as measured by the degree to which adolescents reported paying attention in classes, attending classes, experiencing a sense of challenge in their classes, and exhibiting negative behaviors in school (e.g., getting into a fight, damaging school property). Family routine was positively correlated with paying attention, attending classes, and experiencing a sense of challenge in classes. Further analyses indicated that student engagement in the form of paying attention in class and attending class mediated the relation between family routine and students' achievement. Parental expectations were positively related to attendance, and student attendance mediated the relation between parental expectations and student achievement. Finally, family routine was negatively associated with problem behavior in school, and this relation was mediated by student engagement in the form of paying attention and attending class.

In addition to parental expectations and family routine, parental support and the quality of the parent–child relationship have been associated with student engagement in middle-class African American adolescents (Sirin & Rogers-Sirin, 2005) and at-risk, inner-city African American adolescents (Annunziata, Hogue, Faw, & Liddle, 2006). For example, in a study of about 200 inner-city, African American families, Annunziata and colleagues (2006) examined whether family cohesion and parental support were associated with middle school students' emotional engagement in school. The measure of family cohesion assessed the degree to which the members of their family were close to one another, communicated with and supported one another, and perceived their family to be organized. Both parents and students responded to the items, and the average of their scores represented the family's cohesion score. Similarly, both parents' and students' responses to items regarding parental support for the child (e.g., praising, doing special activities, talking with child) combined to form the parental support score. Hierarchical regression analyses revealed that both family cohesion and parental support were positively related to emotional engagement in school. However, there was a significant interaction between family cohesion and parental support such that when parental support was high, family cohesion was positively correlated with student engagement. Under conditions of low parental support, family cohesion was not associated with student engagement. Subsequent analyses determined that student gender moderated the relations among family cohesion, parental support, and student engagement. For boys, high parental support increased the relation between family cohesion and student engagement; for girls, the interaction was not significant.

Family support and cohesion has also been found to be important for American Indian adolescents (Machamer & Gruber, 1998). In a large study of over 6,000 high school students, including 8% American Indian, 7% Black, and 85% non-Hispanic White adolescents, family connectedness (e.g., family cares about you, parents understand you), student engagement (e.g., school people care about you, like school), and negative school behaviors (e.g., skipping classes, drinking before or during school) were examined. Across groups, adolescents who perceived themselves to be poorly connected to their families were less emotionally engaged in school and more likely to be involved in problem behaviors at school. Compared to their Black and White counterparts, American Indian adolescents had lower scores on family connectedness and student engagement and higher scores on problem behaviors. Machamer and Gruber argued that the discontinuity between the cultural norms of the American Indian people and the school culture (e.g., prohibition against competition among many American Indian communities, avoiding direct eye contact with authority figures) as well as societal changes (e.g., American Indian families moving away from tribal communities) make American Indian adolescents particularly vulnerable to disengagement in school.

Research on racial and ethnic minority parenting brings to light the importance of examining cultural models of education (Gallimore & Goldenberg, 2001; Lareau, 1996). Cultural models are widely shared "understandings of how the world works, or ought to work" (Gallimore & Goldenberg, 2001, p. 47), and there are differences and commonalities across ethnic groups in their conceptions of education, school, and learning. Cultural models of education may include the ideas that parents have about the roles of parents, teachers, and children in education (Lareau). In many Asian cultures, the importance of education is linked to a strong belief in human malleability and the efficacy of working hard and in the importance of bringing honor to one's family (e.g., Ho, 1994). In a study of immigrant parents from Cambodia, Mexico, the Philippines, and Vietnam and US-born parents of Mexican descent and European Americans, Okagaki and Sternberg (1993) found that motivation was an important component of the Asian parents' understanding of intelligence. A child who is intelligent is one who tries hard to get good grades. Belief in the efficacy of hard work and effort is a consistent theme in studies of Asian American students.

In an ethnographic study of immigrant Punjabi Indian and non-Punjabi adolescents in California, Gibson (Gibson, 1987) noted that both the Punjabi students and their parents believed that effort was the determining factor in educational achievement. Based on interviews with Japanese American high school students who were primarily third-generation Japanese Americans, Matute-Bianchi (1986) reported that "[b]elief in diligence, persistence, and hard work—as opposed to inherent ability—as the keys to academic success is the single most commonly shared perception among the Japanese-descent students" (p. 247). In their study of Southeast Asian immigrants, Caplan and his colleagues suggested that three common values—an emphasis on education and achievement, belief in the importance of maintaining a cohesive family, and belief in the efficacy and importance of hard work—served as the foundation for Southeast Asian children's academic achievement (Caplan, Whitmore, & Choy, 1989). Almost all of the Southeast Asian parents (97%) and children (93%) attributed academic success to hard work; in contrast 86% of the parents and 67% of the children identified intellectual ability as causally related to academic achievement. In a comparison of several Asian American subgroups (Chinese, Filipino, Japanese, Korean, Vietnamese, and other Southeast Asian), Mizokawa and Ryckman (1990) found that overall, Asian American students (including elementary, junior high, and high school students) were more likely to attribute academic success and failure to effort than to ability. Chen and Stevenson (1995) observed that relative to Caucasian American students, Asian American high school students were more likely to indicate that doing well in math was the result of studying hard. In addition, Asian American students reported spending more hours studying mathematics outside of class (5.3 h per week) compared to their Caucasian American counterparts (3.2 h per week). Analyses of national data sets have revealed that Asian American students report spending more time working on school work and are more likely to engage in extracurricular classes than other students (Peng & Wright, 1994; Tsang, 1988; Wong, 1990). What role do Asian American parents play in their child's approach to education?

For the most part, it does not appear that Asian American parents spend more time directly helping their children with homework or explicitly talking about school with their children relative to other parents (e.g., Wong, 1990). Several researchers have observed that Asian American parents employ indirect strategies to encourage their children's school achievement, such as structuring the home environment to facilitate the child's learning, rather than directly helping the child with school work (e.g., Caplan et al., 1989; Chao, 2000; Schneider & Lee, 1990). For example, parents may set aside a specific time for the child to do homework and restrict the amount of time the child spends watching television (e.g., Schneider & Lee, 1990). Parents may not want or allow their adolescent to work after school because they believe that the adolescent's "job" is to study for school (e.g., Gibson, 1987). Based on an ethnographic study of third-generation and fourth-generation Japanese Americans, Hieshima and Schneider (1994) noted that even native-born parents' encouragement of schoolwork was indirect. The third-generation Japanese American parents did not directly tell their child what to do; instead, they made indirect comments such as "You sure finished with your homework fast" or "Not much homework tonight?" (p. 322). Schneider and Lee (1990) found that Asian American parents were more likely than European American parents to encourage their child to take private classes in music, language, and computer science and that their children spent more time practicing for their lessons than did European American children. Compared to their European American counterparts, Chinese immigrant parents of primary grade students reported engaging in more "structural parental involvement in school" (Chao, 2000, p. 240; e.g., setting rules for how the child spent time after school and buying extra workbooks or materials to give the child more practice on school tasks) than European American parents. Conversely, European American parents had higher scores on what was called "*managerial* parental involvement in school" (Chao, 2000, p. 240)—activities such as checking homework and attending school functions. It appears that in Asian American homes, an important aspect of socialization for academic achievement is the creation of an overall environment in which discipline, studying, and practice are integral elements of the child's role in multiple contexts. Although for the most part, these studies did not directly assess students' engagement in school, these studies describe a cultural model of education—one that emphasizes (a) that doing well in school is the child's job, (b) that practice and effort are the key to doing well in school, and (c) that the parent's job is to create an environment at home which allows students to spend time studying and to provide students with activities that support education (e.g., giving students books to read or extra math assignments, encouraging music and dance activities that create an expectation for practice and hard work)—that lends itself to supporting engagement in school.

Finally, although much of the research on racial and ethnic minority parenting and student engagement is similar to the broader literature on parenting, researchers have also explored aspects that may be somewhat idiosyncratic to racial and minority parents—cultural socialization and preparation for discrimination. Although this is a relatively new area of research, behavioral scientists are interested in learning if and how cultural socialization may foster children's development (Hughes et al., 2006). As noted earlier, perception of discrimination has generally been found to be negatively associated with student engagement with school, and it appears that for the most part, racial and ethnic identity is positively associated with student engagement. Is it possible that through cultural socialization, parents may protect their children from the negative consequences of discrimination either directly or by fostering children's racial and ethnic identity?

Bennett (2006) surveyed African American adolescents from grades 8 through 12. Of 131 participants, about 40% lived with both parents, 48% lived with one parent, and the others reported living with grandparents or in some other living arrangement. Among the many measures that were collected, students reported on their ethnic identity, racial socialization, and engagement with school. For this study, the student engagement with school measure was a mix of behavioral engagement items (e.g., participating in student government, in an honors club) and school achievement (e.g., being on the honors roll, grade-point average). The measure of racial socialization included items about Black parents teaching their children about racism, families teaching children to be proud to be Black, and schools teaching children about Black history and including signs of Black culture in the classroom. Among other results, Bennett found that racial socialization was positively correlated with ethnic identity which in turn was positively correlated with student engagement with school.

In an elegant study examining the relations among parenting, discrimination, ethnic identity, and engagement, Dotterer et al. (2009) interviewed 148 working and middle-class African American adolescents from two-parent families, along with their mothers and fathers, to explore the relations among experience with discrimination, cultural socialization, preparation for discrimination, ethnic identity, and emotional engagement with school, and school self-esteem. Perception of discrimination was negatively related to emotional engagement and school self-esteem. A series of hierarchical regression analyses were conducted to determine whether cultural socialization, preparation for discrimination, or ethnic identity moderated the relations between discrimination and student engagement and between discrimination and self-esteem. With respect to self-esteem, neither cultural socialization, nor preparation for discrimination, nor ethnic identity moderated the negative relation between discrimination and self-esteem. For student engagement with school, the results were more complicated. Cultural socialization was positively correlated with emotional engagement for boys, but not girls. However, cultural socialization did not moderate the negative relation between discrimination and emotional engagement. Preparation for discrimination was positively associated with emotional engagement in school, but it did not moderate the negative relation between discrimination and emotional engagement. Finally, the analyses with ethnic identity revealed a three-way interaction between ethnic identity, discrimination, and gender, such that ethnic identity moderated the negative relation between discrimination and emotional engagement for girls, but not for boys. Girls who have strong ethnic identities maintain their emotional engagement with school in the context of greater perceived discrimination. However, girls with low ethnic identities have lower emotional engagement in school when discrimination is higher.

Summary There is great diversity in parents' ideas about education, how children learn, what children need to do to succeed in school, and what parents should do to support their child's education (for reviews, see Bornstein, 2002; Okagaki & Bingham, 2010). Many of these beliefs and values ideas appear to be a function of parents' cultural models of education (Gallimore & Goderberg, 2001; Lareau, 1996). Although more research is needed to connect parents' cultural models of education to how they support their child's learning at home, research suggests that ethnic minority parents who are emotionally supportive of their children, have strong and clear academic expectations for their child and establish regular routines, particularly learning or school-related routines in their homes, have children who are more engaged in school. (Annunziata et al., 2006; Murray, 2009; Sirin & Rogers-Sirin, 2005; Taylor & Lopez, 2005).

The Role of Schools: Friends, Teachers, and Instruction

Schools play a major role in children's lives and serve as an important context for their social, emotional, and cognitive development. In this section, we have focused on key aspects of the school context that may be particularly important to the engagement of racial and ethnic minority students. We begin by discussing the research on friendship and peer relationships.

Racial and Ethnic Minority Students' Peer Relationships and Their Engagement in School

As children get older, they spend increasing amounts of time with their friends both in and out of school. As a result, children's friendships and peer relationships begin to play a more central role to their experiences in school (see Chap. 18, this volume), particularly in the areas of school adjustment (Berndt, 1999; Perdue, Manzeske, & Estell, 2009; Ryan, 2000), ethnic identification (Oyserman, Brickman, Bybee, & Celious, 2006; Shin, Daly, & Vera, 2007), and educational aspirations (Antonio, 2004). Because peers and friends encourage some beliefs, values, behaviors, and activities, while rejecting others, they can either play a positive role in an individual's engagement in school by helping a child develop a sense of belonging and affiliation with school (Faircloth & Hamm, 2005; Finn & Voelkl, 1993) or a negative role by contributing to feelings of isolation and disengagement (Oyserman et al., 2003; Rivas-Drake, Hughes, & Way, 2008; Way, Santos, Niwa, & Kim-Gervey, 2008). For racial and ethnic minority youth, friends may serve as a resource for navigating differences between home and school cultures as well as a source of social support that reinforce one's ethnic identification and connection with one's racial or ethnic community (see Way, Becker, & Greene, 2006). In this section, we consider student engagement with school from the perspective of minority students' access to peers of the same race or ethnic groups.

Racial and ethnic group membership is a salient feature in minority children's lives and has been shown to be one characteristic by which children choose and define who their friends are and how they feel about themselves (Bellmore, Nishina, Witkow, Graham, & Juvonen, 2007; Oyserman et al., 2003). For example, in a study of low-income African American, Latino, and Asian American adolescents (Way & Chen, 2000), 73% of ethnic minority students reported having predominately same-race/ethnic group friendship networks, with Asian American students reporting the highest percentage (85%). Similarly, in a study of sixth-grade students (Bellmore et al., 2007), African American, Asian American, Latino, and White middle school students all showed race/ethnic group selection bias in choosing their friends (i.e., they attributed more favorable ratings of acceptance to same-race/ethnic peers). It appeared that the availability of same-race/ethnic group peers influenced students' ratings; students having access to a larger numbers of same-race/ethnic group peers showed a greater selection bias compared to those with less access. Unlike Asian American, Latino, and White students, however, African American students were significantly more likely to nominate a same-race peer as someone who they both did and did not like to spend time with. Although these studies suggest that students generally tend to prefer friends who look like them and come from similar racial-ethnic backgrounds, other research demonstrates that adolescents consider other factors, such as a peer's attitude toward school and participation in extracurricular activities, to be important (Epstein & Karweit, 1983; Ryan, 2000; Shrum, Cheek & Hunter, 1988). For example, Hamm (2000) found that African Americans who attended multiethnic high schools were more likely to have friendships with others who shared their same ethnic group membership as well as other characteristics, such as academic orientation or substance use. In contrast, Asian American and European American students were more likely to have friendships based upon similar academic orientations (measured through a composite variable containing self-reports of effort in completing school work and educational aspirations for future education past high school). The findings from this study are somewhat similar to findings obtained in a study of commonalities between high school best friends. In their study, Tolson and Urberg (1993) found that African American best friendships appear to be less similar on many behaviors and attitudes (e.g., smoking attitudes, in-school activities) than those of European American and Asian American youth. Differences between these studies may be a result of the way that researchers assessed friendships.

For this chapter, the more important question is whether racial and ethnic minority students' friendships are associated with their engagement with school. The limited research that exists on the relation between minority students' access to same-race/ethnic group peers suggests a positive association between access to same-race/ethnic group peers and emotional engagement in school, with many hypothesizing that having access to similar peers may reduce students' overall exposure to racial discrimination (Gonzalez, 2009; Johnson, Crosnoe, & Elder, 2001; Moody, 2001). The relations among school composition (i.e., presence of racial and ethnic minority students), same-race/ethnic group friendships, and emotional engagement, however, is not the same across racial and ethnic groups. For example, in a study using the National Longitudinal Study of Adolescent Health, Ueno (2009) found positive associations between access to same-race/ethnic group peers in school and emotional engagement for Asian and African American students, but not White and Latino students. Positive associations between the presence of same-race/ethnic group friendships and emotional engagement were found for Latino and White students, suggesting for Latino and White students, it is the importance of having friendships that contributes to emotional engagement in school and not simply access to similar peers.

Although minority students' access to same-race/ethnic group peers and friends at school appears to be related to student engagement, the quality of relationship may determine the relative strength of this association. Vaquera (2009) found that compared to students who did not report having a best friend at school, White and Latino high school students who reported having a best friend were more likely to be emotionally engaged and less likely to have behavioral engagement problems (e.g., not being on task in school, not handing in homework). Although few differences in emotional and behavioral engagement persisted across ethnic groups once individual (age, gender, generational status) and school (public, low-achieving school, and proportion of same race) factors were added to the models, students from Mexican and Central/South America reported higher levels of emotional engagement than did White students.

Not surprisingly, racial and ethnic minority students who have access to and relationships with peers and friends who value education and who participate in school activities are more likely to be engaged in school than students without these relationships (Ryan, 2000; Shin et al., 2007). However, they may be less likely to have access to such relationships. Using data from the

National Education Longitudinal Study of 1988 (NELS:88), Ream and Rumberger (2008) found that in general, Mexican American youth were less likely to participate in (a) unorganized academic activities, such as homework and school preparation activities, and (b) organized extracurricular activities, such as athletics or the arts. In addition, Mexican American youth were more likely than their non-Latino White peers to have friends who dropped out of high school and were less likely to have access to friends who valued education (measured by student report of friends attending class regularly, getting good grades, studying, finishing high school, and continuing education past high school). Utilizing a series of structural equation models, Ream and Rumberger found that Mexican American students' homework and school preparation activities were positively associated with school-oriented friendship networks, while these types of behavioral engagement were negatively related to identifying with students who dropped out of school. For both Mexican American and non-Latino White students, participation in athletic activities was positively related to having friends who valued education. For both groups of students, having more access to friends who had dropped out of school was associated with dropping out of school by the 12th grade. Having friends who valued education was correlated with a decrease in dropout rates for non-Latino White students, but not for Mexican American students. On the one hand, these findings suggest that having access to peers who have dropped out of school may increase the likelihood that Mexican American students will also drop out of school. On the other hand, they support the thesis that participation in extracurricular school activities may be a protective factor against future school disengagement (Eccles & Barber, 1999). Although this study highlights the positive relation between students' activities and continued engagement with school, others have noted that limited financial resources may make it challenging for Mexican American adolescents to participate in organized extracurricular activities (Spina, 2000; Updegraff, Kim, Killoren, & Thayer, 2009). Family and work obligations may also make it difficult for these adolescents to complete homework or other school preparation activities.

Three caveats should be considered relative to research on racial and ethnic minority students' friendships and their engagement with school. First, the nature of the schools that students attend constrains or enables access to racial and ethnic friendship experiences. In multiethnic schools in which a large proportion of students are available to form friendships, it may be that individuals are more likely to choose friends based upon similar values, interests, and abilities, rather than simply on the basis of the same ethnic characteristics. However, given the limited research on this subject, it is unclear if this threshold hypothesis is true. Second, multiple types of peer social networks and possible friendship systems exist in and out of schools that may exert an influence on student engagement. Best friends, regular friends, and peer networks exert social pressure on the student (see Brown, Hamm, Herman, & Heck, 2008), and the ways in which these relationships may be associated with student engagement with school may differ. This leads to a third point, not all friendships are created equally (Flores-Gonzalez, 2002). Some friendships and peer relationships may lead children to identify with and become more engaged in school while others may encourage disengagement. Given the complexity of these issues and the limited research to date, more work is needed to understand the ways in which racial and ethnic minority students' peer relationships are related to their engagement in school.

Teachers' Beliefs, Teacher-Child Relationships, and Instructional Practices

In what ways are teachers' beliefs about and interactions with racial and ethnic minority students related to minority students' engagement with school? In general, researchers have observed positive associations between teachers' relationships with their students and children's engagement and achievement in school (e.g., Birch & Ladd, 1997; Decker, Dona, & Christenson, 2007; Griffith, 2002; Hughes & Kwok, 2007; Mashburn & Pianta, 2006; Murray & Greenberg, 2000; Shaunessy & McHatton, 2009;

Urden & Schoenfelder, 2006; Wentzel, 1997). The student-teacher relationship has been hypothesized to be one of the most important components of the learning process (Garcia, Agbemakplido, Abdella, Lopez, & Registe, 2006; Hamre & Pianta, 2006). A positive teacher-child relationship may be particularly important for racial and ethnic minority students who may need support from teachers in order to successfully navigate school and classroom norms, which may differ from those of the family culture (Au, 1998; D'Amato, 1993; Heath, 1983). In this section, we first consider research examining racial or ethnic matching between teachers and their students. Second, we examine how teachers' perceptions of racial and ethnic minority students relate to teachers' expectations for social and academic behavior. Finally, we discuss the research examining teachers' instructional practices as they relate to students' cultural backgrounds.

As noted earlier, the public school population in the USA is remarkably diverse; children of color in kindergarten through high school represent about 44% of the public school enrollment (U.S. Department of Education, 2009). In stark contrast to this diversity is the homogeneity of the teacher population. Of the three million teachers in public elementary and secondary education, the vast majority (83%) are White (U.S. Department of Education, 2007). In this section, we consider the importance of having a racial or ethnic match between teachers and students for children's achievement and engagement. Although relatively little research has directly examined this issue, there is some research examining the relation between teacher-student match on race/ethnicity.

In a study of African American eighth-grade students, Finn and Voelkl (1993) observed that African American eighth graders who were in schools with fewer minority teachers reported lower emotional engagement scores (e.g., feelings of being welcomed, perception of a supportive school environment, attachment to a teacher) compared to peers who were in schools with higher percentages of minority teachers. Conversely, in schools in which there were higher percentages of minority teachers, White students reported lower emotional engagement scores compared to White students who were in school with low percentages of minority teachers. Using the National Longitudinal Study of Adolescent Health database, Crosnoe, Johnson and Elder (2004) obtained similar findings with respect to the relation between the proportion of White teachers at a school and students' bonding with teachers (e.g., how students felt about teachers, whether teachers treated students fairly). In this study, the proportion of White teachers in the school was positively related to White students' ratings of emotional engagement, but was negatively related to ratings of emotional engagement for Latino girls and African American boys and girls (Crosnoe et al., 2004). However, using the same data set, Johnson et al. (2001) found no relation between the proportion of White or minority teachers at schools and students' behavioral engagement.

There is some evidence that matching racial and ethnic minority college students with university mentors who are of the same race or ethnicity is associated with better behavioral engagement (Campbell & Campbell, 2007). Although there was no difference at the end of their first year in grades or retention in college, 11 years after initial enrollment in college, Latino and African American college students, whose faculty mentors were of the same racial or ethnic group, had attended college for more semesters, accumulated more academic units, and were more likely to have entered a graduate program on campus compared to students whose mentors were of a different race or ethnicity.

Given that the existing research on engagement and teacher-student racial/ethnic match is so limited, we highlight one study that examines the effect of teacher-student racial match on student achievement. To examine the effect of having a teacher of the same race on student achievement, Dee (2004) analyzed data from Project STAR, the Tennessee large-scale randomized field trial of the effects of small class size on student achievement. In Project STAR, teachers and students in kindergarten through third grade were randomly assigned to small classes, regular-size classes or regular-size classes with teacher aides within each of the 79 schools in the study. Dee capitalized on the fact that this random assignment to classes also resulted in students being randomly assigned to either same-race or other-race teachers. For both Black and non-Hispanic White students, assignment to a teacher of the same race resulted in a 3- to 5-percentile-point increase on math and reading achievement test scores (note, the limited numbers of teachers and students from other ethnic groups precluded including them in Dee's analyses). The advantage of having a same-race teacher occurred primarily in regular-size classes (22 students) as opposed to small-size classes (15 students) and with teachers who had been teaching less than 12 years. The effect also appeared to be stronger for students from economically disadvantaged homes. Finally, having a same-race teacher for four consecutive years yielded a cumulative effect of 8-percentile points for reading and nearly 9-percentile points for math achievement test scores in the primary grades.

Dee's findings taken together with the limited findings from other studies (Crosnoe et al., 2004; Finn & Voelkl, 1993) suggest that having a teacher-child racial/ethnic match or higher proportions of minority teachers in schools that have substantial numbers of racial and ethnic minority students may be of benefit for racial and ethnic minority students. Why might having a teacher of the same race or ethnicity benefit a child? According to the cultural discontinuity perspective, differences between the ethnic culture at home and the mainstream culture at school may interfere with student engagement and learning. A teacher who shares a common cultural background may be able to help the child better understand the cultural norms of the school or may be more tolerant of the child acting in accord with his or her cultural norms. Alternatively, another possible mechanism driving the positive associations between teacher-student matching and school experiences is that having a teacher of the same race or ethnic group may provide minority students with a strong role model, which may be particularly important for groups in which high-achieving academic role models are less salient. Research is needed to better understand underlying mechanisms. Some have posited that teachers' beliefs about student achievement contribute to the differences between White students and racial and ethnic minority students' engagement and achievement (e.g., Ferguson, 2003; Kuklinski & Weinstein, 2001; Noguera, 2003; for reviews, see Ferguson, 1998; Good & Brophy, 2000; Good & Nichols, 2001). For example, in a recent meta-analysis of teacher expectations, Tenenbaum and Ruck (2007) found that teachers held more positive expectations for European American children compared to Latino or African American children and higher expectations for the school success of Asian American students relative to European American students.

One way in which teachers' beliefs about students may lead to differences in student engagement with school between White students and racial and ethnic minority students is through the self-fulfilling prophecy hypothesis—if White teachers, as compared to racial and ethnic minority teachers, have more negative perceptions of and expectations for minority students and students live up (or down) to their teacher's perceptions and expectations, then racial and ethnic minority students may do better in school if they have minority teachers. A second hypothesis, which is discussed in more detail below, is that White teachers and minority teachers may treat students differently. Although considerable research has been conducted on teachers' expectations since the late 1960s and has been reviewed by others (e.g., Ferguson, 1998; Good & Brophy, 2000; Good & Nichols, 2001; Tenenbaum & Ruck, 2007), there is less research and mixed findings on White and minority teachers' perceptions and expectations of racial and ethnic minority students. For example, in a study of preservice teachers from an urban university in the Southeastern United States, White preservice teachers, as compared to Black preservice teachers, rated Black elementary school students as being more dependent than their White classmates (Kesner, 2000). In a study of elementary school teachers in an urban school district in the Northeastern United States, Pigott and Cowen (2000) found that ratings of Black elementary school students by both Black and White teachers were more negative than were ratings of White students. However, unlike White teachers, Black teachers were more likely to judge all pupils as being more competent and having fewer problems. Pigott and Cowen suggested that differences in teachers' ratings appear to support the notion that White and Black teachers may have variable perceptions about child competence and appropriate school behavior. Finally, in an examination of teachers' perceptions of students from same or other racial and ethnic groups, Dee (2005) found that students were rated more negatively when they were rated by teachers who were not members of the same racial or ethnic group as the student. However, when the data from each region of the country (North, South, East, and West based on Census classifications) were examined separately, Dee observed that the effect was only statistically significant in the South. These data suggest that conflicting findings in previous research may, at least in part, be due to cultural differences or biases that exist across regions of the country.

There is some research addressing the relation between teachers' expectations and minority students' engagement. Tyler and Boelter (2008) found that low-income African American middle school students' perceptions of teachers' expectations were positively related to self-reported ratings of cognitive, behavioral, and emotional engagement. In a study of African American, Latino, and European American low-income middle school students, Tyler and colleagues (Tyler, Boelter, & Boykin, 2008) examined teachers' perceptions of the degree to which parents' beliefs about education were similar to their own beliefs and students' self-reported cognitive, behavioral, and emotional engagement. White teachers were more likely than African American teachers to perceive parents' endorsement of educational values (e.g., importance of parental role in education, the teaching of literacy) to be different from their own. Regardless of teacher race, a significant negative association emerged between teachers' beliefs and European American, Latino, and African American students' self-reported engagement behaviors, with teachers' perceptions of educational value discontinuity (i.e., differences between themselves and parents) being negatively related to students' ratings of behavioral engagement, but not their cognitive or emotional engagement. Although far from conclusive, these studies suggest that teachers' race and ethnic group membership may be an important variable to consider when examining associations between teachers' expectations and students' experiences at school.

Considerable research indicates that teachers' perceptions and beliefs about racial and ethnic minority students are associated with their interactions with students, which in turn, are related to students' engagement and success in school (Farkas, 2003; Gay, 2000; Hamre & Pianta, 2005; Kozol, 2006; Martin, Fergus, & Noguera, 2010). Although a full review of literature connecting teachers' interactions to student engagement is beyond the scope of this chapter, we briefly consider the relations (a) between the quality of teacher-child relationships and racial and ethnic minority students' engagement and (b) between teachers' pedagogical practices and racial and ethnic minority students' engagement.

The amount of teacher support (often defined as the extent to which teachers' listen to, encourage, and respect students) and the quality of teacher-child relationships may be especially important to racial and ethnic minority students' engagement in school because they may help students navigate differences between home and school environments (Gay, 2000; Heath, 1983), cope with experiences of discrimination, failure, and environmental risk (Faircloth & Hamm, 2005; Garcia-Reid, 2007; Garcia-Reid, Reid, & Peterson, 2005; Gay, 2000; Roeser, Strobel, & Quihuis, 2002), and facilitate positive beliefs about learning and the importance of education (Skinner et al., 2008; Strambler & Weinstein, 2010; Urden & Schoenfelder, 2006). Some research suggests that strong teacher support may compensate for low support at home for Latino students. For example, in a study of low-income Latino middle and high school students, Brewster and Bowen (2004) found that students' perceived support from teachers was negatively associated with students' problem school behavior (i.e., showing up late for school, skipping class) and positively associated with students' emotional engagement (i.e., feelings about school). These associations were maintained even when accounting for family and home support effects. In fact, with regard to student problem behavior, once teacher support was entered into the equation, the relationship between parent support and behavior was no longer significant. In a study of low-income, Latino middle school students, students' ratings of teacher closeness and trust were positively related to students' behavioral engagement, after controlling for student achievement and the quality of the parent–child relationship (Murray, 2009). There was a significant interaction between parent–child and teacher-child relationships such that, having a positive teacher-child relationship seems to compensate for a poor parent–child relationship in terms of students' reports of their school competence.

Although students' positive feelings about their teacher correlate with other aspects of engagement with school, it is important to remember that students' relationships with their teachers are dynamic and change over time. In the Longitudinal Immigration Student Adaptation Study, Green, Rhodes, Hirsch, Suárez-Orozco and Camic (2008) assessed students' reports of their behavioral engagement, related to completing school work, turning in homework, and paying attention in class, over 3 years in a sample of Mexican and Central American immigrant students (Green et al., 2008). Students' perceptions of support from teachers and other adults at school were also assessed in each year. The average level of adult support across the 3 years was calculated for each student, and perceived support for each year was represented as a deviation from the 3 year average. Students' reports of their behavioral engagement changed from year to year, and those changes mirrored changes in their reports of adult support at school. That is, when students perceived adult support to be lower than their average level of support across the 3 years, their self-reported level of behavioral engagement was less. When students felt like they were receiving more support from adults at school, their behavioral engagement was higher.

The studies reviewed here support the general hypothesis that having supportive adult relationships at school is positively correlated with racial and ethnic minority middle and high school students' behavioral and emotional engagement. However, most studies have examined the experience of older students and focused on student-reported measures of engagement. In a recent study with African American and Latino elementary students from low-income backgrounds, Strambler and Weinstein (2010) examined the associations among students' perceptions of teacher caring (e.g., my teacher likes me, my teacher really cares about me), negative teacher feedback (e.g., my teacher makes me feel bad when I do not have the right answer), and students' feelings about school and their behavioral engagement. On average, elementary students rated their teachers as being emotionally supportive, but student ratings of teacher emotional support were not associated with teachers' ratings of student behavioral engagement (e.g., completing class work and homework, listening to and following directions), students' valuing of education (e.g., caring about how one does in school), or students' devaluing of education (e.g., not caring about grades, believing that learning is not important). However, students' perceptions of teachers as negative or unsupportive were positively related to students' academic devaluing. Academic devaluing, in turn, was negatively related to students' math and reading scores, but was not associated with teachers' ratings of behavioral engagement. Although the findings do not directly link teacher negativity to behavioral engagement, they do suggest that, for younger students, who generally like their teachers, instances of negativity and insensitivity may be very salient to children's feelings about school and their achievement.

Teachers' instructional practices may support racial and ethnic minority students' engagement. Teachers who are sensitive to the challenges and needs of their minority students may use interaction styles and pedagogical practices that capitalize on these students' strengths and life experiences and, as a result, benefit students' engagement (Gay, 2000). For example, in a case study of a diverse urban high school in California,

Conchas (2001) observed that teacher interactions and the organizational features of the school appeared to be associated with immigrant and native-born Latino students' emotional engagement with peers at school. In this study, the perceptions of students who participated in different academic programs within the high school (e.g., a health-related career academy, general education program, Advanced Placement Program) were contrasted. Conchas argued that the structure and culture of these academic programs elicited very different attitudes from the students. When a program was racially and ethnically diverse and teachers encouraged students to help each other so that all learned, it appeared that the Latino students were more likely to perceive their peers as being supportive, have cross racial- and ethnic-group friendships and feel empowered to learn (Conchas).

Unfortunately, many curricular approaches implemented with racial and ethnic minority students, particularly those who are poor, have been criticized as being behaviorally based, punitive, and, over time, likely to lead to a decrease in student engagement (Levine, Lowe, Peterson, & Tenoiro, 1995; Varenne & McDermott, 1998). For example, in a case study of a second-grade class with Black, Latino, and White students and a young White teacher, Langhout and Mitchell (2008) documented the teacher's implementation of a discipline strategy (i.e., the use of a behavior chart in which children's cards are pulled by the teacher each time the child misbehaves) and its relation to students' behavioral and emotional disengagement from the learning process. Their analyses show that Black and Latino boys were significantly more likely to have their names moved on the behavioral chart, despite the fact that having one's name moved did not increase or decrease the likelihood of a student's name being pulled in the future (i.e., the discipline technique was not effective at reducing misbehavior). Qualitative analyses suggested that use of the chart was adversely related to Black and Latino boys' behavioral and emotional engagement. Because many of the infractions occurred when the children were excited to participate and call out answers, the teacher's response of telling children to raise their hands and then ignoring their response or pulling the student's card or putting him in time out appeared to result in feelings of rejection and behavioral disengagement (e.g., children cried, stopped participating, or were removed from the group).

As illustrated in the above study, the organization of classroom activities may constrain the formation of teacher-student and student-student relationships because of the frequency of teacher reprimands and determination of who receives attention and assistance from the teacher (Bossert, 1979). In studies of student engagement and the organization of classroom activities, high school students reported being less behaviorally engaged during whole-group instruction as compared to during small group or individual work time (Shernoff, Csikszentmihalyi, Schneider, & Shernoff, 2003). Research on ethnic minority children's early childhood experiences documents that Latino and African American children spend significantly less time in free choice activities and significantly more time in teacher-led assigned time and African American children spend significantly more time engaged in routine activities, such as meals or lining up (Early et al., 2010). The amount of teacher-directed instructional time continues to increase into first grade (La Paro, Rimm-Kaufman, & Pianta, 2006).

The instructional experiences of racial and ethnic minority students in US schools often do not reflect the preferred values and corresponding behaviors that are reflected in the home cultures of many racial and ethnic minority children (Gay, 2000; Gutierrez & Rogoff, 2003; Heath, 1983). For example, sharing, cooperation, and primacy of group needs over individual needs are commonly held values among American Indian People, and competitive behavior is often inhibited (Deyhle, 1995; Sanders, 1987; Yates, 1987). In mainstream schools, which generally emphasize individualism and teacher-directed learning, American Indian children may be perceived as being unmotivated or unengaged because of their unwillingness to compete (Castagno, McKinley, Brayboy, 2008). Differences in rules of speaking, listening, and turn taking in conversations may make it more difficult for American Indian children to participate in classroom activities (Greenbaum, 1985; Sanders, 1987).

Research on African American students also emphasizes the importance of communalism (i.e., belief in a fundamental interdependence of people) to African American students' learning experiences outside of school (Tyler, Boykin, Boelter, & Dillihunt, 2005). Boykin, Tyler and Miller (2005) found that many African American students gravitate toward verve-related learning behaviors, meaning that students demonstrated a preference for higher levels of movement or auditory stimulation. The relationship between verve and student engagement and achievement was demonstrated by Cole and Boykin (2008) in a study examining the role that music and movement experiences might have on children's learning of a story that was read to them and their mood during the experience. In the first experiment, 48 African American children were randomly assigned to one of four treatment conditions, while in the second experiment they were assigned to one of the four conditions or a control condition. Each was read a story and either exposed to (a) syncopated music with movement, (b) syncopated music without movement, (c) nonsyncopated music with movement, (d) nonsyncopated music without movement, or (e) no music and no movement (control; study 2) during the reading. In experiment one, fourth-grade children's ability to recall the story was highest in the syncopated music and movement condition and lowest in the nonsyncopated music without movement condition. In experiment two, fourth graders demonstrated better story recall under the syncopated music and movement condition, but sixth graders performed higher on the story recall task in the nonsyncopated music, low movement condition. In experiment 2 undertaken with 128 fourth- and sixth-grade students, both fourth- and sixth-grade children performed the lowest in the control (no music, no movement) condition. Although more research is needed, these data suggest that younger African American students may benefit from an educational context that incorporates the music and movement of their home culture.

In general, the quality of students' relationships at school and the nature of teacher-student interactions appear to be related to racial and ethnic minority students' engagement and achievement (e.g., Decker et al., 2007; Furrer & Skinner, 2003; Griffith, 2002; Wentzel, 1997). Children who report having supportive teachers are more likely to be engaged in learning engagement behaviors. In addition, in some cases, having a racial or ethnic match between teachers and students may be beneficial to student engagement and subsequent school achievement. This may occur as a result of positive teacher beliefs about children's ability to learn, having an ethnic minority role model in the classroom, or through ethnic minority teachers' ability to possibly create less discontinuity between home and school environments. Unfortunately, given the limited number of studies to date and with few exceptions, their correlational nature, making any causal inferences about these relationships is problematic.

Conclusions

The underachievement of African American, Latino, and Native American students in the United States has been partially attributed to poor engagement in school (e.g., Connell et al., 1994; Steele, 1997). However, the relation between engagement and school achievement is not a simple one. Somewhat paradoxically, social scientists have noted that on some dimensions of engagement, underachieving minority students have indicated stronger engagement relative to their higher achieving peers (e.g., Dotterer et al., 2009; Johnson et al., 2001; Mickelson, 1990; Shernoff & Schmidt, 2008). In some instances, for example, minority students more strongly endorse the value or importance of education compared to White students even though the minority students do less well in school (e.g., Mickelson, 1990; Shernoff & Schmidt, 2008). Similarly, self-report measures of emotional engagement (e.g., belonging, feeling a part of school) may result in different engagement scenarios compared to teacher reports of students' behavioral engagement (Shernoff & Schmidt). In this chapter, we have considered a number of factors that are associated with racial and ethnic minority students' engagement with school, and a number of key themes have emerged.

First, ethnic or cultural membership appears to be a critical feature related to racial and ethnic minority schoolchildren's valuing of, beliefs about, and engagement in school. In contrast to the cultural ecological perspective (e.g., Ogbu, 1986), it appears that having a strong racial or ethnic identity can coexist with or encompass a strong academic identity (e.g., Bingham et al., 2001; Chavous et al., 2003; Smalls et al., 2007). It may be that having a strong ethnic identity along with a bicultural identity—one that maintains that achieving within the mainstream culture is appropriate for members of one's racial or ethnic minority group—is the key to minority students' becoming engaged in school (e.g., Okagaki et al., 2009; Oyserman et al., 2001, 2003). As suggested by social identity theorists and researchers, people belong to multiple groups at any given time; they have multiple social identities. It is the interplay among those social identities that directs behavior. For ethnic minority students, their ethnic, bicultural, and academic identities may work together to support, or be at odds in relation to, the student's motivation for, engagement in, and performance in school.

Second, perception of discrimination generally appears to be negatively associated with students' engagement (Dotterer et al., 2009; Okagaki et al., 1996; Taylor et al., 1994), but this relation may be mediated by students' belief in the instrumental importance of school (Taylor et al.). Belief in the pragmatic importance of education (Bingham et al., 2001; Mickelson, 1990) is positively related to students' engagement and achievement, as is having a bicultural identity, one that includes participation and achievement in the mainstream culture (Bingham et al., 2001; Oyserman et al., 2003). In addition, the negative relation between discrimination and engagement may be moderated by having a strong ethnic identity, at least for girls (Dotterer et al.).

Third, peers, teachers, and parents clearly matter to children's educational experiences. For example, although there is great diversity in parents' ideas about education, how children learn, what children need to do to succeed in school, and what parents should do to support their child's education, parents of racial and ethnic minority youth who have (a) strong and clear academic expectations for their child, (b) predictable family routines, and (c) good relationships with their child are more likely to have children who are engaged in school (Annunziata et al., 2006; Murray, 2009; Sirin & Rogers-Sirin, 2005; Taylor & Lopez, 2005). Similar to parental support at home, peer support at school appears to matter to engagement. Students who have access to same-ethnic peers, have friends who value education, and have peer social support at school, particularly a best friend, appear to do better than students who do not have these peer resources (Brown et al., 2008; Gonzalez, 2009; Ryan, 2000; Shin et al., 2007; Vaquera, 2009). Finally, teachers appear to be a crucial component in ethnic minority students' engagement processes, with the quality of teacher-child relationships, teachers' expectations for ethnic minority students' learning, and teachers' pedagogical practices all appearing to be related to students' engagement or disengagement from the learning process (Crosnoe et al., 2004; Faircloth & Hamm, 2005; Ferguson, 2003; Skinner et al., 2008; Urden & Schoenfelder, 2006).

There is so much that we still do not know about factors that support and inhibit the school engagement of racial and ethnic minority students. Among the most promising lines of research are studies that explicitly examine the relations between engagement with school, ethnicity, and their interactions with multiple factors, such as studies by Dotterer et al. (2009), Murray (2009), and Taylor and colleagues (1994). It is only by systematically looking at the interactions among many factors that we are likely to establish clear understandings of the relations between ethnicity and engagement.

Finally, although many have theorized that cultural discontinuity between children's home and school contexts inhibits racial and ethnic minority students' engagement in school, few have attempted to measure that discontinuity and explicitly examine the link between discontinuity and students' cognitive, emotional, and behavioral engagement. As posited earlier, one reason that teachers perceive minority students to be less engaged in school relative to their peers is because teachers, particularly those who are White, may not understand when students are engaging in behaviors consistent with their home cultures (e.g., Deyhle, 1995; Tyler et al., 2008). We need better identification of the discontinuities between home and school cultures. We need to know which differences matter and how much of that difference actually matters.

Public education in the United States is a complex enterprise. Public schools are responsible for providing an education that will enable students from all backgrounds to learn and succeed. Behavioral scientists may not be able to quickly identify all of the ways in which the cultural norms of ethnic and racial minority groups differ from those of the mainstream culture, but perhaps, we can move with speed toward identifying those differences that may make a substantial difference in the engagement and achievement of racial and ethnic minority students. It is encouraging to find that supportive teacher-child relationships are associated with better engagement among racial and ethnic minority children (e.g., Green et al., 2008; Murray, 2009) and that supportive teacher-child relationships may be able to buffer low support from home (Brewster & Bowen, 2004; Murray). Can researchers expediently take the next steps and identify those behaviors that lead to positive teacher-child relationships for minority students and then train teachers to engage in such behaviors? For the sake of current and future ethnic minority children and youth in US schools, we certainly hope so.

References

Alexander, K. L., Entwisle, D. R., & Bedinger, S. D. (1994). When expectations work: Race and socioeconomic differences in school performance. *Social Psychology Quarterly, 57*(4), 283–299.

Annunziata, D., Hogue, A., Faw, L., & Liddle, H. A. (2006). Family functioning and school success in at-risk, inner-city adolescents. *Journal of Youth and Adolescence, 35*(1), 105–113.

Antonio, A. L. (2004). The influence of friendship groups on intellectual self-confidence and educational aspirations in college. *Journal of Higher Education, 75*, 446–471.

Appleton, J. J., Christenson, S. L., & Furlong, M. J. (2008). Student engagement with school: Critical conceptual and methodological issues of the construct. *Psychology in the Schools, 45*, 369–386.

Arroyo, C. G., & Zigler, E. (1995). Racial identity, academic achievement, and the psychological well-being of economically disadvantaged adolescents. *Journal of Personality and Social Psychology, 69*(5), 902–914.

Au, K. H. (1998). Social constructivism and the school literacy learning of students of diverse backgrounds. *Journal of Literacy Research, 30*, 297–319.

Aud, S., Hussar, W., Planty, M., Snyder, T., Bianco, K., Fox, M., et al. (2010). *The condition of education 2010* (NCES 2010–028). Washington, DC: National Center for Education Statistics, Institute of Education Sciences, U.S. Department of Education.

Bellmore, A. D., Nishina, A., Witkow, M. R., Graham, S., & Juvonen, J. (2007). The influence of classroom ethnic composition on same- and other-ethnicity peer nominations in middle school. *Social Development, 16*, 720–740.

Bennett, M. D., Jr. (2006). Cultural resources and school engagement among African American youths: The role of racial socialization and ethnic identity. *Children and Schools, 28*(4), 197–206.

Bernal, M. E., Saenz, D. S., & Knight, G. P. (1991). Ethnic identity and adaptation of Mexican American youths in school settings. *Hispanic Journal of Behavioral Sciences, 13*(2), 135–154.

Berndt, T. J. (1999). Friends' influence on students' adjustment to school. *Educational Psychologist, 34*, 15–28.

Bingham, G., Helling, M. K., & Okagaki, L. (2001, April). *Ethnic identity and school achievement in Native American students.* Presented at the Biennial Meeting of the Society for Research in Child Development, Minneapolis, MN.

Birch, S. H., & Ladd, G. W. (1997). The teacher-child relationship and children's early school adjustment. *Journal of School Psychology, 35*, 61–79.

Bornstein, M. H. (Ed.). (2002). *Handbook of parenting: Social conditions and applied parenting* (2nd ed., Vol. 4). Mahwah, NJ: Erlbaum.

Bossert, S. (1979). *Tasks and social relationships in classrooms.* Cambridge, England: Cambridge University Press.

Boykin, W. A., Tyler, K. M., & Miller, O. (2005). In search of cultural themes and their expressions in the dynamics of classroom life. *Urban Education, 40*, 521–549.

Brewster, A. B., & Bowen, G. L. (2004). Teacher support and the school engagement of Latino middle and high school students at risk of school failure. *Child and Adolescent Social Work Journal, 21*, 47–67.

Brown, B. B., Hamm, J. V., Herman, M., & Heck, D. J. (2008). Ethnicity and image: Correlates of crowd affiliation among ethnic minority youth. *Child Development, 79,* 529–546.

Buriel, R., & De Ment, T. (1997). Immigration and sociocultural change in Mexican, Chinese, and Vietnamese American families. In A. Booth, A. C. Crouter, & N. Landale (Eds.), *Immigration and the family* (pp. 165–200). Mahwah, NJ: Erlbaum Associates.

Campbell, T. A., & Campbell, D. E. (2007). Outcomes of mentoring at-risk college students: Gender and ethnic matching effects. *Mentoring and Tutoring, 15,* 135–148.

Caplan, N., Whitmore, J. K., & Choy, M. H. (1989). *The Boat People and achievement in American: A study of family life, hard work, and cultural values.* Ann Arbor, MI: The University of Michigan Press.

Carrasquillo, A. L. (1991). *Hispanic children and youth in the United States: A resource guide.* New York: Garland.

Castagno, A. E., McKinley, B., & Brayboy, J. (2008). Culturally responsive schooling for indigenous youth: A review of the literature. *Review of Educational Research, 78,* 941–993.

Chao, R. K. (2000). The parenting of immigrant Chinese and European American mothers: Relations between parenting styles, socialization goals, and parental practices. *Journal of Applied Developmental Psychology, 21*(2), 233–248.

Chavous, T. M., Bernat, D. H., Schmeelk-Cone, K., Caldwell, C. H., Kohn-Wood, L., & Zimmerman, M. A. (2003). Racial identity and academic attainment among African American adolescents. *Child Development, 74*(4), 1076–1090.

Chen, C., & Stevenson, H. W. (1995). Motivation and mathematics achievement: A comparative study of Asian-American, Caucasian-American, and East Asian high school students. *Child Development, 66,* 1215–1234.

Cole, J. M., & Boykin, A. W. (2008). Examining culturally structured learning environments with different types of music-linked movement opportunity. *Journal of Black Psychology, 34,* 331–355.

Conchas, G. Q. (2001). Structuring failure and success: Understanding the variability in Latino school engagement. *Harvard Educational Review, 71*(3), 475–504.

Connell, J. P., Spencer, M. B., & Aber, J. L. (1994). Educational risk and resilience in African-American youth: Context, self, action, and outcomes in school. *Child Development, 65,* 493–506.

Crosnoe, R., Johnson, M. K., & Elder, G. H. (2004). School size and the interpersonal side of education: An examination of race/ethnicity and organizational context. *Social Science Quarterly, 85,* 1259–1274.

D'Amato, J. (1993). Resistance and compliance in minority classrooms. In E. Jacob & C. Jordan (Eds.), *Minority education: Anthropological perspectives* (pp. 181–207). Norwood, NJ: Ablex.

Decker, D. M., Dona, D. P., & Christenson, S. L. (2007). Behaviorally at-risk African American students: The importance of student-teacher relationships for student outcomes. *Journal of School Psychology, 45,* 83–109.

Dee, T. S. (2004). Teachers, race, and student achievement in a randomized experiment. *The Review of Economics and Statistics, 86*(1), 195–210.

Dee, T. S. (2005). A teacher like me: Does race, ethnicity, or gender matter? *The American Economic Review, 95,* 158–165.

Deyhle, D. (1995). Navajo youth and Anglo racism: Cultural integrity and resistance. *Harvard Educational Review, 65*(3), 403–445.

Dotterer, A. M., McHale, S. M., & Crouter, A. C. (2009). Sociocultural factors and school engagement among African American youth: The roles of racial discrimination, racial socialization, and ethnic identity. *Applied Developmental Science, 13*(2), 61–73.

Early, D. M., Iruka, I. U., Ritchie, S., Barbarin, O. A., Winn, D. C., et al. (2010). How do pre-kindergarteners spend their time? Gender, ethnicity, and income as predictors of experiences in pre-kindergarten classrooms. *Early Childhood Research Quarterly, 25,* 177–193.

Eccles, J., & Barber, B. (1999). Student council, volunteering, basketball, or matching band: What kind of extracurricular involvement matters? *Journal of Adolescent Research, 14,* 10–43.

Epstein, J. L., & Karweit, N. (Eds.). (1983). *Friends in school: Patterns of selection and influence in secondary schools.* New York: Academic.

Faircloth, B. S., & Hamm, J. V. (2005). Sense of belonging among high school students representing four ethnic groups. *Journal of Youth and Adolescence, 34,* 293–309.

Fan, X., & Chen, M. (2001). Parental involvement and students' academic achievement: A meta-analysis. *Educational Psychology Review, 13*(1), 1–22.

Farkas, G. (2003). Racial disparities and discrimination in education: What do we know, how do we know it, and what do we need to know? *Teachers College Record, 105*(6), 1119–1146.

Ferguson, R. F. (1998). Teachers' perceptions and expectations and the Black-White test score gap. In C. Christopher & M. Phillips (Eds.), *The Black-White test score gap* (pp. 273–317). Washington, DC: Brookings Institution Press.

Ferguson, R. F. (2003). Teachers' perceptions and expectations and the Black-White test score gap. *Urban Education, 38,* 460–507.

Finn, J. D., & Rock, D. A. (1997). Academic success among students at risk for school failure. *Journal of Applied Psychology, 82,* 221–234.

Finn, J. D., & Voelkl, K. E. (1993). School characteristics related to student engagement. *Journal of Negro Education, 62,* 249–268.

Flores-González, N. (1999). Puerto Rican high achievers: An example of ethnic and academic identity compatibility. *Anthropology & Education Quarterly, 30*(3), 343–362.

Flores-Gonzalez, N. (2002). *School kids/street kids: Identity development in Latino students.* New York: Teachers College Press.

Fordham, S., & Ogbu, J. (1986). Black students' school success: Coping with the "burden of acting White". *Urban Review, 18*(3), 176–206.

Fredricks, J. A., Blumenfeld, P. C., & Paris, A. H. (2004). School engagement: Potential of the concept, state of the evidence. *Review of Educational Research, 74*, 59–109.

Furrer, C., & Skinner, E. (2003). Sense of relatedness as a factors in children's academic engagement and performance. *Journal of Educational Psychology, 95*, 148–162.

Gallimore, R., & Goldenberg, C. (2001). Analyzing cultural models and settings to connect minority achievement and school improvement research. *Educational Psychologist, 36*(1), 45–56.

Garcia, V., Agbemakplido, W., Abdella, H., Lopez, O., & Registe, R. T. (2006). High school students' perspectives of the 2001 No Child Left Behind Act's definition of a highly qualified teacher. *Harvard Educational Review, 76*, 698–724.

Garcia-Reid, P. (2007). Examining social capital as a mechanism for improving school engagement among low income Hispanic girls. *Youth and Society, 39*(2), 164–181.

Garcia-Reid, P., Reid, R. J., & Peterson, N. A. (2005). School engagement among Latino youth in an urban middle school context: Valuing the role of social support. *Education and Urban Society, 37*, 257–275.

Gay, G. (2000). *Culturally responsive teaching. Theory, research, and practice.* New York: Teachers College Press.

Gibson, M. A. (1987). The school performance of immigrant minorities: A comparative view. *Anthropology & Education Quarterly, 18*, 262–275.

Gibson, M. A., & Ogbu, J. U. (Eds.). (1991). *Minority status and schooling: A comparative study of immigrant and involuntary minorities.* New York: Garland.

Gill, S., & Reynolds, A. J. (1999). Educational expectations and school achievement of urban African American children. *Journal of School Psychology, 37*(4), 403–424.

Glanville, J. L., & Wildhagen, T. (2007). The measurement of school engagement: Assessing dimensionality and measurement invariance across race and ethnicity. *Educational and Psychological Measurement, 67*, 1019–1041.

Goldenberg, C., Gallimore, R., Reese, L., & Garnier, H. (2001). Cause or effect? A longitudinal study of immigrant Latino parents' aspirations and expectations, and their children's school performance. *American Educational Research Journal, 38*(3), 547–582.

Gonzalez, R. (2009). Beyond affirmation: How the school context facilitates racial/ethnic identity among Mexican American adolescents. *Hispanic Journal of Behavioral Sciences, 31*, 5–31.

Good, T., & Brophy, J. (2000). *Looking in classrooms* (8th ed.). New York: Longman.

Good, T. L., & Nichols, S. L. (2001). Expectancy effects in the classroom: A special focus on improving the reading performance of minority students in first-grade classrooms. *Educational Psychologist, 36*, 113–126.

Graham, S. (1994). Motivation in African Americans. *Review of Educational Research, 64*, 55–118.

Graham, S., Taylor, A. Z., & Hudley, C. (1998). Exploring achievement values among ethnic minority early adolescents. *Journal of Educational Psychology, 90*(4), 605–620.

Green, G., Rhodes, J., Hirsch, A. H., Suarez-Orozco, C., & Camic, P. M. (2008). Supportive adult relationships and the academic engagement of Latin American immigrant youth. *Journal of School Psychology, 46*, 393–412.

Greenbaum, P. E. (1985). Nonverbal differences in communication style between American Indian and Anglo elementary classrooms. *American Educational Research Journal, 22*, 101–115.

Griffith, J. (2002). A multilevel analysis of the relation of school learning and social environments to minority achievement in public elementary schools. *The Elementary School Journal, 102*, 349–366.

Gutiérrez, K. D., & Rogoff, B. (2003). Cultural ways of learning: Individual traits or repertoires of practice. *Educational Researcher, 32*(5), 19–25.

Halle, T. G., Kurtz-Costes, B., & Mahoney, J. (1997). Family influences on school achievement in low-income, African American children. *Journal of Educational Psychology, 89*(3), 527–537.

Hamm, J. V. (2000). Do birds of a feather flock together? The variable bases for African American, Asian American, and European American adolescents' selection of similar friends. *Developmental Psychology, 36*, 209–219.

Hamre, B. K., & Pianta, R. C. (2005). Can instructional and emotional support in the first-grade classroom make a difference for children at risk of school failure? *Child Development, 76*, 949–967.

Hamre, B. K., & Pianta, R. C. (2006). Student-teacher relationships. In G. G. Bear & K. M. Minke (Eds.), *Children's needs III: Development, prevention, and intervention* (pp. 151–176). Washington, DC: National Association of School Psychologists.

Hao, L., & Bonstead-Bruns, M. (1998). Parent–child differences in educational expectations and the academic achievement of immigrant and native students. *Sociology of Education, 71*(3), 175–198.

Harwood, R. L., Handwerker, W. P., Schoelmerich, A., & Leyendecker, B. (2001). Ethnic category labels, parental beliefs, and the contextualized individual: An exploration of the individualism-sociocentrism debate. *Parenting: Science and Practice, 1*, 217–236.

Heath, S. B. (1983). *Ways with words: Language, life, and work in communities and classrooms.* New York: Cambridge University Press.

Helms, J. E., & Talleyrand, R. M. (1997). Race is not ethnicity. *American Psychologist, 52*(11), 1246–1247.

Hieshima, J. A., & Schneider, B. (1994). Intergenerational effects on the cultural and cognitive socialization of third- and fourth-generation Japanese Americans. *Journal of Applied Developmental Psychology, 15*, 319–327.

Ho, D. Y. F. (1994). Cognitive socialization in Confucian heritage cultures. In P. M. Greenfield & R. R. Cocking (Eds.), *Cross-cultural roots of minority child development* (pp. 285–313). Hillsdale, NJ: Erlbaum Associates.

Hoff, E., Laursen, B., & Tardiff, T. (2002). Socioeconomic status and parenting. In P. M. Greenfield & R. R. Cocking (Eds.), *Cross-cultural roots of minority children development* (pp. 285–313). Hillsdale, NJ: Lawrence Erlbaum Associates.

Hudley, C., & Graham, S. (2001). Stereotypes of achievement striving among early adolescents. *Social Psychology of Education, 5*, 201–224.

Huffman, T. E. (1991). The experiences, perceptions, and consequences of campus racism among Northern Plains Indians. *Journal of American Indian Education, 30*(2), 25–34.

Hughes, J., & Kwok, O. (2007). Influence of student-teacher and parent-teacher relationships on lower achieving readers' engagement and achievement in the primary grades. *Journal of Educational Psychology, 99*, 39–51.

Hughes, D., Rodriguez, J., Smith, E. P., Johnson, D. J., Stevenson, H. C., & Spicer, P. (2006). Parents' ethnic-racial socialization practices: A review of research and directions for future study. *Developmental Psychology, 42*, 747–770.

Johnson, M. K., Crosnoe, R., & Elder, G. H. (2001). Students' attachment and academic engagement: The role of race and ethnicity. *Sociology of Education, 74*, 318–340.

Keefe, S. E., & Padilla, A. M. (1987). *Chicano ethnicity*. Albuquerque, NM: University of New Mexico Press.

Kesner, J. E. (2000). Teacher characteristics and the quality of child-teacher relationships. *Journal of School Psychology, 28*, 133–149.

KewalRamani, A., Gilbertson, L., Fox, M., & Provasnik, S. (2007). *Status and trends in the education of racial and ethnic minorities* (NCES 2007–039). Washington, DC: National Center for Education Statistics, Institute of Education Sciences, U.S. Department of Education.

Kozol, J. (2006). *The shame on the nation: The restoration of apartheid in schooling in America*. New York: Random House.

Kuklinski, M. R., & Weinstein, R. S. (2001). Classroom and developmental differences in a path model of teacher expectancy effects. *Child Development, 72*, 1554–1578.

Laboratory of Comparative Human Cognition. (1982). Culture and intelligence. In R. J. Sternberg (Ed.), *Handbook of human intelligence* (pp. 642–719). Cambridge, UK: Cambridge University Press.

LaFromboise, T., Coleman, H. L. K., & Gerton, J. (1993). Psychological impact of biculturalism: Evidence and theory. *Psychological Bulletin, 114*(3), 395–412.

Langhout, R. D., & Mitchell, C. A. (2008). Engaging contexts: Drawing the link between student and teacher experiences of the hidden curriculum. *Journal of Community and Applied Social Psychology, 18*, 593–614.

La Paro, K., Rimm-Kaufman, S. E., & Pianta, R. C. (2006). Kindergarten to 1st grade: Classroom characteristics and the stability and change of children's classroom experiences. *Journal of Research in Childhood Education, 21*, 189–203.

Lareau, A. (1996). Assessing parent involvement in schooling: A critical analysis. In A. Booth & J. F. Dunn (Eds.), *Family-school links: How do they affect educational outcomes?* (pp. 57–64). Mahwah, NJ: Erlbaum Associates.

Levine, D., Lowe, R., Peterson, B., & Tenorio, R. (Eds.). (1995). *Rethinking schools: An agenda for change*. New York: The New Press.

Libbey, H. P. (2004). Measuring student relationships to school: Attachment, bonding, connectedness, and engagement. *Journal of School Health, 74*, 274–283.

Luster, T., & McAdoo, H. (1996). Family and child influences on educational attainment: A secondary analysis of the High/Scope Perry Preschool data. *Developmental Psychology, 32*(1), 26–39.

Machamer, A. M., & Gruber, E. (1998). Secondary school, family, and educational risk: Comparing American Indian adolescents and their peers. *The Journal of Educational Research, 91*(6), 357–369.

Martin, M., Fergus, E., & Noguera, P. (2010). Responding to the needs of the whole child: A case study of a high-performing elementary school for immigrant children. *Reading and Writing Quarterly, 26*, 195–222.

Mashburn, A. J., & Pianta, R. C. (2006). Social relationships and school readiness. *Early Education and Development, 17*, 151–176.

Matute-Bianchi, M. E. (1986). Ethnic identities and patterns of school success and failure among Mexican-descent and Japanese-American students in a California high school: An ethnographic analysis. *American Journal of Education, 95*, 233–255.

Mickelson, R. (1990). The attitude-achievement paradox among black adolescents. *Sociology of Education, 63*, 44–61.

Miller, D. B. (1999). Racial socialization and racial identity: Can they promote resiliency for African American adolescents? *Adolescence, 34*(135), 493–501.

Miller, L. S. (1995). *An American imperative: Accelerating minority educational advancement*. New Haven, CT: Yale University Press.

Mizokawa, D. T., & Ryckman, D. B. (1990). Attributions of academic success and failure: A comparison of six Asian-American ethnic groups. *Journal of Cross-Cultural Psychology, 21*(4), 434–451.

Moody, J. (2001). Race, school integration, and friendship segregation in America. *The American Journal of Sociology, 107*, 679–716.

Murray, C. (2009). Parent and teacher relationships as predictors of school engagement and functioning among low-income urban youth. *The Journal of Early Adolescence, 29*, 379–404.

Murray, C., & Greenberg, M. T. (2000). Children's relationship with teachers and bonds with school. *Journal of School Psychology, 38*, 423–445.

Noguera, P. A. (2003). The trouble with Black boys: The role and influence of environmental and cultural factors on the academic performance of African American males. *Urban Education, 38*, 431–459.

Ogbu, J. U. (1986). The consequences of the American caste system. In U. Neisser (Ed.), *The school achievement of minority children: New perspectives* (pp. 19–56). Hillsdale, NJ: Lawrence Erlbaum Associates.

Ogbu, J. U. (1992). Understanding cultural diversity and learning. *Educational Researcher, 21*(8), 5–14.

Ogbu, J. U., & Matute-Bianchi, M. D. (1986). Understanding sociocultural factors in education: Knowledge, identity, and adjustment. In *Beyond language: Sociocultural factors in schooling, language, and minority students* (pp. 71–143). California State Department of Education. Los Angeles: Education Dissemination and Assessment Center, California State University, Los Angeles.

Okagaki, L. (2001). Triarchic model of minority children's school achievement. *Educational Psychologist, 36*(1), 9–20.

Okagaki, L., & Bingham, G. E. (2010). Diversity in families: Parental socialization and children's development and learning. In S. L. Christenson & A. L. Reschly (Eds.), *Handbook of school-family partnerships* (pp. 80–100). New York: Routledge/Taylor & Francis Group.

Okagaki, L., & Frensch, P. A. (1998). Parenting and children's school achievement: A multi-ethnic perspective. *American Educational Research Journal, 35*(1), 123–144.

Okagaki, L., Frensch, P. A., & Dodson, N. E. (1996). Mexican-American children's perceptions of self and school achievement. *Hispanic Journal of Behavioral Sciences, 18*, 469–484.

Okagaki, L., Helling, M. K., & Bingham, G. E. (2009). American Indian college students' ethnic identity and beliefs about education. *Journal of College Student Development, 50*(2), 157–176.

Okagaki, L., Izarraraz, L., & Bojczyk, K. (2003, April). *Latino adolescents' ethnic beliefs, orientation to school and emotional well-being.* Presented at the biennial meetings of the Society for Research in Child Development, Tampa, FL.

Okagaki, L., & Moore, D. K. (2000). Ethnic identity beliefs of young adults and their parents in families of Mexican descent. *Hispanic Journal of Behavioral Sciences, 22*(2), 139–162.

Okagaki, L., & Sternberg, R. J. (1993). Parental beliefs and children's early school performance. *Child Development, 64*(1), 36–56.

Osborne, J. W. (1997). Race and academic disidentification. *Journal of Educational Psychology, 89*(4), 728–735.

Oyserman, D., Brickman, D., Bybee, D., & Celious, A. (2006). Fitting in matters: Markers of in-group belonging and academic outcomes. *Psychological Science, 17*, 854–861.

Oyserman, D., Bybee, D., Terry, K., & Hart-Johnson, T. (2004). Possible selves as roadmaps. *Journal of Research in Personality, 38*, 130–149.

Oyserman, D., Harrison, K., & Bybee, D. (2001). Can racial identity be promotive of academic efficacy? *International Journal of Behavioral Development, 25*(4), 379–385.

Oyserman, D., Kemmelmeier, M., Fryberg, S., Brosh, H., & Hart-Johnson, T. (2003). Racial-ethnic self-schemas. *Social Psychology Quarterly, 66*, 333–347.

Peng, S. S., & Wright, D. (1994). Explanation of academic achievement of Asian American students. *The Journal of Educational Research, 87*(6), 346–352.

Perdue, N. H., Manzeske, D. P., & Estell, D. B. (2009). Early predictors of school engagement: Exploring the role of peer relationships. *Psychology in the Schools, 46*, 1084–1097.

Phinney, J. S. (1990). Ethnic identity in adolescents and adults: Review of research. *Psychological Bulletin, 108*, 499–514.

Phinney, J. S. (1992). The multigroup ethnic identity measure: A new scale for use with diverse groups. *Journal of Adolescent Research, 7*(2), 156–176.

Phinney, J. S. (1996). When we talk about American ethnic groups, what do we mean? *American Psychologist, 51*, 918–927.

Pigott, R. L., & Cowen, E. L. (2000). Teacher race, child race, racial congruence, and teacher ratings of children's school adjustment. *Journal of School Psychology, 38*(2), 177–196.

Rampey, B. D., Dion, G. S., & Donahue, P. L. (2009). *NAEP 2008 trends in academic progress* (NCES 2009-479). Washington, DC: National Center for Education Statistics, Institute of Education Sciences, U.S. Department of Education.

Ream, R. K., & Rumberger, R. W. (2008). Student engagement, peer social capital, and school dropout among Mexican American and non-Latino White students. *Sociology of Education, 81*, 109–139.

Rivas-Drake, D., Hughes, D., & Way, N. (2008). A closer look at peer discrimination, ethnic identity, and psychological well-being among urban Chinese American sixth graders. *Journal of Youth and Adolescence, 37*, 12–21.

Roberts, R., Phinney, J., Masse, L., Chen, Y., Roberts, C., & Romero, A. (1999). The structure of ethnic identity in young adolescents from diverse ethnocultural groups. *Journal of Early Adolescence, 19*, 301–322.

Roeser, R., Strobel, K. R., & Quihuis, G. (2002). Studying early adolescents' academic motivation, social-emotional functioning, and engagement in learning: Variable- and person-centered approaches. *Anxiety, Stress, and Coping, 15*, 345–368.

Rogoff, B. (1990). *Apprenticeship in thinking: Cognitive development in social context.* New York: Oxford Press.

Ryan, A. M. (2000). Peer groups as a context for the socialization of adolescents' motivation, engagement and achievement in school. *Educational Psychologist, 35*, 101–111.

Sanders, M. G. (1997). Overcoming obstacles: Academic achievement as a response to racism and discrimination. *Journal of Negro Education, 66*, 83–93.

Sanders, S. (1987). Cultural conflicts: An important factor in academic failures of American Indian students. *Journal of Multicultural Counseling and Development, 15*(2), 81–90.

Schneider, B., & Lee, Y. (1990). A model for academic success: The school and home environment of East Asian students. *Anthropology and Education Quarterly, 21*, 358–377.

Shaunessy, E., & McHatton, P. A. (2009). Urban students' perceptions of teachers: Views of students in general, special, and honors education. *Urban Review, 41*, 486–503.

Shernoff, D. J., Csikszentmihalyi, M., Schneider, B., & Shernoff, E. S. (2003). Student engagement in high school classrooms from the perspective of flow theory. *School Psychology Quarterly, 18*, 158–176.

Shernoff, D. J., & Schmidt, J. A. (2008). Further evidence of an engagement-achievement paradox among U.S. high school students. *Journal of Youth and Adolescence, 37*, 564–580.

Shin, R., Daly, B., & Vera, E. (2007). The relationships of peer norms, ethnic identity, and peer support to school engagement in urban youth. *Professional School Counseling, 10*, 379–388.

Shrum, W., Cheek, N. H., & Hunter, S. M. (1988). Friendship in school: Gender and racial homophily. *Sociology of Education, 61*, 227–239.

Sinner, E., Kindermann, T. A., & Furrer, C. (2009). A motivational perspective on engagement and disaffection: Conceptualization and assessment of children's behavioral and emotional participation in academic activities in the classroom. *Educational and Psychological Measurement, 69*, 493–525.

Sirin, S. R., & Rogers-Sirin, L. (2005). Components of school engagement among African American adolescents. *Applied Developmental Science, 9*(1), 5–13.

Skinner, E., Marchand, G., Furrer, C., & Kindermann, T. (2008). Engagement and disaffection in the classroom: Part of a larger motivational dynamic? *Journal of Educational Psychology, 100*, 765–781.

Smalls, C., White, R., Chavous, T., & Sellers, R. (2007). Racial ideological beliefs and racial discrimination experiences as predictors of academic engagement among African American adolescents. *Journal of Black Psychology, 33*(3), 299–330.

Spencer, M. B., Noll, E., Stotzfus, J., & Harpalani, V. (2001). Identity and school adjustment: Revisiting the "Acting White" assumption. *Educational Psychologist, 36*(1), 21–30.

Spina, S. U. (2000). Violence in schools: Expanding the dialogue. In S. U. Spina (Ed.), *Smoke and mirrors: The hidden context of violence in schools and society* (pp. 1–39). Lanham, MD: Rowman & Littlefield.

Starkey, B. S., & Eaton, S. (2008). *The fear of "Acting White" and the achievement gap: Is there really a relationship?* Charles Hamilton Houston Institute for Race and Justice, Harvard Law School. Downloaded on November 20, 2010, from http://www.charleshamiltonhouston.org/assets/documents/publications/BRIEF%20Acting%20White.pdf

Steele, C. M. (1997). A threat in the air: How stereotypes shape intellectual identity and performance. *American Psychologist, 52*, 613–629.

Steinberg, L., Dornbusch, S. M., & Brown, B. B. (1992). Ethnic differences in adolescent achievement: An ecological perspective. *American Psychologist, 47*(6), 723–729.

Strambler, M. J., & Weinstein, R. S. (2010). Psychological disengagement in elementary school among ethnic minority students. *Journal of Applied Developmental Psychology, 31*, 155–165.

Suarez-Orozco, M. M. (1993). "Becoming somebody": Central American immigrants in U.S. inner-city schools. In E. Jacob & C. Jordan (Eds.), *Minority education: Anthropological perspectives* (pp. 129–143). Norwood, NJ: Ablex.

Sue, S., & Okazaki, S. (1990). Asian-American educational achievement: A phenomenon in search of an explanation. *American Psychologist, 45*(8), 913–920.

Tajfel, H. (1981). *Human groups and social categories: Studies in social psychology*. Cambridge, UK: Cambridge University Press.

Taylor, R. D., Casten, R., Flickinger, S. M., Roberts, D., & Fulmore, C. D. (1994). Explaining the school performance of African-American adolescents. *Journal of Research on Adolescence, 4*(1), 21–44.

Taylor, R. D., & Lopez, E. I. (2005). Family management practice, school achievement, and problem behavior in African American adolescents: Mediating processes. *Applied Developmental Psychology, 26*, 39–49.

Tenenbaum, H. R., & Ruck, M. D. (2007). Are teachers' expectations different for racial minority than for European American students? A meta-analysis. *Journal of Educational Psychology, 99*, 253–273.

Tharp, R. G. (1989). Psychocultural variables and constants: Effects on teaching and learning in schools. *American Psychologist, 44*(2), 349–359.

Tolson, J. M., & Urberg, K. A. (1993). Similarity between adolescent best friends. *Journal of Adolescent Research, 8*, 274–288.

Torres, V. (2004). The diversity among us: Puerto Ricans, Cuban Americans, Caribbean Americans, and Central and South Americans. *New Directions for Student Services, 105*, 5–16.

Trueba, H. T. (1987). *Success or failure: Learning and the language of minority students*. Cambridge, MA: Newbury House.

Tsang, S.-L. (1988). The mathematics achievement characteristics of Asian-American students. In R. R. Cocking & J. P. Mestre (Eds.), *Linguistic and cultural influences on learning mathematics* (pp. 123–136). Hillsdale, NJ: Erlbaum.

Tyler, K. M., & Boelter, C. M. (2008). Linking Black middle school students' perceptions of teachers' expectations to academic engagement and efficacy. *The Negro Educational Review, 59*, 27–44.

Tyler, K. M., Boelter, C. M., & Boykin, A. W. (2008). Linking teachers' perceptions of educational value discontinuity to low-income middle school students' academic engagement and self-efficacy. *Middle Grades Research Journal, 3*(4), 1–20.

Tyler, K. M., Boykin, A. W., Boelter, C. M., & Dillihunt, M. L. (2005). Examining mainstream and Afrocultural value socialization in African American households. *Journal of Black Psychology, 31*, 291–311.

Tyler, K. M., Updah, A. L., Dillihunt, M. L., Beatty-Hazelbaker, R., Conner, T., Gadson, N., et al. (2008). Cultural discontinuity: Toward a quantitative investigation of a major hypothesis in education. *Educational Researcher, 7*, 280–297.

Ueno, K. (2009). Same-race friendships and school attachment: Demonstrating the interaction between personal network and school composition. *Sociological Forum, 24*(3), 515–537.

Updegraff, K. A., Kim, J., Killoren, S. E., & Thayer, S. M. (2009). Mexican American parents' involvement in adolescents' peer relationships: Exploring the role of culture and adolescents' peer experiences. *Journal of Research on Adolescence, 20*, 65–83.

Urdan, T., & Schoenfelder, E. (2006). Classroom effect on student motivation: Goal structures, social relationships, and competence beliefs. *Journal of School Psychology, 44*, 331–349.

U.S. Department of Commerce, Census Bureau. (2001). *The Hispanic population in the United States: Population characteristics* by Melissa Therrien and Roberto R. Ramirez. U.S. Department of Commerce, Economics and Statistics Administration. Washington, DC: U.S. Census Bureau.

U.S. Department of Commerce, U.S. Census Bureau. (1993). *We the American…Hispanics*. Washington, DC: U.S. Department of Commerce, Economics and Statistics Administration, Bureau of the Census.

U.S. Department of Education. (2007). *The condition of education 2007* (NCES 2007–064). U.S. Department of Education, Institute of Education Sciences, National Center for Education Statistics. Washington, DC: U.S. Government Printing Office.

U.S. Department of Education. (2009). *The condition of education 2009* (NCES 2009–081). U.S. Department of Education, Institute of Education Sciences, National Center for Education Statistics. Washington, DC: U.S. Government Printing Office.

U.S. Department of Education, National Center for Education Statistics. (2001a). *English literacy and language minorities in the United States*, NCES 2001–464, by Elizabeth Greenberg, Reynaldo F. Macias, David Rhodes, and Tse Chan. Washington, DC.

Vaquera, E. (2009). Friendship, educational engagement, and school belonging: Comparing Hispanic and White adolescents. *Hispanic Journal of Behavioral Sciences, 31*, 492–514.

Varenne, H., & McDermott, R. (1998). *Successful failure: The school America builds*. Boulder, CO: Westview Press.

Way, N., Becker, B. E., & Greene, M. L. (2006). Friendships among Black, Latino, and Asian American Adolescents in an Urban Context. In L. Balter & C. S. Tamis-LeMonda (Eds.), *Child psychology: A handbook of contemporary issues* (pp. 415–443). New York: Psychology Press.

Way, N., & Chen, L. (2000). Close and general friendships among African American, Latino, & Asian American adolescents from low-income families. *Journal of Adolescent Research, 15*, 274–301.

Way, N., Santos, C., Niwa, E. Y., & Kim-Gervey, C. (2008). To be or not to be: An exploration of ethnic identity development in context. In M. Azmitia, M. Syed, & K. Radmacher (Eds.), The intersection of personal and social identities. *New Directions for Child and Adolescent Development, 120*, 61–79.

Weisner, T. S., Gallimore, R., & Jordan, C. (1988). Unpackaging cultural effects on classroom learning: Native Hawaiian peer assistance and child-generated activity. *Anthropology & Education Quarterly, 19*, 327–353.

Wentzel, K. (1997). Student motivation in middle school: The role of perceived pedagogical caring. *Journal of Educational Psychology, 89*, 411–419.

Witherspoon, K. M. C., Speight, S. L., & Thomas, A. J. (1997). Racial identity attitudes, school achievement, and academic self-efficacy among African American high school students. *Journal of Black Psychology, 23*, 344–357.

Wong, M. G. (1990). The education of white, Chinese, Filipino, and Japanese students: A look at "High School and Beyond". *Sociological Perspectives, 33*(3), 353–374.

Wong, C. A., Eccles, J. S., & Sameroff, A. (2003). The influence of ethnic discrimination and ethnic identification on African American adolescents' school and socioemotinal adjustment. *Journal of Personality, 71*, 1197–1232.

Yates, A. (1987). Current status and future directions of research on the American Indian child. *The American Journal of Psychiatry, 144*, 1135–1142.

Student Engagement: What Is It? Why Does It Matter?

Jeremy D. Finn and Kayla S. Zimmer

Abstract

This chapter considers the relationships of student engagement with academic achievement, graduating from high school, and entering postsecondary schooling. Older and newer models of engagement are described and critiqued, and four common components are identified. Research on the relationship of each component with academic outcomes is reviewed. The main themes are that engagement is essential for learning, that engagement is multifaceted with behavioral and psychological components, that engagement and disengagement are developmental and occur over a period of years, and that student engagement can be modified through school policies and practices to improve the prognoses of students at risk. The chapter concludes with a 13-year longitudinal study that shows the relationships of academic achievement, behavioral and affective engagement, and dropping out of high school.

Student Engagement: What is it? Why does it matter?

This chapter considers the relationships of student engagement with academic achievement, graduating from high school, and entering post-secondary schooling. The concept of engagement has emerged as a way to understand—and improve—outcomes for students whose performance is marginal or poor. The idea that engagement behaviors can be manipulated to enhance educational performance promises significant payoff for students at risk of school failure.

In this chapter, early and more recent models of engagement are described together with the

J.D. Finn (✉)
Graduate School of Education,
The State University of New York at Buffalo,
Buffalo, NY 14260, USA
e-mail: finn@buffalo.edu

K.S. Zimmer
Department of Elementary Education,
St. Bonaventure University, St. Bonaventure,
NY 14778-9800, USA
e-mail: kzimmer@sbu.edu

components of each model. Also, early and more recent research showing the relationship of these components to academic achievement and attainment is summarized. A first look at new longitudinal data on student engagement in grades 4 and 8, academic achievement, and high school graduation is described, showing the longitudinal nature of students' school engagement and disengagement. The chapter concludes by summarizing the reasons to focus on engagement (and disengagement) when addressing problems of low achievement and dropping out. Different terms are used for engagement in this chapter; both *student engagement* and *school engagement* are used to connote *students' engagement in school*.

Engagement and Risk

The recent emphasis on student engagement has evolved along with our understanding of what it means for students to be at risk. The ideas of risk and risk factors derive largely from medicine. The Centers for Disease Control (CDC) defined health risk factors as "events, conditions, and behaviors in the life of any individual modify the probability of occurrence of death and disease for that individual when compared to others …in the [same] general population" (Breslow et al., 1985, p. I-1). As an illustration, risk factors for cardiovascular disease (CVD) that cannot be altered—"conditions"—have been identified in epidemiological studies; these include variables such as gender, ethnicity, family history, and aging. Others risk factors are health outcomes at one point in time—"events"—but become precursors of CVD at later points in time, for example, obesity, hypertension, and hypercholesterolemia.

The parallel to educational risk is clear. Research has identified a number of factors associated with educational failure and dropping out. Status risk factors ("conditions") are sociodemographic characteristics that are difficult or impossible to alter through school-based interventions. Family socioeconomic status (SES), race/ethnicity, whether or not English is spoken in the home, family structure, and early pregnancy/parenthood are all highly related to academic outcomes. Educational risk factors ("events") are educational outcomes at one age/grade that interfere with later academic achievement and educational attainment. Low grades and test performance in the early grades, in-grade retention, and student misbehavior are associated with more severe problems in later grades including school failure and dropping out (see Rumberger & Lim, 2008). Mild forms of school misbehavior in early grades can even escalate to acts of delinquency in later years (Broidy et al., 2003; Loeber & Stouthamer-Loeber, 1998). Dropping out is an educational risk factor—an outcome of earlier school experiences that becomes an obstacle to further schooling.

Like medical risk factors, status and educational risk factors cluster, that is, multiple factors tend to occur in the same individuals (Berenson, 1986; Finn, 1989). The correlations among status risk factors are well documented, and academic risk factors tend to cluster because academic problems in one grade make success in the following grades more difficult (Alexander, Entwisle, & Kabbani, 2001; Rumberger, 2001). For this reason, virtually every discussion of dropping out or delinquency refers to the interdependency with low academic performance, early behavior problems, and gender, race, and SES. The picture presented by status and academic risk factors gives educators little reason to expect that prognoses for at-risk students can be improved.

Research focusing on behavioral risk factors (the "behavior" component of the CDC definition) addresses the question "what do some students at risk due to status or educational risk factors *feel* and *do* to be academically successful?" The attitudes and behaviors that answer this question have been termed school engagement, that is, "the attention…investment, and effort students expend in the work of school" (Marks, 2000, p. 155). Engagement behaviors include the everyday tasks needed for learning, for example, attending school and classes, following teachers' directions, completing in-class and out-of-class assignments, and holding positive attitudes about particular subject areas and about school in general. Because of its direct relationship with academic performance and inverse relationship with negative outcomes, school engagement has been viewed as a protective factor with respect to educational risk (Finn & Rock, 1997; Resnick et al., 1997; Steinberg & Avenevoli, 1998).

Disengaged students are those who do not participate actively in class and school activities, do not become cognitively involved in learning, do not fully develop or maintain a sense of school belonging, and/or exhibit inappropriate or counterproductive behavior. All of these risk behaviors reduce the likelihood of school success. Disengaged students may have entered school without adequate cognitive or social skills, find it difficult to learn basic engagement behaviors, and fail to develop positive attitudes that perpetuate their participation in class, or they may have entered school with marginal or positive habits that become attenuated due to unaddressed academic difficulties, dysfunctional interactions with teachers or administrators, or strong ties to other disengaged students. These students may begin what Rumberger (1987) has described as a gradual process of disengagement often leading to dropping out (see also Wehlage, Rutter, Smith, Lesko, & Fernandez, 1989).

Why Does Engagement Matter?

The engagement/disengagement perspective is helpful to educators searching for strategies to reduce the likelihood of school failure; for these reasons:

- *Engagement behaviors are easily understood by practitioners as being essential to learning.* Further, the relationship between engagement behavior and academic performance is confirmed repeatedly by empirical research.
- *Engagement behaviors can be seen in parallel forms in early and later years.* As a result, dropping out of school can be understood as an endpoint of a process of withdrawal that may have had its beginnings in the elementary or middle grades. Students at risk of school failure or dropping out can be identified earlier rather than later.
- *Remaining engaged—persistence—is itself an important outcome of schooling.* Forms of persistence range from continuing to work on a difficult class problem to graduating from high school to entering and completing post-secondary studies.
- *Engagement behaviors are responsive to teachers' and schools' practices, allowing for the possibility of improving achievement and attainment for students experiencing difficulties along the way.* (See section "Responsiveness to the school and classroom context" in this chapter).

Early and Newer Models of Engagement

Student engagement (and disengagement) was conceptualized in the 1980s as a way to understand and reduce student boredom, alienation, and dropping out. Educators argued that the school setting mediates student involvement and engagement which are, in turn, necessary for learning (Newmann, 1981; Newmann, Wehlage, & Lamborn, 1992; Wehlage et al., 1989). Engagement was defined as "the student's psychological investment in and effort directed toward learning, understanding, or mastering the knowledge, skills, or crafts that academic work is intended to promote" (Newmann, 1992, p. 12).

One set of models emphasized the role of school context. Newmann (1981) argued that only major school reform could reduce student alienation and increase engagement. Six guiding principles were identified as promising: reforms that encourage voluntary choice on the part of students and student participation in policy decisions, maintain clear and consistent educational goals, keep school sizes small, encourage cooperative student–staff relationships, and provide an authentic curriculum. The need for school reform was echoed by Wehlage et al. (1989) who analyzed dropout prevention programs reputed to be effective, concluding that developing a strong sense of community with which students could identify is of paramount importance. As a result of the analysis, a "theory of dropout prevention" was forwarded that asserted: (a) social–cultural conditions and student problems and impediments affect two aspects of student behavior, educational engagement and school membership, and (b) these in turn affect students' educational achievements.

Other models emphasize intrapersonal dynamics. A "self-system process model" was proposed based on the assumption that humans have basic needs for competence, autonomy, and relatedness (Connell, 1990; Connell & Wellborn, 1991). Self-system processes, that is, appraisals of the self in relation to ongoing activity, are generated as a means to evaluate whether these basic needs are being met. If not, internal adjustments regarding the needs may be made. These processes are assumed to develop within an individual throughout the lifespan and to be affected by cultural context and interactions with others.

The action that results from self-system processes may take positive or negative forms, in particular, engagement or disaffection; these, in turn, are followed by the development of skills, social behavior, and adjustment (Connell & Wellborn, 1991; Skinner, Kindermann, Connell, & Wellborn, 2009). The self-system model asserts that schools that support competence, autonomy, and relatedness have higher levels of student engagement and academic success (Connell, Spencer, & Aber, 1994). Empirical studies have documented these relationships in diverse samples of elementary and secondary school children (Connell et al., 1994; Klem & Connell, 2004; Patrick, Skinner, & Connell, 1993).

Participation-Identification Model

A third model had features of both the contextual and intrapersonal views. The participation-identification model (Finn, 1989) explained how behavior and affect interact to impact the likelihood of academic success. The behavioral component (participation) referred to the behaviors students engage in that involve them in the activities of the classroom and school. These include basic learning behaviors (e.g., paying attention to the teacher, responding to teacher's questions, completing assignments), initiative-taking behaviors (e.g., engaging in help-seeking activities, doing more than the minimally required work, suggesting new ways to look at material being taught), and engaging in academic extracurricular activities. Participation also included the social tasks of school, for example, attending classes and school, following classroom rules, interacting positively and appropriate with teachers and peers, and not disrupting the class. The four types of behavior were originally combined under one umbrella (participation) but have been viewed as distinct in more recent work.

The affective component (identification) referred to students' "feelings of being a significant member of the school community, having a sense of inclusion in school…" as well as the "recognition of school as both a social institution and a tool for facilitating personal development" (Voelkl, 1997, p. 296). The first of these has been referred to as "belonging," "school membership," "bonding," "school connectedness," and "attachment" by other researchers. The second was termed "valuing."

The participation-identification model (Fig. 5.1) described a cycle that begins with early forms of student behavior (participation), leading over time to bonding with school (identification) and, in turn, to continued participation. The cycle has been described as follows.

Ideally, a child begins school as a willing participant. He or she is

> …drawn to participate initially by encouragement from home and by classroom activities. Over time, participation continues as long as the individual has the minimal ability needed to perform required tasks and as long as instruction is clear and appropriate. There must be a reasonable probability that the student will experience some degree of academic success. As the student progresses through the grades and autonomy increases, participation and success may be experienced in a variety of ways, both within and outside the classroom. These experiences encourage a student's sense of identification with school and continuing participation. (Finn, 1989, p. 129)

According to the model, behavior in the early grades is considered an important ingredient of school success. The classroom and school context need to be conducive to students' developing a sense of school identification; positive rewards for achievement are especially important. Less-than-successful experiences are inevitable for all children, but the self-sustaining nature of

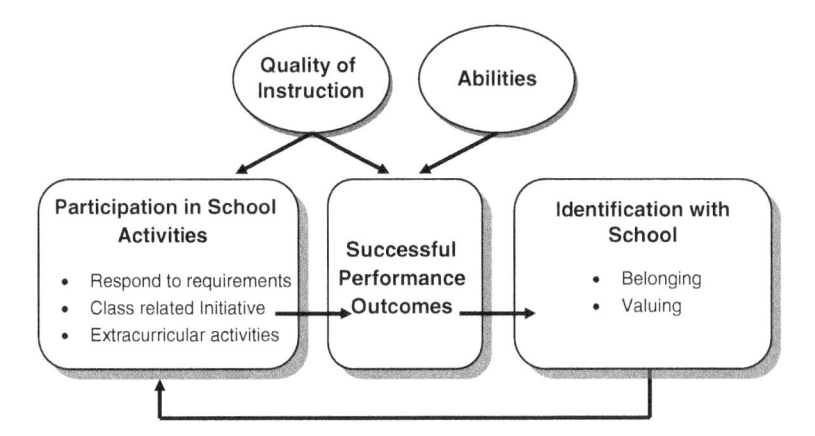

Fig. 5.1 Participation-identification model

the participation-identification cycle serves a protective function that enables students to navigate those situations.

On the negative side,

>…Students lacking the necessary encouragement at home may arrive at school predisposed to nonparticipation and nonidentification. While exceptional teachers may engage the interest of some of these students, others may resist participation, becoming distracted, bored, or restless, avoiding the teachers' attention or failing to respond appropriately to questions. In later years, minimal compliance or total noncompliance with course requirements may persist. Students may refuse to participate in class discussions, turn in assignments late, or arrive late or unprepared for class. As academic requirements become more demanding, this behavior can result in marginal or failing course grades. These students do not have the encouragement to continue participating provided by positive outcomes. If the pattern is allowed to continue, identification with school becomes increasingly unlikely. (Finn, 1989, p. 130)

This sequence of events can lead to disengagement and dropping out, but other avenues can also lead to these outcomes. Some students make reasoned decisions that time off ("stopping out") work or family care is preferable at this point in life. Others may begin school as full participants but encounter obstacles (e.g., disciplinary measures) that cause them to withdraw. Nevertheless, "without a consistent pattern of participation and the reinforcement provided by success experiences, the emotional ingredient needed to maintain a student's involvement or to overcome the occasional adversity is lacking" (p. 130).

The ideas of participation and identification were not as new to educators so much as the way they were assembled into a developmental cycle. The relationship between participation and academic achievement has been studied for decades. Attendance is a well-established factor in academic performance (deJung & Duckworth, 1986; Weitzman et al., 1985). Inattentive and disruptive behavior were identified by psychologist George Spivack and his colleagues as having strong correlations with achievement test scores among students in grades 1 through 6 (r's from 0.15 to 0.74; Swift & Spivack, 1968) and in grades 7 through 12 (r's from 0.26 to 0.32; Swift & Spivack, 1969). The study of "time on task" or "engaged time"—the period of time during which a student is actively engaged in a learning activity—produced a number of studies of the connections between classroom behavior and learning (Anderson, 1975; Berliner, 1990; Fisher et al., 1980). As an example, Anderson (1975) rated students in seventh through ninth grade as being "on task" or "off task" at regular time intervals and calculated the percentage of intervals that each student was on task. This measure yielded correlations between $r=0.59$ and $r=0.66$ with performance in particular math units. Follow-up studies also assessed the context, events, and instructional mode at each time interval in order to understand the factors that promote participation (Anderson & Scott, 1978).

Later research continued to find a strong relationship of participation with academic achievement.

This comes as little surprise given the obvious importance of behavioral engagement for learning class material. One investigation correlated teacher reports of "effort," "initiative-taking," "negative behavior," and "inattentive behavior" with achievement tests in over 1,000 fourth graders (Finn, Pannozzo, & Voelkl, 1995). Correlations with end-of-year achievement scores were all significant at $p<.001$ and in the expected directions; r's ranged from 0.18 to 0.59.

Affective engagement has also been studied for some time. For example, sociologists hypothesized that identification with conventional institutions, including school and the workplace, serves to inhibit misbehavior (Hirschi, 1969; Kanungo, 1979; Liska & Reed, 1985). Affective engagement in this work was termed attachment, involvement, or bonding, and the obverse was termed social isolation or alienation. Research in school settings demonstrated that feelings of alienation are related to delinquency and dropping out and weakly related to academic performance (Elliott & Voss, 1974; Hindelang, 1973; Hirschi, 1969). In the Hirschi and Hindelang studies, large samples of middle- and high school students were administered questionnaires that included indicators of attachment/alienation and a measure of delinquent behavior called "recency." In both studies, the percentage of high-attachment students who were low on recency was substantially greater than the percentage of low-attachment students who were low on recency (e.g., 68% compared to 33% and 64% compared to 34% for two attachment indicators in the Hirschi study). This was interpreted as showing that school attachment inhibits negative behavior.

In the Elliott and Voss (1974) study, over 2,600 high school students responded to questionnaires that yielded measures of normlessness and school isolation. The correlations of normlessness with delinquency ranged from $r=0.59$ to $r=0.63$ and with dropping out from $r=0.30$ to $r=0.32$; the correlations of school isolation with delinquency ranged from $r=0.27$ to $r=0.34$ and with dropping out from $r=0.20$ to $r=0.26$ (all significant at $p<.01$). More recent research indicates that affective engagement is related directly to student behavior and persistence and indirectly to academic achievement (see "Affective engagement" in this chapter).

Newer Models

Other models of engagement have been forwarded in recent years with three, four, or more components (e.g., Appleton, Christenson, Kim, & Reschly, 2006; Darr, Ferral, & Stephanou, 2008; Fredricks, Blumenfeld, & Paris, 2004; Jimerson, Campos, & Greif, 2003; Libbey, 2004; Luckner, Englund, Coffey, & Nuno, 2006; Rumberger & Lim, 2008). Although different terminology makes comparison difficult, four dimensions appear repeatedly. Three correspond to the behavior component of the participation-identification model, and one corresponds to the affective component.

- *Academic engagement* refers to behaviors related directly to the learning process, for example, attentiveness and completing assignments in class and at home or augmenting learning through academic extracurricular activities. Certain minimal "threshold" levels of academic engagement are essential for learning to occur.
- *Social engagement* refers to the extent to which a student follows written and unwritten classroom rules of behavior, for example, coming to school and class on time, interacting appropriately with teachers and peers, and not exhibiting antisocial behaviors such as withdrawing from participation in learning activities or disrupting the work of other students. While a high degree of social engagement may facilitate greater learning, a low degree of social engagement usually interferes with learning, that is, it serves to moderate the connection between academic engagement and achievement.
- *Cognitive engagement* is the expenditure of thoughtful energy needed to comprehend complex ideas in order to go beyond the minimal requirements.[1] Behaviors indicative of cognitive engagement include: asking questions for the

---
[1] Adapted from Fredericks et al. (2004, p. 60).

clarification of concepts, persisting with difficult tasks, reading more than the material assigned, reviewing material learned previously, studying sources of information beyond those required, and using self-regulation and other cognitive strategies to guide learning. High levels of cognitive engagement facilitate students' learning of complex material.

- *Affective engagement* is a level of emotional response characterized by feelings of involvement in school as a place and a set of activities worth pursuing. Affective engagement provides the incentive for students to participate behaviorally and to persist in school endeavors. Affectively engaged students feel included in the school community and that school is a significant part of their own lives (belonging), and recognize that school provides tools for out-of-school accomplishments (valuing).

The components are summarized in Table 5.1. The first three indicate dynamism, or pull or, to use Marks's (2000) term, "investment." Affective engagement provides motivation for the investment of energy the others require. The four components may be exhibited by a student to different extents so it is difficult to label students as "engaged" or "disengaged." But the components tend to be highly intercorrelated so that some students are highly engaged, and others disengaged, on multiple dimensions. This is likely to have a profound effect on their achievement and persistence.

There is a fine line between academic and cognitive engagement. Academic engagement refers to observable behaviors exhibited when a student participates in class work; this was called "participation" in the participation-identification model (Finn, 1989). Cognitive engagement is an internal investment of cognitive energy, roughly speaking, the thought processes needed to attain more than a minimal understanding of the course content.

Measurement Issues

The measures used to assess student engagement usually include *indicators* of engagement or disengagement in addition to questions that address the components directly (see Table 5.1). For example, a self-report instrument for assessing affective engagement might include questions about feelings of belonging (e.g., "I feel connected to my school") plus other questions about relationships with teachers and classmates. An assessment of cognitive engagement might include students' actual recall of the processes a student used to solve a problem plus other behaviors that suggest cognitive engagement (e.g., "Student uses a dictionary or the Internet on his/her own to seek information." Student does more than just the assigned work). These two types of engagement—cognitive and affective—often require indirect measures because of the difficulty of assessing internal states directly (Appleton et al., 2006).

Table 5.1 is intended to define and delimit the components of engagement, but is not intended as an invitation to list every variable correlated with engagement. Some scales that purport to measure engagement include antecedents or consequences of engagement that lie outside the limits of the concept. We agree with Fredricks and colleagues (2004) that students' perceptions of their own abilities, parental support, peer acceptance, teacher expectations, and other difficult-to-change contextual factors should be considered as antecedents. Academic accomplishments and graduating or dropping out are consequences. Even theory-based and well-thought-out scales obfuscate this distinction. One set of instruments includes items about students' perceptions of their peers, mobility, retention in grade, parental support, academic performance, and drug and alcohol use, incorporating both antecedents and outcomes in their definition of engagement (Luckner et al., 2006). Others include questions about the fairness of school rules, the appropriateness of the tests given, parental support, feelings of safety in school, the extent to which school facilitates student autonomy, and the extent to which teachers like and support the student (Appleton et al., 2006; Darr, 2009; Luckner et al., 2006). These may all be antecedents of engagement, but none meets our criteria for engagement itself.

Table 5.1 Components of engagement and their indicators

Engagement component: definition	Primary function	Direct evidence	Other indicators (examples)
Academic (behavioral): observable behaviors related directly to the learning process	Threshold level essential for learning	Observed or self-reported student attentiveness, completing in-class and homework assignments, time on task, academic extracurricular participation	Not required
Social (behavioral): the extent to which a student follows written and unwritten classroom rules of behavior	Moderates the connection between academic engagement and achievement	Observed or self-reported attendance, social and antisocial behaviors, inattentive or disruptive behavior, speaking out of turn, refusing to follow directions	Not required
Cognitive (behavioral internal): the expenditure of thoughtful energy needed to comprehend complex ideas in order to go beyond the minimal requirements	Facilitates learning of complex or challenging material	"Think alouds," where students verbalize their cognitive processes during activity. Students reporting use of cognitive strategies while solving problems or watching a recording of their learning activity. Stimulated recall of cognitive processes	Observed or self-reports of persistence, self-regulation. Questioning of content or "going beyond the minimum" (e.g., using dictionary or Internet to gain further information). Voluntary after-school interaction with teacher
Affective: emotional response characterized by feelings of involvement in school as a place and a set of activities worth pursuing	Provides the incentive for students to participate behaviorally and to persist in school endeavors	Self-reported valuing of school, feelings of acceptance and/or belonging	Self-reports of positive reciprocal relationships with teachers and classmates

Clear definitions are also made difficult by attempts to sweep other terms under one umbrella. Liking for school, boredom, and anxiety are just that—liking for school, boredom, and anxiety (cf. Fredricks et al., 2004); no constructive purpose is served by calling them engagement. Yet some research and several reviews have included these and a plethora of other variables under the engagement umbrella (Jimerson et al., 2003; Libbey, 2004). The issue of definition needs further attention. Engagement models can be used to bolster student performance only to the extent that the components—and engagement itself—are well defined and easy for practitioners to understand.

Motivation and Engagement

The concepts of academic motivation and engagement appear to have much in common, sometimes leading to confusion. Indeed, the National Research Council book *Engaging Schools* (2004) used the terms simultaneously throughout (including a section title "Practices Enhancing Motivation and Engagement") (p. 172), without discussing similarities or differences. Academic motivation, a form germane to educational performance, has been defined as "a general desire or disposition to succeed in academic work and in the more specific tasks of school" (Newmann et al., 1992, p. 13). Affective engagement—but not academic, social, or cognitive engagement—is also an internal state that provides the impetus to participate in certain academic behaviors. According to both motivational and engagement models, the actual behaviors are shaped by the context in which they occur.

Differences between the constructs are largely a matter of focus. Theories of motivation (e.g., Connell & Wellborn, 1991; Maslow, 1970; McClelland, 1985) attribute its source to inner drives to meet underlying psychological needs, for example, the needs for competence, autonomy, and relatedness in the self-system model of Connell and Wellborn. Theories of engagement (e.g., Finn, 1989; Hirschi, 1969; Newmann, 1981; Voelkl, 1997) describe the development of affective engagement as starting with early behavior patterns and external motivators and gradually becoming internalized; the focus is on daily experiences and interactions with others.

Affective engagement is usually viewed more narrowly than is motivation or academic motivation. According to engagement models, it serves as a driving force for a specific set of school-related behaviors and interacts with those behaviors throughout the school years (Appleton et al., 2006; Finn, 1989, 1993; Fredricks et al., 2004; Furrer & Skinner, 2003; Newmann et al., 1992).

The research summarized in this chapter shows that affective engagement is more highly related to behavioral forms of engagement than to academic achievement (see review that follows). Because of its connection with behaviors conducive to learning, it may be more for helpful for understanding and enhancing educational outcomes than the broader concept of motivation.

Responsiveness to the School and Classroom Context

According to the developmental models of engagement of Connell (1990) and Finn (1989), many factors impact school engagement including the school context and the attitudes and behaviors of peers, parents, teachers, and other significant adults. It is outside the purview of this chapter to review the antecedents of engagement. However, it is a basic tenet of the concept that it is responsive to the school and classroom practices. Research listed here has identified aspects of classroom environment (the quality of student-teacher relationships, instructional approaches) and the school environment (school size, safety, rules, and disciplinary practices) found to be important. Each is described in turn.

- Substantial research has linked engagement to teacher warmth and supportiveness (Bergin & Bergin, 2009; Fredricks et al., 2004; Furrer & Skinner, 2003; Hughes, Luo, Kwok, & Lloyd, 2008; Marks, 2000; Skinner & Belmont, 1993;

Voelkl, 1995). In this research, teacher warmth is a collection of attributes including liking and being interested in their students, believing in their capabilities, and listening to their points of view. Supportive teachers show respect for each student as an individual, hold clear and consistent expectations for student behavior, and provide academic assistance for students who need it, including those who have been absent for any reason.

- Instructional approaches that require student-student interactions (e.g., cooperative learning), encourage discussion, or support the expression of students' viewpoints (e.g., use of dialogue) have been found to facilitate student engagement (Guthrie & Wigfield, 2000; Johnson, Johnson, Buckman, & Richards, 1985; Osterman, 2000; Ryan & Patrick, 2001; Wang & Holcombe, 2010). Strategies that promote in-depth inquiry and metacognition have both been found to be related to increased student engagement. These include authentic instruction in which students use inquiry to construct meaning with value beyond the classroom (Newmann, 1992; Rotgans & Schmidt, 2011) and cognitive strategy use (Greene & Miller, 1996; Guthrie & Davis, 2003).
- Organizational features of the school including school size are related to student engagement. Early studies of high school size found that smaller schools were associated with increased student participation, satisfaction and attendance, and social participation as a young adult (Lindsay, 1982, 1984). Since that time, a plethora of studies has confirmed the small school—high engagement connection (Cotton, 1996; Lee & Smith, 1993, 1995; National Research Council and Institute of Medicine, 2004). Research on small learning communities (SLCs) shows that small-school dynamics can be produced even when school buildings have large enrollments (US Department of Education, 2001). This work has found positive impacts of SLCs on various forms of student engagement (e.g., Darling-Hammond, Ancess, & Ort, 2002; Kemple & Snipes, 2000).
- Perceptions of an unsafe environment and negative school sanctions can lead to student disengagement. Surveys have indicated that teachers in up to one fourth of American schools and students across the board perceived that rules were unclear, too severe, or enforced unevenly (AFT in American Educator, 2008; Voelkl & Willert, 2006; Wehlage & Rutter, 1986). Other studies have shown that student engagement was lower when students felt unsafe or victimized (Marks, 2000; Ripski & Gregory, 2009). Discipline policies perceived as too harsh are related to social forms of disengagement and dropping out (Hyman & Perone, 1998; McNeely, Nonnemaker, & Blum, 2002), while unfairness or apparent unfairness with which rules are enforced is related to behavioral and affective disengagement (Ma, 2003; Marks, 2000; Ripski & Gregory, 2009). Fair treatment by school staff has been described as fundamental to the development of identification with school (Newmann et al., 1992).

Several interventions to increase engagement have been tried and found to be effective. For example, First Things First (Connell & Klem, 2006) is a school-wide program that attempts to increase engagement at all grade levels by improving instruction and relationships between teachers and students. The Child Development Project (Battistich, Watson, Solomon, Schaps, & Solomon, 1991) attempts to create close-knit communities in classrooms and schools, thereby promoting several forms of student engagement. Both programs have been evaluated and shown to have positive results. (See Voelkl, 2012).

Engagement and Achievement/Attainment

Recent years have produced many studies of the relationships between engagement and educational outcomes. In this section, we summarize research conducted from the 1990s to the present in three categories: (1) Research showing the importance of engagement/disengagement to learning when both are observed simultaneously. This research demonstrates that behavioral risk is a major factor in producing academic risk. (2) Research that examined the relationship between engagement/disengagement in earlier grades and academic achievement and attainment in later years. This research shows that, without intervention, behavioral risk and academic risk grow in tandem through the grades. (3) Research showing that school engagement can overcome the obstacles presented by status and academic risk factors, that is, engagement can *protect* students from harm that may accrue.

The Importance of Engagement to Learning

Academic Engagement

Students across grade levels who exhibit academic engagement behaviors, such as paying attention, completing homework and coming to class prepared, and participating in academic curricular activities, achieve at higher levels than their less academically engaged peers. These behaviors are especially important for students who face obstacles due to status risk factors such as coming from a low-income home or having a first language other than English.

Studies of inattentiveness continue to find strong correlations between students' achievement and their ability to ignore distractions, persevere on tasks, and act purposefully. A classic study of academic engagement (Rowe & Rowe, 1992) examined the attentiveness and achievement of over 5,000 children aged 5–14. Data were grouped by age (5–6, 7–8, 9–11, and 12–14 years old), but regardless of age group or other risk factors including SES and gender, significant negative correlations were found between lack of attention and reading achievement scores (r's from -0.87 to -0.48). The effects were further shown to be reciprocal: path coefficients showed that inattentive behaviors in the classroom had strong, negative effects on reading achievement and low reading achievement scores led to increased inattentiveness. Reciprocal effects were also found in a longitudinal study of low-achieving first- through third-grade students (Hughes et al., 2008). These results offer partial support for the developmental cycle postulated by Finn (1989).

Some studies combined ratings of attentiveness with other forms of classroom engagement. Across all age groups, and regardless of the approach taken, substantial correlations are found with students' academic performance. For example, in a study of 1,013 fourth graders (Finn et al., 1995), teachers rated the students on the Student Participation Questionnaire (SPQ) (see Appendix for complete questionnaire). The 28-item instrument questionnaire yields multi-item scale scores for "effort," "initiative-taking," "disruptive behavior," and "inattentive behavior" (Finn, Folger, & Cox, 1991). The effort scale included items such as "student pays attention," "student completes assigned seatwork," and "student is persistent when confronted with difficult problems"; inattentive behavior included items such as "student is withdrawn/uncommunicative," "student does not seem to know what is going on in class," and "student loses, forgets, or misplaces materials." Scale reliabilities ranged from 0.89 to 0.94.

In this study, the correlations of effort and initiative with achievement tests at the end of the school year, controlling for race, gender, and classrooms, ranged from $r=0.40$ to $r=0.59$; correlations of inattentive behavior with achievement ranged from $r=-0.52$ to $r=-0.34$. All correlations were significant at $p<.001$.[2] Further, students classified as high on inattentiveness had test scores that were substantially lower than those of nonproblematic and disruptive students.

Student- and teacher-reported engagement was correlated with classroom grades in a study of third- through sixth-grade students (grades averaged across subject areas) (Furrer & Skinner, 2003). The engagement measure included ratings of effort, attention, and persistence. While both

---

[2] Correlations for the other scales are discussed under Cognitive Engagement and Social Engagement.

correlations were significant, the correlation was higher for teacher reports of academic engagement ($r=0.57$) than for student self-reported academic engagement ($r=0.33$).

Engagement-achievement connections have been examined in the upper grades with some inconsistent findings. In a study of 586 ethnically and socioeconomically diverse tenth and 12th graders, students' self-reports yielded a total score comprised of concentration (engagement) and interest and enjoyment (not engagement); the reliability of the total scale was $\alpha=0.64$ (Shernoff & Schmidt, 2008). The total was a significant but modest predictor of students' GPAs for the entire sample ($\beta=0.11$). When the data were disaggregated by race/ethnicity, the total was significantly but negatively related to GPAs among Black students ($\beta=-0.42$). No further analysis or explanation for the negative relationship was reported.

Two studies used data from nationwide samples of students, one based on eighth grade students who participated in the National Educational Longitudinal Study of 1988 (NELS:88) (Finn, 1993) and one based on tenth grade students who participated in the Educational Longitudinal Study of 2002 (ELS:2002) (Ripski & Gregory, 2009). In the latter study, a measure of behavioral engagement was constructed from teacher ratings of students on five behaviors from the Student Participation Questionnaire; the reliability of the scale was $\alpha=.76$. Significant positive correlations were found between engagement and reading and mathematics test scores ($r=0.36$ and $r=0.39$, respectively). The data were not disaggregated by race/ethnicity. These results were consistent with those from Finn, which reported strong positive relationships between engagement and achievement tests in reading, mathematics, history, and science for all students combined.

Homework

Academic engagement in the form of homework completion was examined in relationship to academic performance in two studies (Cooper, Jackson, Nye, & Lindsay, 2001; Cooper, Valentine, Nye, & Lindsay, 1999). The amount of homework completed had small but statistically significant correlations with teacher-assigned grades among elementary students in second and fourth grades ($n=214$, $r=0.23$) and among middle- and high school students ($n=424$, $r=0.26$). Other correlations were nonsignificant, including those between homework and standardized test scores in upper-grade students, and homework with attitudes toward homework (like/interest) and beliefs about homework (helps me learn) among elementary students. The effects of homework on academic achievement need further study to understand the types of homework that may be most useful and the impact of teachers' grading or not grading homework.

Extracurricular Activities

In general, research on extracurricular activities has produced mixed results with respect to academic achievement (Feldman & Matjasko, 2005). However, when the nature of the activities is considered, a more consistent pattern emerges. Participation in academically oriented extracurricular activities, a form of academic engagement, is significantly related to academic achievement. In contrast, the relationship between athletics and achievement is generally nonsignificant, and correlations are significant but smaller when athletic and academic activities are combined.

Studies that focus on academic extracurricular activities are few and far between. A 7-year longitudinal study of 1,259 Michigan school children included measures of involvement in a limited set of academic activities, 4-year high school GPAs, and enrollment in a full-time college program (Eccles & Barber, 1999). Although the measures were limited, the regression coefficients for the two outcomes were small but statistically significant at $p<.01$ ($\beta=0.11$ for GPA, $\beta=0.13$ for full-time college), with statistical controls for gender, socioeconomic status, and student ability.

One of the most in-depth analyses used NELS:88 data for eighth- and tenth-grade girls (Chambers & Schreiber, 2004). In this study, in-school academic extracurricular activities (ISAO) were disaggregated from other forms. The all-girl sample may not have been a severe limitation because girls are significantly overrepresented in academic activities (Eccles & Barber, 1999). Participation in ISAO was the total number of academic activities, out of 16, in which a student participated. This was entered into multilevel regressions controlled for socioeconomic status and other forms of school activity. ISAO had significant positive impacts on academic achievement ($p<.001$) in all four subject areas at both grade levels when all students were considered together. When the data were disaggregated by race/ethnicity, the associations between ISAO and academic achievement were nonsignificant for African American and Latina eighth-grade girls. With only one exception, all relationships for tenth-grade girls were positive and significant regardless of race/ethnicity or subject. This study provided evidence that academic extracurricular activities have a weaker relationship with achievement in eighth grade than in tenth grade. In tenth grade, there is often a larger set of choices, and students tend to self-select either academic or nonacademic extracurricular activities.

When academic and nonacademic extracurricular activities were studied together, small-to-moderate but statistically significant correlations with academic achievement were found. For example, in a separate study using the eighth-grade data from NELS:88, all extracurricular activities considered together had weak but significant correlations with achievement in mathematics, reading, and science (Gerber, 1996). Again, race/ethnicity was an important factor: White students had higher correlations of extracurricular activities to achievement (r's from 0.16 to 0.23) than did their African American peers (r's from 0.07 to 0.13). Other research has produced similar results for students in grades 6 through 12 (Cooper et al., 1999) and for students in grades 10 and 12 (Marsh, 1992; Marsh & Kleitman, 2002). The latter also found significant small-to-moderate effects of high school extracurricular participation on university enrollment ($r=0.27$) and months spent in a university ($r=0.30$).

Qualitative and quantitative studies of the relationship of athletic activities with achievement and high school graduation (Booker, 2004; Chambers & Schreiber, 2004; Melnick & Sabo, 1992) have generally found nonsignificant associations for most students studied. However, some significant relationships were found in specific subgroups. For example, Melnick and Sabo used High School and Beyond (HS&B) to study the relationships of athletic participation with grades and graduation/dropping out among African American and Hispanic male and female students from three urbanicities. When significant interactions were discovered with urbanicity, 12 separate regressions were run for each dependent variable. Weak but significant relationships between athletic participation and grades were found among suburban African American males ($\beta=0.20$) and rural Hispanic females ($\beta=0.10$). Athletics and graduation were weakly but significantly associated among rural Black males ($\beta=0.23$), rural Hispanic females ($\beta=0.17$), and suburban Hispanic males ($\beta=0.14$). From the small number and spottiness of the significant results, the authors concluded that "athletic participation has very little academic impact on minority youth" (p. 302).

In contrast, Chambers and Schreiber's (2004) study of eighth- and tenth-grade girls revealed a significant negative relationship between sports participation and reading achievement; racial ethnic groups were not disaggregated in this study. Despite the inconsistent findings, researchers have argued that sports may be one of the few remaining forms of engagement for students at risk of total disengagement (Finn, 1989; Pittman, 1991; Yin & Moore, 2004). This hypothesis is best tested through a closer look at individual students, perhaps in a qualitative study.

Social Engagement

The written and unwritten rules of behavior, when violated, often reduce academic performance. Most research on classroom social behavior is framed in the negative, that is, one or another form of misbehavior. In this section, we focus on attendance and common forms of indiscipline, for example, disrupting the class, failure to participate in class discussions, refusing to follow directions, disrespectful behavior, and fighting.

Attendance

...omes as little surprise that school attendance ...highly related to academic achievement; time lost from exposure to teachers and teaching can only reduce the opportunity for learning. In a study of all Ohio public schools, Roby (2004) found strong significant correlations between attendance and achievement in grades 4, 6, 9, and 12 (r's from 0.54 to 0.78). The 18 urban schools with the highest all-tests-passed rates on the Ohio test of Proficiency at fourth grade had higher average attendance (95.6%) than the attendance average at the 18 urban schools with the lowest pass rates (89.6%), a highly statistically significant difference. The author estimated that a school of 400 students with a 93% attendance rate, the average for Ohio, lost 25,200 h of student instructional time per year.

The association is also strong at the student level. For example, African American freshmen's absenteeism was significantly and negatively correlated to GPAs ($r=-0.64$) in an urban high-risk high school (Steward, Steward, Blair, Hanik, & Hill, 2008). While noting that absences from school in general are negatively correlated to achievement, Gottfried (2009) differentiated between excused and unexcused absences in an investigation of second through fourth graders. The large-scale study of students in Philadelphia found that, as students trended toward more unexcused than excused absences, their grades on SAT 9 reading and math standardized tests declined. Students with 100% of their absences excused performed higher on the reading test than students with 100% unexcused absences regardless of the total number of absences. However, even excused absences began to negatively affect achievement when students reached 20 absences per year. While the author's approach was informative, the children in the study were approximately 7–9 years old and, presumably, did not make their own decisions about attending school. The author speculated that high unexcused absences were indicative of negative family environments. The issue is sufficiently provocative that we believe the study should have delved into the actual reasons for these absences.

Classroom Social (and Antisocial) Behavior

Researchers have given little attention to the antecedents and consequences of "ordinary" classroom misbehaviors except for those attributable to child psychopathology. This is despite the facts that most students misbehave one time or another and that certain classroom and school conditions may actually promote misbehavior. Ordinary misbehavior (e.g., speaking out of turn, leaving one's seat during class, refusing to follow directions, being late to class or school, talking back to the teacher, using an electronic device) interferes with teaching and learning and can potentially interrupt all students' engagement in the classroom.

In a unique study of social engagement, sixth- and seventh-grade students were asked to nominate classmates who exhibited two prosocial behaviors (e.g., shares, cooperates) and three antisocial behaviors (e.g., breaks rules) (Wentzel, 1993). Two composite scores were obtained for each student by combining the ratings in such a way as to make them comparable; these were also validated by comparing them to teacher ratings of the same students. Correlation and regression analysis showed significant relationships of both scores with grades and standardized achievement tests (correlations from $r=0.35$ to $r=0.55$) even when gender, ethnicity, absenteeism, student IQ, family structure, and teacher preference for the students were included in the equations.

In the Finn et al. (1995) study of fourth graders (above), the disruptive scale was comprised of four items: the student "acts restless, is often unable to sit still," "needs to be reprimanded," "annoys or interferes with peers' work," and "talks with classmates too much." The scale had correlations from $r=-0.29$ to $r=-0.18$ with norm-referenced and criterion-referenced achievement tests when race, gender, and teachers were controlled statistically; all were significant at $p<.001$. The decrement in achievement scores for students who were high on the disruptive behavior scale was statistically significant but not as large as the decrement due to being high on the inattentive scale. Antisocial behavior of eighth graders, defined similarly, was also found to be correlated significantly with mathematics and reading test scores, with and without statistical control for demographic characteristics (see "A study of behavioral and affective engagement in school and dropping out" in this chapter).

Cognitive Engagement

Studies of cognitive engagement and achievement have yielded mixed results, in part due to different methods of assessing internal processes. Direct assessments are accomplished by asking students to report the processes they use to learn course material, and indirect assessments use indicators that can be reported in paper-and-pencil form or observed by teachers. A direct approach was proposed by Benjamin Bloom: stimulated recall (Bloom & Broder, 1958) is a method through which events are recorded and then played back to students at a time shortly after the events occurred. During playback, the recordings are paused at critical moments, such as when a problem is posed or solved, and participants are asked to retell their thoughts or conscious actions. Stimulated recall was used later to gather data on cognitive engagement during reading and math lessons (Juliebo, Malicky, & Norman, 1998; Peterson, Swing, Stark, & Waas, 1984). To reduce bias due to the delay between the events and the time of recall, "think alouds" were developed in which verbal reports are given concurrently with the cognitive event (Afflerbach & Johnston, 1984). Think alouds, however, require cognitive effort that may detract from learning the material itself.

Indirect methods of assessment rely on observable indicators that a high level of cognitive engagement has occurred, for example, students' initiative-taking, undertaking more difficult assignments, discussing class material with the teacher after school. The Student Participation Questionnaire (Finn et al., 1991) includes teacher ratings of student initiative-taking (e.g., "Student attempts to do his/her work thoroughly and well, rather than just trying to get by") and cognitive tool use (e.g., "Student goes to dictionary, encyclopedia, or other reference on his/her own to seek information"). Self-report instruments include the Metacognitive Awareness of Reading Strategies Inventory (Mokhtari & Reichard, 2002) with items such as "I decide what to read closely and what to ignore" and "I take notes while reading to help me understand what I read."

In a pivotal study of students' cognitions, Peterson and colleagues (1984) used three approaches in collecting information on cognitive engagement of fifth-grade students: stimulated recall, videotapes of student behavior, and student questionnaires. In terms of on-task behavior, the researchers found that teacher observations were less highly correlated with student achievement ($r=0.10$) than were stimulated recall measures (r's from 0.21 to 0.33) or the attending subscale of the cognitive processing questionnaire ($r=0.48$). The analysis of cognitive functioning led the authors to conclude that "students with higher levels of attention were not merely listening passively; rather, they were more actively processing the material than students with lower attention" (p. 504).

Studies of self-regulation and use of cognitive strategies in elementary and higher grades yield significant results for some measures and not for others. In a study of 42 kindergarten and second-grade students, teacher-rated failure to self-regulate was not associated with lower reading scores in kindergarten but became a significant influence (r's from 0.37 to 0.51) on reading achievement in second grade (Howse, Lange, Farran, & Boyles, 2003). Data collection in the study also included teacher ratings of cognitive engagement indicators and a direct measure based on a computerized self-regulation task that required that the child continue to work at a job on one part of the screen while distracters were presented (SRTC-AV; Kuhl & Kraska, 1993). The SRTC-AV by itself did not correlate significantly with achievement scores for any group of students in the study.

Likewise, a combination of assessments was used to access cognitive engagement during reading by 492 ethnically diverse fourth graders (Wigfield et al., 2008). Included in this study were three measures that reflect cognitive engagement. First, teachers rated students on a short questionnaire that included three academic engagement questions and one about the use of cognitive strategies. Also, a question-writing task involved students reviewing information in a science packet and then writing as many "good questions" as possible on the topic. Questions were graded with a rubric that considered both number of questions generated and complexity of the questions written. Both variables had moderate-to-high significant correlations with scores on the Gates MacGinitie Test of Reading Comprehension: the teacher report ($r=0.57$) and the question-writing task ($r=0.74$).

In high school, English students' use of deep cognitive strategies (e. g., putting ideas in one's own words and self-regulation of what is and is not understood) was significantly correlated with classroom grades ($r=0.33$) (Greene, Miller, Crowson, Duke, & Akey, 2004), as were seventh- and eighth-graders' general strategy use in English ($r=0.14$) (Wolters & Pintrich, 1998). Cognitive strategies were also correlated to math achievement ($r=0.11$) and social studies ($r=0.22$) When the middle school students reported the use of regulatory strategies such as planning and monitoring, significant and moderate correlations between self-regulation and achievement were found ($r=0.23$ to $r=0.30$). Self-regulation appeared to have a somewhat greater effect on achievement then does general strategy use.

Although we reviewed a limited number of studies, the use of self-regulation and cognitive strategies was correlated with academic achievement in all but the youngest (kindergarten) students. Both direct and indirect measures of cognitive engagement were notable in their relationships to achievement among students in fourth and higher grades. It is possible that measures of cognitive engagement cannot capture the nuances of cognitive functioning among very young students, or, as suggested by some psychologists, the skills involved in cognitive engagement have not yet crystallized in 5- or 6-year-olds.

Affective Engagement

Like cognitive engagement, affective engagement is often assessed through external indicators rather than the internal states they reflect. In the case of affect, this leads to a wide range of measures including some that seem remote from the definition of the construct. Unlike all other forms of engagement, however, the preponderance of research suggests that affective engagement is related *indirectly* to academic achievement (See Voelkl, 2012). It appears instead to affect other forms of engagement (academic, social, cognitive) which, in turn, affect learning (Osterman, 2000).

The relationships of feelings of belonging and valuing with academic achievement, motivation, and academic and social engagement in grades 6 through 8 were examined in studies by Goodenow (1993a, 1993b) and Voelkl (1997). In these studies, affective engagement was assessed through student self-report measures. Generally, small or inconsistent positive correlations were found with grades and standardized achievement tests. In the Voelkl study, identification with school was more strongly correlated with student participation than with achievement. A large-scale study of students in grades 7 through 12 used data from the National Longitudinal Study of Adolescent Health (ADD Health) (McNeely et al., 2002). The data included a measure of school connectedness together with a number of student and school characteristics. Although grade point average was significantly related to student connectedness, the strongest predictor of school connectedness of all individual characteristics was skipping school (behavioral engagement). In a mixed-method study of 61 African American high school students, Booker (2004, 2007) also found little to link a sense of belonging to achievement. Participants' self-reports of school belonging on questionnaires counted for little or no variation in their achievement. This was corroborated by interviews. One student, when asked about the importance of sense of community in their school replied: "How is my achievement [related]? …don't think it really matters about that [belongingness]…the majority of people here are cool" (Booker, 2004, p. 138). Ninety-two percent of all student comments echoed this sentiment.

On the other hand, affective engagement is associated with a range of psychological and behavioral outcomes (Maddox & Prinz, 2003; Osterman, 2000). Students who report high levels of belonging or identification with school also display higher levels of motivation and effort than do students who report lower levels of belonging or identification (Goodenow, 1993a, 1993b; Goodenow & Grady, 1993). The correlation of scores on Goodenow's Psychological Sense of School Membership (PSSM) scale with expectations for school success in a sample of 301 urban junior high school students was $r=0.42$ $(p<.001)$ (Goodenow, 1993b). Differences in average PSSM scores among high-, medium-, and low-effort teacher ratings in a sample of 454 suburban middle-school students were statistically significant at the .001 level; effect sizes between adjacent groups were both approximately 0.5σ (estimated from results in the published report).

Low levels of belonging or identification are associated with negative behaviors including academic cheating (Voelkl & Frone, 2004), school misbehavior and discipline measures (Stewart, 2003), drug and alcohol use on school grounds (Hawkins, Catalano, & Miller, 1992; Voelkl & Frone, 2000), delinquent and antisocial behaviors (Maddox & Prinz, 2003), and high-risk health behaviors including suicidality, violence (Resnick et al., 1997), and dropping out of school (Jessor, Turbin, & Costa, 1998; Rumberger & Lim, 2008). A study of sixth- and seventh-grade students found that after controlling for family relations, effortful control, earlier conduct problems, and gender, school connectedness was negatively related to subsequent conduct problems (Loukas, Roalson, & Herrera, 2010). The interactions in the study also showed that connectedness offset the adversity presented by poor family relations or effortful control, that is, connectedness served as a protective factor.

Valuing

The belief that school provides the individual with useful outcomes may also be related to behavioral engagement and indirectly to learning, although the research base is rather sparse. The valuing component of affective engagement is distinct from general valuing of education. In an analysis of different meanings of valuing, Mickelson (1990) found that "concrete" school attitudes such as the belief that schooling pays off with good jobs were associated with positive school outcomes for Black students. More abstract attitudes were not, for example, the belief that "If everyone gets a good education, we can end poverty" (p. 51).

Concrete attitudes, or "utility," are a prominent part of Eccles's expectancy-value model of student decision-making (see Wigfield & Eccles, 2000). Research based on the model has demonstrated consistently that utility is related to students' choices and behavior. The perceived utility of school and particular courses may be important in sustaining students' participation in school—sometimes despite frustration and failure.

Student perceptions of the present and future value of literacy (reading and English) has an increasing, although still modest, effect on student achievement in the upper grades. In a study of over 5,000 students in 92 schools, perceived usefulness of reading had nonsignificant relationships with achievement among children 5–11 years of age (r's from 0.00 to 0.09) but became a weak but significant factor among students from 12 to 14 years of age ($r=0.11$) (Rowe & Rowe, 1992). Although not compared to prior years, sophomore, junior, and senior high school students' perceptions of the value of English for future goals had higher correlations with course grades ($r=0.25$ for all students combined) (Greene et al., 2004).

These findings are consistent with the participation-identification model (Finn, 1989), which proposes that identification with school (or disidentification) develops over time as a function of behavioral engagement accompanied by academic success (or failure) experiences. The model proposes further that the development of positive feelings of school belonging and valuing helps perpetuate productive behavioral engagement and academic performance.

Summary

Many studies of engagement bundle the components in various ways and some fail to provide information about the composition of their measures. Nevertheless, the picture is clear: the effects of behavioral engagement on educational accomplishments are consistently statistically significant and moderate to strong—no matter what student populations are studied, control variables taken into account or, for the most part, the composition of the measures. The effect of affective engagement on achievement is less consistent, but its relationships with behavioral engagement and high school graduation are consistently positive.

Engagement Predicts Later Achievement and Attainment

Studies of engagement show that early patterns of behavior affect students' performance in later grades. Most of these studies used large-scale longitudinal data collected on urban populations, and assessed combinations of the four types of engagement.

Longitudinal studies have identified students who are at risk of dropping out for reasons other than status risk factors. The study with the longest duration was a 14-year longitudinal study of 790 Baltimore City school children that began in first grade (Alexander, Entwisle, & Horsey, 1997). Attendance and engagement behaviors (academic, prosocial, and antisocial behaviors) were assessed in first grade by examining school. As expected, early scholastic achievement and status risk factors were predictive of dropping out. In addition, students high on the engagement scale were significantly more likely to graduate than their less-engaged peers (odds ratio=2.4). Attendance, more than tardiness or antisocial behaviors, was particularly important; first graders who missed 16 days of school were 30% less likely to graduate than students who missed 10 days or fewer. Alexander et al. concluded that habits of engagement formed at this early stage were shown to have enduring effects on student attainment.

The importance of attendance was underscored in other research that included attendance with measures of antisocial behavior, for example, studies of a large sample of sixth-grade students in Philadelphia (Balfanz, Herzog, & Iver, 2007) and eighth-grade students in Houston (Kaplan, Peck, & Kaplan, 1995). In the Philadelphia study, four warning flags of school problems in sixth grade were identified (absenteeism, suspensions for poor behavior, low math or reading scores). Of these, attendance rates of 80% or less were the most predictive of failure to graduate on time or in the following year.

A 9-year longitudinal study followed ethnically and socioeconomically diverse children from kindergarten through eighth grade (Ladd & Dinella, 2009). Students were identified as having either stable (high or low) or changing (increasing or decreasing) levels of engagement. Students who exhibited stable but poor combined engagement behaviors (e.g., school avoidance, not following rules, defiance) from first through third grade made less academic progress through eighth grade than did those who had stable but higher combined engagement. First graders with equivalent achievement had markedly different trajectories if they were increasingly behaviorally engaged, as opposed to those who decreased in behavioral engagement, ultimately resulting in lower grades on achievement tests for decreasingly engaged eighth graders. Thus, students with either high stable engagement or increasing engagement had higher levels of achievement in eighth grade than their less-engaged peers.

Beyond High School

Postsecondary outcomes have been found to be affected by engagement in elementary and high school. Using national longitudinal data (NELS:88) on students when they were in grades 8 through 12 and of college age, Finn (2006) examined three sets of predictors: demographic characteristics (status risk variables), high school achievement and attainment (academic risk variables), and measures of school engagement (behavioral risk variables). Four composites were formed for each participant in high school reflecting academic participation (extracurricular participation), social engagement (attendance, classroom behavior) and affective engagement (students' perceptions of the usefulness of school subjects).

In regressions that controlled for status and academic risk factors, attendance and classroom behavior were significantly related to all three postsecondary variables studied: entering a postsecondary program, the number of credits earned, and completing a postsecondary program (odds ratios of 1.2–1.5). Participation in extracurricular activities was related to entering a postsecondary institution (odds ratio of 1.4), but not to credits earned or completion of program. The affective measure, perceived usefulness of school subjects, was not related to any postsecondary outcome. When employment and income were examined at age 26, the results were weak or nonsignificant. Only 2 out of 12 possible relationships were significant, those of high school attendance with current employment and classroom behavior with consistency of employment. For the most part, engagement in high school did not impact employment as a young adult.

Research done in Chicago schools corroborated these findings (Ou, Mersky, Reynolds, & Kohler, 2007) and extended the conclusions to adult criminal behavior by age 24. A troublemaking composite score (social engagement) in grades 3 through 6 was a significant predictor of incarceration and conviction (odds ratios of 1.4 and 1.5, respectively). Neither academic engagement nor attendance was significantly related to the income or measures of criminal behavior (conviction or incarceration).

Summary

The principle that continuing engagement throughout from the earliest grades onward is important to high school graduation and participation in postsecondary education. Academic and social engagement stand out as especially salient, although we could not locate any predictive studies of cognitive engagement and found only one recent study that included affective engagement

Engagement Mediates the Effects of Status and Academic Risk Factors

Resilient students are those who can overcome the barriers posed by status or academic risk factors to achieve acceptable outcomes. The study of resilience is important to help identify the factors that distinguish these individuals from their less successful peers in order to apply those principles to other students at risk. Research has shown that school engagement in the early, middle, and upper grades all contribute to student resilience.

Students who were considered at risk in grades 1 through 6 due to home factors (57% poverty, 42% single parent households, school in a high-crime neighborhood) participated in an evaluation of the Seattle Social Development Project ($n=643$) (Hawkins, Guo, Hill, Battin-Pearson, & Abbott, 2001). The 18 participating schools were assigned to one of three conditions: full intervention in grades 1 through 6 designed specifically to increase student engagement, late intervention in grades 5 and 6 only, and a control (no intervention). Each year from age 13 to age 18, teachers rated students on academic, cognitive, and affective dimensions of engagement. At age 13 and every subsequent age, the groups showed substantial differences with the order full intervention group having the highest engagement and the control group the lowest. The groups diverged, and differences became larger still in the period from 16 to 18 years. Further, the engaged-at-18 students had higher GPAs, a lower history of arrests, fewer instances of dropping out, and less cigarette, alcohol, and drug use than did the other groups.

Several studies explored engagement and resilience during transitions from elementary to middle or junior high school. A study of 62 African American students from low-income homes noted a significant drop in GPAs between fifth ($M=2.25$) and sixth grade ($M=2.05$), but affective engagement was shown to protect against this drop (Gutman & Midgley, 2000). After controlling for psychological characteristics, home background, and prior achievement, a high sense of school belonging combined with high parental involvement was related to elevated sixth grade GPAs; the mean GPA in sixth grade for students with high affective engagement was approximately 3.2.

A second study examined the adverse effects of parent and teacher "role strains," that is, pressure placed on adolescents by parents' and teachers' expectations (de Bruyn, 2005). In a Dutch study of 749 students just entering secondary school, role strain negatively impacted academic achievement ($r=-0.19$ to $r=-0.36$). A measure of academic engagement was shown to mediate these effects; students high on the scale had higher achievement despite the role strain they felt. In all, academic engagement increased the prediction of academic achievement from $R^2=0.09$ to $R^2=0.36$. Academic engagement and achievement in the study were highly correlated ($r=.50$). Both studies demonstrated the roles of home and school factors in bolstering student resilience across school transitions.

A nationwide American study was based on a high-risk sample of eighth graders who participated in the NELS:88 longitudinal survey. The sample comprised 1,803 African American and Hispanic students who attended public schools and lived in homes in the lower half of the SES distribution, based on a composite of parents' education, parents' occupations, and household income (Finn & Rock, 1997). Students were classified into three groups based on academic performance in eighth and tenth grade and dropout status in 12th grade: a small group of resilient completers (8.4%) with math and reading test scores at or above the 40th percentile for all students, self-reported GPA's of "half B's and half C's" or better, and who would graduate with their class at the culmination of 12th grade; nonresilient completers who did not meet the achievement criteria but were still in school in 12th grade; and nonresilient dropouts who were reported as having left without graduating. Seven academic and social engagement measures were recorded for each student (three teacher-reported, four student-reported), plus sports and academic extracurricular activities.

Even when the analysis controlled for demographic factors, self-esteem, and locus of control, resilient completers were significantly higher than both groups of nonresilient students on five out of six measures of social and academic engagement, that is, lower rates of absenteeism, higher levels of classroom effort and homework, and fewer behavior problems. Differences were large, with effect sizes for the significant variables ranging from 0.47σ to 0.84σ. Only student self-reports of being prepared for class and participation in sports and academic curricular activities did not relate to student resilience.

A Study of Behavioral and Affective Engagement and Dropping Out[3]

Little if any research has explored the development of engagement and its relationship to achievement over time, and even less has examined the connection between affective engagement and dropping out of school. This study, based on the participation-identification model (Finn, 1989), was designed to investigate dropping out as a developmental process related to students' behavioral and affective engagement in grades 4 and 8. We used a unique data set in which achievement scores were recorded from kindergarten through eighth grade, engagement measures were obtained at several intervals, and high school graduation was later recorded. The three primary research questions were (1) Is

---

[3] A partial version of this report was presented to the American Educational Research Association (Pannozzo, Finn, & Boyd-Zaharias, 2004). The authors are grateful to Gina Pannozzo for her excellent work and contributions to the execution of the study.

behavioral engagement (academic and social) in grades 4 and 8 related to graduation/dropping out of high school above and beyond the effects of academic achievement during the same time period? (2) Is affective engagement in grade 8 related to graduation/dropping out? (3) Does affective engagement explain graduation/dropping out above and beyond the effects of behavioral engagement? The results presented here represent a first look at this database.

Procedures

Participants

Participants in this study were a subset of students who participated in Tennessee's Project STAR, a longitudinal class-size reduction experiment. Students entered the study in kindergarten or first grade and were followed through high school. To be included in this study, they were required to have graduation/dropout information from high school transcripts or State Department of Education records and to have been rated on the grade-4 and/or grade-8 engagement instruments. The final sample of 2,728 students was similar to the full STAR sample of 11,600 students in all ways except the sample for this study had a higher percentage of White/Asian students (74.9% compared to 63.1%) and a higher percentage of students not eligible for free lunches (55.3% compared to 44.0%). Free lunch and race/ethnicity served as control variables in all analyses.

In each phase of the analysis, the sample included students who had key variables in grade 4 and/or grade 8. The fourth grade sample consisted of 1,421 students from 123 schools and the eighth-grade sample had 2,191 students from 119 schools. There were 753 students with both grade-4 and grade-8 data.

Measures

Achievement score composites in reading and math were derived for each student in grades K through 3 and in grades 6 through 8, respectively. Each composite was the first principal component of norm-referenced and criterion-referenced tests administered in the respective subject in spring of each school year.

Academic and social engagements were measured through teacher ratings of individual students on the Student Participation Questionnaire (SPQ; see Appendix) (Finn et al., 1991). Fourth-grade teachers completed a questionnaire in November for up to ten randomly chosen students in her class. Eighth-grade reading and mathematics teachers completed a shortened version of the questionnaire (14 of the same items), yielding two ratings of each student. For this study, two subscales were created from the SPQ, one that measured academic engagement as defined in Table 5.1 (e.g., paying attention, participating in class discussion, completing assignments) and one that measured social/antisocial engagement (e.g., needing to be reprimanded, acting restless, interfering with classmates' work). In fourth grade, these scales had 16 and 7 items, respectively; scale reliabilities were $\alpha=0.95$ and $\alpha=0.85$. The eighth-grade scales had 6 and 5 items, respectively; scale reliabilities were $\alpha=0.89$ and $\alpha=0.81$.

Identification with school was assessed with the Identification with School Questionnaire (Voelkl, 1996) given to students in grade 8. The questionnaire is comprised of 16 items that assess students' sense of belonging in and valuing of school. Belonging items include "I feel proud of being a part of this school" and "The only time I get attention in school is when I cause trouble." Valuing of school includes items such as "School is one of the most important things in my life" and "I can get a good job even if my grades are bad." Confirmatory factor analysis of the scale indicated that it is best scored as a single dimension (Voelkl, 2012). For this study, the reliability of the total scale was $\alpha=0.84$.

Analysis

The three research questions were answered through a series of two-level multilevel logistic regression analyses using the HLM program (Raudenbush, Bryk, & Congdon, 2000) with graduate/dropout as the dependent variable. In all analyses, student variables were centered around the school mean, and school variables were

Table 5.2 Variables used in HLM analysis for each research question

Level of data	Variables	Question (1)	Question (2)	Question (3)
Level-1 (students)	*Dependent variable*			
	Graduate/dropout from high school	X	X	X
	Independent variables			
	Grade 4 academic engagement	X[a]		
	Grade 8 academic engagement	X[b]		X
	Grade 4 social engagement	X[a]		
	Grade 8 social engagement	X[b]		X
	Grade 8 affective engagement[c]		X	X
	Gender	X	X	X
	Race ethnicity			
	White/Asian students–minority students	X	X	X
	Free-lunch eligibility	X	X	X
	Reading achievement composite Grades K-3	X[a]		
	Reading achievement composite Grades 6–8	X[b]	X	X
	Mathematics achievement composite Grades K-3	X[a]		
	Mathematics achievement composite Grades 6–8	X[b]	X	X
Level-2 (schools)	School urbanicity			
	Suburban/urban schools–inner-city schools	X	X	X
	Rural schools–inner-city schools	X	X	X
	School enrollment	X	X	X

[a]Used in grade-4 analysis only
[b]Used in grade-8 analysis only
[c]Identification with school

grand-mean-centered. All effects were treated as fixed except for the student and school intercepts, which were treated as random. A type-1 error rate (α) of .01 was used throughout.

Each analysis was conducted with two runs of HLM. The first run included all the main effects listed in Table 5.2 for the particular question. In the second run, specific interactions were added to the model: the interactions of each engagement scale in the respective analysis with gender and free-lunch eligibility (student-level interactions) and with school enrollment (student-by-school-level interactions). These interactions indicate whether the effects of engagement on graduating/dropping out varied as a function of gender, family income groups, or school enrollment. For effects that involved more than a single independent variable (i.e., academic achievement, academic and social engagement, urbanicity), a blockwise test was conducted to see if the pair of variables were jointly related to graduation/dropping out before tests of the individual variables were conducted.

Tests of significance reveal whether a relationship is statistically reliable, but tell little about whether effects are weak or strong. A strength-of-effect measure in logistic regression is the odds ratio. If the independent variable is dichotomous (e.g., female/male), the odds ratio is the odds that a member of the first group (female) would graduate from high school divided by the odds that a member of the second group (male) would graduate. Odds ratios much below 1.0 or much above 1.0 indicate strong effects; 1.0 would be obtained if the odds for both groups were the same. Odds below 1.0 are sometimes "inverted" to make them easier to understand. For example, if the odds for the first group are one third as large as the odds for the second group, the ratio would be 0.33, which is a bit awkward to think about. It is simpler to say that the odds for the second group are three times that of the first group; this is $1.0 \div 0.33 = 3.0$. If the independent variable is continuous (e.g., academic, social, or affective engagement), the odds ratio is the change in odds associated with a one-standard deviation change

Table 5.3 Graduation rates of sample by demographic characteristics

Variable	Fourth grade ($n=1,421$)	Eighth grade ($n=2,141$)
Gender		
Male	82.6	81.8
Female	91.4	89.3
Race/ethnicity		
White/Asian	89.5	87.4
Minority	78.0	80.9
Free lunch		
Yes	78.7	76.2
No	93.8	92.8
All	87.1	85.8

Results

The percentage of students who graduated from high school was 87.1% in the fourth-grade sample and 85.8% in the eighth-grade sample (Table 5.3). For both samples, graduation rates were higher for females than for males, for Asian/White students than for minority students, and for students who were not eligible for free or reduced-price lunches.

The correlations among the main variables of the study (Table 5.4) are consistent. With the exception of eighth-grade reading with identification, all correlations were significant at $p<.01$. In both grades, academic and social engagement were moderately positively correlated with reading and mathematics, with stronger correlations for academic engagement than for social engagement (r's from 0.44 to 0.54 for academic engagement, r's from 0.33 to 0.36 for social). Academic and social engagement were moderately and positively correlated with high school graduation (r's from 0.23 to 0.32). Identification with school in eighth grade had lower correlations with achievement ($r=0.04$ and $r=0.09$) and with dropping out ($r=0.09$) but larger correlations with academic and social engagement ($r=0.26$ and $r=0.22$). in the particular engagement measure. Odds ratios are presented together with significance levels for each independent variable in the regressions.

Is Behavioral Engagement in Grades 4 and 8 Related to Graduation/Dropping Out of High School?

In this study, we asked whether behavioral engagement in fourth grade was related to graduation/dropping out. The analysis had statistical controls for other precursors of dropping out (race/ethnicity, SES, and academic achievement in prior grades).

The fourth-grade and eighth-grade analyses produced similar results for background characteristics (Table 5.5). In general, students in suburban/urban and rural schools were two to three times more likely to graduate than were students in inner-city schools (odds ratios from 2.1 to 3.2). Neither the enrollment of students' elementary schools nor their eighth-grade schools was significantly related to high school dropout rates. Data from both grades indicated that females were more likely to graduate from high school than were males (Table 5.3), but the difference was only marginally significant in eighth grade. Students not eligible for free or reduced lunches were approximately three times as likely to graduate from high school as were students who were eligible ($1 \div 0.33$ and $1 \div 0.34$ for fourth and eighth grade, respectively). In eighth grade, White students were less likely to graduate than were minority students (opposite the direction in Table 5.3). This was an artifact of the distribution of minority students among schools; many schools had one to three minority students with a graduation rate of 100%.

Behavioral engagement and graduation/dropout. The correlations of academic and social engagement with graduation were small to moderate but statistically significant (Table 5.4). The regressions revealed that, as a set, academic and social engagement in fourth and eighth grades were significantly related to high school completion (Table 5.5). When the two forms of behavioral engagement were viewed separately, only academic participation was statistically significant in fourth grade. The odds ratio indicated that a one-standard deviation increase in academic engagement scale in fourth grade would double a student's odds of graduating (odds ratio=2.1). Social behavior did not add to the prediction of

Table 5.4 Correlations among academic, social, and affective engagement, achievement, and graduation

Variable	Academic engagement	Social engagement	Reading achievement	Mathematics achievement	Identification with school[a]	Graduation[b]
Academic engagement	–	0.72**	0.54**	0.52**	N/A	0.29**
Social engagement	0.71**	–	0.36**	0.34**	N/A	0.22**
Reading achievement	0.44**	0.33**	–	0.78**	N/A	0.21**
Mathematics achievement	0.50**	0.33**	0.79**	–	N/A	0.23**
Identification with school[a]	0.26**	0.22**	0.04*	0.09**	–	N/A
Graduation[b]	0.31**	0.32**	0.27**	0.26**	0.09**	–

Note: Correlations for fourth grade are presented above the diagonal, and correlations for eighth grade are presented below the diagonal
*$p<.05$; **$p<.01$
[a] Not assessed in fourth grade
[b] 1 = graduation, 0 = dropout

Table 5.5 Summary of multilevel logistic regression analysis for graduation/dropout with academic and social engagement in grades 4 and 8

	Grade 4		Grade 8	
Predictor variable	Beta	Odds ratio[a]	Beta	Odds ratio[a]
School level				
Enrollment	.001*	1.00	4.2×10^{-4}	
Suburban/urban–inner city	.719*	2.05	.964**	2.62
Rural–inner city	1.173***	3.23	.770*	2.16
Student level				
Behavioral engagement[b]	**≤.001**		**≤.001**	
Academic	.053***	2.05	.123***	1.69
Social	.002		.111**	1.34
Female–male	.614**	1.85	.316*	1.37
White/Asian–minority	−.159		−1.221***	0.30
Free lunch (yes–no)	−1.078***	0.34	−1.112***	0.33
Achievement[b]	**.114**		**≤.001**	
Reading composite	−.251		.227	
Mathematics composite	.352	1.37	.252	
Student level interactions				
Gender × engagement[b]	**.093**		**>.500**	
Academic	.022		.032	
Social	−.104*		−.061	
Free-lunch × engagement[b]	**>.500**		**.348**	
Academic	.007		.072	
Social	−.014		.101	
Student × school interactions				
Engagement × enrollment[b]	**>.500**		**.348**	
Academic	2.5×10^{-4}		3.4×10^{-4}	
Social	-2.2×10^{-4}		-1.1×10^{-4}	

Note: School- and student-level main effects tested first (not controlling for interactions). Interactions tested in separate analyses, controlling for main effects
*$p<.05$; **$p<.01$; ***$p<.001$
[a] Odds ratios for significant effects computed from main-effect analysis
[b] Bolded values are *p* values for blockwise test of the pair of variables

Table 5.6 Summary of multilevel logistic regression analysis for graduation/dropout including identification with school

Predictor variable	Without behavioral engagement		With behavioral engagement	
	Beta	Odds ratio[a]	Beta	Odds ratio[a]
School level				
Enrollment	4.4×10^{-4}		4.2×10^{-4}	
Suburban/urban–inner city	.950**	2.59	.969**	2.64
Rural–inner city	.844**	2.33	.773**	2.17
Student level				
Behavioral engagement[b]			**≤.001**	
Academic			.120***	1.67
Social			.109**	1.33
Identification with school	.037**	1.26	.011	
Female–male	.555***	1.74	.295	
White/Asian–minority	−1.151***	0.32	−1.211***	0.30
Free lunch (yes–no)	−1.131***	0.32	−1.121***	0.33
Achievement[b]	**≤.001**		**≤.001**	
Reading composite	.223*	1.26	.234	
Mathematics composite	.550***	1.79	.247	
Student level interactions				
Gender × identification with school	−.013		N/A	
Free-lunch × identification with school	−.021		N/A	
Student × school interactions				
Enrollment × identification	-5.1×10^{-4}		N/A	

Note: School- and student-level main effects tested first (not controlling for interactions). Interactions tested in separate analyses, controlling for main effects
*$p < .05$. **$p < .01$. ***$p < .001$
[a] Odds ratios for significant effects computed from main-effect analysis
[b] Bolded values are *p* values for blockwise test of the pair of variables

high school graduation at this point in students' schooling.

Students' academic and social behaviors in eighth grade, considered independently and jointly, were significantly related to graduation. The odds ratios for the two separate measures were 1.69 and 1.34, respectively. That is, a one-standard deviation increase in academic engagement increased the odds of graduating from high school by 69%; a one-standard deviation increase in social engagement increased the odds of graduating by 34%. These results were obtained even after academic achievement, and individual student and school characteristics were controlled statistically. Of the two, academic engagement appeared consistently more important than social engagement.

The interactions of behavioral engagement with school enrollment, gender, and free lunch were all nonsignificant. That is, the impact of academic and social participation on graduating/dropping out is approximately the same for males and females, higher and lower SES students, and in smaller and larger schools.

Is Affective Engagement in Grade 8 Related to Graduation/Dropping Out?

By the time the students reached eighth grade, they had undergone many experiences that could affect their chances of completing high school, for example, transition from elementary grades to middle or junior high school, a series of academic successes and/or failures, changes in school, and changes in attitudes to school. All of these can promote or discourage the development of identification with school.

The correlation between identification with school and graduation/dropping out in Table 5.4

was small but statistically significant ($r=0.09$, $p<.01$). The regression analysis (Table 5.6) showed a statistically significant positive effect as well. Students who identified more positively with school were more likely to graduate than were students with lower levels of identification. A one-standard deviation increase in identification in eighth grade increased the odds of graduating by 26% (odds ratio=1.26), above and beyond the effects of academic achievement in grades 6 through 8 and student and school characteristics. Affective engagement appeared to be an important factor in sustaining a student's persistence through high school, although the effect was not as strong as that of behavioral engagement (Table 5.5).

None of the interactions of identification with gender, free-lunch eligibility, and school enrollment were statistically significant. The impact of identification with school on the likelihood of graduating was similar for male and female students, students from higher- and lower-SES homes, and smaller and larger schools alike.

Does Affective Engagement Explain Graduation/Dropping Out Above and Beyond Behavioral Engagement?

The measures of affective and behavioral engagement in eighth grade were significantly correlated with each other ($r=0.26$ and $r=0.22$). Of these, behavioral engagement (academic and social) had higher correlations with achievement and dropping out than did affective engagement. In a regression analysis of eighth-grade data, the blockwise test of both behavioral measures, and of each individual measure, was virtually unchanged by the addition of identification with school to the model (right-hand portion of Table 5.6). That is, above and beyond identification with school, and above and beyond actual school performance, the academic and social behaviors of eighth graders continued to contribute to high school graduation. A one-standard deviation increase in academic engagement increased the odds of attaining a high school diploma by 67% (odds ratio=1.67) and a one-standard deviation increase in social engagement by 33% (odds ratio=1.33).

Can a similar conclusion be drawn for affective engagement? When behavioral engagement was included in the model, the effect of identification with school became nonsignificant. Although affective engagement alone was correlated with whether or not students graduated or dropped out of high school, it contributed less, if anything, above and beyond observable academic and social behaviors. Consistently with research cited in this chapter, it appears that identification with school affected academic achievement and attainment indirectly through its impact on students' classroom behavior.

Summary and Discussion

The results of the study are summarized in Table 5.7. Academic and social engagement in fourth and eighth grade contributed to students' decisions to remain in school and graduate or to leave school early. Academic engagement predominated; its connection with high school graduation is stronger than that of social participation. These connections were robust, that is, they were found to be significant when achievement levels and affective engagement in eighth grade were controlled statistically, and the absence of significant interactions with gender, SES, or school location indicates that it applies similarly to subgroups of students.

Students who are academically and socially engaged in school are likely to have higher achievement and to receive positive responses from teachers for their work and behavior. These forms of reinforcement help students maintain habits of high engagement throughout the grades, leading to school completion. Students who are not engaged academically or who exhibit negative social behaviors create academic risk: they have lower achievement levels and are more likely to experience frustration and to receive negative responses from teachers. Continued nonengagement, accompanied by low or failing

Table 5.7 Summary of regression analysis for predicting graduation/dropping out

Question/variable(s)	Odds ratios and p values	
	Grade 4	Grade 8
Question 1: Is behavioral engagement in grades 4 and 8 related to graduation/ dropping out of high school?		
Answer 1: Yes, in both grades		
Behavioral engagement (academic and social)	$p<.001$[a]	$p<.001$[a]
Unique effect of academic engagement	2.1**	1.7**
Unique effect of social engagement	NS	1.3*
Question 2: Is affective engagement in grade 8 related to graduation/dropping out?		
Answer 2: Yes, weak association		
Affective engagement (identification with school)	–	1.3*
Question 3: Does affective engagement explain graduation/ dropping out above and beyond behavioral engagement?		
Answer 3: No		
Behavioral engagement controlling for affective engagement	–	$p<.001$[a]
Unique effect of academic engagement	–	1.7**
Unique effect of social engagement	–	1.3*
Affective engagement controlling for behavioral engagement	–	NS

Note: Odds ratios only given for significant effects
NS not statistically significant
*$p<.01$; **$p<.001$
[a]Tests of pairs of predictors (no odds ratios)

grades and negative responses from teachers, increases the likelihood of dropping out.

Exactly how affective engagement and other school-related attitudes influence achievement and persistence is not clear. The data of this study indicated that identification with school may promote academic and social engagement. However, it had a weak correlation with dropping out when considered by itself and did not contribute to dropping out above the impact of observable behavior. More research on the role of affective engagement is needed.

Much remains to be done with the data. The same variables would benefit for being assembled into an inclusive structural equation model in which direct and indirect effects of the independent variables on dropping out and the effects of the independent variables on one another could be examined simultaneously. Other variables could also be considered including characteristics of the teachers and the schools. The analysis is continuing.

Implications: Student Engagement and Disengagement

It is well supported by empirical research that engagement is a precursor to academic achievement and attainment. Further, forms of engagement are intuitive, observable, and easily understood by teachers as being important to learning. The impact of engagement is both direct (e.g., paying attention or completing assignments) and indirect (e.g., antisocial behavior that disrupts instruction thus interfering with learning opportunities). The research reviewed in this chapter shows that (a) engagement has a concurrent impact on academic achievement. The connection is likely to be reciprocal, that is, high achievement is likely to promote continuing engagement and low achievement is likely to discourage further engagement; (b) engagement in early and middle grades is predictive of achievement and attainment in later grades, even up through the postsecondary years; and

(c) engagement behaviors and attitudes can help students overcome the obstacles presented by status and academic risk factors, including factors associated with behavior problems outside of school.

Unfortunately, many students fail to become fully engaged, and others begin to disengage at some point during their schooling. This can lead to academic problems, mild and severe forms of misbehavior, and attenuated school careers. Status and academic risk factors are sometimes used as explanations for these problems, for example, students' attitudes are poor ("blame the student"), single parents, parents who do not monitor their children's behavior or who are not involved with school activities are at the root of the problem ("blame the family"), and/or friends or street life are not conducive to staying in school ("blame the community").

The engagement/disengagement perspective acknowledges that behavioral risk is at least partially situated in the school and classroom and thus partially under our control. It assumes that engagement develops over a period of years—an assumption supported by empirical data presented in this chapter. This view has strong implications for educators: efforts to prevent disengagement should be targeted toward the elementary and middle grades as well as high school. Unlike the status- and academic-risk explanations, attention is focused on behaviors that are wholly or partially manipulable and responsive to school and classroom practices.

This perspective also emphasizes that engagement is multifaceted, although scholars have somewhat different views about what the components are. The four components presented in this chapter—academic, social, cognitive, and affective—are ingredients common to multiple definitions; they avoid ingredients outside the concept of engagement, and they are conceptually distinct. Each plays a different role in supporting academic outcomes, and each, if weak or lacking, contributes to academic or behavior problems or early school leaving.

At this point in time, extensive research into the antecedents or consequences of academic and social engagement is unlikely to produce much in the way of new understandings. The research discussed in this chapter and the other chapters in this book show that a very large knowledge base is already in place.

In contrast, three areas need further research and development. First, *research on cognitive engagement* is disjointed and needs to be assembled into a consistent explanatory framework. Most studies have been conducted in specific academic subjects, leaving questions about commonalities unanswered. For example, is cognitive engagement subject specific or do students have general propensities to become cognitively engaged (or not engaged) in all subjects? If so, what is the nature of these propensities and how can they be assessed? How do students develop the capacity to be cognitively engaged and how do they remain cognitively engaged outside a specific setting? And finally, how is the learning that results from cognitive engagement different from learning without the in-depth thinking it requires? A theoretical perspective that brings diverse findings together into one broad framework would be informative.

Second, we have limited understanding of *how affective engagement develops*. On one hand, research has explored the relationship of academic achievement with specific forms of affect, for example, liking for school and school subjects, liking the teacher(s), academic motivation, frustration, and boredom. On the other hand, the theory and research summarized in this chapter indicate that early transitory forms of affect evolve into more stable forms in later grades. To our knowledge, no study has examined this assertion in depth or in its entirety.

There is pressing need for research that (a) assesses various forms of affect experienced in early grades to examine the relationships among them, (b) examines stability and change in affect as students mature, and the experiences that affect stability and change, and (c) examines the relationship between affect that is more transitory and affect that is more trait-like and generalizes across settings within schools or between one school and the next school a student attends. This research would need to be longitudinal and incorporate both quantitative and qualitative approaches.

The third area in need of further work involves application more than theory: *creating more complete ways to identify students at risk of nonengagement or disengagement.* The approach advocated most widely is to consider the characteristics of students and their school experiences. This is exemplified in the What Works Clearinghouse's dropout prevention guide (Dynarski et al., 2008). The first recommendation, of seven, is "Utilize data systems that… help identify individual students at high risk of dropping out" (p. 10); the recommendation is accompanied by a list of student risk factors such as academic problems, truancy, behavior problems, retentions, and academic and social performances.

This approach does not give adequate attention to the school context. In this chapter, we have identified four conditions of the school setting that promote engagement—teacher warmth and supportiveness, instructional approaches that encourage student participation, small school size, and a safe environment with fair and effective disciplinary practices—and there are more. When these conditions are less than optimal, or lacking altogether, the likelihood of student disengagement goes up. To date, there have been few if any attempts to assess the classroom and school context in addition to student characteristics to identify the threats to student engagement. A package of assessments for this purpose would involve observations of students in the school setting, observations of teacher-student interactions (with specific foci), and reactions from students themselves. It would help guide interventions to make classrooms and schools more conducive to student engagement.

Appendix

Fourth Grade

Student Participation Questionnaire

The codes in parentheses indicate the subscale to which the item belongs:

	Subscale reliability
E = Effort	.94
I = Initiative	.89
N = Nonparticipatory behavior	.89
V = Value	.68

The sign (+, −) indicates the direction of scoring. Items marked "−" should be reverse-scored before summing the items in the subscale.
(Items 29–31 are not part of these subscales).

Notes:
The items in this questionnaire have been combined in different ways for use in different research studies.

This questionnaire is in the public domain and may be used without permission. Notification to the author is requested.

The eighth-grade version of the questionnaire is available from the author upon request.

Fourth Grade

Student Participation Questionnaire

Student's Name:_____
_____

Below are items that describe children's behavior in school. Please consider the behavior of the student named above over the last 2–3 months. Circle the number that indicates how often the child exhibits the behavior. Please answer every item.

Thank you for your time. Please enclose the teacher/class information sheet and all the questionnaires—those completed and not complete—in the envelope provided and return it to your principal.

	This student:	Never		Sometimes		Always
(E+)	1. pays attention in class	1	2	3	4	5
(E+)	2. completes homework on time	1	2	3	4	5
(E+)	3. works well with other children	1	2	3	4	5
(E−)	4. loses, forgets, or misplaces materials	1	2	3	4	5
(E−)	5. comes late to class	1	2	3	4	5
(I+)	6. attempts to do his/her work thoroughly and well, rather than just trying to get by	1	2	3	4	5
(N+)	7. acts restless, is often unable to sit still	1	2	3	4	5
(I+)	8. participates actively in discussions	1	2	3	4	5
(E+)	9. completes assigned seat work	1	2	3	4	5
(V+)	10. thinks that school is important	1	2	3	4	5
(N+)	11. needs to be reprimanded	1	2	3	4	5
(N+)	12. annoys or interferes with peers' work	1	2	3	4	5
(E+)	13. is persistent when confronted with difficult problems	1	2	3	4	5
(E−)	14. does not seem to know what is going on in class	1	2	3	4	5
(I+)	15. does more than just the assigned work	1	2	3	4	5
(I−)	16. is withdrawn, uncommunicative	1	2	3	4	5
(E+)	17. approaches new assignments with sincere effort	1	2	3	4	5
(V−)	18. is critical of peers who do well in school	1	2	3	4	5
(I+)	19. asks questions to get more information	1	2	3	4	5
(N+)	20. talks with classmates too much	1	2	3	4	5
(E−)	21. does not take independent initiative, must be helped to get started, and kept going on work	1	2	3	4	5
(E−)	22. prefers to do easy problems rather than hard ones	1	2	3	4	5
(V−)	23. criticizes the importance of the subject matter	1	2	3	4	5
(E+)	24. tries to finish assignments even when they are difficult	1	2	3	4	5
(I+)	25. raises his/her hand to answer a question or volunteer information.	1	2	3	4	5
(I+)	26. goes to dictionary, encyclopedia, or other reference on his/her own to seek information	1	2	3	4	5
(E−)	27. gets discouraged and stops trying when encounters an obstacle in schoolwork, is easily frustrated	1	2	3	4	5
(I+)	28. engages teacher in conversation about subject matter before or after school, or outside of class	1	2	3	4	5
	29. attends other school activities such as athletic contests, carnivals, and fund-raising events	1	2	3	4	5
	30. The student's overall academic performance is	Above average 1		Average 2		Below average 3
	31. Does this student attend special education classes outside of your classroom?			No 1		Yes 2

References

Afflerbach, P. P., & Johnston, P. (1984). Research methodology: On the use of verbal reports in reading research. *Journal of Reading Behavior, 14*, 307–322.

Alexander, K. L., Entwisle, D. R., & Horsey, C. S. (1997). From first grade forward: Early foundations of high school dropout. *Sociology of Education, 70*, 87–107.

Alexander, K. L., Entwisle, D. R., & Kabbani, N. S. (2001). The dropout process in life course perspective: Early risk factors at home and school. *Teachers College Record, 103*, 760–822.

American Federation of Teachers. (2008). We asked, you answered. *American Educator, 32*(2), 6–7.

Anderson, L. W. (1975). Student involvement in learning and school achievement. *California Journal of Educational Research, 26*(2), 53–62.

Anderson, L. W., & Scott, C. C. (1978). The relationship among teaching methods, student characteristics, and student involvement in learning. *Journal of Teacher Education, 29*(3), 52–57.

Appleton, J. J., Christenson, S. L., Kim, D., & Reschly, A. L. (2006). Measuring cognitive and psychological engagement: Validation of the student engagement instrument. *Journal of School Psychology, 44*, 427–445.

Balfanz, R., Herzog, L., & Iver, D. J. M. (2007). Preventing student disengagement and keeping students on the graduation path in urban middle-grades schools: Early identification and effective interventions. *Educational Psychologist, 42*, 223–235.

Battistich, V., Watson, M., Solomon, D., Schaps, E., & Solomon, J. (1991). The Child Development Project: A comprehensive program for the development of prosocial character. In W. M. Kurtines & J. L. Gewirtz (Eds.), *Handbook of moral behavior and development* (Vol. 3, pp. 1–34). Hillsdale, NJ: Erlbaum.

Berenson, G. S. (1986). Evolution of cardiovascular risk factors in early life: Perspectives on causation. In G. S. Berenson (Ed.), *Causation of cardiovascular risk factors in children: Perspectives on cardiovascular risk in early life* (pp. 1–26). New York: Raven.

Bergin, C., & Bergin, D. (2009). Attachment in the classroom. *Educational Psychology Review, 21*, 141–170.

Berliner, D. C. (1990). *The nature of time in schools: Theoretical concepts, practitioner perceptions*. New York: Teachers College Press.

Bloom, B. S., & Broder, L. (1958). *Problem-solving processes of college students*. Chicago: The University of Chicago Press.

Booker, K. C. (2004). Exploring school belonging and academic achievement in African American adolescents. *Curriculum and Teaching Dialogue, 6*(2), 131–143.

Booker, K. C. (2007). Likeness, comfort, and tolerance: Examining African American adolescents' sense of school belonging. *The Urban Review, 39*, 301–317.

Breslow, L., Fielding, J., Afifi, A. A., Coulson, A., Kheifets, L., Valdiviezo, N., et al. (1985). *Risk factor update project: Final report* (Contract No. 200–80–0527). Atlanta, GA: U.S. Department of Health and Human Services, Centers for Disease Control, Center for Health Promotion and Education.

Broidy, L. M., Nagin, D. S., Tremblay, R. E., Bates, J. E., Brame, B., Dodge, K. A., et al. (2003). Developmental trajectories of childhood disruptive behaviors and adolescent delinquency: A six-site, cross-national study. *Developmental Psychology, 39*, 222–245.

Chambers, E. A., & Schreiber, J. B. (2004). Girls' academic achievement: Varying associations of extracurricular activities. *Gender and Education, 16*, 327–346.

Connell, J. P. (1990). Context, self and action: A motivational analysis of self-system processes across the life span. In D. Cicchetti & M. Beeghly (Eds.), *The self in transition: Infancy to childhood* (pp. 61–97). Chicago: University of Chicago Press.

Connell, J. P., & Klem, A. M. (2006). First things first: What it takes to make a difference. In R. W. Smith (Ed.), *Time for change: New visions for high school* (pp. 15–40). Cresskill, NJ: Hampton Press.

Connell, J. P., Spencer, M. B., & Aber, J. L. (1994). Educational risk and resilience in African-American youth: Context, self, action, and outcomes in school. *Child Development, 65*, 493–506.

Connell, J. P., & Wellborn, J. G. (1991). Competence, autonomy, and relatedness: A motivational analysis of self-system processes. In M. R. Gunnar & L. A. Sroufe (Eds.), *Self processes and development: The Minnesota symposia on child development* (Vol. 23, pp. 43–77). Hillsdale, NJ: Erlbaum.

Cooper, H., Jackson, K., Nye, B., & Lindsay, J. J. (2001). A model of homework's influence on the performance evaluations of elementary school students. *The Journal of Experimental Education, 69*, 181–199.

Cooper, H., Valentine, J. C., Nye, B., & Lindsay, J. J. (1999). Relationships between five after-school activities and academic achievement. *Journal of Educational Psychology, 91*, 369–378.

Cotton, K. (1996). *School size, school climate, and student performance* (Close-up No. 20, Series X). Portland, OR: School Improvement Research Service, Northwest Regional Educational Laboratory.

Darling-Hammond, L., Ancess, J., & Ort, S. (2002). Reinventing high school: Outcomes of the Coalition Campus Schools Project. *American Educational Research Journal, 39*, 639–673.

Dar, C, (2009). The *Me and My School* survey. In J. Morton (Ed.), *Engaging young people in learning: why does it matter and what can we do?* (pp.85–100). Wellington NZ: NZCER press.

Darr, C., Ferral, H., & Stephanou, A. (2008, January). *The development of a scale to measure student engagement*. Paper presented at the Third International Rasch Measurement Conference, Perth, Western Australia.

de Bruyn, E. H. (2005). Role strain, engagement and academic achievement in early adolescence. *Educational Studies, 31*(1), 15–27.

deJung, J. K., & Duckworth, K. (1986, April). *Measuring student absences in the high schools*. Paper presented at the annual meeting of the American Educational Research Association, San Francisco, CA.

Dynarski, M., Clarke, L., Cobb, B., Finn, J., Rumberger, R., & Smink, J. (2008). *Dropout prevention: A practice guide* (NCEE 2008–4025). Washington, DC: National Center for Education Evaluation and Regional Assistance, Institute of Education Sciences, U.S. Department of Education.

Eccles, J. S., & Barber, B. L. (1999). Student council, volunteering, basketball, or marching band: What kind of extracurricular involvement matters? *Journal of Adolescent Research, 14*, 10–43.

Elliott, D. S., & Voss, H. L. (1974). *Delinquency and dropout*. Lexington, MA: D. C. Heath.

Feldman, A. F., & Matjasko, J. L. (2005). The role of school-based extracurricular activities in adolescent development: A comprehensive review and future directions. *Review of Educational Research, 75*, 159–210.

Finn, J. D. (1989). Withdrawing from school. *Review of Educational Research, 59*, 117–142.

Finn, J. D. (1993). *School engagement and students at risk* (NCES report 93–470). Washington, DC: U.S. Department of Education, National Center for Education Statistics.

Finn, J. D. (2006). *The adult lives of at-risk students: The roles of attainment and engagement in high school* (NCES 2006–328). Washington, DC: U. S. Department of Education, National Center for Educational Statistics.

Finn, J. D., Folger, J., & Cox, D. (1991). Measuring participation among elementary grade students. *Educational and Psychological Measurement, 51*, 393–402.

Finn, J. D., Pannozzo, G. M., & Voelkl, K. E. (1995). Disruptive and inattentive-withdrawn behavior and achievement among fourth graders. *The Elementary School Journal, 95*, 421–434.

Finn, J. D., & Rock, D. A. (1997). Academic success among students at risk for school failure. *Journal of Applied Psychology, 82*, 221–234.

Fisher, C. W., Berliner, D. C., Nikola, N., Filby, R. M., Cahen, L. C., & Dishaw, M. M. (1980). Teaching behaviors, academic learning time, and student achievement: An overview. In C. Denham & A. Lieberman (Eds.), *Time to learn* (pp. 7–32). Washington, DC: U.S. Department of Education, National Institute of Education.

Fredricks, J. A., Blumenfeld, P. C., & Paris, A. H. (2004). School engagement: Potential of the concept, state of the evidence. *Review of Educational Research, 74*, 59–109.

Furrer, C., & Skinner, E. (2003). Sense of relatedness as a factor in children's academic engagement and performance. *Journal of Educational Psychology, 95*, 148–162.

Gerber, S. B. (1996). Extracurricular activities and academic achievement. *Journal of Research & Development in Education, 30*(1), 42–50.

Goodenow, C. (1993a). Classroom belonging among early adolescent students: Relationships to motivation and achievement. *The Journal of Early Adolescence, 13*(1), 21–43.

Goodenow, C. (1993b). The psychological sense of school membership among adolescents: Scale development and educational correlates. *Psychology in the Schools, 30*, 79–90.

Goodenow, C., & Grady, K. E. (1993). The relationship of school belonging and friends' values to academic motivation among urban adolescent students. *The Journal of Experimental Education, 62*, 60–71.

Gottfried, M. A. (2009). Excused versus unexcused: How student absences in elementary school affect academic achievement. *Education Evaluation and Policy Analysis, 31*, 392–415.

Greene, B. A., & Miller, R. B. (1996). Influences on achievement: Goals, perceived ability and cognitive engagement. *Contemporary Educational Psychology, 21*, 181–192.

Greene, B. A., Miller, R. B., Crowson, H. M., Duke, B. L., & Akey, K. L. (2004). Predicting high school students' cognitive engagement and achievement: Contributions of classroom perceptions and motivation. *Contemporary Educational Psychology, 29*, 462–482.

Guthrie, J. T., & Davis, M. H. (2003). Motivating struggling readers in middle school through an engagement model of classroom practice. *Reading & Writing Quarterly: Overcoming Learning Difficulties, 19*(1), 59–85.

Guthrie, J. T., & Wigfield, A. (2000). Engagement and motivation and reading. In P. Kamil, P. D. Mosenthal, P. D. Pearson, & R. Barr (Eds.), *Handbook of reading research* (Vol. III, pp. 403–424). Mahwah, NJ: Lawrence Erlbaum.

Gutman, L. M., & Midgley, C. (2000). The role of protective factors in supporting the academic achievement of poor African American students during the middle school transition. *Journal of Youth and Adolescence, 29*, 223–248.

Hawkins, J. D., Catalano, R. F., & Miller, J. Y. (1992). Risk and protective factors for alcohol and other drug problems in adolescence and early adulthood: Implications for substance abuse prevention. *Psychological Bulletin, 112*, 64–105.

Hawkins, J. D., Guo, J., Hill, K. G., Battin-Pearson, S., & Abbott, R. D. (2001). Long-term effects of the Seattle Social Development intervention on school bonding trajectories. *Applied Developmental Science, 5*, 225–236.

Hindelang, M. J. (1973). Causes of delinquency: A partial replication and extension. *Social Problems, 20*, 471–487.

Hirschi, T. (1969). *Causes of delinquency*. Berkeley, CA: University of California Press.

Howse, R. B., Lange, G., Farran, D. C., & Boyles, C. D. (2003). Motivation and self-regulation as predictors of achievement in economically disadvantaged young children. *The Journal of Experimental Education, 71*, 151–174.

Hughes, J. N., Luo, W., Kwok, O.-M., & Loyd, L. K. (2008). Teacher-student support, effortful engagement, and achievement: A 3-year longitudinal study. *Journal of Educational Psychology, 100*, 1–14.

Hyman, I. A., & Perone, D. C. (1998). The other side of school violence: Educator policies and practices that may contribute to student misbehavior. *Journal of School Psychology, 36*, 7–27.

Jessor, R., Turbin, M. S., & Costa, F. M. (1998). Risk and protection in successful outcomes among disadvantaged adolescents. *Applied Developmental Science, 2*, 194–208.

Jimerson, S. R., Campos, E., & Greif, J. L. (2003). Toward an understanding of definitions and measures of school engagement and related terms. *California School Psychologist, 8*, 7–27.

Johnson, D. W., Johnson, R. T., Buckman, L. A., & Richards, P. S. (1985). The effect of prolonged implementation of cooperative learning on social support within the classroom. *The Journal of Psychology, 119*, 405–411.

Juliebo, M., Malicky, G. V., & Norman, C. (1998). Metacognition of young readers in an early intervention programme. *Journal of Research in Reading, 21*, 24–35.

Kanungo, R. N. (1979). The concepts of alienation and involvement revisited. *Psychological Bulletin, 86*, 119–138.

Kaplan, D. S., Peck, B. M., & Kaplan, H. B. (1995). A structural model of dropout behavior: A longitudinal analysis. *Applied Behavioral Science Review, 3*, 177–193.

Kemple, J. J., & Snipes, J. C. (2000). *Career academics: Impacts on students' engagement and performance in high school*. New York: Manpower Demonstration Research Corporation.

Klem, A. M., & Connell, J. P. (2004). Relationships matter: Linking teacher support to student engagement and achievement. *Journal of School Health, 74*, 262–273.

Kuhl, J., & Kraska, K. (1993). Self-regulation: Psychometric properties of a computer-aided instrument. *German Journal of Psychology, 17*, 11–24.

Ladd, G. W., & Dinella, L. M. (2009). Continuity and change in early school engagement: Predictive of children's achievement trajectories from first to eighth grade? *Journal of Educational Psychology, 101*, 190–206.

Lee, V. E., & Smith, J. B. (1993). Effects of school restructuring on the achievement and engagement of middle-grade students. *Sociology of Education, 66*, 164–187.

Lee, V. E., & Smith, J. B. (1995). Effects of high school restructuring and size on early gains in achievement and engagement. *Sociology of Education, 68*, 241–270.

Libbey, H. P. (2004). Measuring student relationships to school: Attachment, bonding, connectedness, and engagement. *Journal of School Health, 74*, 274–283.

Lindsay, P. (1982). The effect of high school size on student participation, satisfaction, and attendance. *Educational Evaluation and Policy Analysis, 4*, 57–65.

Lindsay, P. (1984). High school size, participation in activities, and young adult social participation: Some enduring effects of schooling. *Educational Evaluation and Policy Analysis, 6*, 73–83.

Liska, A. E., & Reed, M. D. (1985). Ties to conventional institutions and delinquency: Estimating reciprocal effects. *American Sociological Review, 50*, 547–560.

Loeber, R., & Stouthamer-Loeber, M. (1998). Juvenile aggression at home and at school. In D. S. Elliot, B. Hamburg, & K. R. Williams (Eds.), *Violence in American schools: A new perspective* (pp. 84–126). New York: Cambridge University Press.

Loukas, A., Roalson, L. A., & Herrera, D. E. (2010). School connectedness buffers the effects of negative family relations and poor effortful control on early adolescent conduct problems. *Journal of Research on Adolescence, 20*, 13–22.

Luckner, A. E., Englund, M. M., Coffey, T., & Nuno, A. A. (2006). Validation of a global measure of school engagement in early and middle adolescence. In M. M. Englund (Chair.), *Adolescent engagement in school: Issues of definition and measurement* symposium conducted at the biennial meeting of the Society for Research on Adolescence, San Francisco, CA.

Ma, X. (2003). Sense of belonging to school: Can schools make a difference? *The Journal of Educational Research, 96*, 340–349.

Maddox, S. J., & Prinz, R. J. (2003). School bonding in children and adolescents: Conceptualization, assessment, and associated variables. *Clinical Child and Family Psychology Review, 6*, 31–49.

Marks, H. M. (2000). Student engagement in instructional activity: Patterns in the elementary, middle and high school years. *American Educational Research Journal, 37*, 153–184.

Marsh, H. W. (1992). Extracurricular activities: Beneficial extension of the traditional curriculum or subversion of. *Journal of Educational Psychology, 84*, 553–562.

Marsh, H. W., & Kleitman, S. (2002). Extracurricular school activities: The good, the bad, and the nonlinear. *Harvard Educational Review, 72*, 464–514.

Maslow, A. (1970). *Motivation and personality* (2nd ed.). New York: Harper & Row.

McClelland, D. C. (1985). *Human motivation*. Dallas, TX: Scott Foresman.

McNeely, C. A., Nonnemaker, J. M., & Blum, R. W. (2002). Promoting school connectedness: Evidence from the National Longitudinal Study of Adolescent Health. *Journal of School Health, 72*, 138–146.

Melnick, M. J., & Sabo, D. F. (1992). Educational effects of interscholastic athletic participation on African-American and Hispanic youth. *Adolescence, 27*, 295–308.

Mickelson, R. A. (1990). The attitude-achievement paradox among black adolescents. *Sociology of Education, 63*, 44–61.

Mokhtari, K., & Reichard, C. A. (2002). Assessing students' metacognitive awareness of reading strategies. *Journal of Educational Psychology, 94*, 249–259.

National Research Council and The Institute of Medicine [NRC & IOM]. (2004). *Engaging schools: Fostering high school students' motivation to learn.* Washington, DC: The National Academies Press.

Newmann, F. M. (1981). Reducing student alienation in high schools: Implications of theory. *Harvard Educational Review, 51,* 546–564.

Newmann, F. M. (1992). *Student engagement and achievement in American secondary schools.* New York: Teachers College Press.

Newmann, F. M., Wehlage, G. G., & Lamborn, S. D. (1992). The significance and sources of student engagement. In F. M. Newmann (Ed.), *Student engagement and achievement in American secondary schools* (pp. 11–30). New York: Teachers College Press.

Osterman, K. F. (2000). Students' need for belonging in the school community. *Review of Educational Research, 70,* 323–367.

Ou, S. R., Mersky, J. P., Reynolds, A. J., & Kohler, K. M. (2007). Alterable predictors of educational attainment, income, and crime: Findings from an inner-city cohort. *The Social Service Review, 81,* 85–128.

Pannozzo, G. M., Finn, J. D., & Boyd-Zaharias, J. (2004, April). *Behavioral and affective engagement in school and dropping out.* Paper presented at the annual meeting of the American Educational Research Association, San Diego, CA.

Patrick, B., Skinner, E., & Connell, J. (1993). What motivates children's behavior and emotion? Joint effects of perceived control and autonomy in the academic domain. *Journal of Personality and Social Psychology, 65,* 781–791.

Peterson, P. L., Swing, S. R., Stark, K. D., & Waas, G. A. (1984). Students' cognitions and time on task during mathematics instruction. *American Educational Research Journal, 21,* 487–515.

Pittman, R. B. (1991). Social factors, enrollment in vocational/technical courses, and high school dropout rates. *The Journal of Educational Research, 84,* 288–295.

Raudenbush, S. W., Bryk, A. S., & Congdon, R. T. (2000). *HLM 5 for Windows.* Lincolnwood, IL: Scientific Software International, Inc.

Resnick, M. D., Bearman, P. S., Blum, R. W., Bauman, K. E., Harris, K. M., Jones, J., et al. (1997). Protecting adolescents from harm: Findings from the national longitudinal study on adolescent health. *Journal of the American Medical Association, 278,* 823–832.

Ripski, M. B., & Gregory, A. (2009). Unfair, unsafe, and unwelcome: Do high school students' perceptions of unfairness, hostility, and victimization in school predict engagement and achievement? *Journal of School Violence, 8,* 355–375.

Roby, D. E. (2004). Research on school attendance and student achievement: A study of Ohio schools. *Educational Research Quarterly, 28*(1), 3–14.

Rotgans, J. I., & Schmidt, H. G. (2011). Situational interest and academic achievement in the active-learning classroom. *Learning and Instruction, 21*(1), 58–67.

Rowe, K. J., & Rowe, K. S. (1992). The relationship between inattentiveness in the classroom and reading achievement: Part A: Methodological issues. *Journal of the American Academy of Child and Adolescent Psychiatry, 31,* 349–356.

Rumberger, R. W. (1987). High school dropouts: A review of issues and evidence. *Review of Educational Research, 57,* 101–121.

Rumberger, R. W. (2001, January). *Why students drop out of school and what can be done.* Paper presented at the forum Dropouts in America: How severe is the problem? What do we know about intervention and prevention? Cambridge, MA: Harvard University, Civil Rights Project.

Rumberger, R. W., & Lim, S. A. (2008). *Why students drop out of school: A review of 25 years of research* (Project Report No. 15). Santa Barbara, CA: University of California, California Dropout Research Project.

Ryan, A. M., & Patrick, H. (2001). The classroom social environment and changes in adolescents' motivation and engagement during middle school. *American Educational Research Journal, 38*(2), 437–460.

Shernoff, D., & Schmidt, J. (2008). Further evidence of an engagement-achievement paradox among U.S. high school students. *Journal of Youth and Adolescence, 37,* 564–580.

Skinner, E. A., & Belmont, M. J. (1993). Motivation in the classroom: Reciprocal effect of teacher behavior and student engagement across the school year. *Journal of Educational Psychology, 85,* 571–581.

Skinner, E., Kindermann, T., Connell, J., & Wellborn, J. (2009). Engagement and disaffection as organizational constructs in the dynamics of motivational development. In *Handbook of motivation at school* (pp. 223–245). New York: Routledge/Taylor & Francis Group.

Steinberg, L., & Avenevoli, S. (1998). Disengagement from school and problem behavior in adolescence: A developmental-contextual analysis of the influences of family and part-time work. In R. Jessor (Ed.), *New perspectives in adolescent risk behavior* (pp. 392–424). New York: Cambridge University Press.

Steward, R. J., Steward, A. D., Blair, J., Hanik, J., & Hill, M. F. (2008). School attendance revisited: A study of urban African American students' grade point averages and coping strategies. *Urban Education, 43,* 518–536.

Stewart, E. A. (2003). School social bonds, school climate, and school misbehavior: A multilevel analysis. *Justice Quarterly, 20,* 575–604.

Swift, M. S., & Spivack, G. (1968). The assessment of achievement-related classroom behavior: Normative, reliability and validity data. *Journal of Special Education, 2,* 137–153.

Swift, M. S., & Spivack, G. (1969). Achievement-related classroom behavior of secondary school normal and disturbed students. *Exceptional Children, 35,* 677–684.

US Department of Education. (2001). *An overview of smaller learning communities in high schools.* Washington, DC: Office of Elementary and Secondary Education and Office of Vocational and Adult Education.

Voelkl, K. E. (1995). School warmth, student participation, and achievement. *The Journal of Experimental Education, 63*, 127–138.

Voelkl, K. E. (1996). Measuring students' identification with school. *Educational and Psychological Measurement, 56*, 760–770.

Voelkl, K. E. (1997). Identification with school. *American Journal of Education, 105*, 294–318.

Voelkl, K. E. (2012). School identification. In S. L. Christenson, A. L. Reschly, & C. Wylie (Eds.), *Handbook of research on student engagement* (pp. 193–218). New York: Springer.

Voelkl, K. E., & Frone, M. R. (2000). Predictors of substance use at school among high school students. *Journal of Educational Psychology, 92*, 583–592.

Voelkl, K. E., & Frone, M. R. (2004). Academic performance and cheating: Moderating role of school identification and self-efficacy. *The Journal of Educational Research, 97*, 115–122.

Voelkl, K. E., & Willert, H. J. (2006). Alcohol and drugs in schools: Teachers' reactions to the problem. *Phi Delta Kappan, 88*(1), 37–40.

Wang, M., & Holcombe, R. (2010). Adolescents' perceptions of school environment, engagement, and academic achievement in middle school. *American Educational Research Journal, 47*, 633–662.

Wehlage, G. G., & Rutter, R. A. (1986). Dropping out: How much do schools contribute to the problem? *Teachers College Record, 87*, 374–392.

Wehlage, G. G., Rutter, R. A., Smith, G. A., Lesko, N., & Fernandez, R. R. (1989). *Reducing the risk: Schools as communities of support*. Philadelphia: Falmer Press.

Weitzman, M., Klerman, L. V., Lamb, G. A., Kane, K., Geromini, K. R., Kayne, R., et al. (1985). Demographic and educational characteristics of inner city middle school problem absence students. *The American Journal of Orthopsychiatry, 55*, 378–383.

Wentzel, K. R. (1993). Does being good make the grade? Social behavior and academic competence in middle school. *Journal of Educational Psychology, 85*, 357–364.

Wigfield, A., & Eccles, J. S. (2000). Expectancy-value theory of achievement motivation. *Contemporary Educational Psychology, 25*, 68–81.

Wigfield, A., Guthrie, J. T., Perencevich, K. C., Taboada, A., Klauda, S. L., McRae, A., et al. (2008). Role of reading engagement in mediating effects of reading comprehension instruction on reading outcomes. *Psychology in the Schools, 45*, 432–445.

Wolters, C. A., & Pintrich, P. R. (1998). Contextual differences in student motivation and self-regulated learning in mathematics, English and social studies classrooms. *Instructional Science, 26*, 27–47.

Yin, Z., & Moore, J. B. (2004). Re-examining the role of interscholastic sport participation in education. *Psychological Reports, 94*(3, Pt 2), 1447–1454.

Part I Commentary: So What Is Student Engagement Anyway?

Jacquelynne Eccles and Ming-Te Wang

Abstract

This chapter, by the esteemed motivation scholar Jacque Eccles and Ming-Te Wang, provides a commentary on the five chapters in Part I. The authors offered additional critique of the issues raised by authors in this part, as well as their perspectives on future directions for the engagement construct. In addition, Eccles and Wang described links between the theories of engagement and the Expectancy-Value Theoretical Model of Achievement-Related Behavior espoused by Eccles.

These chapters provide excellent overviews of the current thinking in the broad field of engagement. Doing the commentary has provided us with a great opportunity to think through our own take on student engagement as a concept. We have been working closely for the last year on a series of papers most directly related to the Frederick et al.'s (Fredricks, Blumenfeld, & Paris, 2004) perspective on school engagement. Both of us have been less involved with the work on engagement growing out of Finn's participation-identification theory and the work on dropout prevention and whole school reform. Reading all five of these chapters with an eye toward writing this commentary has helped me (Eccles) put this collaborative work into a much larger framework. We both thoroughly enjoyed reading each of these chapters and came away from reading them much better informed about engagement theory (ET) and its incredible importance for our thinking about school success and school reform. By and large, the authors of each of the chapters did an admirable job of summarizing the extant theory and research relevant to their chapter as well as critiquing the field and proposing important and promising future directions. Our goal was not to repeat their conclusions but to offer additional critiques and future directions as well as to expand the range of theoretical perspectives considered to be relevant to the general idea of school and classroom engagement.

We have divided our comments into several parts. In the first, we comment directly on each of the five chapters and end with a few summary comments on the full set of chapters. In the second part, we discuss our thinking on the general topic of these five chapters – what is student engagement? In the third part, I (Eccles) discuss my view on the link between general ET and my own work on school success. I focus

J. Eccles (✉) • M.-T. Wang
Institute for Social Research, University of Michigan,
Ann Arbor, MI, USA
e-mail: jeccles@umich.edu; wangmi@umich.edu

more specifically on the links I see between general ET and the Eccles et al. (1983) expectancy-value theoretical model of achievement-related behavior (EEVT).

Comments on Specific Chapters

These five chapters provide a very broad review of the ways in which student engagement (SE) has been conceptualized, defined, and measured as well as a comprehensive review of the extant literature on the association of SE with school achievement. The chapters represented a breadth of perspectives and approaches to the study of SE that will open the eyes of all but the most well-versed reader. This is even truer of the entire volume, which includes perspectives from several fields outside of educational and developmental psychology. The diversity of fields represented makes it likely that most readers will be exposed to previously unknown work. In addition, the looser format of an edited volume allowed the authors to expand more freely in their writing than is normally allowed in the tight confines of a journal article. Because the intended audience of this volume includes both researchers and practitioners, many authors also discussed applied aspects of their work that rarely appear in published research articles. Thus, reading these chapters will provide readers with broader insights into the research than is possible in journal accounts of their scientific findings.

This part begins with an overview chapter by Reschly and Christenson (2012). In this chapter, they discuss the conceptual haziness that has emerged in this field as the definition of SE has broadened. They point out the need for greater clarity. They also point out the overlap between four basic theories of engagement and discuss the important relevance of ET for designing and evaluating school intervention efforts aimed at reducing school dropout. The chapter provides an excellent introduction to this part by laying the groundwork for the other four chapters. We reiterate several of Reschly and Christenson's critiques about the definition of SE in our discussion.

Finn and Zimmer (2012) provide an even more extensive review of the research most directly linked to Finn's perspective on ET. Although not entirely the case, much of the research they review has emerged either from Finn's early participation-identification theory or from work on dropout prevention and school misbehavior. Reading this chapter made it clear to us that two fairly parallel lines of research on school success have been going over the last 20–30 years: (1) the work grounded in ET and linked closely to dropout prevention and at-risk populations – a tradition that includes scholars like Finn, Newmann, Wehlage, Reschly, and Rumburger (see the chapters by Reschly and Christenson and by Finn and Zimmer for extensive reviews of this tradition) – and (2) the work grounded in psychological motivation theory that is more closely linked to academic motivation within the classroom learning context – a tradition that includes scholars associated with self-determination theory, achievement goal theory, achievement motivation theory, attribution theory, self-efficacy theory, and expectancy-value theory of achievement (e.g., scholars such as Anderman, Bandura, Blumenfeld, Connell, Deci, Dweck, Eccles, Elliott, Meece, Midgley, Pintrich, Roeser, Schunk, Skinner, and Wigfield; see Wigfield, Eccles, Schiefele, Roeser, & Davis-Kean, 2006 for a full review of this tradition). Scholars in each of these traditions have tried to understand the psychological characteristics that underlie both academic success and failure. In each tradition, a wide variety of constructs has emerged and extensive research has documented the association of these various constructs with indicators of school success, ranging from basic learning to school completion. What is clear in reading Finn and Zimmer is how separate these two traditions have been from each other despite a quite common goal. As members of the second of these two traditions, we greatly appreciated the breadth of Finn and Zimmer's review of the work from the first tradition. We also appreciated the clear implication of this work for school interventions.

Skinner and Pitzer (2012) provide an excellent overview of an alternative theory of engagement

– one based in the second tradition alluded to in the previous paragraph – self-determination theory (SDT). This model stresses the importance of intrinsic motivation and the ways in which social contextual features facilitate the emergence of intrinsic motivation to engage in a task. In this sense, SDT focuses attention on the precursors of behavioral engagement and assumes that positive engagement is most likely when the context provides opportunities for individuals to fulfill their needs for competence, belonging, and autonomy. Skinner and Pitzer further hypothesize that teacher warmth, adequate structure, and support for autonomy are the three contextual features mostly likely to meet these needs and thus facilitate engagement. Although Skinner and Pitzer begin by stressing their view that "engagement is the outward manifestation of motivation," they then enlarge their definition of engagement to bring it more in line with the broader view of SE salient in all five of these chapters. They do this by including both a behavioral and an emotional component to their definition of engagement. By so doing, they increase the overlap between SDT and ET substantially. They add to the ET theorists' view of engagement a theoretical perspective on the immediate contextual precursors most likely to influence behavioral and cognitive engagement in the classroom. They also add a very thoughtful discussion of disengagement as a key construct and discuss the types of coping behaviors that will either facilitate or undermine learning and achievement. By bringing in these ideas, they focus attention on classroom-level engagement in learning activities, and they acknowledge that disengagement might be an appropriate coping response in some contexts.

Not surprisingly, we like this chapter very much because we are quite familiar and comfortable with Skinner and Pitzer's way of framing their approach to the issue of motivation, engagement, and learning. We particularly like their emphasis on engagement as the behavioral manifestation of motivation. We would add to this the idea that engagement is also the behavioral manifestation of social and personal identities (see Eccles, 2009, and later part in this commentary).

By so doing, we are broadening Skinner and Pitzer's perspective to include something akin to Finn's notion of identification and to the kinds of identity-based self-system beliefs discussed by Bingham and Okagaki (2012) and to a more limited extent by Mahatmya, Lohman, Matjasko, and Farb (2012).

Mahatmya et al. (2012) provide a developmental perspective on student engagement. They link the ideas associated with notions of developmental tasks and developmental stages to age-related changes in the three types of engagement proposed by Fredricks et al. (2004): behavioral, emotional, and cognitive. This chapter is much more speculative than the other four chapters in this part because there has been less research and less theorizing about developmental changes in engagement. As noted by these authors, the most developmental work directly related to the idea of student engagement is the work done by Eccles, Midgley, and their colleagues under the notion of stage-environment fit (see Eccles et al., 1993). Hopefully, this chapter will stimulate such work in the future.

We do have one concern about the chapter that should be voiced as a cautionary note, given the early state of this line of scholarship. To their credit, the authors try to bring in thinking from the new neuroscience of brain growth and development. It is important that we take the cognitive neuroscience perspective seriously as we consider developmental changes in things like student engagement. But we are uncomfortable with the use of terms like "more cognitive engagement" rather than a different type of cognitive engagement to describe the nature of such changes. For example, they say, "during adolescence, individuals experience rapid physical maturation as well as rapid development of cognitive skills. …Thus, the ability to become cognitively engaged with school is greater during adolescence compared to both early and middle childhood." Although the first statement may be correct (however, early brain development is pretty rapid and major neurological changes are also going on in the age 5–7 shift), the second is very controversial and may not be true. It is not even clear to us what evidence one would look at to demonstrate that the "ability to become cognitively engaged is greater during adolescence." This depends on what is defined as cognitive engagement. To the extent that cognitive engagement includes the mental behaviors associated with learning, then it is not clear to us that learning to read and write evidences less cognitive engagement than learning algebra. These two learning tasks may require different types of cognitive engagement, and the brain maturation occurring during adolescence may allow for different and more conscious forms of cognitive engagement than were available during early and middle childhood. At this point, we need to be cautious when using terms like "more" rather than "different," particularly if we are talking about the extent to which individuals use their "full capacity" to be cognitively engaged at each point in development as our marker of individual differences in the extent of cognitive engagement.

Finally, Bingham and Okagaki (2012) provide a very comprehensive review of the literatures aimed at understanding ethnicity and student engagement. Essentially, this chapter focuses on the more distal precursors of student engagement. They draw on several theoretical frameworks and research traditions, including SDT, ET, critical race theory, various sociocultural theories, ecological theories, person-environment fit theories, collective identity theories, social psychological perspective of race, discrimination, and identity and social developmental theories of contextual influences. This makes for a very rich chapter, particularly because they have skillfully interweaved these various theoretical frameworks to help us understand very subtle nuances in ethnic differences in student engagement. Thus, this chapter, like Skinner and Pitzer (2012), focuses on the precursors of engagement, focusing in particular on the three categories of engagement set out by Fredricks et al. (2004). We wish they had been more specific when they reported the findings of various studies as to exactly which subtypes of engagement was actually measured and when engagement was measured as opposed to learning and achievement.

General Comments on This Part

As noted earlier, each of these five chapters provides the reader with solid overviews of the literature related to student engagement at school within the frame of the chapter. In each of these five chapters, the authors also point out a variety of future directions that could help us better understand student engagement. We agree with the authors that developing (1) a more integrative developmental-contextual approach to investigate the individual and contextual factors that predict student engagement, and (2) appropriate instruments to measure student engagement at different levels is critical. To develop appropriate theories, we agree with the authors that it is important to revisit current relevant theories, such as SDT, person-environment fit theory, flow theory, and expectancy-value theory, for more integrated insights into the nature of and influences on student engagement.

A related approach could be to synthesize or modify existing theories. The chapter by Skinner and Pitzer (2012) on the self-system model of motivational development is an excellent example of such an approach. Yet another approach for studying SE would be to build new models or theories that could be applied to classroom settings as well as to situations outside the classroom. Such models or theories could focus more on person-centered approaches. For example, they could focus on the ways in which behavior, emotion, and cognition develop as coordinated engagement-related processes in some individuals but as more disconnected aspects of engagement in others. These person-centered patterns cannot easily be studied using the kinds of linear or hierarchical conceptualizations presented in these five chapters. New approaches might also use patterns of engagement over time to explain and predict effective learning experiences within multiple contexts across time.

There is also a great need for better measures and methods of study, particularly after more comprehensive theories of SE and learning have emerged. We cannot know whether we are improving student engagement unless we can measure it accurately and appropriately. Neither can we design good programs to improve SE until we better understand which aspects of student engagement influence which aspects of learning and performance for which students. In addressing complex questions such as how different types of SE are involved in learning, we need to think carefully about such measurement issues as (1) how we define the constructs that we are measuring or recording, (2) how we achieve internal and external validity, and (3) how we interpret our findings. Such measurement and interpretation issues will necessarily include *multiple perspectives*, *multiple methods*, and *multiple levels*. Student engagement processes are relational and dynamic; they involve ongoing interaction between individuals and contexts. The different components of engagement cannot be wholly captured by collecting data from individuals' self-reports. The use of multiple methods (e.g., survey and interviews) and multiple informants (e.g., teacher, student, and parent) to assess SE would offer a more comprehensive and diverse perspective. However, we also need to be cautious about relying on teacher or parent reports of internal processes linked to emotion and cognitive engagement, particularly if we then use these measures to predict outcomes that are also generated by the teacher (e.g., course grades).

Moreover, it is important to include and distinguish the different levels (e.g., classroom versus school building, as discussed by Skinner and Pitzer, 2012) and different time frames of student engagement (e.g., in-the-moment task engagement versus longer term engagement/commitment to a particular subject area, as discussed by Finn and Zimmer (2012) and by Reschly and Christenson (2012)). Many of the existing engagement measures are quite general, rarely focusing on specific tasks, situations, or subjects. Incorporating domain-specific measures will help to determine to what extent engagement represents a general tendency and to what extent it is content specific. Innovative methods such as the experience sampling method or daily diary methods, for example, could help us capture the moment-to-moment experiences of different subtypes of engagement and then over time how these moment-to-moment experiences of engagement congeal into more integrated "engagement" in a specific subject area or a more global attachment to an institutional setting like a school building. Such methods might also allow us to study the ways in which and for whom "engagement" in a school institution leads to greater moment-to-moment engagement in particular courses.

What Is Engagement?

There is no doubt that "engagement" is currently a very hot topic in the broad field of school achievement. But what is engagement? This is the topic of the five chapters in this part of this handbook. Each of the chapters deals with this issue in one way or another. However, after reading all five, we were still left unsure and unsatisfied. First, it is critical that we understand that the answer to this question is definitional. We can define student engagement in any way we would like, and how we define it will determine its usefulness for various communities. Defining it broadly will make it more useful for the policy making and educated lay thinker communities but less useful for the research and scholarly community. Defining it narrowly will have the opposite effect. Defining it broadly will increase the overlap of engagement with other theories and research literatures, making its unique contribution less clear. Defining it narrowly will force "engagement" scholars to make its unique contribution and value-added clear. The chapters by Reschly and Christenson (2012), Finn and Zimmer (2012), and Skinner and Pitzer (2012) all deal directly with this issue. However, at times, it seemed as though the terms student engagement, and school engagement, were being used rather loosely to mean everything that is good about an individual's relationship with his or her school. To the extent that this is true, then the hypothesis that engagement improves achievement seems rather circular because doing well in school both increases engagement and is used as evidence that engagement is high.

Policy makers and lay educational pundits love broad terms like engagement that appear to "explain" everything: "Students are not doing well because they are not engaged. So let's increase engagement and they will do better." But what exactly is engagement? What should be the specific focus of an intervention to increase engagement? If "engagement" encompasses everything from feeling like one belongs in the school to doing one's homework, or to participating in the school band, then almost anything we do to improve schools can be seen as an intervention to increase engagement. As scientists, we find this level of generality unsatisfying because it encompasses everything and anything that is related to students' and teachers' functioning in the school context. Probably the most concrete example of what we are talking about here is in the debate alluded to in several of the chapters about whether to include the concept of motivation as part of engagement. Those who prefer a broad, inclusive definition of engagement seem comfortable including motivational concepts such as affect, liking, feelings of belonging, and valuing within the definition of affective engagement. In contrast, Skinner and Pitzer (2012) prefer a more restricted definition of engagement, such as "the behavioral manifestation of motivation," that makes the concept of engagement distinct from the many other related concepts. We agree that a more precise definition will make "engagement" easier to measure and study as well as to be related to other theories of achievement and learning. At several points in their chapter, Finn and Zimmer (2012) also seem to prefer a more limited notion of engagement that focuses on behavior (both overt and covert mental behaviors), but then they also appear to be quite comfortable with a much broader definition. Reschly and Christenson (2012) also discuss this tension in their chapter.

It is important to note that the same problem exists in the field of achievement motivation. The tension between broad, inclusive versus more specific perspectives pervades this area of psychology as well. For example, Finn and Zimmer (2012) cite Newmann and colleagues' definition of motivation in their discussion of the possible overlap between the terms engagement and motivation: to quote, "Academic motivation ... has been defined as 'a general desire or disposition to succeed in academic work and in the more specific tasks of school'." As experts in achievement motivation as it applies to motivation in school contexts, we find such a broad definition unsatisfying. On the one hand, such a broad definition is very useful in discussions with policy makers and practitioners because it orients them to the broad domain of motivation as contrasted with other broad domains such as achievement or problem behaviors. On the other hand, it is not particularly useful for discussions among researchers and for increasing our fundamental understanding of human behavior in school contexts.

There is a subfield of educational psychology that focuses specifically on academic motivation. The scholars in this field have spent the last 50 years building a taxonomy of various beliefs, attitudes, needs, and emotions that comprise academic motivation. They have demonstrated the following: (1) The various components of academic motivation influence different aspects of achievement in schools; (2) these components are influenced by different contextual features and experiential histories; (3) as a consequence of 1 and 2, different intervention strategies are needed for the various components, and these different interventions will influence different aspect of school-related behaviors; (4) the developmental patterns associated with these various components differ; and (5) the salience of these different components in motivating behavior differ across developmental time and social context (see Wigfield et al., 2006).

Given these specific facts regarding academic motivation and a very broad definition of engagement, it is impossible to address the question of whether motivation should be seen as part of engagement or vice versa. The answer is both yes and no depending on which part of each elephant one is touching – in other words, "It depends." For example, at the most general level, we can say motivation influences behavior which, in turn, influences subsequent outcomes or A $\rightarrow$ B$\rightarrow$ C, with A=motivation, B=behavior, and

C = let us say learning. C of course could also be high school graduation, GPA, etc. Such a model seems quite satisfying because it is general and because it makes clear the mediating role of behavior. In this general case, one could say that B is engagement. If so, then motivation leads to engagement; motivation is thus a precursor of engagement rather than a part of engagement, and engagement mediates the relationship between motivation and school success. There are elements of this general model in each of the chapters, and ample evidence to support its validity is provided in each chapter.

But when affective engagement is considered to be a form of engagement, then the distinction between A, B, and C begins to blur. This problem is further exacerbated when one takes a developmental perspective, as is explicitly acknowledged by both Finn in his participation-identification model (1989) and Skinner and Pitzer (2012) in their conceptual model of engagement and disengagement in the classroom. In Finn's model, for example, participation in various aspects of school leads to success experiences which in turn lead to identification with school which then influences subsequent participation. Similar iterative processes are assumed in most models of achievement motivation and behavior and are at the core of such fundamental and classic developmentally focused psychological theories as conditioning, internalization, and social learning. The problem stems from the fact that these iterative processes make it very difficult to keep our definitions of A, B, and C distinct. Is identification part of engagement or the result of engagement or the precursor of future engagement?

This general 3-component model is even more problematic as we expand our definition of what fits into A, B, and C. As these general categories of constructs become more inclusive, the likelihood of making incorrect or at least not well-informed specific predictions increases. For example, if we select the desire to become a great singer as our indicator of A, the participation in extracurricular activities for B, and the learning of the content in specific courses for C, then it is quite unlikely that the study will confirm the prediction. We pick this extreme example to illustrate a more general point that is not so extreme: Confirmation of specific predictions depends on the specifics of the predictions. And it is in the specifics that clear definitions really matter. So, for example, policy makers have asked researchers to demonstrate that extracurricular activities affect academic achievement in large part because the research community has argued that student engagement is important for school success, and then we have included participation in extracurricular activities as part of our definition of school engagement. As is pointed out in several of these chapters, there is evidence that participation in extracurricular activities is weakly but significantly associated with GPA in some studies, for some programs, and for some populations. Thus, at a quite general level, these studies provide support for the general prediction that engagement in extracurricular activities influences achievement. But why does this association exist? Here the specifics matter, and they matter when one tries to develop an intervention designed, let us say, to increase the learning of the academic content being taught at school or students' performance on high-stakes tests. Why would we expect, for example, that increasing opportunities for participation in extracurricular activities would lead to better understanding of algebra or a foreign language, or science? We can certainly generate a logic model for why this might be so. For example, getting students to come to school and attend their classes might increase the likelihood of their learning algebra. But this will depend on the extent to which increased feelings of belonging at school actually influence the students' specific cognitive and behavioral engagement with algebra while they are in their algebra class. It will also depend on the extent to which the teachers are providing the type of high-quality algebra instruction that is necessary to help many formerly disengaged students master algebra. Thus, we need to be very careful when we make broad claims about the likely impact of various engagement-focused interventions on different indicators of school success. We need detailed logic models that lay out the likely connections between our interventions and the outcomes we hope to influence.

Otherwise, we are at risk of proving that some very well-designed interventions aimed at increasing school attendance have little impact on content mastery in specific courses. Additionally and perhaps even more importantly, is increasing options, for example, to participate in high-quality extracurricular activities, the most efficient or least expensive way to increase this type of academic performance? We are not saying that such programs are not useful for increasing other aspects of school success; the evidence reviewed indicates that some are and some are not. What we are saying is that we need to be careful and rigorous in our operationalization of concepts like engagement, as well as in our design of appropriate interventions for specific outcomes. In other words, uncovering the right engagement-related interventions requires us to look very closely at the specifics of terms A, B, and C in our general formula.

We are also not saying that the authors of these five chapters have not made similar points. They absolutely have in both these chapters and their other writings. What we are saying is that we need to be very mindful of the need for precision in our definitions and conceptualizations if we really want to change the various subcomponents of students' "engagement" in different aspects of their schooling experiences. If our goal is to reduce dropout rates, then increasing the salience and number of reasons students have to stay in school until graduation may be the most efficient strategy. If our goal is to increase science or math or English literacy and understanding, then we should probably focus on more specific targeted strategies within these classrooms. We worry that using a single phrase like "increasing engagement" for both of these types of intervention strategies decreases the likelihood that the most efficient strategies will be picked for these two very different types of "outcomes." It also increases the likelihood that people will want evaluators of extracurricular activities to assess standardized test scores as a reasonable indicator of the effectiveness of the extracurricular activities, even though there may be nothing going on in these activities that should influence test scores.

These examples illustrate another concern we have with defining what engagement is – a concern very well-articulated by Skinner and Pitzer (2012). This concern focuses on the need to be more specific about what level of engagement we are talking about. In Fig. 2.1, Skinner and Pitzer (2012) provide a very informative picture of the various levels at which the term engagement has been used as well as the types of outcomes likely to be associated with changes in engagement at each level. Keeping such distinctions salient in our discussions is critical to prevent misunderstandings regarding the effectiveness of interventions and overgeneralizations of our findings.

These dilemmas are exacerbated even more when we move beyond motivation as the "A" construct in the generalized 3-component model outlined above. When we let A stand for all precursors of engagement (B), then we have a very general model of human development that overlaps with many theories and is probably too general to be of great scientific significance. Although at the general level, it is bound to be true; at the specific level, it is not particularly useful for either theory testing or intervention design. It becomes a variation of the truism that good things lead to good things, which lead, in turn, to other good things, except when they do not. As noted by all of the authors, it is essential that we keep the distinction between precursors of engagement and indicators of engagement very clear. But, as also noted by the authors and by us in this commentary, achieving this task is often hard to do when one is operating at the psychological or personal level. It is easier when one is looking at social contextual precursors of either engagement or school success, as is evident in the chapters by Bingham and Okagaki (2012) and by Mahatmya et al. (2012). Bingham and Okagaki (2012), in particular, provide an excellent overview of the research linking the many contextual features of families, schools, neighborhoods, and peer groups that both co-occur with ethnic group membership and likely influence engagement, and thus may explain ethnic group differences in both engagement and school success. Mahatmya et al. (2012) discuss the ways in which various contextual features in combination with individual-level developmental changes might influence age-related changes in various indicators of engagement. As is clear in each of these chapters, various family and school contextual features have been shown to be precursors of the psychological processes linked to both motivation and engagement (see other chapters in this volume as well). Similarly, most psychological theories of human development would agree that these psychological processes mediate the associations between distal contextual characteristics and school success. At the general level, this has to be true, except when it is not. The dilemma is finding out when it is true, when it is not, and why. The answers to these questions will come by being very specific about which A, B, and C constructs are being considered.

In closing this part, let us stress how much we sympathize with engagement theorists about each of these dilemmas because these same issues pervade the field of motivation as well. These are inherent problems in various models of motivated behavior as well. We bring it up here just to point out how difficult these definitional issues can be and why we need to be as clear as possible about what we mean by various terms at each point in our discussions. Both engagement and motivational theorists within both the educational psychology and the educational sociology traditions would like to have quite general theories of behavior and achievement in school contexts – theories that explain a broad range of behaviors and educational outcomes. Certainly, the motivational theorists associated with three motivational theoretical systems dominant today (self-determination theory, achievement goal theory, and the Eccles et al. expectancy-value theory) have this goal, as do the theorists associated with engagement theory described in these five chapters. To have such a general theory, one needs to have very broad definitions of one's core constructs. Similarly, to inspire policy makers and educational pundits, one needs sexy and overgeneralized core constructs. But to design effective interventions and move our theoretical understanding forward, we need to be much more specific.

We see the efforts to articulate the various subtypes of "engagement" as akin to the efforts in motivation to break the global construct down into its operative subcomponents. Such microtheorizing is critical in both fields. We also find it very interesting, but not surprising, that the overlap between these more global theoretical frameworks becomes clearer and more salient as this microtheorizing proceeds in both frameworks. The overlap is particularly salient when one adopts a developmental orientation for one's theorizing: From a general developmental perspective, these two general frameworks for understanding school success are very similar in both their explanatory mechanisms and their recommendations for general and specific school reforms. But even more importantly, this microtheorizing is making the unique contributions of these two frameworks clearer, as well as the ways in which the unique constructs within each of these frameworks articulate with each other over developmental time.

Links Between Engagement Theory and the Eccles et al. Expectancy-Value Theory of Achievement-Related Behaviors

Now let us turn to a more specific discussion of the link of engagement theory to one quite similar theory of school achievement: the Eccles et al. expectancy-value theoretical model (EEVT). We focus on this theory because it is not discussed to any great extent in any of the other chapters in this book. The other major theories of motivated behavior in academic settings are discussed extensively in Skinner and Pitzer (2012) and Finn and Zimmer (2012) and the set of chapters in Part II of this handbook.

There are two ways in which Eccles' theoretical frameworks connect to ET. First, the general EEVT model was designed to explain individual and group differences in individuals' decisions to engage in, and the extent of their actual engagement in, various achievement-related activities. Here the overlap is quite explicit. The second overlap relates to Eccles and Midgley's extension of the EEVT into their stage-environment fit theory of motivation. We discuss each of these in turn.

Eccles began her career interested in the question of why males and females engage in different types of achievement-related behaviors in various spheres of life including school, extracurricular activities, educational and occupational choices, and achievement-related avocational behaviors and contexts. Her initial studies focused on why females were less likely than males to aspire to careers in STEM, and as a result, to be less likely than males to enroll in advanced math and physical science courses in secondary school and college. To address this question, Eccles and her colleagues (see Eccles [Parsons] et al., 1983; Meece et al., 1982) developed a socio-cultural embedded expectancy value theoretical model of task choice/engagement – the Eccles et al. expectancy-value theoretical model (EEVT) – and applied it to students' course-taking decisions. Eccles and her colleagues have since used this model to guide their research into a much broader question: Why does anyone do anything? Although they typically used terms like behavioral choices, persistence, and achievement when describing their major dependent measures or outcomes, Eccles has always included the idea of engagement in her set of major dependent measures. When doing so, she was referring to both the behavioral and cognitive aspects of engagement as defined by Fredericks et al. and to behavioral engagement as defined by Skinner et al. rather than to sense of belonging to the institution in which the activities are placed. I (Eccles) would put emotional engagement as either an antecedent of behavioral/cognitive engagement (i.e., anticipated positive or negative emotional arousal resulting from engagement) or an emotional reaction to being engaged in doing the task.

My (Eccles) general perspective was heavily influenced by three broad theoretical perspectives: (1) The life course view that both personal agency and social structure are prime forces in life span development; (2) the social processes underlying socialization and internalization; and (3) the person-environment fit perspective that people fare best and are likely to be most engaged when they are in contexts that meet their psychological needs. I felt that bringing together these three perspectives would provide a comprehensive theoretical approach to task choice and behavioral engagement. The focus on personal agency led me to expectancy-value theoretical perspectives on task choice and task engagement. The focus on socialization and internalization led me to a focus on the ways in which external forces and context become a part of the individuals' expectations for success and subjective task values across a wide array of tasks. Finally, the person-environment fit perspective led me to theorize about those aspects of the context that would increase or decrease the expectations and values of the individuals' deciding to engage in various tasks or contexts. Thus, the person-environment fit perspective focused my and Carol Midgley's attention on the link between the nature of contexts and the needs of the persons; we assumed that motivation would be highest when the demands of the task fit well with both the person's sense of agency (in this case, their expectations of success) and the values, needs, and goals of the individual. In this way, the theoretical approach adopted by my colleagues and me is quite consistent with the approaches guiding both ET and SDT.

The EEVT general model that emerged is illustrated in Fig. 6.1. Our ultimate goal was to predict task choice and intensity of task engagement. The task could be as focused as doing a homework assignment or as broad as being engaged at school with sufficient intensity to lead to graduation. We argued that such engagements would be directly predicted by two major psychological constructs: expectations of success and perceived/subjective task value. Thus, the most proximal precursors of engagement where beliefs that are commonly thought to be part of modern achievement motivational theories. We then specified the more distal psychological and social processes likely to influence these proximal beliefs. Thus, like Skinner and Pitzer (2012), Finn and Zimmer (2012) and Bingham and Okagaki (2012), most of our theorizing has focused on the precursors of engagement rather than on the definition of engagement itself. We put both engagement and achievement in our outcome box. However, like both engagement and SDT theorists (e.g., Finn & Zimmer, 2012; Reschly & Christenson, 2012; Skinner &

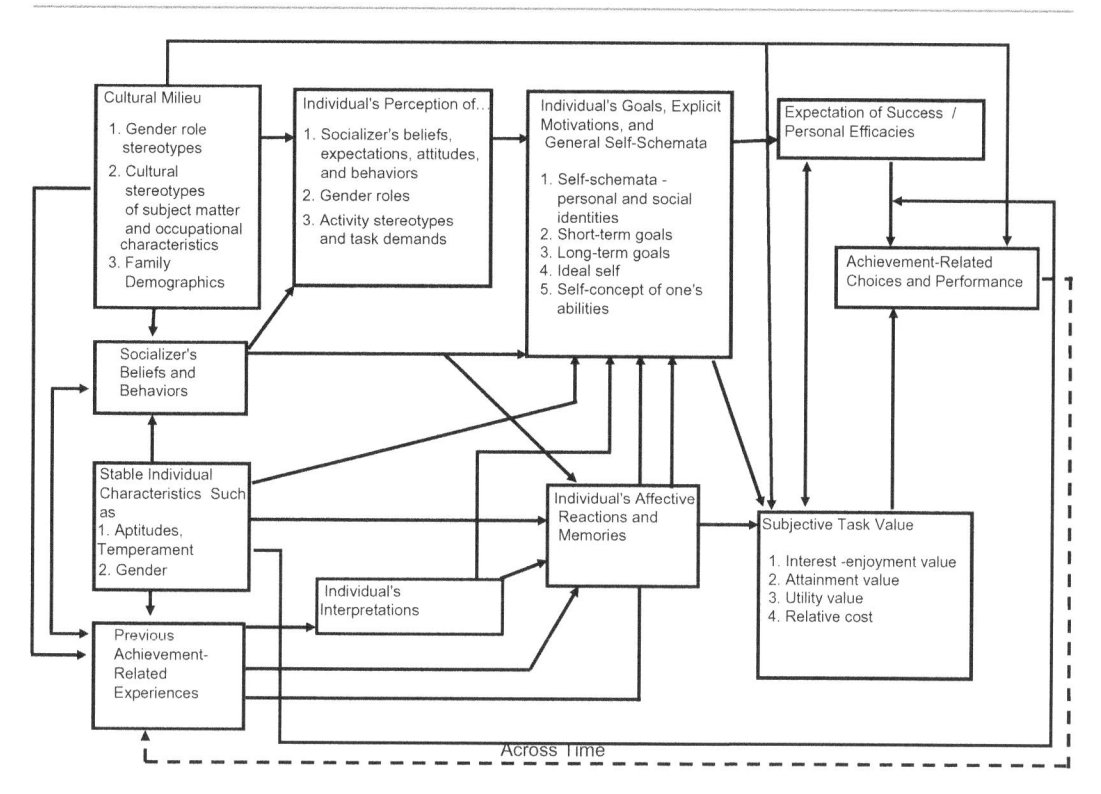

Fig. 6.1 Eccles et al. Expectancy-value model of achievement behaviors

Pitzer, 2012; Finn & Zimmer, 2012), we consider our larger perspective to be a general theory of motivated behavior that helps understand individual and group differences in school achievement. We differ more in the labels for specific constructs than in the overarching goal of the theoretical system.

Perhaps the aspect of EEVT that overlaps most with ET is the role of affect and of determinants of subjective task value. Because we are developmentalists, we see affect as both a precursor and a consequence of engagement rather than as a part of engagement. Like Finn in his participation-identification model (1989), we proposed that success (or failure) experiences in various settings create emotional reactions, which over time accumulate within the person to form stable positive (or negative) feelings about similar settings and activities, which, in turn both raise (or lower) the value one attaches to these settings and, to the extent that these association become part of the person's core self-beliefs or self-schema, increase identification with or attachment to the institutional settings in which such activities take place. We include such experiences in the box labeled affective memories and the link of these memories to the box labeled self-related beliefs. We further assume that these beliefs increase the subjective task value of engaging in tasks in such settings.

We also believe that subjective task value is composed of beliefs about how enjoyable the task will be, how useful the task is for fulfilling one's various short- and long-term goals, how well the task helps one manifest one's personal needs and both personal and social identities, and finally how much engaging in the task costs in terms of time, effort, energy, external assets, and the ability to engage in other tasks either more or less directly related to one's personal and social needs and goals. These same ideas are evident in all of the five chapters in this part. For example, they overlap with (1) what Skinner and Pitzer (2012) include under emotion and cognitive orientation in Fig. 2.2; (2) what both Finn and Zimmer (2012) and Reschly and Christenson (2012) include under the rubrics of affective engagement, cognitive engagement, and school identification; and (3) what Martin 2012 (chapter in this volume) refers to as adaptive cognitions. However, EEVT places greater emphasis on the role of both personal and social identities and short- and long-term goals as key mediators of engagement through their influence on the individual's hierarchies of subjective task values. The central role of personal and social identities has become a major focus on my work over the last 10–15 years (see Eccles 2009), as I have extended the model to look at racial identities as well as more personal identities that underlie what we labeled attainment value. By focusing on these dimensions of the self, we have expanded the range of self-related characteristics that might influence engagement through their impact on perceived person-environment fit and thus subjective task value.

We also place greater emphasis than such motivational theoretical frameworks as SDT or AGT on the social or more distal precursors of engagement. In this way, we are more like Bingham and Okagaki (2012) in our orientation than we are like Skinner and Pitzer (2012), and Finn and Zimmer (2012). However, like Skinner and Pitzer (2012), Finn and Zimmer (2012), Mahatmya et al. (2012), and Reschly and Christenson (2012), we are very interested in interventions designed to increase engagement. This has lead us to focus, in the various extensions of the EEVT, on those characteristics of the school, family, and peer groups that influence school-related task engagement through increasing the perceived subjective task value of these tasks or activities. Like Mahatmya et al. (2012), we have been particularly interested in those aspects of the changing school context that may underlie the declines in many students' interest in engaging in school academic-related task as they move into and through primary and secondary school.

This concern with social precursors lead Eccles and Midgley to take a closer look at developmental changes in both expectations for success in and the subjective task value associated with the learning aspects of classroom experiences. Our own longitudinal data from the 1980s showed major declines in the students' expectations for and interest in various school subjects as they moved from elementary school into secondary school. Carol Midgley and I became intrigued by what might be going on to explain these differences. We decided that the decline reflected changes in the kinds of experiences the students were having in their classrooms. We predicted that students on average experienced what we called a developmentally inappropriate shift in the types of classroom and teacher characteristics as they moved into secondary school, leading to increasingly poor fit between the needs of many adolescents and the opportunities provided by their school. We called this perspective stage-environment fit or misfit (Eccles & Midgley, 1989; Eccles et al., 1993).

Much like SDT, we argued that individuals thrive best in classrooms that meet their personal and social needs. Like SDT, we argued (1) that students have a strong need to feel competent if they are to maintain high expectations for success and (2) that students need to have positive relationships with their teachers for a variety of reasons. We felt that maintaining this sense of competence would become more difficult for many adolescents, particularly in large schools where their teachers are working with so many other students, because their academic deficits would make mastery of the material being taught more difficult. We felt that this problem would be further exacerbated by an increased focus on social comparative grading. Similar to SDT, we also argued that adolescents, in particular, have a growing need for greater autonomy and self-direction, while at the same a growing need to have close relationships with nonfamilial adults. We also argued that they need the chance to try new, challenging tasks, activities, and contexts in an environment that also provides a strong safety net. Finally, we argued that the emergence of more well-articulated personal and social identities would increase the need for opportunities to explore activities directly related to these identities – thus increasing the importance of the relevance of the material they were learning for the subjective task value they would attach to various courses and activities in the secondary school setting. Directly related, the emergence of more well-articulated social identities would increase the salience of ethnic relevance and peer group norms. Thus, like Bingham and Okagaki (2012), we argued that ethnic compatibility and sensitivities would become increasingly important during the secondary school years. Many of these same points were discussed by Lohman et al. (2012). Thus, we see many overlaps between the work associated with Eccles and her colleagues and the work being done by theorists in the engagement theory tradition.

General Conclusions

In summary, there is substantial overlap across the various general theories of motivated behavior in the school context discussed in these five chapters, in the other chapters in this handbook, and in our commentary. At the most general level, this overlap suggests that we are converging on a shared theoretical framework across both the psychology and the sociology of education. Thus, it is not surprising that the measures used to assess engagement itself as well as its precursors and consequences are quite similar to the measures used to assess various key constructs in these other theories – a point well made by Reschly and Christenson (2012) and by Finn and Zimmer (2012). Finally, and also not surprisingly, much of the research presented in these chapters provides support for the basic tenets of each of the theories of motivated behavior discussed in this commentary and in the other chapters in this book.

At the more specific level, it is important that we compare and contrast the details of each of these theories in order to determine the most powerful and the most easily controlled influences on school engagement. It is also important that we find the places where these theories and approaches make different predictions and then test these varying hypotheses. Such research is critical to both the research and policy/practice communities. Thus, it is critical that we focus on both the similarities and the differences among these various theoretical approaches as we move forward on both the theoretical and applied fronts.

References

Bingham, G. E., & Okagaki, L. (2012). Ethnicity and student engagement. In S. L. Christenson, A. L. Reschly, & C. Wylie (Eds.), *Handbook of research on student engagement* (pp. 65–95). New York: Springer.

Eccles, J. (2009). Who am I and what am I going to do with my life? Personal and collective identities as motivators of action. *Educational Psychologist, 44*(2), 78–89.

Eccles, J. S., & Midgley, C. M. (1989). Stage/environment fit: Developmentally appropriate classrooms for early adolescents. In R. E. Ames & C. Ames (Eds.), *Research on motivation in education: Goals and cognitions* (Vol. 3, pp. 139–186). New York: Academic Press.

Eccles, J. S., Midgley, C., Buchanan, C. M., Wigfield, A., Reuman, D., & Mac Iver, D. (1993). Development during adolescence: The impact of stage/environment fit. *American Psychologist, 48*, 90–101.

Eccles (Parsons), J., Adler, T. F., Futterman, R., Goff, S. B., Kaczala, C. M., Meece, J. L., & Midgley, C. (1983). Expectancies, values and academic behaviors. In J. Spence (Ed.), *Achievement and achievement motivation* (pp. 75–146). San Francisco: W.H. Freeman and Co.

Finn, J. D. (1989). Withdrawing from school. *Review of Educational Research, 59*, 117–142.

Finn, J. D., & Zimmer, K. (2012). Student engagement: What is it? Why does it matter? In S. L. Christenson, A. L. Reschly, & C. Wylie (Eds.), *Handbook of research on student engagement* (pp. 97–131). New York: Springer.

Fredricks, J. A., Blumenfeld, P. C., & Paris, A. H. (2004). School engagement: Potential of the concept, state of the evidence. *Review of Educational Research, 74*, 59–109.

Mahatmya, M., Lohman, B. J., Matjasko, J. L., & Farb, A. F. (2012). Engagement across developmental periods. In S. L.Christenson, A. L. Reschly, & C. Wylie (Eds.), *Handbook of research on student engagement* (pp. 45–63). New York: Springer.

Meece, J. L., Eccles-Parsons, J., Kaczala, C. M., Goff, S. E., & Futterman, R. (1982). Sex differences in math achievement: Toward a model of academic choice. *Psychological Bulletin, 91*, 324–348.

Reschly, A. L., & Christenson, S. L. (2012). Jingle, jangle, and conceptual haziness: Evolution and future directions of the engagement construct. In S. L. Christenson, A. L. Reschly, & C. Wylie (Eds.), *Handbook of research on student engagement* (pp. 3–19). New York: Springer.

Skinner, E. A., & Pitzer, J. R. (2012). Developmental dynamics of student engagement, coping, and everyday resilience. In S. L.Christenson, A. L. Reschly, & C. Wylie (Eds.), *Handbook of research on student engagement* (pp. 21–44). New York: Springer.

Wigfield, A., Eccles, J. S., Schiefele, U., Roeser, R. W., & Davis-Kean, P. (2006). Development of achievement motivation. In N. Eisenberg (Ed.), *Handbook of child psychology* (6th edition, Vol. 3, pp. 933–1002). New York: Wiley.

Part II

Engagement as Linked to Motivational Variables

A Self-determination Theory Perspective on Student Engagement*

Johnmarshall Reeve

Abstract

This chapter pursues three goals. First, it overviews self-determination theory (SDT). SDT is a macrotheory of motivation comprised of five interrelated minitheories—basic needs theory, organismic integration theory, goal contents theory, cognitive evaluation theory, and causality orientations theory. Each minitheory was created to explain specific motivational phenomena and to address specific research questions. Second, the chapter uses the student-teacher dialectical framework within SDT to explain how classroom conditions sometimes support but other times neglect and frustrate students' motivation, engagement, and positive classroom functioning. Third, the chapter highlights student engagement. In doing so, it overviews recent classroom-based, longitudinally designed research to reveal three new and important functions of student engagement—namely, that student engagement fully mediates and explains the motivation-to-achievement relation, that changes in engagement produce changes in the learning environment, and that changes in engagement produce changes in motivation, as students' behavioral, emotional, cognitive, and agentic engagements represent actions taken not only to learn but also to meet psychological needs. The chapter concludes with implications for teachers and with suggestions for future research.

---

*This research was supported by the WCU (World Class University) Program funded by the Korean Ministry of Education, Science and Technology, consigned to the Korea Science and Engineering Foundation (Grant no. R32-2008-000-20023-0).

J. Reeve (✉)
Department of Education, Korea University,
Anam-Dong, Seongbuk-Gu Seoul, 136-701 Korea
e-mail: reeve@korea.ac.kr

Watch as a student engages herself in a learning activity. What catches your eye? What really matters in terms of whether she will learn something new or develop her skills? What unseen motivational processes contribute to and explain her attention, effort, emotionality, strategic thinking, and sense of initiative and agency? As you watch the ebb and flow of her engagement, can you predict what will happen next? Can you predict what she will and will not do in the coming minute? If you were to provide some assistance (the way a teacher might), what would you say? What would you do?

Using the eyes and experience of the teacher and using the theory and tools of the researcher, the present chapter reflects on these questions to pursue three goals. First, the chapter overviews self-determination theory (SDT). SDT is a theory of motivation that helps researchers and practitioners alike to understand and enhance not only student motivation but also the engagement that arises out of that motivation. It is a macrotheory of motivation comprised of five interrelated mini-theories, including basic needs theory, organismic integration theory, goal contents theory, cognitive evaluation theory, and causality orientations theory (Ryan & Deci, 2002; Vansteenkiste, Niemiec, & Soenens, 2010). Second, using an SDT perspective, the chapter explains how classroom conditions sometimes support but other times interfere with students' motivation, engagement, and positive school functioning. The focus in this discussion will be on the student-teacher dialectical framework that is embedded within an SDT analysis. Third, the chapter highlights student engagement. Recent classroom-based, longitudinally designed research has produced several new and important insights into defining, understanding, and promoting students' engagement. In the discussion of these new findings, particular emphasis will be paid to the functions of student engagement.

Three Questions

To help readers compare, contrast, and integrate the various chapters of the *Handbook of Research on Student Engagement*, the editors asked each contributing author team to address the following three questions:
1. What are your definitions of engagement and motivation, and how do you differentiate between the two?
2. What overarching framework or theory do you use to study and explain engagement or motivation?
3. What is the role of context in explaining engagement or motivation?

What Is Engagement? What Is Motivation? How Do You Differentiate the Two?

Engagement refers to the extent of a student's active involvement in a learning activity, a definition borrowed from Wellborn's (1991) pioneering work on the subject. The definitional emphasis on "learning activity" is important because the present chapter focuses rather narrowly on engagement as a task- or domain-specific event, as the student is engaged in a particular learning activity (for a matter of minutes) or in a particular course (for a matter of months).

Engagement is a multidimensional construct. As depicted in Fig. 7.1, engagement features four distinct, but highly intercorrelated, aspects. Each of these four aspects will be discussed in depth in the chapter, but for now recall the observational episode from the opening paragraph in which you might find yourself observing a student reading, practicing, or playing. From the perspective of the present chapter, making a judgment of how actively involved the student was in the learning activity would involve assessments of her concentration, attention, and effort (behavioral engagement), the presence of task-facilitating emotions such as interest and the absence of task-withdrawing emotions such as distress (emotional engagement), her usage of sophisticated rather than superficial learning strategies (cognitive engagement), and the extent to which she tries to enrich the learning experience rather than just passively receive it as a given (agentic engagement).

Motivation refers to any force that energizes and directs behavior (Reeve, 2009a). Energy gives behavior its strength, intensity, and persistence. Direction gives behavior its purpose and

```
                    ┌─────────────────────────┐
                    │      Engagement         │
                    │ during a Learning Activity │
                    └─────────────────────────┘
```

Behavioral Engagement	Emotional Engagement	Cognitive Engagement	Agentic Engagement
• On-task attention and concentration. • High effort. • High task persistence.	• Presence of task-facilitating emotions (e.g., interest, curiosity, and enthusiasm). • Absence of task-withdrawing emotions (e.g., distress, anger, frustration, anxiety, and fear).	• Use of sophisticated, deep, and personalized learning strategies (e.g., elaboration). • Seeking conceptual understanding rather than surface knowledge. • Use of self-regulatory strategies (e.g., planning).	• Proactive, intentional, and constructive contribution into the flow of the learning activity (e.g., offering input, making suggestions). • Enriching the learning activity, rather than passively receiving it as a given.

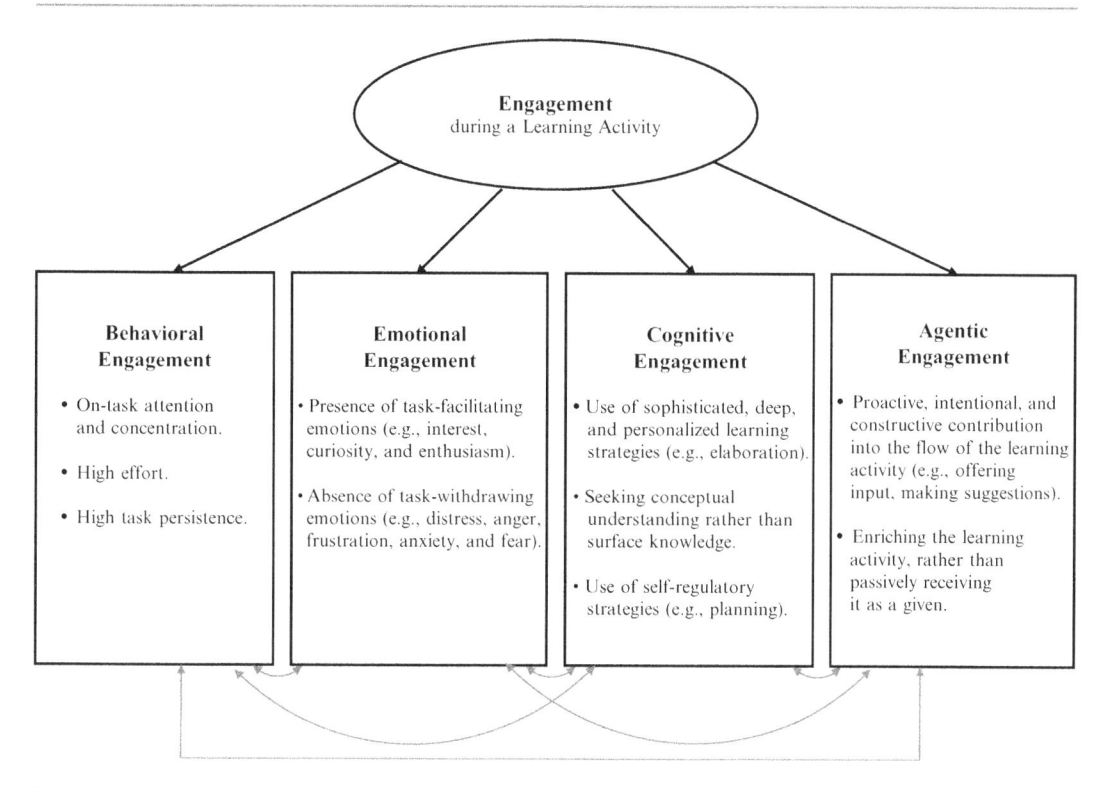

Fig. 7.1 Four interrelated aspects of students' engagement during a learning activity

goal-directedness. While motivation arises from many different sources (e.g., needs, cognitions, emotions, environmental events), it is viewed in the present chapter from a needs-based perspective within the self-determination theory framework; hence, motivation is equated with students' psychological need satisfaction. That is, students who perceive themselves to be acting with a sense of autonomy, competence, and relatedness during the learning activity experience high-quality motivation, while those who have these three needs neglected or frustrated during instruction experience low-quality motivation.

The distinction between the two constructs is that motivation is a private, unobservable psychological, neural, and biological process that serves as an antecedent cause to the publically observable behavior that is engagement. While motivation and engagement are inherently linked (each influences the other), those who study motivation are interested in engagement mostly as an outcome of motivational processes, whereas those who study engagement are interested mostly in motivation as a source of engagement. So, motivation is the relatively more private, subjectively experienced cause, while engagement is the relatively more public, objectively observed effect.

What Overarching Framework Informs Your Understanding of Motivation and Engagement?

Self-determination theory provides the overarching theoretical framework to guide my research questions and empirical study of both motivation and engagement. A particular emphasis is placed on the student-teacher dialectical framework embedded within SDT. Both of these frameworks will be presented in the present chapter.

What Is the Role of Context in Explaining Engagement or Motivation?

Students have needs, goals, interests, and values of their own, and these motivations sometimes manifest themselves in a context-free way, as when a student adopts a mastery goal orientation across all achievement contexts. These motivations also express themselves when student are alone, as when an adolescent clicks on a web page, finds it interesting, and reads about the topic for hours, all in the privacy of his or her personal time on a computer. When students are in the classroom, however, context matters. In the classroom, students live and interact in a social world that offers supports for and threats against their needs, goals, interests, and values. In the classroom, the teacher and the learning environment are so instrumental in supporting versus frustrating student motivation and engagement that it almost does not make sense to refer to "student" engagement because it cannot be separated or disentangled from the social context in which it occurs. That is, every student's classroom engagement is invariably a joint product of his or her motivation and classroom supports versus thwarts.

This view on the role of context in motivation and engagement foreshadows three implications. First, to flourish, student motivation and student engagement need supportive conditions, especially supportive student-teacher relationships. Second, the role of the teacher (or the classroom context more generally) is not to create or manufacture student motivation or engagement. Rather, the teacher's role is to support the student motivation and engagement that is already there and to do so in a way that allows for high- (rather than low-) quality motivation and engagement. Third, it is only partially valid to think of the relations among social context, motivation, engagement, and student outcomes in a linear fashion (i.e., social context → motivation → engagement → outcomes) because one also needs to think about these relations in a reciprocal way.

Self-determination Theory

Self-determination theory (SDT) is a theory of motivation that uses traditional empirical methods to build its theory and to inform its classroom applications. The theory, which has been 40 years in the making, assumes that all students, no matter their age, gender, socioeconomic status, nationality, or cultural background, possess inherent growth tendencies (e.g., intrinsic motivation, curiosity, psychological needs) that provide a motivational foundation for their high-quality classroom engagement and positive school functioning (Deci & Ryan, 1985a, 2000; Reeve, Deci, & Ryan, 2004; Ryan & Deci, 2000, 2002; Vansteenkiste et al., 2010). While other motivation theories explain how students' expectations, beliefs, and goals contribute to their classroom engagement, self-determination theory is unique in that it emphasizes the instructional task of *vitalizing* students' inner motivational resources as the key step in facilitating high-quality engagement (Reeve & Halusic, 2009). That is, SDT identifies the inner motivational resources that all students possess, and it offers recommendations as to how teachers can involve, nurture, and vitalize these resources during the flow of instruction to facilitate high-quality student engagement (Niemiec & Ryan, 2009).

The theory acknowledges that students sometimes lack self-motivation, display disaffection, and act irresponsibly. To resolve this seeming paradox of possessing inner motivational resources on the one hand yet displaying disaffection on the other, SDT research identifies the classroom conditions that support and vitalize students' inner motivational resources versus those that neglect, undermine, and thwart them (Deci & Ryan, 1985a; Reeve et al., 2004; Ryan & Deci, 2000). In doing so, SDT addresses how students' inner resources interact with classroom conditions to result in varying levels of students' engagement.

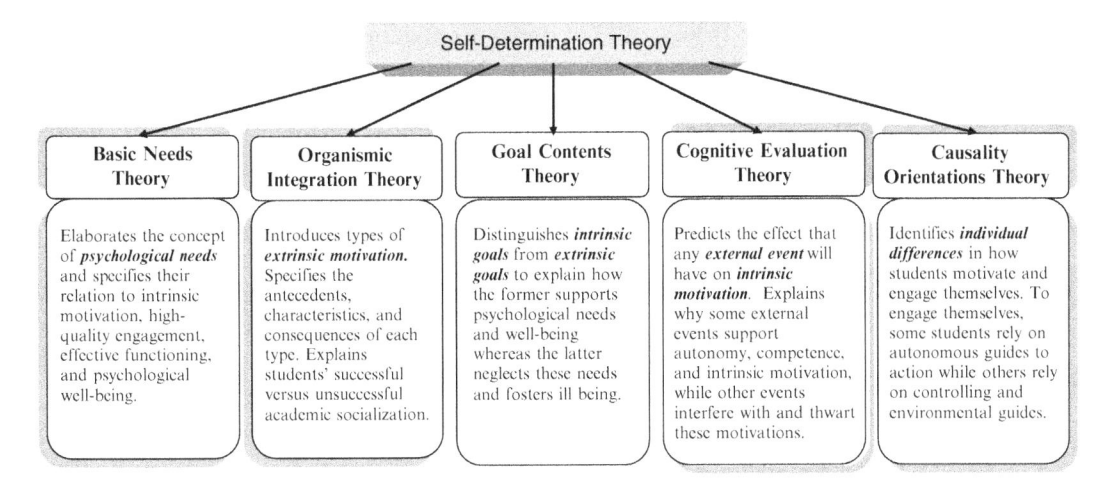

Fig. 7.2 Five minitheories of self-determination theory and the motivational phenomena each was developed to explain

As SDT research has advanced, different motivational phenomena (e.g., intrinsic motivation) and different research questions (e.g., how do extrinsic rewards affect intrinsic motivation?) have emerged and required empirical study. As summarized in Fig. 7.2, five minitheories emerged to explain these motivational phenomena and to answer their associated research questions. *Basic needs theory* focuses on psychological needs as inherent inner motivational resources and specifies their foundational and nutriment-like relation to students' motivation, high-quality engagement, effective functioning, and psychological well-being. *Organismic integration theory* focuses on internalization and why students initiate socially important, but not intrinsically motivating, behaviors. It represents SDT's theory of extrinsic motivation, specifies types of extrinsic motivation, and explains students successful versus unsuccessful academic socialization. *Goal contents theory* focuses on the "what" of motivation—what goals students strive for—to distinguish intrinsic from extrinsic goals. This minitheory explains how intrinsic goals support psychological need satisfaction and foster well-being and also how extrinsic goals neglect psychological needs and foster ill-being. *Cognitive evaluation theory* explains how external events (e.g., rewards, feedback) affect intrinsic motivational processes, as external events sometimes support but other times interfere with and thwart students' psychological needs and perceptions of autonomy and competence. *Causality orientations theory* highlights individual differences in how students motivate themselves. To initiate and sustain their classroom engagement, some students tend to rely on autonomous and self-determined guides to action, while others tend to rely on controlled and environmentally determined guides.

Basic Needs Theory

Basic needs theory identifies the three psychological needs of autonomy, competence, and relatedness as the source of students' inherent and proactive intrinsically motivated tendency to seek out novelty, pursue optimal challenge, exercise and extend their capabilities, explore, and learn. *Autonomy* is the psychological need to experience behavior as emanating from and as endorsed by the self; it is the inner endorsement of one's behavior (Deci & Ryan, 1985a). Students experience autonomy need satisfaction to the extent to which their classroom activity affords them opportunities to engage in learning activities with an internal locus of causality, sense of psychological freedom, and perceived choice over their actions (Reeve, Nix, & Hamm, 2003). *Competence* is the need to be effective in one's pursuits and interactions with the environment. It reflects the inherent desire to exercise one's capacities and, in doing so, to seek out and master environmental challenges (Deci, 1975). *Relatedness* is the need to establish close emotional bonds and secure attachments with others. It reflects the desire to be emotionally connected to and interpersonally involved in warm, caring, and responsive relationships (Deci & Ryan, 1991). Students experience relatedness need satisfaction to the extent to which they relate to others in an authentic, caring, and reciprocal way (Ryan, 1993).

Basic needs theory contributes to the overarching SDT framework in three important ways. First, basic needs theory identifies the origin of students' active nature in the three psychological needs (Deci & Ryan, 2000). In this way, basic needs theory presents psychological need satisfaction as its unifying principle (Vansteenkiste et al., 2010), as psychological needs energize engagement and are conceptualized as psychological nutriments that the daily life events need to fulfill if one is to be psychologically, physically, and socially well. Second, basic needs theory explains *why* students sometimes show active engagement in learning activities but other times show a passive or even antagonistic involvement, as need satisfaction promotes active engagement, whereas the neglect and thwarting of these needs anticipates various manifestations of disaffection (Deci & Ryan, 2000; Reis, Sheldon, Gable, Roscoe, & Ryan, 2000; Sheldon, Ryan, & Reis, 1996). Third, the three needs provide the basis for predicting a priori which aspects of the classroom environment will be supportive versus undermining of students' engagement—namely, those conditions that affect students' perceptions of autonomy, competence, and relatedness (Deci, Koestner, & Ryan, 1999). This study of how teachers support students' autonomy has been the foundation of my own program of research on teachers' autonomy-supportive versus controlling motivating styles (e.g., Reeve, 2009b) as well as others' research on competence support and relatedness support (e.g., Skinner & Belmont, 1993).

Organismic Integration Theory

Organismic integration theory recognizes that students engage in many behaviors that are inherently interesting or enjoyable. It is probably the case that most behaviors students engage in at school are extrinsically motivated and enacted as a means to an outcome that is separate from the engaged task itself, such as practicing a musical instrument to develop skill or to please a teacher, rather than simply enjoying the playing itself. Organismic integration theory explains under which conditions students do, do not, and only sort of acquire, internalize, and integrate extrinsic motivational processes into the self-motivation system. It proposes that students are naturally and volitionally inclined to internalize aspects of their social surroundings and to integrate some of these values and ways of behaving as acquired motivations. That is, students want to internalize societal norms, rules, and behaviors; indeed, they proactively seek out such opportunities. The motivation to internalize societal prescriptions ("do this") and proscriptions ("don't do that") exists because students naturally want to discover new ways to increase their competence in the social world and to relate the self more closely to others (e.g., shared values, shared goals, greater sense of community). To the extent that students internalize and integrate healthy external regulations (i.e., achieve "organismic integration"), they experience greater autonomy and show relatively more positive functioning in the relevant domain, including the school context (Ryan, 1993; Ryan & Connell, 1989).

According to organismic integration theory, extrinsic motivation (unlike intrinsic motivation) is a differentiated construct. Different types of extrinsic motivation are associated with different degrees of autonomous motivation. To be autonomous is not so much to be free from external forces; rather, students experience autonomy in accordance with how much they personally endorse the value and significance of the way of thinking or behaving. Because students feel varying degrees of ownership of their beliefs and behaviors, the four types of extrinsic motivation can be conceptualized along a unipolar continuum of autonomous motivation.

External regulation is the least autonomous type of extrinsic motivation. It exists as a contingency-based "in order to" type of motivation in which the student engages in an activity in order to obtain a reward or in order to avoid a punishment. With external regulation, the personal value of the behavior itself is very low. *Introjected regulation* is slightly autonomous extrinsic motivation. With introjected regulation, the student complies with external requests to affirm or maintain self-worth in the eyes of others or to silence a self-esteem threat (avoid feeling guilty or ashamed). Both external regulation and introjected regulation are associated with an external perceived locus of causality, sense of pressure, and perceived obligation (i.e., controlled motivation). Moving up the ladder of autonomous types of extrinsic motivation, *identified regulation* represents an autonomous type of extrinsic motivation. With identified regulation, the student sees value in the external regulation ("that is important, useful") and willingly transforms it into a self-endorsed (internalized) regulation that has a sense of choice and personal commitment behind it. *Integrated regulation* is the most autonomous type of extrinsic motivation. It occurs as the student evaluates and brings an identification into coherence with other aspects of the self-system, as when "studying hard on this assignment" is brought into the "I'm a scholar" sense of self. Integrated regulation approximates intrinsic motivation in its degree of self-determination, though the two motivational constructs clearly differ, as integrated regulation is based on the importance of the activity and requires considerable reflection and self-awareness, whereas intrinsic motivation is based on interest in the activity and emerges spontaneously. Both identified regulation and integrated regulation are associated with an internal perceived locus of causality, sense of psychological freedom, and perceived choice (i.e., autonomous motivation).

In adding organismic integration theory to the SDT framework, SDT ceased contrasting intrinsic motivation against extrinsic motivation and now distinguishes between autonomous motivation and controlled motivation (Vansteenkiste et al., 2010). Organismic integration theory nicely complements basic needs theory in the overall SDT framework, as basic needs theory identifies students' inherent motivational resources, whereas organismic integration theory identifies students' acquired motivational resources.

Goal Contents Theory

Organismic integration theory was created to answer questions of *why* people engage in uninteresting activities—why does he study? Why does he participate in class? Why does he do his homework? In contrast, goal contents theory was created to answer questions of *what* people strive to attain—what is his goal while studying? What is her goal as she participates in class? Goal contents theory arose out of the distinction between intrinsic and extrinsic goals (or intrinsic and extrinsic aspirations) and out of the finding that the differing goal content affects motivation and well-being in different ways (Ryan, Sheldon, Kasser, & Deci, 1996; Vansteenkiste, Lens, & Deci, 2006). Specifically, engagement in pursuit of intrinsic goals such as personal growth and deeper interpersonal relationships affords basic need satisfactions and thus enhances effort and psychological well-being, whereas engagement in pursuit of extrinsic goals such as enhanced status, increased popularity, or material success neglects basic need satisfactions and therefore foreshadows ill-being (e.g., anxiety, depression, and physical symptoms).

Importantly, engagement in pursuit of extrinsic goals undermines learning and well-being even for those who actually attain their extrinsic goals (Niemiec, Ryan, & Deci, 2009; Vansteenkiste et al., 2006; Vansteenkiste, Timmermans, Lens, Soenens, & Van den Broeck, 2008). So, psychological need satisfaction and psychological well-being do not depend so much on whether people attain the goals they seek as much as they depend on what people seek to attain in the first place—intrinsic or extrinsic goal content. This conclusion stands in contrast to all other theories of student motivation that argue that the pursuit and attainment of valued goals is central to students' psychological well-being (e.g., expectancy x valence theory, social cognitive theory).

According to goal contents theory, the pursuit and attainment of intrinsic goals fosters deeper learning, better performance, enduring persistence, and greater psychological well-being than does the pursuit of extrinsic goals (Vansteenkiste, Simons, Lens, Sheldon, & Deci, 2004a; Vansteenkiste et al., 2004b; Vansteenkiste et al., 2006) because intrinsic goals tap into and vitalize students' inner motivational resources in ways that extrinsic goals do not. The pursuit and attainment of extrinsic goals does not foster these motivational and well-being benefits and is, in fact, typically counterproductive.

Cognitive Evaluation Theory

Cognitive evaluation theory explains how and why external events such as rewards or praise affect intrinsic motivation. Intrinsically motivated behaviors are those that are initiated and maintained by the spontaneous satisfactions students experience while engaged in an activity. The two inherent satisfactions within intrinsic motivation are feeling autonomous and feeling competent, though relatedness satisfaction may also play a role in intrinsic motivation (Ryan & Deci, 2000). According to cognitive evaluation theory, any external event that affects students' perceived autonomy or perceived competence will necessarily affect their intrinsic motivation.

According to the theory, all external events (e.g., tests, rewards, grades, scholarships, deadlines, written feedback on a paper) have two functional aspects: a controlling aspect and an informational aspect (Deci & Ryan, 1980, 1985a), and it is the relative salience of the controlling versus informational aspect of the event that determines its effect on intrinsic motivation. The *controlling aspect* of an external event pressures students toward a specific outcome or toward a specific way of behaving. That is, students experience a reward as a controlling event if the reward is offered in exchange for compliant behavior (e.g., "If you come to class on time, then I will give you a special privilege."). Controlling external events diminish intrinsic motivation, whereas noncontrolling external events preserve autonomy and maintain intrinsic motivation. The *informational aspect* of an external event communicates competence feedback. That is, students experience a reward as an informational event if the reward is offered to communicate competent or improved functioning (e.g., "Because your punctuality has improved so much, you have earned a special privilege."). Informational, competence-enhancing external events increase intrinsic motivation, whereas competence-undermining external events (e.g., criticism) decrease it.

Cognitive evaluation theory is a crucial mini-theory in the overall SDT framework (and the first to emerge; Deci & Ryan, 1980) because it specifies how classroom conditions can enhance and support students' intrinsic motivational processes or undermine and thwart them. For instance, some common classroom autonomy thwarts are surveillance (Lepper & Greene, 1975), deadlines (Amabile, DeJong, & Lepper, 1976), imposed rules and limits (Koestner, Ryan, Bernieri, & Holt, 1984), imposed goals (Mossholder, 1980), directives/commands (Reeve & Jang, 2006), competition (Deci, Betley, Kahle, Abrams, & Porac, 1981), and evaluation (Ryan, 1982). Some common classroom autonomy and competence supports are choice (Katz & Assor, 2007), opportunities for self-direction (Reeve et al., 2003), explanatory rationales (Reeve, Jang, Hardre, & Omura, 2002), acknowledgement of feelings (Koestner et al., 1984), encouragement (Reeve & Jang, 2006), and positive feedback (Ryan). As will become a crucial point later in the chapter, the interpersonal climate in which the external event is administered—autonomy supportive or controlling—predicts additional important variance in intrinsic motivation, even to the point that the same external event will have different effects on intrinsic motivation when applied in an autonomy-supportive versus controlling way—for instance, autonomy-supportive versus controlling praise (Ryan), autonomy-supportive versus controlling rewards (Ryan, Mims, & Koestner, 1983), autonomy-supportive versus controlling limits on behavior (Koestner et al., 1984), and autonomy-supportive versus controlling competitions (Reeve & Deci, 1996).

Causality Orientations Theory

Causality orientations theory describes personality-level individual differences in students' orientations toward the motivational forces that cause their behavior (Deci & Ryan, 1985b). In the classroom, some students tend to adopt an orientation in which they rely on autonomous or self-determined guides—interests, personal goals, and self-endorsed values—for the initiation and regulation of their classroom activity, while other students tend to adopt an orientation in which they rely on controlling guides—environmental incentives, social prescriptions, and pressuring internal language—for the initiation and regulation of their classroom activity. To the extent that students rely on self-determined sources of motivation to guide their plans and actions, they embrace an autonomy causality orientation; to the extent that students rely on controlled sources of motivation to guide their plans and actions, they embrace a control causality orientation.

Whereas cognitive evaluation theory reflects the social psychology of self-determination theory, causality orientations theory reflects a personality approach. In examining students' motivation and engagement from a personality perspective, it is important to distinguish students' causality orientation dispositions from other types of personality dispositions such as the widely studied Big Five personality traits. Whereas the Big Five traits are stable and biologically rooted core dimensions of personality, causality orientations are surface individual differences that are relatively malleable and influenced by socialization experiences (Vansteenkiste et al., 2010). Also, causality orientations theory suggests that each student possesses both causality orientations within the personality. What makes individual differences in causality orientations is the relative degree to which the two causality orientations are endorsed, as some students dispositionally endorse a highly autonomous causality orientation as they rely heavily on intrinsic motivation, integrated regulation, and identified regulation as sources of motivation but only lightly or occasionally on external regulation and introjected regulation, while other students dispositionally endorse a highly controlled causality orientation as they rely heavily on external regulation and introjected regulation as sources of motivation but only lightly or occasionally on intrinsic motivation, integrated regulation, and identified regulation.

Individual differences in causality orientations are important because they foreshadow students' adjustment outcomes, as students with autonomy causality orientations tend to display greater self-esteem, greater self-awareness, more mature ego development, and less self-derogation, while students with control causality orientations tend to display greater daily stress, defensiveness, and public self-consciousness (Deci & Ryan, 1985b). By adding the personality perspective to complement the other four minitheories, causality orientations theory completes the overall SDT framework.

Student-Teacher Dialectical Framework Within SDT

The starting point to understand student motivation and engagement within a SDT perspective is to appreciate that students possess inner motivational resources that allow them to be fully capable of engaging themselves constructively in the learning environment. The learning environment, in turn, features conditions that tend either to support or to thwart the inner motivational resources that students bring with them as they walk into the school and into the classroom. Hence, student motivation and the learning environment affect one another, as students tap into their inherent motivational resources to change the learning environment even as they simultaneously receive and internalize new sources of motivation from the learning environment. This reciprocal relation between student and teacher lies at the center of the student-teacher dialectical framework within SDT. To the extent that students are able to express themselves, pursue their interests and values, and acquire constructive new sources of motivation, the dialectical outcome of student-teacher interactions will be synthesis, resulting in greater student autonomy, engagement, and well-being. But if

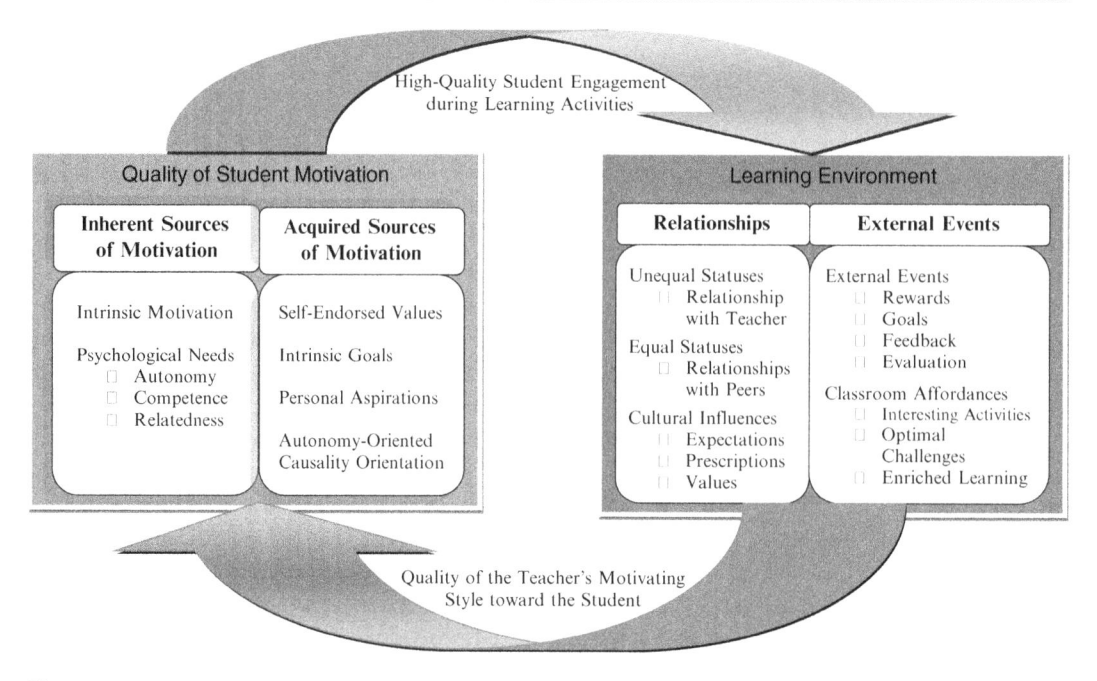

Fig. 7.3 Student-teacher dialectical framework within self-determination theory

controlling classroom events interfere with and thwart students' autonomous engagement, synthesis will be impaired, interpersonal conflict will arise, new sources of motivation will be rejected, and less optimal student outcomes will result.

The dialectical framework appears in Fig. 7.3. The box on the left hand side of the figure represents the quality of the student's motivation during instruction, as informed by SDT's basic needs theory, organismic integration theory, and causality orientations theory. According to basic needs theory, students' inherent sources of motivation include those that are universal across cultures, genders, and backgrounds, including intrinsic motivation and the three psychological needs of autonomy, competence, and relatedness. According to organismic integration theory, students' acquired sources of motivation include those that are internalized through cultural experience and self-reflections that vary from student to student, including self-endorsed values, intrinsic goals, and personal aspirations. According to causality orientations theory, students' acquired sources of motivation further include the disposition-like individual differences of general causality orientations.

As shown in the large upper arrow in the figure, high-quality student engagement arises out of the quality of the student's inherent and acquired sources of motivation and out of the twin desires to interact effectively with the environment and to grow as a person and as a learner. The twofold purpose of the large upper arrow is to communicate that student engagement, first, arises out of and expresses the underlying quality of students' inner motivational resources and, second, feeds forward to affect changes in the learning environment.

The box on the right hand side of the figure represents various aspects of the learning environment. As explained by cognitive evaluation theory, some classroom influences are specific external events, such as rewards, classroom goal structures, feedback, evaluations, and the Friday-afternoon vocabulary quiz. Because of its ubiquity, goals represent particularly important external events in the classroom, and goal contents theory explains when goals support versus interfere with students' motivation, engagement, and well-being. Other classroom influences are interpersonal relationships, including those with teachers, peers, parents, and school administrators as well as more general affiliations with school-related groups, communities, organizations, or the nation in general. All of these relationships have implications for students' motivation, but empirical research on the student-teacher dialectical framework within SDT focuses special attention on those relationships in which people of high status or expertise attempt to motivate or socialize people of lower status or lesser expertise, as with parents relating to children (Grolnick, 2003), coaches relating to athletes (Mageau & Vallerand, 2003), and teachers relating to students (Reeve, 2009b). Other classroom influences are social and cultural forces such as the learning climate (e.g., home schooling; Cai, Reeve, & Robison, 2002) or high-stakes testing policies (Ryan & LaGuardia, 1999).

Finally, as shown in the large lower arrow in the figure, external events and interpersonal relationships that collectively comprise the learning environment provide students with opportunities, hindrances, and an overall climate in which their self-motivation develops (Ryan & LaGuardia, 1999). The most constant aspect of the learning environment is the quality of the teacher's motivating style. And the most important aspect of the teacher's motivating style toward students is whether that style is autonomy supportive or controlling, as students develop autonomous motivations when teachers are autonomy supportive, while they develop controlled motivations when teachers are controlling (Reeve, 2009b).

The student-teacher dialectical framework within SDT was first proposed in 2004, and it was built on experimental studies and cross-sectional survey investigations that largely examined how one variable within the framework affected another. For example, an extensive body of research has accumulated to understand how extrinsic rewards (Deci et al., 1999), interpersonal feedback (Ryan et al., 1983), and the teachers' motivating style (Deci, Schwartz, Sheinman, & Ryan, 1981) affect student motivation, just as an extensive body of empirical research has accumulated to understand how psychological needs (Skinner & Belmont, 1993), intrinsic goals (Vansteenkiste et al., 2004a), and causality orientations (Deci & Ryan, 1985b) affect students' engagement and learning outcomes.

More recently, classroom-based, longitudinally designed research investigations have been undertaken to test the student-teacher dialectical framework as a whole.

Figure 7.4 shows the research design and theoretical predictions from one classroom-based, longitudinally designed, data-based study that was specifically undertaken to test the student-teacher dialectical framework as a whole (Jang, Kim, & Reeve, 2011). Students' perceptions of their teacher's motivating style and self-reports of their own motivation, and engagement, and their objective class-specific achievement were assessed in three waves—at the beginning, middle, and end of the semester. The three downward-slopping boldface lines in Fig. 7.4 represent separate predictions from the student-teacher dialectical framework as (1) the teacher's motivating style affects midsemester changes in students' motivation, as defined by the extent of students' psychological need satisfaction, (2) changes in students' motivation during the course affect corresponding changes in how engaged versus disengaged students are, and (3) changes in student engagement over the course of the semester predict gains versus losses in students' achievement, controlling for students' anticipated achievement at the beginning of the course.

Each of the five boldface lines from Fig. 7.4 parallels an important feature within the student-teacher dialectical framework depicted in Fig. 7.3. Specifically, the path from teacher-provided autonomy support at Time 1 to changes in students' motivation (need satisfaction) at Time 2 in Fig. 7.4 represents the lower U-shaped arrow in Fig. 7.3. The path from student motivation at Time 2 to student engagement at Time 3 in Fig. 7.4 represents the upper rainbow-shaped arrow in Fig. 7.3. In addition, Fig. 7.4 depicts three important extensions of the student-teacher dialectical framework. Each new path will be highlighted in the third section of the present chapter, but each is introduced here. The path from student engagement at Time 3 to students' end-of-course achievement in Fig. 7.4 explains the first new function of student engagement—namely, that it predicts students' positive outcomes, including achievement. The upward-slopping path from student engagement

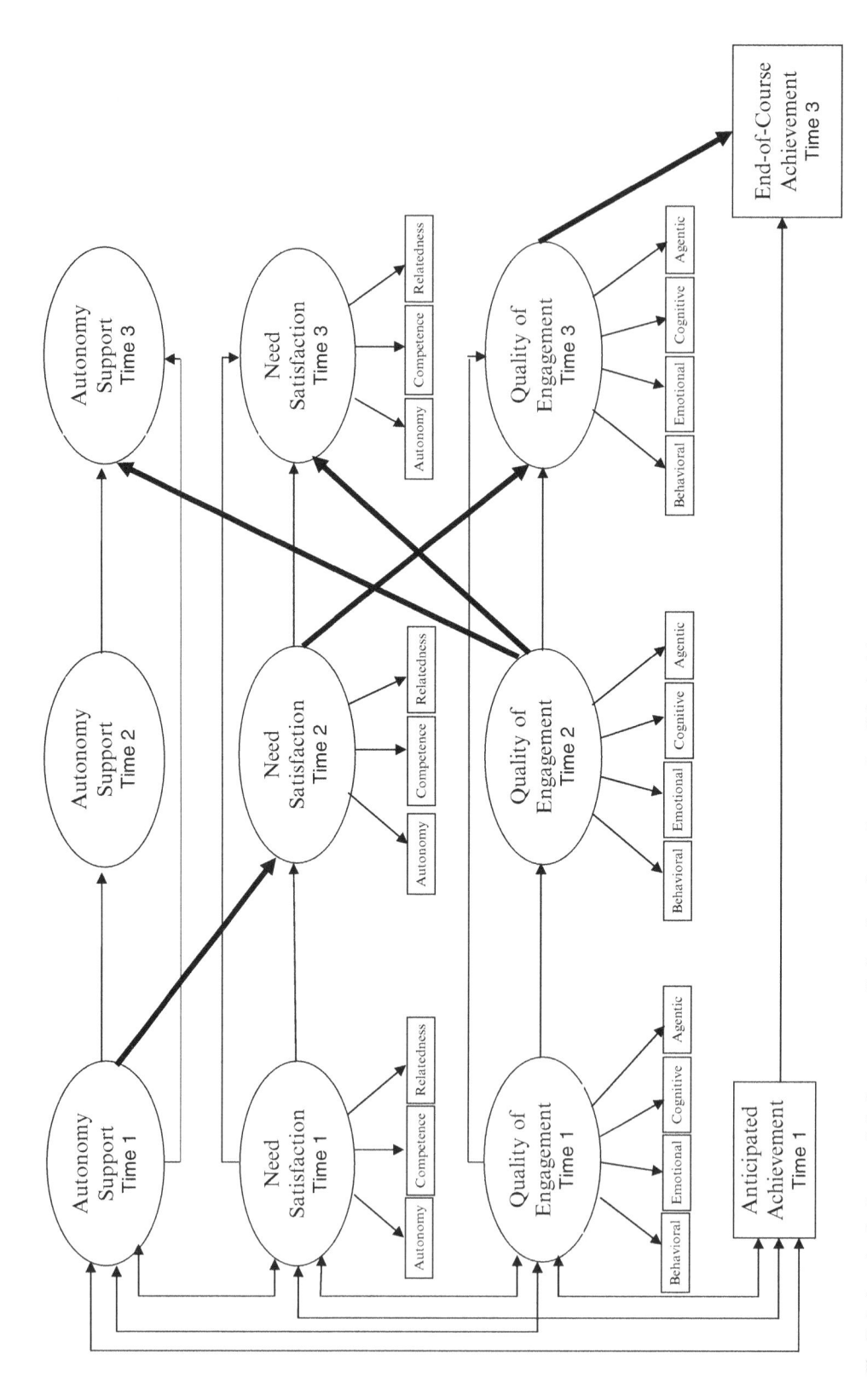

Fig. 7.4 Longitudinal research design to test predictions from the student-teacher dialectical framework

at Time 2 to teacher-provided autonomy support at Time 3 explains the second new function of student engagement—namely, that it predicts constructive changes in the learning environment. The upward-slopping path from student engagement at Time 2 to changes in students' motivation (need satisfaction) explains the third new function of student engagement—namely, that it predicts constructive changes in students' own motivation.

Student Engagement Within the SDT Dialectical Framework

Among those who study the relation between student motivation and student engagement, a general consensus has emerged to characterize engagement as a three-component construct featuring behavioral (on-task attention, effort, persistence, lack of conduct problems), emotional (presence of interest and enthusiasm, absence of anger and boredom), and cognitive (strategic learning strategies, active self-regulation) aspects (Fredricks, Blumenfeld, & Paris, 2004; Jimerson, Campos, & Grief, 2003; National Research Council [NRC], 2004). Echoing this three-component conceptualization, SDT-based research investigations routinely assess these same engagement constructs (e.g., Reeve, Jang, Carrell, Jeon, & Barch, 2004; Skinner & Belmont, 1993). For instance, Skinner and her colleagues (2009) showed how autonomous motivation leads to behavioral engagement and to emotional engagement, while Vansteenkiste and colleagues (2005) showed how autonomous motivation leads to deep rather than to superficial learning (i.e., cognitive engagement).

While each of these three aspects of engagement is certainly important to understanding student engagement, this three-component model of student engagement represents only an incomplete understanding—not an incorrect one, just an incomplete one. The reason why any conceptualization of student engagement as a three-component construct is an incomplete one can be understood through the earlier-presented student-teacher dialectical framework. That is, any focus on students' behavioral, emotional, and cognitive engagement during a learning activity unwittingly embraces a unidirectional flow of instructional activity from the teacher to the student, as the teacher says "Here is an assignment for you" and students respond with some display of behavioral, emotional, and cognitive engagement. What is missing from such a conceptualization of student engagement can be seen in the large upper arrow in Fig. 7.3. That rainbow-shaped arrow represents student engagement in general, but it specifically represents students' constructive contribution into the flow of the instruction they receive, as students try to enrich and personalize that instruction. To understand this process of how students enrich learning activities, we proposed the concept of agentic engagement, and we proposed it as a fourth aspect that was distinct from—yet also highly intercorrelated with—the original three aspects (as through exploratory and confirmatory factor analyses; Reeve & Tseng, 2011).

Agentic engagement refers to students' intentional, proactive, and constructive contribution into the flow of the instruction they receive. It is assessed with both behavioral observation (Reeve et al., 2004) and self-report (Reeve & Tseng, 2011), with questionnaire items such as "During class, I express my preferences and opinions" and "I let the teacher know what I'm interested in." Conceptually, agentic engagement is the process in which students proactively try to create, enhance, and personalize the conditions and circumstances under which they learn. For instance, upon hearing the learning objective for the day (e.g., "Today, class, we are going to learn about Mendel's experiments on heredity."), an agentically engaged student might offer input, make a suggestion, express a preference, contribute something helpful, seek clarification, request an example, ask for a say in how problems will be solved, or a 100 other constructive and personalizing acts that functionally enhance the conditions under which the student learns. Such agentic engagement arises out of students' high-quality motivation, and it potentially affects changes in the learning environment (i.e., the upper arrow in Fig. 7.3).

Why Agentic Engagement Needs to Be Added as a Fourth Aspect of Student Engagement

The present chapter is likely to be the only chapter in the handbook to mention the concept of agentic engagement. For this reason, its value to both researchers and practitioners needs to be explained, as does it status as a potential fourth aspect of engagement.

As teachers provide them with learning activities, students clearly react by displaying varying levels of involvement (engagement) in the learning activities they receive. That is, when the teacher asks students to analyze a poem, students will show varying levels of attention, put forth much or only little effort, enjoy or feel anxious about the activity, and utilize deep and conceptual learning strategies or rely on only superficial ones. The existing concepts of behavioral engagement, emotional engagement, and cognitive engagement nicely capture the extent to which students differentially react to teacher-provided learning activities. Such a linear model (teacher presents a learning activity → students more or less engage themselves → student learn in proportion to their engagement) overlooks students' agentic involvement in the learning process. In actuality, students not only react to learning activities but they proact on them—enriching them (e.g., transforming them into something more interesting or optimally challenging), modifying them (e.g., seeking to learn with a partner rather than alone), personalizing them (e.g., generating options, communicating preferences), and even creating or requesting the learning opportunity in the first place, rather than merely reacting to them as a given (Bandura, 2006). Stated differently, engaged involvement includes not only reacting to the learning task one has been given by showing more or less persistence, enjoyment, and strategic thinking, but it also means initiating a process in which the student generates options that expand his or her freedom of action and increase the chance for that student to experience both strong motivation and meaningful learning.

Three Newly Discovered Functions of Student Engagement

Student engagement is important, and this is so for many reasons. Student engagement is important because it makes learning possible, as it is difficult to imagine learning a foreign language or mastering a musical instrument without considerable engagement. Student engagement is important because it predicts how well students do in school, including the academic progress they make or fail to make (Ladd & Dinella, 2009). Student engagement is also important because it is a relatively malleable student characteristic than is unusually open to constructive influences, such as a teacher's support (Birch & Ladd, 1997). Student engagement is further important because it affords teachers the moment-to-moment feedback they need during instruction to assess how well their efforts to motivate students are working, as there is no better telltale signal about student's private motivation than their public engagement. But all of these reasons, important as they are, are fairly well known.

If you accept agency as a fourth aspect of engagement, however, three new and important functions of engagement emerge, as illustrated graphically in Fig. 7.5. Figure 7.5 mirrors the earlier-presented student-teacher dialectical framework from Fig. 7.3, though it expands on the concept and functions of student engagement within that framework. In comparing Figs. 7.3 and 7.5, notice what has changed is that the single upper rainbow-shaped arrow in Fig. 7.3 has been differentiated into three distinct upper arrows in Fig. 7.5.

The first new function, depicted in the vertical arrow arising out of the quality of student motivation and extending to the newly added "Positive Student Outcomes" box, is that student engagement directly causes positive student outcomes. Of course, many researchers argue this point, as can be seen throughout the pages in this handbook. But what is new and important about this first new function of student engagement is the rather strong assertion that engagement fully mediates

7 A Self-determination Theory Perspective on Student Engagement

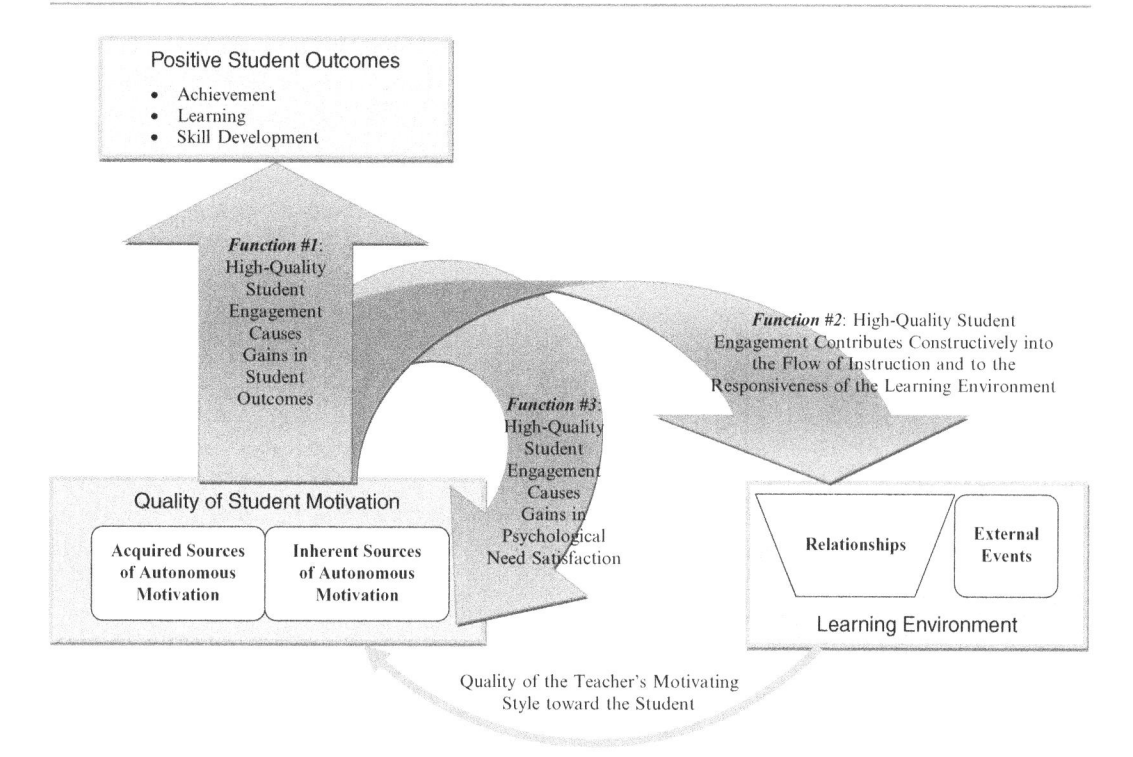

Fig. 7.5 Three new functions of student engagement within the student-teacher dialectical framework

and explains the motivation-to-outcomes relation, as will be discussed in the next section. The second new function, depicted in the rightmost, rainbow-shaped arrow extending to the learning environment, is that student engagement affects the future quality of the learning environment, especially its flow of instruction, the external events it provides, and the teacher's motivating style. The third new function, depicted in the centermost arrow that circles back into student motivation, proposes that the extent of a student's active involvement in a learning activity affects his or her subsequent motivation toward that same activity—that increases in student engagement feedback to enrich future student motivation, just as declines in student engagement feedback to impoverish it.

New Function #1: Engagement Fully Mediates the Motivation-to-Achievement Relation

Part—and probably most—of the reason that educators embrace student engagement as such an important educational construct is because it anticipates and predicts the sort of positive student outcomes identified in the upper left box in Fig. 7.5, such as academic achievement, course grades, learning, and skill development. That is, engagement bridges students' motivation to highly valued outcomes. In statistical terms, this is to say that engagement mediates the motivation-to-achievement relation. This is not, however, a controversial assertion (see Skinner & Belmont, 1993), as researchers who focus on a range of student motivations—including autonomous motivation (Black & Deci, 2000), self-efficacy (Multon, Brown, & Lent, 1991), and achievement goal orientations (Greene & Miller, 1996)—routinely show that motivation exerts a direct effect on achievement. It becomes controversial (and hence worthy of future research), however, with the assertion that engagement *fully mediates* and explains the motivation-to-achievement relation (Reeve & Tseng, 2011). That is, when student engagement is considered as a predictor of students' positive school outcomes, the direct effect that student motivation has on student achievement drops to zero.

Two features differentiate our research showing that engagement fully mediates the motivation-to-achievement relation from others' research showing a direct effect of motivation on achievement. First, we include agentic engagement within our conceptualization of student engagement, whereas others do not. When engagement is operationally defined as students' behavioral, emotional, and cognitive engagement, we often find that some residual variance in end-of-course achievement remains unexplained. Each of these three aspects of engagement does function as an important (though partial) mediator to explain end-of-course achievement, but the significant direct effect of motivation often remains—the direct effect of motivation on achievement is reduced, but it is not eliminated. This means that motivation is contributing to achievement in a way that is not fully explained by students' behavioral, emotional, and cognitive engagement. It is only when we add agentic engagement as a fourth component that engagement fully mediates and explains the motivation-to-achievement relation (Reeve & Tseng, 2011). The reason why agentic engagement explains unique variance in student achievement (or other outcomes, such as skill development or learning) is because it is through agentic acts such as making suggestions, asking questions, and personalizing lessons that students find ways to enrich and to adapt the lessons they receive into improved opportunities for learning, skill development, and achievement to occur. Hence, agentic engagement contributes achievement-enabling behaviors that the behavioral, emotional, and cognitive aspects of engagement fail to capture.

This is both a new hypothesis and a new finding, so the finding that engagement fully mediates the motivation-to-achievement relation will need to be replicated before it might advance from a tentative hypothesis to a reliable principle. However, we have now tested for this full mediation effect twice and found the effect both times (Reeve & Cheon, 2011; Reeve, Lee, Kim, & Ahn, 2011). In both studies, we operationally defined student motivation as the extent of students' psychological need satisfaction (i.e., autonomy, competence, and relatedness) during instruction. We further operationally defined student engagement in a way that was consistent with Fig. 7.1 (the four-aspect conceptualization of engagement) and student achievement as end-of-course grade. Both studies used a longitudinal research design and structural equation modeling to show that the significant direct effect that beginning-of-course motivation had on end-of-course achievement was fully explained by the mediating variable of engagement. In one of the studies (Reeve & Cheon, 2011), we expanded our conceptualization of students' positive outcomes to include not only end-of-course achievement but also skill development, a research strategy that allowed us to test for the full mediating effect of engagement on student outcomes in general rather than on student achievement in particular. This study investigated middle-school students in Korea taking classes in physical education, and student engagement fully mediated the effect that motivation had on both outcomes.

A second feature that makes our research different from previous research (besides including agentic engagement) is that we operationally defined student motivation as the extent of psychological need satisfaction during instruction. When student motivation is conceptualized in this way, several studies have now shown that student engagement fully mediates the effect that student motivation has on their positive end-of-course outcomes (Reeve & Cheon, 2011; Reeve & Tseng, 2010; Reeve et al., 2011). Recognizing this, we expanded our conceptualization of student motivation in two studies beyond the self-determination theory framework (i.e., psychological need satisfaction) to include both academic efficacy and mastery goal orientation. We did this because we wanted to assess the generalizability of our assertion that engagement fully mediates and explains the direct effect of motivation (in general) on student outcomes. Both studies that included academic efficacy (as assessed by the PALS questionnaire) showed that engagement fully mediated the effect that academic efficacy had on student achievement (Reeve & Cheon, 2010; Reeve et al., 2011) and also on student skill development (Reeve & Cheon, 2011).

One study assessed students' mastery goal orientation as a third operational definition of student motivation (Reeve et al., 2011). In this study with Korean middle- and high-school students enrolled in a wide range of courses, engagement did not fully mediate the mastery goal-to-achievement main effect. We found this result surprising, as it challenges our assertion that engagement fully mediates the effect that motivation in general has on achievement. We will return to this issue in the Future Research section at the end of the chapter.

New Function #2: Engagement Changes the Learning Environment

Adding agency as a new component of student engagement paints a fuller picture of how students really engage themselves in learning activities. Recognizing that students (sometimes) proactively, intentionally, and constructively contribute into the instruction they receive clarifies how students learn and profit from classroom learning opportunities—or even how they create new learning opportunities for themselves. What agentically engaged students are doing (that agentically disengaged students are not doing) is offering input, personalizing and enriching the lesson, and modifying and adapting it into an improved opportunity for learning.

Such agency is the ideal complement to a teacher's autonomy-supportive motivating style, just as the lack of student agency is the ideal complement to a teacher's controlling style. That is, agency involves students asking questions, expressing opinions, and communicating interests, while autonomy support involves teachers creating the classroom conditions in which students feel free to ask questions, express opinions, and pursue interests. What adding the concept of agentic engagement can do for any view of student motivation (e.g., need satisfaction, self-efficacy, personal goals, possible selves, individual interests, and mastery goal orientation) is to draw greater attention to students' intentional, proactive, and origin-like motivational involvement in learning activities.

The empirical evidence to support the second (rainbow-shaped) arrow in Fig. 7.5 has been mixed. One the one hand, laboratory research shows that experimentally manipulated levels of how engaged versus disengaged a student is in a learning activity causally affects the teacher's subsequent motivating style toward that student (Pelletier & Vallerand, 1996). That is, teachers generally react to student displays of high-quality engagement with a more autonomy-supportive motivating style, while they react to student displays of disengagement with a more controlling style (Pelletier, Seguin-Levesque, & Legault, 2002; Skinner & Belmont, 1993). Our own research, however, has not always found this engagement-to-motivating style causal effect in naturally occurring classrooms. We sometimes find that changes in student engagement during the course of the semester do not cause subsequent changes in the teachers' end-of-course motivating style (Jang et al., 2011). The biggest difference between the hypothesis-confirming experimental research and our hypothesis-questioning classroom research is likely the student-teacher ratio difference, as the ratio is 1:1 in the laboratory experiments but something like 30:1 in classroom studies. For this reason, the "relationships" variable within the Learning Environment box in Fig. 7.5 is drawn with an open-ended funnel shape. The funnel shape communicates the teacher's need to be attuned to classroom expressions of high-quality engagement, especially to expressions of agentic engagement. Teachers might become more attuned to students' engagement, for instance, by listening, by asking students as to what they would like to do, and by communicating perspective-taking comments (Reeve & Jang, 2006).

New Function #3: Engagement Changes Motivation

Another new, interesting, and important finding to emerge out of our recent longitudinal classroom-based investigations of the student-teacher dialectic is the consistent finding that changes in the quality of students' engagement during the course of the semester predict gains versus declines in students' end-of-semester motivation (i.e., psychological need satisfaction). This effect that changes in engagement make on subsequent changes in motivation appears in Fig. 7.5 as the circular arrow in which changes in the quality of students' engagement loop back to predict subsequent changes in the quality of students' motivation. That is, students' motivation (the "Quality of Student Motivation" box in the figure) is both a cause and a consequence of student engagement. The role of this third new function of engagement is to highlight the causal role that changes in engagement contribute to changes in motivation.

The hypothesis that changes in engagement cause changes in motivation is premised on the idea that students can take action to meet their own psychological needs. According to SDT, the needs for autonomy, competence, and relatedness provide the psychological nutriments necessary for positive psychological well-being. That is, students need autonomy, competence, and relatedness experiences to be well. This assertion has received considerable empirical support. For instance, research participants reliably report having a "good day" (feeling joyful, enthusiastic) when they experience high levels of daily autonomy, competence, and relatedness, while they just as reliably report having a "bad day" (feeling distress, anger) when they experience low (or frustrated) levels of daily autonomy, competence, and relatedness (Kasser & Ryan, 1993, 1996; Sheldon et al., 1996). But to experience autonomy, competence, and relatedness, one first has to take action and actually engage in environmental transactions that are capable of producing such experiences and feelings (e.g., read a book, exercise with friends, try something new). Thus, high-quality engagement in what one is doing would seem necessary to produce need-satisfying and positive subjective experiences.

We have tested for this "changes in engagement causes changes in motivation" effect twice, and we have found the effect both times (Jang et al., 2011; Reeve et al., 2011). In both studies, student motivation was operationally defined as the extent of psychological need satisfaction, while student engagement was operationally defined in a way that was consistent with the four-component depiction in Fig. 7.1. Both studies used a full longitudinal design and structural equation modeling to test the hypothesis [i.e., the boldface upward-slopping arrow in Fig. 7.4 that extends from engagement at Time 2 to motivation (need satisfaction) at Time 3]. That path in Fig. 7.4 does not look the same as the slopping arrow from Fig. 7.5, but the effect and the interpretation are the same—changes in the quality of engagement predict (and temporally cause) changes in the quality of motivation.

Consider why this new function of engagement might be important to future engagement research. In an SDT framework, changes in students' psychological need satisfaction occur in response to the teacher's motivating style. That is, when teachers relate to students in autonomy-supportive ways, students experience greater autonomy, competence, and relatedness, and when teachers relate to students in controlling ways, they experience lesser autonomy, competence, and relatedness. Again, this is a reliable finding (Black & Deci, 2000; Deci et al., 1981; Jang, Reeve, Ryan, & Kim, 2009; Ryan & Grolnick, 1986). But the findings from the longitudinal classroom-based investigations summarized above confirm a second reliable source of changes in students' course-related motivation— namely, changes in students' course-related engagement. In fact, these studies find that changes in student engagement is a stronger predictor of end-of-course motivation than is the quality of the teacher's motivating style (in terms of the magnitude of the two respective *beta* coefficients predicting end-of-course motivation; Jang et al., 2011). This means that students can take action to meet their own psychological needs and to enhance the quality of their own motivation. This also means that students can be (and are) architects of their own motivation, at least to the extent that students can be architects of their own course-related behavioral, emotional, cognitive, and agentic engagement.

Implications for Teachers

If you are a teacher and have invested your behavioral, emotional, and cognitive engagement in reading and reflecting on the chapter to this point, it is now time to give you an opportunity to agentically voice your interests and hopes for the chapter. Accordingly, the chapter now turns to two key implications for teachers.

The first implication is to recommend that teachers work to increase their capacity to practice a more autonomy-supportive motivating style toward their students. Generally speaking, autonomy support is whatever a teacher says and does during instruction to facilitate students' perceptions of autonomy and experiences of psychological need satisfaction. More specifically, an autonomy-supportive motivating style is the interpersonal sentiment and behavior teachers provide to identify, vitalize, and develop their students' inner motivational resources during instruction (Assor, Kaplan, & Roth, 2002; Reeve, 2009b; Reeve et al., 2004). It is important because it predicts students' constructive motivation, engagement, and functioning in a reliable way, as discussed earlier. It is also important because, like student engagement, a teacher's motivating style is malleable. While it is true that teachers' naturally occurring motivating styles (controlling, neutral, or autonomy supportive) tend to remain fairly consistent throughout the school year, it is also true that teachers can learn how to be more autonomy supportive toward students. Intervention training programs have shown that teachers can learn how to be more autonomy supportive and also that such a change in one's motivating style endures well beyond the initial training experience (Su & Reeve, 2011). In these intervention studies, teachers randomly assigned into an experimental group participate in a training program that, first, tells them what autonomy support is and how beneficial it typically is for students and, second, provides them with the modeling, scaffolding, and "how-to" problem-solving discussions they need to be able to support students' autonomy during classroom practice. This research is important for the purposes of the present chapter because it shows that (1) teachers can learn how to become more autonomy supportive and (2) the more autonomy supportive they become, the more high-quality engagement their students show (e.g., Reeve et al., 2004). Stated differently, the first recommendation seeks to offer teachers a reliable path to enhancing student engagement—namely, adopt a more autonomy-supportive motivating style toward students.

The second implication is to recommend that teachers intentionally monitor and enhance students' classroom engagement. Monitoring and enhancing students' motivation and engagement is an important skill, but these are also difficult responsibilities for teachers to fulfill on a reliable basis. Monitoring students' motivation and engagement is difficult not only because classrooms are large, fluid, and diverse environments but also because motivation is a private, subjective, and unobservable student experience. That is, teachers cannot objectively see their students' underlying psychological need satisfaction, self-efficacy, interest, goal orientation, etc. The instructional task of monitoring what is unobservable and only privately experienced (i.e., student motivation) would seem overly difficult. In contrast to motivation, however, student engagement is a relatively public, objective, and observable classroom event. That is, teachers can see whether or not a student is paying attention, putting forth effort, enjoying class, solving problems in a sophisticated way, and contributing constructively into the flow of instruction. The instructional task of monitoring what is observable and publically expressed (i.e., student engagement) would seem possible.

To test this logic, we asked a group of middle- and high-school Korean teachers who taught a wide range of different subject matters to rate each student in their class on how motivated and how engaged the teacher thought the student was (Lee & Reeve, 2011). In particular, we asked these teachers to rate their students on three aspects of motivation—psychological need satisfaction, self-efficacy, and mastery goal orientation—and on four aspects of engagement—behavioral engagement, emotional engagement, cognitive

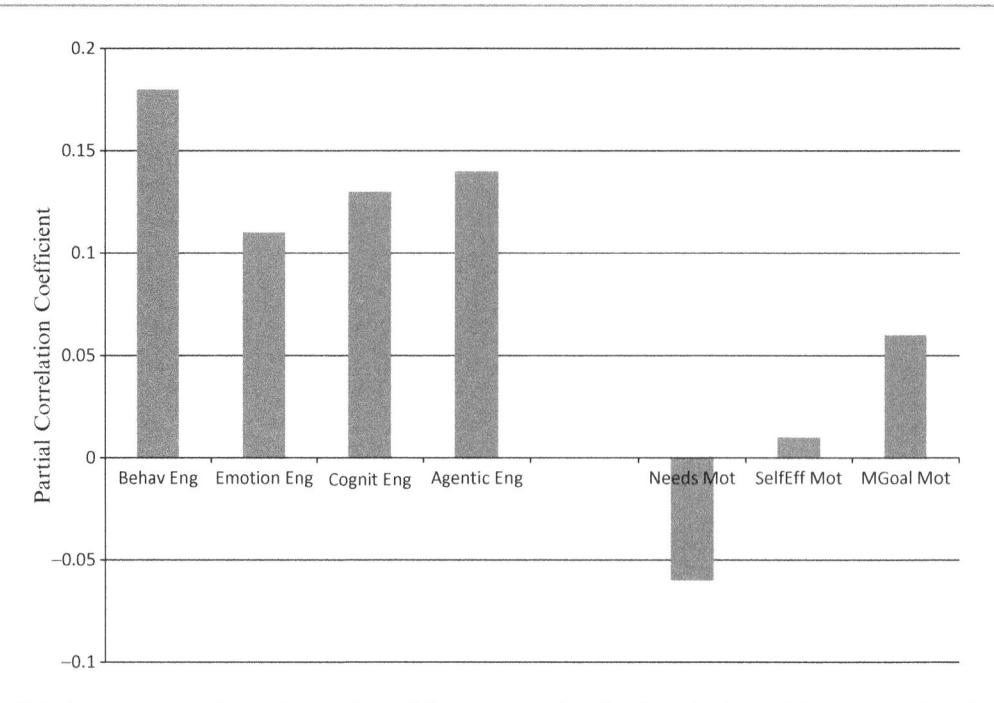

Fig. 7.6 Accuracy scores for teachers' ratings of three aspects of students' motivation and four aspects of students' engagement

engagement, and agentic engagement. At the same time, we asked the students of these teachers to self-report the same three aspects of their course-related motivation and the same four aspects of their course-related engagement, using previously validated questionnaires. How accurate teachers were in rating their students' motivation and engagement appears in Fig. 7.6.

Accuracy scores were determined with partial correlation statistics that showed the association between each teacher rating and each student self-report after partialling out variance attributable to student achievement. It was necessary to partial out student achievement scores because teachers generally rate high-achieving students as more motivated and as more engaged than they rate low-achieving students. Looking at the composite scores only, teacher rated their students' motivation unreliably ($pr=-.03$, ns) but their students' engagement reliably ($pr=.13$, $p<.05$), as reported in Lee and Reeve (2011). The bars in Fig. 7.6 show the partial correlations observed for each of the four aspects of engagement (on the left side of the figure) and for each of the three aspects of motivation (on the right side of the figure). Overall, results were clear: Teacher ratings of their students' motivation were inaccurate, while teachers' ratings of their students' engagement were accurate. Further, teachers' inaccuracy scores did not depend on the type of student motivation they rated, just as teacher accuracy scores did not depend on the type of student engagement they rated.

The data summarized in Fig. 7.6 are important because they suggest that the instructional effort to monitor students' motivation is probably too difficult (because it is a private, unobservable student experience), while the instructional effort to monitor students' engagement is probably manageable (because it is a public, observable student behavior). We are not suggesting that student motivation is not important, and we are not suggesting that teachers not think about how to facilitate it. After all, student motivation is the key variable underlying and causing students' classroom engagement. Instead, we recommend that teachers allocate a significant proportion of their attention during instruction to the effort of monitoring and enhancing students' engagement. Doing so allows teachers to invest their attention on the variable that changes students' academic lives for the better—namely, high-quality student engagement.

Future Research

The present chapter relied on a pair of well-established theoretical perspectives—namely, SDT and the student-teacher dialectical framework within SDT—to present three new ideas about the nature and function of student engagement. Each one of these ideas is both new and somewhat controversial, so each requires extensive future research to assess its reliability, validity, and potential contribution to the larger literature on student engagement.

The first new finding that requires extensive future research is the definitional claim that student engagement is better conceptualized as a four-component construct than as a three-component construct. The difference between the two conceptualizations is that the four-component conceptualization includes agentic engagement, whereas the three-component conceptualization excludes it. This future research will need to examine both the conceptual status of agentic engagement as well as its assessment procedures. In terms of conceptualizing agentic engagement, Reeve and Tseng (2011) proposed five defining features of the construct: (1) it is proactive in that it occurs before or during the learning activity; (2) it is intentional in that agentic engagement is both deliberate and purposive; (3) it attempts to enrich the learning activity by making the learning experience more personal, more interesting, more challenging, or more valued; (4) it contributes constructive input into the planning or ongoing flow of the teacher's instruction; and (5) it does not connote teacher ineffectiveness or incompetence. In terms of assessing agentic engagement, researchers currently assess the construct either by having trained raters score students' agency from the Hit-Steer Observation System (for illustrations see, Jang, Reeve, & Deci, 2010; Koenig, Fielder, & deCharms, 1977; Reeve et al., 2004) or from a five-item self-report scale (Reeve & Tseng, 2011). As clarity emerges as to the nature and function of students' agentic engagement during learning activities, future research will be better positioned to improve the assessment of the construct. Part of that empirical effort will be to better assess the construct, and part of the empirical effort will be to better distinguish agentic engagement both from similar constructs (e.g., instructional help seeking) and from the other three aspects of engagement.

The second new finding that requires extensive future research is the functional claim that student engagement serves purposes beyond those that are already well established and understood. Specifically, the SDT perspective suggests three new and important functions of student engagement—namely, that student engagement fully mediates and explains the motivation-to-achievement relation, that changes in student engagement produce changes in the learning environment, and that changes in student engagement produce changes in student motivation, as students' behavioral, emotional, cognitive, and agentic engagement represents action taken to meet their psychological needs. The validity of the claim that student engagement fully mediates and explains the motivation-to-achievement relation may boil down to how the engagement construct itself is conceptualized and assessed. As emphasized above, when engagement is conceptualized and assessed as a four-component construct, student engagement does seem to consistently and fully mediate the direct effect that motivation has on students' positive outcomes. If this rather strong assertion does not eventually hold up to future analysis, there will still be important insights to gain from asking the question as to what effect motivation has on student outcomes that lies outside of its effect on engagement. It is actually rather difficult to think of a path from motivation to achievement that does not go through student engagement, though both social engagement and an improved teacher-student relationship might be two candidates. The idea that student motivation might improve the teacher-student relationship is nicely captured by the student-teacher dialectical framework within SDT, though our recent evidence suggests rather strongly that what affects the quality of the student-teacher relationship during learning activities is more the publically observable engagement that students show and less the privately experienced motivation they harbor.

Finally, the finding that changes in student engagement produce changes in student motivation requires extensive future study. It is an exciting finding that students can take self-initiated action—in terms of their behavioral, emotional, cognitive, and agentic engagements—to meet their psychological needs. The reason this finding has such potential to improve our understanding of the functions of student engagement is partly because the effect of engagement on students' motivation seems to be as strong as the effect of the teacher's motivating style on student motivation and partly because it illustrates empirically that students can be architects of their own motivation—for better or for worse.

References

Amabile, T. M., DeJong, W., & Lepper, M. R. (1976). Effects of externally-imposed deadlines on subsequent intrinsic motivation. *Journal of Personality and Social Psychology, 34*, 92–98.

Assor, A., Kaplan, H., & Roth, G. (2002). Choice is good, but relevance is excellent: Autonomy-enhancing and suppressing teaching behaviors predicting students' engagement in schoolwork. *British Journal of Educational Psychology, 27*, 261–278.

Bandura, A. (2006). Toward a psychology of human agency. *Perspectives on Psychological Science, 1*, 164–180.

Birch, S. H., & Ladd, G. W. (1997). The student-teacher relationship and children's early school adjustment. *Journal of School Psychology, 35*, 61–79.

Black, A. E., & Deci, E. L. (2000). The effects of instructors' autonomy support and students' autonomous motivation on learning organic chemistry: A self-determination theory perspective. *Science Education, 84*, 740–756.

Cai, Y., Reeve, J., & Robinson, D. T. (2002). Home schooling and teaching style: Comparing the motivating styles of home school and public school teachers. *Journal of Educational Psychology, 94*, 372–380.

Deci, E. L. (1975). *Intrinsic motivation*. New York: Plenum.

Deci, E. L., Betley, G., Kahle, J., Abrams, L., & Porac, J. (1981). When trying to win: Competition and intrinsic motivation. *Personality and Social Psychology Bulletin, 7*, 79–83.

Deci, E. L., Koestner, R., & Ryan, R. M. (1999). A meta-analytic review of experiments examining the effects of extrinsic rewards on intrinsic motivation. *Psychological Bulletin, 125*, 627–668.

Deci, E. L., & Ryan, R. M. (1980). The empirical exploration of intrinsic motivational processes. In L. Berkowitz (Ed.), *Advances in experimental social psychology* (Vol. 13, pp. 39–40). New York: Academic Press.

Deci, E. L., & Ryan, R. M. (1985a). *Intrinsic motivation and self-determination in human behavior*. New York: Plenum.

Deci, E. L., & Ryan, R. M. (1985b). The General Causality Orientations Scale: Self-determination in personality. *Journal of Research in Personality, 19*, 109–134.

Deci, E. L., & Ryan, R. M. (1991). A motivational approach to self: Integration in personality. In R. Dienstbier (Ed.), *Nebraska symposium on motivation: Perspectives on motivation* (Vol. 38, pp. 237–288). Lincoln: University of Nebraska Press.

Deci, E. L., & Ryan, R. M. (2000). The "what" and "why" of goal pursuits: Human needs and the self-determination of behavior. *Psychological Inquiry, 11*, 227–268.

Deci, E. L., Schwartz, A., Sheinman, L., & Ryan, R. M. (1981). An instrument to assess adult's orientations toward control versus autonomy in children: Reflections on intrinsic motivation and perceived competence. *Journal of Educational Psychology, 73*, 642–650.

Fredricks, J. A., Blumenfeld, P. C., & Paris, A. H. (2004). School engagement: Potential of the concept, state of the evidence. *Review of Educational Research, 74*, 59–109.

Greene, B. A., & Miller, R. B. (1996). Influences on achievement: Goals, perceived ability, and cognitive engagement. *Contemporary Educational Psychology, 21*, 181–192.

Grolnick, W. S. (2003). *The psychology of parental control: How well-meant parenting backfires*. Mahwah, NJ: Erlbaum.

Jang, H., Kim, E., & Reeve, J. (2011). *Longitudinal test of self-determination theory in a school context*. Manuscript submitted for publication

Jang, H., Reeve, J., & Deci, E. L. (2010). Engaging students in learning activities: It is not autonomy support or structure but autonomy support and structure. *Journal of Educational Psychology, 102*, 588–600.

Jang, H., Reeve, J., Ryan, R. M., & Kim, A. (2009). Can self-determination theory explain what underlies the productive, satisfying learning experiences of collectivistically-oriented Korean adolescents? *Journal of Educational Psychology, 101*, 644–661.

Jimerson, S. J., Campos, E., & Grief, J. L. (2003). Toward an understanding of definitions and measures of school engagement and related terms. *The California School Psychologist, 8*, 7–27.

Kasser, T., & Ryan, R. M. (1993). A dark side of the American dream: Correlates of financial success as a central life aspiration. *Journal of Personality and Social Psychology, 65*, 410–422.

Kasser, T., & Ryan, R. M. (1996). Further examining the American dream: Differential correlates of intrinsic and extrinsic goals. *Personality and Social Psychology Bulletin, 22,* 280–287.

Katz, I., & Assor, A. (2007). When choice motivates and when it does not. *Educational Psychology Review, 19,* 429–442.

Koenig, S. S., Fielder, M. L., & deCharms, R. (1977). Teacher beliefs, classroom interaction and personal causation. *Journal of Applied Social Psychology, 7,* 95–114.

Koestner, R., Ryan, R. M., Bernieri, F., & Holt, K. (1984). Setting limits on children's behavior: The differential effects of controlling versus informational styles on intrinsic motivation and creativity. *Journal of Personality, 52,* 233–248.

Ladd, G. W., & Dinella, L. M. (2009). Continuity and change in early school engagement: Predictive of children's achievement trajectories from first to eighth grade? *Journal of Educational Psychology, 101,* 190–206.

Lee, W., & Reeve, J. (2011). *Teacher accuracy in judging students' motivation and engagement.* Manuscript for publication.

Lepper, M. R., & Greene, D. (1975). Turning play into work: Effects of adult surveillance and extrinsic rewards on children's intrinsic motivation. *Journal of Personality and Social Psychology, 31,* 479–486.

Mageau, G. A., & Vallerand, R. J. (2003). The coach-athlete relationship: A motivational model. *Journal of Sports Science, 21,* 883–904.

Mossholder, K. W. (1980). Effects of externally mediated goal setting on intrinsic motivation: A laboratory experiment. *Journal of Applied Psychology, 65,* 202–210.

Multon, K. D., Brown, S. D., & Lent, R. W. (1991). Relation of self-efficacy beliefs to academic outcomes: A meta-analytic investigation. *Journal of Counseling Psychology, 38,* 30–38.

National Research Council. (2004). *Engaging schools: Fostering high school students' motivation to learn.* Washington, DC: The National Academies Press.

Niemiec, C. P., & Ryan, R. M. (2009). Autonomy, competence, and relatedness in the classroom: Applying self-determination theory to educational practice. *Theory and Research in Education, 7,* 133–144.

Niemiec, C. P., Ryan, R. M., & Deci, E. L. (2009). The path taken: Consequences of attaining intrinsic and extrinsic aspirations in post-college life. *Journal of Research in Personality, 43,* 291–306.

Pelletier, L. G., Seguin-Levesque, C., & Legault, L. (2002). Pressure from above and pressure from below as determinants of teachers' motivation and teaching behaviors. *Journal of Educational Psychology, 94,* 186–196.

Pelletier, L. G., & Vallerand, R. J. (1996). Supervisors' beliefs and subordinates' intrinsic motivation: A behavioral confirmation analysis. *Journal of Personality and Social Psychology, 71,* 331–340.

Reeve, J. (2009a). *Understanding motivation and emotion* (5th ed.). Hoboken, NJ: Wiley.

Reeve, J. (2009b). Why teachers adopt a controlling motivating style toward students and how they can become more autonomy supportive. *Educational Psychologist, 44,* 159–175.

Reeve, J., & Cheon, S. H. (2011). *Interrelations among teachers' motivating styles and students' motivation, engagement, and skill development in a physical education context.* Manuscript submitted for publication.

Reeve, J., & Deci, E. L. (1996). Elements of the competitive situation that affect intrinsic motivation. *Personality and Social Psychology Bulletin, 22,* 24–33.

Reeve, J., Deci, E. L., & Ryan, R. M. (2004). Self-determination theory: A dialectical framework for understanding the sociocultural influences on student motivation. In D. McInerney & S. Van Etten (Eds.), *Research on sociocultural influences on motivation and learning: Big theories revisited* (Vol. 4, pp. 31–59). Greenwich, CT: Information Age.

Reeve, J., & Halusic, M. (2009). How K-12 teachers can put self-determination theory principles into practice. *Theory and Research in Education, 7,* 145–154.

Reeve, J., & Jang, H. (2006). What teachers say and do to support students' autonomy during learning activities. *Journal of Educational Psychology, 98,* 209–218.

Reeve, J., Jang, H., Carrell, D., Jeon, S., & Barch, J. (2004). Enhancing high school students' engagement by increasing their teachers' autonomy support. *Motivation and Emotion, 28,* 147–169.

Reeve, J., Jang, H., Hardre, P., & Omura, M. (2002). Providing a rationale in an autonomy-supportive way as a strategy to motivate others during an uninteresting activity. *Motivation and Emotion, 26,* 183–207.

Reeve, J., Lee, W., Kim, H., & Ahn, H. S. (2011). *Longitudinal test of the hypothesis that student engagement fully mediates the motivation-to-achievement relation.* Manuscript submitted for publication.

Reeve, J., Nix, G., & Hamm, D. (2003). Testing models of the experience of self-determination in intrinsic motivation and the conundrum of choice. *Journal of Educational Psychology, 95,* 375–392.

Reeve, J., & Tseng, C.–M (2011). Agency as a fourth aspect of students' engagement during learning activities. *Contemporary Educational psychology, 36,* 257–267.

Reis, H. T., Sheldon, K. M., Gable, S. L., Roscoe, J., & Ryan, R. M. (2000). Daily well-being: The role of autonomy, competence, and relatedness. *Personality and Social Psychology Bulletin, 26,* 419–435.

Ryan, R. M. (1982). Control and information in the intrapersonal sphere: An extension of cognitive evaluation theory. *Journal of Personality and Social Psychology, 43,* 450–461.

Ryan, R. M. (1993). Agency and organization: Intrinsic motivation, autonomy and the self in psychological development. In J. Jacobs (Ed.), *Nebraska symposium on motivation: Developmental perspectives on motivation* (Vol. 40, pp. 1–56). Lincoln, NE: University of Nebraska Press.

Ryan, R. M., & Connell, J. P. (1989). Perceived locus of causality and internalization: Examining reasons for acting in two domains. *Journal of Personality and Social Psychology, 57,* 749–761.

Ryan, R. M., & Deci, E. L. (2000). Self-determination theory and the facilitation of intrinsic motivation, social development, and well-being. *American Psychologist, 55,* 68–78.

Ryan, R. M., & Deci, E. L. (2002). An overview of self-determination theory: An organismic-dialectical perspective. In E. L. Deci & R. M. Ryan (Eds.), *Handbook of self-determination research* (pp. 3–33). Rochester, NY: University of Rochester Press.

Ryan, R. M., & Grolnick, W. S. (1986). Origins and pawns in the classroom: Self-report and projective assessments of individual differences in children's perceptions. *Journal of Personality and Social Psychology, 50*, 550–558.

Ryan, R. M., & LaGuardia, J. G. (1999). Achievement motivation within a pressured society: Intrinsic and extrinsic motivation to learn and the politics of school reform. In T. Urdan (Ed.), *Advances in motivation and achievement* (Vol. 11, pp. 45–85). Greenwich, CT: JAI Press.

Ryan, R. M., Mims, V., & Koestner, R. (1983). Relation of reward contingency and interpersonal context to intrinsic motivation: A review and test using cognitive evaluation theory. *Journal of Personality and Social Psychology, 45*, 736–750.

Ryan, R. M., Sheldon, K. M., Kasser, T., & Deci, E. L. (1996). All goals are not created equal: An organismic perspective on the nature of goals and their regulation. In P. M. Gollwitzer & J. A. Bargh (Eds.), *The psychology of action: Linking cognition and motivation to behavior* (pp. 7–26). New York: Guilford Press.

Sheldon, K. M., Ryan, R. M., & Reis, H. T. (1996). What makes for a good day? Competence and autonomy in the day and in the person. *Personality and Social Psychology Bulletin, 22*, 1270–1279.

Skinner, E. A., & Belmont, M. J. (1993). Motivation in the classroom: Reciprocal effects of teacher behavior and student engagement across the school year. *Journal of Educational Psychology, 85*, 571–581.

Skinner, E. A., Kindermann, T. A., & Furrer, C. J. (2009). A motivational perspective on engagement and disaffection: Conceptualization and assessment of children's behavioral and emotional participation in academic activities in the classroom. *Educational and Psychological Measurement, 69*, 493–525.

Su, Y.-L., & Reeve, J. (2011). A meta-analysis of the effectiveness of intervention programs designed to support autonomy. *Educational Psychology Review, 23*, 159–188.

Vansteenkiste, M., Lens, W., & Deci, E. L. (2006). Intrinsic versus extrinsic goal contents in self-determination theory: Another look at the quality of academic motivation. *Educational Psychologist, 41*, 19–31.

Vansteenkiste, M., Niemiec, C. P., & Soenens, B. (2010). The development of the five mini-theories of self-determination theory: An historical overview, emerging trends, and future directions. *Advances in motivation and achievement: The decade ahead: Theoretical perspectives on motivation and achievement, 16A*, 105–167.

Vansteenkiste, M., Simons, J., Lens, W., Sheldon, K. M., & Deci, E. L. (2004a). Motivating learning, performance, and persistence: The synergistic role of intrinsic goals and autonomy support. *Journal of Personality and Social Psychology, 87*, 246–260.

Vansteenkiste, M., Simons, J., Lens, W., Soenens, B., & Matos, L. (2005). Examining the impact of extrinsic versus intrinsic goal framing and internally controlling versus autonomy-supportive communication style upon early adolescents' academic achievement. *Child Development, 76*, 483–501.

Vansteenkiste, M., Simons, J., Lens, W., Soenens, B., Matos, L., & Lacante, M. (2004b). "Less is sometimes more": Goal-content matters. *Journal of Educational Psychology, 96*, 755–764.

Vansteenkiste, M., Timmermans, T., Lens, W., Soenens, B., & Van den Broeck, A. (2008). Does extrinsic goal framing enhance extrinsic goal oriented individuals' learning and performance? An experimental test of the match-perspective vs. self-determination theory. *Journal of Educational Psychology, 100*, 387–397.

Wellborn, J. G. (1991). *Engaged and disaffected action: The conceptualization and measurement of motivation in the academic domain.* Unpublished doctoral dissertation, University of Rochester, Rochester.

Achievement Goal Theory, Conceptualization of Ability/Intelligence, and Classroom Climate

Eric M. Anderman and Helen Patrick

Abstract

In this chapter, we examine relations between achievement goal theory and student engagement. Achievement goal theorists generally examine two types of goals (mastery and performance goals), each of which has been conceptualized as having both approach and avoid components. After reviewing the history and development of achievement goal theory and describing the current four-factor model, we examine correlates of achievement goal orientations; these include students' beliefs about intelligence, academic achievement, and engagement (cognitive, emotional, and behavioral). We then review research on classroom goal structures; we specifically examine how classroom contexts, as conceptualized through goal orientation theory, are related to student engagement. We also review instructional practices that are related to both mastery and performance goal structures and how those practices are related to academic achievement.

Achievement goal theory is a framework that is used to explain and study academic motivation. The theory became particularly prominent during the 1980s and 1990s and has emerged as one of the most accepted and supported theories in the field of educational psychology (Elliot, 1999; Maehr & Zusho, 2009). Currently, achievement goal theory informs both educational research and classroom practice, given its strong empirical support. Relevant to the present chapter, achievement goal theory has been, and continues to be, a predominant perspective used to understand students' engagement in academics.

In the present chapter, we review many aspects of achievement goal theory. In addition to describing the theory and its relation to valued educational outcomes, we also argue that achievement goal theory is related in important ways to student engagement. Although the constructs utilized by achievement goal theorists differ from the constructs used by researchers who study

E.M. Anderman
School of Educational Policy and Leadership,
The Ohio State University, Columbus, OH, USA
e-mail: eanderman@ehe.osu.edu

H. Patrick (✉)
Department of Educational Studies,
Purdue University, West Lafayette, IN, USA
e-mail: hpatrick@purdue.edu

engagement, there is much overlap. We believe that a more thorough examination and possible integration of research conducted by achievement goal theorists and by engagement researchers will lead to a broader and more conceptually useful understanding of academic motivation.

The Basic Tenets of Achievement Goal Theory

Achievement goal theory has a rich history within the field of motivation. This history includes both the original development of the theory, as well as more recent subtle changes in the ways in which goal theory constructs are operationalized. These changes are reflected in research examining correlates of achievement goal orientations; indeed, as measurement of goal orientations has changed over time, results of research examining the relations of goal orientations to other outcomes also have evolved.

Historical Development of Achievement Goal Theory

The study of achievement goal orientations formally began in the late 1970s, although many aspects of the theory can be traced back to much earlier conceptions of achievement motivation. Researchers at the University of Illinois were particularly prominent in early developments of the theory. In particular, Martin Maehr, Carole Ames, John Nicholls, and Carol Dweck all were influential in early work on goal orientation theory.

As we will review in this chapter, the theory has developed and changed in quite remarkable ways during the past three decades. The theory, which was originally conceptualized in terms of two types of goal orientations, has blossomed into a robust theoretical framework that now includes the original conceptions of goal orientations, as well as numerous additional distinctions between subtypes. Originally, the theory focused predominantly on students' personal goal orientations (i.e., the reasons that students give for engaging personally in specific tasks). Researchers identified two types—"mastery" (i.e., a focus on understanding and personal improvement) and "performance" (i.e., a focus on outperforming others), although different researchers used different names. There was also some consideration, however, of students' perceptions of what is emphasized in their classrooms or schools in terms of reasons for engaging in schoolwork and the meaning of success (i.e., classroom goal structures; Ames, 1984). Although personal goal orientations continue to receive most attention, consideration of classroom goal structures has become more prevalent, consistent with the greater attention to the role of social contexts in motivational research (Anderman & Anderman, 2000; Meece, Anderman, & Anderman, 2006; Midgley, 2002).

As we will review later, goal theorists also draw strongly from the approach/avoid distinctions often made in psychology (Elliot, 1999; Elliot & Covington, 2001). Approach and avoidance motivations are distinguished by whether or not behavior is directed by desirable (*approach*) or undesirable (*avoid*) potential outcomes. As research on achievement goal theory progressed over the past two decades, in particular, psychometric studies focusing on the measurement of goal orientations have drawn in significant ways from approach/avoid distinctions (Elliot & Harackiewicz, 1996).

In addition, numerous methodological developments over the past few decades have enhanced our understanding of achievement goal orientations. Whereas many of the original studies used survey methodology to examine students' personal goal orientations, later studies have included classroom observations, discourse analyses, multilevel models, experimental designs, and mixed-method approaches. These methodological advances have allowed motivation researchers to understand the nature of achievement goals more fully, as well as their many correlates.

Variations in Operationalizations of Goal Orientations

Personal goal orientations have been defined and operationalized differently by various researchers.

Although we use the terms "mastery" and "performance" to broadly characterize goal orientations, it is important to note that a variety of developments have occurred over the years. Maehr (1984) called his version of mastery goals "task goals," which he defined as focusing on (a) an individual's involvement with a specific task and (b) an individual's perceptions of his or her competence at the task. Maehr noted in particular that when individuals hold task goals, "social comparisons of performance are remote or are virtually nonexistent" (Maehr, 1984, p. 129). In contrast, Maehr defined "ego goals"—his version of performance goals—in terms of being able to exceed a standard of performance, particularly as related to the performance of other individuals. Interestingly, Maehr distinguished ego goals from "extrinsic goals," which he described as a separate class of goals that are related to earning rewards (e.g., money or a prize) that are not directly aligned with the reasons why an individual would engage with a given task in the first place.

Nicholls (1989) described students' goals as motivational orientations; he labeled the two dimensions as task orientation and ego orientation. The specific types of survey items that he and his colleagues developed to measure these orientations focused on whether students feel "pleased" when they accomplish certain tasks. For example, a student with a high task orientation is a student who feels pleased when he or she works hard, tries hard, and understands the material. In contrast, a student with a high ego orientation feels pleased when he or she feels superior to others and beats others (Nicholls, Cobb, Wood, Yackel, & Patashnick, 1990). In contrast, Ames' (1987) descriptions of goal orientations were influenced by earlier work by Maehr and Nichols. She described task-oriented students as those who "are interested in developing their ability and gaining mastery," and ego-oriented students as those who "want to demonstrate that they have ability" (Ames, 1987, p. 127).

Dweck and her colleagues distinguished between learning (analogous to mastery) and performance goals and argued that learners frame their responses to and interpretations of events based on these goals (Dweck & Leggett, 1988; Elliott & Dweck, 1988). Learning goals are described as goals "in which individuals are concerned with increasing their competence," whereas performance goals are described as goals "in which individuals are concerned with gaining favorable judgments of their competence" (Dweck & Leggett, 1988, p. 256).

In summary, although a variety of terms have been used to describe these two broad classes of goals, we have chosen to refer to these goals as "mastery" and "performance" goals for the remainder of this chapter. All of the various definitions suggest that when students pursue mastery goals, they are interested in truly mastering the task, they are concerned with gaining competence, and they are willing and eager to exert effort in order to achieve mastery. In contrast, when students pursue performance goals, they are interested in demonstrating their ability relative to others, in outperforming others, and in being judged by others as being competent at academic tasks.

Current Four-Factor Model of Achievement Goal Theory

The mastery/performance distinction has been studied by many researchers, for many years (see Anderman & Wolters, 2006; Urdan, 1997, for reviews). However, in the mid-1990s, several researchers argued that the distinction between approach and avoid orientations also should be considered within a goal orientation framework. Elliot and Harackiewicz (1996) noted that some of the early work by achievement goal researchers such as Dweck and Nicholls did distinguish between approach and avoid forms of performance goals, but these distinctions were lost in later definitions.

A trichotomous framework for achievement goals suggests that in addition to mastery goals, a distinction should be made between performance-approach and performance-avoid goals (Elliot, 1999). Elliot and Harackiewicz (1996) initially conducted experiments in which participants were asked to solve puzzles using mastery goals, performance-approach goals, and performance-avoid goals. Participants in the performance-approach condition were informed that students who solve the puzzles more successfully than other students at the same university "have good puzzle solving ability" (p. 468); in contrast, students in the performance-avoid condition were told that if they solved fewer puzzles than others, they would demonstrate that they "have poor puzzle solving ability" (p. 468). Results indicated that participants in the performance-avoid condition displayed lower intrinsic motivation toward the puzzles than those in the performance-approach condition.

Midgley and her colleagues developed a widely used measure of achievement goals, the *Patterns of Adaptive Learning Survey* (PALS) (Midgley et al., 2000). Initially, separate measures of performance-approach and performance-avoid goal orientations were developed (Middleton & Midgley, 1997). Using a large sample of middle school students, Middleton and Midgley demonstrated that performance goals could be separated into performance-approach and performance-avoid goal orientations. They operationalized performance-approach goals in terms of students (a) wanting to do better than other students in their class and (b) wanting to demonstrate that they are more competent than others; in contrast, performance-avoid goals were operationalized in terms of wanting to avoid appearing incompetent or "dumb." Skaalvik (1997) also examined different types of performance goals. Specifically, using a sample of Norwegian sixth and eighth grade students, Skaalvik developed a measure of self-enhancing ego orientation (similar to a performance-approach goal orientation) and a measure of a self-defeating ego orientation (similar to a performance-avoid goal orientation).

The approach/avoid distinction was also applied to mastery goal orientation, resulting in a 2×2 framework for achievement goals (Elliot & McGregor, 2001). In this model, mastery goals are broken down into mastery-approach and mastery-avoid goals, matching the separation of performance-approach and performance-avoid goals. The new addition to the model was the mastery-avoid construct. A student who endorses mastery-avoid goals wants to avoid misunderstanding or losing a sense of competence. The 2×2 model has been supported in both North American (Conroy, Elliot, & Hofer, 2003) and international samples (Bong, 2009).

Currently, goal orientation theorists generally support the 2×2 model. Nevertheless, the validity of mastery-avoid goals has been questioned (e.g., Sideridis & Mouratidis, 2008). Specifically, some researchers question whether individuals actually think about mastery-avoid goals in real-life situations. Ciani and Sheldon (2010) conducted a qualitative study in which they interviewed Division I college baseball players about their endorsement of mastery-avoid goals while playing baseball. Although players endorsed both high and low levels of mastery-avoid goals, when players who endorsed mastery-avoid goals were probed about these beliefs, results suggested that the players actually were referring to mastery-approach goals in many cases. Ciani and Sheldon suggested that one of the reasons for this may be that it is difficult to truly get study participants to understand the nuances of what a "mastery-avoid" goal is, using a survey instrument.

In addition, some research suggests some students may have difficulty distinguishing between performance-approach and performance-avoid goals. For example, Urdan and Mestas (2006) conducted an interview study with 53 high school seniors who all reported high levels of performance-avoid goals (as determined by responses to a survey). Students were probed about their responses to various survey items. Results indicated that students often did not easily distinguish between performance-approach and performance-avoid goals. In addition, students indicated that they pursue performance goals for a variety of different reasons (e.g., to look smart, to please parents, to look smart to one's peers, or simply because students enjoyed competition). Additional work on the measurement, interpretation, and predictive validity of mastery-avoid goal orientation will be an important area for future research.

Correlates of Goal Orientations

Much of the research conducted over the past two decades by achievement goal theorists has focused on relations between students' goal orientations and a variety of academic outcomes, including implicit beliefs about intelligence, academic achievement, and numerous aspects of engagement. In the following sections, we review the major findings of these studies.

Goal Orientations and Beliefs About Intelligence

Carol Dweck and her colleagues have examined students' beliefs about intelligence and how those beliefs are related to a variety of academic outcomes (Dweck, 2000). When students endorse an entity theory of intelligence, they believe that their intellectual abilities are fixed (i.e., generally unchangeable); in contrast, when students endorse an incremental view of intelligence, they believe that their intellectual abilities are malleable (Dweck & Leggett, 1988). Research generally indicates that incremental beliefs about intelligence are associated with a host of adaptive outcomes, including self-regulated learning (Dweck & Master, 2008), academic achievement (Blackwell, Trzesniewski, & Dweck, 2007), and the utilization of remedial (as opposed to defensive) strategies when self-esteem is threatened (Nussbaum & Dweck, 2008).

Beliefs about intelligence also have been examined in relation to goal orientations. Research generally indicates that when students believe that intelligence is incremental, they are likely to endorse mastery goals; in contrast, when students believe that intelligence is fixed and unchangeable, they are likely to adopt performance goals (Dweck & Leggett, 1988). Although a variety of studies have revealed similar relations between implicit theories of intelligence and goal orientations, some studies have failed to replicate these findings (e.g., Dupeyrat & Marine, 2005).

Goal Orientations and Academic Achievement

Academic achievement often is regarded as one of the most important educational outcomes. Researchers and practitioners have been particularly interested in the relations of goal orientations to achievement since academic achievement is greatly valued as an indicator of educational performance (Anderman, Anderman, Yough, & Gimbert, 2010; Hattie & Anderman, in press).

Relations between goal orientations and academic achievement are somewhat inconsistent. Although reasons are not clear, much depends on how student achievement is measured. Achievement can be measured in a variety of ways (e.g., scores on standardized tests, teacher-made tests, or teacher-assigned grades that may or may not include homework or conduct) and do not necessarily reflect students' real understanding. A mastery goal orientation, with its accompanying thoughtfulness and strategic effort, is only likely to be important if achievement tests require students to demonstrate deep understanding; if simple memorization is sufficient to score well, then a mastery goal orientation is not likely to be related differentially to test scores or grades. Furthermore, a very strong desire to outscore others may lead students to having inflated achievement scores through means such as cheating.

Mastery Goal Orientation

In a comprehensive study examining over 90 peer-reviewed articles that addressed the relations of achievement goals to academic achievement, Linnenbrink-Garcia, Tyson, and Patall (2008) reported that mastery goals appear sometimes to be beneficial for academic achievement, as expected theoretically. For example, Bong (2009) found positive correlations between upper elementary and middle school students' mastery-approach goals and math achievement. However, across studies, results are somewhat mixed; numerous studies have not shown the expected positive direct relations between mastery goals and achievement (Ames & Archer, 1988; Anderman & Johnston, 1998; Barron &

Harackiewicz, 2001; Daniels et al., 2009; Elliot & Church, 1997; Elliot & McGregor, 2001; Harackiewicz, Barron, Carter, Lehto, & Elliot, 1997; Pintrich, 2000a; Skaalvik, 1997).

In addition, results of several studies indicate that mastery goals are sometimes indirectly related to achievement. Specifically, mastery goals often are predictive of mediators, such as affect or certain types of behaviors, that are in turn related to achievement. Thus, students who endorse mastery goals are more likely to either engage in achievement-promoting behaviors or experience affect that is related to achievement. For example, in one study, adolescents who reported being mastery-oriented toward current events were more likely to engage in news-seeking behaviors outside of school; in turn, these behaviors were directly and positively predicted knowledge of current events (Anderman & Johnston, 1998). In another study, mastery orientation, although not directly predictive of achievement, was related inversely to indicators of negative affect (e.g., boredom, anxiety), which in turn were related to lower academic achievement (Daniels et al., 2009).

Performance Goal Orientation

The relations between performance-approach goals and academic achievement are fairly consistent for college students. In many studies, the adoption of performance-approach goals is related to high achievement (Church, Elliot, & Gable, 2001; Daniels et al., 2009; Elliot & Church, 1997; Elliot & McGregor, 2001; Elliot, McGregor, & Gable, 1999; Harackiewicz et al., 1997).

For younger students, a similar pattern is found in some studies, although relations at times are not as strong. For example, Bong (2009) reported a low (.19) correlation between performance-approach goals and achievement for students in middle school and lower elementary grades, but no relation for middle and upper elementary students. Wolters (2004) found a weak positive relation between performance-approach goals and math grades in middle school students. Some of these differential relations may at least in part be explained by how researchers operationalize goal orientations on survey instruments. When items in goal measures are assessed differently, research results may vary (Hulleman, Schrager, Bodmann, & Harackiewicz, 2010).

Considering relations between performance-approach orientation and achievement for students as a whole may also mask possible differential relations depending on student characteristics. For example, there has been concern about the long-term outcomes for performance-approach oriented students who seem to do well in the short term (Midgley, Kaplan, & Middleton, 2001): What happens when these students move to a new, more competitive, or challenging environment (e.g., a larger school, a class with more advanced content or more high-achieving students)? One possibility is that students accustomed to outperforming others and being viewed that way by other people, but who are not confident about maintaining their rank, will move to an avoidance focus. This was what Middleton, Kaplan, and Midgley (2004) found. Specifically, sixth graders' performance-approach orientation predicted a performance-avoid orientation in seventh grade, but only for students with high self-efficacy in sixth grade. That is, students who were concerned with outscoring others and who felt confident of their abilities were more likely, as they progressed through middle school, to become more focused on protecting their image and not looking incompetent compared to other students. This is concerning, given the poor outcomes associated with a performance-avoid orientation.

Performance-avoid goal orientations are consistently and negatively related to achievement. These results have been documented for both college students (e.g., Elliot et al., 1999) and younger adolescents (e.g., Middleton & Midgley, 1997; Wolters, 2004).

Goal Orientations and Engagement

Since we use goal orientation theory as our framework for explaining motivation and engagement, it is important to distinguish how we are defining goal orientations and how we are defining engagement. As noted by Appleton, Christenson, and Furlong (2008), the phrase "academic engagement" needs empirical and conceptual clarification; similar arguments have been made regarding the need for the clarification of terms in the motivation field in general (Murphy & Alexander, 2000) and within goal theory specifically (Pintrich, 2000b). For our review of the relations between goal orientations and engagement, we have adopted the model described by Fredricks, Blumenfeld, and Paris (2004). In that model, the construct of engagement is described as being multidimensional; specifically, engagement consists of behavioral, emotional, and cognitive forms of engagement. Cognitive engagement refers to learners' willingness to exert the necessary effort to understand and master complex phenomena; emotional engagement refers to learners' positive and negative affective reactions to aspects of schooling; and behavioral engagement refers to actual participation in specific activities that are related to achievement (Fredricks et al., 2004, p. 60). Specifically, the definitions of engagement provided by Fredricks and her colleagues imply that students are engaged while they are working on a specific task; thus, a student is cognitively engaged when he or she is exerting appropriate effort while completing a task; a student's emotional engagement with a task is operationalized in terms of her affective reactions to the task (while engaging with the task); and a student's behavioral engagement with the task is operationalized in terms of her actual behaviors during the task. Goal orientations, in contrast, are operationalized in terms of the goals that students have toward tasks *both prior to and during task participation*. Thus, in our conceptualization of the relations between goal orientations and engagement, the specific goal orientation that a student holds for a particular task will determine the quality of the student's engagement with the task (Ames, 1992a, 1992b). For example, when a student is highly mastery goal–oriented toward a particular task, the quality of cognitive, emotional, and behavioral engagement will likely be adaptive for learning (because the student's goal is task mastery, which requires high levels of engagement). Indeed, evidence from studies examining students' effective strategy usage and goal orientations supports this since the adoption of mastery goals is related to more effective academic strategy usage (Graham & Golan, 1991; Nolen, 1988). In the following sections, we describe the relations of each type of engagement to goal orientations.

Cognitive Engagement

The types of goal orientations that students adopt are related to the kinds of cognitive and self-regulatory strategies they use when engaged with academic tasks. Results of numerous studies indicate that when students focus on mastery, they tend to be willing to think deeply and broadly about their academic work; they use effective learning and self-regulatory strategies, including monitoring their comprehension and thinking about how current academic tasks are related to previously learned information (e.g., Anderman & Young, 1994; Graham & Golan, 1991; Nolen & Haladyna, 1990; Pintrich & De Groot, 1990; Wolters, 2004). For example, Nolen (1988), in an early study, found that both general and task-specific mastery (task) goal orientations were related positively to middle students' use of both deep-processing strategies (e.g., figuring out how new information fits with prior knowledge, monitoring one's comprehension) and surface-level strategies (e.g., memorizing words, rehearsing information). More recent research with a large sample of South Korean adolescents, measuring both mastery-approach and mastery-avoid orientations, indicated that both were related positively to use of cognitive strategies (rehearsal, elaboration, and organizational strategies) and more adaptive self-regulation, although the associations with mastery-avoid goals were weaker (Bong, 2009).

The evidence for students holding a performance goal orientation is more mixed, although no study has identified positive links between performance-avoid goals and cognitive engagement. In Nolen's (1988) study, students' adoption of performance (ego) goals was either unrelated or negatively related to their use of deep-processing strategies and either unrelated or positively related to using surface-level strategies; approach and avoid orientations were not yet differentiated. Bong (2009) found that performance-approach goals were related to greater use of cognitive strategies and more adaptive self-regulation, whereas performance-avoid goals were not. When students are focused on their relative performance and are busy thinking about ability differences, they simply may not have the cognitive resources to devote to the use of effective cognitive and self-regulatory strategies.

Emotional Engagement

Several researchers have examined the relations between goal orientations and various indicators of emotional engagement, such as affect and motivation. Results generally indicate that mastery goals are related to positive affect about school (e.g., Roeser, Midgley, & Urdan, 1996) and different aspects of motivation, such as intrinsic motivation, positive self-concept, and self-efficacy (e.g., Murayama & Elliot, 2009). However, the relations of performance goals to affect and motivation are somewhat mixed.

Daniels et al. (2009) examined the relations between emotions, goal orientations, and achievement in a large sample of college students. Results indicated that feelings of hopefulness were related positively to both mastery- and performance-approach goals, whereas feelings of helplessness were inversely related to mastery goals, but unrelated to performance goals. Skaalvik (1997) examined the relations between mastery (task) goals, self-defeating ego goals (i.e., performance-avoid goals), and self-enhancing ego goals (i.e., performance-approach goals), and several measures of affect. Results indicated that the adoption of mastery goals was related positively to self-esteem, and negatively to math anxiety. The adoption of performance-approach goals was related weakly and positively to self-esteem, and weakly and negatively to math anxiety. The adoption of performance-avoid goals was related negatively to self-esteem and positively to both math and verbal anxiety.

Recent research suggests that the achievement goals of early adolescents may be predicted by parental involvement and control (i.e., related to numerous aspects of students' lives, not just academics), as well as anxiety and depression during the elementary school years. In a recent study, Duchesne and colleagues examined a longitudinal sample of 498 early adolescents (Duchesne & Ratelle, 2010). Students reported their perceptions of general parental involvement and control and completed measures of anxiety and depression at the end of the sixth grade in elementary school; students then reported their achievement goals during the following year, at the end of the first year of middle school (seventh grade). Results indicated that mastery goals were predicted by perceptions of parental involvement; however, anxiety mediated the relation between perceptions of parents as controlling and performance goals (combined approach and avoid). Specifically, students who perceived their parents as controlling experienced greater anxiety; anxiety in turn positively predicted performance goals.

Behavioral Engagement

The goal orientations that students adopt are also associated with a range of behaviors evident in the classroom. For example, a mastery orientation is associated with positive academic behaviors, such as expending effort (Miller, Greene, Montalvo, Ravindran, & Nichols, 1996), discussing schoolwork with other students (Patrick, Ryan, & Kaplan, 2007), engaging in relevant activities outside of school (Anderman & Johnston, 1998), and seeking help when needed (Ryan & Pintrich, 1997). Conversely, a performance orientation is related to avoiding seeking needed help (Ryan & Pintrich) and being disruptive during lessons (Ryan & Patrick, 2001).

Summary

Achievement goal theory has developed into a robust, empirically supported framework for examining student motivation. The types of goal orientations that students adopt are related in important ways to their achievement, affect, beliefs about the nature of intelligence, and cognitive/self-regulatory strategy use. Goal orientations also are related to cognitive, emotional, and behavioral engagement. Although goal orientations represent cognitions that are related to behavior, goals are influenced by the social contexts in which students participate. In the next section, we examine the relations between social contexts and achievement goals.

Classroom Goal Structures

A particularly important aspect of achievement goal theory is its attention to the educational contexts within which students are, or are supposed to be, engaged. This is because, according to goal theory, students' motivation is influenced not only by their individual personal characteristics, beliefs, and achievement histories, but also by the contexts in which they learn. Within these environments, students' construals of what is valued in terms of schooling and what constitutes achievement and success influence their goal orientations and therefore play a significant role in affecting the nature and quality of engagement in learning tasks (Ames, 1992b; Maehr, 1984; Nicholls, 1989). We focus here on research within goal theory that addresses an especially critical and salient educational context—classrooms.

During the considerable amount of time students spend in classrooms, they construct meaning systems or schema about the purpose and meaning of schooling and academics from their experiences and perceptions of what is emphasized in the classroom. These perceptions of what is emphasized are termed *classroom goal structures* (Ames, 1984, 1992b). Specifically, classroom goal structures encompass students' subjective perceptions of the meaning of academic tasks, competence, success, and purposes for students' engaging in schoolwork. From a goal theory perspective, classroom goal structures represent a powerful empirical tool that can be used to examine the roles of classroom contexts in student motivation (Meece et al., 2006).

Personal mastery and performance goal orientations, reviewed in the previous section, have parallels in classroom mastery and performance goal structures. Accordingly, a classroom *mastery goal structure* involves a perception that learning and understanding are valued and that success is indicated by personal improvement. A classroom *performance goal structure* involves a perception that achievement and success entail outperforming others or surpassing normative standards (Ames, 1992b). Classroom goal structures are usually measured by student self-report surveys, predominantly with scales from the *Pattern of Adaptive Learning Survey* (PALS; Midgley et al., 1996, 2000). Just as mastery and performance goal orientations are orthogonal, so too are classroom goal structures. That is, classrooms may be high in both mastery and performance goal structure, high in just one, low in both, or any other configuration.

Classroom goal structures are not "objective" characteristics but instead depend on how individual students perceive and give meaning to their classroom experiences (Ames, 1992b). Because students' individual past and current experiences and interpretations contribute to their current perceptions, students in the same class will not necessarily perceive the classroom goal structures in the same way (Ames, 1992b). Adding to variability in perceptions, students in the same classroom are often treated differently and therefore do not even experience the same educational context (Brophy, 1985; Turner & Patrick, 2004).

Teachers play a potent role in contributing to the classroom goal structures through explicit and implicit messages about the purpose of school activities, what counts as learning, and the role of student talk and through the norms and rules they establish for student behavior. These norms begin from the first days of the school year—indeed, they are particularly explicit at this time when teachers introduce and socialize students to their philosophies and beliefs. Early teacher practices foreshadow significant differences in mastery and performance classroom goal structures, both after a few months and near the end of the year (Patrick, Anderman, Ryan, Edelin, & Midgley, 2001; Patrick, Turner, Meyer, & Midgley, 2003).

Classroom Mastery Goal Structure

A classroom mastery goal structure involves a perception that students' real learning and understanding, rather than just memorization, are valued and that success is accompanied by effort and indicated by personal improvement. Thus, a classroom mastery goal structure emphasizes an incremental theory of ability (Ames, 1992b). Theoretically, perceptions of a classroom mastery goal structure influence students' invoking a mastery goal orientation for themselves in that context; that is, students are likely to focus on their own improvement and understanding when these aspects are emphasized. Mastery goal orientation, in turn, is believed to influence students' optimal effort, affect, use of adaptive learning strategies, and, ultimately, achievement (Ames, 1992b). There is a considerable body of empirical studies that provide support for these tenets, as we discuss next.

Associations with Student Engagement

A classroom mastery goal structure constitutes a holistic system of meanings. Accordingly, it is associated with all aspects of engagement—emotional (e.g., enjoyment, interest, efficacy, commitment), cognitive (e.g., thoughtfulness, use of learning strategies, self-regulation), and behavioral (e.g., effort, persistence, asking for help). From both theoretical and practical standpoints, all aspects of engagement should be high in classrooms that are perceived as emphasizing mastery. Specifically, when the overarching focus in the classroom is perceived as increasing each student's understanding and skill, with success gauged by personal improvement (i.e., classroom mastery structure), it is adaptive and beneficial for students to be fully and thoroughly engaged with those tasks.

Emotional Engagement

Students' perceptions that their teacher and classroom emphasize mastery are related significantly to their personal mastery goal orientation (Nolen & Haladyna, 1990; Wolters, 2004). Also, given that *all* students can be successful when success is viewed as personal improvement, students tend to experience positive affect and motivational beliefs in mastery goal structured classrooms. Specifically, a perceived classroom mastery goal structure is related positively to students' positive school-related affect (Ames & Archer, 1988; Anderman, 1999; Kaplan & Midgley, 1999), feelings of belonging at school (Anderman, 2003; Anderman & Anderman, 1999; Stevens, Hamman, & Olivarez, 2007), and desire to follow the school's expectations (i.e., social responsibility goal; Anderman & Anderman). Students in these environments express adaptive motivational beliefs, such as self-efficacy and intrinsic motivation (Fast et al., 2010; Murayama & Elliot, 2009; Wolters, 2004). Moreover, students express more positive views about their schoolwork, such as preference for challenge (Ames & Archer, 1988), the usefulness of learning strategies (Nolen & Haladyna, 1990), satisfaction with their learning (Nolen, 2003), and adaptive coping responses after failure (Kaplan & Midgley, 1999), compared to those in settings with low classroom mastery goal structure.

Cognitive Engagement

Not surprisingly, given students' positive affect and motivation, they tend to be more cognitively engaged in classrooms with a high (compared to low) classroom mastery goal structure. Specifically, a classroom mastery goal structure is associated positively with the use of effective cognitive strategies (e.g., elaboration) and metacognitive strategies (e.g., planning, monitoring, regulating) (Ames & Archer, 1988; Wolters, 2004), just as personal mastery goal orientation is.

Behavioral Engagement

Underscoring the close connections of emotional and cognitive engagement with behavior, classroom mastery goal structure is related positively to many forms of adaptive behavioral engagement. This is because working to learn the material is likely to pay off for students if all can experience success, rather than just a few. Classrooms that are perceived, on average, as having a high (compared to low) mastery goal structure tend to have students who expend effort, persist with tasks (Wolters, 2004), and use adaptive help-seeking strategies such as asking for explanations but not answers (Karabenick, 2004). They also have the lowest average rates of maladaptive student behaviors, including not asking for help when it is needed (Karabenick, 2004;

Ryan, Gheen, & Midgley, 1998), self-handicapping (i.e., purposefully withdrawing effort; Midgley & Urdan, 2001; Urdan & Midgley, 2003), being disruptive (Kaplan, Gheen, & Midgley, 2002), procrastinating (Wolters, 2004), and cheating (Murdock, Hale, & Weber, 2001).

Classroom Performance Goal Structure

A classroom performance goal structure conveys to students that learning is predominantly a means of achieving recognition and prestige, and it is characterized by relative ability comparisons among students. Success is indicated by outperforming others or surpassing normative standards (Ames, 1992b). An integral characteristic of classroom performance goal structure is that students are compared to each other, with an inherent assumption that this hierarchy is relatively stable and reflects some aspect of students' ability. That is, it reflects an entity view of intelligence (Dweck, 2000).

A classroom performance goal structure is different from an extrinsic goal structure; the latter conveys that the purpose of engaging in academic tasks is to gain external incentives; however, the success of any one student does not affect the success of others (see Urdan, 1997). That is, if students are graded on a curve, with grades indicating relative position, a classroom performance goal structure is invoked; however, if grades (or other incentives) are very salient but do not signify students' relative placement, a classroom extrinsic goal structure is involved.

After the recognition that personal performance goal orientations could be separated, theoretically and empirically, into approach and avoidance dimensions, some researchers have made the same distinction with classroom performance goal structure (e.g., Karabenick, 2004; Murayama & Elliot, 2009). That is, they suggest that some performance-focused classrooms emphasize approach characteristics, such as scoring better than others, whereas others emphasize avoidance characteristics, such as not doing worse than others. However, we do not find this distinction to be meaningful in classrooms, like it is for individuals' personal orientations. During naturalistic classroom observations, we see teachers suggesting, implicitly or explicitly, that students who score the highest are "smarter" or more able than are those with lower scores; however, we have not observed teachers or classrooms promoting either a distinguishable approach or avoidance orientation. We think that students in performance-focused classrooms evaluate, perhaps subconsciously, their likelihood of being ranked highly. If they view outperforming others as realistic, they will likely take an approach orientation, and if they are pessimistic about their chances of outscoring others, they will instead likely adopt an avoidance orientation. Therefore, a general classroom performance goal structure may invoke some students taking a performance-approach orientation and others in the same classroom being performance-avoid oriented.

Associations with Student Engagement

Perceiving a classroom performance goal structure is associated with affective, cognitive, and behavioral engagement. In contrast to the mixed findings associated with a personal performance-approach goal orientation, perceiving a classroom performance goal structure is generally associated with students' beliefs and behaviors that are less conducive, and often detrimental, to learning and achievement. We review this research briefly next.

Emotional Engagement

Students' perceptions that their teacher and classroom emphasize relative ability comparisons (i.e., have a high classroom performance goal structure) are related to the adoption of personal performance-approach and/or performance-avoid goals (Wolters, 2004). A pervasive focus on how students "stack up" against each other can provoke students to focus on the outcomes of their efforts, rather than the process of learning. This state of affairs is not comfortable for many students, not just those near the bottom of the achievement continuum, and therefore students tend to experience negative affect and motivational beliefs in these types of classrooms. Students in classrooms with a strong performance goal structure tend to express more negative affect about school (Ames & Archer, 1988; Anderman, 1999; Kaplan & Midgley, 1999), and less sense of belonging at school (Anderman & Anderman, 1999), compared to those in classrooms with low perceived performance goal structure. Similarly, students view teachers of performance-focused classrooms as less fair (Murdock, Miller, & Kohlhardt, 2004) and more to blame for student dishonesty (Murdock, Miller, & Goetzinger, 2007), compared to teachers of mastery-focused classrooms. Students' intrinsic motivation and academic self-concepts are related inversely to classroom performance goal structure (Ames & Archer, 1988; Murayama & Elliot, 2009). There is also greater use of maladaptive coping strategies after failure, such as denial or projecting blame onto other people or events (Kaplan & Midgley, 1999) or attributing failures to one's own lack of ability (Ames & Archer, 1988).

Cognitive Engagement

There is some evidence indicating that perceiving a classroom as being focused on ability differences is related to lower academic achievement. Anderman and Midgley (1997) examined the relations between perceptions of classroom performance goal structures and end-of-year grades both before and after the transition from elementary school into middle school. Results in both English and math classes indicated that when students perceived a classroom performance goal structure, their end-of-year grades after the transition were lower in both subjects than they had been a year previously. This is related in part to the fact that grading practices often become more focused on relative ability of students after the middle school transition (Eccles & Midgley, 1989; Midgley, Anderman, & Hicks, 1995). Similar patterns of relations between perceptions of classroom performance goal structures and achievement have been reported in other studies as well (e.g., Anderman & Anderman, 1999).

Behavioral Engagement

When classrooms are perceived as emphasizing a hierarchy of ability and students' relative position within that hierarchy, students are likely to report engaging in behaviors that are not conducive, and often detrimental, to learning. With an emphasis on outcomes but not process, students may feel encouraged to disregard *how* they come to outscore others and be concerned only that they *do*. Consistent with this, cheating is most prevalent in classrooms with a high performance goal structure (Anderman, Griesinger, & Westerfield, 1998; Murdock et al., 2004). In performance-structured classrooms, students who are not successful at a task immediately may be unlikely to continue trying, given both that a hierarchy of ability tends to invoke an entity view of ability, and high effort without success is suggestive of low ability. As posited, classroom performance goal structure is related inversely to students' task persistence (Wolters, 2004).

Furthermore, in classrooms with a performance goal structure, students who are pessimistic about their chances of placing near the top of the hierarchy may find ways to avoid engaging in schoolwork and therefore protect their self-worth by not providing evidence that their ability is lower than their classmates'. Again, research supports this premise. Classrooms perceived, on average, as being highly performance-focused tend to have the highest rates of students not seeking help when they need it (Ryan et al., 1998), procrastinating (Wolters, 2004), self-handicapping (Midgley & Urdan, 2001; Urdan, 2004; Urdan, Midgley, & Anderman, 1998), and being disruptive (Kaplan et al., 2002; Ryan & Patrick, 2001).

Findings of associations between classroom performance goal structures and student achievement have been mixed across studies. For example, classroom performance goal structure has been related inversely to test scores (Nolen, 2003), but not related to grades (Wolters, 2004). Researchers have long noted, however, that the different ways that achievement is measured, including differences among teachers in how grades are assigned and differences between standardized assessments and teacher-assigned grades, make for difficulties with conducting research on these relations. In addition, grade-level differences in assessment procedures (e.g., developmental differences in grading practices across elementary and high school settings) compound these difficulties.

Teacher Practices Associated with Classroom Goal Structures

Classroom Mastery Goal Structure

Because a classroom mastery goal structure represents a particularly adaptive learning environment, goal theorists recommend that teachers create mastery goal–focused classrooms (e.g., Midgley, 1993). To this end, researchers have identified teacher practices associated with a classroom mastery goal structure. Importantly, classroom mastery goal structure is established by a coherent *set of practices* that together communicate a consistent perspective toward learning and task engagement; isolated practices are generally not sufficient to influence students' overall meaning systems.

The holistic approach to creating a mastery goal–structured classroom was first represented by Ames' (1990, 1992a) conceptual framework, where she organized teaching principles and strategies associated with a classroom mastery goal structure into six categories. This framework, represented by the acronym TARGET (see Epstein, 1983), is comprised of the academic task, authority, recognition, grouping, evaluation, and time. Specifically, *tasks* should be meaningful, challenging, and interesting, and there should be a range of task options available so that ability differences are not accentuated. The teacher should share *authority* and responsibility for rules and decisions with the students. *Recognition* should be available to all students, should involve progress or effort, and there should be few opportunities for social comparison among students. *Grouping* should be flexible and heterogeneous, and students should not be grouped by ability. *Evaluation* should be criterion-referenced, not made public, and grades and test scores should be interpreted in terms of improvement and effort. And, finally, there should be flexible use of *time* in the classroom and opportunities for student self-pacing. As mentioned, Ames was clear that practices within all six categories must be integrated in order for a classroom mastery goal structure to be evident (see also Maehr & Anderman, 1993).

Support for the relevance and utility of TARGET has come from multimethod studies, whereby survey measures were triangulated with classroom observations or students' responses to open-ended questions (Meece, 1991; Patrick & Ryan, 2008; Patrick et al., 2001). However, two other facets of classrooms associated with mastery goal structure have also been identified: social relationships and pedagogical practices.

A sizable body of research has documented the importance of social relationship features for perceptions of classroom mastery goal structure. Teachers in high mastery-focused classrooms appear to promote a more interpersonally positive climate and engage in more motivationally supportive interactions (e.g., encouraging and supporting students' persistence, using humor, showing enthusiasm) compared to teachers in low mastery-focused classrooms (Patrick et al., 2001, 2003; Turner et al., 2002). Teacher support (for students' learning and for students as people), mutual respect, positive affect, and teacher enthusiasm are salient in high, but not low, mastery-focused classrooms (Miller & Murdock, 2007; Patrick et al., 2001, 2003; Turner et al., 2002). Those findings have led to the revised acronym TARGETS. That is, for classroom mastery goal structure, in addition to features of the other six categories, *social relationships* should be respectful, supportive of students both socioemotionally and academically, and convey positive affect about both students and the content to be learned.

There is also evidence that teachers' pedagogical approaches comprise another category of practices associated with a classroom mastery goal structure (e.g., Murdock et al., 2004; Patrick & Ryan, 2008). For example, students report that the extent to which teachers make efforts to explain the material to them, help them understand, and use a variety of approaches as necessary influences their views of the classroom's mastery goal structure (Patrick & Ryan, 2008). Observational studies support this finding. High, but not low, mastery-focused teachers use active instructional approaches and adapt instruction to their students' developmental levels (Meece, 1991) and engage in academic press (Anderman, Andrzejewski, & Allen, 2011). They also provide supportive instructional discourse, or scaffolding, comprised of negotiating with students what academic tasks involve and transferring responsibility for tasks to students in accordance with their capabilities (Turner et al., 2002).

Classroom Performance Goal Structure

There has been less interest in identifying teacher practices associated with classroom performance goal structure than with classroom mastery goal structure. One reason is the possibility that the crucial element of learning environments is a high classroom mastery goal structure, regardless of the extent of classroom performance goal structure (Midgley, 2002; Midgley et al., 2001). Nevertheless, it may be valuable to identify practices associated with classroom performance goal structure, given its associations with negative indicators of students' engagement; to decrease the prevalence of practices that contribute to perceptions of a performance focus, it is necessary to know the specific practices involved. In addition, classroom mastery and performance goal structures can be perceived simultaneously within the same classroom (Midgley, 2002). For example, a science teacher can emphasize the importance of effort and persistence in order to understand and master a principle (mastery), but the same teacher can also simultaneously emphasize grades and relative ability (performance).

From classroom observation studies, it appears that teachers perceived as having a high performance focus emphasize formal assessments, grades, and students' relative performance to a substantially greater extent than do low performance-focused teachers (Patrick et al., 2001). That information, however, is considerably less than what is known about the aforementioned practices related to classroom mastery goal structure. This relative paucity of information is consistent with the argument that a focus on external incentives (i.e., classroom extrinsic goal structure) is more prevalent and salient to students than are messages about relative performance or ability (Brophy, 2005). Perhaps, ubiquitous societal messages about outscoring others do more to promote students' performance goal orientation than do more proximal teacher classroom practices.

Summary

Students' perceptions of classroom goal structures are related to valued motivational outcomes. Perceptions of a classroom mastery goal structure are generally related to beneficial outcomes, whereas perceptions of a classroom performance goal structure are related to a mixed array of outcomes. In terms of the relations of classroom goal structures to engagement, the goal structure that is perceived in the classroom is related to the quality of engagement evidenced by the student. As we have reviewed, perceptions of classroom mastery and performance goal structures are related to cognitive, emotional, and behavioral engagement in different ways. The fact that classroom goal structures are related to the types of instructional practices used by teachers in classrooms suggests that changes in instructional practices may yield benefits for student engagement.

Conclusion

In this chapter, we have reviewed the relations between personal achievement goals, classroom goal structures, and academic engagement. Whereas motivation researchers who study achievement goals and researchers who study academic engagement operationalize and discuss constructs in different ways, there is substantial and important overlap. Future research that draws upon both achievement goal theory and research on student engagement will be fruitful, particularly in terms of developing interventions designed to more fully engage students with academic tasks.

We briefly reviewed the history of the development of achievement goal theory, and we noted that the measurement of achievement goal constructs has changed in subtle yet important ways over the past three decades (for more comprehensive reviews, see Elliot, 2005, and Maehr & Zusho, 2009). We then examined the relations of personal goal orientations to a variety of educational outcomes, including achievement, strategy usage, and affect. We noted in particular that the relations between personal goal orientations and achievement are complex. Finally, we reviewed research on classroom goal structures. We noted in particular that facets of classroom contexts that are controlled by teachers (i.e., instructional practices) affect students' perceptions of classroom goal structures, which in turn affect the types of personal goal orientations that students adopt.

Throughout this chapter, we have noted that the two main classes of achievement goals (mastery and performance) are related to engagement in different ways. Engagement researchers typically discuss three distinct forms of engagement (behavioral, emotional, and cognitive) (Fredricks et al., 2004). Although these three forms of academic engagement differ, all forms of engagement focus on students' involvement with academic tasks (either behaviorally, emotionally, or cognitively).

Goal orientation theorists also are concerned with students' involvement with academic tasks. When students pursue mastery goals, the students' goal is to truly learn or "master" the task. Goal orientations can be adopted by students for many types of learning, including specific activities (e.g., a particular science lab experiment), more general academic tasks (e.g., book reports), or subject domains (e.g., mathematics) (Anderman & Anderman, 2010; Anderman & Wolters, 2006). From an engagement perspective, students who hold mastery goals are likely to be more cognitively, emotionally, and behaviorally engaged with tasks because the overarching "goal" is task mastery. In contrast, when students pursue various types of performance goals, the goal is to demonstrate one's ability at the task, or, in the case of avoidance goals, to avoid appearing incompetent at the task. When students hold such goals, their engagement may not be as deep as with mastery goals; rather, students may engage with the task at more of a surface level in order to merely demonstrate ability.

For example, a student who holds an avoidance goal may avoid extensive cognitive engagement with a task (i.e., spend little time on the actual task), in order to preserve the appearance of competence. Specifically, the student might perceive that spending a great deal of time engaged with a task would make the student "look dumb" to his or her classmates; therefore, although extensive cognitive engagement might be beneficial to the student, such engagement may be avoided in order to preserve appearances.

Future research examining more specifically the relations between the various forms of engagement and goal orientations will be important. In particular, research that examines students' goals and engagement while students are participating in actual academic tasks may be particularly fruitful. Studies that utilize the experience sampling method (e.g., Shernoff, 2010), where students report on their motivation and engagement during actual task participation, may be especially useful. In addition, it will be particularly important to address developmental shifts in motivation and engagement. Given that much research indicates that goal orientations and classroom goal structures change as students move from elementary schools into middle schools (e.g., Anderman & Midgley, 1997), it will be important to examine changes in the relations between goals and engagement across developmental shifts.

In summary, both achievement goal orientation researchers and engagement researchers can benefit greatly from collaborative efforts. Although achievement goal researchers and engagement researchers use different terminologies and constructs, we all are concerned with students' involvement with academic tasks. As these two lines of research continue to develop, a convergence and sharing of ideas should lead to richer interventions for students and more effective training for teachers.

References

Ames, C. (1984). Competitive, cooperative, and individualistic goal structures: A cognitive-motivational analysis. In R. Ames & C. Ames (Eds.), *Research on motivation in education: Vol. 1. Student motivation* (pp. 177–207). New York: Academic.

Ames, C. (1987). The enhancement of student motivation. In M. Maehr & D. Kleiber (Eds.), *Advances in motivation and achievement: Vol. 5. Enhancing motivation* (pp. 123–148). Greenwich, CT: JAI Press.

Ames, C. (1990, April). *Achievement goals and classroom structure: Developing a learning orientation in students*. Paper presented at the annual meeting of the American Educational Research Association, Boston, MA.

Ames, C. (1992a). Achievement goals and the classroom motivational climate. In D. H. Schunk & J. L. Meece (Eds.), *Student perception in the classroom* (pp. 327–348). Hillsdale, NJ: Lawrence Erlbaum Associates.

Ames, C. (1992b). Classrooms: Goals, structures, and student motivation. *Journal of Educational Psychology, 84*, 261–271.

Ames, C., & Archer, J. (1988). Achievement goals in the classroom: Students' learning strategies and motivation processes. *Journal of Educational Psychology, 80*, 260–267.

Anderman, E. M., & Anderman, L. H. (2010). *Classroom motivation*. Columbus, OH: Merrill/Prentice Hall.

Anderman, E. M., Anderman, L. H., Yough, M. S., & Gimbert, B. J. (2010). Value added models of assessment: Implications for motivation and accountability. *Educational Psychologist, 45*, 123–137.

Anderman, E. M., Griesinger, T., & Westerfield, G. (1998). Motivation and cheating during early adolescence. *Journal of Educational Psychology, 90*, 84–93.

Anderman, E. M., & Johnston, J. (1998). Television news in the classroom: What are adolescents learning? *Journal of Adolescent Research, 13*, 73–100.

Anderman, E. M., & Midgley, C. (1997). Changes in achievement goal orientations, perceived academic competence, and grades across the transition to middle level schools. *Contemporary Educational Psychology, 22*, 269–298.

Anderman, E. M., & Wolters, C. (2006). Goals, values, and affect: Influences on student motivation. In P. Alexander & P. Winne (Eds.), *Handbook of educational psychology* (2nd ed., pp. 369–389). Mahwah, NJ: Lawrence Erlbaum Associates.

Anderman, E. M., & Young, A. J. (1994). Motivation and strategy use in science: Individual differences and classroom effects. *Journal of Research in Science Teaching, 31*, 811–831.

Anderman, L. H. (1999). Classroom goal orientation, school belonging, and social goals as predictors of students' positive and negative affect following the transition to middle school. *Journal of Research and Development in Education, 32*, 89–103.

Anderman, L. H. (2003). Academic and social perceptions as predictors of change in middle school students' sense of school belonging. *The Journal of Experimental Education, 72*, 5–22.

Anderman, L. H., & Anderman, E. M. (1999). Social predictors of changes in students' achievement goal orientations. *Contemporary Educational Psychology, 25*, 21–37.

Anderman, L. H., & Anderman, E. M. (2000). Considering contexts in educational psychology: Introduction to the special issue. *Educational Psychologist, 35*, 67–68.

Anderman, L. H., Andrzejewski, C. E., & Allen, J. L. (2011). How do teachers support students' motivation and learning in their classrooms? *Teachers College Record 113*(5) 969–1003. http://www.tcrecord.org. ID Number: 16085.

Appleton, J. J., Christenson, S. L., & Furlong, M. J. (2008). Student engagement with school: Critical conceptual and methodological issues of the construct. *Psychology in the Schools, 45*, 369–386.

Barron, K. E., & Harackiewicz, J. M. (2001). Achievement goals and optimal motivation: Testing multiple goal models. *Journal of Personality and Social Psychology, 80*, 706–722.

Blackwell, L. S., Trzesniewski, K. H., & Dweck, C. S. (2007). Implicit theories of intelligence predict achievement across an adolescent transition: A longitudinal study and an intervention. *Child Development, 78*, 246–263.

Bong, M. (2009). Age-related differences in achievement goal orientation. *Journal of Educational Psychology, 101*, 879–896.

Brophy, J. (2005). Goal theorists should move on from performance goals. *Educational Psychologist, 40*, 167–176.

Brophy, J. E. (1985). Teacher-student interaction. In J. B. Dusek (Ed.), *Teacher expectancies* (pp. 303–328). Hillsdale, NJ: Lawrence Erlbaum Associates.

Church, M. A., Elliot, A. J., & Gable, S. L. (2001). Perceptions of classroom environment, achievement goals, and achievement outcomes. *Journal of Educational Psychology, 93*, 43–54.

Ciani, K. D., & Sheldon, K. M. (2010). Evaluating the mastery-avoidance goal construct: A study of elite college baseball players. *Psychology of Sport and Exercise, 11*, 127–132.

Conroy, D. E., Elliot, A. J., & Hofer, S. M. (2003). A 2 x 2 achievement goals questionnaire for sport: Evidence for factorial invariance, temporal stability, and external validity. *Journal of Sport and Exercise Physiology, 25*, 456–476.

Daniels, L. M., Stupnisky, R. H., Pekrun, R., Hanyes, T. L., Perry, R. P., & Newall, N. E. (2009). A longitudinal analysis of achievement goals: From affective antecedents to emotional effects and achievement outcomes. *Journal of Educational Psychology, 101*, 948–963.

Duchesne, S., & Ratelle, C. (2010). Parental behaviors and adolescents' achievement goals at the beginning of middle school: Emotional problems as potential mediators. *Journal of Educational Psychology, 102*, 497–507.

Dupeyrat, C., & Marine, C. (2005). Implicit theories of intelligence, goal orientation, cognitive engagement, and achievement: A test of Dweck's model with returning to school adults. *Contemporary Educational Psychology, 30*, 43–59.

Dweck, C. S. (2000). *Self-theories: Their role in motivation, personality, and development*. Philadelphia: Psychology Press.

Dweck, C. S., & Leggett, E. L. (1988). A social-cognitive approach to motivation and personality. *Psychological Review, 95*, 256–273.

Dweck, C. S., & Master, A. (2008). Self-theories motivate self-regulated learning. In D. H. Schunk & B. J. Zimmerman (Eds.), *Motivation and self-regulated learning: Theory, research, and applications* (pp. 31–51). Mahwah, NJ: Lawrence Erlbaum Associates.

Eccles, J. S., & Midgley, C. (1989). Stage-environment fit: Developmentally appropriate classrooms for young adolescents. In C. Ames & R. Ames (Eds.), *Research on motivation in education: Goals and cognitions* (Vol. 3, pp. 139–186). New York: Academic.

Elliot, A. J. (1999). Approach and avoidance motivation and achievement goals. *Educational Psychologist, 34*, 169–189.

Elliot, A. J. (2005). A conceptual history of the achievement goal construct. In A. J. Elliot & C. S. Dweck (Eds.), *Handbook of competence and motivation* (pp. 52–72). New York: Guilford.

Elliot, A. J., & Church, M. A. (1997). A hierarchical model of approach and avoidance achievement motivation. *Journal of Personality and Social Psychology, 72*, 218–232.

Elliot, A. J., & Covington, M. V. (2001). Approach and avoidance motivation. *Educational Psychology Review, 13*, 73–92.

Elliot, A. J., & Harackiewicz, J. M. (1996). Approach and avoidance achievement goals and intrinsic motivation: A mediational analysis. *Journal of Personality and Social Psychology, 70*, 461–475.

Elliot, A. J., & McGregor, H. A. (2001). A 2 x 2 achievement goal framework. *Journal of Personality and Social Psychology, 80*, 501–519.

Elliot, A. J., McGregor, H. A., & Gable, S. (1999). Achievement goals, study strategies, and exam performance: A mediational analysis. *Journal of Educational Psychology, 91*, 549–563.

Elliott, E. S., & Dweck, C. S. (1988). Goals: An approach to motivation and achievement. *Journal of Personality and Social Psychology, 54*, 5–12.

Epstein, J. L. (1983). Longitudinal effects of family-school-person interactions on student outcomes. In A. C. Kerckhoff (Ed.), *Research in sociology of education and socialization: Vol. 4. Personal change over the life course* (pp. 101–127). Greenwich, CT: JAI Press.

Fast, L. A., Lewis, J. L., Bryant, M., Bocian, K. A., Cardullo, R. A., Rettig, M., et al. (2010). Does math self-efficacy mediate the effect of the perceived classroom environment on standardized math test performance? *Journal of Educational Psychology, 102*, 729–740.

Fredricks, J. A., Blumenfeld, P. C., & Paris, A. H. (2004). School engagement: Potential of the concept, state of the evidence. *Review of Educational Research, 74*, 59–109.

Graham, S., & Golan, S. (1991). Motivational influences on cognition: Task involvement, ego involvement, and depth of information processing. *Journal of Educational Psychology, 83*, 187–194.

Harackiewicz, J. M., Barron, K. E., Carter, S. M., Lehto, A. T., & Elliot, A. J. (1997). Predictors and consequences of achievement goals in the college classroom: Maintaining interest and making the grade. *Journal of Personality and Social Psychology, 73*, 1284–1295.

Hattie, J., & Anderman, E. M. (2011). *International handbook of student achievement*. New York: Routledge.

Hulleman, C. S., Schrager, S. M., Bodmann, S. M., & Harackiewicz, J. M. (2010). A meta-analytic review of achievement goal measures: Different labels for the same constructs or different constructs with similar labels? *Psychological Bulletin, 136*, 422–449.

Kaplan, A., Gheen, M., & Midgley, C. (2002). The classroom goal structure and student disruptive behavior. *British Journal of Educational Psychology, 72*, 191–211.

Kaplan, A., & Midgley, C. (1999). The relationship between perceptions of the classroom goal structure and early adolescents' affect in school: The mediating role of coping strategies. *Learning and Individual Differences, 11*, 187–212.

Karabenick, S. A. (2004). Perceived achievement goal structure and college student help seeking. *Journal of Educational Psychology, 96*, 569–581.

Linnenbrink-Garcia, L., Tyson, D. F., & Patall, E. A. (2008). When are achievement goal orientations beneficial for academic achievement? A closer look at moderating factors. *International Review of Social Psychology, 21*, 19–70.

Maehr, M. L. (1984). Meaning and motivation: Toward a theory of personal investment. In R. Ames & C. Ames (Eds.), *Research on motivation in education: Student motivation* (Vol. 1, pp. 115–143). New York: Academic.

Maehr, M. L., & Anderman, E. M. (1993). Reinventing schools for early adolescents: Emphasizing task goals. *The Elementary School Journal, 93*, 593–610.

Maehr, M. L., & Zusho, A. (2009). Achievement goal theory: The past, present, and future. In K. R. Wentzel & A. Wigfield (Eds.), *Handbook of motivation at school* (pp. 77–104). New York: Routledge.

Meece, J., Anderman, E. M., & Anderman, L. H. (2006). Classroom goal structure, student motivation, and academic achievement. In S. T. Fiske, A. E. Kazdin, & D. L. Schacter (Eds.), *Annual review of psychology: Vol. 57*. Stanford, CA: Annual Reviews.

Meece, J. L. (1991). The classroom context and students' motivational goals. In M. L. Maehr & P. Pintrich (Eds.), *Advances in motivation and achievement: Vol. 7: Goals and self-regulatory processes* (pp. 261–286). Greenwich, CT: JAI Press.

Middleton, M. J., Kaplan, A., & Midgley, C. (2004). The change in middle school students' achievement goals in mathematics over time. *Social Psychology of Education, 7*, 289–311.

Middleton, M. J., & Midgley, C. (1997). Avoiding the demonstration of lack of ability: An underexplored aspect of goal theory. *Journal of Educational Psychology, 89*, 710–718.

Midgley, C. (1993). Motivation and middle level schools. In M. L. Maehr & P. R. Pintrich (Eds.), *Advances in motivation and achievement: Vol. 8. Motivation and adolescent development* (pp. 217–274). Greenwich, CT: JAI Press.

Midgley, C. (Ed.). (2002). *Goals, goal structures, and patterns of adaptive learning*. Mahwah, NJ: Lawrence Erlbaum Associates.

Midgley, C., Anderman, E. M., & Hicks, L. H. (1995). Differences between elementary and middle school teachers and students: A goal theory approach. *Journal of Early Adolescence, 15*, 90–113.

Midgley, C., Kaplan, A., & Middleton, M. J. (2001). Performance-approach goals: Good for what, for whom, under what circumstances, and at what cost? *Journal of Educational Psychology, 93*, 77–86.

Midgley, C., Maehr, M. L., Hicks, L., Roeser, R., Urdan, T., Anderman, E. M., et al. (1996). *The Patterns of Adaptive Learning Survey (PALS)*. Ann Arbor, MI: University of Michigan.

Midgley, C., Maehr, M. L., Hruda, L. A., Anderman, E., Anderman, L., Gheen, M., et al. (2000). *Manual for the Patterns of Adaptive Learning Scale*. Ann Arbor, MI: University of Michigan.

Midgley, C., & Urdan, T. (2001). Academic self-handicapping and achievement goals: A further examination. *Contemporary Educational Psychology, 26*, 61–75.

Miller, A. D., & Murdock, T. B. (2007). Modeling latent true scores to determine the utility of aggregate student perceptions as classroom indicators in HLM: The case of classroom goal structures. *Contemporary Educational Psychology, 32*, 83–104.

Miller, R. B., Greene, B. A., Montalvo, G. P., Ravindran, B., & Nichols, J. D. (1996). Engagement in academic work: The role of learning goals, future consequences, pleasing others, and perceived ability. *Contemporary Educational Psychology, 21*, 388–422.

Murayama, K., & Elliot, A. J. (2009). The joint influence of personal achievement goals and classroom goal structures on achievement-relevant outcomes. *Journal of Educational Psychology, 101*, 432–447.

Murdock, T. B., Hale, N. M., & Weber, M. J. (2001). Predictors of cheating among early adolescents: Academic and social motivations. *Contemporary Educational Psychology, 26*, 96–115.

Murdock, T. B., Miller, A., & Goetzinger, J. (2007). Effects of classroom context variables on university students' judgments about cheating: Mediating and moderating processes. *Social Psychology of Education, 106*, 141–169.

Murdock, T. B., Miller, A., & Kohlhardt, J. (2004). Effects of classroom context variables on high school students' judgments of the acceptability and likelihood of cheating. *Journal of Educational Psychology, 96*, 765–777.

Murphy, P. K., & Alexander, P. A. (2000). A motivated exploration of motivation terminology. *Contemporary Educational Psychology, 25*, 3–53.

Nicholls, J. G. (1989). *The competitive ethos and democratic education*. Cambridge, MA: Harvard University Press.

Nicholls, J. G., Cobb, P., Wood, T., Yackel, E., & Patashnick, M. (1990). Assessing students' theories of success in mathematics: Individual and classroom differences. *Journal for Research in Mathematics Education, 21*, 109–122.

Nolen, S. B. (1988). Reasons for studying: Motivational orientations and study strategies. *Cognition and Instruction, 5*, 269–287.

Nolen, S. B. (2003). Learning environment, motivation, and achievement in high school science. *Journal of Research in Science Teaching, 40*, 347–368.

Nolen, S. B., & Haladyna, T. M. (1990). Motivation and studying in high school science. *Journal of Research in Science Teaching, 27*, 115–126.

Nussbaum, A. D., & Dweck, C. S. (2008). Defensiveness versus remediation: Self-theories and modes of self-esteem maintenance. *Personality and Social Psychology Bulletin, 34*, 599–612.

Patrick, H., Anderman, L. H., Ryan, A. M., Edelin, K., & Midgley, C. (2001). Teachers' communication of goal orientations in four fifth-grade classrooms. *The Elementary School Journal, 102*, 35–58.

Patrick, H., & Ryan, A. M. (2008). What do students think about when evaluating their classroom's mastery goal structure? An examination of young adolescents' explanations. *The Journal of Experimental Education, 77*, 99–123.

Patrick, H., Ryan, A. M., & Kaplan, A. (2007). Early adolescents' perceptions of the classroom social environment, motivational beliefs, and engagement. *Journal of Educational Psychology, 99*, 83–98.

Patrick, H., Turner, J. C., Meyer, D. K., & Midgley, C. (2003). How teachers establish psychological environments during the first days of school: Associations with avoidance in mathematics. *Teachers College Record, 105*, 1521–1558.

Pintrich, P. R. (2000a). Multiple goals, multiple pathways: The role of goal orientation in learning and achievement. *Journal of Educational Psychology, 92*, 544–555.

Pintrich, P. R. (2000b). An achievement goal theory perspective on issues in motivation terminology, theory, and research. *Contemporary Educational Psychology, 25*, 92–104.

Pintrich, P. R., & De Groot, E. (1990). Motivational and self-regulated learning components of classroom academic performance. *Journal of Educational Psychology, 82*, 33–40.

Roeser, R. W., Midgley, C., & Urdan, T. C. (1996). Perceptions of the school psychological environment and early adolescents' psychological and behavioral functioning in school: The mediating role of goals and belonging. *Journal of Educational Psychology, 88*, 408–422.

Ryan, A. M., Gheen, M., & Midgley, C. (1998). Why do some students avoid asking for help? An examination of the interplay among students' academic efficacy, teacher's social-emotional role and classroom goal structure. *Journal of Educational Psychology, 90*, 528–535.

Ryan, A. M., & Patrick, H. (2001). The classroom social environment and changes in adolescents' motivation and engagement during middle school. *American Educational Research Journal, 38*, 437–460.

Ryan, A. M., & Pintrich, P. R. (1997). "Should I ask for help?" The role of motivation and attitudes in adolescents' help seeking in math class. *Journal of Educational Psychology, 89*, 329–341.

Shernoff, D. J. (2010). Engagement in after-school programs as a predictor of social competence and academic performance. *American Journal of Community Psychology, 45*, 325–337.

Sideridis, G. D., & Mouratidis, A. (2008). Forced choice versus open-ended assessments of goal orientations: A descriptive study. *International Review of Social Psychology, 21*, 219–248.

Skaalvik, E. M. (1997). Self-enhancing and self-defeating ego orientation: Relations with task and avoidance orientation, achievement, self-perceptions, and anxiety. *Journal of Educational Psychology, 89*, 71–81.

Stevens, T., Hamman, D., & Olivarez, A. (2007). Hispanic students' perception of White teachers' mastery goal orientation influences sense of school belonging. *Journal of Latinos and Education, 6*, 55–70.

Turner, J. C., Midgley, C., Meyer, D. K., Gheen, M., Anderman, E., Kang, Y., et al. (2002). The classroom environment and students' reports of avoidance behaviors in mathematics: A multi-method study. *Journal of Educational Psychology, 94*, 88–106.

Turner, J. C., & Patrick, H. (2004). Motivational influences on student participation in classroom learning activities. *Teachers College Record, 106*, 1759–1785.

Urdan, T. (1997). Achievement goal theory: Past results, future directions. In M. L. Maehr & P. R. Pintrich (Eds.), *Advances in motivation and achievement* (Vol. 10, pp. 99–141). Greenwich, CT: JAI Press.

Urdan, T. (2004). Predictors of academic self-handicapping and achievement: Examining achievement goals, classroom goal structures, and culture. *Journal of Educational Psychology, 96*, 251–264.

Urdan, T., & Mestas, M. (2006). The goals behind performance goals. *Journal of Educational Psychology, 98*, 354–365.

Urdan, T., & Midgley, C. (2003). Changes in the perceived classroom goal structure and pattern of adaptive learning during early adolescence. *Contemporary Educational Psychology, 28*, 524–551.

Urdan, T. C., Midgley, C., & Anderman, E. M. (1998). The role of classroom goal structure in students' use of self-handicapping strategies. *American Educational Research Journal, 35*, 101–122.

Wolters, C. A. (2004). Advancing achievement goal theory: Using goal structures and goal orientations to predict students' motivation, cognition, and achievement. *Journal of Educational Psychology, 96*, 236–250.

School Identification

Kristin E. Voelkl

Abstract
This chapter provides a framework for understanding the integral role of school identification in shaping students' social and learning behavior. In the first part of this chapter, the components of identification (belonging and valuing) are described from a theoretical perspective. Next, the development of identification in students is described, and contextual factors that affect the development of identification are highlighted. These contextual factors are: association with similar others, feelings of safety, being treated fairly, and teacher supportiveness. A model is forwarded that relates identification to student behavior and learning. Finally, behavioral correlates of school identification that explain the direct and indirect relationships of identification with students' academic success are presented. Three assumptions underlie the position taken in this chapter. First, identification with school is "affective"; that is, it involves emotion more than cognition, and it is comprised of a particular set of attitudes toward school and school work. Second, these attitudes shape student behavior and vice versa. Third, identification with school develops over time so that its precursors may be seen in the early grades.

It comes as no surprise that positive behavior is associated with positive attitudes. This relationship is particularly important in the context of school or employment where productive behavior is a consequence of maintaining positive attitudes toward the institution. In school, positive attitudes may be expressed in many forms such as liking, acceptance, attachment, valuing, and perceived supportiveness. Taken together, these attitudes may result in the development of a bond or sense of identification with the institution and positive outcomes are likely to follow. On the other hand, students who fail to develop a positive emotional bond with school are likely to disengage, exhibit dysfunctional behavior, and withdraw from school (Finn, 1989; Hawkins, Catalano, & Miller, 1992; Maddox & Prinz, 2003; Rumberger & Lim, 2008; Voelkl & Frone, 2000, 2004).

K.E. Voelkl, Ph.D. (✉)
Department of Adolescence Education,
Canisius College, Buffalo, NY 14208, USA
e-mail: finnk@canisius.edu

This chapter provides a framework for understanding the integral role of school identification in shaping students' social and learning behavior. In the first part of this chapter, the components of identification are described from a theoretical perspective. Next, the development of identification in students is described, and contextual factors that affect the development of identification are highlighted. A model is forwarded that relates identification to student behavior and learning. Finally, empirical data that support the model are summarized: behavioral correlates of school identification that explain the direct and indirect relationships of identification with students' academic success are presented.

Three assumptions underlie the position taken in this chapter. First, identification with school is "affective"; that is, it involves emotion more than cognition, and is comprised of a particular set of attitudes toward school and school work. Second, these attitudes, like attitudes generally, help shape student behavior and vice versa. Third, identification with school develops over time so that only its precursors may be seen in the early grades. Identification is not internalized in early grades, but becomes established over time under appropriate conditions. Empirical evidence for the second and third assumptions is summarized in the sections that follow.

Identification as a Form of Engagement

Nearly two decades ago, Finn (1989) proposed one of the earliest models of student engagement. The participation-identification model was an attempt to explain how the interplay of school attitudes and behaviors affects the likelihood of academic success. In this two-component model, participation referred to behaviors that engage students in learning activities and keep students on-task. Identification referred to students' attitudes about school, in particular, feelings of belongingness and valuing. Belongingness was students' sense of being a part of the school environment and that school is an important part of their own experience. Valuing was the extent to which students value success in school-relevant goals. According to the model, dropping out of school is a developmental process that ensues when students fail to participate in school or classroom activities and fail to identify with school.

More contemporary views of engagement have broadened the model to include additional dimensions and terms, for example, academic engagement (Appleton, Christenson, Kim, & Reschly, 2006; Johnson, Crosnoe, & Elder, 2001), social or conduct engagement (Hughes, Luo, Kwok, & Loyd, 2008; Pannozzo, Finn, & Boyd-Zaharias, 2004), cognitive engagement (Appleton et al., 2006; Fredricks, Blumenfeld, & Paris, 2004; Greene, Miller, Crowson, Duke, & Akey, 2004), affective engagement (Jimerson, Campos, & Greif, 2003), psychological engagement (Appleton et al., 2006; Christenson et al., 2008; Rumberger & Lim, 2008), and emotional engagement (Connell, Spencer, & Aber, 1994; Fredricks et al., 2004; Ladd & Dinella, 2009). The first three terms correspond to the behavioral component in the participation-identification model, that is, behaviors related directly to the learning process and to classroom behavior, and cognitive efforts beyond a minimal investment in learning.

The remaining terms describe affect, that is, attitudes and emotions associated with school and school work. Educators agree that affective engagement in school is important, but research has not clarified its exact role in the learning process. This chapter focuses on affective engagement, showing how affect develops over time as a result of many interactions and experiences including academic performance. Further, affect predicts academic achievement because of its impact on school and classroom behavior (i.e., behavioral engagement) which, in turn, affects learning.

In this chapter, identification is viewed as an intrinsic form of achievement motivation that encourages students to engage in appropriate learning behaviors. Achievement motivation is a "general desire or disposition to succeed in academic work and in the more specific tasks of school" (Newmann, Wehlage, & Lamborn, 1992, p. 13). Motivated students exert effort and persist on academic tasks. Affectively, they enjoy and are eager to approach learning tasks, are optimistic about the chances of success, and take pleasure in their academic work. Beyond the extrinsic reinforcements provided by teachers and parents, students are motivated by internal factors, in particular, individual needs, values, and goals (for a comprehensive review, see Stipek, 2004). Internalized achievement values arise from precepts conveyed by parents and teachers that achievement is valued. Over time, most students internalize these values and make them their own. Identification with school is regarded as intrinsic motivation, that is, an internal desire to achieve, develop competencies, and take pleasure in academic success. When internal motivation is weak, students are less likely to engage in learning and have successful school experiences.

The Components of Identification

The framework for studying identification as an affective form of student engagement is rooted in psychological theories of human needs (Maslow, 1968) and in theory that explains individuals' need to experience a sense of community (McMillan, 1996; McMillan & Chavis, 1986). Sense of community is a "feeling that members have of belonging, a feeling that members matter to one another and to the group, and a shared faith that members' needs will be met through their commitment to be together" (McMillan & Chavis, 1986, p. 9). Individuals also share a need to feel their actions are worthwhile and to have a sense of competence and positive self-regard.

Both needs are reflected in the components of identification in Finn's (1989) model, that is, belonging and valuing. Both components derive from basic human needs, and both can motivate productive learning behavior. The lion's share of research to date has focused on sense of belonging and closely allied concepts including psychological investment (Newmann et al., 1992), relatedness (Connell & Wellborn, 1991), school membership (Goodenow, 1993), school connectedness (Libbey, 2004; Whitlock, 2006), and school attachment (Mouton & Hawkins, 1996), among other terms. Jimerson et al. (2003) discussed similarities and differences among the terms as suggested by the actual measures used in research studies. This component rests on classic psychological theory asserting that individuals have a fundamental need to belong to groups and institutions (Baumeister & Leary, 1995; Maslow, 1968). Outside the home, school and the work place are the most salient institutions for most youth.

Humans also have a need to feel that their actions are worthwhile, that is, of value. This assumption too is based in classical psychological theories asserting that individuals have a need for feelings of competence (Bandura, 1977; Connell & Wellborn, 1991; Deci & Ryan, 2000) and self-esteem based on competence (Maslow, 1968). Both of these needs rest on the assumption that the arena in which a person is competent is important—of value—to the individual or to other people. Valuing can be experienced as a personal sense of fulfillment ("It gives me pleasure" or "I get praise for doing this") or in practical terms as a means to an end, that is, goal attainment. The reason behind the value, however, is less important for identification than the value attribution itself. A person may pursue an activity because of its perceived importance or rationalize that an activity at which she/he is competent is of value, but in either case, it is accompanied by a sense of fulfillment or being worthwhile.

The Need to Belong

Belongingness has been defined as "feelings that one is a significant member of the school community, is accepted and respected in school, has a sense of inclusion in school, and includes school as part of one's self-definition" (Voelkl, 1996, p. 762). The bidirectional nature of belongingness is described by Whitlock (2006) as "[belongingness] is conceptualized as something not merely received (e.g., 'To what extent do you feel cared for?') but reciprocated as well (e.g., 'To what extent do you care about your school?')" (p. 15). Several attempts have been made to compare the terms that have been used in place of or in addition to belongingness (Jimerson et al., 2003; Libbey, 2004; O'Farrell & Morrison, 2003). By and large, these analyses conclude that behind the multiple definitions, there are multiple similar constructs, each arising from a particular measurement instrument. There is little point in reiterating these analyses here; they are complex and tend to change as new terms enter the field. Instead, this chapter discusses only studies that match the definitions of belonging and/or valuing as used here. It was discovered, however, that most measures of belongingness yield similar correlations with other educational variables (Goodenow, 1993; McNeely, Nonnemaker, & Blum, 2002; Rumberger & Lim, 2008; Voelkl, 1997).

The importance of a sense of belonging can be traced back at least to the classic work of Maslow (1968) who proposed a hierarchy of innate human needs: physiological (e.g., food, shelter), safety (e.g., security, peace), love (e.g., relationships, bonds with others), esteem (e.g., efficacy, mastery), knowledge (e.g., understanding), esthetic (e.g., order, beauty), and self-actualization (e.g., avocation). The first four levels were classified as "deficiency needs," deemed essential for physical and psychological well-being.

Maslow's assertion about the importance of nutrition, safety, and emotional bonds has implications for student success. Recognizing that students who are hungry tend to perform poorly, the US Department of Agriculture provides lunch subsidies for student from low-income homes (Institute of Medicine, 2010). Similarly, federal initiatives such as the Safe and Drug-Free Schools Act of 1990, the Gun-Free School Zones Act of 1990, and the widespread implementation of zero-tolerance policies demonstrate the recent emphasis placed on the health and safety of students in public schools (Cornell & Mayer, 2010).

As with food and safety, the need to feel that one is part of a group or institution also shapes behavior. In their extensive review of belongingness, Baumeister and Leary (1995) summarized evidence that humans are naturally driven toward establishing and sustaining bonds with others. To satisfy this drive, there is a need for frequent, positive personal interactions in the context of long-term, caring relationships. They also provide evidence that the deprivation of belongingness is associated with a broad range of psychological, behavioral, and health problems (Deci, Vallerand, Pelletier, & Ryan, 1991; Newmann, 1981; Ryan, 1995).

These ideas have been used to explain motivation and behavior in the work place and in school. For several decades, management researchers have studied job involvement of employees, that is, "the degree to which a person is identified psychologically with his work" (Rabinowitz & Hall, 1977, p. 266). Identification was indicated by the extent to which success or failure on the job affects an individual's self-esteem. Indeed, successes and failures can affect a fundamental trait like self-esteem only in individuals who feel that the work place is an important part of their own self-definition (i.e., belongingness). The phrases "work engagement" and "job embeddedness" have also been used in place of job involvement, although some researchers have explained that there are subtle differences among the terms (e.g., Halbesleben & Wheeler, 2008; Kanungo, 1982; Saleh & Hosek, 1976; Simpson, 2009).

Despite the use of different terms, empirical research in the workplace has supported two common principles. First, sense of belonging is impacted by structural and interpersonal features of the work place such as management style, workplace safety, and autonomy (Harter, Schmidt, & Keyes, 2003; Kahn, 1990; Lawler & Hall, 1970). Second, sense of belonging is associated with employee job performance, satisfaction, and intention to stay or leave (Kanungo, 1979; Simpson, 2009).

These conclusions apply to students and schools as well, where sense of belonging has been viewed in terms of "school community." A community is both a territorial or geographic unit (a "place") and a set of human relationships (McMillan & Chavis, 1986; Osterman, 2000). According to McMillan and Chavis, community membership serves four major purposes for the individual, "shared emotional connection," "influence," "integration and fulfillment of needs," and "membership," the feeling of belonging. "[I]n a community, the members feel that the group is important to them and that they are important to the group" (Osterman, 2000, p. 324).

Likewise, this two-part description is the basis of Voelkl's (1996) definition of belongingness.

Outside the home, youth spend large amounts of time at school and in classes—from an early age onward. They establish relationships with fellow students and teachers and, for those who succeed, experience the achievements and rewards that ensue. These experiences promote a sense of connectedness or belonging with the institution itself, that is, "the place" (McMillan & Chavis, 1986; Sarason, Pierce, & Sarason, 1990). School is where students come to be with their friends, to participate in organized academic and social group activities, and receive encouragements or discouragements for their successes and failures. Building on McMillan and Chavis's concept of four functions of communities, researchers have proposed that sense of belonging is enhanced in schools where students are active and frequent participants in the learning process, where students develop feelings of academic and social competence, and where students' needs for autonomy, for engaging in challenging activities, and for a social comfort zone are met (Bateman, 2002).

The need for belongingness, then, can be fulfilled by the school community. In turn, through its impact on motivation and behavior, students' feelings of belonging can facilitate academic persistence and performance. According to classic sociological theory, the school serves a normative function, encouraging and reinforcing behavior like that of others in the same setting (Elliott & Voss, 1974; Hirschi, 2005; Polk & Halferty, 1972; Seeman, 1975). Social control theory proposes that bonds to institutions are accompanied by sensitivity to the opinions and behaviors of others and a tendency to emulate those opinions and behaviors. When the behaviors of others are positive and goal-oriented, belongingness provides incentive for students to work hard for the same goals, that is, grades and continuing progress. When the bond fails to develop or is broken, individuals may reject the legitimacy of the institution and perceive it as unfair and alienating. In an often-cited study of these principles, Hirschi documented a causal chain of events from poor school performance to weakened bonds with school to juvenile delinquency.

The connections between students' sense of community and behavioral engagement have been confirmed in a number of empirical studies (Furrer & Skinner, 2003; Royal & Rossi, 1996) and are reviewed in the final section of this chapter. Education researchers have also proposed that a sense of membership in home and school settings serves a protective function that offsets the negative effects of social handicaps (e.g., poverty or a language other than English being spoken at home) (Connell et al., 1994; Finn & Rock, 1997; Maddox & Prinz, 2003; Marcus & Sanders-Reio, 2001; Resnick, Harris, & Shew, 1997). Using home interview data from the National Longitudinal Study of Adolescent Health, Resnick et al. (1997) found that parent-family connectedness and school connectedness reduced the likelihood of a host of health risk factors among 7th through 12th graders including emotional distress and suicidality, drug and alcohol use, sexual activity, and violence. School connectedness was associated (negatively) with adolescent emotional distress and suicidality. Connell and colleagues forwarded a model of contextual and personal factors, including attachment to peers in school and emotional engagement in school on outcomes including attendance, grades, and disciplinary measures. Three studies of 10–16-year-old African-American adolescents were conducted to test these models. Although specific relationships differed among the studies, they all showed that combinations of personal connectedness and emotional engagement were associated with positive education outcomes despite that many of the participants were from low-income homes.

When the need for belonging is not satisfied, diminished motivation, impaired development, and alienation may follow (Connell & Wellborn, 1991; Furrer & Skinner, 2003; see Juvonen, 2006). Sense of belonging may fail to develop as a student matures or be attenuated by experiences encountered in school, for example, unfair or disproportionate discipline or close association with peers who decide to leave school. The educational harm that students can suffer in these situations include emotional and behavioral withdrawal and dropping out.

The Need for Personal and Practical Value

Valuing is feeling that school and school outcomes have personal importance and/or practical importance, that is, that they are worthwhile (Anderman & Wolters, 2006; Eccles et al., 1983; Schiefele, 1999; Wigfield & Eccles, 1992). Personal importance can evolve from an internal sense of fulfillment (e.g., interest, enjoyment, satisfaction from completing school tasks) or external sources (e.g., satisfactory grades, encouragement from teachers or parents). Practical importance is the recognition that school experiences have utility in attaining future goals (e.g., a high school diploma, a particular job, or access to postsecondary schooling).

Theory and empirical research support that students are most likely to be engaged, to expend more effort in the classroom, and to persist in learning tasks when they place high value on schoolwork (Eccles, 2008; Pintrich & De Groot, 1990). To the extent that values have been internalized by a student, they are an intrinsic motivator of behavior and engagement (Deci & Ryan, 1985; Deci et al., 1991). Indeed, one of the earliest theories of achievement motivation proposed that one's tendency to approach success (or avoid failure) is partially a function of the internalized incentive value of success or failure (Atkinson, 1964). More contemporary models show that achievement-related behaviors are related to the value of a task, which is a function of the perceived qualities of the task and the person's needs, goals, and self-perception (Eccles et al., 1983).

Research on values as motivators recognizes the distinction of personal and practical values of school. According to the expectancy-value model of achievement forwarded by Eccles et al. (1983), "subjective task value" is based on perceptions of the task to be performed, namely, its attainment value, intrinsic or interest value, and utility value. Attainment value is the personal importance of doing well on a task. Interest value is the inherent, immediate enjoyment or pleasure derived from engaging in the activity, and utility value is the importance of the task for current and future goals. Students in early elementary grades do not reliably distinguish between the three types of values, but are able to do so by the fifth grade (Wigfield & Eccles, 1992). All three, however, can influence students' task choices, persistence, and performance. Tests of the model showed that students' perception of the usefulness of a subject was related to intentions to enroll in future course work, and that task values predicted career choices and course plans to enroll in math, physics, and English (Eccles & Wigfield, 2002; Eccles et al., 1983). Among middle school students, peer group influence has been related to intrinsic but not utility value. The between-group HLM model accounted for 46% of the variance between peer groups in average intrinsic value. Students with peers who disliked school showed decreased enjoyment of school (intrinsic value) over the school year compared with students who spent time with friends who liked school. However, peer group did not influence student beliefs about the usefulness or importance of school (utility value) in their lives (Ryan, 2001).

In an attempt to explain the attitude-achievement disparity for African-American students, Mickelson (1990) distinguished between concrete and abstract attitudes. Concrete attitudes (practical values) represent the perception of one's probable returns on education from the opportunity structure in society. Abstract attitudes represent the dominant ideology of society that education will bring opportunity. She found that, for African-American students, abstract attitudes were unrelated to GPA, but the more students valued schooling as a realistic means toward future success (concrete values), the higher their performance in school. In addition, research by Schiefele (1991, 1999) showed that individual interest or enjoyment of a topic (personal value) was associated with more meaningful processing of text, use of deep-level learning strategies, and perception of skills. His review of evidence found that although interest was only moderately related to deep-level learning, the relations were stronger than the correlation between interest and surface-level learning (below the .30 level).

In sum, research and theory support the idea that other forms of engagement, and academic success, are related to beliefs about school activities being worthwhile. Valuing has both a personal dimension and a practical dimension; both provide intrinsic motivation for student engagement. The personal dimension reflects a student's feelings that schoolwork is rewarding because s/he receives pleasure from doing it. For example, a first-grade student values learning to read because she finds the activity fun and feels pride when she demonstrates competence. The practical dimension reflects the student's belief that schoolwork is associated with the attainment of future goals. For example, a high school student values learning new math concepts because she believes that math skills are important for entrance to college. Following their review of research on intrinsic motivation in education, Deci et al. (1991) summarized the combined impact of values on behavior as follows: "For students to be actively engaged in the educational endeavor, they must value learning, achievement, and accomplishment even with respect to topics and activities they do not find interesting… When the value of an activity is internalized, people do not necessarily become more interested in the activity…but they do become willing to do it because of its personal value" (p. 338).

Connections Between Attitudes and Behavior

Social psychologists have long studied the link between attitudes and behaviors and have concluded that the relationship is likely to be reciprocal. The influence of behaviors on attitudes is explained in terms of two prominent theories: cognitive dissonance theory (Festinger, 1957) and the closely related self-perception theory (Bem, 1972). In simple terms, dissonance theory postulates that people who become aware they have behaved in a manner that conflicts with their beliefs tend to form or change their attitudes to be consistent with behavior. For example, an engaged student who enters a high school with a high dropout rate may be influenced by peers to skip school and eventually stop attending altogether. This student has become disengaged from school, and his attitudes are likely to become congruent with his behavior. Experimental research on the impact of behavior on attitudes has shown extensive support for these theories (Olson & Stone, 2005).

Behavior also shapes attitudes through a sequence of events linking the two. A restless student or one with short attention span may attract the teacher's attention due to his/her behavior. If the teacher reacts to the behavior rather than to learning, this may lead to punishment followed by resentment and dislike for school on the student's part. A classic example of this was described by Bernstein and Rulo (1976) who explained the possible consequences of undiagnosed learning problems. If the student is not following the material being presented, she/he may exhibit inappropriate behavior. The more attention teachers pay to the behavior, the further behind the student becomes academically, bringing with it frustration and negative attitudes toward school.

It is also commonly acknowledged that behavior is guided by attitudes. The "model of reasoned action" (Ajzen & Fishbein, 2005) asserts that behavior is rational and follows from intentions which, in turn, are shaped by attitudes and beliefs. Salient beliefs and attitudes include the perceived likely consequences of the behavior, and the perceived approval or disapproval of the behavior by respected others. Empirical studies support the connections among the components of this model (Ajzen & Fishbein).

Whether or not the assumption of rationality is correct, the principle of attitudes shaping behavior is seen in many arenas. The needs that underlie students' identification with school in particular—needs for belonging and valuing—are strong motivators of school and classroom behavior and misbehavior (see, e.g., Eccles & Wigfield, 2002; Furrer & Skinner, 2003; Pannozzo et al., 2004; Royal & Rossi, 1996; Voelkl, 1997). Students who have positive attitudes about school are more engaged in school, and those who do not like school are more likely to be disengaged or withdraw (Connell & Wellborn, 1991; Fredricks et al., 2004).

The Development of School Identification

This section discusses the role of identification as a mediator of student behavior. Figure 9.1 is a pictorial representation of theory and research on the development of identification and the ways in which it becomes associated with academic achievement. According to this view, students do not begin schooling with established feelings of school identification. Instead, identification is portrayed as having its roots in relatively simple attitudes developed in the early grades. Over time, early attitudes become crystallized, and the need for external motivators is replaced increasingly by the student's own intrinsic motivation. According to Ryan (1995), through a process of internalization, behaviors that were motivated by external requirements become matters of personal choice instead.

In the early years of school, some behaviors are required and others are encouraged. Parents take students to school, and teachers require them to sit in their seats and follow directions, but responding to questions and even completing assignments (academic engagement) have some level of discretion to them. Also, students learn to cope with having to wait their turn, working well with others, and the teacher-student power structure (social engagement). All of these behaviors are reinforced by extrinsic motivators including teacher praise and encouragement, gold stars, awards, candy, and stickers. It should be noted, however, that the use of rewards for motivating learning is controversial (e.g., Cameron & Pierce, 1994). Early behaviors are accompanied by basic emotional reactions such as liking the teacher, having fun with peers, feelings of safety, and having pride in a picture drawn or work sheet completed.

As students progress through the grades, they exhibit new forms of academic and social engagement. They take increased initiative and persist in completing their school work and establish relationships with teachers and friendships with peers. Peer relationships contribute increasingly to the sense of belonging. As behaviors become habits and habits continue to be reinforced from

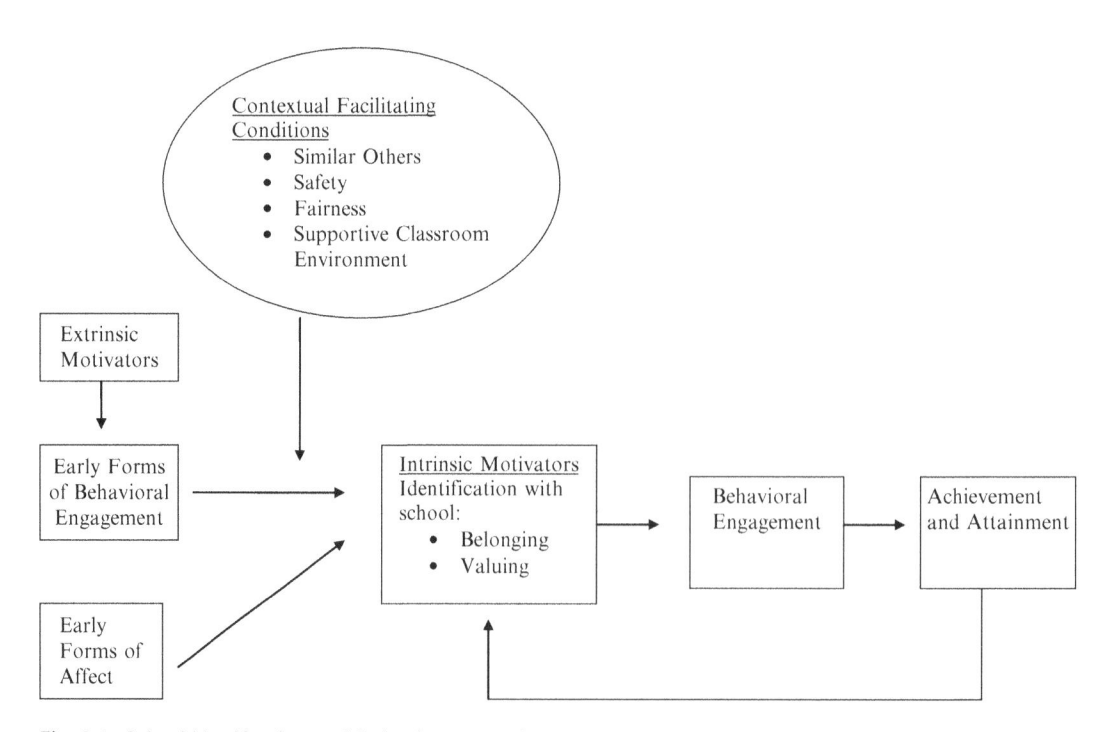

Fig. 9.1 School identification model: development and consequences

teachers and parents or by a personal sense of accomplishment, students increase their sense of belongingness and the value they attribute to school and academic performance. For students who establish patterns of consistent classroom engagement, external motivators are gradually replaced by well-learned behaviors and internal motivation.

Over time and under appropriate conditions, identification with school crystallizes and provides internal motivation for continued academic, social, and cognitive engagement. Because of the academic outcomes that follow, the behavior is reinforced by grades, praise from parents and teachers, recognition from classmates, and also by personal pride and sense of ownership of the skills acquired. Students form deeper emotional bonds with school if they feel accepted by peers, respected and supported by teachers, and perceive that their accomplishments are recognized. That is, continued positive behavior helps solidify students' identification with school (the reverse arrow in Fig. 9.1).

The model portrayed in Fig. 9.1 carries with it three assumptions about student development. First, identification (or disidentification) with school develops over a period of time as the result of numerous interactions, achievements, and other related experiences. The precursors of identification (or disidentification) can be seen in earlier grades. In later grades, when motivation derives more from internal sources, identification with school has a continuing impact on student behavior. That is, students do not begin schooling with a well-developed sense of identification, but early behaviors lead to early affect which, in turn, leads to continued or modified behavior reinforced by more well-developed identification with school.

Second, the development of sense of identification is mediated by contextual factors ("appropriate conditions"), namely, similarity to others in a common setting, perceptions of being safe in school, fair distribution of discipline and recognition for accomplishments, and caring teachers who provide academic and personal support. All of these can be altered, if necessary, to improve school outcomes.

Third, identification with school is ultimately a set of affective responses or attitudes likely to have greater impact on other attitudes or on in-school and out-of-school behaviors than directly on academic achievement. To the extent that attitudes impact learning behavior, the development of school identification can facilitate academic success. On the other hand, the failure to identify with school can create insurmountable obstacles to high performance.

Other developmental models that include identification with school or its correlates have been proposed. These include a social development model used to predict adverse outcomes (e.g., antisocial behavior, substance use, delinquency) from individuals' social bonds with other individuals (Catalano & Hawkins, 1996), and a general model of interpersonal, intrapsychic, and behavioral influences on educational outcomes (Connell et al., 1994). The reciprocal nature of identification and school outcomes was given more attention in a longitudinal study of students as they progressed from seventh to ninth grade (Kaplan, Peck & Kaplan, 1995). Beginning with a large sample of seventh graders attending junior high schools in a Houston school district, the authors found that negative academic outcomes (grades over the previous 7 years) tended to lead to perceived rejection by teachers followed by association with negative peers who, in turn, contributed to further negative academic experiences (grades in junior high school). The study did not identify observable processes that could be altered by school practices to improve students' academic prognoses.

Contextual Factors That Facilitate Identification

Children spend large amounts of time in school where contextual factors play an important role in shaping student motivation. Interpersonal relationships in the classroom, among peers and between students and teachers, are important elements that help individuals meet their basic needs of belonging and valuing. Research has identified four contextual conditions that affect the likelihood a student will identify with school: association with similar others, feelings of safety, being treated fairly, and being supported by teachers. To the extent that each condition is absent, the likelihood that identification will develop is reduced, along with the probability that students will remain behaviorally engaged. These conditions can be altered by changing classroom and school practices. But much of the responsibility lies in the hands of teachers who are in a unique position to impact feelings of safety, fairness, and student support.

Similar Others

It has long been understood that individuals tend to form relationships with those similar to themselves, whether similarity is based on physical characteristics (e.g., age, weight, racial-ethnic background), social characteristics (e.g., religious origins, attitudes and interests, sexual orientation), or common characteristics of the setting, for example, a common power structure or shared goals and activities (Byrne, 1997; Pearson, Muller, & Wilkinson, 2007; Schug, Yuki, Horikawa, & Takemura, 2009; Ueno, 2009).

When youngsters are free to choose among peers, research has shown that two mechanisms are at work: selection of those similar to oneself and the homogenizing influence of those who are already in one's proximity. However, the classroom lacks the element of personal choice. De facto, it is populated by students who share many characteristics and who are also subject to common underlying dynamics, which can be characterized as "crowds, praise, and power" (Jackson, 1990). Students learn together the implications of being one of many, needing to share space and time, needing to wait for other students to finish their work, take their turns, and give their answers. Most class activities are based on a system of evaluations and rewards for the products students produce; in general, some will be praised highly and others less so, but for responses to the same learning tasks. Finally, the classroom is controlled by one person, and all students are required to behave in accordance with that person's authority.

The same conclusion would be drawn from a school-as-community perspective. Many schools and classes serve as cohesive groups, that is, groups in which members are tied together by many shared characteristics—including shared values—and have an affinity for one another as well as for the group as a whole (Homans, 1974; McMillan & Chavis, 1986). Cohesive groups tend to exert pressure for individuals to conform to group expectations, creating even more similarity among participants. This has been demonstrated over several decades with activities ranging from forming opinions to interpreting ambiguous stimuli to completing questionnaires (Hogg, 1992; Shaw, 1976). From either view, similarity among students in a class or school tends to "draw students in" and foster their identification with the institution and its activities (Bateman, 2002; Royal & Rossi, 1996).

The classroom would appear to be an intense environment for fostering student identification with school. Yet despite the structural similarity of the classroom and social pressure toward similarity, many students do not become strongly identified with school. Some of this may be attributable to school practices that create conspicuous dissimilarities among students. Retaining a student in grade who is then older than most of his/her classmates may cause emotional distress and behavioral or emotional withdrawal (Resnick et al., 1997). Discipline practices that remove individual students from the class group are also likely to interfere with students' sense of identification. On the other hand, looping, or keeping, the same class together for several years can serve increase students' identification with school.

Feeling Safe

When students do not feel physically safe, feelings of belongingness are less apt to develop, while feelings of being safe facilitate the likelihood of identifying with school. This connection has been documented empirically. A mixed-methods study of 350 eighth-, tenth-, and 12th-grade students in the northeastern United States explained school connectedness in terms of a number of structural and process variables including perceived safety (Whitlock, 2006). The correlation of the two scales for the full sample was .29 (significant at the .01 level), and in the regression, the contribution of safety was significant at the .05 level independently of a host of other variables included in the analysis.

Some fairly common circumstances raise concerns about safety, namely, teachers' lack of control over students' behavior, the presence of gangs or gang measures in the school, and witnessing or being the victim of bullying. Research has connected bullying to identification with school. For example, a group of 517 students in sixth through eighth grade were administered a questionnaire that included a school attachment scale, and scales that assessed the student's attitudes toward bullying, whether friends engaged in acts of bullying, and the students own history of bullying others (Cunningham, 2007). The correlations between attachment and the three bullying scales ranged from .25 to .41 and were statistically significant at the .01 level. Based on the bullying scales and additional information, the students were classified as "bully," "victim," or "neither" (a comparison group). The highest mean on school attachment was obtained by the comparison group, and the lowest mean attachment was obtained by the victims; victims had significantly lower attachment to school than did bullies or the comparison students.

A British study of 364 students in years four through six of primary school provided self-reports of being bullied, of their perceived relationships with the teacher, and of their perceived safety in the classroom and on the playground (Boulton et al., 2009). All participants completed the questionnaires in small groups with a researcher present. The teacher relationship scale included several school bonding questions, for example, "I can talk to my teacher about anything" and "My teacher makes sure I am OK." The main analysis focused on predicting perceived safety, but the correlations reported showed that being bullied was significantly negatively correlated with perceived safety in the classroom and playground and also with the quality of the relationship with the teacher.

Given the salience of unsafe environments to students, it is no surprise that the findings of studies of safety and identification, as well as other forms of engagement, are consistently positive (Bateman, 2002; Ripski & Gregory, 2009). Any safety-related issue that causes a student to be wary and hesitant when going to school is likely to reduce the strength of connection between students and the institution if not between students and their teachers and peers. Eccles et al. (1993) proposed that adolescents, in particular, need to feel safe and have a "zone of comfort" as they transition to from elementary to middle or junior high school.

In the classroom, safety may be construed in another way, namely, safety from ridicule and public criticism. Studies of the perceived supportiveness of teachers sometimes allude to "feeling welcome and safe in the classroom," but few, if any, studies have examined the relationship of this form of safety with identification with school directly.

Fair Treatment

Fair treatment is essential to a student's developing strong identification with school (Newmann et al., 1992), but inequities can occur in several forms. Schools' discipline practices may be unclear, disproportionate to the infraction, or administered unevenly across student groups. Or students may perceive that teachers are biased against them based on personal characteristics such as race, ethnicity, gender, appearance, or ability. Both of these create barriers to the development of a sense of belongingness.

Research reports have documented students' perceptions of negative treatment by teachers and other school staff based on race (e.g., Irvine, 1986; Kailin, 1999; Thompson, 2002). For example, Leitman, Binns, and Unni (1995) found that 64% of nonminority students reported encouragement by teachers or counselors to take high school mathematics and science, compared to 49% of African-American students. Few, if any, studies have documented whether teachers' actual behavior is consistent with the perceptions or the impact of the perceptions on student attitudes and behavior. Nevertheless, the perceptions themselves may stand in the way of students' feelings of belonging in class or in school generally. According to Steele (1997), African-American students experience disidentification from school because they must contend with negative stereotypes about their academic abilities. "Stereotype threat" arises for African-American students when they are placed in a predicament (e.g., test taking) where they may be treated stereotypically or face the prospect of conforming to the negative stereotype (i.e., intellectual inferiority). This threat pressures students to disidentify from school so as to remove this domain from their self-identity and to avoid the risk of confirming the negative stereotype.

Discipline policies may be unclear to both teachers and students. In a survey of K-12 teachers commissioned by the American Federation of Teachers, 11% of teachers reported that their schools did not have a clearly stated discipline policy, and an additional 50% reported that the policy in effect was not enforced consistently (American Federation of Teachers, 2008). Likewise, a survey of junior high and high school teachers found that 27% did not think their school's drug policy was clear to staff, and 25% did not think it was enforced fairly (Voelkl & Willert, 2006). In terms of students' views, 31% of a national sample of eighth graders reported that their school's discipline was unfair (Rumberger, 1995). A recent survey of school crime and safety reported that 17% of students aged 12–18 felt that school punishment for rule breaking was inconsistent (U.S. Department of Justice, 2007). And several studies have documented that many students—both minorities and whites—perceive that harsher discipline measures are administered to minority than to white students (Skiba, Peterson, & Williams, 1997; Wayman, 2002; Wehlage & Rutter, 1986). In one national study of students in grades six through 12, 9% of white students regarded school rules as unfair compared to 18% of black students (U.S. Department of Justice).

The discipline practices of school hold a lot of potential for alienating students. Unduly harsh punishments (e.g., out-of-school suspensions; zero-tolerance policies) create rifts between students and school and cause students to be absent physically and emotionally. Students who perceive that their everyday behavior can result in punishment are less likely than their peers to identify with school. Indeed, one large-scale study of students in grades 7 through 12, using a self-report measure of school belonging, documented that "connectedness is lower in schools that expel a student temporarily or permanently for infractions more serious than cheating or smoking" (McNeely et al., 2002, p. 140). This is not to say that harsh punishments are not needed, but the circumstances under which they are used should be reasonable, stated clearly, and administered equitably across student groups. Care-based disciplinary practices may be more effective in maintaining school connectedness than are the traditional punishment-based practices (Cassidy, 2005; McCloud, 2005).

If rules and consequences are not stated clearly or not disseminated, then teachers "or administrators" disciplinary actions can be or appear inequitable. "[S]tudents may experience school staff as lacking in consistency or impartiality" (Ripski & Gregory, 2009, p. 369). With these negative perceptions, students are less likely to form bonds with teachers that could dampen their sense of identification with school in general (Pianta, 1999). Using data on sixth- and eighth-grade students in a province-wide survey in New Brunswick, Ma (2003) used multilevel modeling to predict eighth-grade students' sense of belonging from student and school characteristics including students' perceptions of the disciplinary climate of the school (e.g., rules are clear, consistent, and fair). The analysis showed a particularly large impact of school climate on sense of belonging among schools, with an effect size of 5.70 with all other student and school variables included in the analysis. Although perceptions of the disciplinary climate were collected from each student, the analysis included the mean climate rating for each school. Thus, this effect describes differences among schools. The results for variability among students' perceptions would have differed from this.

A Supportive Class Environment

Students need to be in caring, supportive class environments to develop and maintain a sense of identification with school. This principle has been echoed many times over by practitioners and researchers alike (Pianta, 1999). Positive relationships with teachers and peers are necessary to create a positive environment, but teachers are primary in establishing relationships with students, setting the tone in the classroom, providing personal and academic support, and encouraging positive student-student relationships. From a student's perspective, teachers serve as authority figures to be respected, provide a feeling of being a worthwhile and welcome member of the school community, and give reinforcement for personal and academic accomplishments.

The importance of teachers and peers for identification has been confirmed by countless empirical studies. And many of the same teacher qualities that impact identification also affect other school-related attitudes, student behavior, and academic achievement. These are discussed in two broad groupings: teacher qualities that shape their direct relationships with students and behaviors that impact the classroom community which, in turn, affect individual students.

Teachers' Relationships with Students

Teachers provide encouragement to students in three important ways: by showing concern for students' welfare and supporting their school efforts, by articulating clear norms and expectations for students, and by encouraging student autonomy. In early grades, caring teachers come to know each student personally and distribute praise and rewards to all students. These teachers often provide a reason for a child to want to go to school and to try hard to do assigned work. Teachers' encouragement contributes to students' school identification above and beyond support and encouragement from home (Battistich, Solomon, Kim, Watson, & Schaps, 1995; Brewster & Bowen, 2004; Hughes & Kwok, 2007).

In middle grades, supportive teachers may help young adolescents over the hurdles of striving for independence despite the increased structure and impersonality presented by middle or junior high school (Eccles et al., 1993). In later grades, they can encourage students to persist when faced with difficult tasks, serving a protective function against failure (Furrer & Skinner, 2003; Hudley & Daoud, 2007; Newmann et al., 1992; Ryan & Patrick, 2001). Supportive teachers also encourage students to engage in prosocial behavior with other students, which is likely to benefit all students socially and academically (Wentzel, 1997).

Throughout, teachers' expressions of support are likely to be interpreted as a sign of caring. A caring, supportive teacher can impact students' identification with school. In a study of 300 eighth-grade students, Roeser, Midgley, and Urdan (1996) assessed aspects of the school context including close teacher-student relationships, feelings of belonging, affective outcomes of schooling, and academic achievement. The statistical association of student-teacher relationships with belonging was robust: the simple correlation between the two was .35, which remained significant when prior achievement and demographic variables were controlled statistically. Belonging, in turn, was related significantly to all other affective outcomes and achievement with correlations ranging from .17 to .52.

Several programs have been designed to improve student-teacher relationships including First Things First, a school reform program intended to improve relationships and improve instruction by reallocating school resources to achieve these ends (Institute for Research and Improvement in Education, 2002). An evaluation of First Things First in elementary and middle schools was conducted using a comprehensive measure of teacher caring and support and a composite measure of behavioral engagement and identification with school (Klem & Connell, 2004). Students who received optimal levels of teacher support were more likely to be engaged than were students receiving low levels of teacher support. In elementary grades, students with optimal support were 89% more likely to be engaged than were students with low levels of support; middle school students with optimal support were almost three times more likely to be engaged, and those with low levels of support were 68% more likely to be disengaged. The authors concluded that high levels of teacher support are a resource that students may or may not take advantage of, while low levels of support are a liability.

Teachers also support students by setting clear standards for academic and social behavior and holding students to those standards (Yowell, 1999). The importance of clear expectations was highlighted in a study of 144 third- through fifth-grade students (Skinner & Belmont, 1993). The researchers assessed teacher involvement with students, structure (including clear expectations), support for autonomy, and student engagement including both behavioral and emotional reactions. Although the study did not include indicators of school identification, it showed that teacher-provided structure in the classroom was related to students' engagement across the school year. Further, teachers who provided less support and structure were viewed as less consistent and more coercive (Deci et al., 1991; Reeve, Bolt, & Cai, 1999).

Consistent expectations for all students are also important. If teachers hold differential expectations and display differential treatment for some students based on gender, race/ethnicity, or achievement levels, this can reduce students' trust or receptivity to the teacher as a source of support, motivation, and feelings of belonging. This has been found empirically among African-American students (Chavous, Rivas-Drake, Smalls, Griffin, & Cogburn, 2008; Felice, 1981) and students of Hispanic origin (Rubie-Davies, 2006). In interviews with 56 high school students (Davidson & Phelan, 1999), students were critical of teachers who expressed differential expectations for academic or economic futures across ethnic or racial lines. If teachers hold lower expectations for some students than for others, this can translate into less optimal interactions with those students, poorer academic performance, and disidentification from school.

Appreciating each student as an individual and promoting their individual predispositions supports school identification. This is shown by teachers who respect students' uniqueness and encourage their autonomy (McNeely et al., 2002; Perry, Turner, & Meyer, 2006; Ryan & Patrick, 2001; Skinner & Belmont, 1993; Wang & Holcombe, 2010). In the Skinner-Belmont (1993) study, support for the autonomy of third- through fifth-grade students was significantly related to engagement across the school year. In the study of high schoolers, Davidson and Phelan (1999) found that students were more engaged in classrooms where they felt they were respected for their unique capabilities and interests, and where teachers were supportive of individual autonomy.

Teachers' Impact on the Classroom Community

Teachers can play a role in promoting positive interactions between students and their peers and in creating a caring classroom community. The powerful effects of peers on students' behavior, work habits, and values—especially when youngsters enter adolescence—are well established. For students entering their teen years, the influences of peers may even override those of parents. In school, the presence of positive support from peers can increase identification, and the absence of peer support can hinder its development (Connell & Wellborn, 1991; Ladd, Kochenderfer, & Coleman, 1996; Radziwon, 2003).

Negative peer influences can lead a student to disidentify and engage in dysfunctional behavior. Interestingly, in a study of 331 seventh-grade students in one urban school, Ryan (2001) found that peers affected students' intrinsic value for school (defined to include several elements of belongingness) more than its utility value: "Students who 'hung out' with a group of friends who disliked school showed a greater decrease in their own enjoyment of school over the course of the school year" (p. 1146). Students who engage in destructive behavior may lead others down that path. To the extent that teachers can encourage positive student behavior, these harmful effects can be avoided.

Some research suggests that working in groups increases affinity among students. Interviews with elementary students elicited a number of positive comments about working together including that they learn better themselves and help other students learn (Allen, 1995).

Instructional strategies that create close working groups include cooperative learning and dialogue. Cooperative learning increases student-student interactions and affects learning conditions (cooperative instead of competitive). Research shows that the improvements due to cooperative learning include increases in interpersonal attraction, more prosocial interactions, and enhanced feelings of belongingness (Johnson, Johnson, Buckman, & Richards, 1985; Osterman, 2000).

Dialogue, also a component of cooperative learning, is discussion among students that allows each participant to express their own feelings and opinions while working on learning tasks. Although research is sparse, arguments presented by Osterman (2000) indicate that dialogue in the classroom gives students the opportunity to express themselves to their classmates and to discover that they are accepted by others; it is a mechanism for enhancing belongingness. A study of eighth-graders' perceptions of the classroom environment (Ryan & Patrick, 2001) revealed that teachers' attempts to promote interactions in the classroom were themselves related to increased student motivation and engagement.

The culture of the classroom community generally is also important (Bateman, 2002; Battistich, Solomon, Watson, & Schaps, 1997; McMillan & Chavis, 1986; Osterman, 2000). Research on school communities and students' psychological sense of community are based on the assumption that the basic needs for belonging and valuing are best met in cohesive, caring group settings with a shared purpose. This follows from Battistich et al.'s (1997) description of a "caring school community." The Child Development Project (CDP) is an attempt to create classroom and school communities that enhance behavioral and affective engagement. CDP encourages students to collaborate with other students, help other students, discuss the experiences of others, reflect on their own behavior, develop appropriate prosocial behavior, and take responsibility for personal decision-making (Battistich et al.). The intervention is implemented largely by teachers with support from others.

The original evaluation showed that CDP increased fourth- through sixth-grade students' perceptions of sense of community, an affective measure that includes components of identification with school, with effect sizes from one-third to one-half standard deviation (Solomon, Watson, Battistich, Schaps, & Delucchi, 1992). Continuing research led to the conclusion that students' engagement was affected, not only by individual classrooms, but by school community in general. Paramount among the empirical results was the finding that the classroom practices included in the CDP program were related to students' sense of community and, in turn, "a positive orientation toward school and learning, including attraction to school…task orientation toward learning, educational aspirations, and trust in a respect for teachers" (p. 143). Further, caring school communities appeared to be most beneficial for the neediest students.

The Correlates of School Identification

School identification has been examined in numerous educational and psychological studies, usually in the form of separate components (belonging or valuing). Recent research on the connection of identification with school outcomes is summarized in this section. Some studies purport to measure belonging, bonding, attachment, or connectedness but on close examination do not assess these constructs as defined in this chapter. They are not included in this summary. The studies show that identification with school, being an affective construct, is more directly related to other attitudes and behaviors than it is to academic achievement or attainment. However, the consistency and strength of the association of identification with student behavior is impressive.

The mechanisms through which identification is connected to different outcomes may vary. Identification has been shown to have a direct link with behavioral engagement, with positive identification (internal motivation) prompting positive academic and social behavior (Voelkl, 1997). Misbehavior out of school may result from weakened bonds to school which would serve otherwise to control students' behavior. And identification may be related to academic achievement indirectly through its impact on engagement in the classroom.

Although many studies consider identification in its positive forms (i.e., more identification associated with better behavior), some examine low levels of identification or disidentification and their consequences. This is seen in the connection between identification with in-school misbehavior and out-of-school misbehavior (e.g., substance use or delinquency). These consequences are of greater concern to educators.

Identification and Behavioral Engagement

Research has shown that students who identify with school are more likely than others to engage in classroom activities, follow written and unwritten rules of behavior, and invest more energy in understanding academic subject matter. It is little surprise that the connections are found consistently in school-based research: classroom behavior is the most proximal outcome of identification of those discussed in this chapter.

Several studies have used Voelkl's (1996) Identification with School scale. The 16-item self-report instrument assesses both belonging and valuing. The instrument was pilot tested on over 3,500 eighth-grade students. Confirmatory factor analysis showed that it could be scored as two separate belonging and valuing subscales or as one combined identification scale; the choice would depend on the particular context in which it was being used. Scale reliabilities were .76 and .73 for the two subtests and .84 for total identification scores.

In one longitudinal study (Voelkl, 1997), academic achievement was assessed in 1,335 fourth- and seventh-grade students, and participation in learning activities and identification were assessed in eighth grade. Of all the demographic and educational variables in the study, identification was correlated most strongly with classroom participation (.30). In an analysis predicting identification from the other variables, participation had the largest standardized regression weight, which was statistically significant above and beyond all other measures. These findings are mirrored in other studies of identification and classroom participation (Leithwood & Jantzi, 1999; Pannozzo et al., 2004).

Other studies focused on belongingness. In one, over 1,000 students in three high schools were administered a self-report sense of community scale and a questionnaire regarding their behavioral engagement (e.g., class cutting, thoughts of dropping out, perceptions of class disruptiveness, and preparedness) (Royal & Rossi, 1996). The zero-order correlations of sense of community with all engagement behaviors were positive and statistically significant in each high school. Depending on the engagement behavior, correlations ranged from .17 to .56. In a separate study, school membership was found to be related to time spent on homework among middle school students (Hagborg, 1998). And several studies have found identification to be related to extracurricular participation, but the results were less consistent than those for classroom participation (Eccles & Barber, 1999; Leithwood & Jantzi, 1999)

Conversely, research has shown that low levels of identification affect negative in-school behaviors. For example, in a study of over 800 students in grades 3 through 12, Hill and Werner (2006) used self-report questionnaires to assess levels of affiliative orientation (need for affiliation), school attachment, and aggression. Aggression was the frequency of a number of aggressive acts, out of seven, the student displayed in the past semester. In this study, school attachment was directly (negatively) related to aggression and also mediated the connection between affiliative orientation and aggression.

Both aspects of identification (belonging and valuing) were assessed in studies of school misbehavior, which the authors called "school delinquency" (Jenkins, 1995; Payne, 2008; Stewart, 2003). In one study (Jenkins) middle school students responded to a self-report measure of school commitment. School delinquency was comprised of three indicators: school crime, school misconduct, and nonattendance. School commitment (i.e., valuing educational goals) was a strong predictor of all measures of delinquency even when a number of background characteristics were taken into account. In a separate study of high school students, Payne measured identification through two scales: attachment and commitment. The study also included a third "belief" scale, but this particular scale does not fall within the definition of identification in this chapter. Delinquency was the number of in-school crimes, out of 13, committed in the past 12 months. Both components of identification were significant: "students who are more attached to their school and teachers…are less likely to engage in delinquency" (Payne, 2008, p. 447).

Identification with school has also been found to be connected with particular types of misbehavior, specifically bullying, cheating, and alcohol use during the school day. A study of "bullies, victims, and bully victims" (Cunningham, 2007) examined bullying and school bonding in a sample of sixth- through eighth-grade students in Catholic schools. Students who were neither bullies nor bullied had the highest average bonding scores. Both groups of victims had the lowest scores, indicating to the authors that being bullied puts students at risk for disidentification from school.

A study of high school students' academic cheating (Voelkl & Frone, 2004) yielded a strong correlation ($-.43$) of the Identification with School scale with self-reported cheating (defined as cheating on tests, not doing one's own homework, and plagiarism). The results also revealed an interaction between identification and academic performance: students who were less identified with school and who had low achievement scores had the highest rates of cheating of all groups studied. In a separate study of aggression and vandalism at school, Voelkl and Frone (2003) administered lengthy questionnaires to 208 high school students that included measures of aggression and vandalism, in-school and out-of-school alcohol use, the Identification with School scale, and other academic and personality measures. In-school alcohol use, the main focus of the study, was related to aggression and vandalism, but out-of-school use was not. Identification with school was (negatively) significantly related to both outcomes even when demographic and personality factors were controlled statistically. The size of the effects was $-.27$ and $-.32$ standard deviations for aggression and vandalism, respectively.

The connection of identification with school with student behavior and misbehavior is found consistently. In no study reviewed except those concerning extracurricular activities was the relationship nonsignificant or could it be considered weak. For the most part, this consistency is found with regard to out-of-school behavior as well.

Identification and Out-of-School Misbehavior

Students who develop positive bonds with school are more likely to succeed in school and refrain from delinquent behavior. Conversely, students who reject school norms are more likely to engage in antisocial behavior (Maddox & Prinz, 2003; Simons-Morton, Crump, Haynie, & Saylor, 1999). Several theories have been forwarded to explain the impact of school attitudes on misbehavior. Jessor and Jessor's (1977) problem behavior theory asserted that due to underlying motives, perceptions, and attitudes, behaviors are linked across contexts. Thus, problem behaviors in one context tend to be related to problem behavior in other contexts. According to this logic, the association of identification with in-school behavior would extend to out-of-school settings. Also, according to social control theory, individuals are more likely to commit delinquent acts when ties to conventional social institutions such as school are weakened (Hirschi, 1969). Thus, students who devalue teachers' expectations, do not value educational goals, and regard school rules as unfair are more likely to commit delinquent acts (Jenkins, 1995; Krohn & Massey, 1980).

Evidence for the association between school bonds and out-of-school problem behavior has focused largely on substance use and delinquency. Maddox and Prinz (2003) conducted an extensive review of conceptualizations, measurements, and theories of school bonding. The authors concluded that despite the multitude of definitions and measures of bonding, higher levels of school bonding have been found consistently to be related to less substance use and delinquency. School bonding was identified as an important target for intervention in order to protect against negative outcomes and promoting positive outcomes.

Classic sociological work identified identification with school as an important antecedent of juvenile delinquency. Hirschi (1969) used questionnaires to assess attachment to school, parents, and peers, and self-reported delinquency in a sample of 1,200 adolescent boys. In this study, attachment to delinquent friends was found to be associated with delinquency, and delinquency was inversely related to attachment to school. Elliott and Voss (1974) studied over 2,600 students from ninth grade onward, assessing disidentification in the form of "normlessness" and "school isolation." Both factors were related significantly to serious delinquent acts and dropping out of school. Correlations for normlessness ranged from .30 to .52, and from .20 to .30 for school isolation.

In a more recent national study, Resnick et al. (1997) analyzed data from the Add Health survey that included measures of connectedness and a range of negative behaviors. Connectedness was defined as perceiving fair treatment from teachers, closeness to others, and belonging. The authors of this study identified school connectedness as a protective factor for both adolescent substance use and violence. Among both middle school and high school students, perceived school connectedness was associated with less frequent cigarette use, alcohol use, and marijuana use. Also, higher levels of school connectedness were associated with lower levels of violence such as physical fighting and weapon use.

In a review of research on adolescent substance use, Hawkins et al. (1992) identified four contextual and 13 individual risk factors associated with the use of alcohol and other illicit substances. School factors included academic failure and low commitment to school; commitment was considered as liking for school, perceived relevance of course work (valuing), educational expectations, truancy, and time spent on homework. All of the reviewed evidence demonstrated that lower commitment to school was associated with higher levels of drug use.

Shears, Edwards, and Stanley (2006) examined the relationship between school bonding as a "protective factor" and substance use in a national study of students in grades 7 through 12. The measure of school bonding included the degree to which students liked school and their teachers, felt their teachers liked them, and regarded school as fun. Two measures of use were assessed for each substance (alcohol, marijuana, inhalant, amphetamine): having ever tried the substance and level of involvement with each substance. The study revealed that for all substances, greater school bonding was associated with lower odds of having tried the substance and lower levels of involvement. Bonding was found to be more protective for female, white, and Mexican-American students and for students living in isolated rural communities.

The assumption that schools vary in their impacts on substance use lead Henry and Slater (2007) to study the effect at the school level. Using a national sample of students in middle and junior high schools, they examined the effects of both student-level and school-level indicators of school attachment on five measures of alcohol use. A composite measure of school attachment included feelings of liking school and teachers, sense of belongingness, and academic success. Using multilevel modeling, the findings showed that students' own level of school attachment was significantly associated with recent alcohol use, intention to use alcohol, beliefs about peer use, and favorable attitudes toward alcohol use. In addition, a strong contextual effect of school attachment was found. Attending schools where students were more attached was associated with lower odds of recent or anticipated future alcohol use, a decreased perception that students in their school use alcohol, and a stronger belief that alcohol use is detrimental to life aspirations.

While much of the research on adolescent substance use has measured general use (not tied to any particular setting), Voelkl and colleagues have focused use during the school day (Voelkl, 2004; Voelkl & Frone, 2000; Voelkl, Willert, & Marable, 2003). Data from national and local investigations indicate that anywhere between 6% and 25% of adolescents in the USA reported using alcohol or marijuana during school hours (Voelkl et al., 2003). Teachers and principals are also aware that their schools are not drug free (Heaviside, Rowand, Williams, & Farris, 1998; Mansfield, Alexander, & Farris, 1991; Voelkl & Willert, 2006).

According to Voelkl et al. (2003), substance use in school is largely a function of the degree to which students feel identified with or disidentified from their school and also the degree to which schools provide the opportunity to use drugs. This hypothesis was tested empirically in an investigation of personal and situational predictors of substance use in school (Voelkl & Frone, 2000). The results confirmed the hypotheses; identification with school was significantly related to both alcohol and marijuana use at school, but the effect was moderated by ease of use. That is, school identification was negatively related to alcohol and marijuana use among students who perceived they had ample opportunity to use these substances at school without being caught. When students felt they were likely to be caught, school identification was unrelated to either type of substance.

Identification and Academic Achievement/Attainment

Research on the components of identification with school has typically found weak or indirect relationships with academic achievement. This is consistent with the framework depicted in Fig. 9.1; behavioral engagement is shown as intervening between identification and achievement. Relatively, little research has explored the relationship between dropping out of school and identification although the theory and the limited data indicate that students who become disidentified from school have increased odds of dropping out.

Despite inconsistent findings in general, some studies found significant positive linkages between a component of identification and academic achievement (Goodenow, 1993; Hagborg, 1998; LeCroy & Krysik, 2008). Goodenow developed the 18-item psychological sense of school membership (PSSM) questionnaire and tested it in three samples of fifth- through eighth-grade students. The correlation between PSSM scores and measures of achievement in the three studies were .36, .55, and .33, respectively. All were statistically significant at the .001 level. Hagborg developed a shortened form of the PSSM and tested it with 120 middle school students. This study also revealed a significant correlation (.35) between PSSM scores and grade point averages.

Other studies discovered that the relationship between belonging and achievement was more complex. Ladd and Dinella (2009) followed 383 children from kindergarten through eighth grade, obtaining measures of school liking-avoidance in first through third grade and academic achievement in first through eighth grade. The authors called school liking "emotional engagement." Although it does not fit the definition of identification with school used in this chapter, the items appear to reflect aspects of identification, and the study added an important consideration—the continuity of affect over several years. In a set of sophisticated analyses, the authors concluded that "average levels of school liking-avoidance during the primary grades predicted growth in achievement" (p. 200) over the 8-year period. If identification with school is related directly to academic achievement, it may be long-term growth of identification rather than identification at one point in time that is important.

Wang and Holcombe (2010) used data on over 1,000 adolescents from the Maryland Adolescent Development in Context Study to test structural equation models of the relationships among students' perceptions of the school environment (seventh grade), school engagement (eighth grade), and grade point average (GPA) at the end of eighth grade. The engagement measures were indicators of school participation, the use of self-regulation strategies, and identification with school, the latter including belonging and valuing items. Two conclusions emerged from the study regarding identification and achievement. First, the direct paths from the three engagement measures to GPA were statistically significant with school identification having the strongest impact of the three. Second, the connections between perceptions of the school environment and GPA were mediated by school identification. It can be concluded from this study that there are both direct and indirect effects of identification on academic achievement.

These studies stand in contrast to others that show only weak, inconsistent, or indirect relationships. For example, Goodenow (1993) reported that the correlations between school membership and grades were lower than those between membership and motivation (as measured by expectations for success and valuing schoolwork). Voelkl (1997) found that identification was more strongly correlated with student participation than with grades; the latter ranged from .02 to .13. Ma (2003) found a negative correlation in grade 6 and a positive correlation in grade 8. Strambler and Weinstein (2010) assessed valuing and devaluing of academic subjects in a sample of elementary-grade African-American and Latino students. They reported that devaluing was significantly related to lower standardized achievement test scores in language arts and math, but valuing was not significantly related to either.

Research on identification and graduation/dropping out also introduces some complexities. For example, a longitudinal Canadian survey of over 13,000 seventh- through 11th-grade students attending low-SES high schools administered measures of behavioral and affective engagement (identification with school) (Archambault, Janosz, Morizot, & Pagani, 2009). The analysis revealed that, of the three, behavioral disengagement was the most highly associated with dropping out. Above and beyond that, dropouts tended to have low scores on multiple types of engagement including school identification. In a separate study of over 2,000 eighth-grade students, Pannozzo et al. (2004) compiled teacher ratings of students' academic and social engagement, reading and mathematics achievement, identification with school, and graduation/dropout status 4 years later. The correlation between identification with school and graduation/dropping out was small but statistically significant (.09). However, in several regressions predicting dropping out from behavioral engagement and school identification, Pannozzo et al. found the effect of identification was reduced to nonsignificance. Even though dropping out is often described as a gradual process of disengagement from school, both of these studies indicate that behavioral engagement is the most important.

Based on a review of a large number of studies of affective engagement and school achievement published through 1999, Osterman (2000) concluded "There is little evidence demonstrating that sense of belonging is directly related to achievement, but there is substantial evidence showing or suggesting that sense of belonging influences achievement through its effects on [behavioral] engagement" (p. 341). More recent achievement studies and studies using newer methodology tended to find positive relationships, but the inconsistencies remain to be resolved. The research on identification and dropping out suggests that identification with school has an indirect effect on graduation, if any. These linkages require further study to understand the processes by which identification may be related to these particular outcomes.

Conclusion

This chapter provides a theoretical perspective on students' identification with school and accompanying empirical evidence. Several themes emerge from this chapter. School identification is as an affective form of engagement comprised of students' sense of belonging in school and feeling that school is valuable. Both components are based on psychological theory that asserts that humans have basic needs to belong and to feel their actions are worthwhile. A host of affective responses to school have been identified as forms of student engagement (Jimerson et al., 2003; Libbey, 2004; Maddox & Prinz, 2003). Terms such as interest, liking, boredom, and motivation have also been used to conceptualize students' relationship with school (Fredricks et al., 2004). Although considerable progress has been made on distinguishing among these concepts, more research is needed on how these affective responses are related and how they are measured.

It is important to distinguish between simple emotional responses to school (e.g., liking school) and more complex psychological responses. Indeed, children who have internalized the value of doing well in school may work on tasks that are less interesting and for which no external rewards are expected (Deci et al., 1991; Ryan, Connell, & Grolnick, 1992).

Identification with school has not evolved when children enter school. Rather, identification develops over a period of time in response to academic accomplishments and failures, and to interactions with parents, peers, and teachers. Identification is preceded by elementary forms of affect (e.g., regarding school as fun, enjoying school) and extrinsic rewards (e.g., stickers, praise) which can lead to early forms of behavioral engagement (e.g., attending school, completing homework). In addition, appropriate school conditions—feelings of safety, being treated fairly, and being supported by teachers—are important factors that help shape students' identification and engagement behaviors. Over time, identification becomes an internal source of motivation for continued engagement in school.

More research is needed to understand the process by which identification becomes internalized. Longitudinal studies or overlapping cohort studies would be particularly useful for understanding the maturation of attitudes and behaviors. Because individual needs change as students progress from elementary to middle school, research should identify critical age periods when attitudes toward school are most vulnerable (Eccles et al., 1993). To what extent are external rewards important to students in elementary, middle, and high school? Is it possible to develop a sense of identification with school in middle school after years of negative attitude/behavior patterns have been established? Finally, work is needed to understand the roles of contextual factors such as a welcoming school environment, student and faculty composition, availability of help for students who need it, and safety in the development of school identification. This knowledge would be particularly important to educators and administrators. Future research should assess the degree to which each factor can be measured as strong, moderate, or weak in a particular school. With proper school conditions and appropriate support, most students can develop the internal motivation that drives school behavior and school success.

References

Ajzen, I., & Fishbein, M. (2005). The influence of attitudes on behavior. In D. Albarracin, B. T. Johnson, & M. P. Zanna (Eds.), *The handbook of attitudes* (pp. 173–221). Mahwah, NJ: Lawrence Erlbaum Associates.

Allen, J. (1995). Friends, fairness, fun, and the freedom to choose: Hearing student voices. *Journal of Curriculum and Supervision, 10*, 286–301.

American Federation of Teachers. (2008). We asked, you answered. *American Educator, 32*(2), 6–7.

Anderman, E. M., & Wolters, C. A. (2006). Goals, values, and affect: Influences on student motivation. In P. A. Alexander & P. H. Winne (Eds.), *Handbook of educational psychology* (pp. 369–389). Mahwah, NJ: Lawrence Erlbaum Associates.

Appleton, J. J., Christenson, S. L., Kim, D., & Reschly, A. L. (2006). Measuring cognitive and psychological engagement: Validation of the student engagement instrument. *Journal of School Psychology, 44*, 427–445.

Archambault, I., Janosz, M., Morizot, J., & Pagani, L. (2009). Adolescent behavioral, affective, and cognitive engagement in school: Relationship to dropout. *Journal of School Health, 79*, 408–415.

Atkinson, J. W. (1964). *An introduction to motivation*. Princeton, NJ: Van Nostrand.

Bandura, A. (1977). Self-efficacy: Toward a unifying theory of behavioral change. *Psychological Review, 84*, 191–215.

Bateman, H. V. (2002). Sense of community in the school: Listening to students' voices. In A. T. Fisher, C. C. Sonn, & B. J. Bishop (Eds.), *Psychological sense of community: Research, applications, and implications* (pp. 161–179). New York: Academic/Plenum publishers.

Battistich, V., Solomon, D., Kim, D., Watson, M., & Schaps, E. (1995). Schools as communities: Poverty levels of student populations, and students' attitudes, motives, and performance: A multilevel analysis. *American Educational Research Journal, 32*, 627–658.

Battistich, V., Solomon, D., Watson, M., & Schaps, E. (1997). Caring school communities. *Educational Psychologist, 32*, 137–151.

Baumeister, R. F., & Leary, M. R. (1995). The need to belong: Desire for interpersonal attachments as a fundamental human motivation. *Psychological Bulletin, 117*, 497–529.

Bem, D. J. (1972). Self perception theory. In L. Berkowitz (Ed.), *Advances in experimental social psychology* (Vol. 6, pp. 1–62). New York: Academic.

Bernstein, S., & Rulo, J. H. (1976). Learning disabilities and learning problems: Their implications for the juvenile justice system. *Juvenile Justice, 27*, 43–47.

Boulton, M. J., Duke, E., Holman, G., Laxton, E., Nicholas, B., Spells, R., et al. (2009). Associations between being bullied, perceptions of safety in classroom and playground, and relationship with teacher among primary school pupils. *Educational Studies, 35*, 255–267.

Brewster, A. B., & Bowen, G. L. (2004). Teacher support and the school engagement of Latino middle and high school students at risk of school failure. *Child and Adolescent Social Work Journal, 21*, 47–67.

Byrne, D. (1997). An overview (and underview) of research and theory within the attraction paradigm. *Journal of Social and Personal Relationships, 14*, 417–431.

Cameron, J., & Pierce, W. D. (1994). Reinforcement, reward, and intrinsic motivation: A meta-analysis. *Review of Educational Research, 64*, 363–423.

Cassidy, W. (2005). From zero tolerance to a culture of care. *Education Canada, 45*(3), 40–42.

Catalano, R., & Hawkins, J. (1996). *Delinquency and crime: Current theories*. New York: Cambridge University Press.

Chavous, T. M., Rivas-Drake, D., Smalls, C., Griffin, T., & Cogburn, C. (2008). Gender matters, too: The influences of school racial discrimination and racial identity on academic engagement outcomes among African American adolescents. *Developmental Psychology, 44*, 637–654.

Christenson, S. L., Reschly, A. L., Appleton, J. J., Berman, S., Spanjers, D., & Varro, P. (2008). Best practices in fostering student engagement. In A. Thomas & J. Grimes (Eds.), *Best practices in school psychology V* (pp. 1099–1120). Washington, DC: National Association of School Psychologists.

Connell, J. P., Spencer, M. B., & Aber, J. L. (1994). Educational risk and resilience in African American youth: Context, self, action, and outcomes in school. *Child Development, 65*(2), 493–506.

Connell, J., & Wellborn, J. (1991). Competence, autonomy, and relatedness: A motivational analysis of self-system processes. In M. Gunnar & L. Sroufe (Eds.), *Self processes in development. Minnesota symposia on child psychology* (Vol. 23, pp. 43–77). Chicago: University of Chicago Press.

Cornell, D. G., & Mayer, M. J. (2010). Why do school order and safety matter? *Educational Researcher, 39*, 7–15.

Cunningham, N. J. (2007). Level of bonding to school and perceptions of the school environment by bullies, victims, and bully victims. *Journal of Early Adolescence, 27*, 457–478.

Davidson, A. L., & Phelan, P. (1999). Students' multiple worlds: An anthropological approach to understanding students' engagement with school. In T. Urdan (Ed.), *Advances in motivation and achievement* (Vol. 11, pp. 233–273). Stamford, CT: JAI.

Deci, E. L., & Ryan, R. M. (1985). *Intrinsic motivation and self-determination in human behavior*. New York: Plenum.

Deci, E. L., & Ryan, R. M. (2000). The "what" and "why" of goal pursuits: Human needs and the self-determination of behavior. *Psychological Inquiry, 11*, 227–268.

Deci, E. L., Vallerand, R. J., Pelletier, L. G., & Ryan, R. M. (1991). Motivation and education: The self-determination perspective. *Educational Psychologist, 26*, 325–346.

Eccles, J. S. (2008, June). *Can middle school reform increase high school graduation rates?* (California Dropout Research Policy Brief #12). Santa Barbara, CA: University of California.

Eccles, J. S., & Barber, B. L. (1999). Student council, volunteering, basketball, or marching band: What kind of extracurricular involvement matters? *Journal of Adolescent Research, 14*, 10–43.

Eccles, J. S., Midgley, C., Wigfield, A., Buchanan, C. M., Reuman, D., Flanagan, C., et al. (1993). Development during adolescence: The impact of stage-environment fit on young adolescents' experiences in schools and in families. *American Psychologist, 48*, 90–101.

Eccles, J. S., & Wigfield, A. (2002). Motivational beliefs, values, and goals. *Annual Review of Psychology, 53*, 109–132.

Eccles (Parsons), J., Adler, T. F., Futterman, R., Goff, S. B., Kaczala, C. M., Meece, J. L., et al. (1983). Expectancies, values, and academic behaviors. In J. T. Spence (Ed.), *Achievement and achievement motives: Psychological and sociological approaches* (pp. 75–146). San Francisco, CA: W.H. Freeman.

Elliott, D. S., & Voss, H. L. (1974). *Delinquency and dropout*. Lexington, MA: D.C. Health.

Felice, L. G. (1981). Black student dropout behavior: Disengagement from school rejection and racial discrimination. *The Journal of Negro Education, 50*, 415–424.

Festinger, L. (1957). *A theory of cognitive dissonance*. Evanston, IL: Row, Peterson.

Finn, J. D. (1989). Withdrawing from school. *Review of Educational Research, 59*, 117–142.

Finn, J. D., & Rock, D. A. (1997). Academic success among students at risk for school failure. *Journal of Applied Psychology, 82*, 221–234.

Fredricks, J. A., Blumenfeld, P. C., & Paris, A. H. (2004). School engagement: Potential of the concept, state of the evidence. *Review of Educational Research, 74*, 59–109.

Furrer, C., & Skinner, E. (2003). Sense of relatedness as a factor in children's academic engagement and performance. *Journal of Educational Psychology, 95*, 148–162.

Goodenow, C. (1993). The psychological sense of school membership among adolescents: Scale development and educational correlates. *Psychology in the Schools, 30*, 79–90.

Greene, B. A., Miller, R. B., Crowson, H. M., Duke, B. L., & Akey, K. L. (2004). Predicting high school students' cognitive engagement and achievement: Contributions of classroom perceptions and motivation. *Contemporary Educational Psychology, 29*, 462–482.

Hagborg, W. J. (1998). An investigation of a brief measure of school membership. *Adolescence, 33*, 461–468.

Halbesleben, J. R. B., & Wheeler, A. R. (2008). The relative roles of engagement and embeddedness in predicting job performance and intention to leave. *Work & Stress, 22*, 242–256.

Harter, J. K., Schmidt, F. L., & Keyes, C. L. M. (2003). Well-being in the workplace and its relationship to business outcomes: A review of the Gallup studies. In C. L. Keyes & J. Haidt (Eds.), *Flourishing: The positive person and the good life* (pp. 205–224). Washington, DC: American Psychological Association.

Hawkins, J. D., Catalano, R. F., & Miller, J. Y. (1992). Risk and protective factors for alcohol and other drug problems in adolescents and early adulthood: Implications for substance abuse prevention. *Psychological Bulletin, 112*, 64–105.

Heaviside, S., Rowand, C., Williams, C., & Farris, E. (1998). *Violence and discipline problems in U.S. public schools: 1996–97 (NCES 98–030)*. Washington, DC: U.S. Department of Education, National Center for Education Statistics.

Henry, K. L., & Slater, M. D. (2007). The contextual effect of school attachment on young adolescents' alcohol use. *Journal of School Health, 77*, 67–74.

Hill, L. G., & Werner, N. E. (2006). Affiliative motivation, school attachment, and aggression in school. *Psychology in the Schools, 43*, 231–246.

Hirschi, T. (1969). *Causes of delinquency*. Berkeley, CA: University of California Press.

Hirschi, T. (2005). *Causes of delinquency*. New Brunswick, NJ: Transaction Publishers.

Hogg, M. A. (1992). *The social psychology of group cohesiveness: From attraction to social identity*. New York: New York University Press.

Homans, G. C. (1974). *Social behavior: Its elementary forms*. New York: Harcourt Brace Jovanovich.

Hudley, C., & Daoud, A. (2007). High school students' engagement in school: Understanding the relationship to school context and student expectations. In F. Salili & R. Hoosain (Eds.), *Culture motivation and learning: A multicultural perspective* (pp. 365–389). New York: Information Age.

Hughes, J., & Kwok, O.-M. (2007). Influence of student-teacher and parent-teacher relationships on lower achieving readers' engagement and achievement in the primary grades. *Journal of Educational Psychology, 99*, 39–51.

Hughes, J. N., Luo, W., Kwok, O.-M., & Loyd, L. K. (2008). Teacher-student support, effortful engagement, and achievement: A 3-year longitudinal study. *Journal of Educational Psychology, 100*, 1–14.

Institute for Research and Improvement in Education. (2002). *First Things First's approach to small learning communities: An overview*. Philadelphia: Institute for Research and Reform in Education.

Institute of Medicine. (2010). *School meals: Building blocks for healthy children*. Washington, DC: The National Academies Press.

Irvine, J. J. (1986). Teacher-student interactions: Effects of student race, sex, and grade level. *Journal of Educational Psychology, 78*, 14–21.

Jackson, P. W. (1990). *Life in classrooms*. New York: Teachers College Press.

Jenkins, P. H. (1995). School delinquency and school commitment. *Sociology of Education, 68*, 221–239.

Jessor, R., & Jessor, S. L. (1977). *Problem behavior and psychosocial development: A longitudinal study of youth*. New York: Academic.

Jimerson, S. R., Campos, E., & Greif, J. L. (2003). Toward an understanding of definitions and measures of school engagement and related terms. *California School Psychologist, 8*(7), 27.

Johnson, D. W., Johnson, R. T., Buckman, L. A., & Richards, P. S. (1985). The effect of prolonged implementation of cooperative learning on social support within the classroom. *The Journal of Psychology, 119*, 405–411.

Johnson, M. K., Crosnoe, R., & Elder, G. H. (2001). Students' attachment and academic engagement: The role of race and ethnicity. *Sociology of Education, 74*, 318–340.

Juvonen, J. (2006). Sense of belonging, social bonds, and school functioning. In P. A. Alexander & P. H. Winne (Eds.), *Handbook of educational psychology* (pp. 655–674). Mahwah, NJ: Erlbaum.

Kahn, W. A. (1990). Psychological conditions of personal engagement and disengagement at work. *Academy of Management Journal, 33*, 692–724.

Kailin, J. (1999). How white teachers perceive the problem of racism in their schools: A case study in "liberal" Lakeview. *Teachers College Record, 100*, 724–750.

Kanungo, R. N. (1979). The concept of alienation and involvement revisited. *Psychological Bulletin, 86*, 119–138.

Kanungo, R. N. (1982). Measurement of job and work involvement. *Journal of Applied Psychology, 67*, 341–349.

Kaplan, D. S., Peck, B. M., & Kaplan, H. B. (1995). A structural model of dropout behavior: A longitudinal analysis. *Applied Behavioral Science Review, 3*, 177–193.

Klem, A. M., & Connell, J. P. (2004). Relationships matter: Linking teacher support to student engagement and achievement. *Journal of School Health, 74*, 262–273.

Krohn, M., & Massey, J. (1980). Social control and delinquent behavior: An examination of the elements of the social bond. *The Sociological Quarterly, 21*, 529–543.

Ladd, G. W., & Dinella, L. M. (2009). Continuity and change in early school engagement: Predictive of children's achievement trajectories from first to eighth grade? *Journal of Educational Psychology, 101*, 190–206.

Ladd, G. W., Kochenderfer, B. J., & Coleman, C. C. (1996). Friendship quality as a predictor of young children's early school adjustment. *Child Development, 67*, 1103–1118.

Lawler, E. E., & Hall, D. T. (1970). Relationship of job characteristics to job involvement, satisfaction, and intrinsic motivation. *Journal of Applied Psychology, 54*, 305–312.

LeCroy, C. W., & Krysik, J. (2008). Predictors of academic achievement and school attachment among Hispanic adolescents. *Children and Schools, 30*, 197–209.

Leithwood, K., & Jantzi, D. (1999). The relative effects of principal and teacher sources of leadership on student engagement in school. *Educational Administration Quarterly, 35*, 679–706.

Leitman, R., Binns, K., & Unni, A. (1995). Uninformed decisions: A survey of children and parents about math and science. *NACME Research Letter, 5*, 1–9.

Libbey, H. P. (2004). Measuring student relationships to school: Attachment, bonding, connectedness, and engagement. *Journal of School Health, 74*, 274–283.

Ma, X. (2003). Sense of belonging in school: Can schools make a difference? *The Journal of Educational Research, 96*, 340–349.

Maddox, S. J., & Prinz, R. J. (2003). School bonding in children and adolescents: Conceptualization, assessment, and associated variables. *Clinical Child and Family Psychology Review, 6*, 31–49.

Mansfield, W., Alexander, D., & Farris, E. (1991). *Teacher survey on safe, disciplined, and drug-free schools (NCES 91–091)*. Washington, DC: U.S. Department of Education, National Center for Education Statistics.

Marcus, R. F., & Sanders-Reio, J. (2001). The influence of attachment on school completion. *School Psychology Quarterly, 16*, 427–444.

Maslow, A. H. (1968). *Toward a psychology of being*. New York: Van Nostrand Reinhold.

McCloud, S. (2005). From chaos to consistency. *Educational Leadership, 62*(5), 46–49.

McMillan, D. W. (1996). Sense of community. *Journal of Community Psychology, 24*, 315–325.

McMillan, D. W., & Chavis, D. M. (1986). Sense of community: A definition and theory. *Journal of Community Psychology, 14*, 6–23.

McNeely, C. A., Nonnemaker, J. M., & Blum, R. W. (2002). Promoting school connectedness: Evidence from the National Longitudinal Study of Adolescent Health. *Journal of School Health, 72*, 138–146.

Mickelson, R. A. (1990). The attitude-achievement paradox among black adolescents. *Sociology of Education, 63*, 44–61.

Mouton, S. G., & Hawkins, J. (1996). School attachment: Perspectives of low-attached high school students. *Educational Psychology, 16*, 297–304.

Newmann, F. M. (1981). Reducing student alienation in high schools: Implications of theory. *Harvard Educational Review, 51*, 546–564.

Newmann, F. M., Wehlage, G. G., & Lamborn, S. D. (1992). The significance and sources of student engagement. In F. M. Newmann (Ed.), *Student engagement and achievement in American secondary schools*. New York: Teachers College Press.

O'Farrell, S. L., & Morrison, G. M. (2003). A factor analysis exploring school bonding and related constructs among upper elementary students. *The California School Psychologist, 8*, 53–72.

Olson, J. M., & Stone, J. (2005). The influence of behavior on attitudes. In D. Albarracin, B. T. Johnson, & M. P. Zanna (Eds.), *The handbook of attitudes* (pp. 223–272). Mahwah, NJ: Lawrence Erlbaum Associates.

Osterman, K. F. (2000). Students' need for belonging in the school community. *Review of Educational Research, 70*, 323–367.

Pannozzo, G. M., Finn, J. D., & Boyd-Zaharias, J. (2004, April). *Behavioral and affective engagement in school and dropping out*. Paper presented at the American Educational Research Association Conference, San Diego, CA.

Payne, A. A. (2008). A multilevel analysis of the relationships among communal school organization, student bonding, and delinquency. *Journal of Research in Crime and Delinquency, 45*, 429–455.

Pearson, J., Muller, C., & Wilkinson, L. (2007). Adolescent same-sex attraction and academic outcomes: The role of school attachment and engagement. *Social Problems, 54*, 523–542.

Perry, N. E., Turner, J. C., & Meyer, D. K. (2006). Classrooms as contexts for motivating learning. In P. A. Alexander & P. H. Winne (Eds.), *Handbook of educational psychology* (2nd ed., pp. 327–348). Mahwah, NJ: Lawrence Erlbaum Associates.

Pianta, R. C. (1999). *Enhancing relationships between children and teachers*. Washington, DC: American Psychological Association.

Pintrich, P. R., & De Groot, E. V. (1990). Motivational and self-regulated learning components of classroom academic performance. *Journal of Educational Psychology, 82*, 33–40.

Polk, K., & Halferty, D. (1972). School cultures, adolescent commitments, and delinquency: A preliminary study. In K. Polk & W. E. Schafer (Eds.), *Schools and delinquency* (pp. 70–90). Englewood Cliffs, NJ: Prentice Hall.

Rabinowitz, S., & Hall, D. T. (1977). Organizational research on job involvement. *Psychological Bulletin, 84*, 265–288.

Radziwon, C. D. (2003). The effects of peers' beliefs on 8th grade students' identification with school. *Journal of Research in Childhood Education, 17*, 236–249.

Reeve, J., Bolt, E., & Cai, Y. (1999). Autonomy-supportive teachers: How they teach and motivate students. *Journal of Educational Psychology, 91*, 537–548.

Resnick, M. D., Harris, K. M., & Shew, M. (1997). Protecting adolescents from harm: Findings from the National Longitudinal Study on Adolescent Health. *Journal of the American Medical Association, 278*, 823–832.

Ripski, M. B., & Gregory, A. (2009). Unfair, unsafe, and unwelcome: Do high school students' perceptions of unfairness, hostility, and victimization in school predict engagement and achievement? *Journal of School Violence, 8*, 355–375.

Roeser, R. W., Midgley, C., & Urdan, T. C. (1996). Perceptions of the social psychological environment and early adolescents' psychological and behavioral functioning in school: The mediating role of goals and belonging. *Journal of Educational Psychology, 88*, 408–422.

Royal, M. A., & Rossi, R. J. (1996). Individual-level correlates of sense of community: Findings from workplace and school. *Journal of Community Psychology, 24*, 395–416.

Rubie-Davies, C. M. (2006). Teacher expectations and student self-perceptions: Exploring relationships. *Psychology in the Schools, 43*(5), 37–552.

Rumberger, R. W. (1995). Dropping out of middle school: A multilevel analysis of students and schools. *American Educational Research Journal, 32*, 583–625.

Rumberger, R. W., & Lim, S. A. (2008). *Why students drop out of school: A review of 25 years of research* (Project Report No. 15). Santa Barbara, CA: University of California, California Dropout Research Project.

Ryan, A. M. (2001). The peer group as a context for the development of young adolescent motivation and achievement. *Child Development, 72*, 1135–1150.

Ryan, A. M., & Patrick, H. (2001). The classroom social environment and changes in adolescents' motivation and engagement during middle school. *American Educational Research Journal, 38*, 437–460.

Ryan, R. (1995). Psychological needs and the facilitation of integrative processes. *Journal of Personality, 63*, 397–427.

Ryan, R., Connell, J., & Grolnick, W. (1992). When achievement is not intrinsically motivated: A theory of internalization and self-regulation in school. In K. Boggiano & T. Pittman (Eds.), *Achievement and motivation: A social developmental perspective* (pp. 167–188). Cambridge, UK: Cambridge University Press.

Saleh, S. D., & Hosek, J. (1976). Job involvement: Concepts and measurements. *Academy of Management Journal, 19*, 213–224.

Sarason, B. R., Pierce, G. R., & Sarason, I. G. (1990). Social support: The sense of acceptance and the role of relationships. In B. R. Sarason, I. G. Sarason, & G. R. Pierce (Eds.), *Social support: An interactional view* (pp. 95–128). New York: John Wiley.

Schiefele, U. (1991). Interest, learning, and motivation. *Educational Psychologist, 26*, 299–323.

Schiefele, U. (1999). Interest and learning from text. *Scientific Studies of Reading, 3*, 257–279.

Schug, J., Yuki, M., Horikawa, H., & Takemura, K. (2009). Similarity attraction and actually selecting similar others: How cross-societal differences in relational mobility affect interpersonal similarity in Japan and the USA. *Asian Journal of Social Psychology, 12*, 95–103.

Seeman, M. (1975). Alienation studies. In A. Inkeles (Ed.), *Annual review of sociology* (Vol. 1, pp. 91–123). Palo Alto, CA: Annual Reviews, Inc.

Shaw, M. E. (1976). *Group dynamics: The psychology of small group behavior* (2nd ed.). New York: McGraw-Hill.

Shears, J., Edwards, R. W., & Stanley, L. R. (2006). School bonding and substance use in rural communities. *Social Work Research, 30*, 6–18.

Simons-Morton, B. G., Crump, A. D., Haynie, D. L., & Saylor, K. E. (1999). Student-school bonding and adolescent problem behavior. *Health Education Research, 14*, 99–107.

Simpson, M. R. (2009). Engagement at work: A review of the literature. *International Journal of Nursing Studies, 46*, 1012–1024.

Skiba, R. J., Peterson, R. L., & Williams, T. (1997). Office referrals and suspension: Disciplinary intervention in middle schools. *Education and Treatment of Children, 20*, 295–315.

Skinner, E. A., & Belmont, M. J. (1993). Motivation in the classroom: Reciprocal effects of teacher behavior and student engagement across the school year. *Journal of Educational Psychology, 85*, 571–581.

Solomon, D., Watson, M., Battistich, V., Schaps, E., & Delucchi, K. (1992). Creating a caring community: Educational practices that promote children's prosocial development. In F. K. Oser, A. Dick, & J.-L. Patry (Eds.), *Effective and responsible teaching: The new synthesis* (pp. 383–396). San Francisco: Jossey-Bass.

Steele, C. M. (1997). A threat in the air: How stereotypes shape intellectual identity and performance. *American Psychologist, 52*, 613–629.

Stewart, E. A. (2003). School social bonds, school climate, and school misbehavior: A multilevel analysis. *Justice Quarterly, 20*, 575–604.

Stipek, D. (2004). Motivation and instruction. In D. C. Berliner & R. C. Calfee (Eds.), *Handbook of educational psychology* (pp. 85–113). Mahwah, NJ: Lawrence Erlbaum Associates.

Strambler, M. J., & Weinstein, R. S. (2010). Psychological disengagement in elementary school among ethnic minority students. *Journal of Applied Developmental Psychology, 31*(155), 165.

Thompson, G. L. (2002). *African-American teens discuss their schooling experiences*. Westport, CT: Bergin & Garvey.

Ueno, K. (2009). Same-race friendships and school attachment: Demonstrating the interaction between personal network and school composition. *Sociological Forum, 24*, 515–537.

U.S. Department of Justice, Bureau of Justice Statistics. (2007). *School crime supplement to the National crime victimization survey*. Retrieved Dec 15, 2010, from http://nces.ed.gov/surveys/ssocs/tables/scs_2007_tab_04.asp.

Voelkl, K. (2004). School characteristics related to in-school substance use. *Research in the Schools, 11*, 22–33.

Voelkl, K. E. (1996). Measuring students' identification with school. *Educational and Psychological Measurement, 56*, 760–770.

Voelkl, K. E. (1997). Identification with school. *American Journal of Education, 105*, 294–318.

Voelkl, K. E., & Frone, M. R. (2000). Predictors of substance use at school among high school students. *Journal of Educational Psychology, 92*, 583–592.

Voelkl, K., & Frone, M. R. (2003). Predictors of aggression at school: The effect of school-related alcohol use. *NASSP Bulletin, 87*, 38–54.

Voelkl, K., & Frone, M. R. (2004). Academic performance and cheating: Moderating role of school identification and self-efficacy. *The Journal of Educational Research, 97*, 115–122.

Voelkl, K., & Willert, J. H. (2006). Alcohol and drugs in schools: Teachers' reactions to the problem. *Phi Delta Kappan, 88*, 37–40.

Voelkl, K., Willert, J. H., & Marable, M. A. (2003). Substance use in schools. *Educational Leadership, 60*, 80–84.

Wang, M., & Holcombe, R. (2010). Adolescents' perceptions of school environment, engagement, and academic achievement in middle school. *American Educational Research Journal, 47*, 633–662.

Wayman, J. C. (2002). Student perceptions of teacher ethnic bias: A comparison of Mexican-American and non-Latino white drop outs and students. *The High School Journal, 85*(1), 27–37.

Wehlage, K., & Rutter, R. A. (1986). Dropping out: How much do schools contribute to the problem? *Teachers College Record, 3*, 374–392.

Wentzel, K. (1997). Student motivation in middle school: The role of perceived pedagogical caring. *Journal of Educational Psychology, 89*, 411–419.

Whitlock, J. L. (2006). Youth perceptions of life at school: Contextual correlates of school connectedness in adolescence. *Applied Developmental Science, 10*, 13–29.

Wigfield, A., & Eccles, J. S. (1992). The development of achievement values: A theoretical analysis. *Developmental Review, 12*, 265–310.

Yowell, C. (1999). The role of the future in meeting the challenge of Latino school dropouts. *Educational Foundations, 13*, 5–28.

Self-Efficacy as an Engaged Learner

Dale H. Schunk and Carol A. Mullen

Abstract

Student underachievement brought about by low academic motivation is a major factor contributing to school dropout. Motivation affects students' *engagement*, or how their cognitions, behaviors, and affects are energized, directed, and sustained during academic activities. According to Bandura's social cognitive theory, *self-efficacy* (perceived capabilities for learning or performing actions at designated levels) is a key cognitive variable influencing motivation and engagement. The conceptual framework of social cognitive theory is described to include the roles played by vicarious, symbolic, and self-regulatory processes. We discuss how self-efficacy affects motivation through goals and self-evaluations of progress and how various contextual factors may influence self-efficacy. Research is described that relates self-efficacy to underachievement and dropout. This chapter concludes with programs designed to raise school success and recommendations for future research.

School dropout is a major issue in the USA. It is estimated that in the 50 largest US cities, the dropout rate is almost 50%, with 3.5–6 million students dropping out of high school each year (Bloom, 2010; Bloom & Haskins, 2010). Although dropout affects youth from all backgrounds, culturally ethnic and immigrant students are disproportionately represented: "The dropout rate is 6% for whites, 12% for blacks, and 12% for Hispanics" (Bloom, 2010, p. 91). Dropout incurs a major economic loss, likely totaling more than $3 trillion over the next decade (PR Newswire, 2009). Dropout also perpetuates such social problems as unemployment, underemployment, welfare, teen pregnancy, and incarceration (PR Newswire, 2009).

Underlying these widespread problems is the disengagement of urban youth in their learning and success (U.S. Department of Education, 2008).

D.H. Schunk, Ph.D. (✉)
Department of Teacher Education and Higher Education,
The University of North Carolina at Greensboro,
Greensboro, NC 27412, USA
e-mail: dhschunk@uncg.edu

C.A. Mullen, Ph.D.
Department of Educational Leadership and Cultural Foundations, The University of North Carolina at Greensboro, Greensboro, NC 27412, USA
e-mail: camullen@uncg.edu

Approximately 72% of high school students who perform poorly are from lower-income families, and 53% of English-language learners are underperforming (Cuban, 2010). These trends of dropout and underachievement continue at the postsecondary level, with disproportionate attrition among undergraduates from nontraditional groups, including culturally ethnic students, immigrants, and nontraditional students (e.g., older, part-time; Smedley, Myers, & Harrell, 1993; Zajacova, Lynch, & Espenshade, 2005).

Many factors contribute to school dropout, but a major one is underachievement brought about by low academic motivation. As used in this chapter, *motivation* refers to the process whereby goal-directed activities are energized, directed, and sustained (Schunk, Pintrich, & Meece, 2008). Motivation is a complex process that can be affected by personal factors (e.g., individuals' thoughts, beliefs, and emotions) and contextual factors, such as classrooms, peer groups, and community and home influences.

Herein we present the case that low academic motivation perpetuates poor engagement in learning and that certain strategies and interventions can make a difference in the education of America's youth. By *engagement*, we mean the manifestation of students' motivation, or how their cognitions, behaviors, and affects are energized, directed, and sustained during learning and other academic activities (Skinner, Kindermann, Connell, & Wellborn, 2009). Although different theoretical approaches explain student motivation and engagement, we utilize Bandura's (1977b, 1986, 1997, 2001) *social cognitive theory* of psychological functioning, which emphasizes that much human learning and behavior occur in social environments. By interacting with others, people learn knowledge, skills, strategies, beliefs, norms, and attitudes. Students act in accordance with their beliefs about their capabilities and the expected outcomes of their actions. Social cognitive researchers have explored the operation and outcomes of cognitive and affective processes hypothesized to underlie motivation (Pintrich, 2003; Schunk & Pajares, 2009).

Our interest is in a key social cognitive variable: *self-efficacy,* or one's perceived capabilities for learning or performing actions at designated levels (Bandura, 1977a, 1997). Research has shown that a higher sense of self-efficacy can positively affect learning, achievement, self-regulation, and motivational outcomes such as individuals' choices of activities, effort, persistence, and interests (Bandura, 1997; Pajares, 1996; Schunk & Pajares, 2009; Usher & Pajares, 2008). Self-efficacious students are motivated and engaged in learning, which promotes their competence as learners. Conversely, a lower sense of self-efficacy for learning and performing well in school can negatively affect students' motivation and engagement (Pajares, 1996), increasing the risk of underachievement and dropout. Teachers who help students experience success by fostering their development of skills, learning strategies, and a positive outlook on life and their future can positively impact self-efficacy in their classrooms (McInerney, 2004; Miller & Brickman, 2004).

Despite the solid foundation of self-efficacy research pertaining to school-aged children and school-to-work interventions, fewer scholars have assessed its relevance for urban youth struggling at school. Given that school dropout affects youth from all backgrounds but particularly those who are culturally and economically disadvantaged, the self-efficacy of urban youth has undeniable importance (Mullen & Schunk, 2011). Self-efficacy has been identified as a predictor of adolescent success in life (Perry, DeWine, Duffy, & Vance, 2007).

Examining the predictors of academic self-efficacy in ethnic adolescents to include resiliency and persistence despite hardships and obstacles, perceived control over one's own successes, and school and community engagement, will contribute to the emerging literature on this topic (Vick & Packard, 2008). Our particular focus is the roles of personal and contextual factors on disadvantaged adolescents' academic motivation.

We next describe the conceptual framework of social cognitive theory and the key roles played by vicarious, symbolic, and self-regulatory processes. We then discuss self-efficacy and the process whereby self-efficacy affects motivation through goals and self-evaluations of progress, as well as how self-efficacy can affect student engagement and how contextual factors may influence self-efficacy. The research evidence presented relates self-efficacy to underachievement and dropout. We also briefly highlight some programs designed to enhance school success through such means as school engagement, community activism, and career decision-making. Recommendations for future research conclude this chapter.

Conceptual Framework

Reciprocal Interactions

A central tenet of Bandura's (1977b, 1986, 1997, 2001) social cognitive theory is that human behavior operates within a framework of *triadic reciprocality* involving interactions among personal factors (e.g., cognitions, beliefs, skills, affects), behaviors, and social/environmental factors (Fig. 10.1). These interacting influences can be demonstrated using self-efficacy as the personal factor. Regarding the interaction of self-efficacy and behavior, studies have shown that self-efficacy influences achievement behaviors such as task choice, effort, persistence, and use of effective learning strategies (person→behavior; Schunk & Pajares, 2009). These behaviors also affect self-efficacy. As students perform tasks and observe their learning progress, self-efficacy for continued learning is enhanced (behavior→person).

Many students with learning disabilities hold low self-efficacy for performing well (Licht & Kistner, 1986). The link between personal and contextual factors is seen when individuals react to these students based on attributes typically associated with them (e.g., low skills) rather than based on their actual capabilities (person→social/environment). In turn, environmental feedback can affect self-efficacy, such as when teachers encourage students by communicating, "I know you can do this" (social/environment→person).

The link between behaviors and environmental factors is evident in many instructional sequences. Environmental factors can direct behaviors, such as when teachers point to a display and say, "Look here," which students do with little conscious effort (social/environment→behavior). Behaviors can alter learners' instructional environments. When students give incorrect answers, teachers are apt to reteach the material, temporarily discontinuing the lesson (behavior→social/environment).

Social cognitive theory presents a view of human *agency* in which individuals proactively engage in creating their own career and life trajectories (Schunk & Pajares, 2005). They hold beliefs that allow them to exert control over their thoughts, feelings, and actions. In reciprocal fashion, people influence and are influenced by their actions and environments. But the scope of this reciprocal influence is broader than individuals because they live in social environments. *Collective agency* refers to people's shared beliefs about what they are capable of accomplishing as a group. Groups, too, affect and are affected by their actions and environments.

Vicarious, Symbolic, and Self-Regulatory Processes

Social cognitive theory stresses that people possess capabilities that distinguish them from others and motivate them to strive for a sense of agency (Bandura, 1986). Among the most prominent of these are vicarious, symbolic, and self-regulatory processes.

Vicarious processes. Much human learning occurs *vicariously* through observing modeled performances (e.g., live, filmed symbolic; Bandura, 1977b). The capability for learning vicariously allows individuals to acquire beliefs, cognitions,

Person ↔ Behavior

Person ↔ Social/Environment

Social/Environment ↔ Behavior

Fig. 10.1 Reciprocal interactions in social cognitive theory

affects, skills, strategies, and behaviors from observations of others in their social environments and vicariously via media outlets, which saves time because learning is not demonstrated when it occurs. This capability also allows people to shape their lives because they proactively select environmental features (e.g., individuals, materials) to which they want to attend. Thus, students who want to become teachers enroll in education programs and put themselves in situations where they can learn vicariously, such as by observing and working with classroom teachers.

Symbolic processes. Symbolic processes involve language, mathematical and scientific notation, iconography, and cognition. These processes help people adapt to and alter their environments (Bandura, 1986). They use symbolic processes when they formulate thoughts and take action and, perhaps unconsciously, to guide their actions. Cognitively in tune, students do not simply react to events but rather resolve issues and generate new courses of action. Symbolic processes also foster verbal and written communications, which further promotes learning.

Self-regulatory processes. Social cognitive theory assigns a prominent role to *self-regulation,* or the processes individuals use to activate and sustain their behaviors, cognitions, and affects that are focused on attaining goals (Zimmerman, 2000). People regulate their behaviors to conform to their internal standards and goals. Before embarking on a task, individuals determine their goals and what strategies to use, and they feel self-efficacious about performing well. As they engage in tasks, they monitor their performances, assess their progress toward goals, and decide whether their strategy needs adjusting. As tasks are completed, they reflect on their experiences, make modifications, and determine next steps. Believing they have learned and made progress strengthens their self-efficacy and motivates further learning. People who are continually engaged while learning are apt to be self-regulated (Schunk & Pajares, 2009; Zimmerman & Cleary, 2009).

Self-Efficacy

Self-efficacy is a key personal factor in social cognitive theory, which postulates that achievement depends on interactions among behaviors, personal factors, and social/environmental conditions (Perry et al., 2007). *Academic self-efficacy,* or the perceived confidence in one's ability to execute actions for attaining academic goals, plays a crucial role in adolescent motivation and learning. Self-efficacy is hypothesized to influence behaviors and environments and be affected by them (Bandura, 1986, 1997). Self-efficacy affects choice of tasks, effort, persistence, and achievement. Research in academic settings shows that students who feel efficacious about learning tend to be competent and engaged and are likely to set learning goals, use effective learning strategies, monitor comprehension, evaluate goal progress, and create supportive environments (Schunk & Pajares, 2005). In turn, self-efficacy is influenced by the outcomes of behaviors (e.g., goal progress, achievement) and by inputs from the environment (e.g., feedback from teachers, comparisons with peers). Individuals' self-efficacy impacts motivation and learning, as well as decisions and events that affect their lives (Schunk & Pajares, 2009).

Sources of Information About Self-Efficacy

Information for assessing one's self-efficacy is acquired from actual performances, observations of others (vicarious experiences), social persuasion, and physiological indexes (Table 10.1; Bandura, 1997). Because these are tangible indicators of individuals' capabilities, one's performances constitute the most reliable information (Schunk & Pajares, 2009). Interpretations of one's performances as successful raise self-efficacy whereas perceived failures may lower it, although an occasional failure or success should not have much impact.

Table 10.1 Self-efficacy sources and consequences

Sources of self-efficacy information
- Mastery experiences (actual performances)
- Vicarious (modeled) experiences
- Forms of social persuasion
- Physiological indexes

Consequences of self-efficacy
- Motivational outcomes (task choice, effort, persistence)
- Learning
- Achievement
- Self-regulation

Interpretations of one's performances are important, along with the performances themselves. Individuals engage in metacognitive mediation by thinking of areas of their learning such as planning and problem-solving. In a study of college undergraduates (mixed gender, no race specified), Coutinho (2008) found that students' metacognition and self-efficacy influenced their performances.

Individuals acquire information about their capabilities through social comparisons with others (Bandura, 1997). Similarity to others is a cue for gauging one's self-efficacy (Schunk, 1995). Observing others succeed can raise observers' self-efficacy and motivate them to try the task at hand because they are apt to believe that if others can achieve, they can as well. But a vicarious increase in self-efficacy can be negated by subsequent difficulties. Persons who observe peers fail may believe they lack competence, which can dissuade them from attempting the task.

People also may assess self-efficacy when they receive persuasive information from others (e.g., "I know you can do this"; Bandura, 1997); however, such persuasion must be credible for people to believe that success is attainable. Although positive feedback can raise individuals' self-efficacy, the effects will not endure if they subsequently perform poorly (Schunk & Pajares, 2009).

Physiological and emotional reactions such as anxiety and stress also provide input about self-efficacy (Bandura, 1997). Strong emotional reactions can signal anticipated success or failure. When people experience negative thoughts and fears about their capabilities (e.g., feeling nervous when thinking about taking a test), those affective reactions can lower self-efficacy (Zajacova et al., 2005). Conversely, when people feel less stressful (e.g., anxiety subsides while taking a test), they may experience higher self-efficacy for performing well.

Sources of self-efficacy information do not automatically affect self-efficacy (Bandura, 1997). Individuals interpret the results of events, and these interpretations generate information on which judgments are based (Schunk & Pajares, 2009). Some ways that research has shown to effectively build students' self-efficacy are to have students set difficult but attainable goals and assess their own goal progress (mastery experiences), allow students to observe models similar to themselves learning skills (vicarious experiences), and provide students with feedback that links their learning progress to their diligently applying a learning strategy (social persuasion; Schunk, 1995).

Important as it is, self-efficacy is not the only influence on behavior; no amount of it will produce a competent performance when requisite skills are lacking (Schunk & Pajares, 2009). Also important are *outcome expectations* (beliefs about the likely consequences of actions; Bandura, 1997) and *values* (perceptions of the importance and utility of learning and acting in given ways; Wigfield, Tonks, & Eccles, 2004). Even students who feel efficacious about performing well in school may disengage from learning if they do not value it or believe that negative outcomes may result, such as rejection by peers. Assuming the activation of requisite skills, positive values, and outcome expectations, self-efficacy is a key determinant of individuals' motivation, learning, self-regulation, and achievement (Schunk & Pajares, 2009).

Consequences of Self-Efficacy

Self-efficacy has diverse effects on various motivational outcomes associated with student engagement, including task choice, effort, and persistence (Bandura, 1997; Pajares, 1996; Schunk & Pajares, 2005, 2009; Table 10.1).

Individuals typically select tasks and activities at which they feel competent. Self-efficacy can affect how much cognitive and physical effort people expend on an activity, how long they persist when they encounter difficulties, and their levels of learning and achievement. Students with high self-efficacy tend to set challenging goals, work diligently, persist in the face of failure, and recover their sense of self-efficacy after setbacks. As a consequence, they develop higher levels of competence. In contrast, those with low self-efficacy may set easier goals, expend minimal effort, disassociate as difficulties arise, and feel dejected by failure, all of which negatively affect engagement and learning.

Goals and Self-Evaluations of Progress

Social cognitive theory highlights the importance of various symbolic processes for motivation. Among the most critical are self-efficacy, goals, and self-evaluations of goal progress, which work together to enhance motivation and engagement in learning.

Goals, or what people are consciously trying to attain, are symbolic processes that instigate and sustain actions. Because goals do not affect behavior without commitment, learners must commit to attempting goals (Locke & Latham, 2002). As learners work on a task, they compare their current performance with their specific goals. Positive self-evaluations of progress strengthen self-efficacy and sustain motivation. A perceived discrepancy between present performance and the goal may create dissatisfaction, which can propel effort. Goals motivate learners to expend the effort necessary and persist at the task (Locke & Latham, 2002), resulting in better performance and enhanced engagement.

Although goals are motivational catalysts, their effects depend on their properties: specificity, proximity, and difficulty. Goals that include specific performance standards are more likely to activate self-evaluations of progress and enhance self-efficacy and motivation than are general goals (e.g., "Do your best"; Bandura, 1986). Specific goals are a better indicator of the kind of effort needed to succeed and evaluate progress. Goals also are distinguished by how far they project into the future. Because it is easier to determine progress toward goals that are closer at hand, proximal (short-term) goals enhance self-efficacy and motivation better than do distant (long-term) goals (Bandura & Schunk, 1981).

Goal difficulty, which refers to the level of task proficiency required as assessed against a standard, influences the effort people expend. In general, learners work harder to attain more challenging goals; however, perceived difficulty and motivation do not bear an unlimited positive relation to one another. Goals that students believe are overly trying can obstruct motivation because they hold low self-efficacy for attaining them. Learners are apt to feel self-efficacious for attaining goals that they perceive as difficult but attainable.

A distinction can be drawn between learning and performance goals. A *learning goal* refers to what knowledge, behavior, skill, or strategy students are to acquire, and a *performance goal* refers to what task is to be completed. These goals can have differential effects on achievement behaviors (Anderman & Wolters, 2006). Learning goals motivate by focusing and sustaining attention on both processes and strategies that help students acquire competence and new skills. Self-efficacy is substantiated as they work on the task and assess their progress (Schunk, 1996).

In contrast, performance goals focus attention on completing tasks. They may not highlight the value of the processes and strategies underlying task completion or raise self-efficacy for learning. As they engage in tasks, students may not compare their present and past performances to determine progress. Performance goals can lead to social comparisons with the work of others to determine progress. These comparisons can lower self-efficacy when students experience learning difficulties, which adversely affects motivation and engagement in learning.

Research supports these hypothesized effects of learning and performance goals. Schunk and Ertmer (1999) conducted two studies with college undergraduates as they worked on computer projects. Students received the goal of learning computer applications or the goal of performing them. In the first study, half of the students in each goal condition evaluated their learning progress midway through the instructional program. The learning goal led to higher self-efficacy, self-judged progress, and self-regulatory competence and strategy use. The opportunity to self-evaluate progress promoted self-efficacy. In the second study, self-evaluation students assessed their progress after each instructional session. Frequent self-evaluation produced comparable results when linked with a learning or performance goal. These results suggest that multiple self-evaluations of learning progress can raise motivation and achievement outcomes.

Self-Efficacy and Student Engagement

Engaged Learning

Student engagement in learning reflects cognitive, behavioral, and affective variables that encompass aspects of motivation and self-regulation (Schunk, 1995; Zimmerman, 2000). Among cognitive variables, students engaged in learning have a sense of self-efficacy for learning. They hold positive outcome expectations and value the learning. They set goals and evaluate their progress, and they decide what they believe are effective strategies for learning the material and succeeding. They focus their attention on the task and strive to avoid distraction.

Students who are engaged also display productive achievement behaviors. They create work environments conducive to learning. Disadvantaged students must especially endeavor to overcome barriers where they lack necessary materials and equipment. While engaged with tasks, students expend effort and persist when they encounter difficulties. If they become stuck, they seek help (e.g., teachers, parents, peers, manuals). Engaged learners self-monitor to ensure good use of time. They may keep records of their accomplished tasks and what remains to be done.

Affective variables include creating and maintaining a positive attitude toward learning. Engaged learners value learning; by succeeding, they experience a sense of pride. They are strategic about learning and know how to keep themselves from becoming discouraged. For example, if they cannot answer the easier questions on a test, they change their strategy by moving onto questions they can answer and reassuring themselves that they are making progress while internally checking their understanding.

Self-efficacy comes into play at all points in engaged learning. Prior to starting on a task, students hold a sense of self-efficacy for learning (Schunk, 1995). Their self-efficacy is substantiated as they work on tasks and observe the progress being made toward their goal. Self-efficacy helps to keep students motivated and engaged in learning activities. Students who feel efficacious about learning but perceive that their progress is inadequate make adjustments to improve their learning (e.g., changing strategy, seeking help, improving one's environment). Such modifications help foster engagement in learning.

Contextual Influences

As noted, self-efficacy is affected by contextual factors such as familial, sociocultural, and educational influences that are critical for engaged learning.

Familial influences. Families influence self-efficacy in different ways, such as through their capital. *Capital* includes resources and assets (Bradley & Corwyn, 2002), primarily material resources (e.g., income), human resources (e.g., education), and social resources (e.g., networks). *Cultural capital* refers to the wealthy norm reflected in an accumulation of specific types of knowledge, skills, and abilities that are acquired by families and valued in school settings (e.g., technological resources such as computers in the home; Yosso, 2005). Children are motivated to learn when the home has activities and materials that arouse their curiosity and offer challenges that can be met (Schunk & Pajares, 2009). Parents who are better educated and have social connections are apt to stress education and enroll their children in school and extramural programs that foster their self-efficacy and learning.

Families that foster a responsive and supportive environment, encourage exploration and stimulate curiosity, and facilitate learning experiences accelerate their children's intellectual development. Because mastery experiences constitute a powerful source of self-efficacy information, parents who arrange for their children to experience mastery in concert with their personal interests are apt to develop efficacious youngsters (Schunk & Pajares, 2009). Activities conducive to learning may include playing a musical instrument or a sport in which children have the freedom to explore. In contrast, parents can negatively affect their children's academic competence and achievement through such behaviors as providing rewards extrinsic to academic tasks, making unrealistic demands, avoiding conflict arising from learning expectations, and not valuing self-directed learning (Borkowski & Thorpe, 1994).

Another means of influence is vicariously through role models. Family members who model ways to cope with difficulties, persistence, and effort strengthen their children's self-efficacy. Family members also provide persuasive information. Parents who encourage their children to try different activities as appropriate to their ages facilitate their capability for welcoming challenges and meeting them (Schunk & Pajares, 2009).

The plight of delayed adulthood affects self-efficacy as well. Western societies now have a longer transition to adulthood and thus a prolonged time for youth to finish school, become employed, and start families (Settersten & Ray, 2010). Youth from impoverished backgrounds do not meet these adult milestones at the same rate as their more privileged peers. Modern families can experience undue stress where their youth remain semidependent for different types of assistance. Youth from low-income families receive approximately 70% less material assistance than those in the top quarter of the income distribution (Settersten & Ray, 2010).

Sociocultural influences. A major factor associated with self-efficacy and achievement is socioeconomic status. Borkowski and Thorpe (1994) reviewed empirical studies and found that students from lower-income families tend to lack positive visions of themselves over time and as related to school, career, and life. Metacognitive processing of information and development are fostered as longer-term goals are formed (e.g., "future time perspective"), and self-schemas (e.g., "possible selves") are imagined (Borkowski & Thorpe, 1994; Shell & Husman, 2001). Future time perspective is not a self-schema per se, but these two concepts share similarities. Notably, future time perspective is implicit in an individual's capability for projecting possible selves into the near and distant future (Miller & Brickman, 2004; Shell & Husman, 2001; Simons, Vansteenkiste, Lens, & Lacante, 2004).

For example, students who relate to their school subjects in the context of what they want to become (e.g., lawyer, teacher) improve their mental competence and engagement in learning goals and tasks (Shell & Husman, 2001). Based on their study involving almost 200 primarily White undergraduate students, Shell and Husman found that students' future time beliefs (i.e., relative importance of attaining immediate versus long-term future outcomes) were associated with higher self-efficacy, achievement, and study time and effort.

Youth and children from different sociocultural backgrounds must be guided to express future-oriented conceptions of themselves (possible selves) and of society (Borkowski & Thorpe, 1994). The idea is that the present self imagines the future, envisioning a future self to orient current choices and behaviors. Notably, short- and long-range goals are critical building blocks for the development of possible selves, which represent goals and opportunities for making executive decisions about the future (Borkowski & Thorpe, 1994; Oyserman & James, 2009). Teachers who have a future time perspective can influence engagement and motivate students by explaining the "future importance of their present behavior" in fostering ideas of development, identity, and community (Simons et al., 2004, p. 122). While student goal setting needs to be clear and specific, future goals—and especially their anticipated benefits—also play a role in motivation (Bandura, 1986). Optimal outcomes can be increased where students understand that their "current task engagement is instrumental to attain a future goal" (Simons et al., p. 122). Intrinsic benefits (e.g., personal development) and extrinsic benefits (e.g., career satisfaction) can increase overall motivation by way of instructional interventions that change individuals' limited attitudes toward their future and time.

Teachers engage their students by taking into account each individual's capacity to think about the future and by being attuned to their discovery process. One direction for personal development involves integrating the meaning or instrumental value of activities into one's concept of self (Husman & Lens, 1999). Importantly, as Miller and Brickman (2004) attest, teachers exert sociocultural influence as role models when they help students understand what possibilities can be acted upon in their environment and when they assist with problem-solving in such areas as limited knowledge of one's context and goal setting for achieving future goals. On the other hand, teachers must be aware of students' impressions of or beliefs about negative teacher bias and/or obstacles to learning. Teachers can exert a positive influence by changing the classroom environment, modifying their instructional or interpersonal strategies, or addressing students' individual goals (Miller & Brickman, 2004).

Possible selves is a concept that places value on unrealized but better selves and habits or orientations that learners wish to possess. Habits such as persistence, flexibility, and civic centering are high-level ideas that should be integrated in the early stages of students' education (Settersten & Ray, 2010). Because a gap exists between the present self that dwells on what is and the possible self on what can be, individuals mentally strain to see the future. In a 5-year study of the motivational levels of Native Americans and White Americans, McInerney, Hinkley, Dowson, and Van Etten (1998) found that middle schoolers generally experienced difficulty in imagining the future (e.g., employability and other long-term goals). Students may need to be encouraged to connect their present and future goals by determining an instrumental route to the future (McInerney, 2004). McInerney et al. (1998) found that some of the middle schoolers, by the time they reached high school, became more receptive to imagining their futures and projecting themselves into colleges and jobs.

Peers constitute another sociocultural influence. With development, peers become important influences on self-efficacy (Schunk & Meece, 2006). Parents who steer their children toward efficacious peers provide opportunities for vicarious increases in self-efficacy. When children observe their peers succeed, they are likely to experience higher self-efficacy and motivation.

Social influence also operates through *peer networks*, or groups of friends and others with whom students associate. Students who belong to networks tend to be similar (Cairns, Cairns, & Neckerman, 1989), which enhances the likelihood of influence by modeling. Networks help define students' opportunities for interactions and observations of others' interactions, as well as their access to activities. Over time, network members tend to become even more similar, as in the case of racially and psychologically identified members. Some researchers, such as Arroyo and Zigler (1995) who studied African American and White peer groups in urban high schools, have found that the "racial identification" can "impact academic achievement and affective states" where members believe that others hold a negative perception of their group (p. 912). The African American participants reported having lessened their identification and engagement with their racial group, concerned about jeopardizing the approval of nonmembers.

Peer groups promote motivational socialization when perceived in reassuring ways. Changes in children's motivation across the school year are predicted by their peer group membership (Kindermann, McCollam, & Gibson, 1996). Children affiliated with highly motivated groups change positively, whereas those in less motivated groups change negatively. Steinberg, Brown, and Dornbusch (1996) tracked students throughout their high school years, finding that those with similar grades but affiliated with academically oriented crowds achieved more than those affiliated with less academically inclined peers. Peer group academic socialization can influence the academic self-efficacy of individual members and their groups (Schunk & Pajares, 2009).

Another influence on academic self-efficacy is perceived stress and anxiety. Stress has the potential to depress students' self-efficacy, especially among disadvantaged college populations (e.g., nontraditional, immigrant, and minority; Zajacova et al., 2005) and urban high school students (Gillock & Reyes, 1999). Although stress affects performance, self-efficacy has been shown to be the stronger influence, as demonstrated by Pajares and Kranzler (1995) who found that mathematics anxiety exerted a weaker influence than self-efficacy on high school students' mathematical performances. Zajacova et al. assessed self-efficacy and the stress of freshmen immigrant and minority college students. While they found that social stress did not seem to have a negative effect on the students' GPA and credits, stress did seem to have an effect, albeit marginal, on persistence and enrollment.

Researchers have emphasized the important role of self-efficacy in alleviating the effect of stressors on perceived stress and academic success (Pajares & Kranzler, 1995; Zajacova et al., 2005). Minority and immigrant students experience "acculturative stress," making them more susceptible to social stress than native-born and White students (Zajacova et al., 2005). For such reasons, King (2005) argued that despite the increasing diversity within their classrooms, many African American and Hispanic students feel disengaged and culturally segregated.

Educational influences. Self-efficacy has been explored in various educational domains and among individuals differing in age, developmental level, and cultural background. Researchers have established that self-efficacy influences individuals' motivation, achievement, and self-regulation (Bandura, 1997; Pajares, 1997; Schunk & Pajares, 2009; Stajkovic & Luthans, 1998). Multon, Brown, and Lent (1991) found that self-efficacy accounted for 14% of the variance in academic performance. Stajkovic and Luthans (1998) determined that self-efficacy resulted in a 28% gain in performance. Schunk (1981) obtained evidence that self-efficacy exerted a direct effect on children's achievement and persistence in mathematics. Additionally, Pajares and Kranzler (1995) found that mathematics self-efficacy had a direct effect on performance and that it mediated the influence of mental ability on performance.

Experimental research has shown that instructional and social practices that convey to students that they are making progress and becoming competent learners raise self-efficacy, motivation, and achievement (Schunk & Pajares, 2009). Some beneficial instructional and social practices are having students pursue proximal and specific goals, using social models in instruction, providing feedback indicating competence, having students self-monitor and evaluate their learning progress, and teaching students to use metacognitive strategies while learning (Coutinho, 2008; Schunk & Ertmer, 2000). Other benefits on students' self-efficacy occur from role models who provide encouragement of and high expectations for achievement, a feeling of control over and empowerment within one's environment, and rewards for doing well in school (Jonson-Reid, Davis, Saunders, Williams, & Williams, 2005; Miller & Brickman, 2004).

Research also shows that competence beliefs such as self-efficacy, as well as academic motivation, often decline as students advance through school (Eccles, Wigfield, & Schiefele, 1998; Jacobs, Lanza, Osgood, Eccles, & Wigfield, 2002). However, a few studies caution that the attitudinal and developmental patterns of young adolescents defy tidy summarization (McInerney, 2004). This widely reported decline has been attributed to such factors as increased competition, more norm-referenced grading, less teacher attention on individual student progress, and stresses associated with school transitions (Schunk & Meece, 2006). These and other school problems, including teacher bias and obstacles to learning (Miller & Brickman, 2004), can negatively affect the development of academic self-efficacy, especially among those who are poorly prepared to cope with academic challenges and first-generation college students (i.e., those whose parents are not college graduates; Majer, 2009). Rigid sequences of instruction frustrate some students, and lower-ability groupings can weaken the self-efficacy of members. Classrooms in which students are allowed to socially compare their work can have the unintended effect of lowering self-efficacy for those who judge themselves deficient.

Periods of transition in schooling also can affect self-efficacy (Schunk & Meece, 2006). Because elementary students remain with the same teacher and peers for most of the day, teachers can better provide focused attention and feedback on their individual progress. In middle school, though, children move among rooms for subjects and are exposed to new peers. Learning often is rote, evaluation becomes normative, and teacher attention to individual progress lessens (McInerney, 2004). The expanded social reference group and the shift in evaluation standards require students to reassess their academic capabilities and regulate their learning, which can lower self-efficacy for some.

Educational influences on self-efficacy also vary depending on the sociodemographics of the institution. Allen (1992) reviewed studies that investigated educational advantage and disadvantage as linked to type of institution and race. While historically Black colleges and universities (HBCUs) have fewer educational resources than many predominately White institutions, the self-efficacy and competence of African American students at HBCUs often is higher. For example, they earn higher grades and are more academically socialized, better psychologically adjusted, and more culturally aware than their counterparts at White institutions. On White college campuses, African American males may display lower academic motivation, in contrast with African American females, whereas at HBCUs, African American males exhibit less anxiety about their peer networks and role. The African American females' experience on White campuses is thought to be mixed, though, with acceleration in their assertiveness and competence due to a decrease in the need to cultivate relationships with same-race males, on the one hand, and feeling socially isolated and even ostracized, on the other. Hence, educational institutions can play a significant role in the acculturative stress and adaptation of culturally ethnic and disadvantaged students.

Self-Efficacy and Underachievement

The role of self-efficacy in student underachievement and dropout is receiving much attention (Alexander, Entwisle, & Kabbani, 2001; Hardre & Reeve, 2003; Lee & Burkam, 2003; Rumberger & Thomas, 2000). Factors contributing to underachievement and dropout are varied. These include poorly developed academic and social skills, little interest in school subjects, classrooms that stress competition and ability social comparisons, low perceived value of school learning, little sense of belonging or relatedness to the school environment, and no sense of purpose or vision of the future (Alexander et al., 2001; McInerney, 2004; Meece, Anderman, & Anderman, 2006; Wentzel, 2005). Students' involvement and participation in school depend in part on how much the environment promotes their perceptions of autonomy and relatedness, which in turn can influence self-efficacy and achievement (Hymel, Comfort, Schonert-Reichl, & McDougall, 1996). Parents, teachers, and peers affect students' feelings of autonomy and relatedness, and peer groups exert increasing influence during adolescence (Kindermann, 2007; Steinberg et al., 1996).

We have discussed how low self-efficacy can weaken motivation and lessen engagement in learning. But high self-efficacy does not automatically translate into strong motivation and deep engagement. Students who feel efficacious about learning but disconnected from the school environment or mainstream society may be unmotivated and disengaged. Families supporting youth who have low motivation to succeed and who are disengaged from school, other educational institutions, and military and service programs are particularly burdened. Families with low incomes and educational levels would benefit from new kinds of institutions that can help fulfill this necessary role of provider and motivator, as well as civic pathway to lifelong success (Gibbons & Shoffner, 2004; Settersten & Ray, 2010).

Socially, structurally, and historically, students who have been socialized through caste systems (i.e., segregated schools and neighborhoods) have had to overcome multiple challenges to nourish developing belief systems that support achievement and self-efficacy (Cuban, 2010). Disadvantaged students' academic self-efficacy and engagement are "deeply entangled in histories of segregation, desegregation, and resegregation" (Cuban, 2010, p. 204), and the negative consequences of school desegregation on Black families have been documented (Horsford, 2010). Cuban's analysis of school district reforms and leadership is associated with failed initiatives across the USA. Given the discriminatory forces at work in socially stratified hierarchical systems, lower socioeconomic status and personal cognitive deficits, then, are only part of a multifaceted problem that drives underachievement and engagement. Other researchers also have viewed the poor academic performance of students of color, particularly African Americans and Hispanics, as perpetuated by systems of inequity and other social ills that make academic efforts seem futile and penalizing (Horsford, 2010). To succeed academically and vocationally in mainstream communities, disadvantaged students have had to minimize their associations with same-race peers, unlike privileged White students (Arroyo & Zigler, 1995; Cuban, 2010).

Intervention as seen in the forms of social policies and second-chance programs have been in effect for years; however, many of these are restrictive in scope and problem-based, not developmental (Bloom, 2010). They often have not assessed students' self-efficacy. These programs should also focus on ethnic identity issues and prevention orientation at the high school level or earlier to not only be more effective but also have a lasting effect (Bloom, 2010). Engagement strategies for assisting high-risk dropout populations (e.g., immigrants, disabled, young mothers, foster care youth, and youth offenders) include identity development, paid work, internships, job training, community service, and life skills.

Some of these components appear to be evidenced in YouthBuild and Service and Conservation Corps, and other programs. The Challenge and City Year programs engage participants in residential building projects and team-based civic work. For high school and middle school students, the Advancement Via Individual Determination (AVID) program found in 45 US states and 15 countries prepares students, including first-generation populations, for 4-year colleges (Chapel Hill–Carrboro City Schools, 2009). Strategies that the AVID program uses include developing analytic thinking, improving organizational skills, providing tutoring support, and exposing students to higher education institutions, all of which have the potential of raising self-efficacy and motivation. We suspect that these programs might benefit from thorough evaluation of their effect on participants' self-efficacy. Studies of community college students indicate that success interventions are necessary for facilitating the academic self-efficacy of diverse first-generation students (Majer, 2009).

Despite the importance of such societal interventions, their degree of effectiveness has yet to be established. Some postdropout programs select the most motivated and competent individuals, making high-risk dropouts especially difficult to engage in any organized way (Bloom, 2010). While the long-term effects of such programs are unknown, consolidated efforts across communities and the USA are needed. Such programs would gain from becoming more inclusive, cohesive, and intensive enough to engage youth over a long period.

Future Research Directions

There is much evidence that self-efficacy relates to achievement outcomes including motivation and engagement. Students who hold a sense of self-efficacy for learning and performing well are apt to be engaged, competent learners.

But our discussion also raises many issues. We recommend more research, especially on contextual factors and influences, students from different cultures, and high-performing schools.

Contextual Influences on Self-Efficacy

Self-efficacy—a personal factor—can affect and be influenced by contextual factors. Enhancing students' self-efficacy, motivation, and engagement requires that we understand how contextual variables operate.

We have noted that school transitions (e.g., middle school to high school) bring about many changes in learning contexts. Research is needed that explores which contextual factors affect self-efficacy and how students combine the influences of these new contexts with their prior experiences to arrive at self-efficacy judgments. New practical knowledge can inform the design of effective learning environments at school, home, and elsewhere.

Social factors are crucial. Students who lack a sense of belonging within their school environment are at risk for underachievement and dropout. Research on factors that affect students' sense of belonging will suggest ways to improve their self-efficacy and engagement in learning. For example, one self-efficacy-enhancing strategy involves activating possible selves by envisioning one's future and understanding the links between present and later goals (Borkowski & Thorpe, 1994; Jonson-Reid et al., 2005). Thus, high school students who want to become medical doctors might picture themselves using science and mathematics in their work as doctors, which underscores the importance of their studying in their current courses. We encourage probing of academic self-efficacy among African American students and other non-White student populations. Research can investigate their self-conceptions and possible selves, perceived influences on their self-images and learning, and experiences of academic identification and disassociation (Kerpelman, Eryigit, & Stephens, 2008).

Political factors are yet another important contextual variable. For example, school districts have been urged to systematically analyze the effects of policies aimed at increasing student achievement (Cuban, 2010). Studies of changes in test scores by both racial and socioeconomic status need to follow from district-level policy implementation, with a focus on students' self-efficacy resulting from standardized testing. As another example, districts will need to anticipate the effect on student self-efficacy of new assignment plans that enforce attendance zones closer to students' homes. Critics argue that such initiatives undermine achievement by resegregating schools and confining ethnic students to their own neighborhoods (Cuban, 2010).

Cross-Cultural Research

More needs to be known about students from different cultures and countries. Most self-efficacy studies have focused on students from the USA without sufficient attention on issues of diversity, especially as related to learning and engagement. Cross-cultural studies will expand understanding of the operation and generality of self-efficacy. Klassen's (2004b) review of 20 cross-cultural studies found that although self-efficacy was lower for non-Western students (e.g., Asian and Asian-immigrant students) than for Western students (e.g., Western Europe, Canada, USA), the more modest self-efficacy expressed by non-Western students predicted academic outcomes better than the higher self-efficacy of Western students. Klassen posited that immigration status and political factors can modify the mean self-efficacy of a cultural group.

Research that focuses on culturally ethnic students' experiences at different types of institutions is also needed, especially when unemployment and underemployment are on the increase (Allen, 1992). Hand in hand with this focus is that of social policies and programs that can address in a more specific way not only the lower achievement and higher attrition for African American college students but also what types of interventions and resources foster ethnic students' self-efficacy and success (Allen, 1992). As Jonson-Reid et al. (2005) attest, given that research on self-efficacy has mostly focused on White students at predominately White institutions, we need a better understanding of African American youths' sense of self-efficacy, in addition to strategies that foster a belief in the value of education.

Cultural dimensions such as individualism and collectivism may influence the relation of self-efficacy to academic outcomes (Oettingen & Zosuls, 2006). Kim and Park (2006) argued that theories that emphasize individualistic values—such as self-efficacy—cannot explain the high achievement of East Asian students. Instead, the Confucian-based socialization practices that promote close parent–child relationships seem responsible for high levels of self-regulatory, relational, and social efficacy. In these cultures, relational efficacy (i.e., perceived competence in family and social relations), as well as social support from parents, may influence students' academic performances. Self-efficacy may be more other-oriented in some non-Western (particularly Asian) cultures than in Western cultures (Klassen, 2004a). In short, cross-cultural research has implications for educational practices, especially given the influx of immigrants in US schools.

Self-Efficacy in High-Performing Schools

High-performing schools create a positive environment for learning and support teachers and students so that learning can occur. The literature on high-performing schools focuses on their effects on student achievement and teacher satisfaction (Muncey & McQuillan, 1993; Sizer, 1992). We recommend that self-efficacy researchers devote attention to the features of high-performing schools that contribute to students' and teachers' self-efficacy.

Some characteristics of high-performing schools that should have positive effects on self-efficacy are parental involvement, supportive learning environments, and smooth transitions between grades and levels (Maehr & Midgley, 1996; Muncey & McQuillan, 1993; Sizer, 1992). Research directions include examining the influence of these and other factors to determine how they create and build self-efficacy for learners.

Another area deserving attention is the self-efficacy of low-income students who have transitioned to better schools and are being socialized in new surroundings within school districts that favor economic integration. Kahlenberg (2004) contended that lower-income students who attend middle-class and high-performing schools can feel out of place because their peers have clearer goals for their learning and are better prepared and more academically engaged. The culture of the school is unfamiliar to the lower-income population in other respects as well, in that parents are likely more active in the school's programs, and teachers generally are better qualified. Ways to raise the self-efficacy of low-income students in such environments could benefit from research that is attuned to this practical focus.

Conclusion

Social cognitive theory stresses learning from the social environment. The conceptual focus of Bandura's theory postulates reciprocal interactions among personal, behavioral, and social/environmental factors. Self-efficacy is a critical personal factor that can affect motivation, engagement, learning, and achievement. Self-efficacy is shaped by personal, cultural, and social factors, making learning and achievement complex sociocultural phenomena.

Attention to ways of building students' skills and self-efficacy will help more learners become academically motivated and engaged in learning. These outcomes should help to diminish the pervasive problem of student underachievement and dropout. Important questions remain to be addressed by researchers and school leaders, which will refine theory, expand practical knowledge, and help prepare better-educated citizens. Finally, we urge legislators to advocate more strongly for interventions that promote student success, with the goals of alleviating the nation's dropout problem and increasing educational opportunities for all youth.

References

Alexander, K., Entwisle, D., & Kabbani, N. (2001). The dropout process in life course perspective: Early risk factors at home and school. *Teachers College Record, 103*, 760–822.

Allen, W. R. (1992). The color of success: African-American college student outcomes at predominately White and historically Black public colleges and universities. *Harvard Educational Review, 62*(1), 26–44.

Anderman, E. M., & Wolters, C. A. (2006). Goals, values, and affects: Influences on student motivation. In P. A. Alexander & P. H. Winne (Eds.), *Handbook of educational psychology* (2nd ed., pp. 369–389). Mahwah, NJ: Erlbaum.

Arroyo, C. G., & Zigler, E. (1995). Racial identity, academic achievement, and the psychological well-being of economically disadvantaged adolescents. *Journal of Personality and Social Psychology, 69*(5), 903–914.

Bandura, A. (1977a). Self-efficacy: Toward a unifying theory of behavioral change. *Psychological Review, 84*, 191–215.

Bandura, A. (1977b). *Social learning theory*. Englewood Cliffs, NJ: Prentice Hall.

Bandura, A. (1986). *Social foundations of thought and action: A social cognitive theory*. Englewood Cliffs, NJ: Prentice Hall.

Bandura, A. (1997). *Self-efficacy: The exercise of control*. New York: Freeman.

Bandura, A. (2001). Social cognitive theory: An agentic perspective. *Annual Review of Psychology, 52*, 1–26.

Bandura, A., & Schunk, D. H. (1981). Cultivating competence, self-efficacy, and intrinsic interest through proximal self-motivation. *Journal of Personality and Social Psychology, 41*, 586–598.

Bloom, D. (2010). Programs and policies to assist high school dropouts in the transition to adulthood. *The Future of Children, 20*(1), 89–108.

Bloom, D., & Haskins, R. (2010). Helping high school dropouts improve their prospects [policy brief]. *The Future of Children, 20*(1), 1–8. Retrieved April 19, 2010, from www.futureofchildren.org

Borkowski, J. G., & Thorpe, P. K. (1994). Self-regulation and motivation: A life-span perspective on underachievement. In D. H. Schunk & B. J. Zimmerman (Eds.), *Self regulation of learning and performance: Issues and educational applications* (pp. 45–73). Hillsdale, NJ: Erlbaum.

Bradley, R. H., & Corwyn, R. F. (2002). Socioeconomic status and child development. *Annual Review of Psychology, 53*, 371–399.

Cairns, R. B., Cairns, B. D., & Neckerman, J. J. (1989). Early school dropout: Configurations and determinants. *Child Development, 60*, 1437–1452.

Chapel Hill–Carrboro City Schools. (2009, July 10). *AVID: Decade of college dreams*. Retrieved April 20, 2010, from http://www2.chccs.k12.nc.us/education/components/scrapbook/default.php?sectiondetailid=73208&

Coutinho, S. (2008). Self-efficacy, metacognition, and performance. *North American Journal of Psychology, 10*(1), 165–172.

Cuban, L. (2010). *As good as it gets: What school reform brought to Austin*. Cambridge, MA: Harvard University Press.

Eccles, J. S., Wigfield, A., & Schiefele, U. (1998). Motivation to succeed. In W. Damon (Series Ed.) & N. Eisenberg (Vol. Ed.), *Handbook of child psychology: Vol. 3. Social, emotional, and personality development* (5th ed., pp. 1017–1095). New York: Wiley.

Gibbons, M. M., & Shoffner, M. F. (2004). Prospective first-generation college students: Meeting their needs through social cognitive career theory. *Professional School Counseling, 8*(1), 91–97.

Gillock, K. L., & Reyes, O. (1999). Stress, support, and academic performance of urban, low-income, Mexican–American adolescents. *Journal of Youth and Adolescence, 28*(2), 259–282.

Hardre, P., & Reeve, J. (2003). A motivational model of rural students' intentions to persist in, versus drop out of, high school. *Journal of Educational Psychology, 95*, 347–356.

Horsford, S. D. (2010). Black superintendents on educating Black students in separate and unequal contexts. *Urban Review, 42*(1), 58–79.

Husman, J., & Lens, W. (1999). The role of the future in student motivation. *Educational Psychologist, 34*(2), 113–125.

Hymel, S., Comfort, C., Schonert-Reichl, K., & McDougall, P. (1996). Academic failure and school dropout: The influence of peers. In J. Juvonen & K. R. Wentzel (Eds.), *Social motivation: Understanding children's school adjustment* (pp. 313–345). Cambridge, England: Cambridge University Press.

Jacobs, J. E., Lanza, S., Osgood, D. W., Eccles, J. S., & Wigfield, A. (2002). Changes in children's self-competence and values: Gender and domain differences across grades one to twelve. *Child Development, 73*, 509–527.

Jonson-Reid, M., Davis, L., Saunders, J., Williams, T., & Williams, J. H. (2005). Academic self-efficacy among African American youths: Implications for school social work practice. *Children and Schools, 27*(1), 5–14.

Kahlenberg, R. D. (2004). *America's untapped resource: Low-income students in higher education*. Washington, DC: Century Foundation Press.

Kerpelman, J. L., Eryigit, S., & Stephens, C. J. (2008). African American adolescents' future education orientation: Associations with self-efficacy, ethnic identity, and perceived parental support. *Journal of Youth and Adolescence, 37*, 997–1008.

Kim, U., & Park, Y. S. (2006). Factors influencing academic achievement in collectivist societies: The role of self-, relational, and social efficacy. In F. Pajares & T. Urdan (Eds.), *Self-efficacy beliefs of adolescents* (pp. 267–286). Greenwich, CT: Information Age Publishing.

Kindermann, T. A. (2007). Effects of naturally existing peer groups on changes in academic engagement in a cohort of sixth graders. *Child Development, 78*, 1186–1203.

Kindermann, T. A., McCollam, T. L., & Gibson, E., Jr. (1996). Peer networks and students' classroom engagement during childhood and adolescence. In J. Juvonen & K. R. Wentzel (Eds.), *Social motivation: Understanding children's school adjustment* (pp. 279–312). Cambridge, England: Cambridge University Press.

King, J. E. (2005). *Black education: A transformative research and action agenda for the new century*. New York: Routledge.

Klassen, R. M. (2004a). A cross-cultural investigation of the efficacy beliefs of south Asian immigrant and Anglo Canadian nonimmigrant early adolescents. *Journal of Educational Psychology, 96*, 731–742.

Klassen, R. M. (2004b). Optimism and realism: A review of self-efficacy from a cross-cultural perspective. *International Journal of Psychology, 39*, 205–230.

Lee, V. E., & Burkam, D. T. (2003). Dropping out of high school: The role of school organization and structure. *American Educational Research Journal, 40*, 353–393.

Licht, B. G., & Kistner, J. A. (1986). Motivational problems of learning-disabled children: Individual differences and their implications for treatment. In J. K. Torgesen & B. W. L. Wong (Eds.), *Psychological and educational perspectives on learning disabilities* (pp. 225–255). Orlando, FL: Academic.

Locke, E. A., & Latham, G. P. (2002). Building a practically useful theory of goal setting and task motivation: A 35-year odyssey. *American Psychologist, 57*, 705–717.

Maehr, M. L., & Midgley, C. (1996). *Transforming school cultures*. Boulder, CO: Westview Press.

Majer, J. M. (2009). Self-efficacy and academic success among ethnically diverse first-generation community college students. *Journal of Diversity in Higher Education, 2*(4), 243–250.

McInerney, D. M. (2004). A discussion of future time perspective. *Educational Psychology Review, 16*(2), 141–151.

McInerney, D. M., Hinkley, J., Dowson, M., & Van Etten, S. (1998). Aboriginal, Anglo, and immigrant Australian students' motivational beliefs about personal academic success: Are there cultural differences? *Journal of Educational Psychology, 90*, 621–629.

Meece, J. L., Anderman, E. M., & Anderman, L. H. (2006). Classroom goal structure, student motivation, and academic achievement. *Annual Review of Psychology, 57*, 487–503.

Miller, R. B., & Brickman, S. J. (2004). A model of future-oriented motivation and self-regulation. *Educational Psychology Review, 16*(1), 9–33.

Mullen, C. A., & Schunk, D. H. (2011). The role of professional learning community in dropout prevention. *AASA Journal of Scholarship and Practice, 8*, 26–29.

Multon, K. D., Brown, S. D., & Lent, R. W. (1991). Relation of self-efficacy beliefs to academic outcomes: A meta-analytic investigation. *Journal of Counseling Psychology, 38*, 30–38.

Muncey, D., & McQuillan, P. (1993). Preliminary findings from a five-year study of the Coalition of Essential Schools. *Phi Delta Kappan, 74*, 486–489.

Oettingen, G., & Zosuls, C. (2006). Self-efficacy of adolescents across culture. In F. Pajares & T. Urdan (Eds.), *Self-efficacy beliefs of adolescents* (pp. 245–266). Greenwich, CT: Information Age Publishing.

Oyserman, D., & James, L. (2009). Possible selves: From content to process. In K. D. Markman, W. M. P. Klein, & J. A. Suhr (Eds.), *Handbook of imagination and mental simulation* (pp. 373–394). New York: Psychology Press.

Pajares, F. (1996). Self-efficacy beliefs in achievement settings. *Review of Educational Research, 66*, 543–578.

Pajares, F. (1997). Current directions in self-efficacy research. In M. Maehr & P. R. Pintrich (Eds.), *Advances in motivation and achievement* (Vol. 10, pp. 1–49). Greenwich, CT: JAI Press.

Pajares, F., & Kranzler, J. (1995). Self-efficacy beliefs and general mental ability in mathematical problem-solving. *Contemporary Educational Psychology, 20*(4), 426–443.

Perry, J. C., DeWine, D. B., Duffy, R. D., & Vance, K. S. (2007). The academic self-efficacy of urban youth: A mixed-methods study of a school-to-work program. *Journal of Career Development, 34*, 103–126.

Pintrich, P. R. (2003). A motivational science perspective on the role of student motivation in learning and teaching contexts. *Journal of Educational Psychology, 95*, 667–686.

PR Newswire. (2009). *Panel discussion on crisis of high school dropouts and cost to our economy*. Retrieved April 18, 2010, from http://www.forbes.com/feeds/prnewswire/2010/02/24/prnewswire201002241350PR_NEWS_USPR____DC60266.html

Rumberger, R. W., & Thomas, S. L. (2000). The distribution of dropout and turnover rates among urban and suburban high schools. *Sociology of Education, 73*(1), 39–67.

Schunk, D. H. (1981). Modeling and attributional effects on children's achievement: A self-efficacy analysis. *Journal of Educational Psychology, 73*, 93–105.

Schunk, D. H. (1995). Self-efficacy and education and instruction. In J. E. Maddux (Ed.), *Self-efficacy, adaptation, and adjustment: Theory, research, and application* (pp. 281–303). New York: Plenum Press.

Schunk, D. H. (1996). Goal and self-evaluative influences during children's cognitive skill learning. *American Educational Research Journal, 33*, 359–382.

Schunk, D. H., & Ertmer, P. A. (1999). Self-regulatory processes during computer skill acquisition: Goal and self-evaluative influences. *Journal of Educational Psychology, 91*, 251–260.

Schunk, D. H., & Ertmer, P. A. (2000). Self-regulation and academic learning: Self-efficacy enhancing interventions. In M. Boekaerts, P. R. Pintrich, & M. Zeidner (Eds.), *Handbook of self-regulation* (pp. 631–649). San Diego, CA: Academic.

Schunk, D. H., & Meece, J. L. (2006). Self-efficacy development in adolescence. In F. Pajares & T. Urdan (Eds.), *Self-efficacy beliefs of adolescents* (pp. 71–96). Greenwich, CT: Information Age Publishing.

Schunk, D. H., & Pajares, F. (2005). Competence perceptions and academic functioning. In A. J. Elliot & C. S. Dweck (Eds.), *Handbook of competence and motivation* (pp. 85–104). New York: Guilford Press.

Schunk, D. H., & Pajares, F. (2009). Self-efficacy theory. In K. R. Wentzel & A. Wigfield (Eds.), *Handbook of motivation at school* (pp. 35–53). New York: Routledge.

Schunk, D. H., Pintrich, P. R., & Meece, J. L. (2008). *Motivation in education: Theory, research, and applications* (3rd ed.). Upper Saddle River, NJ: Pearson Education.

Settersten, R. A., Jr., & Ray, B. (2010). What's going on with young people today? The long and twisting path to adulthood. *The Future of Children, 20*(1), 19–41.

Shell, D. F., & Husman, J. (2001). The multivariate dimensionality of personal control and future time perspective beliefs in achievement and self-regulation. *Contemporary Educational Psychology, 26,* 481–506.

Simons, J., Vansteenkiste, M., Lens, W., & Lacante, M. (2004). Placing motivation and future time perspective theory in a temporal perspective. *Educational Psychology Review, 16*(2), 121–139.

Sizer, T. (1992). *Horace's compromise: Redesigning the American high school.* Boston: Houghton Mifflin.

Skinner, E. A., Kindermann, T. A., Connell, J. P., & Wellborn, J. G. (2009). Engagement and disaffection as organizational constructs in the dynamics of motivational development. In K. R. Wentzel & A. Wigfield (Eds.), *Handbook of motivation at school* (pp. 223–245). New York: Routledge.

Smedley, B. D., Myers, H. F., & Harrell, S. P. (1993). Minority-status stresses and the college adjustment of ethnic minority freshmen. *Journal of Higher Education, 64*(4), 434–452.

Stajkovic, A. D., & Luthans, F. (1998). Self-efficacy and work-related performances: A meta-analysis. *Psychological Bulletin, 124,* 240–261.

Steinberg, L., Brown, B. B., & Dornbusch, S. M. (1996). *Beyond the classroom: Why school reform has failed and what parents need to do.* New York: Simon & Schuster.

U.S. Department of Education. (2008). *Dropout prevention* (pp. 1–66). [Institute of Education Sciences]. Retrieved March 14, 2010, from http://ies.ed.gov/ncee/wwc/pdf/practiceguides/dp_pg_090308.pdf

Usher, E. L., & Pajares, F. (2008). Sources of self-efficacy in school: Critical review of the literature and future directions. *Review of Educational Research, 78,* 751–796.

Vick, R. M., & Packard, B. W.-L. (2008). Academic success strategy use among community-active urban Hispanic adolescents. *Hispanic Journal of Behavioral Sciences, 30*(4), 463–480.

Wentzel, K. R. (2005). Peer relationships, motivation, and academic performance at school. In A. J. Elliot & C. S. Dweck (Eds.), *Handbook of competence and motivation* (pp. 279–296). New York: Guilford Press.

Wigfield, A., Tonks, S., & Eccles, J. S. (2004). Expectancy value theory in cross-cultural perspective. In D. M. McInerney & S. Van Etten (Eds.), *Big theories revisited* (pp. 165–198). Greenwich, CT: Information Age Publishing.

Yosso, T. J. (2005). Whose culture has capital? A critical race theory discussion of community cultural wealth. *Race, Ethnicity, and Education, 8*(1), 69–91.

Zajacova, A., Lynch, S. M., & Espenshade, T. J. (2005). Self-efficacy, stress, and academic success in college. *Research in Higher Education, 46*(6), 677–706.

Zimmerman, B. J. (2000). Attaining self-regulation: A social cognitive perspective. In M. Boekaerts, P. R. Pintrich, & M. Zeidner (Eds.), *Handbook of self-regulation* (pp. 13–39). San Diego, CA: Academic.

Zimmerman, B. J., & Cleary, T. J. (2009). Motives to self-regulate learning: A social cognitive account. In K. R. Wentzel & A. Wigfield (Eds.), *Handbook of motivation at school* (pp. 247–264). New York: Routledge.

A Cyclical Self-Regulatory Account of Student Engagement: Theoretical Foundations and Applications

Timothy J. Cleary and Barry J. Zimmerman

Abstract

Educators have long been interested in understanding the variables or factors underlying student motivation and desire to engage in and regulate their academic behaviors. In this chapter, we delineate a social-cognitive theoretical framework of self-regulatory engagement that integrates a set of highly related yet distinctive constructs such as motivation, engagement, and metacognition. Central to our self-regulation framework is a cyclical feedback loop, a process that operates in a temporal sequence (before, during, and after a learning activity) and is largely cognitive in nature. We also draw a distinction between the "will" of students to engage in learning and the "skill" with which they regulate or self-manage their level of engagement. The historical evolution and the conceptual and empirical advantages of cyclical feedback loops will be emphasized along with a description of various academic intervention programs designed to teach "cyclical" thinking and strategic behaviors to academically at-risk students. Finally, an innovative alternative assessment approach, called self-regulated learning microanalysis, is presented to illustrate how researchers and practitioners can reliably and accurately capture students' regulatory engagement in particular contexts and settings.

Introduction

Educators have long been interested in understanding the factors underlying student motivation or desire to engage and regulate their academic behaviors and functioning. In fact, recent survey research shows that school psychologists and regular and special education teachers report student motivation, self-regulatory skills, and self-determination to be critical professional development areas of interest (Agran, Snow, & Swaner, 1999; Cleary, 2009; Cleary & Zimmerman, 2006; Coalition for Psychology in Schools and Education, 2006). This line of research further indicates that these areas are important to school-based professionals because of the relatively high frequency with which they encounter youth exhibiting these deficits as well as their lack of formal training and clinical skills to work effectively with disengaged or poorly regulated youth (Cleary, 2009; Cleary, Gubi, & Prescott, 2010a; Wehmeyer, Agran, & Hughes, 2000). Although different lines of research separately target constructs such as self-regulation, engagement, and motivation, it is important to note that these types of constructs are highly related and complementary. As a result, presenting a theoretical framework integrating all of these terms can be quite valuable and informative to both researchers and practitioners. Accordingly, a primary goal of this manuscript is to delineate a theoretical framework that integrates motivation, engagement, and self-regulation to describe the process through which students initiate and sustain a high level of investment in school-based learning activities.

Historically, engaged students have been defined as those who "concentrate on their work, are enthusiastic about it, and are deeply interested in academic content" (Pressley & McCormick, 1995, p. 328). More recently, researchers have conceptualized engagement as a multidimensional concept that extends across various behavioral, academic, cognitive, and emotional or psychological domains (Christenson et al., 2008; Fredricks, Blumenfeld, & Paris, 2004). Christenson and colleagues have argued that these broadly defined engagement categories can be further understood as either an observable indicator, such as academic (e.g., task completion, work productivity) and behavioral engagement (e.g., class participation), or as an internal process, such as students' self-reflection and evaluation of the effectiveness of a learning strategy (i.e., cognitive engagement) or their perceptions of connectedness and belongingness to school (i.e., affective or emotional engagement). Christenson's engagement model also posits that these observable and covert forms of engagement are best understood within the social context or milieu in which they occur. Thus, the extent to which students engage in learning activities may vary depending on the classroom environments or school contexts in which they learn – a key similarity with many self-regulation models (Boekaerts, Pintrich, & Zeidner, 2000).

Although engagement is a broad multidimensional construct, we will devote particular attention to cognitive engagement, that is, the process through which students become cognitively and strategically invested in learning. As with most definitions of engagement reported in the literature, cognitive engagement is a loosely defined construct encapsulating students' use of cognitive strategies and regulatory processes and or the extent to which their perceptions of interest and value stimulate their attention and immersion into the learning process (Bandura, 1986; Corno & Mandinach, 1983; Eccles & Wigfield, 2002; Pintrich & de Groot, 1990). Although these general depictions of cognitive engagement provide clear examples of what a cognitively engaged student might look like, they do not comprehensively describe the dynamic process through which students initially become engaged in learning and sustain this level of investment over time. From our perspective, self-regulation theories can address this conceptual gap because such models delineate a clearly defined "process" account of student learning, emphasizing the role of cognitive and metacognitive subprocesses as well as the related motivation beliefs impacting these processes (Zimmerman & Cleary, 2006; Zimmerman & Labuhn, 2011).

Self-Regulation, Cognitive Engagement, and Motivation

Self-regulation researchers have long been interested in studying the mechanisms through which individuals engage in strategic thinking or the manner in which they cognitively manage their learning (Bandura, 1986; Boekaerts et al., 2000; Carver & Scheier, 2000; Winne & Perry, 2000). The self-regulation literature is replete with theoretical frameworks explaining cognitive engagement, although most models differ in terms of essential processes, sources of motivation, and impact of social environment (Mace, Belfiore, & Hutchinson, 2001; Puustinen & Pulkkinen, 2001; Weinstein, Husman, & Dierking, 2000; Winne & Hadwin, 1998; Zimmerman & Schunk, 2001). For example, operant theories typically emphasize reinforcement as a key motivational influence on regulatory behaviors, whereas phenomenological perspectives highlight self-actualization as the major driving force (Mace et al., 2001; McCombs, 2001). Furthermore, information processing theorists pay particular attention to how individuals process, store, and transfer information through the use of cognitive strategies and tactics (Winne & Hadwin), whereas social-cognitive theoretical models tend to highlight individuals' self-motivational beliefs, such as self-efficacy, task interest and value, and goal orientation, as well as the types of self-evaluations, attributions, and self-reactions students make following learning (Bandura, 1997; Pintrich, 2000; Schunk, 2001).

Despite these differences, several researchers have noted the conceptual overlap among these models. In fact, Puustinen and Pulkkinen (2001) noted, "In sum, the differences in the definitions become blurred and when one examines the models in more detail, suggesting that it is the relative weight given to the component parts, more than the components themselves, that varies from one model to another" (p. 280). Of particular importance to our attempt to link the constructs of cognitive engagement and self-regulated learning (SRL) is that most theorists describe self-regulation in terms of a cyclical feedback loop that is largely cognitive in nature (Schmitz & Wiese, 2006; Schunk, 2001; Winne, 2001; Zimmerman, 2000). These loops tend to function in a temporal sequence (i.e., before, during, and after dimensions) as students engage in specific academic tasks. For example, to understand the SRL engagement of a student attempting to solve algebraic expression problems, researchers would seek to examine the extent to which this student plans or approaches these types of problems (before), directs attention to use and monitor specific strategies while solving math problems (during), and uses internal or external feedback to reflect on the effectiveness of their strategies (after). Although the phases of this sequential feedback loop have been labeled in different ways, such as preaction, action, and postaction (Schmitz & Wiese, 2006) or forethought, performance control, and self-reflection (Zimmerman, 2000), they all delineate a strategic process of thinking that guides planning, performance, and evaluation to optimize academic success.

In this manuscript, we seek to accomplish several objectives. First, we highlight the primary features of a social-cognitive account of SRL engagement, emphasizing a cyclical feedback loop as the key foundational component. Although self-regulation clearly involves the integration of cognition, affect, behavior, and environmental factors, our model of engagement will be discussed primarily relative to the cognitive and metacognitive dimensions. Accordingly, we use the terms SRL engagement and cognitive engagement interchangeably throughout the manuscript.

Our second objective involves highlighting the connection between student motivation and self-regulation. In our model, we include motivation and self-regulation as a set of interrelated processes operating within a single framework. Social cognitive researchers have described motivation as a process in which goal-directed behavior is initiated and sustained (Schunk, Pintrich, & Meece, 2008). Motivation has often been operationally defined in behavioral terms, such as effort, persistence, and choice of activities (Multon, Brown, & Lent, 1991; Schunk, 1981; Zimmerman, 1995). In our account, these motivated behaviors are distinguished from the motivation beliefs, such as self-efficacy, task interest, and goal orientation, which influence such behaviors. Thus, students' beliefs of personal capabilities and their interest in learning do not only influence one's behavioral engagement or investment in learning but also the extent to which one engages cognitively in the cyclical feedback loop of self-regulation (Zimmerman & Cleary, 2006). In essence, our model of self-regulated learning engagement distinguishes between the "will" of student to engage in learning (as highlighted by self-motivation beliefs) and the "skill" with which one regulates or self-manages his or her level of engagement (as described by the cyclical loop).

Third, we provide some illustrative examples of school-based academic interventions that directly teach students this strategic cycle of thought and action as they perform different academic activities, such as writing, performing math, or studying. Fourth, we detail an alternative assessment methodology called SRL microanalysis, specifically designed to capture the dynamic, context-specific dimension of cognitive engagement. Finally, we highlight key areas of future research.

Overview of a Social-Cognitive Perspective of Engagement

Our model of cognitive engagement is grounded in a social-cognitive perspective of self-regulated functioning. In general, social-cognitive theory places primary importance on reciprocal determinism; that is, human functioning involves reciprocal interactions among environment, person (beliefs, affect), and behavior. Bandura argued, however, that cognition, and in particular an individual's beliefs of personal agency or efficacy, is the primary factor underlying the proactive and self-directed nature of human behavior (Bandura, 1986, 2001). Bandura also emphasized that humans will use various types of cognitive processes to regulate their behaviors and performance, such as self-observation, self-judgments, and self-reactions. Thus, from this perspective, in order to understand the nature or causal impetus underlying students' investment in learning, one needs to consider these cognitive variables.

Consistent with recent models of engagement, social-cognitive theorists emphasize situation dependence or context specificity (Bandura, 1997; Christenson et al., 2008; Urdan & Midgley, 2003). Thus, the extent to which students become cognitively or strategically immersed in learning activities will vary across academic settings and situational demands. This premise has been established empirically (Cleary & Chen, 2009; Hadwin, Winne, Stockley, Nesbit, & Woszczyna, 2001; Urdan & Midgley, 2003; Winne & Jaimeson-Noel, 2002). For example, Hadwin et al. (2001) found that the types of strategies that students employ during learning varied across three types of academic tasks – reading for learning, completing a brief essay, and studying for an exam. Furthermore, Cleary and Chen found that the relationship between student motivation and self-regulation with math achievement was stronger in more demanding and academically challenging learning contexts than in less demanding settings (e.g., honors versus regular math courses).

Of particular relevance to our model of engagement is that social-cognitive models emphasize the importance of cyclical feedback loops. As will be discussed in the following section, cyclical feedback loops are particularly useful because they underscore the essential processes that prompt individuals to initiate and sustain cognitive engagement during learning (Cleary, Zimmerman, & Keating, 2006; Schunk, 2001). We now turn to presenting a formal definition of SRL engagement as well as the historical evolution of the cyclical model serving as the centerpiece of this definition.

SRL Engagement as a Cyclical Feedback Loop

Social-cognitive researchers have defined self-regulation as self-generated thoughts, feelings, and behaviors that are strategically oriented or directed toward the attainment of personal goals (Schunk, 2001). Although some researchers equate cognitive engagement to characteristics of self-regulation, it is important to note that self-regulation is more than a cognitive construct. It also involves the intentional enactment of overt behaviors, such as using strategies during learning or self-recording the number of incorrectly solved homework problems, and the management of environmental or internal constraints during learning. As previously discussed, the source of these behaviors involves students' self-efficacy beliefs, their level of interest in a task or the inherent value of that task, or their beliefs regarding why they are engaging in learning. For the purposes of this manuscript, however, our definition of SRL engagement focuses heavily on the notion of being cognitively and strategically engaged in learning. In short, SRL engagement is defined as the extent to which individuals think strategically before, during, and after performance on some learning activity. From our perspective, SRL engagement is not an all or nothing phenomenon but rather exists along a continuum across and within each of the three phases. Given the importance of the feedback loop to our definition of cognitive engagement, we will provide a brief overview of the historical evolution of this loop as well as a rationale detailing why adherence to such a framework is informative and valuable.

Historical Aspects of the Cyclical Feedback Loop

Historically, models of self-regulation have included some type of feedback loop to explain the process by which individuals manage their learning (Carver & Scheier, 2000; Miller, Galanter, & Pribham, 1960; Powers, 1973). Theorists espoused the importance of negative feedback loops, whereby an individual seeks to reduce a discrepancy between a goal state and current level of performance. According to this formulation, a person's initial performance level is first tested against a standard. If the feedback is "negative," indicating that a discrepancy still exists, then an individual will be motivated to decrease this aversive state by recursively self-correcting or adapting one's efforts to learn until that discrepancy is sufficiently diminished. Once a student reaches his or her standard, his or her engagement in the activity will cease until a new discrepancy between a target and goal is identified, typically in an entirely different domain or for a different task (Carver & Scheier, 2000).

The distinction between closed and open feedback loops is not a trivial one. Closed loops are based on the negative feedback principle illustrated previously. Thus, it is assumed that individuals simply attempt to reduce performance discrepancies against a fixed standard and will disengage after the goal is attained. Although some current models of self-regulation, such as information processing, emphasize negative or "closed" feedback loops, social-cognitive accounts embrace open feedback models, recognizing that individuals will often seek to expand their knowledge or skills and to redefine one's standards of success.

In the 1980s, Bandura postulated an open cyclical feedback loop based on three recursive social-cognitive processes: self-observation, self-judgment, and self-reactions. Self-observation is a regulatory process that typically occurs during performance or learning and involves attending to and tracking specific aspects of performance, such as quantity, accuracy, or quality, as well as the personal and environmental conditions surrounding that performance (Bandura, 1986; Zimmerman & Paulsen, 1995). Bandura cautioned that information generated via self-observation will do little to impact behavioral or strategic change unless one first effectively judges or evaluates one's performance. Self-judgment involves the conclusions one draws about performance outcomes, regarding success or failure as well as the reasons for these performance attainments. The quality of one's self-reactions is critically important in our model of SRL engagement because they impact the extent to which students will seek to initiate new cycles of regulated learning.

Current Conceptualization of the Cyclical Feedback Loop

Zimmerman (2000) expanded Bandura's model to a more comprehensive and descriptive three-phase cyclical loop (see Fig. 11.1). From this perspective, engagement in regulatory or strategic learning consists of three sequential phases: forethought (i.e., processes that precede efforts to

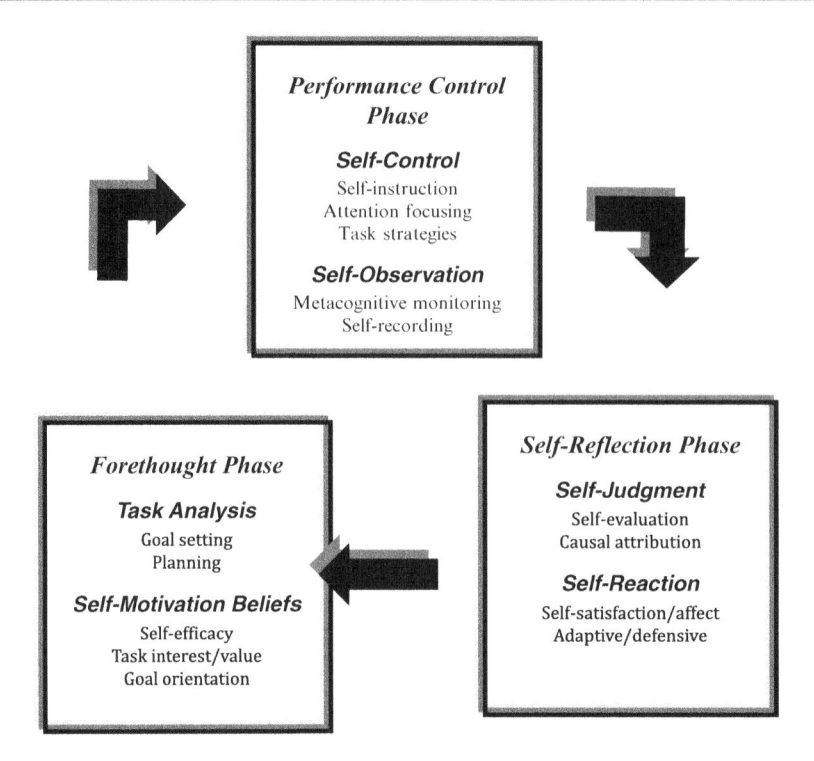

Fig. 11.1 Phases and processes of self-regulation (From Zimmerman & Campillo (2003), p. 239. Reprinted with permission)

```
                    ┌─────────────────────────────┐
                    │   Performance Control       │
                    │         Phase               │
                    │                             │
                    │      Self-Control           │
                    │     Self-instruction        │
                    │    Attention focusing       │
                    │      Task strategies        │
                    │                             │
                    │    Self-Observation         │
                    │  Metacognitive monitoring   │
                    │       Self-recording        │
                    └─────────────────────────────┘

  ┌─────────────────────────────┐     ┌─────────────────────────────┐
  │     Forethought Phase       │     │    Self-Reflection Phase    │
  │                             │     │                             │
  │      Task Analysis          │     │       Self-Judgment         │
  │       Goal setting          │     │       Self-evaluation       │
  │         Planning            │     │      Causal attribution     │
  │                             │     │                             │
  │   Self-Motivation Beliefs   │     │       Self-Reaction         │
  │       Self-efficacy         │     │   Self-satisfaction/affect  │
  │     Task interest/value     │     │      Adaptive/defensive     │
  │      Goal orientation       │     │                             │
  └─────────────────────────────┘     └─────────────────────────────┘
```

learn or perform), performance control (i.e., processes occurring during learning efforts), and self-reflection (i.e., processes occurring after learning or performance) (Zimmerman, 2000). These phases are hypothesized to be interdependent so that changes in forethought processes impact performance control, which, in turn, influence self-reflection phase processes. Relative to our definition of SRL engagement, we are primarily concerned with the extent to which individuals become cognitively engaged in learning, with particular emphasis placed on students' selection, use, and reflection on the effectiveness of learning strategies.

In terms of forethought, highly SRL-engaged students seek to identify the essential requirements of a learning task (task analysis), set outcome, and or process goals (goal setting), and develop learning plans (strategic planning) to achieve one's goals. Students who proactively engage in strategic goal setting and planning prior to learning are more likely to be aware of the subtleties of a learning activity as well as the outcomes they hope to accomplish and methods used to attain these goals (Locke & Latham, 1990; Zimmerman, 2000). It is also important to note that self-motivation beliefs are also considered forethought phase processes and are important because they impact the extent to which students engage in self-control and self-observation processes during learning (Zimmerman & Cleary, 2009).

During learning or performance of an academic task, such as studying for a test or solving math problems, a SRL-engaged learner will utilize various *self-control* phase processes, such as self-instruction, attention-focusing, and task strategies, to optimize their focus on the task and their effort and persistence (Wolters, 2003; Zimmerman, 2000). Thus, a student who proactively develops a strategic plan (e.g., use of cognitive maps, environmental structuring strategies, and time management tactics), prior to studying for a social studies exam, is more likely to enlist strategic cognition during studying, such as making self-statements to prompt implementation of one's study plan or using self-consequences to optimize one's motivation to use these strategies (Wolters, 2003).

During learning, a SRL-engaged student will also utilize various forms of self-observation procedures, such as self-monitoring or self-recording. This regulatory process involves tracking one's task performance and the conditions surrounding it. From an engagement perspective, this process is important because it facilitates error analysis and the capacity to make fine-grained adjustments to one's strategies when not learning effectively. For example, a student who is struggling to learn how to write essays in English class may benefit from cognitively tracking the specific steps of a writing strategy that are challenging (Graham & Harris, 2005). In a cyclical framework, self-monitored feedback helps students strategically reflect on their learning and to make the necessary strategic adjustments to improve task performance.

According to Zimmerman (2000), self-reflection is a multicomponent cognitive process involving various subprocesses, such as self-evaluation, causal attributions, and adaptive inferences. Following performance on some academic activity, students who are highly SRL-engaged will first compare self-monitored or externally provided feedback to some standard in order to judge their level of success. This process is important because it ultimately determines whether students perceive their learning efforts in favorable or unfavorable terms. Following these performance judgments, students who are strategically engaged in learning are more likely to attribute their success and failure to the strategies that they utilized during learning and will seek to make adjustments to their learning tactics in order to improve their future performances (i.e., adaptive inferences) (Cleary et al., 2006; Schunk, 2001). Although students can attribute their successes and failures to other personal and contextual factors that also can be adaptive or helpful for modifying one's behaviors, the key point here is that a hallmark feature of a SRL-engaged learning is exhibiting consistent "thinking in the language of strategies."

Importance and Applications of a Dynamic Feedback Cycle of Engagement

In this section, we underscore the value and importance of conceptualizing cognitive engagement as a cyclical feedback loop. At the outset, it is important to emphasize that Zimmerman's (2000) three-phase model represented a significant theoretical advance over prior models because of its emphasis on forethought processes, such as goal setting and strategic planning. Including forethought in this regulatory loop was important because it reinforced the premise that students have the potential to proactively engage with academic tasks and are not simply reactive organisms to environmentally imposed circumstances (Bandura, 2001). In addition, students who learn to use adaptive forms of forethought will also enhance the quality of their strategic engagement during learning as well as their skill in adaptively reflecting on their performance outcomes. For example, if a student does not strategically plan or develop goals prior to reading a chapter from a science textbook, the student is less likely to implement purposeful, goal-directed strategies when reading the text. A lack of awareness or poor mindfulness of the strategies one uses during learning makes it extremely difficult to evaluate the effectiveness of one's learning methods following learning or performance.

Unfortunately, these reactive types of regulators try to "fix" poorly defined problems in a post hoc fashion, an approach characterized by trial and error learning, ambiguity, frustration, and a reliance on normative comparisons (Zimmerman, 2000; Zimmerman & Kitsantas, 1997). Thus, suppose a 12-year-old middle school student, Betsy, attained an average math quiz grade of 63 on her prior five math quizzes. She is largely unaware of how she should prepare for math quizzes and displays an inconsistent pattern of studying behaviors. Betsy also rarely thinks about the types of grades that she wants to attain, aside from a general, ambiguous belief "to do better." Without a particular standard from which to judge her performance, Betsy is prone to making social comparison types of self-evaluative judgments, such as comparing her quiz performance to that of her classmates. In this scenario, if the math quiz class average was 89 and Betsy attained a 76, she would likely view this performance as a failure and thus not recognize that her score was 13 points higher than the average of her prior math quizzes. Furthermore, because Betsy has very little awareness of her approach or the particular strategies that she uses to learn, it is highly unlikely that she will attribute her "poor performance" to these strategies, further crippling her skill in adjusting or modifying her studying behaviors for future quizzes (Cleary et al., 2006; Zimmerman & Kitsantas, 1997).

In addition to the conceptual advantage of linking forethought, performance, and self-reflection, we would like to highlight three additional points underscoring the utility of this three-phase conceptual framework: (a) integration of motivation and regulatory processes, (b) empirical support for multiphase self-regulation training, and (c) the level of correspondence between the cyclical model and self-regulation intervention programs.

SRL Engagement and Motivation

An important aspect of our cyclical account of engagement is that it integrates metacognition, motivation, and strategic processes and behaviors. Although students can learn powerful learning strategies, such as summarization when reading text or using graphic organizers to learn science material, if students are not motivated to plan out their learning efforts, to use these strategies, or to reflect on the effectiveness of their learning tactics – quite an effortful process – it is highly probable that their overall performance will be greatly diminished. From our perspective, the primary sources underlying students' motivation to initiate and sustain a high level of SRL engagement during learning include a host of self-motivation beliefs, such as self-efficacy, outcome expectations, task interest or valuing, and goal orientation (Eccles & Wigfield, 2002; Pintrich, 2000; Zimmerman, 2000). Collectively, these motivation beliefs have been found to affect the strategic choices that students make, their effort and persistence during learning, as well as the quality of their reflective processes following performance (Schunk & Zimmerman, 2008).

Although space limitations prevent us from providing a comprehensive review of all types of the motivational beliefs (For a comprehensive review see Schunk & Zimmerman, 2008), we will focus specifically on the relationship between students' efficacy beliefs and their cognitive engagement in cyclical phase processes. Self-efficacy is often defined as beliefs about one's capabilities to learn or perform at designated levels and has been shown to be a particularly potent source of motivation (Pajares, 2006). More specifically, these types of beliefs have been shown to not only enhance students' adaptive behaviors, such as effort, persistence, and choice of activities (Bandura, 1986, 1997; Schunk & Pajares, 2004; Zimmerman, 1995), but also to induce and sustain their cognitive engagement in cyclical strategic thinking.

For example, a voluminous literature shows that high perceptions of personal efficacy predict the types and quality of learning goals and choice of strategies that individuals select prior to learning (Cleary & Zimmerman, 2001; Zimmerman & Bandura, 1994; Zimmerman, Bandura, & Martinez-Pons, 1992). Students' beliefs of personal efficacy have also been shown to predict the type and quality of strategies that students use during learning as well as their use of self-control and self-monitoring tactics, all key performance control phase processes (Bandura, Barbaranelli, Caprara, & Pastorelli, 1996; Bouffard-Bouchard, Parent, & Larivee, 1991; Schunk & Swartz, 1993). For example, Schunk and Swartz found that elementary school children who exhibited high levels of self-efficacy following an experimental manipulation were more likely to use writing strategies during follow-up assessments than youth possessing low self-efficacy. Furthermore, Bouffard-Bouchard et al. (1991) found that inducing higher levels of self-efficacy in middle school and high school youth not only impacted their persistence and effort, but also the extent to which they monitored their working time during a verbal concept formation task.

Students who are highly efficacious also tend to set higher self-evaluative standards and will often perceive failure to be the result of controllable or changeable factors, such as effort or strategy use (Bandura, 1997; Cleary & Zimmerman, 2001; Silver, Mitchell, & Gist, 1995; Zimmerman & Bandura, 1994). Clearly, as students' beliefs of personal efficacy increase, there is a greater likelihood that they will engage in the cyclical feedback loop and will focus their cognition on the selection, use, and adaptation of learning strategies.

In addition to motivational beliefs, however, social-cognitive researchers recognize that regulatory subprocesses within the feedback loop also impact student motivation. We will consider a couple of performance- and self-reflection-phase processes to illustrate this point. Relative to the "during" or performance phase of the feedback loop, researchers have shown that various self-control processes, such as self-instruction, self-consequences, and environmental control, can increase students' effort and persistence (Meichenbaum, 1977; Wolters, 1999, 2003; Zimmerman & Martinez-Pons, 1986), particularly when such tactics focus students' attention on process or strategic aspects of learning. Suppose a tenth grade student needs to attain a grade of A on her next math test in order to obtain a personal semester goal of B+ in the course. During math study sessions, the student repeatedly tells herself, "I can do this if I just keep studying what is on the study guide" (self-instruction). She also decided to reward herself with 30 min of TV time following at least 1 h of studying (self-consequences) and to study with a few of her friends who are highly motivated to get into college (environment control). The latter tactic is particularly motivating to this student because it prompts her to visualize the possibility of her going to college, thereby elevating studying behaviors as a valued and important activity (Wolters, 2003).

Self-monitoring is another regulatory process that induces cycles of SRL engagement (Bandura, 1997; Lan, 1998; Schunk, 2001; Shapiro, Durnan, Post, & Skibitsky-Levinson, 2002). Self-monitoring serves an awareness building or informational function in that students obtain data about the frequency, duration, or intensity of their behaviors or cognition. For example, self-observation can motivate youth by conveying enhanced performance over time or by highlighting the conditions under which a particular strategy or behavior is most effective. Using the case example in the preceding paragraph, suppose the student was asked to self-record the number of points lost on her prior three math tests across five different types of problems. Performing this type of self-recording can serve a motivational function if it helps the student to not only isolate patterns of errors that she made but to stimulate reflective thinking to develop solutions to remedy these problems.

Two self-reflection processes that also promote motivation in youth include self-evaluation and causal attributions. Self-evaluation represents the initial cognitive dimension of self-reflection, whereby individuals compare their current performance on a task to some standard or benchmark (Kitsantas & Zimmerman, 2006; Zimmerman, 2000). Many empirically supported self-regulation interventions emphasize the use of mastery or self-related self-evaluation standards, such as improvement from prior performance or a benchmark score of 80% on a test (Butler, 1998; Cleary, Platten, & Nelson, 2008; Fuchs et al., 2003; Graham & Harris, 2005). These types of standards are considered optimal because they shift students' attention and cognition toward indicators of personal progress or the effectiveness of one's learning strategies. In contrast, if students who struggle in school are prompted to make normative comparisons, such as when a teacher publicly displays class grades, their attention and thinking will often shift to variables that are not essential or unrelated to their personal success, such as lack of personal ability (Schunk et al., 2008).

The types of causal attributions students make following performance, and in particular failure outcomes, can also have a major impact on students' motivation to cognitively adapt ineffective learning methods (Borkowski, Weyhing, & Carr, 1988; Clifford, 1986; Weiner, 1986). From a motivational perspective, encouraging students to make internal, controllable, and unstable attributions following failure, such as to effort and strategy use, is adaptive because they sustain students' efficacy beliefs and direct their cognition on the effectiveness of one's methods to learn (Cleary et al., 2006; Kuhl, 1985; Schunk, 1982; Zimmerman & Kitsantas, 1997). In one study examining the self-regulatory characteristics of expert, nonexpert, and novice basketball players in high school, Cleary and Zimmerman (2001) reported that the types of attributions that students make following missed free throws was not only highly predictive of expertise status, but also of the types of cognitive reactions and adaptations players make. For example, players who made strategic attributions following poor free throws were more likely to report making strategic adaptations or modifications prior to taking subsequent shots. Regardless of the domain of interest, individuals who believe that the strategies they use to learn or to perform a task are ineffective (i.e., strategic attributions) will initiate attempts to change these strategies to optimize their learning (i.e., strategic adaptive inferences) (Cleary & Zimmerman, 2001; Cleary et al., 2006; Schunk et al., 2008).

Empirical Advantages of the Cyclical Feedback Loop

A marked advantage of a cyclical model of engagement is its strong empirical support in the literature (Cleary et al., 2006; Schunk & Swartz, 1993; Zimmerman & Kitsantas, 1996, 1997). That is, students who are trained in multiple SRL phase processes, such as forethought and performance control, are more likely to display greater achievement and strategic cyclical thinking than those who are only trained in one of these phases. For example, Zimmerman and Kitsantas conducted a series of studies examining the effects of forethought and performance control training on the self-regulatory skills and dart-throwing proficiency of high school girls. Across studies, a consistent finding was that students who were trained in both goal setting *prior* to dart-throwing practice and self-recording their performance outcomes *during* practice sessions exhibited higher dart-throwing skill, self-efficacy, and satisfaction than those who only engaged in forethought (i.e., goal setting).

In a more recent study, Cleary et al. (2006) examined the additive effects of self-regulatory training on novice basketball players' free-throw shooting skill and self-reflection phase processes during a short practice session. Fifty college students were randomly assigned to either one of three experimental groups, to a practice control group, or to a no-practice control group. Each of the three experimental groups received either three-, two-, or one-phase training in the cyclical feedback loop. Participants assigned to the three-phase condition were instructed to set process goals (forethought phase), to self-record effective shooting processes (performance phase), and to make strategic attributions and adjustments following missed free throws (self-reflection phase). The two-phase group received the same forethought and performance phase training but no self-reflection instruction, whereas the one-phase group only received training in goal setting. The participants in the two control conditions did not receive any self-regulatory instruction.

All five groups received identical shooting strategy instructions to insure that achievement differences were not due to variations in knowledge of shooting technique. Furthermore, all groups (except for the no-practice control group) were given 12 min to practice using the shooting strategy. An important finding was that the three-phase and two-phase groups performed *significantly better* in free-throw shooting than all other groups even though they shot *significantly fewer* free throws during the practice sessions. Fewer shots were taken in the multiphase conditions because participants were required to self-record and or reflect on missed free-throw attempts during the practice session. These results suggest that it was not simply behavioral engagement in routine practice sessions that facilitated success but rather one's cognitive and strategic engagement in the cyclical loop during these practice opportunities. Furthermore, although the three-phase and two-phase groups were highly similar in terms of performance outcomes and adaptive self-regulation processes, the three-phase intervention group exhibited the most adaptive self-reflection profile, exhibited by their strategic attributions and reactions following failure as well as the use of process-oriented self-evaluative criteria to judge their level of success and satisfaction (i.e., personal improvement, use of correct shooting strategy) (Cleary et al., 2006).

Academic Applications of the Cyclical Loop

A final advantage of the SRL cyclical engagement model is that it can serve as the foundation or framework through which researchers and or practitioners develop and implement engagement-related academic interventions. As Zimmerman revealed in a recent interview in the *Journal of Advanced Academics*, one of the reasons why the cyclical model was developed was because it links together the processes that precede, guide, and come after learning. Such a model allows one to examine the causal links among these processes and to also guide intervention development (Bembenutty, 2008). A variety of academic-focused SRL interventions reported in the literature devote primary attention to teaching students how to become engaged in a cyclical process of thought and action across diverse academic tasks.

There are several comprehensive self-regulation intervention programs available in the literature that seek to induce cyclical phase changes in students' cognitive engagement during specific academic tasks (Butler, 1998; Cassel & Reid, 1996; Cleary et al., 2008; Fuchs et al., 2003; Graham & Harris, 2005). Although most authors of these programs do not specifically refer to the dynamic feedback loop as the guiding framework for developing the intervention, it is quite apparent that instruction in cyclical regulatory thought and action is a core focus of these interventions. Our primary goal in this section is not to provide an exhaustive review of all SRL interventions that address elements of the cyclical loop but rather to provide a few illustrative examples of interventions that comprehensively target all three phases of the cognitive loop.

Self-Regulated Strategy Development (SRSD)

Graham and Harris developed the SRSD intervention program over 20 years ago to improve the writing performance of elementary school students (Graham & Harris, 2005; Graham, Harris, & Troia, 1998). In general, SRSD involves a six-step process that actively engages students in the three-phase cyclical process during various types of writing activities. To promote forethought, tutors typically engage students in discussions about their prior knowledge of writing as well as the essential components of specific writing tasks. Students also discuss their current strategies to write and learn how to set process goals, such as learning how to write better essays.

During writing practice sessions, SRSD teachers or tutors explain, model, and prompt students to use a specific writing strategy (i.e., strategies often vary based on writing assignment). Students are typically provided several structured guided practice sessions in which tutors provide hints and feedback to students as they refine their use and application of the writing strategies. During these practice sessions, students are also taught to self-record the number of writing elements included in their essay and to make adaptive self-instruction statements pertaining to problem definition, planning, and self-evaluation (Sexton, Harris, & Graham, 1998). This instructional feature is particularly important as it continually directs students' attention to the essential elements of the writing process and the key tactics to optimize performance across these elements.

To complete the cyclical loop, SRSD instructors prompt students to reflect on their writing performance, such as using criterion-based self-evaluative standards to judge their success (e.g., number of story elements included) and attributing success or failure to effort and or strategy use (Graham et al., 1998).

Strategic Content Learning (SCL)

Butler developed this innovative self-regulation instructional program to enhance the academic achievement, motivation, and regulatory behaviors of college-aged and secondary school students

(Butler, 1998; Butler, Beckingham, & Lauscher, 2005). The program has been administered to college students across multiple content areas, including reading, writing, and math (Butler, 1995, 1998) and to middle school students in math (Butler et al., 2005). Regardless of academic context or developmental level of students, SCL adheres to a largely constructivist framework. Thus, students are encouraged to become active participants in learning, via establishing personal goals, selecting and modifying their learning strategies, and reflecting on the effectiveness of their learning strategies. In addition, consistent with the engagement framework that we present in this manuscript, engaging students in a recursive cycle of cognitive regulatory activities is a core SCL instructional principle.

In terms of forethought, students who receive SCL are typically instructed in task analysis skills, which involve interpreting the basic demands and requirements of specific academic assignments or tasks. Task analysis is crucial in this model because it enables one to purposefully develop strategic plans to accomplish specific goals relative to the task (Butler & Cartier, 2004). SCL tutors will often use strategic questioning to assess students' knowledge of math problems and their use of learning strategies. These activities not only help students become more aware of their learning methods when solving math problems but also help tutors to better understand the types of questions and prompts that are needed to impact and guide students' strategic learning (Butler et al., 2005).

Regarding the performance phase, an important element of math-based SCL is for tutors to continually engage students in interpreting math problems successfully and to prompt them to use and refine their self-generated learning strategies and metacognitive strategies. In one case study, Butler et al. (2005) reported that over the course of SCL instruction, a student generated seven new strategy steps when solving fraction problems, with these tactics increasing in complexity and sophistication over time. In addition, the student became more skillful in describing the nature of her math problem-solving strategies and showed a high level of flexibility when applying these strategies to solve particular math problems.

Self-reflection is naturally infused within each SCL session, whereby students are often encouraged to continually self-evaluate their performance during math problem solving. Students are not only encouraged to evaluate correctness of their answers to problems but to also consider the role and impact of their problem-solving strategies. Accordingly, SCL tutors use attribution and adaptive inference questions in order to prompt students to reflect on the strategic reasons for their success or failure when solving a problem and to consider alternative methods or tactics to improve math performance.

Self-Regulation Empowerment Program (SREP)

A more recent intervention, Self-Regulation Empowerment Program (SREP), was developed to empower at-risk middle school or high school youth to become more strategic, motivated, and regulated during more complex and comprehensive academic activities, such as studying for content-area exams (Cleary et al., 2008; Cleary & Zimmerman, 2004). This approach emphasizes the use of evidence-based learning tactics or strategies that are linked particularly to academic tasks, such as concept maps and mnemonic devices for learning science concepts. This program was borne out of social-cognitive theory and research and thus emphasizes the importance of social change agents, such as teachers and tutors, in cultivating adaptive cognition during instruction (Bandura, 1997; Cleary & Zimmerman, 2004). This instructional program is closely aligned with each of the three phases of the dynamic feedback loop and thus involves training in task analysis, goal setting and strategic planning, self-recording, self-evaluation, strategic attributions, and adaptive inferences.

The initial components of SREP instruction involve enhancing students' awareness of their maladaptive beliefs, such as poor causal attributions (e.g., failure on tests is due to poor ability), and providing explicit instruction in core forethought processes such as task analysis, goal setting, and strategic planning. Similar to most

Self-Regulation Graph

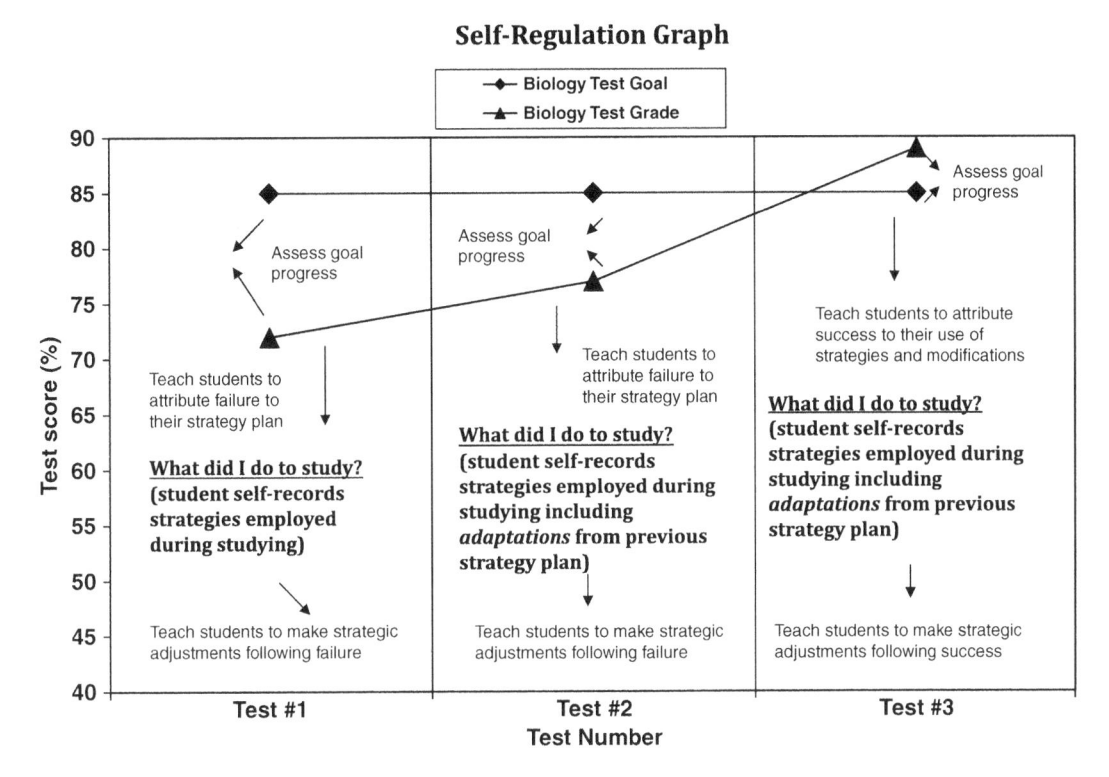

Fig. 11.2 Example of a self-regulation graph used to teach students to evaluate goal progress and to make strategic attributions and adaptive inferences (From Cleary et al. (2008), p. 87. Copyright 2008 by Prufrock Press. Reprinted with permission)

effective self-regulation programs, SREP tutors teach regulatory processes and learning strategies within the context of authentic curriculum materials and content. Thus, students not only learn about the value and importance of goal setting, use of learning strategies, and self-recording, but also the use of these processes to learn specific course material. In addition, primary emphasis is placed on shifting students' attention to powerful learning strategies before, during, and after studying and test performance. In Cleary et al. (2008), given that science was the target content area of interest, the authors elected to utilize concept maps and mnemonic devices as the primary learning strategies to be taught within the cyclical framework (Nesbit & Adesope, 2006).

The primary instructional mechanism through which students are taught to cognitively engage in strategic, cyclical thinking is the use of a self-regulation graph (Cleary et al., 2008; see Fig. 11.2). To stimulate forethought thinking, a SREP tutor, such as a trained graduate student or school support staff, helps students adopt outcome- and process-related goals as well as a specific plan for addressing those goals. On the graph, students are taught to plot their outcome goal and to record the strategic plan that will be used to accomplish their goal. As part of the performance phase dimension, students are encouraged to add, modify, or adjust their strategic plans listed on the graph when appropriate and to self-record their test or exam grades. This self-monitored outcome and process information is used to stimulate self-reflective activities during SREP sessions. Thus, after each test performance, a SREP tutor leads students through a series of self-reflection questions and activities targeting self-evaluation, causal attributions, and adaptive inferences. In terms of self-evaluation, two types of criteria are emphasized: prior performance and forethought goals. Thus, students judge success or failure based on comparing their current performance to both their prior test grades as well as their test grade goal. Both of these types of self-criteria facilitate SRL engagement because they shift students' attention and thinking on their own performance and the strategies linked to this performance.

Finally, SREP tutors also ask students to answer reflection questions targeting attributions ("What is the main reason why you got that grade on the test?") and adaptive inferences ("What do you need to do to improve your next test score?"). Ultimately, the SREP tutors guide students' thinking to focus on the relationship between their performance outcomes and the effort that they displayed in using their strategic plan. In this way, students learn how to make strategic attributions following failure and continuously focus on how to sustain or adapt their methods of learning to attain their personal goals.

Although our review of SRL intervention programs was not exhaustive, it illustrated that a cyclical account of cognitive and strategic engagement can successfully be taught to students across academic tasks and development levels.

SRL Microanalysis: Measuring Cyclical Regulatory Engagement

Consistent with most models of self-regulation, our definition of SRL engagement is best represented by a dynamic, cyclical process that varies across learning contexts and tasks (Bandura, 1997; Hadwin et al., 2001; Schunk, 2001; Winne & Jaimeson-Noel, 2002). This "event" conceptualization of SRL engagement contrasts from "ability" perspectives, the latter of which depicts self-regulation to be a fixed or stable trait-like construct. This conceptual distinction parallels the difference made in the assessment literature regarding *event* and *aptitude* measures of self-regulation (Cleary, 2011; Winne & Perry, 2000; Zimmerman, 2008). Aptitude measures are described as those targeting an enduring attribute of an individual and typically include self-report scales, such as the Learning and Study Strategies Inventory (LASSI) (Weinstein & Palmer, 1990), Motivated Strategies for Learning Questionnaire (MSLQ) (Pintrich, Smith, & Garcia, 1993), and more recently the Strategy Motivation and Learning Strategy Inventory (SMALSI) (Stroud & Reynolds, 2006). Although these measures can capture general aspects of students' self-regulation of learning in a psychometrically reliable way, they may not be well suited to capture the dynamic, context-specific aspects of SRL engagement. Because these measures are typically decontextualized in nature, they do not lend themselves to evaluating the actual "process" of engagement in real time and are interpreted based on aggregated scores and normative criteria (Perry & Winne, 2006; Zimmerman, 2008).

To more accurately and comprehensively evaluate students' engagement in a cycle of thought and action, researchers have developed a variety of alternative measures, such as think-aloud protocols (Greene & Azevedo, 2007), direct observations (Perry, Vandekamp, Mercer, & Nordby, 2002), behavioral traces (Perry & Winne, 2006), and SRL microanalysis (Cleary & Zimmerman, 2001; Kitsantas & Zimmerman, 2002). These assessment approaches are labeled as "event" measures because they seek to target students' thoughts and behaviors as they engage in particular tasks or activities. Consistent with our three-phase model of engagement, an event is considered to be a temporal entity with a before, during, and after component (Cleary, 2011; Winne & Perry, 2000).

A cyclical event assessment method that has been receiving increased attention in recent years is SRL microanalysis (Cleary, 2011; Cleary & Zimmerman, 2001). In short, this approach is grounded in social-cognitive theory and was influenced by various lines of research and clinical practice, including think-aloud protocols, emergence of cognitive-behavioral therapy, and the importance of situation-dependence or specificity (Bandura, 1977; Beck, 1963; Cleary, 2011; Ericsson & Simon, 1980). In short, this methodology is designed to examine students' regulatory beliefs and reactions as they participate in context-specific tasks and activities. This approach differs from typical self-report scales because it entails observing human functioning as it occurs in real time and directly targets the self-motivation beliefs (e.g., self-efficacy) and regulatory processes (e.g., goal setting, attributions) outlined in the three-phase cyclical model (Cleary, 2011; Kitsantas & Zimmerman, 2002). An essential component of this methodology is the use of a structured interview protocol whereby task-specific regulatory questions delineated in the three-phase cyclical loop are administered in a predetermined sequence during a specific activity. In order for questions to fully qualify as SRL microanalytic, they must be directly linked to the phase dimensions of the academic event and thus administered in a temporally appropriate sequence. That is, forethought phase questions are administered "before" an event, performance processes "during" the activity, and self-reflection "after" performance on the event (Cleary, 2011).

To illustrate this process, we will discuss the methodology of two studies that were the first to use SRL microanalysis in a comprehensive fashion. Cleary and Zimmerman (2001) examined forethought (self-efficacy, goal setting, strategic planning) and self-reflection (i.e., attributions, adaptive inferences, satisfaction) differences among expert, nonexpert, and novice high school basketball players as they practiced shooting free throws. The participants were asked to shoot free throws individually at a basket during a 10-min practice session. This activity ultimately served as the event around which microanalytic measures were administered. To examine participants' strategic approach to shooting free throws, the researchers asked participants a series of forethought questions *prior* to the practice session: (a) self-efficacy (e.g., "How sure are you that you can make two shots in a row"), (b) goal setting (e.g., "Do you have a goal when practicing free throws?" "If so what is it?"), and (c) strategy choice (e.g., "What do you need to do to accomplish that goal?").

Although this study did not examine students' performance phase processes, such as self-monitoring or self-control tactics, the participants were asked attribution and adaptive inference questions at two points: following two consecutive missed shots and two consecutive made shots. The attribution question following a missed shot was, "Why do you think you missed those last two shots?", whereas the adaptive inference question involved, "What do you need to do to make the next shot?" These latter two questions were considered microanalytic in nature because they were context- and task-specific (i.e., linked to basketball free throwing), targeted regulatory processes delineated in the three-phase model, and were administered immediately following a specific performance outcome.

Kitsantas and Zimmerman (2002) expanded the scope of SRL microanalysis by including additional microanalytic questions across all three phases: perceived instrumentality and task interest (forethought), self-monitoring (performance), and self-evaluation (self-reflection). This study examined differences across achievement groups relative to volleyball skills. Thus, in addition to goal setting, strategic planning, and self-efficacy beliefs, Kitsantas and Zimmerman also targeted students' level of interest in volleyball serving ("How interesting is serving a volleyball overhand to you on a scale from 0 to 100?") and the importance of volleyball serving ("How important is volleyball serving in attaining your future goals on a scale from 0 to 100?") prior to the volleyball practice session. With respect to self-evaluation, all of the players were asked to report their self-evaluative methods, if any, following a volleyball serving practice session. Consistent with the temporal sequencing of microanalytic methodology, this self-reflection question along with attribution and adaptive inference questions was administered after the practice session to effectively link them to the "after" dimension of the event.

Microanalytic methodology consists of both metric and categorical questions, with most involving single-item scales. The metric questions consist of motivation beliefs, such as self-efficacy, task interest, instrumentality, and satisfaction. Participants rate their responses to these closed-ended questions on a Likert scale, typically ranging from 0 to 100. The categorical microanalytic questions target self-regulation phase processes including goal setting, strategic planning, self-monitoring, self-evaluation, attributions, and adaptive inferences. These questions are open-ended and thus allow participants to provide elaborate or detailed responses to describe their regulatory cognitions. To quantify these variables, two individuals are trained to independently code the responses using a structured scoring rubric (Cleary & Zimmerman, 2001). The interrater reliability of these scales has been shown to be strong as evidenced by Kappa coefficients ranging from .81 to .98 (Cleary, 2011).

Collectively, both the metric and categorical scales have been shown to differentiate experts, nonexperts, and novices across different motoric activities. The predictive validity of microanalytic questions has also been investigated. Kitsantas and Zimmerman (2002) conducted an ex post facto study to examine differences in volleyball serving skill and self-regulatory processes among expert, nonexpert, and novice volleyball players. The authors combined 12 self-regulatory measures into a single scale to predict women's volleyball serving skill score. The authors reported that the scale was highly reliable ($\alpha = 90$) and correlated extremely well with volleyball serving score ($r = .95$); the scale accounted for 90% of the variance in volleyball serving skill.

More recently, researchers have begun to use microanalysis within academic contexts (Cleary et al., 2008; Cleary, Callan, Peterson & Adams, 2011; Zimmerman, Moylan, Hudesman, White, & Flugman, 2008). Cleary et al. (2011) used hierarchical regression analysis to examine the extent to which self-reflection microanalytic questions (attributions, adaptive inferences, and self-evaluation) accounted for a unique amount of variance in final course grades of college students over and above that accounted for by an abbreviated version of the MSLQ. In general, the results indicated that the MSLQ did not account for a negligible amount of a significant amount of variance in final course grade, whereas three self-reflection phase processes, causal attribution, adaptive inferences, and self-evaluative standards accounted for a statistically and clinically significant change in R^2. It is also of interest to note the microanalytic questions exhibited low to non significant corrections with the MSLQ, suggesting that the microanalytic questions measure a different aspect of regulation than that which is measured by self-report scales (Cleary et al., 2011).

Future Research Directions

There are many fruitful lines of research that can be generated based on our cyclical account of cognitive engagement. First, although several SRL academic interventions target various subprocesses within each of the three phases of the feedback loop, very few intervention studies have directly measured the dynamic shifts or changes in students' regulatory processes as they occur during academic activities. To capture these cyclical phase changes, researchers are encouraged to use event measures, such as SRL microanalysis. Using these types of measures will also allow one to draw inferences about the causal links among the specific regulatory processes that promote these sustained cycles of learning. In addition, although the use of SRL microanalysis has recently been utilized in academic contexts (Cleary et al., 2008, 2011), most microanalytic studies have employed motoric tasks. To effectively use microanalysis in academic contexts, researchers need to first identify specific tasks with a clear beginning and end, such as writing an essay, solving math problems, reading a textbook, etc. Then, one can employ SRL microanalytic questions before, during, and after this task to evaluate students' level of cognitive and strategic engagement.

Second, aside from the self-motivation literature, there is a paucity of studies examining the external mechanisms or environmental factors that facilitate or inhibit students' engagement in the cyclical model. Thus, another interesting line of research involves examining the extent to which particular components of instruction, such as the amount of autonomy support or the type, quantity, or quality of feedback provided to students, impact students' cyclical cognitive engagement during learning. Of particular interest is for future research to examine the most effective ways to engage students to continuously self-reflect on their academic progress and performance across key content areas, such as math, science, and English. That is, researchers are encouraged to examine the personal (i.e., cognitive and affective) and environmental factors which either inhibit or facilitate students' skill in adapting and modifying their behaviors following difficulty or failure in school and whether such reflective activities directly change student performance and behavior.

Third, self-efficacy perceptions have been shown to be an important motivational source of students' SRL engagement. Although these beliefs are typically assessed during the forethought phase, research has clearly revealed that they also affect regulatory processes during other phases in the cyclical loop, such as the accuracy of metacognitive monitoring during the performance control phase and self-evaluation judgments during the self-reflection phase (Ramdass & Zimmerman, 2008). The primary implication here is that researchers and practitioners may find it valuable to examine the influence of self-efficacy perceptions on other self-regulatory processes before, during, and after performance in order to evaluate shifts in these beliefs and to more closely examine microanalytic proximal links between efficacy beliefs and regulatory processes.

As a concluding thought, it is important to emphasize the emergent research demonstrating that educators and school psychologists perceive issues of student motivation and self-regulation to be highly valuable and relevant to student performance and to their own professional activities, yet they do not frequently engage in assessment, instructional, or intervention activities relative to these areas (Cleary, 2009; Cleary et al., 2010, 2011; Cleary & Zimmerman, 2006; Grigal, Neubart, Moon, & Graham, 2003; Wehmeyer et al., 2000). It is highly probable that this practice gap is due to a variety of factors, such as educators' limited knowledge of, and potentially limited access to, key assessment tools and intervention programs.

Another reason why both teachers and school psychologists express a strong desire for professional development training in motivation and self-regulation is because the training that they received in graduate school may not have adequately addressed such issues (Cleary, 2009; Cleary et al., 2010). Most school psychology programs in the United States emphasize coursework addressing several key content areas including core psychology topics such as learning and development, academic, behavioral, and mental health interventions, consultation activities, psychoeducational assessment, and professional ethics and behavior (Jimerson & Oakland, 2007). Although information pertaining to student self-management, regulation, and motivation may be embedded within such courses, research suggests that students may not receive enough extensive training in these processes during graduate school. For example, Cleary (2009) found that the average school psychologist reported that their graduate training programs did not adequately prepare them to work with youth exhibiting motivation and self-regulation difficulties. Along the same lines, Wehmeyer et al. (2000) showed that 41% of teachers indicated that a key barrier to providing instruction in self-determination, a closely related concept to self-regulation, was that they did not receive sufficient training or information on how to do so in graduate school (Wehmeyer et al. 2000). In short, although self-regulation intervention programs are highly effective in improving the performance of youth across multiple domains and that such programs help to cultivate adaptive beliefs and cognitive processes, there is much work to be done to ensure that these programs are integrated into the curriculum and services provided by schools.

References

Agran, M., Snow, K., & Swaner, J. (1999). Teacher perceptions of self-determination: Benefits, characteristics, and strategies. *Education and Training in Mental Retardation and Developmental Disabilities, 34*, 293–301.

Bandura, A. (1977). Self-efficacy: Toward a unifying theory of behavior change. *Psychological Review, 84*, 191–215.

Bandura, A. (1986). *Social foundations of thought and action: A social cognitive theory*. Englewood Cliffs, NJ: Prentice-Hall.

Bandura, A. (1997). *Self-efficacy: The exercise of control*. New York: W. H. Freeman.

Bandura, A. (2001). Social cognitive theory: An agentic perspective. *Annual Review of Psychology, 52*, 1–29.

Bandura, A., Barbaranelli, C., Caprara, G. V., & Pastorelli, C. (1996). Multifaceted impact of self-efficacy beliefs on academic functioning. *Child Development, 67*, 1206–1222.

Beck, A. T. (1963). Thinking and depression. *Archives of General Psychiatry, 9*, 324–333.

Bembenutty, H. (2008). The last word: An interview with Barry J. Zimmerman. *Journal of Advanced Academics, 20*, 174–192.

Boekaerts, M., Pintrich, P. R., & Zeidner, M. (Eds.). (2000). *Handbook of self-regulation*. San Diego, CA: Academic.

Borkowski, J. G., Weyhing, R. S., & Carr, M. (1988). Effects of attributional retraining on strategy-based reading comprehension in learning disabled students. *Journal of Educational Psychology, 80*, 46–53.

Bouffard-Bouchard, T., Parent, S., & Larivee, S. (1991). Influence of self-efficacy on self-regulation and performance among junior and senior high-school age students. *International Journal of Behavioral Development, 14*, 153–164.

Butler, D. (1995). Promoting strategic learning by postsecondary students with learning disabilities. *Journal of Learning Disabilities, 28*, 170–190.

Butler, D. (1998). The strategic content learning approach to promoting self-regulated learning: A report of three studies. *Journal of Educational Psychology, 90*, 682–697.

Butler, D. L., Beckingham, B., & Lauscher, H. J. N. (2005). Promoting strategic learning by eighth-grade students struggling in mathematics: A report of three case studies. *Learning Disabilities Research and Practice, 20*, 156–174.

Butler, D. L., & Cartier, S. C. (2004). Promoting effective task interpretation as an important work habit: A key to successful teaching and learning. *Teachers College Record, 106*, 1729–1758.

Carver, C. H., & Scheier, M. F. (2000). On the structure of behavioral self-regulation. In M. Boekaerts, P. Pintrich, & M. Zeidner (Eds.), *Handbook of self-regulation* (pp. 41–84). Orlando, FL: Academic.

Cassel, J., & Reid, R. (1996). Use of a self-regulated strategy intervention to improve word problem-solving skills of students with mild disabilities. *Journal of Behavioral Education, 6*, 153–172.

Christenson, S. L., Reschly, A. L., Appleton, J. J., Berman-Young, S., Spanjers, D. M., & Varro, P. (2008). Best practices in fostering student engagement. In A. Thomas & J. Grimes (Eds.), *Best practices in school psychology* (5th ed., pp. 1099–1119). Bethesda, MD: National Association of School Psychologists.

Cleary, T. J. (2009). School-based motivation and self-regulation assessments: An examination of school psychologist beliefs and practices. *Journal of Applied School Psychology, 25*, 71–94.

Cleary, T. J. (2011). Emergence of self-regulated learning microanalysis: Historical overview, essential features, and implications for research and practice. In B. J. Zimmerman & D. Schunk (Eds.), *Handbook of self-regulation of learning and performance*. New York: Routledge.

Cleary, T. J., & Chen, P. P. (2009). Self-regulation, motivation, and math achievement in middle school: Variations across grade level and math context. *Journal of School Psychology, 47*, 291–314.

Cleary, T. J., Gubi, A., & Prescott, M. (2010). Motivation and self-regulation assessments: Professional practices and needs of school psychologists. *Psychology in the Schools, 47*(10), 985–1002.

Cleary, T. J., Callan, G., Peterson, J., & Adams, T. (2011). Validity of Self-Regulated Learning (SRL) in an academic context. Manuscript submitted for publication.

Cleary, T. J., Platten, P., & Nelson, A. C. (2008). Effectiveness of self-regulation empowerment program with urban high school students. *Journal of Advanced Academics, 20*, 70–107.

Cleary, T. J., & Zimmerman, B. J. (2001). Self-regulation differences during athletic practice by experts, non-experts, and novices. *Journal of Applied Sport Psychology, 13*, 185–206.

Cleary, T. J., & Zimmerman, B. J. (2004). Self-regulation empowerment program: A school-based program to enhance self-regulated and self-motivated cycles of student learning. *Psychology in the Schools, 41*, 537–550.

Cleary, T. J., & Zimmerman, B. J. (2006). Teachers' perceived usefulness of strategy microanalytic assessment information. *Psychology in the Schools, 43*, 149–155.

Cleary, T. J., Zimmerman, B. J., & Keating, T. (2006). Training physical education students to self-regulate during basketball free-throw practice. *Research Quarterly for Exercise and Sport, 77*, 251–262.

Clifford, M. (1986). Comparative effects of strategy and effort attributions. *British Journal of Educational Psychology, 56*, 75–83.

Coalition for Psychology in Schools and Education. (2006). *Report on the teacher needs survey*. Washington, DC: American Psychological Association, Center for Psychology in Schools and Education.

Corno, L., & Mandinach, E. B. (1983). The role of cognitive engagement in classroom learning and motivation. *Educational Psychologist, 18*, 88–108.

Eccles, J. S., & Wigfield, A. (2002). Motivational beliefs, values, and goals. *Annual Review of Psychology, 53*, 109–132.

Ericsson, K. A., & Simon, H. A. (1980). Verbal reports as data. *Psychological Review, 87*, 215–251.

Fredricks, J. A., Blumenfeld, P. C., & Paris, A. H. (2004). School engagement: Potential of the concept, state of the evidence. *Review of Educational Research, 74*, 59–109.

Fuchs, L. S., Fuchs, D., Prentice, K., Burch, M., Hamlett, C. L., Owen, R., et al. (2003). Enhancing third-grade students' mathematical problem solving with self-regulated learning strategies. *Journal of Educational Psychology, 95*, 306–315.

Graham, S., & Harris, H. R. (2005). Improving the writing performance of young struggling writers: Theoretical and programmatic research from the center on accelerating student learning. *The Journal of Special Education, 39,* 19–33.

Graham, S., Harris, K., & Troia, G. A. (1998). Writing and self-regulation: Cases from the self-regulated strategy development model. In D. H. Schunk & B. J. Zimmerman (Eds.), *Self-regulated learning: From teaching to self-reflective practice.* New York: Guilford Press.

Greene, J. A., & Azevedo, R. (2007). Adolescents' use of self-regulatory processes and their relation to qualitative mental model shifts while using hypermedia. *Journal of Educational Computing Research, 36,* 125–148.

Grigal, M., Neubart, D. A., Moon, S. M., & Graham, S. (2003). Self-determination for students with disabilities: Views of parents and teachers. *Exceptional Children, 70,* 97–112.

Hadwin, A. F., Winne, P. H., Stockley, D. B., Nesbit, J. C., & Woszczyna, C. (2001). Context moderates students' self-reports about how they study. *Journal of Educational Psychology, 93,* 477–487.

Jimerson, S. R., & Oakland, T. D. (2007). School psychology in the United States. In S. R. Jimerson, T. D. Oakland, & P. T. Farrell (Eds.), *The handbook of international school psychology.* Thousand Oaks, CA: Sage Publications.

Kitsantas, A., & Zimmerman, B. J. (2002). Comparing self-regulatory processes among novice, non-expert, and expert volleyball players: A microanalytic study. *Journal of Applied Sport Psychology, 14,* 91–105.

Kitsantas, A., & Zimmerman, B. J. (2006). Enhancing self-regulation of practice: The influence of graphing and self-evaluative standards. *Metacognition and Learning, 1,* 201–212.

Kuhl, J. (1985). Volitional mediators of cognitive-behavior consistency: Self-regulatory processes and action versus state orientation. In J. Kuhl & J. Beckman (Eds.), *Action control: From cognition to behavior* (pp. 101–128). West Berlin, Germany: Springer.

Lan, W. Y. (1998). Teaching self-monitoring skills in statistics. In D. H. Schunk & B. J. Zimmerman (Eds.), *Self-regulated learning: From teaching to self-reflective practice* (pp. 86–105). New York: Guilford Press.

Locke, E. A., & Latham, G. P. (1990). *A theory of goal setting and task performance.* Englewood Cliffs, NJ: Prentice-Hall.

Mace, F. C., Belfiore, P. J., & Hutchinson, J. M. (2001). Operant theory and research on self-regulation. In B. J. Zimmerman & D. H. Schunk (Eds.), *Self-regulated learning and academic achievement* (2nd ed., pp. 39–66). Mahwah, NJ: Lawrence Erlbaum Associates.

McCombs, B. L. (2001). Self-regulated learning and academic achievement: A phenomenological view. In B. J. Zimmerman & D. H. Schunk (Eds.), *Self-regulated learning and academic achievement* (2nd ed., pp. 67–123). Mahwah, NJ: Lawrence Erlbaum Associates.

Meichenbaum, D. (1977). *Cognitive-behavior modification: An integrative approach.* New York: Plenum.

Miller, G. A., Galanter, E., & Pribham, K. (1960). *Plans and the structure of behavior.* New York: Holt, Rinehart and Winston.

Multon, K. D., Brown, S. D., & Lent, R. W. (1991). Relation of self-efficacy beliefs to academic outcomes: A meta-analytic investigation. *Journal of Counseling Psychology, 18,* 30–38.

Nesbit, J. C., & Adesope, O. O. (2006). Learning with concept and knowledge maps: A meta-analysis. *Review of Educational Research, 76,* 413–448.

Pajares, F. (2006). Self-efficacy during childhood and adolescence: Implications for teachers and parents. In F. Pajares & T. Urdan (Eds.), *Self-efficacy beliefs of adolescents* (pp. 339–367). Greenwich, CT: Information Age Publishing.

Perry, N. E., VandeKamp, K. O., Mercer, L. K., & Nordby, C. J. (2002). Investigating teacher-student interactions that foster self-regulated learning. *Educational Psychologist, 37,* 5–15.

Perry, N. E., & Winne, P. H. (2006). Learning from learning kits: Study traces of students' self-regulated engagements with Computerized content. *Educational Psychology Review, 18,* 211–228.

Pintrich, P. R. (2000). The role of goal orientation in self-regulated learning. In M. Boekaerts, P. Pintrich, & M. Zeidner (Eds.), *Handbook of self-regulation* (pp. 452–502). Orlando, FL: Academic.

Pintrich, P. R., & de Groot, E. V. (1990). Motivational and self-regulated components of classroom academic performance. *Journal of Educational Psychology, 82,* 33–40.

Pintrich, P. R., Smith, D. A., & Garcia, T. (1993). Reliability and predictive validity of the Motivated Strategies for Learning Questionnaire (MSLQ). *Educational and Psychological Measurement, 53,* 801–813.

Powers, W. T. (1973). *Behavior: The control of perception.* Chicago: Aldine.

Pressley, M., & McCormick, C. B. (1995). *Advanced educational psychology for educators, researchers, and policymakers.* New York: Harper Collins.

Puustinen, M., & Pulkkinen, L. (2001). Models of self-regulated learning: A review. *Scandinavian Journal of Educational Research, 45,* 269–286.

Ramdass, D. H., & Zimmerman, B. J. (2008). Effects of self-correction strategy training on middle school students' self-efficacy, self-evaluation, and mathematics division learning. *Journal of Advanced Academics, 20,* 18–41.

Schmitz, B., & Wiese, B. S. (2006). New perspectives for the evaluation of training sessions in self-regulated learning: Time series analyses of diary data. *Contemporary Educational Psychology, 31,* 64–96.

Schunk, D. H. (1981). Modeling and attributional effects on children achievement: A self-efficacy analysis. *Journal of Educational Psychology, 73,* 93–105.

Schunk, D. H. (1982). Progress self-monitoring: Effects on children's self-efficacy and achievement. *The Journal of Experimental Education, 51,* 89–93.

Schunk, D. H. (2001). Social cognitive theory and self-regulated learning. In B. J. Zimmerman & D. H. Schunk (Eds.), *Self-regulated learning and academic achievement* (2nd ed., pp. 125–151). Mahwah, NJ: Lawrence Erlbaum Associates Publishers.

Schunk, D. H., & Pajares, F. (2004). Self-efficacy in education revisited: Empirical and applied evidence. In D. M. McInerney & S. Van Etten (Eds.), *Big theories revisited* (pp. 115–138). Greenwich, CT: Information Age Publishing.

Schunk, D. H., Pintrich, P. R., & Meece, J. L. (2008). *Motivation in education: Theory, research, and applications* (3rd ed.). Upper Saddle River, NJ: Pearson Education.

Schunk, D. H., & Swartz, C. W. (1993). Writing strategy instruction with gifted students: Effects of goals and feedback on self-efficacy and skills. *Roeper Review, 15*, 225–230.

Schunk, D. H., & Zimmerman, B. J. (Eds.). (2008). *Motivation and self-regulated learning: Theory, research, & applications*. Mahwah, NJ: Lawrence Erlbaum Associates.

Sexton, M., Harris, K. R., & Graham, S. (1998). Self-regulated strategy development and the writing process: Effects on essay writing and attributions. *Exceptional Children, 64*, 295–311.

Shapiro, E. S., Durnan, S. L., Post, E. E., & Skibitsky-Levinson, T. (2002). Self-monitoring procedures for children and adolescents. In M. R. Shinn, H. M. Walker, & G. Stoner (Eds.), *Interventions for academic and behavior problems II: Preventive and remedial approaches* (pp. 433–454). Washington, DC: National Association of School Psychologists.

Silver, W. S., Mitchell, T. R., & Gist, M. E. (1995). Responses to successful and unsuccessful performance: The moderating effect of self-efficacy on the relationship between performance and attributions. *Organizational Behavior and Human Decision Processes, 62*, 286–299.

Stroud, K. C., & Reynolds, C. R. (2006). *School motivation and learning strategy inventory*. Los Angeles, CA: Western Psychological Services.

Urdan, T., & Midgley, C. (2003). Changes in the perceived classroom goal structure and pattern of adaptive learning during early adolescence. *Contemporary Educational Psychology, 28*, 524–551.

Wehmeyer, M. L., Agran, M., & Hughes, C. A. (2000). National survey of teachers' promotion of self-determination and student-directed learning. *The Journal of Special Education, 34*, 58–68.

Weiner, B. (1986). *An attribution theory of motivation and emotion*. New York: Springer.

Weinstein, C. E., Husman, J., & Dierking, D. R. (2000). Self-regulation interventions with a focus on learning strategies. In M. Boekaerts, P. Pintrich, & M. Zeidner (Eds.), *Handbook of self-regulation*. Orlando, FL: Academic.

Weinstein, C. E., & Palmer, D. R. (1990). *Learning and study strategies inventory: High school version user manual*. Clearwater, FL: H&H Publishing Company.

Winne, P. H. (2001). Self-regulated learning viewed from models of information processing. In B. J. Zimmerman & D. H. Schunk (Eds.), *Self-regulated learning and academic achievement: Theoretical perspectives* (2nd ed., pp. 153–189). Mahwah, NJ: Lawrence Erlbaum Associates.

Winne, P. H., & Hadwin, A. F. (1998). Studying as self-regulated learning. In D. J. Hacker, J. Dunlosky, & A. C. Graesser (Eds.), *Metacognition in educational theory and practice* (pp. 279–306). Hillsdale, NJ: Erlbaum.

Winne, P. H., & Jamieson-Noel, D. L. (2002). Exploring students' calibration of self-reports about study tactics and achievement. *Contemporary Educational Psychology, 28*, 259–276.

Winne, P. H., & Perry, N. E. (2000). Measuring self-regulated learning. In M. Boekaerts, P. Pintrich, & M. Zeidner (Eds.), *Handbook of self-regulation*. Orlando, FL: Academic.

Wolters, C. A. (1999). The relation between high school students' motivational regulation and their use of learning strategies, effort, and classroom performance. *Learning and Individual Differences, 11*, 281–299.

Wolters, C. A. (2003). Regulation of motivation: Evaluating an underemphasized aspect of self-regulated learning. *Educational Psychologist, 38*, 189–205.

Zimmerman, B. J. (1995). Self-regulation involves more than metacognition: A social cognitive perspective. *Educational Psychologist, 30*, 217–221.

Zimmerman, B. J. (2000). Attaining self-regulation: A social-cognitive perspective. In M. Boekaerts, P. Pintrich, & M. Zeidner (Eds.), *Handbook of self-regulation* (pp. 13–39). Orlando, FL: Academic.

Zimmerman, B. J. (2008). Investigating self-regulation and motivation: Historical background, methodological developments, and future prospects. *American Educational Research Journal, 45*, 166–183.

Zimmerman, B. J., & Bandura, A. (1994). Impact of self-regulatory influences on writing course attainment. *American Educational Research Journal, 31*, 845–862.

Zimmerman, B. J., Bandura, A., & Martinez-Pons, M. (1992). Self-motivation for academic attainment. *American Educational Research Journal, 31*, 845–862.

Zimmerman, B. J., & Campillo, M. (2003). Motivating self-regulated problem solvers. In J. E. Davidson & R. J. Sternberg (Eds.), *The nature of problem solving*. New York: Cambridge University Press.

Zimmerman, B. J., & Cleary, T. J. (2006). Adolescents' development of personal agency: The role of self-efficacy beliefs and self-regulatory skill. In F. Pajares & T. Urdan (Eds.), *Self-efficacy beliefs of adolescence* (pp. 45–69). Greenwich, CT: Information Age Publishing.

Zimmerman, B. J., & Cleary, T. J. (2009). Motives to self-regulate learning: A social cognitive account. In K. R. Wenzel & A. Wigfield (Eds.), *Handbook of motivation at school* (pp. 247–264). New York: Routledge/Taylor & Francis Group.

Zimmerman, B. J., & Kitsantas, A. (1996). Self-regulated learning of a motoric skill: The role of goal-setting and self-monitoring. *Journal of Applied Sport Psychology, 8*, 60–75.

Zimmerman, B. J., & Kitsantas, A. (1997). Developmental phases in self-regulation: Shifting from process to outcome goals. *Journal of Educational Psychology, 89*, 29–36.

Zimmerman, B. J., & Labuhn, A. S. (2011). Self-regulation of learning: Process approaches to personal development. In K. Harris, S. Graham, & T. Urdan (Eds.), *APA educational psychology handbook*. Volume. 1: Theories, constructs, and critical issues (pp. 397–423). Washington, DC: APA Press.

Zimmerman, B. J., & Martinez-Pons, M. (1986). Development of a structured interview for assessing student use of self-regulated learning strategies. *American Educational Research Journal, 23*, 614–628.

Zimmerman, B. J., Moylan, A., Hudesman, J., White, N., & Flugman, B. (2008, June). *Assessing the impact of self-reflection training with at-risk college students: Error analysis, calibration, and math attainment*. Poster presented at the 2008 Research Conference of the Institute of Education Sciences, U.S. Department of Education, Washington, DC.

Zimmerman, B. J., & Paulsen, A. S. (1995). Self-monitoring during collegiate studying: An invaluable tool for academic self-regulation. In P. Pintrich (Ed.), *New directions in college teaching and learning*. San Francisco, CA: Jossey-Bass, Inc.

Zimmerman, B. J., & Schunk, D. H. (2001). *Self-regulated learning and academic achievement* (2nd ed.). Mahwah, NJ: Lawrence Erlbaum Associates.

Academic Emotions and Student Engagement

Reinhard Pekrun and Lisa Linnenbrink-Garcia

Abstract

Emotions are ubiquitous in academic settings, and they profoundly affect students' academic engagement and performance. In this chapter, we summarize the extant research on academic emotions and their linkages with students' engagement. First, we outline relevant concepts of academic emotion, including mood as well as achievement, epistemic, topic, and social emotions. Second, we discuss the impact of these emotions on students' cognitive, motivational, behavioral, cognitive-behavioral, and social-behavioral engagement and on their academic performance. Next, we examine the origins of students' academic emotions in terms of individual and contextual variables. Finally, we highlight the complexity of students' emotions, focusing on reciprocal causation as well as regulation and treatment of these emotions. In conclusion, we discuss directions for future research, with a special emphasis on the need for educational intervention research targeting emotions.

Emotions are ubiquitous in academic settings. Remember the last time you studied some learning material? Depending on your goals and the contents of the material, you may have enjoyed learning or been bored, experienced flow forgetting time or been frustrated about never-ending obstacles, felt proud of your progress or ashamed of lack of accomplishment. Furthermore, these emotions affected your effort, motivation to persist, and strategies for learning—even if you were unaware of these effects. Similarly, think of the last time you took an important exam. You may have hoped for success, been afraid of failure, or felt desperate because you were unprepared, but you likely did not feel indifferent about it. Again, these emotions likely had profound effects on your motivational engagement, concentration, and strategies used when taking the exam.

Empirical findings corroborate that students experience a wide variety of emotions when attending class, doing homework assignments, and taking tests and exams. For example, in exploratory research on emotions experienced by

R. Pekrun (✉)
Department of Psychology, University of Munich,
Munich, Germany
e-mail: pekrun@lmu.de

L. Linnenbrink-Garcia
Department of Psychology and Neuroscience,
Duke University, Durham, NC, USA
e-mail: llinnen@duke.edu

university students, emotions reported frequently included enjoyment, interest, hope, pride, anger, anxiety, frustration, and boredom in academic settings (Pekrun, Goetz, Titz, & Perry, 2002a). Until recently, these emotions did not receive much attention by researchers, two exceptions being studies on test anxiety (Zeidner, 1998, 2007) and research on causal attributions of success and failure as antecedents of emotions (Weiner, 1985). During the past 10 years, however, there has been growing recognition that emotions are central to human achievement strivings. Emotions are no longer regarded as epiphenomena that may occur in academic settings but lack any instrumental relevance. In this nascent research, affect and emotions are recognized as being of critical importance for students' academic learning, achievement, personality development, and health (Efklides & Volet, 2005; Linnenbrink, 2006; Linnenbrink-Garcia & Pekrun, 2011; Schutz & Lanehart, 2002; Schutz & Pekrun, 2007).

In this chapter, we consider academic emotions and their functions for students' engagement. As noted by Fredricks, Blumenfeld, and Paris (2004; see also Appleton, Christenson, & Furlong, 2008), student engagement is best viewed as a metaconstruct consisting of several components. In line with this view, we define student engagement as a multicomponent construct, the common denominator being that all the components (i.e., types of engagement) comprise active, energetic, and approach-oriented involvement with academic tasks. We distinguish five types of engagement: *cognitive* (attention and memory processes), *motivational* (intrinsic and extrinsic motivation, achievement goals), *behavioral* (effort and persistence), *cognitive-behavioral* (strategy use and self-regulation), and *social-behavioral* (social on-task behavior), as detailed in our later discussion of emotions and engagement. Given our focus on emotions as precursors to these five forms of engagement, emotional engagement (e.g., in terms of enjoyment of learning) is considered as an antecedent of other components of engagement in this chapter.

These five categories of engagement overlap substantially with the three broad categories of behavioral, emotional, and cognitive engagement described by Fredricks et al. (2004); however, we have expanded this framework to clarify the unique ways in which emotions relate to engagement. Specifically, within Fredricks et al.'s broad category of cognitive engagement, we differentiate among motivational, cognitive, and cognitive-behavioral engagement. Our conceptualization of behavioral engagement is similar to that proposed by Fredricks et al.; however, we take a narrower view focusing specifically on effort and persistence. We also extend Fredricks et al.'s framework to include social-behavioral engagement to better capture forms of engagement related to peer-to-peer learning.

Before discussing the relation of emotions to engagement, we begin by outlining different concepts describing students' emotions, including affect, mood, achievement emotions, epistemic emotions, topic emotions, and social emotions. Next, the effects of emotions on the five types of student engagement and resulting academic achievement are addressed. In the third section, we discuss the individual and social origins of students' emotions, including a brief discussion of the relative universality of mechanisms of emotions and engagement across contexts. We conclude by considering principles of reciprocal causation of emotion and engagement and their implications for emotion regulation, treatment of emotions, and the design of learning environments.

Concepts of Academic Emotions

Emotion, Mood, and Affect

In contemporary emotion research, *emotions* are defined as multifaceted phenomena involving sets of coordinated psychological processes, including affective, cognitive, physiological, motivational, and expressive components (Kleinginna & Kleinginna, 1981; Scherer, 2000). For example, a students' anxiety before an exam can be comprised of nervous, uneasy feelings (affective); worries about failing the exam (cognitive); increased heart rate or sweating (physiological); impulses to escape the situation

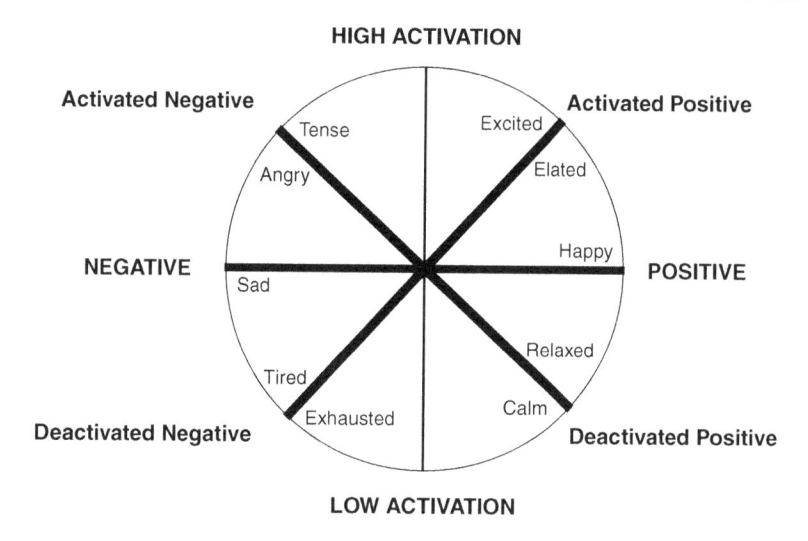

Fig. 12.1 Affective circumplex (Model adapted with permission from Feldman Barrett and Russell [1998], published by the American Psychological Association)

(motivation); and an anxious facial expression (expressive). As compared to intense emotions, *moods* are of lower intensity and lack a specific referent. Some authors define emotion and mood as categorically distinct (see Rosenberg, 1998). Alternatively, since moods show a similar profile of components and similar qualitative differences as emotions (as in cheerful, angry, or anxious mood), they can also be regarded as low-intensity emotions (Pekrun, 2006).

Different emotions and moods are often compiled in more general constructs of *affect*. Two variants of this term are used in the research literature. In the educational literature, affect is often used to denote a broad variety of noncognitive constructs including emotion, but also including self-concept, beliefs, motivation, etc. (e.g., McLeod & Adams, 1989). In contrast, in emotion research, affect refers to emotions and moods more specifically. In this research, the term is often used to refer to omnibus variables of positive versus negative emotions or moods, with *positive affect* being compiled of various positive states (e.g., enjoyment, pride, satisfaction) and *negative affect* consisting of various negative states (e.g., anger, anxiety, frustration). For example, in experimental mood research, most studies have compared the effects of positive versus negative affect on psychological functioning, without further distinguishing between different emotions or moods.

Valence and Activation

Two important dimensions describing emotions, moods, and affect are *valence* and *activation*. In terms of valence, positive (i.e., pleasant) states, such as enjoyment and happiness, can be differentiated from negative (i.e., unpleasant) states, such as anger, anxiety, or boredom. In terms of activation, physiologically activating states can be distinguished from deactivating states, such as activating excitement versus deactivating relaxation. These two dimensions are orthogonal, making it possible to organize affective states in a two-dimensional space. In *circumplex models* of affect, affective states are grouped according to the relative degree of positive versus negative valence and activation versus deactivation (e.g., Feldman Barrett & Russell, 1998; see Fig. 12.1). By classifying affective states as positive or negative, and as activating or deactivating, the circumplex can be transformed into a 2 × 2 taxonomy including four broad categories of emotions and moods (*positive activating*: e.g.,

Table 12.1 A three-dimensional taxonomy of achievement emotions

Object focus	Positive[a]		Negative[b]	
	Activating	Deactivating	Activating	Deactivating
Activity	Enjoyment	Relaxation	Anger Frustration	Boredom
Outcome/ Prospective	Hope Joy[c]	Relief[c]	Anxiety	Hopelessness
Outcome/ Retrospective	Joy Pride Gratitude	Contentment Relief	Shame Anger	Sadness Disappointment

[a] Positive = pleasant emotion
[b] Negative = unpleasant emotion
[c] Anticipatory joy/relief

enjoyment, hope, pride; *positive deactivating:* relief, relaxation; *negative activating:* anger, anxiety, shame; *negative deactivating:* hopelessness, boredom; Pekrun, 2006).

Academic Emotions

In addition to valence and activation, emotions can be grouped according to their object focus (Pekrun, 2006). For explaining the psychological functions of emotions, this dimension is no less important than valence and activation. Specifically, regarding the functions of emotions for students' academic engagement, object focus is critical because it determines if emotions pertain to the academic task at hand or not. In terms of object focus, the following broad groups of emotions and moods may be most important in the academic domain.

General and Specific Mood

Students may experience moods that lack a referent, but may nevertheless strongly influence their performance. Moods can be generalized, being experienced as just positive (pleasant) or negative (unpleasant), without clear differentiation of specific affective qualities. Alternatively, moods can be qualitatively distinct, as in joyful, angry, or fearful mood. While moods, by their very nature, may not be directly tied to a specific academic activity, they nonetheless have the potential to shape the way in which students' engage academically. For instance, a student in a negative mood may have difficulty focusing on the task at hand, thus limiting engagement.

Achievement Emotions

We define achievement emotions as emotions that relate to activities or outcomes that are judged according to competence-related standards of quality. In the academic domain, achievement emotions can relate to academic activities like studying or taking exams and to the success and failure outcomes of these activities. Accordingly, two groups of achievement emotions are activity-related emotions, such as enjoyment or boredom during learning, and outcome-related emotions, such as hope and pride related to success, or anxiety, hopelessness, and shame related to failure. Within the latter category, an important distinction is between prospective emotions related to future success and failure, such as hope and anxiety, and retrospective emotions related to success and failure that already occurred, such as pride, shame, relief, and disappointment. Combining the valence, activation, and object focus (activity versus outcome) dimensions renders a 3 × 2 taxonomy of achievement emotions (Pekrun, 2006; see Table 12.1). To date, research on achievement emotions has focused on outcome emotions such as anxiety, pride, and shame (Weiner, 1985; Zeidner, 2007), but failed to pay sufficient attention to activity emotions such as enjoyment and boredom.

Epistemic Emotions

Emotions can be caused by cognitive qualities of task information and of the processing of such information. A prototypical case is cognitive incongruity triggering surprise and curiosity. As suggested by Pekrun and Stephens (in press), these emotions can be called epistemic emotions since they pertain to the epistemic aspects of learning and cognitive activities. During learning, many emotions can be experienced either as achievement emotions or as epistemic emotions, depending on the focus of attention. For example, the frustration experienced by a student not finding the solution to a mathematical problem can be regarded an epistemic emotion if it is focused on the cognitive incongruity implied by a non-solved problem, and as an achievement emotion if the focus is on personal failure and inability to solve the problem. A typical sequence of epistemic emotions induced by a cognitive problem may involve (1) surprise, (2) curiosity and situational interest if the surprise is not dissolved, (3) anxiety in case of severe incongruity and information that deeply disturbs existing cognitive schemas, (4) enjoyment and delight experienced when recombining information such that the problem gets solved, or (5) frustration when this seems not to be possible (also see Craig, D'Mello, Witherspoon, & Graesser, 2008).

Topic Emotions

During studying or attending class, emotions can be triggered by the contents covered by learning material. Examples are the empathetic emotions pertaining to a protagonist's fate when reading a novel, the emotions triggered by political events dealt with in political lessons, or the emotions related to topics in science class, such as the frustration experienced by American children when they were informed by their teachers that Pluto was reclassified as a dwarf planet (Broughton, Sinatra, & Nussbaum, 2010). In contrast to achievement and epistemic emotions, topic emotions do not directly pertain to learning and problem-solving. However, they can strongly influence students' engagement by affecting their interest and motivation in an academic domain (Ainley, 2007).

Social Emotions

Academic learning is situated in social contexts. Even when learning alone, students do not act in a social vacuum; rather, the goals, contents, and outcomes of learning are socially constructed. By implication, academic settings induce a multitude of social emotions related to other persons. These emotions include social achievement emotions, such as admiration, envy, contempt, or empathy related to the success and failure of others, as well as nonachievement emotions, such as love or hate in the relationships with classmates and teachers (Weiner, 2007). Social emotions can directly influence students' engagement with academic tasks, especially so when learning is situated in teacher-student or student-student interactions. They can also indirectly influence learning by motivating students to engage or disengage in task-related interactions with teachers and classmates (Linnenbrink-Garcia, Rogat, & Koskey, 2011).

Functions for Students' Engagement and Achievement

Cognitive and neuroscientific research has shown that emotions, and affect more broadly, are fundamentally important for human learning and development. Specifically, experimental mood studies have found that affect influences a broad variety of cognitive processes that contribute to learning, such as perception, attention, social judgment, cognitive problem-solving, decision-making, and memory processes (Clore & Huntsinger, 2007, 2009; Loewenstein & Lerner, 2003; Parrott & Spackman, 2000). However, one fundamental problem with much of this research is that it used global constructs of positive versus negative affect or mood but did not attend to the specific qualities of different kinds of affects. As will be detailed below, this implies that it may be difficult and potentially misleading to use the findings for explaining students' emotions and learning in real-world academic contexts. Specifically, as argued both in Pekrun's (1992a, 2006; Pekrun et al., 2002a) cognitive/motivational model of emotion effects and in Linnenbrink-Garcia's research on affect and engagement (Linnenbrink, 2007; Linnenbrink-Garcia et al., 2011; Linnenbrink & Pintrich, 2004), it is not sufficient to differentiate positive from negative affective states but imperative to also attend to the degree of activation implied. As such, the minimum necessary is to distinguish between the four groups of emotions outlined earlier (positive activating, positive deactivating, negative activating, negative deactivating). For example, both anxiety and hopelessness are negative (unpleasant) emotions; however, their effects on students' engagement can differ dramatically, as anxiety can motivate a student to invest effort in order to avoid failure, whereas hopelessness likely undermines any kind of engagement. Even within each of the four categories, however, it may be necessary to further distinguish between distinct emotions. For example, both anxiety and anger are activating negative emotions; however, paradoxically, whereas anxiety is associated with avoidance, anger is related to approach motivation (Carver & Harmon-Jones, 2009).

Emotions can influence students' engagement, which in turn impacts their academic learning and achievement. By implication, as suggested in our earlier work (Linnenbrink, 2007; Linnenbrink & Pintrich, 2004; Pekrun, 1992a, 2006), we regard engagement as a mediator between students' emotions and their achievement. In the following sections, we first summarize research on the relation of emotions to the five types of engagement outlined at the outset (i.e., cognitive, motivational, behavioral, cognitive-behavioral, and social-behavioral engagement). We then outline implications for the effects of different emotions on students' academic achievement.

Cognitive Engagement

In our discussion of cognitive engagement, we focus on cognitive processes related to attention, mood-congruent memory recall, and memory storage and retrieval implying active involvement with academic tasks. Specifically, cognitive engagement refers to the way in which emotions shape cognitive resources and memory processes that are activated automatically (for intentional and more complex cognitive processes, see the section on "Cognitive-behavioral engagement").

Attention and Flow

Emotions consume cognitive resources (i.e., resources of the working memory) by focusing attention on the object of emotion. This effect was first addressed in interference models of test anxiety, which posited that anxiety reduces performance on complex and difficult tasks; this occurs because anxiety involves worries and produces task-irrelevant thoughts that interfere with task completion (e.g., Eysenck, 1997; Wine, 1971; see Zeidner, 1998). For example, while preparing for an exam, a student may fear failure and worry about the consequences of failure, which in turn may distract her attention away from the task. Interference models of anxiety were expanded by H. Ellis' resource allocation model, which postulated that any negative emotions can consume cognitive resources (Ellis & Ashbrook, 1988). Further expanding the perspective, recent studies found that not only negative emotions, but positive emotions as well can reduce working memory resources and attention (Meinhardt & Pekrun, 2003).

However, the resource consumption effect likely is bound to emotions that have task-extraneous objects and produce task-irrelevant thinking, such as affective pictures in experimental mood research, or worries about impending failure on an exam in test anxiety. In contrast, in task-related emotions such as curiosity and enjoyment of learning, the task is the object of emotion. In positive task-related emotions, attention is focused on the task, and working memory resources can be used for task completion. However, it is possible that some positive task-related emotions, such as overexcitement, may also distract attention away from the task. Corroborating these expectations, empirical studies with K-12 and university students found that negative emotions such as anger, anxiety, shame, boredom, and hopelessness were associated with task-irrelevant thinking and reduced flow, whereas enjoyment related negatively to irrelevant thinking and positively to flow (Pekrun, Goetz, Daniels, Stupnisky, & Perry, 2010; Pekrun, Goetz, Perry, Kramer, & Hochstadt, 2004; Pekrun, Goetz, Titz, & Perry, 2002b; Pekrun et al., 2002a; Zeidner, 1998). A similar pattern was observed with more global measures of positive and negative affect for college students (Linnenbrink & Pintrich, 2002a; Linnenbrink, Ryan, & Pintrich, 1999). These findings suggest that students' emotions have profound effects on their attentional engagement with academic tasks.

Mood-Congruent Memory Recall

Memory research has shown that emotions influence storage and retrieval of information. Two effects that are especially important for the academic context are mood-congruent memory recall and retrieval-induced forgetting and facilitation. Mood-congruent retrieval (Parrott & Spackman, 2000) implies that mood facilitates the retrieval of like-valenced material, with positive mood facilitating the retrieval of positive self- and task-related information, and negative mood facilitating the retrieval of negative information. Mood-congruent recall can impact students' motivation. For example, positive mood can foster positive self-appraisals and thus benefit motivation to learn and performance; in contrast, negative mood can promote negative-self appraisals and thus hamper motivation and performance (e.g., Olafson & Ferraro, 2001).

Retrieval-Induced Forgetting and Facilitation

Retrieval-induced forgetting and facilitation are basic functional mechanisms of human learning that currently get widespread attention in cognitive research. Retrieval-induced forgetting implies that practicing some learning material impedes later retrieval of related material that was not practiced, presumably so because of inhibitory processes in memory networks. In contrast, retrieval-induced facilitation implies that practicing enhances memory for related but unpracticed material (Chan, McDermott, & Roediger, 2006). With learning material consisting of disconnected elements, such as single words, retrieval-induced forgetting has been found to occur. For example, after learning a list of words, practicing half of the list can impede memory for the other half. In contrast, facilitation has been shown to occur for connected materials consisting of elements that show strong interrelations. For example, after learning coherent text material, practicing half of the material leads to better memory for the nonpracticed half.

Emotions have been shown to influence retrieval-induced forgetting. Specifically, negative mood can undo forgetting, likely because it can inhibit spreading activation in memory networks which underlies retrieval-induced forgetting (Bäuml & Kuhbandner, 2007). Conversely, it can be expected that positive emotions should facilitate retrieval-induced facilitation since they promote the relational processing of information underlying such facilitation. However, the generalizability of these laboratory findings to academic learning is open to question. If these mechanisms operate under natural conditions as well, they would imply that negative emotions can be helpful for learning lists of unrelated material (such as lists of foreign language vocabulary), whereas positive emotions should promote learning of coherent material.

Motivational Engagement

Motivation refers to processes shaping goal direction, intensity, and persistence of behavior (Heckhausen, 1991; Schunk, Pintrich, & Meece, 2008). Given the active, energetic, and approach-oriented role of these processes in both initiating and sustaining goal-directed academic effort, it is important to consider motivation directed toward task involvement as a form of engagement (for an alternative perspective, see Appleton et al., 2008). Of course, motivational engagement can in turn shape other forms of engagement (e.g., behavioral, cognitive, or cognitive-behavioral engagement), and motivational processes such as interests and values may not always translate into actually initiating and sustaining behavior. Nonetheless, it is useful to consider how emotions shape motivational engagement.

As compared to cognitive effects, the effects of emotions on motivational engagement have been less well studied. However, emotion research traditionally assumed that specific emotions function to trigger and facilitate impulses for specific action and thus play a role in initiating behaviors. Specifically, each of the major negative emotions is associated with distinct action impulses and serves to prepare the organism for action (or nonaction), such as fight, flight, and behavioral passivity in anger, anxiety, and hopelessness, respectively. For positive emotions, motivational consequences are less specific. Likely, one of the functions of positive emotions such as joy and interest is to motivate exploratory behavior and an enlargement of one's action repertoire, as addressed in Fredrickson's (2001) broaden-and-build metaphor of positive emotions.

In the academic domain, emotions can profoundly influence students' motivational engagement. The little empirical evidence available to date suggests that affect influences students' adoption of achievement goals, as addressed in Linnenbrink and Pintrich's (2002b) bidirectional model of affect and achievement goals. Specifically, it has been shown that pleasant emotions can have positive effects, and unpleasant emotions negative effects, on undergraduate students' adoption of mastery-approach goals (Daniels et al., 2009; Linnenbrink & Pintrich, 2002b). In line with this evidence, positive achievement emotions such as enjoyment of learning, hope, and pride have been shown to relate positively to K-12 and university students' interest and intrinsic motivation, whereas negative emotions such as anger, anxiety, shame, hopelessness, and boredom related negatively to these motivational variables (Helmke, 1993; Pekrun et al., 2002a, 2002b, 2004, 2010; Zeidner, 1998).

However, as addressed in Pekrun's (1992a, 2006) cognitive/motivational model of emotion effects, motivational effects may be different for activating versus deactivating emotions. This model posits that activating positive emotions (e.g., joy, hope, pride) promote motivational engagement, whereas deactivating emotions (e.g., hopelessness, boredom) undermine motivational engagement (Pekrun et al., 2010). In contrast, effects are posited to be more complex for deactivating positive emotions (e.g., relief, relaxation) and activating negative emotions (e.g., anger, anxiety, and shame). For example, relaxed contentment following success can be expected to reduce immediate motivation to reengage with learning contents, but strengthen long-term motivation to do so. Regarding activating negative emotions, anger, anxiety, and shame have been found to reduce intrinsic motivation but strengthen extrinsic motivation to invest effort in order to avoid failure, especially so when expectations to prevent failure and attain success are favorable (Turner & Schallert, 2001). Due to these variable effects on different kinds of motivation, the effects of these emotions on students' overall motivation to learn can be variable as well.

Behavioral Engagement

Behavioral engagement refers to effort and persistence, with an emphasis on the amount or quantity of engagement rather than its quality (Fredricks et al., 2004; Pintrich, 2000). Several psychological models suggest that positive affect leads to behavioral disengagement, either because one is progressing at a sufficient rate toward one's goals (Carver, Lawrence, & Scheier, 1996) or because it signals that all is well and there is no need to engage (Schwartz & Clore, 1996). Other models question this perspective and instead suggest that positive affect frees resources away from a threat, allowing more expansive task-related action (Fredrickson, 2001). Negative emotions such as sadness (for approach goals) and anxiety (for avoidance goals) may signal that one is not making sufficient progress toward one's goals or that there is a threat in the environment, suggesting that they may also contribute to intensified effort (Carver et al., 1996).

However, these perspectives do not consider the interplay between valence and activation and thus may not fully capture the way in which emotions shape behavioral engagement in academic settings. As noted, activating versus deactivating emotions can exert different effects on students' motivation. By implication, the effects on resulting effort and persistence can differ as well. There is general support that positive activating emotions such as enjoyment of learning are positively associated with effort (Ainley, Corrigan, & Richardson, 2005; Efklides & Petkaki, 2005; Pekrun et al., 2002a, 2002b; Pekrun, Frenzel, Goetz, & Perry, 2007), and that negative deactivating emotions such as hopelessness and boredom are negatively associated with effort (Linnenbrink, 2007; Pekrun et al., 2002a, 2010). In contrast, effects have been shown to be more variable for negative activating emotions such as anger, anxiety, and shame. These emotions often show negative overall correlations with effort, but in some cases, they may support behavioral engagement as they can serve to energize students (Linnenbrink, 2007; Pekrun et al., 2002a; Turner & Schallert, 2001).

Cognitive-Behavioral Engagement

Cognitive-behavioral engagement refers to complex cognitive processes that are intentionally instigated by the learner, including cognitive problem-solving, use of cognitive and metacognitive learning strategies, and self-regulation of learning. These processes are similar to what Fredricks et al. (2004) referred to as cognitive engagement. We use the term cognitive-behavioral engagement to differentiate these processes both from automatic cognitive processes described earlier and from pure quantity of effort as reflected by behavioral engagement.

Problem-Solving

Experimental mood research has shown that positive and negative moods impact problem-solving. Specifically, experimental evidence suggests that positive mood promotes flexible, creative, and holistic ways of solving problems and a reliance on generalized, heuristic knowledge structures (Fredrickson, 2001; Isen, Daubman & Nowicki, 1987). Conversely, negative mood has been found to promote focused, detail-oriented, and analytical ways of thinking (Clore & Huntsinger, 2007, 2009). A number of theoretical explanations have been proffered for these findings. For example, in mood-as-information approaches, it is assumed that positive affective states signal that all is well (e.g., sufficient goal progress), whereas negative states signal that something is wrong (e.g., insufficient goal progress; e.g., Bless et al., 1996). "All is well" conditions imply safety and the discretion to creatively explore the environment, broaden one's cognitive horizon, and build new actions, as addressed by Fredrickson's broaden-and-build theory of positive emotions. In contrast, "all is *not* well" conditions may imply a threat to well-being and agency, thus making it necessary to focus on these problems in analytical, cognitively cautious ways. Furthermore, positive emotions may facilitate flexible problem-solving via increasing brain dopamine levels (Ashby, Isen, & Turken, 1999), and negative moods may promote effort investment and performance on analytical tasks by inducing a need for "mood repair" (e.g., Schaller & Cialdini, 1990).

Learning Strategies

Judging from the experimental evidence on problem-solving, positive activating emotions such as enjoyment of learning should facilitate use of flexible, holistic learning strategies like elaboration and organization of learning material or critical thinking. Negative emotions, on the other hand, should sustain more rigid, detail-oriented learning, like simple rehearsal of learning material. Correlational evidence from studies with university students generally supports this view (Linnenbrink & Pintrich, 2002a; Pekrun et al., 2002a, 2004). However, for deactivating positive and negative emotions, these effects may be less pronounced. Deactivating emotions, like relaxation or boredom, may produce shallow information processing rather than any more intensive use of learning strategies.

Metastrategies and Self-Regulation

Self-regulation of learning includes the use of metacognitive, metamotivational, and metaemotional strategies (Wolters, 2003) making it possible to adopt goals, monitor and regulate learning activities, and evaluate their results in flexible ways, such that learning activities can be adapted to the demands of academic tasks. An application of these strategies presupposes cognitive flexibility. Therefore, it can be assumed that positive emotions foster self-regulation and the implied use of metastrategies, whereas negative emotions can motivate the individual to rely on external guidance. Correlational evidence from studies with university students is generally in line with these propositions (Linnenbrink & Pintrich, 2002a; Pekrun et al., 2002a, 2004, 2010). However, the reverse causal direction may also play a role in producing such correlations—self-regulated learning may instigate enjoyment, and external directions for learning may trigger anxiety.

Social-Behavioral Engagement

With the growing emphasis on constructivist forms of learning, student-student interactions have become increasingly important in shaping students' learning and achievement. Within these settings, students must engage socially with their peers. This type of social engagement includes behavioral engagement, such as engaging in discussion or listening to one's peers (Fredricks et al., 2004), but it can also include higher-order quality forms of social participation such as working cohesively, respectfully, and supporting other students' learning. Thus, we use the term social-behavioral engagement to refer to a range of social forms of engagement around academic tasks including participation with peers as well as higher-quality social interactions (Linnenbrink-Garcia et al., 2011). Social-behavioral engagement is distinct from other forms of engagement such as emotional engagement, which is focused more on students' emotions in relation to learning tasks, and on feelings of belonging which refer to a sense of general connectedness with peers, teachers, or the school (see Appleton et al., 2008). In this way, social-behavioral engagement includes support for high-quality social interactions that directly facilitate students' engagement and learning within peer-to-peer learning contexts through collaboration.

Instructional settings that require interactions with peers may present unique emotional challenges and evoke strong emotional responses (Crook, 2000; Do & Schallert, 2004; Jarvenoja & Jarvela, 2009; Linnenbrink-Garcia et al., 2011; Wosnitza & Volet, 2005). This is not surprising, especially given the key role that social agents play in shaping emotions across time (Denzin, 1984; Frenzel, Goetz, Lüdtke, Pekrun, & Sutton, 2009; Schutz, Hong, Cross, & Osbon, 2006). As such, we consider the interplay between emotions and social-behavioral engagement both in terms of direct peer-to-peer interactions as well as online peer interactions.

Direct Interaction

There is growing evidence that emotions relate to social-behavioral engagement in direct peer interaction, in both laboratory and field-based research involving small groups and class discussion. This research generally suggests that positive emotions such as feeling happy or calm promote social-behavioral engagement including active listening, supporting one's peers, and increasing group cohesion, while negative deactivating states, such as feeling tired, undermine engagement (Bramesfeld & Gasper, 2008; Do & Schallert, 2004; Linnenbrink-Garcia et al., 2011). Linnenbrink-Garcia et al. (2011) also found that both activated (tense) and deactivated (tired) negative affective states were associated with decreased social-behavioral engagement in the form of social loafing or allowing the other students during small group work to do all the work. Moreover, within small group settings, negative emotions seemed to sustain negative cycles of group interactions such as disrespecting other group members and discouraging their participation. However, this research also suggests that the interplay between emotions and social-behavioral engagement is complex, such that negative emotions can at times support rather than undermine social-behavioral engagement (Do & Schallert, 2004; Linnenbrink-Garcia et al., 2011).

Online Interaction

Studies analyzing online discussions and group work also suggest that emotions and social engagement are related (Nummenmaa & Nummenmaa, 2008; Vuorela & Nummenmaa, 2004; Wosnitza & Volet, 2005). For example, in a study of undergraduates working in an asynchronous web environment (e.g., students post comments and discuss ideas but are not required to interact in real time), social interactions were more likely to evoke emotional responses, as compared with other aspects of the learning environment such as the online web program or the technology (Vuorela & Nummenmaa). There was no relation between mean levels of emotion with social-behavioral engagement; however, students who had more variability (ranging from pleasant to unpleasant emotions) were found to engage more in the online exchange.

In sum, there is growing evidence that emotions are related to social-behavioral engagement when students work with their peers on academic tasks.

Broadly speaking, positive emotions seem to support social-behavioral engagement, while negative emotions can undermine it. However, with social-behavioral engagement as well, it is important to note that the nature of these relations is complex, suggesting the need to consider reciprocal and cyclical relations between emotions and social-behavioral engagement.

Academic Achievement

Since many different mechanisms of engagement can contribute to the functional effects of emotions, the overall effects on students' academic achievement are inevitably complex and may depend on the interplay between different mechanisms, as well as between these mechanisms and task demands. Nevertheless, it seems possible to derive inferences from the existing evidence and the above considerations.

Positive Emotions

Traditionally it was assumed that positive emotions, notwithstanding their potential to foster creativity, are often maladaptive for performance as a result of inducing unrealistically positive appraisals triggered by mood-congruent retrieval, fostering nonanalytical information processing, and making effort expenditure seem unnecessary by signaling that everything is going well (Aspinwall, 1998; Pekrun et al., 2002b). From this perspective, "our primary goal is to feel good, and feeling good makes us lazy thinkers who are oblivious to potentially useful negative information and unresponsive to meaningful variations in information and situation" (Aspinwall, 1998, p. 7).

However, as noted, positive mood has typically been regarded as a unitary construct in experimental mood research. As argued earlier, such a view is inadequate because it fails to distinguish between activating versus deactivating moods and emotions. As detailed in Pekrun's (2006) cognitive/motivational model, *deactivating* positive emotions, like relief or relaxation, may well have the negative performance effects described for positive mood, whereas *activating* positive emotions, such as task-related enjoyment or pride, should have positive effects.

The evidence cited earlier suggests that enjoyment preserves cognitive resources and focuses attention on the task; promotes relational processing of information; induces intrinsic motivation; and facilitates use of flexible learning strategies and self-regulation, thus likely exerting positive effects on overall performance under many task conditions. In contrast, deactivating positive emotions, such as relief and relaxation, can reduce task attention; can have variable motivational effects by undermining current motivation while at the same time reinforcing motivation to reengage with the task; and can lead to superficial information processing, thus likely making effects on overall achievement more variable.

Related empirical evidence is scarce, but supports the view that activating positive emotions can enhance achievement. Specifically, enjoyment of learning was found to correlate moderately positively with K-12 and college students' academic performance (Helmke, 1993; Pekrun et al., 2002a, 2002b). Furthermore, students' enjoyment, hope, and pride correlated positively with college students' interest, effort invested in studying, elaboration of learning material, and self-regulation of learning, in line with the view that these activating positive emotions can be beneficial for students' academic agency (Pekrun et al., 2002a, 2002b). Consistent with evidence on discrete emotions, general positive affect has also been found to correlate positively with students' cognitive engagement (Linnenbrink, 2007). However, some studies have found null relations between activating positive emotions (or affect) and individual engagement and achievement (Linnenbrink, 2007; Pekrun, Elliot, & Maier, 2009). Also, caution should be exercised in interpreting the reported correlations. Linkages between emotions and achievement are likely due not only to performance effects of emotions, but also to effects of performance attainment on emotions, implying reciprocal rather than unidirectional causation.

Negative Activating Emotions

As noted, emotions such as anger, anxiety, and shame produce task-irrelevant thinking, thus reducing cognitive resources available for task purposes, and undermine students' intrinsic motivation. On the other hand, these emotions can induce motivation to avoid failure and facilitate the use of more rigid learning strategies. By implication, the effects on resulting academic performance depend on task conditions and may well be variable, similar to the proposed effects of positive deactivating emotions. The available evidence supports this position.

Specifically, it has been shown that *anxiety* impairs performance on complex or difficult tasks that demand cognitive resources, such as difficult intelligence test items, whereas performance on easy, less complex, and repetitive tasks may not suffer or is even enhanced (Hembree, 1988; Zeidner, 1998, 2007). In line with experimental findings, field studies have shown that test anxiety correlates moderately negatively with students' academic performance. Typically, 5–10% of the variance in students' achievement scores is explained by self-reported anxiety (Hembree, 1988; Zeidner, 1998). Again, in explaining the correlational evidence, reciprocal causation of emotion and performance has to be considered. Linkages between test anxiety and achievement may be caused by effects of success and failure on the development of test anxiety, in addition to effects of anxiety on achievement. The scarce longitudinal evidence available suggests that test anxiety and students' achievement are in fact linked by reciprocal causation across school years (Meece, Wigfield, & Eccles, 1990; Pekrun, 1992b). Furthermore, correlations with performance variables have not been uniformly negative across studies. Zero and positive correlations have sometimes been found, in line with our view that anxiety can exert ambiguous effects. Anxiety likely has deleterious effects in many students, but it may facilitate overall performance in those who are more resilient and can productively use the motivational energy provided by anxiety.

Few studies have addressed the effects of negative activating emotions other than anxiety. Similar to anxiety, *shame* related to failure showed negative overall correlations with college students' academic achievement and negatively predicted their exam performance (Pekrun et al., 2004, 2009). However, as with anxiety, shame likely exerts variable effects (Turner & Schallert, 2001). Similarly, while achievement-related *anger* correlated negatively with academic performance in a few studies (Boekaerts, 1993; Pekrun et al., 2004), the underlying mechanisms may be complex and imply more than just negative effects. In a study by Lane, Whyte, Terry, and Nevill (2005), depressed mood interacted with anger experienced before an academic exam, such that anger was related to improved performance in students who reported no depressive mood symptoms—presumably because they were able to maintain motivation and invest necessary effort. In sum, the findings for anxiety, shame, and anger support the notion that performance effects of negative activating emotions are complex, although relationships with overall performance are negative for many task conditions and students.

Negative Deactivating Emotions

In contrast to negative activating emotions, negative deactivating emotions, such as boredom and hopelessness, are posited to uniformly impair performance by reducing cognitive resources, undermining both intrinsic and extrinsic motivation, and promoting superficial information processing (Pekrun, 2006). However, in spite of the frequency of boredom experienced by many individuals in school today, this emotion has received scant attention, as has the less frequent, but devastating emotion of achievement-related hopelessness. An exception is experimental research on boredom induced by very simple, repetitive tasks, such as assembly-line, vigilance, or data entry tasks. Boredom was found to reduce performance on these tasks (Fisher, 1993). In education, boredom has been discussed as being experienced by gifted students (Sisk, 1988). The little evidence available corroborates that boredom and hopelessness relate uniformly negatively to students' achievement, in line with theoretical expectations (Goetz, Frenzel, Pekrun, Hall, & Lüdtke, 2007; Maroldo, 1986; Pekrun et al., 2002a, 2004, 2010).

In sum, theoretical expectations, the evidence produced by experimental studies, and findings from field studies imply that students' emotions have profound effects on their engagement and academic achievement. As such, administrators and educators should pay attention to the emotions experienced by students. Most likely, the effects of students' enjoyment of learning are beneficial, whereas hopelessness and boredom are detrimental for engagement. The effects of emotions like anger, anxiety, or shame are more complex, but for the average student, these emotions also have negative overall effects.

Origins of Academic Emotions

Given the relevance of students' emotions for their engagement, it pays to analyze their origins as well. While a more detailed review of the literature is beyond the scope of this chapter, we provide a short overview of current research in this section (for more comprehensive treatments, see Schutz & Pekrun, 2007; Zeidner, 1998). We first address appraisals and achievement goals as individual antecedents of students' emotions, and subsequently the role of learning tasks and social environments.

Appraisals as Proximal Antecedents

Generally, emotions can be caused and modulated by numerous individual factors, including situational perceptions, cognitive appraisals and emotion schemata, neurohormonal processes, and sensory feedback from facial, gestural, and postural expression (Davidson, Scherer, & Goldsmith, 2003; Scherer, Schorr, & Johnstone, 2001). However, the emotions experienced in an academic context pertain to culturally defined demands in settings that are a recent product of civilization. In these settings, the individual has to learn how to adapt to situational demands while preserving individual autonomy—inevitably a process guided by appraisals. As such, cognitive appraisals of task demands, personal competences, the probability of success and failure, and the value of these outcomes likely play a major role in the arousal of academic emotions, and research on the determinants of academic emotions from early on has focused on such appraisals.

Test Anxiety Research
Test anxiety studies were the first to address the appraisal antecedents of students' emotions. In these studies, appraisals concerning threat of failure have been addressed as causing anxiety. In terms of R. S. Lazarus' transactional stress model (Lazarus & Folkman, 1984), threat in a given achievement setting is evaluated in terms of the likelihood and subjective importance of failure ("primary appraisal") and in terms of possibilities to cope with this threat ("secondary appraisal"). A student may experience anxiety when her primary appraisal indicates that failure on an important exam is likely, and when her secondary appraisal indicates that this threat is not sufficiently controllable. Empirical research confirms that test anxiety is closely related to perceived lack of control over performance. Specifically, numerous studies have shown that K-12 and postsecondary students' self-concept of ability, self-efficacy expectations, and academic control beliefs correlate negatively with their test anxiety (Hembree, 1988; Pekrun et al., 2004; Zeidner, 1998).

Attributional Theory
In attributional theories explaining emotions following success and failure, perceived control plays a central role as well. In B. Weiner's (1985, 2007) approach, attributions of success and failure to various causes are held to be primary determinants of these emotions, except "attribution-independent" emotions which are directly instigated by perceptions of success or failure (happiness and sadness/frustration for success and failure, respectively). Pride is assumed to be aroused by attributions of success to internal causes (i.e., causes located within the person, such as ability and effort). Shame is seen to be instigated by failure attributed to internal causes that are uncontrollable (like lack of ability), and gratitude and anger by attributions of success and failure, respectively, to external causes that are under control by others. The stability of perceived causes is posited to be important for hopefulness and hopelessness regarding future performance. Findings from scenario studies asking students how they, or others, might

react to success and failure were largely in line with Weiner's propositions, as were findings from correlational field studies (Heckhausen, 1991; Weiner, 1985).

Control-Value Theory

While test anxiety theories and attributional theories have addressed outcome emotions pertaining to success and failure, they have neglected activity-related emotions. In Pekrun's (2006; Pekrun et al., 2007) control-value theory of achievement emotions, core propositions of the transactional stress model and attributional theories are revised and expanded to explain a broader variety of emotions. The theory posits that achievement emotions are induced when the individual feels in control of, or out of control of, achievement activities and outcomes that are subjectively important—implying that appraisals of control and value are the proximal determinants of these emotions (e.g., Goetz, Frenzel, Stoeger, & Hall, 2010). Control appraisals pertain to the perceived controllability of actions and outcomes, as implied by related causal expectations (self-efficacy expectations and outcome expectations), causal attributions, and competence appraisals. Value appraisals relate to the subjective importance of these activities and outcomes.

Different combinations of control and value appraisals are proposed to instigate different achievement emotions. Prospective, anticipatory joy and hopelessness are expected to be triggered when there is high perceived control (joy) or a complete lack of perceived control (hopelessness). For example, a student who believes he has the necessary resources to get an A+ on an important exam may feel joyous about the prospect of receiving such a grade. Conversely, if he believes he is incapable of preventing to fail the exam, he may experience hopelessness. Prospective hope and anxiety are instigated when there is uncertainty about control, the attentional focus being on anticipated success in the case of hope, and on anticipated failure in the case of anxiety. For example, a student who is unsure about being able to master an important exam may hope for success, fear failure, or both. Similarly, retrospective pride, shame, gratitude, and anger are also seen to be induced by appraisals of control and value.

Regarding activity emotions, enjoyment of achievement activities is proposed to depend on a combination of positive competence appraisals and positive appraisals of the intrinsic value of the action (e.g., studying) and its reference objects (e.g., learning material). For example, a student is expected to enjoy learning if she feels competent to meet the demands of the learning task and values the learning material. If she feels incompetent, or is disinterested in the material, studying is not enjoyable. Anger and frustration are aroused when the intrinsic value of the activity is negative (e.g., when working on a difficult project is perceived as taking too much effort which is experienced as aversive). Finally, boredom is experienced when the activity lacks any intrinsic incentive value (Pekrun et al., 2010).

Nonreflective Induction of Emotions

Importantly, emotions need not always be mediated by conscious appraisals. Rather, recurring appraisal-based induction of emotions can become automatic and nonreflective over time. When academic activities are repeated over and over again, appraisals and the induction of emotions can become routinized to the extent that there is no longer any conscious mediation of emotions—or no longer any cognitive mediation at all (Reisenzein, 2001). In the procedural emotion schemata established by routinization, situation perception and emotion are directly linked such that perceptions can automatically induce the emotion (e.g., the mere smell of a chemistry lab inducing joy). However, when the situation changes or attempts are made to change the emotion (as in psychotherapy), appraisals come into play again.

The Role of Achievement-Related Goals and Orientations

To the extent that cognitive appraisals are proximal determinants of achievement emotions, more distal individual antecedents, such as gender or achievement-related beliefs, should affect these emotions by first influencing appraisals (Fig. 12.2;

```
Environment          Appraisal           Emotion         Engagement +
                                                         Achievement
```

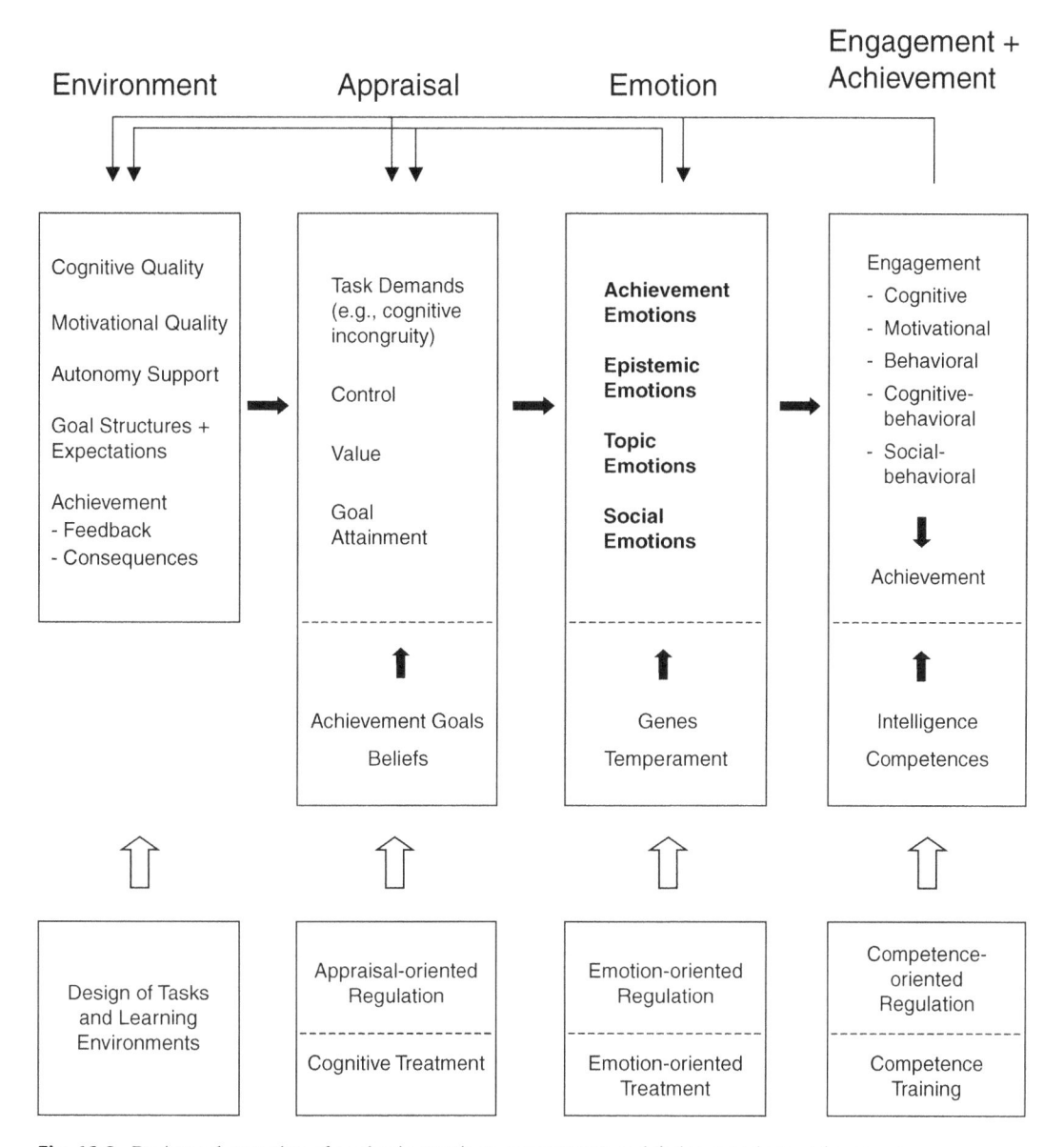

Environment	Appraisal	Emotion	Engagement + Achievement
Cognitive Quality	Task Demands (e.g., cognitive incongruity)	**Achievement Emotions**	Engagement - Cognitive
Motivational Quality			- Motivational
Autonomy Support	Control	**Epistemic Emotions**	- Behavioral - Cognitive-behavioral
Goal Structures + Expectations	Value	**Topic Emotions**	- Social-behavioral
Achievement - Feedback - Consequences	Goal Attainment	**Social Emotions**	Achievement
	Achievement Goals Beliefs	Genes Temperament	Intelligence Competences
Design of Tasks and Learning Environments	Appraisal-oriented Regulation Cognitive Treatment	Emotion-oriented Regulation Emotion-oriented Treatment	Competence-oriented Regulation Competence Training

Fig. 12.2 Reciprocal causation of academic emotions, engagement, and their antecedents and outcomes

Pekrun, 2006). This can also be assumed for the influence of achievement-related goals and goal orientations which are thought to direct attentional focus in the course of achievement activities. Specifically, these goals and orientations provide a lens through which individuals interpret and respond to achievement-related settings (Dweck & Leggett, 1988). *Achievement goals* can be defined as the competence-relevant aims that individuals strive for in achievement settings (Elliot, 2005), with different goals being related to different definitions of achievement. In mastery goals, achievement is judged by intraindividual standards or absolute criteria; in performance goals, achievement is judged by normative standards comparing performance across individuals. *Achievement goal orientations* are broader cognitive schemas that comprise achievement goals as well as associated reasons to pursue these goals (Maehr & Zusho, 2009;

Pintrich, 2000). Mastery goal orientations focus on developing competence and learning, whereas performance goal orientations focus on demonstrating competence, often in relation to the others (Dweck & Leggett). Researchers have also proposed that these primary goals and orientations can be further differentiated into approach and avoidance dimensions (Elliot, 1999; Elliot & McGregor, 2001; Pintrich, 2000). In this way, individuals can strive toward success or away from failure, resulting in four possible goals and goal orientations (mastery-approach, mastery-avoidance, performance-approach, performance-avoidance; for a recent revision of this framework, see Elliot, Murayama, & Pekrun, 2011).

As achievement-related goals and goal orientations are central to achievement motivation (Dweck & Leggett, 1988; Elliot & McGregor, 2001; Nicholls, 1984), understanding their relations with emotions is of specific importance for explaining students' engagement. The relation can be explained by assuming that different goals and orientations focus attention on different aspects of current academic activities, thus promoting different kinds of appraisals. Specifically, goals can promote appraisals of the controllability and value of achievement, and of the rate of progress toward goal attainment. Furthermore, they can differentially focus the individual on the task versus the self.

In terms of controllability and value, Pekrun's (2006; Pekrun, Elliot, & Maier, 2006; Pekrun et al., 2009) control-value theory implies that mastery goals should focus attention on the controllability and positive values of task activities, thus promoting positive activity emotions such as enjoyment of learning and reducing negative activity emotions such as boredom. Performance-approach goals should focus attention on the controllability and positive values of success, thus facilitating positive outcome emotions such as hope and pride, and performance-avoidance goals should focus attention on the uncontrollability and negative value of failure, thus inducing negative outcome emotions such as anxiety, shame, and hopelessness.

In terms of the rate of progress toward goal attainment, Linnenbrink and Pintrich's (2002b; Linnenbrink, 2007; Tyson, Linnenbrink-Garcia, & Hill, 2009) bidirectional model of goals and affect proposes that mastery goals promote perceptions of progress toward success since progress is judged relative to one's own improvement, thus facilitating emotions such as elation and happiness. Performance-approach goals are thought to promote emotions such as sadness for the many individuals who perceive insufficient progress toward success due to competition with others, and happiness for those who do perceive sufficient progress; performance-avoidance goals promote perceptions of moving away from or toward failure, thus facilitating relief or anxiety, respectively. Both performance-approach and performance-avoidance goals are proposed to be associated with anxiety, due to the heightened focus on the self. As such, performance-approach goal orientations in particular should be associated with a range of emotions including elation, happiness, sadness, and anxiety, depending both on perceived progress and the salience of the self. Overall, the predictions derived from the two models are complementary and largely consistent, with few exceptions such as differences in the proposed links for hopelessness and sadness (see Pekrun & Stephens, 2009; Tyson et al., 2009).

The available evidence corroborates that students' goals affect their emotions. Relations between achievement goals and omnibus variables of general positive and negative affect tend to lack consistency (Linnenbrink & Pintrich, 2002b; Pekrun et al., 2006, 2009); however, there are fairly clear linkages with discrete achievement emotions, especially for mastery and performance-avoidance goals. The relation between performance-avoidance goals and test anxiety is best documented, but recent research also shows consistent relations for mastery goals and activity emotions (positive for enjoyment, negative for boredom) and for performance goals and outcome emotions other than anxiety, such as pride, shame, and hopelessness (Daniels et al., 2009; Linnenbrink, 2007; Linnenbrink & Pintrich, 2002b; Mouratidis, Vansteenkiste, Lens, & Auweele, 2009; Pekrun et al., 2006, 2009). The close relation between achievement-related goals and subsequent emotions also implies that emotions can function as mediators of the effects of achievement goals on engagement and achievement. For example, in research by Linnenbrink et al. (1999), general negative affect was a mediator of mastery goal effects on task performance. Similarly, in studies by Elliot and McGregor (1999) and Pekrun et al. (2009), performance-avoidance goals predicted anxiety which in turn was a negative predictor of achievement, implying that anxiety mediated the effects of performance-avoidance goals on achievement.

The Influence of Tasks and Environments

The impact of task design and learning environments on students' emotions is largely unexplored, with the exception of research on the antecedents of test anxiety (see Wigfield & Eccles, 1990; Zeidner, 1998, 2007) and task interest/enjoyment (e.g., Deci & Ryan, 1987). Lack of structure and clarity in classroom instruction and exams, as well as excessively high task demands, relate positively to students' test anxiety. These effects are likely mediated by students' perceptions of low control and resulting expectancies of failure (Pekrun, 1992b). Furthermore, the format of tasks has been found to be relevant. Open-ended formats (e.g., essay questions) seem to induce more anxiety than multiple-choice formats, likely due to higher working memory demands which are difficult to meet when memory capacity is used for worrying about failure (Shaha, 1984; Zeidner, 1987). In contrast, giving individuals the choice between tasks, relaxing time constraints, and giving second chances in terms of retaking tests have been found to reduce test anxiety, presumably so because perceived control is enhanced under these conditions (Zeidner, 1998). These findings are in line with research demonstrating that task structures that function to promote autonomy and a sense of control are positively related to intrinsic motivation, cognitive flexibility, positive affect, and well-being (e.g., Deci & Ryan, 1987).

Regarding social environments, high achievement expectancies from important others, negative feedback after performance, and negative consequences of poor performance (e.g., public humiliation) show moderate to strong positive correlations with students' test anxiety (Pekrun, 1992b; Zeidner, 1998). Also, individual competition in classrooms is positively related to students' anxiety, presumably because competition reduces expectancies for success and increases the importance of avoiding failure (Wigfield & Eccles, 1990). In contrast, in K-12 research, social support from parents and teachers and a cooperative classroom climate have been found to be uncorrelated with students' test anxiety scores (Hembree, 1988). Negative feedback loops of support and anxiety may account for this surprising noncorrelation. Social support can alleviate anxiety (negative effect of support on anxiety), but anxiety can provoke support in the first place (positive effect of anxiety on support), thus yielding an overall zero correlation.

The quality of tasks, expectations from significant others, and functional importance of achievement likely influence academic emotions other than anxiety as well. Related evidence is largely lacking to date. The following factors may be relevant for a broad variety of academic emotions (see Fig. 12.2).

Cognitive Quality

The cognitive quality of classroom instruction and tasks as defined by their structure, clarity, and potential for cognitive stimulation likely has a positive influence on perceived competence and the perceived value of tasks (e.g., Cordova & Lepper, 1996), thus positively influencing students' emotions and engagement. Specifically, the cognitive quality of tasks in terms of inducing appropriate levels of cognitive incongruity may be of primary importance for the arousal of epistemic emotions such as surprise and curiosity. In addition, the relative difficulty of tasks can influence perceived control, and the match between task demands and competences can influence subjective task value, thus also influencing emotions. If demands are too high or too low, the incentive value of tasks may be reduced to the extent that boredom is experienced (Acee et al., 2010; Csikszentmihalyi, 1975; Pekrun et al., 2010).

Motivational Quality

Teachers and peers deliver both direct and indirect messages conveying academic values. Two ways of inducing emotionally relevant values in indirect ways may be most important. First, if tasks and environments are shaped such that they meet students' needs, positive activity-related emotions should be fostered. For example, learning environments that support cooperation should help students fulfill their needs for social relatedness, thus making working on academic tasks more enjoyable and promoting their social engagement as discussed earlier. Second, teachers' own enthusiasm in dealing with tasks can facilitate the adoption of achievement values and related emotions (Frenzel et al., 2009; Turner, Meyer, Midgley, & Patrick, 2003). Observational learning and emotional contagion may be prime mechanisms mediating these effects (Hatfield, Cacioppo, & Rapson, 1994).

Autonomy Support

Tasks and environments supporting autonomy can increase perceived control and, by meeting needs for autonomy, the value of related achievement activities (Tsai, Kunter, Lüdtke, Trautwein, & Ryan, 2008). However, these beneficial effects likely depend on the match between individual competences and needs for academic autonomy, on the one hand, and the affordances of these environments, on the other. In case of a mismatch, loss of control and negative emotions could result.

Goal Structures and Social Expectations

Different standards for defining achievement can imply individualistic (mastery), competitive (normative performance), or cooperative goal structures (Johnson & Johnson, 1974). The goal structures provided in academic settings conceivably influence emotions in two ways. First, to the extent that these structures are adopted, they influence individual achievement goals (Murayama & Elliot, 2009) and any emotions influenced by these goals (Kaplan & Maehr, 1999; Roeser, Midgley, & Urdan, 1996). Second, goal structures determine relative opportunities for experiencing success and perceiving control, thus influencing control-dependent emotions. Specifically, competitive goal structures imply, by definition, that some individuals have to experience failure, thus inducing negative outcome emotions such as anxiety and hopelessness in these individuals. Similarly, the demands implied by an important other's unrealistic expectancies for achievement can lead to negative emotions resulting from reduced subjective control.

Feedback and Consequences of Achievement

Cumulative success can strengthen perceived control, and cumulative failure can undermine control. In environments involving frequent assessments, performance feedback is likely of primary importance for the arousal of academic emotions. In addition, the perceived consequences of success and failure are important, since these consequences affect the instrumental value of achievement outcomes. Positive outcome emotions (e.g., hope for success) can be increased if success produces beneficial long-term outcomes (e.g., future career opportunities) and provided sufficient contingency between one's own efforts, success, and these outcomes. Negative consequences of failure (e.g., unemployment), on the other hand, may increase achievement-related anxiety and hopelessness (Pekrun, 1992b).

In sum, individual antecedents as well as social environments and academic tasks shape students' academic emotions and, consequently, any emotion-dependent engagement with learning. Environments, goals, and appraisals can induce, prevent, and modulate students' emotions, and they can shape their objects and contents. Depending on individual goals and the learning environment provided, students' academic life can be infused with positive affect and joyful task engagement, or with anxiety, frustration, and boredom. However, the strong impact of tasks and the social environment does not imply that basic mechanisms linking students' emotions with their engagement vary as a function of task and social context. Rather, these mechanisms seem to be pretty stable across contexts (Pekrun, 2009). For example, concerning the context provided by different task domains, students' emotions experienced in mathematics, science, and languages differed in mean levels across domains, but showed equivalent internal structures and linkages with academic achievement across domains in recent research with high school students (Goetz et al., 2007). Similarly, in a cross-cultural comparison of Chinese and German high school students' emotions in mathematics, Frenzel, Thrash, Pekrun, and Goetz (2007) found that mean levels of emotions differed between cultures, with Chinese students reporting more achievement-related enjoyment, pride, anxiety, and shame, and less anger in mathematics. However, the functional linkages of these emotions with perceived control, important others' expectations, and academic achievement in mathematics were equivalent across cultures. Most likely, the general functions of emotions for students' engagement and achievement described earlier are universal across different task domains, social environments, and cultural contexts.

Reciprocal Causation, Emotion Regulation, and Therapy

Academic emotions influence students' engagement and achievement, but achievement outcomes are expected to reciprocally influence appraisals, emotions, and the environment (Pekrun, 2006; see Fig. 12.2). As such, academic emotions, their antecedents, and their effects are thought to be linked by reciprocal causation over time. Reciprocal causation may involve a number of feedback loops, including the following three that may be especially important. First, learning environments shape students' appraisals and emotions, as argued earlier, but these emotions reciprocally affect students' learning environments and the behavior of teachers and classmates. For example, teachers' and students' enjoyment of classroom instruction are likely linked in reciprocal ways, emotional contagion being one of the mechanisms producing these links (see Frenzel et al., 2009). Second, emotions impact students' engagement, and engagement affects students' emotions. For example, enjoyment of learning can facilitate students' self-regulation and use of creative learning strategies, as outlined earlier.

Creative, self-directed involvement with tasks may in turn promote students' enjoyment, suggesting that students' enjoyment and their strategy use are reciprocally linked. Similarly, emotions influence students' motivational engagement in terms of adopting various achievement goals, but these goals reciprocally influence students' emotions (Linnenbrink & Pintrich, 2002b). Third, by impacting engagement, students' emotions have an influence on their achievement. Academic achievement outcomes and feedback on these outcomes, however, are primary forces shaping students' emotions, again suggesting reciprocal causation.

In line with perspectives of dynamical systems theory (Turner & Waugh, 2007), it is assumed that such reciprocal causation can take different forms and can extend over fractions of seconds (e.g., in linkages between appraisals and emotions), days, weeks, months, or years. Positive feedback loops likely are commonplace (e.g., in reciprocal linkages between teachers' and students' enjoyment as cited earlier), but negative feedback loops can also be important (e.g., when failure on an exam induces anxiety in a student, and anxiety motivates the student to successfully avoid failure on the next exam).

Reciprocal causation has implications for the regulation of academic emotions, for the treatment of excessively negative emotions, and for the design of "emotionally sound" (Astleitner, 2000) learning environments. Since emotions, their antecedents, and their effects can be reciprocally linked over time, emotions can be regulated and changed by addressing any of the elements involved in these cyclic feedback processes. Regulation and treatment can target (a) the emotion itself (*emotion-oriented* regulation and treatment, such as using drugs and relaxation techniques to cope with anxiety or employing interest-enhancing strategies to reduce boredom; Sansone, Weir, Harpster, & Morgan, 1992); (b) the control and value appraisals underlying emotions (*appraisal-oriented* regulation and treatment; e.g., attributional retraining, Ruthig, Perry, Hall, & Hladkyj, 2004); (c) the competences determining individual agency (*competence-oriented* regulation and treatment; e.g., training of learning skills); and (d) tasks and learning environments (*design of tasks and environments*).

Emotion regulation and ways to treat excessive negative academic emotions have mainly been studied for test anxiety and related test emotions (e.g., Davis, DiStefano, & Schutz, 2008). Specifically, test anxiety treatment is among the most successful psychological therapies available, effect sizes often being above $d=1$ (Hembree, 1988; Zeidner, 1998). Empirical evidence on ways to regulate and modify academic emotions more generally is still largely lacking to date, with few exceptions (c.f., Nett, Goetz, & Hall, 2010).

Conclusion

As argued in this chapter, emotions are critically important for students' engagement with academic tasks. This is likely true for all major types of cognitive, motivational, and behavioral engagement contributing to students' academic success. However, much of the research supporting this conclusion has been conducted by cognitive psychologists, social psychologists, and neuroscientists in laboratory studies and is far removed from the reality of academic contexts. Except for studies examining test anxiety, which has been a popular construct in educational research since the 1950s (Zeidner, 1998), research on students' emotions in real-world academic settings is clearly in a nascent stage. Educational research is just beginning to acknowledge the importance of affect and emotions.

To better understand the role of emotions for engagement in school, we suggest several areas for future research. First, researchers should investigate a variety of forms of emotions (mood, achievement, epistemic, topic, social) that may be relevant in educational contexts. There is a growing body of research on achievement emotions, but relatively little research on epistemic emotions or social emotions. We still know very little about how emotions emerge in response to specific task elements or in relation to social interactions in the classroom. Given the close proximity of epistemic and social emotions to the learning activity itself, studying emotions at this level may be especially fruitful for understanding how emotions shape engagement in school. Second, diverse theoretical definitions have plagued emotion research in other fields. Thus, we urge researchers conducting research on emotions in educational settings to be clear about how they define emotions within the context of education and to carefully match the theoretical conceptualization of emotions with their assessment instruments. Third, within the field of psychological neuroscience, great strides have been made in understanding the neurological bases for emotions and their link to other aspects of neurological functioning (c.f., Davidson, Pizzagalli, Nitschke, & Kalin, 2003; Immordino-Yang, McColl, Damasio, & Damasio, 2009). Researchers studying emotions in the classroom should be aware of the implications of this research, especially with respect to the implicit aspects of emotions and the way in which emotions shape underlying cognitive processing. Fourth, as noted earlier, the reciprocal aspects of emotions are often neglected. Yet the models we discussed highlight the dynamic quality of emotions and engagement. Future research needs to develop better methods for unpacking these dynamic relations across time.

Finally, if we are to truly understand the role of emotions in classroom settings, we need to design learning environments that are emotionally adaptive for students and test the effectiveness of these environments. As yet, the few attempts to design academic environments that foster students' positive academic emotions have met with partial success at best (e.g., Glaeser-Zikuda, Fuss, Laukenmann, Metz, & Randler, 2005). The limited success may be due, at least in part, to the need for additional research about which emotions are especially beneficial in educational settings. Nevertheless, the success story of test anxiety research suggests that future research can be successful in developing ways to shape academic settings so that adaptive student emotions fostering students' engagement are promoted and maladaptive emotions prevented.

References

Acee, T. W., Kim, H., Kim, H. J., Kim, J.-I., Chu, H. R., & Kim, M. (2010). Academic boredom in under- and over-challenging situations. *Contemporary Educational Psychology, 35*, 17–27.

Ainley, M. (2007). Being and feeling interested: Transient state, mood, and disposition. In P. A. Schutz & R. Pekrun (Eds.), *Emotion in education* (pp. 147–163). San Diego, CA: Academic.

Ainley, M., Corrigan, M., & Richardson, N. (2005). Students, tasks and emotions: Identifying the contribution of emotions to students' reading of popular culture and popular science texts. *Learning and Instruction, 15*, 433–447.

Appleton, J. J., Christenson, S. L., & Furlong, M. J. (2008). Student engagement with school: Critical conceptual and methodological issues of the construct. *Psychology in the Schools, 45*, 369–386.

Ashby, F. G., Isen, A. M., & Turken, A. U. (1999). A neuropsychological theory of positive affect and its influence on cognition. *Psychological Review, 106*, 529–550.

Aspinwall, L. (1998). Rethinking the role of positive affect in self-regulation. *Motivation and Emotion, 22*, 1–32.

Astleitner, H. (2000). Designing emotionally sound instruction: The FEASP-approach. *Instructional Science, 28*, 169–198.

Bäuml, K.-H., & Kuhbandner, C. (2007). Remembering can cause forgetting – but not in negative moods. *Psychological Science, 18*, 111–115.

Bless, H., Clore, G. L., Schwarz, N., Golisano, V., Rabe, C., & Wölk, M. (1996). Mood and the use of scripts: Does a happy mood really lead to mindlessness? *Journal of Personality and Social Psychology, 71*, 665–679.

Boekaerts, M. (1993). Anger in relation to school learning. *Learning and Instruction, 3*, 269–280.

Bramesfeld, K. D., & Gasper, K. (2008). Happily putting the pieces together: A test of two explanations for the effects of mood on group-level information processing. *British Journal of Social Psychology, 47*, 285–309.

Broughton, S. H., Sinatra, G. M., & Nussbaum, M. (2011). "Pluto has been a planet my whole life!" Emotions, attitudes, and conceptual change in elementary students' learning about Pluto's reclassification. Manuscript submitted for publication.

Carver, C. S., & Harmon-Jones, E. (2009). Anger is an approach-related affect: Evidence and implications. *Psychological Bulletin, 135*, 183–204.

Carver, C. S., Lawrence, J. W., & Scheier, M. F. (1996). A control-process perspective on the origins of affect. In L. L. Martin & A. Tesser (Eds.), *Striving and feeling: Interactions among goals, affect, and self-regulation* (pp. 11–52). Mahwah, NJ: Lawrence Erlbaum Associates.

Chan, C. K., McDermott, K. B., & Roediger, H. L. (2006). Retrieval-induced facilitation: Initially nontested material can benefit from prior testing. *Journal of Experimental Psychology. General, 135*, 533–571.

Clore, G. L., & Huntsinger, J. R. (2007). How emotions inform judgment and regulate thought. *Trends in Cognitive Sciences, 11*, 393–399.

Clore, G. L., & Huntsinger, J. R. (2009). How the object of affect guides its impact. *Emotion Review, 1*, 39–54.

Cordova, D. I., & Lepper, M. R. (1996). Intrinsic motivation and the process of learning: Beneficial effects of contextualization, personalization, and choice. *Journal of Educational Psychology, 88*, 715–730.

Craig, S. D., D'Mello, S., Witherspoon, A., & Graesser, A. (2008). Emote aloud during learning with AutoTutor: Applying the Facial Action Coding System to cognitive-affective states during learning. *Cognition and Emotion, 22*, 777–788.

Crook, C. (2000). Motivation and the ecology of collaborative learning. In R. Joiner, K. Littleton, D. Faulkner, & D. Miell (Eds.), *Rethinking collaborative learning* (pp. 161–178). London: Free Association Books.

Csikszentmihalyi, M. (1975). *Beyond boredom and anxiety*. San Francisco: Jossey-Bass.

Daniels, L. M., Stupnisky, R. H., Pekrun, R., Haynes, T. L., Perry, R. P., & Newall, N. E. (2009). A longitudinal analysis of achievement goals: From affective antecedents to emotional effects and achievement outcomes. *Journal of Educational Psychology, 101*, 948–963.

Davidson, R. J., Pizzagalli, D., Nitschke, J. B., & Kalin, N. H. (2003). Parsing the subcomponents of emotion and disorders of emotion: Perspectives from affective neuroscience. In R. J. Davidson, K. R. Scherer, & H. H. Goldsmith (Eds.), *Handbook of affective sciences* (pp. 8–24). Oxford, UK: Oxford University Press.

Davidson, R. J., Scherer, K. R., & Goldsmith, H. H. (Eds.). (2003). *Handbook of affective sciences*. Oxford, UK: Oxford University Press.

Davis, H. A., DiStefano, C., & Schutz, P. A. (2008). Identifying patterns of appraising tests in first-year college students: Implications for anxiety and emotion regulation during test taking. *Journal of Educational Psychology, 100*, 942–960.

Deci, E. C., & Ryan, R. M. (1987). The support of autonomy and the control of behavior. *Journal of Personality and Social Psychology, 53*, 1024–1037.

Denzin, N. K. (1984). A new conception of emotion and social interaction. In N. K. Denzin (Ed.), *On understanding emotion* (pp. 49–61). San Francisco: Jossey-Bass.

Do, S. L., & Schallert, D. L. (2004). Emotions and classroom talk: Toward a model of the role of affect in students' experiences of classroom discussions. *Journal of Educational Psychology, 96*, 619–634.

Dweck, C. S., & Leggett, E. L. (1988). A social-cognitive approach to motivation and personality. *Psychological Review, 95*, 256–273.

Efklides, A., & Petkaki, C. (2005). Effects of mood on students' metacognitive experiences. *Learning and Instruction, 15*, 415–431.

Efklides, A., & Volet, S. (Eds.). (2005). Feelings and emotions in the learning process [Special issue]. *Learning and Instruction, 15*, 377–515.

Elliot, A. J. (1999). Approach and avoidance motivation and achievement goals. *Educational Psychologist, 34*, 169–189.

Elliot, A. J. (2005). A conceptual history of the achievement goal construct. In A. J. Elliot & C. S. Dweck (Eds.), *Handbook of competence and motivation* (pp. 52–72). New York: Guilford Press.

Elliot, A. J., & McGregor, H. (1999). Test anxiety and the hierarchical model of approach and avoidance achievement motivation. *Journal of Personality and Social Psychology, 76*, 628–644.

Elliot, A. J., & McGregor, H. A. (2001). A 2 × 2 achievement goal framework. *Journal of Personality and Social Psychology, 80*, 501–519.

Elliot, A. J., Murayama, K., & Pekrun, R. (2011). A 3 x 2 achievement goal model. *Journal of Educational Psychology, 103*, 632-648.

Ellis, H. C., & Ashbrook, P. W. (1988). Resource allocation model of the effect of depressed mood states on memory. In K. Fiedler & J. Forgas (Eds.), *Affect, cognition, and social behavior*. Toronto, Canada: Hogrefe International.

Eysenck, M. W. (1997). *Anxiety and cognition*. Hove, UK: Psychology Press.

Feldman Barrett, L., & Russell, J. A. (1998). Independence and bipolarity in the structure of current affect. *Journal of Personality and Social Psychology, 74*, 967–984.

Fisher, C. D. (1993). Boredom at work: A neglected concept. *Human Relations, 46*, 395–417.

Fredricks, J. A., Blumenfeld, P. C., & Paris, A. H. (2004). School engagement: Potential of the concept, state of the evidence. *Review of Educational Research, 74*, 59–109.

Fredrickson, B. L. (2001). The role of positive emotions in positive psychology: The broaden-and-build theory of positive emotions. *American Psychologist, 56*, 218–226.

Frenzel, A. C., Goetz, T., Lüdtke, O., Pekrun, R., & Sutton, R. E. (2009). Emotional transmission in the classroom: Exploring the relationship between teacher and student enjoyment. *Journal of Educational Psychology, 101*, 705–716.

Frenzel, A. C., Thrash, T. M., Pekrun, R., & Goetz, T. (2007). Achievement emotions in Germany and China: A cross-cultural validation of the Academic Emotions Questionnaire-Mathematics (AEQ-M). *Journal of Cross-Cultural Psychology, 38*, 302–309.

Glaeser-Zikuda, M., Fuss, S., Laukenmann, M., Metz, K., & Randler, C. (2005). Promoting students' emotions and achievement – Instructional design and evaluation of the ECOLE-approach. *Learning and Instruction, 15*, 481–495.

Goetz, T., Frenzel, A. C., Pekrun, R., Hall, N. C., & Lüdtke, O. (2007). Between- and within-domain relations of students' academic emotions. *Journal of Educational Psychology, 99*, 715–733.

Goetz, T., Frenzel, A. C., Stoeger, H., & Hall, N. C. (2010). Antecedents of everyday positive emotions: An experience sampling analysis. *Motivation and Emotion, 34*, 49–62.

Hatfield, E., Cacioppo, J. T., & Rapson, R. L. (1994). *Emotional contagion*. New York: Cambridge University Press.

Heckhausen, H. (1991). *Motivation and action*. New York: Springer.

Helmke, A. (1993). Die Entwicklung der Lernfreude vom Kindergarten bis zur 5. Klassenstufe [Development of enjoyment of learning from kindergarten to grade 5]. *Zeitschrift für Pädagogische Psychologie, 7*, 77–86.

Hembree, R. (1988). Correlates, causes, effects, and treatment of test anxiety. *Review of Educational Research, 58*, 47–77.

Immordino-Yang, M., McColl, A., Damasio, H., & Damasio, A. (2009). Neural correlates of admiration and compassion. *Proceedings of the National Academy of Sciences of the United States of America, 106*(19), 8021–8026.

Isen, A. M., Daubman, K. A., & Nowicki, G. P. (1987). Positive affect facilitates creative problem solving. *Journal of Personality and Social Psychology, 52*, 1122–1131.

Jarvenoja, H., & Jarvela, S. (2009). Emotion control in collaborative learning situations: Do students regulate emotions evoked by social challenges? *British Journal of Educational Psychology, 79*, 463–481.

Johnson, D. W., & Johnson, R. T. (1974). Instructional goal structure: Cooperative, competitive or individualistic. *Review of Educational Research, 4*, 213–240.

Kaplan, A., & Maehr, M. L. (1999). Achievement goals and student well-being. *Contemporary Educational Psychology, 24*, 330–358.

Kleininna, P. R., & Kleininna, A. M. (1981). A categorized list of emotion definitions, with suggestions for a consensual definition. *Motivation and Emotion, 5*, 345–379.

Lane, A. M., Whyte, G. P., Terry, P. C., & Nevill, A. M. (2005). Mood, self-set goals and examination performance: The moderating effect of depressed mood. *Personality and Individual Differences, 39*, 143–153.

Lazarus, R. S., & Folkman, S. (1984). *Stress, appraisal, and coping*. New York: Springer.

Linnenbrink, E. A. (Ed.). (2006). Emotion research in education: Theoretical and methodological perspectives on the integration of affect, motivation, and cognition [Special issue]. *Educational Psychology Review, 18*(4), 315–341.

Linnenbrink, E. A. (2007). The role of affect in student learning: A multi-dimensional approach to considering the interaction of affect, motivation, and engagement. In P. A. Schutz & R. Pekrun (Eds.), *Emotion in education* (pp. 107–124). San Diego, CA: Academic.

Linnenbrink, E. A., & Pintrich, P. R. (2002a). The role of motivational beliefs in conceptual change. In M. Limon & L. Mason (Eds.), *Reconsidering conceptual change: Issues in theory and practice* (pp. 115–135). Dordrecht, The Netherlands: Kluwer Academic Publishers.

Linnenbrink, E. A., & Pintrich, P. R. (2002b). Achievement goal theory and affect: An asymmetrical bidirectional model. *Educational Psychologist, 37*, 69–78.

Linnenbrink, E. A., & Pintrich, P. R. (2004). Role of affect in cognitive processing in academic contexts. In D. Dai & R. Sternberg (Eds.), *Motivation, emotion, and cognition: Integrative perspectives on intellectual functioning and development* (pp. 57–87). Mahwah, NJ: Lawrence Erlbaum.

Linnenbrink, E. A., Ryan, A. M., & Pintrich, P. R. (1999). The role of goals and affect in working memory functioning. *Learning and Individual Differences, 11*, 213–230.

Linnenbrink-Garcia, L., & Pekrun, R. (2011). Students' emotions and academic engagement: Introduction to special issue. *Contemporary Educational Psychology, 36*(1), 1–3.

Linnenbrink-Garcia, L., Rogat, T. M., & Koskey, K. L. (2011). Affect and engagement during small group instruction. *Contemporary Educational Psychology, 36*, 13–24.

Loewenstein, G., & Lerner, J. S. (2003). The role of affect in decision making. In R. J. Davidson, K. R. Scherer, & H. Hill Goldsmith (Eds.), *Handbook of affective sciences* (pp. 619–642). Oxford, UK: Oxford University Press.

Maehr, M. L., & Zusho, A. (2009). Achievement goal theory: The past, present, and future. In K. R. Wentzel & A. Wigfield (Eds.), *Handbook of motivation at school* (pp. 77–104). New York: Routledge/Taylor & Francis Group.

Maroldo, G. K. (1986). Shyness, boredom, and grade point average among college students. *Psychological Reports, 59*, 395–398.

McLeod, D. B., & Adams, V. M. (Eds.). (1989). *Affect and mathematical problem solving: A new perspective*. New York: Springer.

Meece, J. L., Wigfield, A., & Eccles, J. S. (1990). Predictors of math anxiety and its influence on young adolescents' course enrollment intentions and performance in mathematics. *Journal of Educational Psychology, 82*, 60–70.

Meinhardt, J., & Pekrun, R. (2003). Attentional resource allocation to emotional events: An ERP study. *Cognition and Emotion, 17*, 477–500.

Mouratidis, A., Vansteenkiste, M., Lens, W., & Auweele, Y. V. (2009). Beyond positive and negative affect: Achievement goals and discrete emotions in the elementary physical education classroom. *Psychology of Sport and Exercise, 10*, 336–343.

Murayama, K., & Elliot, A. J. (2009). The joint influence of personal achievement goals and classroom goal structures on achievement-relevant outcomes. *Journal of Educational Psychology, 101*, 432–447.

Nett, U. E., Goetz, T., & Hall, N. C. (2010). Coping with boredom in school: An experience sampling perspective. *Contemporary Educational Psychology, 36*, 49–59.

Nicholls, J. G. (1984). Achievement motivation: Conceptions of ability, subjective experience, task choice, and performance. *Psychological Review, 91*, 328–346.

Nummenmaa, M., & Nummenmaa, L. (2008). University students' emotions, interest and activities in a web-based learning environment. *British Journal of Educational Psychology, 78*, 163–178.

Olafson, K. M., & Ferraro, F. R. (2001). Effects of emotional state on lexical decision performance. *Brain and Cognition, 45*, 15–20.

Parrott, W. G., & Spackman, M. P. (2000). Emotion and memory. In M. Lewis & J. M. Haviland-Jones (Eds.), *Handbook of emotions* (2nd ed., pp. 476–490). New York: Guilford Press.

Pekrun, R. (1992a). The impact of emotions on learning and achievement: Towards a theory of cognitive/motivational mediators. *Applied Psychology, 41*, 359–376.

Pekrun, R. (1992b). Expectancy-value theory of anxiety: Overview and implications. In D. G. Forgays, T. Sosnowski, & K. Wrzesniewski (Eds.), *Anxiety: Recent developments in self-appraisal, psychophysiological and health research* (pp. 23–41). Washington, DC: Hemisphere.

Pekrun, R. (2006). The control-value theory of achievement emotions: Assumptions, corollaries, and implications for educational research and practice. *Educational Psychology Review, 18*, 315–341.

Pekrun, R. (2009). Global and local perspectives on human affect: Implications of the control-value theory of achievement emotions. In M. Wosnitza, S. A. Karabenick, A. Efklides, & P. Nenniger (Eds.), *Contemporary motivation research: From global to local perspectives* (pp. 97–115). Cambridge, MA: Hogrefe.

Pekrun, R., & Stephens, E. J. (in press). Academic emotions. In K. R. Harris, S. Graham, & T. Urdan (Eds.), *APA educational psychology handbook* (Vol. 2). Washington, DC: American Psychological Association.

Pekrun, R., Elliot, A. J., & Maier, M. A. (2006). Achievement goals and discrete achievement emotions: A theoretical model and prospective test. *Journal of Educational Psychology, 98*, 583–597.

Pekrun, R., Elliot, A. J., & Maier, M. A. (2009). Achievement goals and achievement emotions: Testing a model of their joint relations with academic performance. *Journal of Educational Psychology, 101*, 115–135.

Pekrun, R., Frenzel, A., Goetz, T., & Perry, R. P. (2007). The control-value theory of achievement emotions: An integrative approach to emotions in education. In P. A. Schutz & R. Pekrun (Eds.), *Emotion in education* (pp. 13–36). San Diego, CA: Academic.

Pekrun, R., Goetz, T., Daniels, L. M., Stupnisky, R. H., & Perry, R. P. (2010). Boredom in achievement settings: Control-value antecedents and performance outcomes of a neglected emotion. *Journal of Educational Psychology, 102*, 531–549.

Pekrun, R., Goetz, T., Perry, R. P., Kramer, K., & Hochstadt, M. (2004). Beyond test anxiety: Development and validation of the Test Emotions Questionnaire (TEQ). *Anxiety, Stress, and Coping, 17*, 287–316.

Pekrun, R., Goetz, T., Titz, W., & Perry, R. P. (2002a). Academic emotions in students' self-regulated learning and achievement: A program of qualitative and quantitative research. *Educational Psychologist, 37*, 91–106.

Pekrun, R., Goetz, T., Titz, W., & Perry, R. P. (2002b). Positive emotions in education. In E. Frydenberg (Ed.), *Beyond coping: Meeting goals, visions, and challenges* (pp. 149–174). Oxford, UK: Elsevier.

Pekrun, R., & Stephens, E. J. (2009). Goals, emotions, and emotion regulation: Perspectives of the control-value theory of achievement emotions. *Human Development, 52*, 357–365.

Pintrich, P. R. (2000). The role of goal orientation in self-regulated learning. In M. Boekarts, P. R. Pintrich, &

M. Zeidner (Eds.), *Handbook of self-regulation: Theory, research and applications* (pp. 451–502). San Diego, CA: Academic.

Reisenzein, R. (2001). Appraisal processes conceptualized from a schema-theoretic perspective. In K. R. Scherer, A. Schorr, & T. Johnstone (Eds.), *Appraisal processes in emotion* (pp. 187–201). Oxford, UK: Oxford University Press.

Roeser, R. W., Midgley, C., & Urdan, T. C. (1996). Perceptions of the school psychological environment and early adolescents' psychological and behavioral functioning in school: The mediating role of goals and belonging. *Journal of Educational Psychology, 88*, 408–422.

Rosenberg, E. L. (1998). Levels of analysis and the organization of affect. *Review of General Psychology, 2*, 247–270.

Ruthig, J. C., Perry, R. P., Hall, N. C., & Hladkyj, S. (2004). Optimism and attributional retraining: Longitudinal effects on academic achievement, test anxiety, and voluntary course withdrawal in college students. *Journal of Applied Social Psychology, 34*, 709–730.

Sansone, C., Weir, C., Harpster, L., & Morgan, C. (1992). Once a boring task always a boring task? Interest as a self-regulatory mechanism. *Journal of Personality and Social Psychology, 63*, 379–390.

Schaller, M., & Cialdini, R. B. (1990). Happiness, sadness, and helping: A motivational integration. In R. Sorrentino & E. T. Higgins (Eds.), *Handbook of motivation and cognition: Foundations of social behavior* (Vol. 2, pp. 265–296). New York: Guilford Press.

Scherer, K. R. (2000). Emotions as episodes of subsystems synchronization driven by nonlinear appraisal processes. In I. Granic & M. D. Lewis (Eds.), *Emotion, development, and self-organization: Dynamic systems approaches to emotional development* (pp. 70–99). New York: Cambridge University Press.

Scherer, K. R., Schorr, A., & Johnstone, T. (Eds.). (2001). *Appraisal processes in emotion*. Oxford, UK: Oxford University Press.

Schunk, D. H., Pintrich, P. R., & Meece, J. L. (2008). *Motivation in education: Theory, research, and applications* (3rd ed.). Upper Saddle River, NJ: Merrill Prentice Hall.

Schutz, P. A., Hong, J. Y., Cross, D. I., & Osbon, J. N. (2006). Reflections on investigating emotion in educational activity settings. *Educational Psychology Review, 18*, 343–360.

Schutz, P. A., & Lanehart, S. L. (Eds.). (2002). Emotions in education [Special issue]. *Educational Psychologist 37*(2), 67-135.

Schutz, P. A., & Pekrun, R. (Eds.). (2007). *Emotion in education*. San Diego, CA: Academic.

Schwartz, N., & Clore, G. L. (1996). Feelings and phenomenal experiences. In E. T. Higgins & A. W. Kruglanski (Eds.), *Social psychology: Handbook of basic principles* (pp. 433–465). New York: The Guilford Press.

Shaha, S. H. (1984). Matching-tests: Reduced anxiety and increased test effectiveness. *Educational and Psychological Measurement, 44*, 869–881.

Sisk, D. A. (1988). The bored and disinterested gifted child: Going through school lockstep. *Journal for the Education of the Gifted, 11*, 5–18.

Tsai, Y.-M., Kunter, M., Lüdtke, O., Trautwein, U., & Ryan, R. M. (2008). What makes lessons interesting? The role of situational and individual factors in three school subjects. *Journal of Educational Psychology, 100*, 460–472.

Turner, J. C., Meyer, D. K., Midgley, C., & Patrick, H. (2003). Teacher discourse and sixth graders' reported affect and achievement behaviors in two high-mastery/high-performance mathematics classrooms. *The Elementary School Journal, 103*, 357.

Turner, J. E., & Schallert, D. L. (2001). Expectancy-value relationships of shame reactions and shame resiliency. *Journal of Educational Psychology, 93*, 320–329.

Turner, J. E., & Waugh, R. M. (2007). A dynamical systems perspective regarding students' learning processes: Shame reactions and emergent self-organizations. In P. A. Schutz & R. Pekrun (Eds.), *Emotions in education* (pp. 125–145). San Diego, CA: Academic.

Tyson, D. F., Linnenbrink-Garcia, L., & Hill, N. E. (2009). Regulating debilitating emotions in the context of performance: Achievement goal orientations, achievement-elicited emotions, and socialization contexts. *Human Development, 52*, 329–356.

Vuorela, M., & Nummenmaa, L. (2004). Experienced emotions, emotion regulation and student activity in a web-based learning environment. *European Journal of Psychology of Education, 19*, 423–436.

Weiner, B. (1985). An attributional theory of achievement motivation and emotion. *Psychological Review, 92*, 548–573.

Weiner, B. (2007). Examining emotional diversity in the classroom: An attribution theorist considers the moral emotions. In P. A. Schutz & R. Pekrun (Eds.), *Emotion in education* (pp. 73–88). San Diego, CA: Academic.

Wigfield, A., & Eccles, J. S. (1990). Test anxiety in the school setting. In M. Lewis & S. M. Miller (Eds.), *Handbook of developmental psychopathology: Perspectives in developmental psychology* (pp. 237–250). New York: Plenum Press.

Wine, J. D. (1971). Test anxiety and the direction of attention. *Psychological Bulletin, 76*, 92–104.

Wolters, C. A. (2003). Regulation of motivation: Evaluating an underemphasized aspect of self-regulated learning. *Educational Psychologist, 38*, 189–205.

Wosnitza, M., & Volet, S. (2005). Origin, direction and impact of emotions in social online learning. *Learning and Instruction, 15*, 449–464.

Zeidner, M. (1987). Essay versus multiple choice type classroom exams: The students' perspective. *The Journal of Educational Research, 80*, 352–358.

Zeidner, M. (1998). *Test anxiety: The state of the art*. New York: Plenum.

Zeidner, M. (2007). Test anxiety in educational contexts: What I have learned so far. In P. A. Schutz & R. Pekrun (Eds.), *Emotion in education* (pp. 165–184). San Diego, CA: Academic.

Students' Interest and Engagement in Classroom Activities

Mary Ainley

Abstract

This chapter focuses on interest as a key motivational construct for investigating the relation between motivation and engagement. The emphasis is on identifying the links between the underlying interest processes and students' participation in achievement activities. It is suggested that a dynamic systems perspective with its emphasis on the individual as a self-organizing system provides a productive framework for future developments in understanding the sets of processes that support engagement. Central in this analysis will be an examination of the microprocess level to identify the process variables that combine in different patterns of student engagement. Addressing the relation between motivation and engagement at the microprocess level puts a major emphasis on the immediate context of the task and the broader classroom. However, these are nested within expanding contexts of school and community cultures, and the relation between interest processes and engagement in achievement activities will be considered within the framework of investigations into patterns of interest and engagement using data from the PISA 2006 international survey of science achievement.

At the beginning of this century, Hidi and Harackiewicz (2000) reviewed research on achievement goals and interest to address the issue of how educators might motivate the academically unmotivated. At one point in their review, Hidi and Harackiewicz stated that "All children have interests, motivation to explore, to engage, but not all children have academic interests and motivation to learn to the best of their abilities in school" (p. 168). This statement foreshadows a number of the questions that will be addressed in this chapter. It points to a range of motivations that can be seen in students and acknowledges that there may be a mismatch between students' motivation and what is required to achieve within school contexts. In this chapter, I explore the relation between students' interest and engagement in classroom activities.

It is clear from the recent literature that a lot of attention has been given to researching the

M. Ainley, Ph.D. (✉)
Psychological Sciences, University of Melbourne,
Melbourne, VIC, 3010 Australia
e-mail: maryda@unimelb.edu.au

motivation of achievement. As Fredricks, Blumenfeld, and Paris (2004) pointed out, the literature on motivation in education is more extensive and has more precise distinctions drawn within component categories than has been typical in the engagement literature. One strand in the motivation literature takes the form of research into the functioning of specific, tightly defined variables, for example, achievement goals (Hulleman & Senko, 2010; Sideridis, 2009). Another strand explores interconnections and overlaps between pairs of motivational variables, for example, interest and self-efficacy (Hidi & Ainley, 2007), and sets of motivation variables, (Murphy & Alexander, 2000). Yet another strand focuses attention on how these variables and interconnections between variables play out in classrooms and other schooling contexts (Boekaerts, de Koning, & Vedder, 2006; Turner, 2010; Wosnitza & Volet, 2009). In this chapter, I focus attention on the motivation construct of *interest* and use contemporary directions in the understanding of interest to explore relations between students' interest and engagement in classroom activities. My exploration will be organized in terms of the three key questions posed to the handbook authors:

1. What is your definition of engagement and motivation, and how do you differentiate the two?
2. What overarching framework or theory do you use to study and explain engagement and motivation?
3. What is the role of context in explaining engagement or motivation?

On Definition

Across most areas of educational research, there are differences in definition and differences in emphasis within definitions of motivation and engagement, and these contribute to the challenge of the debate. Over the last two decades, the literatures on both interest and engagement have witnessed a large growth in volume. The interest literature struggled with conceptual issues in the early 1990s and the bulk of references in education over the last decade have taken the broad distinction between situational and individual interest as a starting point. On the other side, some of the major reviews synthesizing the debate on engagement have been published more recently and are presenting some degree of consensus on the need to distinguish between types, components, or indicators of engagement. For example, Jimerson, Campos, and Greif (2003) summarized the findings of their review of engagement and associated terms such as "school bonding" and "school attachment" by distinguishing three dimensions: affective, behavioral, and cognitive. Fredricks et al. (2004) referred to the multifaceted nature of engagement specifying behavioral, emotional, and cognitive facets: a "multidimensional construct that unites the three components in a meaningful way" (p. 60). Skinner, Furrer, Marchand, and Kindermann (2008) separated factors that are "outside of the construct" as facilitators of engagement from features that are "inside the construct," that is, are indicators of engagement, or part of the essential character of engagement. The two included in their model are behavioral and emotional indicators but with acknowledgement that cognitive facets of engagement could be added to the model. While there seems to be general agreement concerning the tripartite dimensionality of engagement, there is also recognition of potential overlaps between behavioral, emotional, and cognitive aspects of engagement.

When it comes to the place of interest in these models, for Fredricks et al. (2004), interest is one of the variables grouped as emotional engagement along with values and emotions. Cognitive engagement includes "motivation, effort, and strategy use" (p. 64). Using somewhat different groupings, the taxonomy proposed by Christenson and Reschly (Appleton, Christenson, Kim, & Reschly, 2006; Reschly & Christenson, 2006) includes motivational concepts concerned with values and goals as cognitive engagement, while psychological engagement includes feelings of belonging, identification, and interpersonal relationships. Following this taxonomy, interest falls within the cognitive engagement domain.

At the same time as these distinctions are articulated, reviews of the engagement literature qualify their analysis with the caveat that there are overlaps between the groupings, and the classification of concepts such as interest and motivation highlight some of the difficulty in developing a single taxonomy of engagement that encompasses all of the relevant perspectives. While Fredricks et al. (2004) separate interest as a subset of emotional engagement and motivation as a subset of cognitive engagement, this chapter identifies interest as a subset of motivation, and this is consistent with the general understanding in the motivation literature. However, the overlaps within the engagement literature highlight the need for close scrutiny of these constructs and the relations between them.

Turning the Lens on Engagement

For my analysis of the engagement side of the relation, the starting point is a dictionary definition (*The Australian Oxford Paperback Dictionary*, 1999). Engagement and the associated verb "to engage" have a range of meanings that go far beyond the educational domain. All of the meanings, including those to do with betrothal, drawing battle lines, and employment, involve being occupied in an activity, for example, being engaged in conversation. However, whether used as the verb "to engage" or the noun "engagement," to convey meaning unambiguously, the term requires further specification of the activity that is occupying the subject's time and attention. Sometimes, in the educational research literature, the referent for engagement is explicit, for example, student engagement with school (Appleton et al., 2006, p. 427), engagement in instructional activity (Marks, 2000, p. 172), styles of engagement with learning (Ainley, 1993, p. 395), or engagement in school life (Linnakylä & Malin, 2008, p. 585). Sometimes, the activity is not specified although with knowledge of the context often the activity is clear by implication. However, the referent needs to be explicit to avoid the vagueness and overinclusiveness that can come with terms like engagement. Jimerson et al. (2003) make a similar point from their review of usage of terms associated with school engagement: terms such as "school bonding" and "school attachment." Jimerson et al. found that often these terms were not defined and the meaning of the term had to be deduced from the content of the measures used.

But, back to the dictionary definition. An additional meaning in general dictionary definitions comes from the field of mechanics, more specifically, the operation of gears. Gears engage or interlock for the purpose of moving the parts of a machine. The metaphor can be pursued further. Gears used for driving a car can be mapped onto levels of engagement in classroom activities. For example, top gear represents the level of being fully engaged. Low gear and neutral gear are indicative of lower levels of engagement, minimal activity and marking time, respectively. The metaphor can be followed through into disengaged behavior and to dropping out of school, which map onto reverse gear. Hence, engagement as a construct for understanding involvement in education, irrespective of educational level, implies connection between students and the activities of schooling; it implies participation whether that is measured as attendance (e.g., Willms, 2003), participation in extracurricular activities (e.g., Fullarton, 2002), completion of homework, attitudes to school, student-teacher relationships, and sense of belonging (e.g., Linnakylä & Malin, 2008; Willms, 2003).

Distinguishing Motivation and Engagement

One way of distinguishing motivation and engagement is to identify motivation as underlying psychological process and engagement as a descriptor for the level of involvement or connection between person and activity:

> Motivation is about *energy* and *direction*, the reasons for behavior, why we do what we do. Engagement describes *energy in action*, the connection between person and activity. (Russell, Ainley, & Frydenberg, 2005)

The same point distinguishing underlying psychological motivational processes from engagement as motivated action has been used and elaborated further by Appleton et al. (2006). They suggested that "one can be motivated but not actively engage in a task. Motivation is thus necessary, but not sufficient for engagement" (p. 428). It is important to notice here that the implication for the meaning of the term engagement is that the individual has connected with the content of the task (top gear) rather than simply performing the activity mechanically or pretending to perform the activity (low gear). Hence, describing students' engagement with learning mathematics implicates motivation for the activity, just as describing students' disengagement or disaffection with learning mathematics implicates lack of motivation for the activity.

Turning the Lens on Interest

To this point, the discussion has used the more general term motivation, and this sets the context for specific attention to the relation between interest, as a specific type of motivation, and engagement. Interest researchers and writers (see e.g., Hidi, 1990, 2006; Krapp, 2005; Rathunde & Csikszentmihalyi, 1993) often take Dewey's writings as a reference point for their definitions. Referring to interest, Dewey asserted that "the root idea of the term seems to be that of being engaged, engrossed, or entirely taken up with some activity because of its recognized worth" (1913, see Boydston, 1979, p. 160). This is "top gear" engagement, and the underlying psychological process is interest.

Consideration of the relation between interest and engagement directs attention to the underlying processes that function to connect learners and learning tasks. At its simplest level, interest is a core psychological process energizing and directing students' interaction with specific classroom activities: a very specific situational engagement. In addition, there are more complex levels of interest identified as individual or personal interest, and these depend on both the immediate situation and students' past experience with relevant learning domains as well as connections with many other forms of participation in schooling. The interest relation expressed in engagement with classroom activities implicates both situational and personal factors to different degrees and in different combinations.

A range of metaphors can be used to help elaborate qualities of connection inherent in the relation between interest and engagement. Two will be explored. The first metaphor is a **hook**. When an activity triggers interest, students readily engage with that activity. It is *as if* the activity or specific features of the activity snare the student, drawing them in to engage. The second metaphor is a **switch** that connects students' existing personal interests with opportunities to express those interests. Rather than being snared into the activity, this metaphor carries the implication that the activity is within the student's range of valued activities and that simply encountering the opportunity to engage switches open connections, and the person immediately engages with the activity.

As with all metaphors, both of these highlight some aspects of interest processes; neither captures the full spectrum. Each metaphor resonates with a different type of interest. Situational interest (Hidi, 1990; Hidi & Renninger, 2006; Krapp, 2005) refers to interest that is triggered or activated by features of a specific situation (the **hook** metaphor). As has been shown in research on situational interest, especially in relation to reading, exposure to a specific text or topic that is novel, or ambiguous (Schraw & Lehman, 2001; Wade, 2001), or that has to do with life and death issues or themes of universal significance (Hidi & Baird, 1988) will trigger arousal, attention, and positive affect which together prompt the person to engage with the text. With physical education activities, it has been shown that situational interest is triggered when students perceive the presence of some basic task features. Features such as novelty, opportunities for exploration and challenge, and instant enjoyment triggered situational interest in physical education tasks (Chen & Ennis, 2004; Sun, Chen, Ennis, Martin, & Shen, 2008). In mathematics classes, Mitchell (1993) reported how novel features of computer presentation of mathematical problems triggered situational interest (catch factors), but these features often did not maintain or hold interest. Perception of certain task features triggers the energy that is then invested in engagement with the activity.

On the other hand, individual interest refers to a positive orientation toward an activity or domain that has value for the person. For example, a young student is known to spend hours reading about "life in the middle ages," to watch any available films depicting stories of heroes from the middle ages, and is known to find the best websites for discovering more about medieval characters. What has been observed is the student's intense engagement with "life in the middle ages." The intensity of involvement and the fact that the student seeks every opportunity to engage and reengage with activities from this domain is an indicator of an individual or personal interest in "life in the middle ages." With this form of interest, it is not that the activity has triggered engagement. Engagement occurs when a person who has accrued knowledge and value for an activity, and who knows they enjoy the activity, perceives an opportunity to reengage. The individual interest in the learning domain ("life in the middle ages") adheres in the legacy of past experience that engenders anticipatory affect and expectations of finding out something important. The **switch** metaphor gives emphasis to the quickening of intention and activity that ensues when the student perceives an opportunity to engage in their valued activity. The complex set of psychological processes subsumed under the individual interest concept emphasize that students' existing interests represent their ways of valuing and interpreting contextual features in relation to potential activities. When there is a match between students' individual interest and specific contextual affordances, students readily embrace the activity expressing enjoyment, concentration, and a desire to find out more.

In short, when there is little or no existing interest relation between person and task, something needs to happen to start the forging of a link; specific situational features are the hook that initiates activity. On the other hand, when the student has an existing positively valued organization or schema, an individual interest, perceiving an opportunity for congruent activities can be sufficient for activity to occur. Opportunity is the switch that opens the connection between student and activity.

This exposition would be incomplete without consideration of another set of circumstances where interest has been shown to energize engagement. A form of interest with different origins is illustrated in findings reported by Sansone who has explored students' behavior when constrained to perform a boring task which involved copying a letter matrix (Sansone & Thoman, 2005; Sansone, Weir, Harpster, & Morgan, 1992). Confronted with this type of condition (an uninteresting task but contextual reasons for staying with the task), students used self-generated strategies to enhance their interest in the task and so maintained engagement. This form of interest is akin to situational interest, but there is no hook from the task. The student reorganizes or reconstructs their perception of the task, so there is some aspect of it that is ambiguous, uncertain, or has new meaning. Alternatively, the student may generate interest in the task through reshaping their perception of it to fit with personal meanings and interests.

In sum, whether it is situational interest, or individual interest, or a form of self-generated interest serving a self-regulatory function, interest is an important source of the energy and direction that sustains engagement with classroom activities.

Theoretical Orientation

In this section, we explore the implications of a dynamic systems perspective for understanding the relation between interest and students' engagement in classroom activities. By referring to a dynamic systems perspective, we are drawing on a set of theories loosely grouped as dynamic systems theories (see Lewis & Granic, 2000). One of the basic proposals in these theories is that an individual's behavior is best represented as a self-organizing system whereby pattern and internal organization emerge from the interactive experience of the individual in a changing environment (Thelen & Smith, 2006). From their research into perceptual, motor, and cognitive systems in infants and young children, Thelen and Smith suggested that self-organization can be observed in the "patterns assembled for task-specific purposes whose form and stability depended on both the immediate and more distant history of the system" (p. 284). Within the educational domain, Jörg, Davis, and Nickmans (2007) have suggested that this general perspective on behavior is equally appropriate for the learning sciences. They suggest that complexity is central in this paradigm. It involves dealing with concepts such as interactivity, reciprocal interactions, and connectivity, and more attention to these aspects of learning will advance understanding to support student learning. Dynamic systems concepts are gaining wider currency in the educational literature and are being applied to explore particular educational phenomena, for example, the consequences for learning processes when students experience academic shame (Turner & Waugh, 2007).

If we apply a dynamic systems perspective to the motivation of achievement behavior, each motivational construct can be viewed as an organization of psychological processes such as feelings, thoughts, and action tendencies. A student's current state of motivation is a unique organization of immediate experiences interacting with their history of experiences in relation to a specific learning situation. Students come to a new learning situation with active organizations or motivation schema. These are likely to include components such as achievement goals, interest, and competency beliefs. In addition, experiences that have occurred immediately prior to the new learning situation become part of the schema. At any point in time, the motivation schemas currently active play a part in the system of factors that influence how an individual student reacts to a new situation.

At the simplest level in any new situation, the student has a perception of the task which may or may not align with the intentions of the task designer. Task perceptions are likely to involve a distinct combination of expectations of what the task is about, anticipatory feelings, and estimates of what actions and effort might be required. However, because learning tasks are never completely novel, these perceptions will also draw on existing schemas with their inherent organization of feelings, thoughts, and action tendencies, and this adds to individual variability. In short, awareness and perception of particular properties of a new situation activates schemas that are organized units combining perceptions activated by the new situation and associated elements from existing motivational schemas. Such schemas guide students' behavior in relation to the new learning situation.

Process Schemas and Task Engagement

Some findings from a recent study illustrate this interdependence of past, present, and individual variability in students' engagement with a classroom activity. A range of variables, including mood, interest, achievement goal orientation, and students' assessment of their confidence and satisfaction with their performance on the task, were monitored as students worked online to complete an open-ended problem task (see Ainley, 2007; Ainley, Flowers, & Patrick, 2005). Before commencing the task, students completed a mood scale adapted from a short form of the positive and negative affect schedule (PANAS, Watson & Clark, 1994). This was repeated at the end of the session. Using cluster analysis techniques, three mood profiles were identified: a *happy* group with a profile of higher than average positive affect and lower than average negative affect, an *unhappy* group whose profile indicated low negative affect coupled with lower than average positive affect, and an *anxious* group distinguished by a profile of very high negative affect and low positive affect.

The same three mood profiles were identified at the end of the session. However, there were a number of students who changed their mood status. One third of the students reporting the *unhappy* profile at the start had changed (20 of 61 students), and at end of the task were reporting a mood profile that classified them with the *happy* group. Contrasting this group with those who maintained their *unhappy* mood profile provided an opportunity to investigate student characteristics and task responses that were associated with a change in mood while working on the problem scenario.

The students whose mood became more positive across the task had more positive personal achievement goal orientations as measured by an initial self-report. After the task was explained, self-reports of task interest and confidence about their performance were recorded. There was no significant difference between the group whose *unhappy* mood changed and the group with no change from their *unhappy* mood. However, what differed between these groups were their on-task responses to working on the problem scenario. A probe part way into the task asked students to report on their goal at that specific moment. Students whose mood became more positive reported higher on-task salience of both mastery and performance-approach goals. They were more likely to record higher ratings for the goals of understanding what they were doing (mastery: "right now my aim is to understand and learn as much as I can") and showing they could outperform other students (performance-approach: "right now my aim is to show I can do better than other students") than were the students whose mood did not change. Interest also increased across the task. In addition, post-task reflections from students whose mood changed reported a stronger sense of achieving their goals and feeling satisfied with the quality of their submitted answer. Hence, engagement with the new learning situation involved a complex interaction of initial and on-task mood changes, feelings of competence, and on-task goals, and one of the important components was interest.

The Role of Interest

A number of current theories of development focus on the adaptive significance of positive emotions. For example, Fredrikson's (2001) broaden-and-build theory of positive emotions proposes that positive emotions, interest, joy, and contentment are key factors in knowledge acquisition and creativity. More recently, Izard (2007) has drawn attention to the pervasive role that interest plays in a wide range of complex human behavior.

> Its (i.e., interest) ubiquity is further enhanced by its effectiveness in engaging and sustaining the individual in person-environment interactions that facilitate exploration, learning and constructive endeavours. (Izard, 2007, p. 272)

In his earlier writings, Izard (1977) used the construct of affective-cognitive structures to highlight the system of processes that through experience becomes organized around basic emotions. Beginning in infancy, the emotion of interest as an immediate positive state is triggered by small changes in the perceptual field. Interest engages an infant with the world of objects and leads to exploration; the brightly colored object that moves or emits a new sound is approached, inspected, and manipulated. With each new experience, these basic organizations of affect and cognition are expanded and reorganized. In the more recent formulations, these are referred to as emotion schemas, and within this model, interest schemas involve integrated systems of ideas and feelings (Izard, 2007). These propositions concerning the way that interest is implicated in a wide range of human behavior underscore the significance of understanding the development of interest schema for students' engagement with classroom activities.

Therefore, when we examine the concept of interest, we expect to find variation in the component processes and in relations between component processes at different levels of organization of interest schema. These variable patterns reflect the experiences that have built students' interest schemas, and so it is reasonable to expect common experiences within groups of students as well as experiences that are unique to individual students. In a recent paper, Frenzel, Dicke, Goetz, and Pekrun (2009) have demonstrated how the content of the meaning of interest varies when 5th grade and 9th grade students rate their interest in mathematics. Affective terms were prominent for both groups of students, but older students also included references to value and competency aspects. As has been argued previously, "part of the challenge for interest research is to identify those combinations of affect and cognitions functioning as interest schema at different levels of interest development" (Ainley, 2010, p. 237).

In what follows, some of our current understandings of interest schema specifically as they relate to the relation between interest and engagement will be elaborated.

Interest: Developmental Phases and Stages

Interest is not a unitary construct. Some of the most recent perspectives from educational research that are informative for identifying psychological processes that constitute interest are the models describing phases (Hidi & Renninger, 2006), or stages (Krapp, 2003), in interest development. Situational interest, defined as interest triggered by a specific situation, is the simplest form of interest, and both of these models conceptualize situational interest as the first step in the development of individual or personal interest.

Hidi and Renninger's (2006) four-phase model of interest development describes a sequence extending from the initial triggering of a situational interest through to a well-developed individual interest. At the most basic level, a newly *triggered situational interest* involves arousal of affect and focused attention toward the object triggering interest. If the situation is completely novel, this is the beginnings of a new schema. However, most educational contexts are not completely novel, and so elements of past experience with related situations are also aroused and have the potential to become part of the developing interest organization or schema. Further, interaction with and exploration of the new situation with associated feelings and thoughts allow dimensions of those feelings and new knowledge to become part of the developing interest schema. If this continues over time or is repeated a number of times across a relatively short period, the triggered situational interest develops into a *maintained situational interest*. The implication here is that there is a more stable organization of feeling, knowledge, and experience that makes up the interest schema. The initial positive affect may now be more differentiated and involve a combination of emotions. It is conceivable that negative emotion may sometimes be part of these schemas. More knowledge about the situation has been incorporated into the interest schema, and this extension in time makes it more likely that the interest schema will be triggered again in further similar situations. Continued opportunities to engage with the domain entail new and varied experiences. Each outcome adds to the developing interest schema, and over time, the schema becomes an important area of activity for the person. The interest schema is starting to take on the character of an individual interest or personal orientation, and this type of self-sustaining organization or schema is referred to in the four-phase model as an *emerging individual interest*. This phase of interest development is characterized by positive feelings, an accrued body of knowledge, and a sense that this domain is personally important and valued. The final developmental level is a *well-developed individual interest* and is identified by the depth of value, knowledge, and feeling that the person has for the domain and by independent seeking of opportunities for reengagement.

Krapp (2003) has proposed a similar model but distinguishes only three stages: "awakened or triggered" and "stabilized" stages of situational interest and individual interest. The underlying developmental trajectory is similar, but more emphasis is placed on value and feeling components as the core of individual interest.

Although these phases or stages define a developmental progression, it is possible for development to be terminated as interest in the situation lapses or dies. For example, when we next encounter the student who was passionate about "life in the middle ages," we observe that they have ignored the latest release movie set in the middle ages, that they have closed down their links to previously frequented middle ages websites, and that they have stopped reading books on "life in the middle ages." Their former passionate individual interest has lapsed. In addition, under certain circumstances, interest development may regress and revert to a simpler form. For example, our student who had the passionate interest in "life in the middle ages" may have their former interest activated when they see an advertisement for a new movie set in the middle ages, but they no longer seek out sources of information as they did previously. Their former individual interest appears to have reverted to a situational interest. Interest can still be triggered by certain events, such as the movie advertisement, but they no longer independently seek opportunities for reengagement.

Both the Hidi and Renninger (2006) and the Krapp (2003) models of interest development sketch distinguishing features for interest at each of the phases or stages of development. However, applying this framework to support student engagement with classroom activities requires ways to identify some of the richness and variability of the affective and cognitive dimensions that make up students' interest schemas. This issue has recently been taken up in relation to a particular applied educational issue: the problem of engaging students with challenging behavior in productive classroom learning activities. Ely and colleagues (Ely, Ainley, & Pearce, 2010) are using innovative software to develop a system for profiling the component processes distinguishing students' interest schemas. In particular, the tool has been designed to identify phases of interest development to assist teachers. Providing this level of detail about students' interests should assist teachers in their endeavors to establish and maintain students' engagement with classroom activities especially with students who might otherwise be uncommunicative.

Prototype software (MINE: Ely et al., 2010) has been developed and is being tested with young adolescent students. Using an interactive exploratory environment populated with approximately 60 "interest cells," students are able to explore the interest space in a way that allows them to discover ideas, activities, or "stuff" that they may not have previously encountered and might be interested in, as well as other familiar ideas, activities, and "stuff" that they may be interested in already. Students are asked to select a basket of at least three interests. Importantly, these interests may represent anything from newly triggered situational interests to well-developed individual interests. After choosing their basket of interests, participants use rating scales and open-ended comments to provide an in-depth profile of affective, cognitive, and experiential aspects of their selected interests. At the theoretical level, the interest profiles are being used to give further definition to some of the affective and cognitive dimensions associated with interest at the different phases of development. At the applied level, they will be used to inform curriculum design and development with the objective of supporting engagement in productive classroom activities for students with challenging behavior.

In short, interest is not a unitary construct. Knowledge of the phases of interest development and the psychological processes that go to make up specific interest schema at all phases of interest development will provide greater insight into ways that all students can be supported to engage with classroom activities.

Interest and Processes That Contribute to Engagement

In this section, we describe findings from studies using a general research design that involves students working on tasks constructed to highlight how interest and associated processes relate to some of the more readily observed indicators of students' engagement with learning tasks. Individual projects have recruited students as young as 5th grade and from secondary classes up to and including 10th grade. The number of participants has varied between 100 and 300 students, and while most of the studies referred to have been conducted with Australian students, some projects have included groups of Canadian students (see e.g., Ainley, Hidi, & Berndorff, 2002). Two general types of task have been used, one a reading task, the other an open-ended problem scenario requiring students to generate a solution which they present with supporting reasons. Both types of tasks are administered using interactive computer software, and the underlying structure of the software allows monitoring of students' decisions about the extent and direction of their actions. Hence, decisions and level of task activity are the indicators of engagement, while specific probes and questions concerning processes such as interest, other emotions, task efficacy, and task difficulty allow parallel self-report monitoring of key psychological process variables.

For the reading tasks, texts were divided into three, sometimes four, sections and were presented through a sequence of computer screens. Students were in control of the text screens, and the simple click of a button labeled "NEXT" allowed them to move to the next screen. When a student chose to move on, a screen asked whether they wanted to read more about the topic or to quit. From the sequence of possible choices, an index of persistence (number of text sections accessed) was generated. Initial interest in the topic as measured by a 5-point Likert rating was predictive of this index of persistence with the reading task (see Ainley, Hidi et al., 2002). The same pattern of findings has been replicated in a number of similar studies using other texts and separate groups of secondary school students from 7th to 8th grades (Ainley, Corrigan, & Richardson, 2005) and from 10th grade (Ainley, Hillman, & Hidi, 2002). Interest is one of the variables that powers decisions about engaging and maintaining engagement with classroom activities.

Individual Interest and Trajectories of On-Task Interest

As has been argued throughout this chapter, interest in a task is dynamic, and so the level of task interest and its relation with engagement, even for a task that is limited to the relatively short time duration of a single class lesson, may involve changing patterns of relations between process variables. The structure of these research tasks has allowed these changing reactions to be monitored and recorded.

Most of the tasks we have used have asked students to make ratings of their individual interest in domains related to the task prior to finding out details of the task. Across all of the studies, we have found a significant predictive relation between measures of individual interest and on-task interest. For the reading tasks, individual interest in content domains related to specific text content was positively related to the level of interest triggered by the text title and with initial interest responses to the text (Ainley, Corrigan et al., 2005; Ainley, Hidi et al., 2002; Ainley, Hillman et al., 2002). As might be expected, the strength of these associations differed for different content domains and different text topics. For example, with groups of 7th and 8th graders, individual interest in the domain of social issues was a significant predictor of how much interest was triggered by the Body Image text topic and individual interest in the domain of sports predicted interest in the Formula 1 Racing text topic (see Ainley, Corrigan et al., 2005).

In addition, recording students' self-report ratings in the real-time sequence of task performance has allowed mapping of trajectories of interest. As described above, when students were able to decide after each section of text whether to continue or to quit, levels of on-task interest were predictive of these decisions. In other tasks, students were not given this choice, allowing the trajectory of successive states of interest to be plotted. Consistent with the basic character of interest as a quality of relation between student and the text, there was considerable variation in these trajectories. In one study (Buckley, Hasen, & Ainley, 2004), female secondary students were presented with a set of texts dealing with social and political issues. The interest trajectory in response to a text dealing with euthanasia indicated that interest in the text was high and was maintained across all three text sections. On the other hand, in the same study, a text on ecotourism initially drew moderate interest ratings, but over successive text sections, the level of interest declined significantly. In addition to the variability in trajectory related to the text content, there were differences in interest trajectories related to students' general patterns of individual interest. Students with strong individual interest in social and political issues generally recorded higher interest trajectories across successive text sections than did students whose individual interests were in areas such as sports and popular music.

Recent findings reported by Rotgans and Schmidt (2011) support our findings. In their research with polytechnic students, task interest measures (referred to as situational interest) were administered five times during a problem-based learning program. Each problem involved teams of five students working on that problem over a whole day. Tutors observed and recorded students' achievement-related classroom behaviors including "participation, teamwork, presentation skills, and self-directed learning" (p. 5). Situational interest was significantly related to patterns of achievement-related classroom behavior, but at the same time, there was considerable variability in interest levels across the five measurement points.

Similar patterns in the variability of the trajectories of on-task interest to those observed with the reading tasks have been found in our studies using problem scenarios. The problem scenario software was designed to present students with an open problem where their task is to explore sets of information and to use the products of their research to construct a solution to the problem and give reasons to support their solution. At critical points in the task, students respond to probes monitoring aspects of what they were thinking and feeling. Most commonly, the probes have been programmed to appear immediately after students had been introduced to the problem details and instructions, after students have been working on the problem for about 10 minutes, and then the final probe appears immediately after a student has submitted their answer.

As expected, the levels of interest recorded reflect task content. For example, our fantasy detective problem presented to 9th grade students indicated a moderately high level of interest which was maintained across the whole task (see Ainley, Buckley, & Chan, 2009). However, when further problems were presented to the same students but with content related to the social issues being researched as part of a course on research skills, the overall level of interest barely reached the midpoint of the 5-point interest rating scale. Across the course of these tasks, the overall level of interest appeared to decrease.

As has already been asserted, individual variability is part of what is expected of dynamic systems, and these data lend themselves to identification of trajectories of interest development across the task. Within the student cohorts, subgroup trajectories have been identified using cluster analysis. For the fantasy detective problem, three trajectories were identified representing high, medium, and low interest. When problem tasks based on curriculum issues have been used with successive cohorts of 9th grade students, most of the problem scenario data sets have generated two trajectories: a medium-interest trajectory showing the interest level maintained and sometimes increasing across the task and a second low-interest trajectory starting with low interest in the task and most often decreasing as the task progressed.

In summary, the strongest impression from inspection of these trajectories across a number of student cohorts has been that students' initial reaction to the task sets a direction for their level of engagement. Students who initially responded with low interest generally stayed at that level. These were often students who came to the task with little individual interest in the domain. If there was a change, it was often in the direction of their interest decreasing further. On the other hand, students who responded with moderate or high interest were likely to maintain that interest, and if there was change interest increased.

This pattern is consistent with the findings of Skinner and colleagues who reported trajectories of achievement motivation across a number of years of schooling suggesting that "In general, these dynamics seem to be amplifying, in that children who start out motivationally rich maintain their engagement as the year(s) progress, whereas children who start out motivationally poor tend to become more disengaged over time" (Skinner et al., 2008, p. 765). These diverging trajectories suggest that more attention needs to be directed to understanding the dynamics of reactivity to classroom activities. For students who do not come with strong individual interest in the content domains of schooling and do not have their interest triggered by the classroom activities set for them, there is little evidence of engagement.

While this was the overall impression from these studies, there were also signs of individual variability associated with different topics. Overall, students who were identified with the medium-interest trajectory maintained this status across similar tasks. The same was also generally the case for the low-interest trajectory groups. However, just as with the mood study reported earlier where a small number of students were responsive to the task and developed more positive mood as they engaged with the task, in the cohort of 9th grade students working on social issues problems, there were a number of students who showed a different interest status on different tasks. Students who were in the low-interest trajectory on the first task recorded similar low interest at the first measurement point when completing another problem scenario approximately 3 months later. However, as the second task progressed, interest ratings for these students increased to the extent that their overall profile was more like the medium-interest group.

A major implication that emerges from these findings is that interest and its relation to students' engagement with classroom activities is a dynamic system that draws on more enduring individual interests while at the same time being responsive to the particular contents of the immediate task.

Interest in Combination with Other Emotions

Another component of the dynamic system of interest-related processes associated with task engagement is the emotion states aroused simultaneously with interest. Along with variations in levels of task interest, it is likely that there are changes in emotions that students experience while working on a single task. One of the probes included in the problem scenario tasks used in our research asked how students were feeling at the three critical points: before commencing, mid-task, and after the task was finished. Sets of face icons representing achievement emotions as described by Pekrun and colleagues (Pekrun, Goetz, Titz, & Perry, 2002) were presented, and students selected an icon to indicate "How are you feeling right now?" This was followed by an intensity rating for the selected icon. To illustrate the differences in emotions students report across a task and how these experiences are linked with interest in the task, the results from a cohort of 9th grade students who completed the fantasy detective problem are shown in Fig. 13.1. The figure shows the successive emotion states for the three interest trajectories identified in that cohort of students: low, moderate, and high interest. The panel of icons included an icon for neutral, and this was selected by a large proportion of students but with decreasing frequency as the task progressed. Students in the moderate-interest cluster were more likely to select *neutral* across the whole task, and the major deviation from this pattern was the choice of *relieved* at the end of the task. The patterns for the high-interest and low-interest groups show some important contrasts. The high-interest group was more likely to choose an emotion icon rather than selecting *neutral*, and their choices were more likely to be for positive emotions such as *happy* and *hopeful*, while the low-interest group, when not choosing *neutral*, was more likely to choose negative emotions such as *sad*, *angry*, and *hopeless*.

As can be seen in these pattern of emotions associated with the interest trajectories, other achievement emotions vary systematically with interest and are part of the system of psychological processes that energize and direct task engagement.

Interest in Combination with Other Motivation Variables: Achievement Goals

Further evidence that the relation between interest and engagement involves a dynamic system connecting interest with a range of psychological processes can be seen in the findings we have reported relating trajectories of interest with achievement goals. Achievement goal orientations have been linked with interest by a number of researchers. In particular, in longitudinal studies of achievement in college students (Harackiewicz, Barron, Tauer, & Elliot, 2002), interest has been demonstrated to mediate the influence of mastery goals on academic achievement. At the task level, through tracking on-task achievement goals and interest, we have demonstrated (Ainley & Patrick, 2006) that general achievement goals predict congruent on-task

A High Interest Group

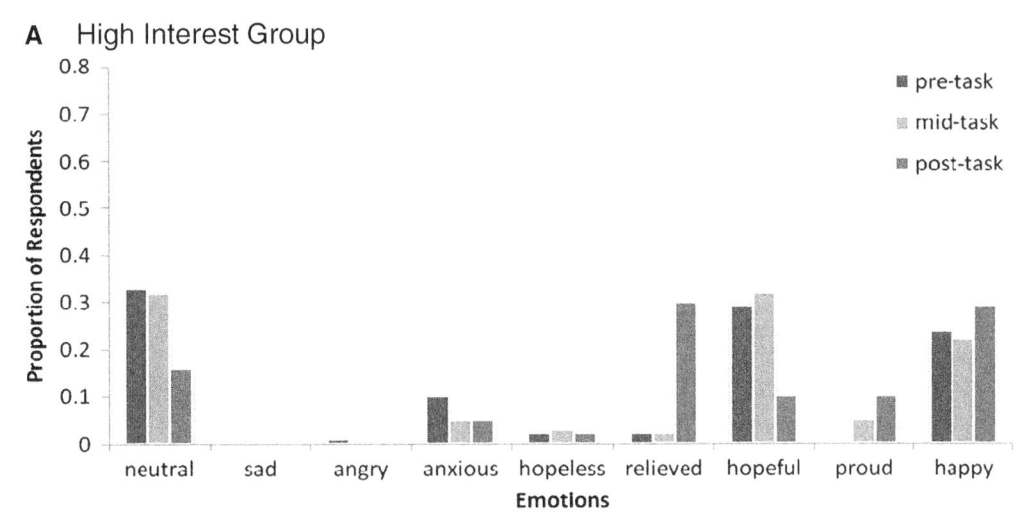

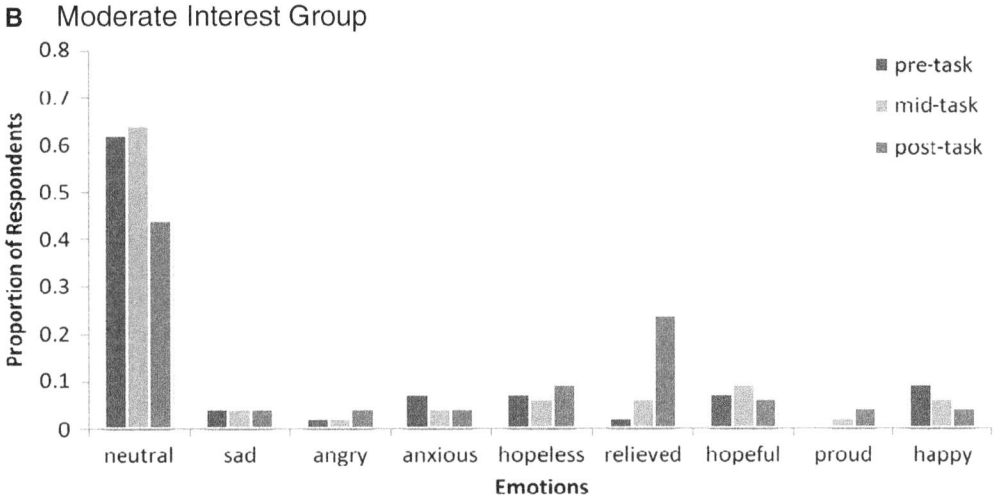

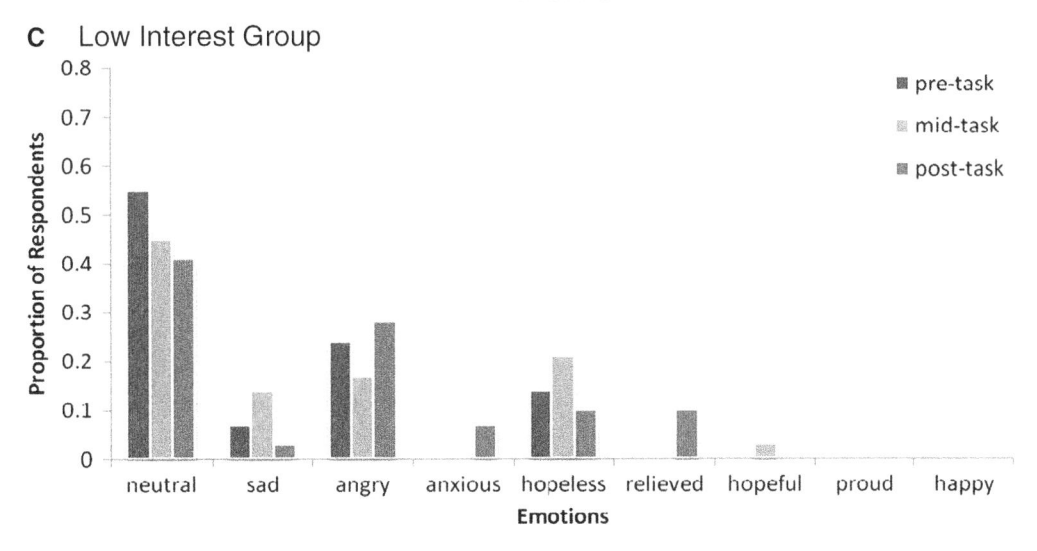

B Moderate Interest Group

C Low Interest Group

Fig. 13.1 Profiles of emotions for high (*panel A*)-, moderate (*panel B*)-, and low (*panel C*)-interest trajectory groups showing emotions recorded pre-task, mid-task, and post-task

achievement goals and that both mastery and performance goals measured as on-task goals are associated with levels of interest as the task progresses. Across a number of research programs, the relations between these variables are increasingly being represented as interactive and cyclic systems with each variable being both predictor and outcome, rather than as simple linear relations (see e.g., Harackiewicz, Durik, Barron, Linnenbrink-Garcia, & Tauer, 2008; Tapola, Dayez, & Veermans, 2009).

The dynamic model of classroom engagement and disaffection developed by Skinner and colleagues (Skinner et al., 2008) also represents levels of interaction among sets of processes that underpin what is observed as classroom engagement and disaffection. In particular, their representation of the internal dynamic or system allows for simultaneous feedback and interaction between what they define as engaged behavior, disaffected behavior, engaged emotion, and disaffected emotion. Of particular significance for this approach is their modeling of the contingency between these components across two measurement points within the school year for cohorts of 5th, 6th, and 7th graders. This dynamic system operates within a broader system linking aspects of the school context and the individual student's self-system represented in their analysis by components of autonomy, competence, and relatedness. It is my contention that a similar systems approach is needed to allow for ways that the complexity of the components of the external system, for example, interactive loops between the relatedness, competence, and autonomy, also interact with the internal system dynamics.

A range of evidence has been described supporting the contention that the relation between interest and engagement is most productively viewed as a dynamic system. The classroom tasks we have focused on have generally been individual activities. The inclusion of classroom peers working together on a problem adds to the complexity of the system as separate individual systems adjust their dynamic to the functional requirements of the joint working arrangements. Rotgans and Schmidt (2011) collected measures of situational interest and achievement-related behaviors from students working in teams and reported on the dynamic of interest development across the task for individual students. Consideration of the relation between interest and engagement requires parallel consideration of a broad network of variables both within the time frame of a classroom activity but also going beyond to include broader personal orientations and characteristics as well as a myriad of contextual factors.

Context and Relations Between Interest and Engagement

In this final section, I consider relations between interest and engagement and focus on the nested contexts within which learning occurs. The title for this chapter refers to classroom activities, and in most of the research program I have been describing, the emphasis has been on the microprocess level exploring the dynamics of interest and its role in classroom learning. The research tasks we have used include activities that are similar to the tasks students encounter in their classes, and our research tools have monitored and recorded sequences of action and reaction in real time. This has provided rich data from which to view ways that a variety of psychological processes interact and combine with interest to influence students' engagement with classroom activities. However, this is only one level of the dynamic system that is the student in their environment.

Following the ecological model of Bronfenbrenner, first articulated as an approach to the study of human development (Bronfenbrenner, 1992; Bronfenbrenner & Morris, 1998), it is informative to view the individual learner and their world as a microsystem embedded within layers of ever more general contexts that have the potential to influence a student's life space including their opportunities for learning and academic development. In this section, we describe some findings from analyses (Ainley & Ainley, 2011a, 2011b) of international science achievement data (OECD, 2007), to consider whether relations between interest and engagement differ according to the different contexts represented by countries with varied historical and cultural traditions.

The Macrocontext and Relations Between Interest and Engagement

Over the last two decades, there have been a number of important research findings that highlight how broad social and cultural contexts influence students' achievement and development. Strong family traditions and cultural values have been associated with differences in achievement favoring Asian-American students (Asakawa & Csikszentimihalyi, 1998). Other studies have shown that cultural values impact on students' perception of choice (Iyengar & Lepper, 1999) and the meaning of achievement goals (Dekker & Fischer, 2008). In addition, it is clear from Larson and Verma's (1999) review of patterns of work and leisure for children and adolescents around the world that time in school and opportunities for educational achievement vary across countries.

The studies we describe now had the broad goals of testing relations between interest and engagement as well as determining whether the structure of these relations was consistent for students from countries with different historical and cultural traditions. Decisions for selection of the comparison countries were made using Inglehart's cultural world map (Inglehart & Baker, 2000; Inglehart & Welzel, 2005). According to Inglehart and colleagues, two orthogonal value factors underlie the patterns of responses that have been gathered in the World Values Surveys and European Surveys (1981–1982; 1990–1991; 1995–1998). The first dimension consists of an orientation to authority which contrasts more *traditional* values emphasizing religion and obedience to traditional authorities, with *secular-rational* values where family and social values are viewed as relative rather than absolute and where deference to religious authority is not a high priority. The second dimension contrasts *survival* values where the physical and economic security of the community is central to values, with *self-expression* where values such as subjective well-being, individual autonomy, and personal quality of life are prominent concerns. From this cultural map, four countries were chosen to represent the four quadrants formed by the intersection of these two dimensions. The four countries were Sweden (secular-rational/self-expression), Estonia (secular-rational/survival), USA (traditional/self-expression), and Colombia (traditional/survival). The other criterion for selection was that the country had participated in the Programme for International Student Assessment (PISA) 2006 (OECD, 2007). These data on the science achievement of 15-year-old students, included a student questionnaire, with a number of scales measuring variables that are pertinent for understanding relations between interest and engagement. This provided an opportunity to test some of the relations between interest and engagement as represented in the four-phase model of interest development and to test whether the same relations between the variables operated for students from countries representing different cultural contexts.

Interest and Engagement in PISA 2006

All of the PISA 2006 measures have been designed and trialed by international teams to ensure that the measurement model is robust across countries. Interest in science was the special focus of PISA 2006, and a set of attitudinal items covering a range of aspects of how students feel and think about science were administered (OECD, 2007, 2009). Hidi and Renninger's (2006) four-phase model of interest development identifies the components of individual interest as positive affect, knowledge, and value. We chose measures from the PISA 2006 student questionnaires to represent these components and to test their relations with individual interest.

The main achievement measure in PISA 2006 is a measure of students' science knowledge. In addition, a student questionnaire included a measure of general interest in learning science which asked how much interest students had in learning about a range of science domains, a measure of enjoyment of science, and a measure of personal value of science focusing specifically on ways that science might be of value to them personally.

As outlined in an earlier section, a key feature of the behavior associated with an individual interest is that the student seeks opportunities to engage and reengage with content from their interest domain. Hence, an important motivation for the modeling studies (Ainley & Ainley, 2011a, 2011b) was to test the relations: firstly, among knowledge, value, and enjoyment of science and their relations with the general interest in learning science measure, and secondly to model the relations between these variables and engagement variables.

Several measures from PISA 2006 represented aspects of engagement. The first was a scale asking about current participation in out-of-school science activities such as projects, watching television programs about science, and reading about science. The second was a scale called future-oriented motivation to learn science and was designed to measure "how many students actually intended to continue their interest in science," that is, intentions for future engagement. Items referred to future science careers, studies in science, and participation in science projects. These two scales provided a measure of current engagement and intentions for future engagement.

Using AMOS 7.0 (see Arbuckle, 2005), we tested a number of models to determine the best fit depicting relations between the variables representing general interest in learning science, science knowledge, value of science, and enjoyment of science, and their combined predictive relations with current engagement and intended future engagements (Ainley & Ainley, 2011a). The final model gave an acceptable fit (Byrne, 2001) for all four countries suggesting that the structure of relations between these variables could be represented in the same way across the four countries (RMSEA: Sweden=0.052, USA=0.054, Colombia=0.056, and Estonia=0.076). The strongest coefficients in this model predicted from personal value of science to enjoyment of science, and enjoyment of science predicted each of general interest in learning science, current engagement, and intended future engagements. Additional paths with lower coefficients linked personal value of science with general interest in learning science and the two engagement variables. Hence, the predictive effect of personal value of science on the engagement variables was partially mediated by its relation with enjoyment of science. Simultaneously, general interest in learning science was also linked with the two engagement variables, but again the coefficients were smaller than those linking enjoyment of science with the engagement variables. A very small coefficient linked science knowledge with the enjoyment of science variable. These patterns held for all four of the selected countries, and the full set of coefficients is available in Ainley and Ainley (2011a).

The coefficients were strongest for Sweden and generally smaller for Colombia, with the other two countries in between. For example, the model accounted for 50% of the variance in score on the intended future engagement variable for Sweden and 31% for Colombia. Differences between the patterns of relations for the four countries were seen in the magnitude of the coefficients and of special interest were the science knowledge effects. For Colombia, the predictive relation between science knowledge and the central mediating variable of enjoyment of science was close to zero (−0.01) compared with a coefficient of 0.19 for Sweden. Coefficients for the other countries were in between these two values. These findings support the conclusion that the relations between these variables should be interpreted as a network of interacting processes. In this model, the central mediating variable was enjoyment of science which was strongly correlated with interest in learning science (Colombia 0.43 and Sweden 0.69).

Except for the knowledge scale, all of the measures described so far are based on self-report questionnaires. A feature of the PISA 2006 data collection was the inclusion of what are referred to as embedded interest items. These items were designed to assess the degree to which students were interested in finding out more about the specific science topics that they were working on in the knowledge assessment problems. For example, the content of one of the problem topics concerned tobacco smoking. At the end of the problem questions, students were asked, "How much interest do you have in the following information?" Students were given three statements: "knowing how tar in tobacco reduces lung efficiency," "understanding why nicotine is addictive," and "learning how the body recovers after stopping smoking" (OECD, 2006, p. 164). This measure is informative as it represents students' willingness to reengage with a specific science topic to find out and understand more about it.

Similar modeling techniques were used to test the pattern of relations between the set of predictor variables and the form of engagement represented in the embedded interest scores (Ainley & Ainley, 2011b). Again, we found that our final model mapping the network of relations had acceptable fit for all four countries (RMSEA: Sweden=0.043; USA=0.061; Colombia=0.051; and Estonia=0.039). Again, the coefficients linking the variables were strongest for Sweden and weakest for Colombia, and the proportion of variance in the engagement indicator (embedded interest) predicted by the model varied from 46% for Sweden to 22% for Colombia. The network as represented in the final model showed a sequence linking knowledge of science and personal value of science with the engagement variable through the mediators of firstly, enjoyment of science and secondly, general interest in learning science. There were also some additional direct effects on engagement, but these were relatively small. The main path linked knowledge and value through enjoyment and interest to predict engagement in the form of wanting to reengage with the topic to find out and understand more.

The strength of the relations within the network of science variables differed between samples of students from countries with different historical and cultural traditions. They were strongest in the country chosen to represent countries with secular-rational and self-expression values and weaker in the country chosen to represent more traditional and survival values. However, these analyses do provide evidence that our models linking the set of variables referred to by the PISA researchers as interest in science has been shown to apply beyond the countries where much of the work on motivation and engagement has been conducted. Although limited in scope to an assessment of relations between the specific process variables included in the PISA framework, this evidence supports our major contention that relations between interest in science and engagement with science consist in networks of psychological processes related to learning, including value, enjoyment, and, to a lesser extent, existing knowledge of science.

Conclusion

In this chapter, it has been argued that a useful way to conceptualize the relations between interest and engagement in relation to classroom activities consists in a dynamic self-organizing system. Interest is not static. At all educational levels, activities that are attractive, in terms of color, sound, and movement, novel, complex, or uncertain can be used to trigger students' interest or to capture students' attention. However, this is only the first step to the forms and quality of engagement with classroom activities that are likely to lead to acquisition of knowledge and understanding. Using a dynamic systems perspective, it has been argued that an interest reaction akin to triggered situational interest is the first step in the development of a more extended individual interest. This in turn consists of an organized schema combining knowledge, value, and affect and is manifest in students seeking opportunities to engage and reengage with content from that interest domain (Hidi & Renninger, 2006).

From a systems' perspective, specific localized interest processes are significant as they contribute to the overall configuration of a student's behavior. These extend from the microprocess level, nested within increasingly broader units of process and action, to the macrolevel of the historical, cultural traditions within which that student's educational experiences exist. Approaching interest and engagement in classroom activities from this perspective, at the theoretical level, provides direction for further investigation of the substance and dynamic of interest and its related processes. At the practical level, the challenge is to apply this knowledge to support students' learning. How many of the students in classes characterized as difficult or challenging might become engaged if the content of learning activities connected with their existing interests? Knowledge of situational factors or the **hooks** that can attract students to an activity is part of the story, but for the **gears** to engage and generate forward movement, other processes must come into play. The analyses of PISA data demonstrated how personal value and enjoyment are two key processes that are part of the dynamic system when students express a desire to reengage with content they have been examining. When the content of learning activities pertains to something that is valued and/or is perceived to be enjoyable, students choose to engage and often seek to reengage if given the opportunity. The hook is no longer essential, but opportunities for reengagement with the achievement domain are critical. To a large extent, what we know about the workings of the system of processes that connect students with learning domains relate to individual students or groups of students. Simultaneously, individual students are nested within contexts extending from local friendship groups within their classes to the broader cultural context that surrounds them. At each level, these contexts can influence the development of students' personal interests, values, and access to knowledge and understanding.

Our analysis has specifically focused on relations between interest and engagement and has shown that what is known about the relations between these two constructs necessarily implicates a wider range of psychological processes that together function as dynamic systems whenever students interact with classroom activities.

References

Ainley, M. (1993). Styles of engagement with learning: Multidimensional assessment of their relationship with strategy use and school achievement. *Journal of Educational Psychology, 85*(3), 395–405.

Ainley, M. (2007). Being and feeling interested: Transient state, mood, and disposition. In P. Schutz & R. Pekrun (Eds.), *Emotions and education* (pp. 147–163). Burlington, MA: Academic.

Ainley, M. (2010). Interest in the dynamics of task behavior: Processes that link person and task in effective learning. In T. Urdan & S. A. Karabenick (Eds.), *Advances in motivation and achievement. The decade ahead: Theoretical perspectives on motivation and achievement* (Vol. 16A, pp. 235–264). Bingley, UK: Emerald Group.

Ainley, M., & Ainley, J. (2011a). Interest in science: Part of the complex structure of student motivation in science. *International Journal of Science Education, 33*(1), 51–71.

Ainley, M., & Ainley, J. (2011b). Student engagement with science in early adolescence: The contribution of enjoyment to students' continuing interest in learning about science. *Contemporary Educational Psychology, 36*(1), 4–12.

Ainley, M., Buckley, S., & Chan, J. (2009). Interest and efficacy beliefs in self-regulated learning: Does the task make a difference? In M. Wosnitza, S. A. Karabenick, A. Efklides, & P. Nenniger (Eds.), *Contemporary motivation research: From global to local perspectives* (pp. 207–227). Göttingen, Germany: Hogrefe & Huber.

Ainley, M., Corrigan, M., & Richardson, N. (2005). Students, tasks and emotions: Identifying the contribution of emotions to students' reading of popular culture and popular science texts. *Learning and Instruction, 15*(5), 433–447.

Ainley, M., Flowers, D., & Patrick, L. (2005). *The impact of mood on learning – The impact of task on mood.* Paper presented at the Annual Conference of the European Association for Research in Learning and Instruction (EARLI), Nicosia, Cyprus.

Ainley, M., Hidi, S., & Berndorff, D. (2002). Interest, learning and the psychological processes that mediate their relationship. *Journal of Educational Psychology, 94*(3), 545–561.

Ainley, M., Hillman, K., & Hidi, S. (2002). Gender and interest processes in response to literary texts: Situational and individual interest. *Learning and Instruction, 12*(4), 411–428.

Ainley, M., & Patrick, L. (2006). Measuring self-regulated learning processes through tracking patterns of student interaction with achievement activities. *Educational Psychology Review, 18*(3), 267–286.

Appleton, J. J., Christenson, S. L., Kim, D., & Reschly, A. L. (2006). Measuring cognitive and psychological engagement: Validation of the student engagement instrument. *Journal of School Psychology, 44*(5), 427–445.

Arbuckle, J. (2005). *AMOS 6.0 user's guide*. Chicago, IL: SPSS Inc.

Asakawa, K., & Csikszentimihalyi, M. (1998). The quality of experience of Asian American adolescents in academic activities: An exploration of educational achievement. *Journal of Research on Adolescence, 8*(2), 241–262.

Boekaerts, M., de Koning, E., & Vedder, P. (2006). Goal-directed behavior and contextual factors in the classroom: An innovative approach to the study of multiple goals. *Educational Psychologist, 41*(1), 33–51.

Boydston, J. A. (Ed.). (1979). *John Dewey: The middle works 1899–1924* (Vol. 7: 1912–1914). London: Southern Illinois University Press.

Bronfenbrenner, U. (1992). Ecological systems theory. In R. Vasra (Ed.), *Six theories of child development* (pp. 187–249). London: Jessica Kingsley Publications.

Bronfenbrenner, U., & Morris, P. A. (1998). The ecology of developmental processes. In R. M. Lerner (Ed.), *Handbook of child psychology* (5th ed., Vol. 1: Theoretical models of human development, pp. 535–584). New York: Wiley.

Buckley, S., Hasen, G., & Ainley, M. (2004, November). *Affective engagement: A person-centred approach to understanding the structure of subjective learning experiences*. Paper presented at the Australian Association for Research in Education (AARE), Melbourne, Australia.

Byrne, B. M. (2001). *Structural equation modeling with AMOS*. Mahwah, NJ: Lawrence Erlbaum Associates.

Chen, A., & Ennis, C. D. (2004). Goal, interest, and learning in physical education. *The Journal of Educational Research, 97*(6), 329–338.

Dekker, S., & Fischer, R. (2008). Cultural differences in academic motivation goals: A meta-analysis across 13 societies. *The Journal of Educational Research, 102*(2), 99–110.

Ely, R., Ainley, M., & Pearce, J. (2010). *A new method for identifying dimensions of interest: MINE*. Paper presented at the International Conference on Motivation (ICM), Porto, Portugal.

Fredricks, J. A., Blumenfeld, P. C., & Paris, A. H. (2004). Student engagement: Potential of the concept, state of the evidence. *Review of Educational Research, 74*(1), 59–109.

Fredrickson, B. L. (2001). The role of positive emotions in positive psychology: The broaden-and-build theory of positive emotions. *American Psychologist, 56*(3), 218–226.

Frenzel, A., Dicke, A.-L., Goetz, T., & Pekrun, R. (2009). *Quantitative and qualitative insights into the development of interest in adolescence*. Paper presented at the European Association for Research in Learning and Instruction (EARLI), Amsterdam, The Netherlands.

Fullarton, S. (2002). *Student engagement with school: Individual and school level influences* (LSAY Research Report No. 27). Camberwell, Australia: ACER.

Harackiewicz, J. M., Barron, K. E., Tauer, J. M., & Elliot, A. J. (2002). Predicting success in college: A longitudinal study of achievement goals and ability measures as predictors of interest and performance from freshman year through graduation. *Journal of Educational Psychology, 94*(3), 562–575.

Harackiewicz, J. M., Durik, A. M., Barron, K. E., Linnenbrink-Garcia, L., & Tauer, J. M. (2008). The role of achievement goals in the development of interest: Reciprocal relations between achievement goals, interest, and performance. *Journal of Educational Psychology, 100*(1), 105–122.

Hidi, S. (1990). Interest and its contribution as a mental resource for learning. *Review of Educational Research, 60*(3), 549–571.

Hidi, S. (2006). Interest: A unique motivational variable. *Educational Research Review, 1*(2), 69–82.

Hidi, S., & Ainley, M. (2007). Interest and self-regulation: Relationships between two variables that influence learning. In B. J. Zimmerman & D. H. Schunk (Eds.), *Motivation and self-regulated learning: Theory, research, and applications* (pp. 77–109). Mahwah, NJ: Erlbaum.

Hidi, S., & Baird, W. (1988). Strategies for increasing text-based interest and students' recall of expository texts. *Reading Research Quarterly, 23*(4), 465–483.

Hidi, S., & Harackiewicz, J. M. (2000). Motivating the academically unmotivated: A critical issue for the 21st century. *Review of Educational Research, 70*(2), 151–179.

Hidi, S., & Renninger, K. A. (2006). The four-phase model of interest development. *Educational Psychologist, 41*(2), 111–127.

Hulleman, C. S., & Senko, C. (2010). Up and around the bend: Forecasts for achievement goal theory and research in 2020. In T. Urdan & S. A. Karabenick (Eds.), *Advances in motivation and achievement. The decade ahead: Theoretical perspectives on motivation and achievement* (Vol. 16A, pp. 71–104). Bingley, UK: Emerald Group.

Inglehart, R., & Baker, W. E. (2000). Modernization, cultural change, and the persistence of traditional values. *American Sociological Review, 65*(1), 19–51.

Inglehart, R., & Welzel, C. (2005). *Modernization, cultural change and democracy: The human development sequence*. New York: Cambridge University Press.

Iyengar, S. S., & Lepper, M. R. (1999). Rethinking the value of choice: A cultural perspective on intrinsic motivation. *Journal of Personality and Social Psychology, 76*(3), 349–366.

Izard, C. E. (1977). *Human emotions*. New York: Plenum Press.

Izard, C. E. (2007). Basic emotions, natural kinds, emotion schemas, and a new paradigm. *Perspectives on Psychological Science, 2*(3), 260–280.

Jimerson, S. R., Campos, E., & Greif, J. L. (2003). Toward an understanding of definitions and measures of school engagement and related terms. *The California School Psychologist, 8*(1), 7–27.

Jörg, T., Davis, B., & Nickmans, G. (2007). Towards a new, complexity science of learning and education. *Educational Research Review, 2*(2), 145–156.

Krapp, A. (2003). Interest and human development: An educational-psychological perspective. *Development and Motivation, BJEP Monograph Series, II*(2), 57–84.

Krapp, A. (2005). Basic needs and the development of interest and intrinsic motivational orientations. *Learning and Instruction, 15*(5), 381–395.

Larson, R. W., & Verma, S. (1999). How children and adolescents spend time across the world: Work, play, and developmental outcomes. *Psychological Bulletin, 125*(6), 701–736.

Lewis, M. D., & Granic, I. (Eds.). (2000). *Emotion, development, and self-organization: Dynamic systems approaches to emotional development*. Cambridge, UK: Cambridge University Press.

Linnakylä, P., & Malin, A. (2008). Finnish students' school engagement profiles in the light of PISA 2003. *Scandinavian Journal of Educational Research, 52*(6), 583–602.

Marks, H. M. (2000). Student engagement in instructional activity: Patterns in the elementary, middle, and high school years. *American Educational Research Journal, 37*(1), 153–184.

Mitchell, M. (1993). Situational interest: Its multifaceted structure in the secondary school mathematics classroom. *Journal of Educational Psychology, 85*(3), 424–436.

Murphy, P. K., & Alexander, P. A. (2000). A motivated exploration of motivation terminology. *Contemporary Educational Psychology, 25*(1), 3–53.

OECD. (2006). *Assessing scientific, reading and mathematical literacy: A framework for PISA 2006*. Paris: OECD.

OECD. (2007). *PISA 2006: Science competencies for tomorrow's world* (Vol. 1: Analysis). Paris: OECD.

OECD. (2009). *PISA 2006 technical report*. Paris: OECD.

Pekrun, R., Goetz, T., Titz, W., & Perry, R. P. (2002). Academic emotions in students' self-regulated learning and achievement: A program of qualitative and quantitative research. *Educational Psychologist, 37*(2), 91–105.

Rathunde, K., & Csikszentmihalyi, M. (1993). Undivided interest and the growth of talent: A longitudinal study of adolescents. *Journal of Youth and Adolescence, 22*(4), 385–405.

Reschly, A. L., & Christenson, S. L. (2006). Prediction of dropouts among students with mild disabilities: A case for the inclusion of student engagement variables. *Remedial and Special Education, 27*(5), 276–292.

Rotgans, J. I., & Schmidt, H. G. (2011). Situational interest and academic achievement in the active-learning classroom. *Learning and Instruction, 21*(1), 58–67. doi:10.1016/j.learninstruc.2009.1011.1001.

Russell, J., Ainley, M., & Frydenberg, E. (2005). *Schooling issues digest: Student motivation and engagement.* Canberra, Australia: Australian Government, Department of Education Science and Training.

Sansone, C., & Thoman, D. B. (2005). Interest as the missing motivator in self-regulation. *European Psychologist, 10*(3), 175–186.

Sansone, C., Weir, C., Harpster, L., & Morgan, C. (1992). Once a boring task always a boring task? Interest as a self-regulatory mechanism. *Journal of Personality and Social Psychology, 63*(3), 379–390.

Schraw, G., & Lehman, S. (2001). Situational Interest: A review of the literature and directions for future research. *Educational Psychology Review, 13*(1), 23–52.

Sideridis, G. D. (2009). Normative vs. non-normative performance goals: Effects on behavioral and emotional regulation in achievement situations. In M. Wosnitza, S. A. Karabenick, A. Efklides, & P. Nenniger (Eds.), *Contemporary motivation research: From global to local perspectives* (pp. 321–338). Göttingen, Germany: Hogrefe & Huber.

Skinner, E., Furrer, C., Marchand, G., & Kindermann, T. (2008). Engagement and disaffection in the classroom: Part of a larger motivational dynamic? *Journal of Educational Psychology, 100*(4), 765–781.

Sun, H., Chen, A., Ennis, C. D., Martin, R., & Shen, B. (2008). An examination of the multidimensionality of situational interest in elementary school physical education. *Research Quarterly for Exercise and Sport, 79*(1), 62–70.

Tapola, A., Dayez, J.-B., & Veermans, M. (2009). *Students' experience in a simulation-based science learning task: The role of individual and situational factors.* Paper presented at the European Association for Research in Learning and Instruction (EARLI), Amsterdam, The Netherlands.

The Australian Oxford Paperback Dictionary. (1999). (2nd ed.). Melbourne: Oxford University Press.

Thelen, E., & Smith, L. B. (2006). Dynamic systems theories. In W. Damon & R. M. Lerner (Eds.), *Handbook of child psychology* (6th ed., Vol. 1, pp. 258–312). Hoboken, NJ: Wiley.

Turner, J. C. (2010). Unfinished business: Putting motivation theory to the "classroom test". In T. Urdan & S. A. Karabenick (Eds.), *Advances in motivation and achievement: The decade ahead: Applications and contexts of motivation and achievement* (Vol. 16B, pp. 109–138). Bingley, UK: Emerald Group.

Turner, J. E., & Waugh, R. M. (2007). A dynamical systems perspective regarding students' learning processes: Shame reactions and emergent self-organizations. In P. Schutz & R. Pekrun (Eds.), *Emotions and education* (pp. 125–145). Burlington, MA: Academic.

Wade, S. E. (2001). Research on importance and interest: Implications for curriculum development and future research. *Educational Psychology Review, 13*(3), 243–261.

Watson, D., & Clark, L. A. (1994). Emotions, moods, traits and temperaments: Conceptual distinctions and empirical findings. In P. Ekman & R. J. Davidson (Eds.), *The nature of emotion: Fundamental questions* (pp. 89–93). New York: Oxford University Press.

Willms, J. D. (2003). *Student engagement at school: A sense of belonging and participation. Results from PISA 2000*. Paris: OECD.

Wosnitza, M., & Volet, S. (2009). A framework for personal goals in collaborative learning contexts. In M. Wosnitza, S. A. Karabenick, A. Efklides, & P. Nenniger (Eds.), *Contemporary motivation research: From global to local perspectives* (pp. 49–67). Gottingen, Germany: Hogrefe & Huber.

Part II Commentary: Motivation and Engagement: Conceptual, Operational, and Empirical Clarity

14

Andrew J. Martin

Abstract

A noted scholar in the field of engagement, Andrew Martin, provided commentary on the chapters in Part II. Martin summarized the theories and definitions offered by authors in this part and shared his perspective on motivation and engagement. He argued for the inclusion of disengagement in addition to engagement in future research and discourse in this area. Martin concluded by proposing a framework and analytic model to integrate authors' ideas and to test tenets of various conceptualizations of engagement and motivation.

As discussed by all authors in this part, motivation and engagement are fundamental components of the learning process. Motivation and engagement provide the energy, direction, and skill set required to effectively tackle academic subject matter. Further, being relatively malleable, they are a point of important educational intervention for students, practitioners, and parents/caregivers. This commentary on motivation and engagement summarizes the essence of theories, definitions, factors, and processes presented by authors in this part. Following this, some additional perspectives on motivation and engagement (and disengagement) are presented. The commentary concludes with a proposed framework for integrating central ideas from these chapters and a suggested analytic model that can test many contentions made (here and elsewhere) about motivation and engagement.

Contributions by Part Authors

Perhaps the most difficult task for motivation and engagement researchers relates to conceptual and operational clarity. In each chapter, the authors demarcated motivation and engagement in terms of the theories underpinning them, the factors or constructs relevant to them, and the processes and contexts in which they occur in students' academic lives. Major ideas relevant to each of these are briefly summarized.

A.J. Martin, Ph.D.(✉)
Faculty of Education and Social Work,
University of Sydney, Sydney, NSW, Australia
e-mail: andrew.martin@sydney.edu.au

Theories Explaining and Describing Motivation and Engagement

Conceptual approaches to differentiating motivation and engagement spanned self-determination, goal, attribution, social-cognitive, dynamic systems, humanistic, achievement-motivation, and ecological theories. According to Reeve (2012), self-determination theory (SDT; Ryan & Deci, 2000) focuses on vitalizing students' inner states and thus is centrally concerned with motivation. Anderman and Patrick (2012) emphasize achievement goal theory (Elliot, 1999) describing how this is a useful way to disentangle motivation and engagement – with goals (motivation) being a significant basis for subsequent engagement. In shaping arguments around school identification, Voelkl (2012) draws on theories of human needs (e.g., Maslow, 1968) and perspectives on identification by Finn (1989). Schunk and Mullen (2012) draw on social-cognitive theory (Bandura, 1997, 2001) to articulate a model comprising self-efficacy, motivation, and engagement. In their chapter, two aspects of social-cognitive theory are emphasized: self-efficacy (as a social-cognitive variable) and context (as the social environment in which motivation and engagement occur). Cleary and Zimmerman (2012) also draw on social-cognitive perspectives to describe how environment, person, and behavior interact such that, for example, cognition underlies effective academic behavior. Focusing on emotion, Pekrun and Linnenbrink-Garcia (2012) traverse cognitive, social-cognitive, and achievement theories to differentiate multiple aspects of emotion and their role in the motivation-engagement process. Harnessing dynamic systems (e.g., Lewis & Granic, 2000) and ecological perspectives (Bronfenbrenner, 1992), Ainley (2012) situates interest as a motivational factor impacting subsequent engagement.

Factors Residing Within Motivation and Engagement Frameworks

According to Reeve, motivation comprises "private, unobservable, psychological, neural, and biological" factors, whereas engagement comprises "publicly observable behavior." This inner vs. outer concept is also described by Cleary and Zimmerman, demarcating engagement into observable factors (e.g., behavioral) and internal factors (e.g., cognition and affect) (see also Christenson et al., 2008). Cleary and Zimmerman focus on cognitive engagement that encompasses strategies and regulatory processes and position self-efficacy as a form of motivation that leads to cognitive self-regulatory activity (cognitive engagement).

Anderman and Patrick describe the engagement framework of Fredricks, Blumenfeld, and Paris (2004), disaggregating engagement in affective, cognitive, and behavioral terms. Similarly, Schunk and Mullen describe engagement in terms of affective, cognitive, and behavioral components and motivation in terms of an energizing function that impacts these. Pekrun and Linnenbrink-Garcia extend the cognitive, affective, and behavioral engagement framework to five components: motivational (e.g., goals), cognitive (e.g., attention, memory), behavioral (e.g., effort, persistence), cognitive-behavioral (e.g., self-regulation), and social-behavioral (e.g., social on-task behavior). Pekrun and Linnenbrink-Garcia then focus on emotional engagement and further unpack emotional engagement into affect, mood, achievement emotions, epistemic emotions, topic emotions, and social emotions.

Through the school identification perspective, Voelkl makes a clear distinction between affective and behavioral factors and suggests identification with school as a form of motivation that then leads to engagement in appropriate learning behaviors. Ainley also describes motivation in terms of inner psychological factors and engagement in terms of the level and nature of involvement in an activity. Ainley's focus is on interest and, similar to Voelkl, describes interest in terms of motivation – in contrast to other perspectives that position interest as part of engagement (e.g., see Reschly & Christenson, 2006).

Importantly, in one way or another, all authors recognize an "agentic" perspective on motivation and engagement. For example, Reeve explicitly includes agentic engagement in his framing of engagement and its factors. The social-cognitive model described by Schunk and Mullen also explicitly positions human agency as part of the motivation-engagement process such that students exert control over their cognition, affect, and behavior. Cleary and Zimmerman emphasize students' proactive engagement with tasks – moving beyond "reactive" models of engagement.

The Process of Motivation and Engagement

Striving for clarity in the motivation-engagement domain also requires researchers to articulate the operational process underlying motivation and engagement. At this point, theories, definitions, and factors can be disentangled and tested empirically. Across the chapters, there appears to be broad agreement that motivation underpins engagement and that engagement leads to outcomes such as achievement. Thus, while there may be some disagreement as to what factors are deemed to be motivation and what are seen as engagement, it seems to be the case that motivation is a basis for subsequent engagement.

Based on SDT, Reeve describes how students' inner motivational resources allow them to fully engage in the classroom. Anderman and Patrick point out that motivation occurs both before and during a task whereas engagement is predominantly operational during a task. They describe how goals (motivation) precede students' cognitive engagement (e.g., self-regulation), emotional engagement (e.g., positive affect about school), and behavioral engagement (e.g., effort). Similarly, Cleary and Zimmerman distinguish between the "will" of the student and the "skill" of the student (see also Covington, 1998), with the former indicating motivation and the latter indicating engagement. Thus, for example, motivational beliefs will predict cognitive self-regulation. Schunk and Miller also detail the energizing role of motivation on engagement, with engagement seen as "the manifestation of students' motivation." They also detail the role of self-efficacy in impacting both motivation and engagement and the impact of these processes on achievement.

Other authors unpacked processes relevant to affect, emotion, and interest. For example, Voelkl separates affective school identification from behavioral school identification and argues that affective identification precedes behavioral identification. Voelkl further suggests engagement as a mediator between motivation and achievement. Pekrun and Linnenbrink-Garcia emphasize the role of emotions and detail evidence showing how emotions impact motivational, cognitive, behavioral, cognitive-behavioral, and social-behavioral engagement. They also suggest that engagement mediates the relationship between emotion and achievement. Another argument for the mediating role of engagement is proposed by Ainley who describes how interest (part of motivation) leads to achievement via engagement. Consistent with Hidi and Renninger (2006; see also Krapp, 2005), Ainley further delineates the sequence of interest from an initial triggering of situational interest through to well-established and sustained individual interest.

All authors recognize a loop or reciprocity in which motivation and engagement (and achievement) occur. Reeve notes the reciprocal relationships linking context, motivation, engagement, and outcomes. Cleary and Zimmerman describe a cyclical feedback loop for cognitive engagement (self-regulation) that functions in a temporal sequence comprising cognitive engagement before, during, and after a learning task. Invoking dynamic systems theory (Turner & Waugh, 2007; see also Lewis & Granic, 2000), Pekrun and Linnenbrink-Garcia describe loops in the process as achievement impacts appraisals and emotions relevant to subsequent motivation and engagement. Ainley also invokes the dynamic systems perspective to assist understanding of the relations between interest and engagement.

Context Considerations Relevant to Motivation and Engagement

All authors emphasize the central role of context in formulations of motivation, engagement, and achievement. Reeve points out that for motivation and engagement to flourish, students require a supportive environment, particularly a strong teacher-student relationship. In similar vein, Voelkl identifies contextual conditions central to school identification including being supported by teachers, being treated fairly, and feelings of safety. Under a social-cognitive framework, Cleary and Zimmerman identify situation dependence and context specificity in shaping individual student engagement.

Anderman and Patrick extend the individual-level goal orientation constructs to describe classroom goal structures that are individuals' subjective perceptions of the meaning and purpose of tasks within the classroom. Notably, these goal structures impact students' individual motivation (goals) that then impacts cognitive, behavioral, and emotional engagement and achievement. Pekrun and Linnenbrink-Garcia also draw on goal theory to describe how goal structures impact emotions and emotional engagement. Similar to goal structure concepts, Schunk and Mullen describe how collective agency refers to students' shared beliefs about what they are capable of achieving as a class. In the development of self-efficacy and engagement, they also identify family, sociocultural (e.g., cultural capital), peer, and educational (e.g., instruction) influences. Ainley draws on Bronfenbrenner's (1992) ecological model to describe the layers of contextual influence that impact individual development, including their academic development by way of motivation and engagement.

Future Directions Offered by Authors

Collecting together such a wealth of expertise enables some powerful observations about future directions for motivation and engagement research. Reeve suggests a number of directions for future research, including testing a hypothesized four-factor model of engagement comprising cognition, affect, behavior, and *agency* and demonstrating that changes in these lead to changes in hypothesized outcomes. Anderman and Patrick suggest research into engagement while students are actually carrying out tasks using methods such as experience sampling. They also suggest further exploring developmental shifts and trajectories in students' motivation and engagement. Ainley also indicates the need for longitudinal research into motivation and engagement trajectories. Along similar methodological lines, Voelkl suggests longitudinal research that examines how school identification is internalized and how context influences school identification. Schunk and Mullen also highlight the need for contextual research and the need for cross-cultural studies into learning and engagement.

Cleary and Zimmerman recommend intervention work that tracks shifts (including at the microlevel) in engagement as a function of targeted practice. They also suggest that this research should focus on tasks with a clear beginning and end so as to understand the full process of regulatory engagement within them (e.g., writing an essay). Pekrun and Linnenbrink-Garcia suggest investigating the impact of task design and learning environments on emotions. Also, having identified numerous emotions relevant to the learning process, they urge research that investigates the distinct influence of each on learning and achievement and intervention research seeking to foster positive emotion in the classroom. They also signal the importance of emerging neuroscientific research in shedding further light on emotional engagement as relevant to learning.

Additional Contributions to Motivation and Engagement

In addition to what has been offered in these chapters, it is perhaps useful to recognize other approaches that explicitly integrate motivation and engagement into operationalization and measurement. This author has suggested one such approach – the Motivation and Engagement Wheel – that encompasses diverse motivation and engagement theorizing and research (Martin, 2007, 2009, 2010). The Motivation and Engagement Wheel reflects thinking offered by Pintrich (2003) who identified seven substantive areas for the development of an integrative motivational science. He underscored the importance

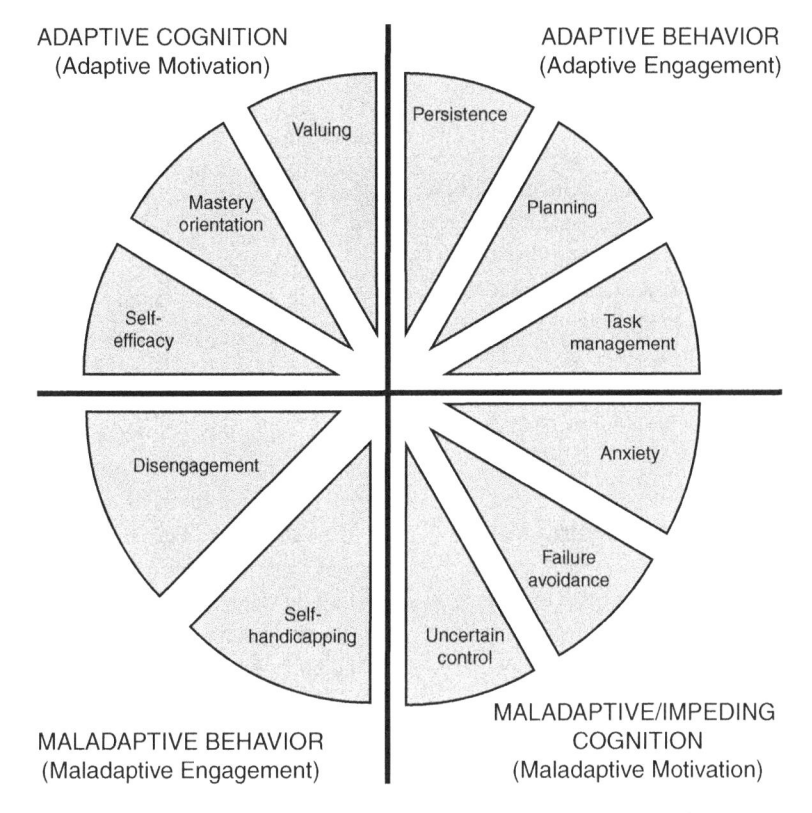

Fig. 14.1 Motivation and Engagement Wheel (Reproduced with permission from Martin 2010)

of considering a model of motivation from salient and seminal theorizing related to: self-efficacy, attributions, valuing, control, self-determination, goal orientation, need achievement, self-regulation, and self-worth. Martin (2007, 2009) identified congruencies across a number of these themes and integrated them into a multidimensional framework representing adaptive and maladaptive cognition and behavior.

This framework – the Motivation and Engagement Wheel – and its accompanying measurement tool, the Motivation and Engagement Scale (MES, see Martin, 2011), comprised four higher-order factors (or clusters) and 11 first-order factors: (1) *adaptive cognition (or adaptive motivation)*, reflecting students' positive attitudes and orientations to academic learning, including (i) self-efficacy, (ii) valuing, and (iii) mastery orientation; (2) *adaptive behavior (or adaptive engagement)*, reflecting students' positive behaviors and engagement in academic learning, including (iv) planned behavior, (v) task management, and (vi) persistence; (3) *impeding/maladaptive cognition (or maladaptive motivation)*, reflecting students' attitudes and orientations inhibiting academic learning, including (vii) anxiety, (viii) failure avoidance, and (ix) uncertain control; and (4) *maladaptive behavior (or maladaptive engagement)*, reflecting students' problematic learning behaviors, including (x) self-handicapping and (xi) disengagement. The wheel is presented in Fig. 14.1.

While seeking to integrate conceptual terrain, there is also a much applied purpose to the wheel. It seeks to articulate a motivation and engagement framework that is readily accessible to practitioners (e.g., teachers, counselors, psychologists), parents/caregivers, and students. In so doing, it attempts to bridge a gap between diverse dimensions of motivation and engagement theorizing on the one hand and, on the other hand, the need for practitioners to draw on the strengths of these dimensions within a parsimonious framework that they can clearly communicate to students and their parents/caregivers (Martin, 2007).

Locating Motivation and Engagement in Time and Space

The set of chapters and other recent perspectives (e.g., the Motivation and Engagement Wheel) provide substantial detail on seminal and emerging theories, concepts, methodologies, and analytical approaches to motivation and engagement. The task now is to distill and synthesize fundamental ideas and contributions in a way that assists conceptual and operational clarity. One approach is to consider motivation and engagement in time and space.

The Sequence × Space Learning Map

Considering each contribution in this part, it is evident that two primary dimensions consistently emerge. One dimension relates to the sequence of learning-related factors. The other dimension relates to the space in which the learning-related factors operate. These dimensions are presented in Fig. 14.2, referred to here as a Sequence × Space Learning Map. The horizontal axis represents sequence, and the vertical axis represents space.

The lower end of the sequence axis reflects learning antecedents (e.g., motivation), and the upper end reflects learning consequences (e.g., achievement). Between the lower and upper ends are mediators such as engagement (as suggested in most chapters in this part). The lower end of the space axis reflects the individual (e.g., student). The space axis is then progressively represented by classroom and school levels. Taken together, this Sequence × Space Learning Map seeks to synthesize some of the major conceptual and operational arguments represented in this chapter. It specifies the ordering of motivation and engagement in determining achievement and the level/s at which these processes play out.

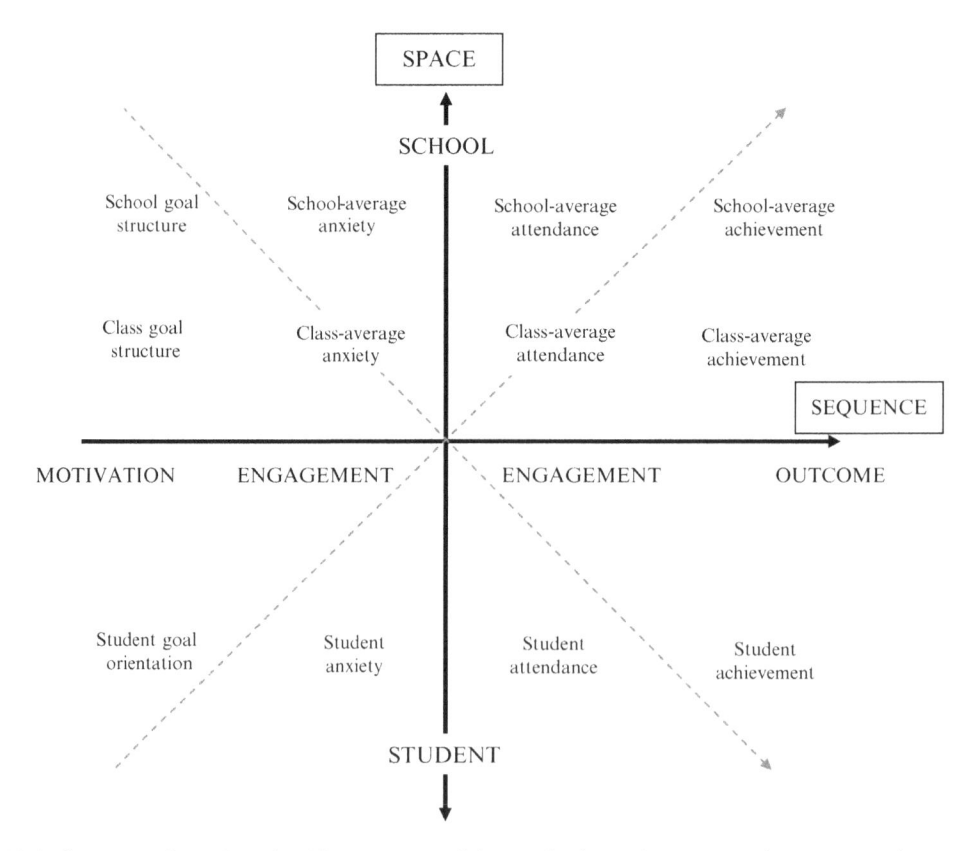

Fig. 14.2 Sequence × Space Learning Map – conceptualizing motivation and engagement in sequence and space

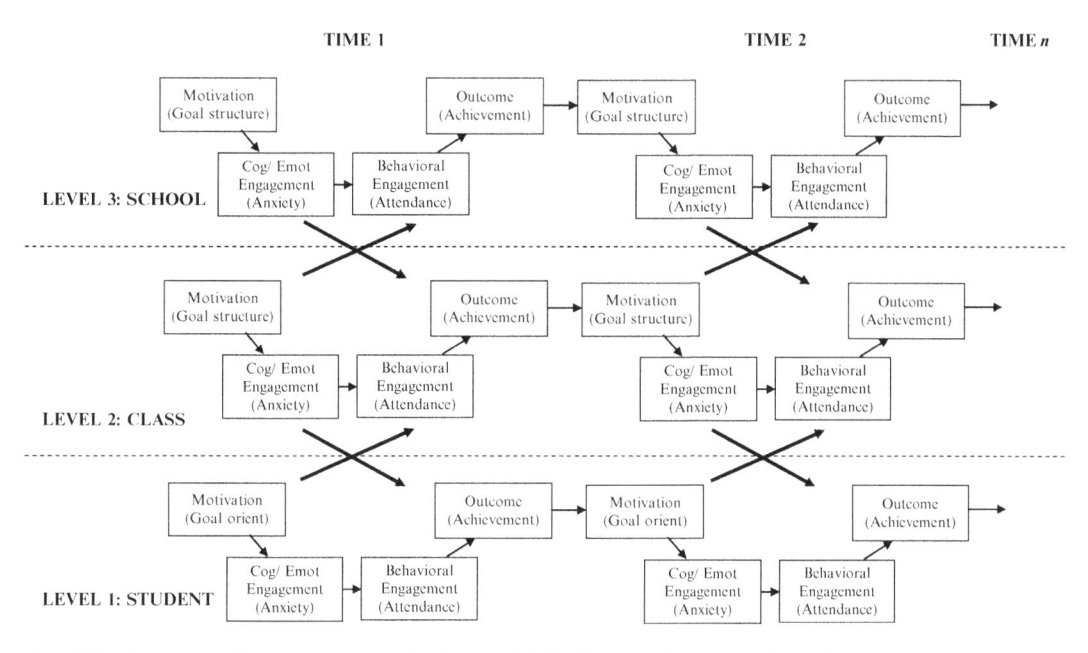

Fig. 14.3 Sequence × Space Learning Analysis – empirically investigating motivation and engagement sequence and space

To illustrate, four factors from the part are plotted in the Sequence × Space Learning Map. At far left is motivation represented by student goals and classroom and school goal structures. Further along is emotional/cognitive (depending on an author's perspective) engagement represented by student anxiety and anxiety at classroom and school levels. Further again is behavioral engagement represented by student attendance and also by class- and school-average attendance numbers/patterns. Following from attendance is student achievement as well as class- and school-average achievement.

Consistent with most accounts in this part, there is a feedback loop (indicated by an arrow) on the sequence axis, indicating that achievement then impacts motivation. There are feedback loops at both ends of the space axis, indicating that context impacts the individual and the individual impacts context. There are also diagonal axes indicating that motivation, engagement, and achievement impact each other across sequence and space. For example, class-level goal structure (motivation) impacts subsequent student-level anxiety (cognitive/emotional engagement).

The Sequence × Space Learning Analysis

The Sequence × Space Learning Map offers conceptual and operational integration of core motivation and engagement constructs. This map can also be used to specify a Sequence × Space Learning Analysis that tests major arguments and processes relevant to motivation, engagement, and achievement.

As Fig. 14.3 shows, the Sequence × Space Learning Analysis is a multilevel design with student at level 1, classroom at level 2, and school at level 3. It comprises motivation, engagement, and achievement measures at each level on the space axis. It is longitudinal in terms of the sequence of motivation, engagement, and achievement and also in terms of feedback loops across time. Parameters operate across sequence and space with student-level factors, for example, predicting class- and school-level factors.

The Sequence × Space Learning Analysis can be adapted to differentiate or expand the sequence and space axes. For example, authors in this part frequently referred to microanalysis of processes inherent in their models. In this case, the sequence axis would be further differentiated into subelements, and these elements can be plotted in Fig. 14.3 and tested accordingly. Conversely, the sequence axis can be expanded to test processes across years – particularly important for understanding the developmental nature of engagement and motivation. Other authors commented on national and international contexts. In this case, the space axis would be expanded to the country level, such as in PISA datasets. Or the space axis can be further differentiated to encompass intraindividual factors such as genetics and neural profiles – a direction suggested by Pekrun and Linnenbrink-Garcia.

What of Disengagement?

It is also worth observing that across the set of contributions, disengagement received relatively little *direct* attention (though it was implied throughout all chapters). Across approximately 70,000 words of text in seven chapters, the word "disengagement" ("disengag*") was used about 20 times. In contrast, the word "engagement" ("engag*") was used approximately 900 times. In important ways, this differential is quite understandable in a volume focusing on "engagement." On the other hand, one could be forgiven to expect somewhat greater direct attention to its counterpart, "disengagement," and its relations/juxtaposition with motivation. Is this because we tend to see engagement and disengagement on a unidimensional continuum? Is low (or no) engagement simply disengagement? Is shared variance between disengagement and motivation the same as that between engagement and motivation?

In very recent work, Martin, Anderson, Bobis, Way, and Vellar (2011) argue that learning, motivation, and achievement require attention to both engagement and disengagement. Although the two are significantly correlated, it appears that they explain unique variance in the academic process and thus should be addressed in complementary but distinct ways. They conceptualize and operationalize persistence at school in terms of the joint forces of "switching on" (engagement) and "switching off" (disengagement). To the extent that this is the case, there will be implications of this multidimensional engagement/disengagement perspective for theorizing and analyses involving motivation, learning, and achievement.

Engagement and Disengagement: A Shared Responsibility

A major message from these chapters is that engagement logically follows from a constellation of contextual (e.g., teacher) and student factors. Put another way, it seems that engagement is a rational response to contextual and individual influences. It is good to know that this is the case because it enables the logical development of targeted educational intervention to promote engagement. It also underscores the need for action on the part of practitioners (e.g., teachers, psychologists, counselors), parents/caregivers, and students – a shared responsibility frequently emphasized in the chapters in this part. A necessary corollary to this is that we must also conclude that disengagement is a rational response to contextual and individual influences. In some ways, this is a more challenging notion. It means that disengagement is a shared responsibility – and for various reasons, practitioners (e.g., teachers, psychologists, counselors), parents/caregivers, and students may have difficulty recognizing and/or accepting this.

The authors in this part of this volume have clearly demonstrated that sharing the responsibility for engagement and disengagement will promote positive academic pathways. They have identified specific factors, processes, and ideas practitioners, parents/caregivers, and students can harness to make this happen. Thanks to these authors – and also the researchers and work on which they draw – there is a solid conceptual and empirical basis for optimism as we support students' learning through school and beyond.

References

Ainley, M. (2012). Students' Interest and engagement in classroom activities. In S. L. Christenson, A. L. Reschly, & C. Wylie (Eds.), *Handbook of research on student engagement* (pp. 283–302). New York: Springer.

Anderman, E. M., & Patrick, H. (2012). Achievement goal theory, conceptualization of ability/intelligence, and classroom climate. In S. L. Christenson, A. L. Reschly, & C. Wylie (Eds.), *Handbook of research on student engagement* (pp. 173–191). New York: Springer.

Bandura, A. (1997). *Self-efficacy: The exercise of control*. New York: Freeman.

Bandura, A. (2001). Social cognitive theory: An agentic perspective. *Annual Review of Psychology, 52*, 1–26.

Bronfenbrenner, U. (1992). Ecological systems theory. In R. Vasra (Ed.), *Six theories of child development* (pp. 187–249). London: Jessica Kingsley Publications.

Christenson, S. L., Reschly, A. L., Appleton, J. J., Berman-Young, S., Spanjers, D. M., & Varro, P. (2008). Best practices in fostering student engagement. In A. Thomas & J. Grimes (Eds.), *Best practices in school psychology* (5th ed., pp. 1099–1119). Bethesda, MD: National Association of School Psychologists.

Cleary, T. J., & Zimmerman, B. J. (2012). A cyclical self-regulatory account of student engagement: theoretical foundations and applications. In S. L. Christenson, A. L. Reschly, & C. Wylie (Eds.), *Handbook of research on student engagement* (pp. 237–257). New York: Springer.

Covington, M. V. (1998). *The will to learn: A guide for motivating young people*. New York: Cambridge University Press.

Elliot, A. J. (1999). Approach and avoidance motivation and achievement goals. *Educational Psychologist, 34*, 169–189.

Finn, J. D. (1989). Withdrawing from school. *Review of Educational Research, 59*, 117–142.

Fredricks, J. A., Blumenfeld, P. C., & Paris, A. H. (2004). Student engagement: Potential of the concept, state of the evidence. *Review of Educational Research, 74*, 59–109.

Hidi, S., & Renninger, K. A. (2006). The four-phase model of interest development. *Educational Psychologist, 41*, 111–127.

Krapp, A. (2005). Basic needs and the development of interest and intrinsic motivational orientations. *Learning and Instruction, 15*, 381–395.

Lewis, M. D., & Granic, I. (Eds.). (2000). *Emotion, development, and self-organization: Dynamic systems approaches to emotional development*. Cambridge, UK: Cambridge University Press.

Martin, A. J. (2007). Examining a multidimensional model of student motivation and engagement using a construct validation approach. *British Journal of Educational Psychology, 77*, 413–440.

Martin, A. J. (2009). Motivation and engagement across the academic lifespan: A developmental construct validity study of elementary school, high school, and university/college students. *Educational and Psychological Measurement, 69*, 794–824.

Martin, A. J. (2010). *Building classroom success: Eliminating academic fear and failure*. London: Continuum.

Martin, A. J. (2011). *The motivation and engagement scale* (11th ed.). Sydney: Lifelong Achievement Group (www.lifelongachievement.com).

Martin, A. J., Anderson, J., Bobis, J., Way, J., & Vellar, R. (2011). Switching on and switching off in mathematics: An ecological study of future intent and disengagement amongst middle school students. *Journal of Educational Psychology*. 10.1037/a0025988.

Maslow, A. H. (1968). *Toward a psychology of being*. New York: Van Nostrand Reinhold.

Pekrun, R., & Linnenbrink-Garcia, L. (2012). Academic emotions and student engagement. In S. L. Christenson, A. L. Reschly, & C. Wylie (Eds.), *Handbook of research on student engagement* (pp. 259–282). New York: Springer.

Pintrich, P. R. (2003). A motivational science perspective on the role of student motivation in learning and teaching contexts. *Journal of Educational Psychology, 95*, 667–686.

Reeve, J. (2012). A self-determination theory perspective on student engagement. In S. L. Christenson, A. L. Reschly, & C. Wylie (Eds.), *Handbook of research on student engagement* (pp. 149–172). New York: Springer.

Reschly, A. L., & Christenson, S. L. (2006). Prediction of dropouts among students with mild disabilities: A case for the inclusion of student engagement variables. *Remedial and Special Education, 27*, 276–292.

Ryan, R. M., & Deci, E. L. (2000). Self-determination theory and the facilitation of intrinsic motivation, social development, and well-being. *American Psychologist, 55*, 68–78.

Schunk, D. H., & Mullen, C. A. (2012). Self-efficacy as an engaged learner. In S. L. Christenson, A. L. Reschly, & C. Wylie (Eds.), *Handbook of research on student engagement* (pp. 219–235). New York: Springer.

Turner, J. E., & Waugh, R. M. (2007). A dynamical systems perspective regarding students' learning processes: Shame reactions and emergent self-organizations. In P. A. Schutz & R. Pekrun (Eds.), *Emotions in education* (pp. 125–145). San Diego, CA: Academic.

Voelkl, K. E. (2012). School identification. In S. L. Christenson, A. L. Reschly, & C. Wylie (Eds.), *Handbook of research on student engagement* (pp. 193–218). New York: Springer.

Part III

Engagement and Contextual Influences

Parental Influences on Achievement Motivation and Student Engagement

15

Janine Bempechat and David J. Shernoff

Abstract

Underachievement and school disengagement have serious consequences, both at individual and societal levels. In this chapter, we adopt a strength-based perspective to examine the multiple ways in which parents foster achievement motivation and student engagement. Our theoretical orientation is grounded in Bronfenbrenner's (1977) ecological systems theory in which the child is situated at the center of increasingly distal and interconnected spheres of influence, from family and school to community and societal institutions. Given the increasingly diverse composition of our nation's schools, we place a premium on understanding how varied ethnic and cultural models of learning and socialization, particularly among low-income families, differentially influence parents' educational socialization strategies and how these come to affect children's developing achievement-related beliefs and behaviors. We examine several theoretical models of engagement, motivation, and parental involvement and highlight some notable research efforts that seek to explain parents' roles in fostering motivation and engagement. We then share several models of innovative programs that have experienced success in creating authentic partnerships between parents, children, schools, and communities toward the goal of stemming the tide of underachievement and disengagement.

J. Bempechat, Ed.D. (✉)
Department of Psychology and Human Development,
Wheelock College, Boston, MA, USA
e-mail: jbempechat@wheelock.edu

D.J. Shernoff, Ph.D.
Department of Leadership, Educational Psychology,
and Foundations, Northern Illinois University,
DeKalb, IL, USA
e-mail: dshernoff@niu.edu

The Role of Parents in Student Motivation and Engagement

Underachievement and school disengagement have serious consequences, both at individual and societal levels. Disengagement often manifests in a gradual cycle of withdrawal from schooling, culminating in school dropout for large numbers of youth (Finn, 1989). On some estimates, over one million (or 30%) of all ninth graders in the USA fail to graduate from high school, with the dropout (nongraduation) rate approaching 50–55% in some urban communities (Alliance for Excellent Education, 2009; Toppo, 2010). This dropout rate includes students from states in which graduation is dependent on both the successful completion of the 4-year high school curriculum and the state-administered high school leaving or exit examination. Currently, 17, or just over one-third of states, mandate such an exit exam.[1]

Problems associated with underachievement and disengagement are perhaps the most intense for students who live in poverty. Among US children under 18 years of age, 39% live in poverty, disproportionate numbers of which are from ethnic minority groups (i.e., 60% of African American, 61% of Latino, 30% of Asian American, and 26% of Caucasian children; Cauthen & Fass, 2008). Immigrant students and children of immigrants face additional challenges of acculturation (García Coll & Marks, 2009; Suárez-Orozco, Suárez-Orozco, & Todorova, 2008). Low-income children are more likely than their middle-class peers to live in poor neighborhoods with higher rates of crime, violence, and unemployment (Brooks-Gunn, Linver, & Fauth, 2005; Leventhal, Fauth, & Brooks-Gunn, 2005). In such neighborhoods, children's schools are likely to be of lower quality, characterized by less qualified teachers and higher teacher turnover than in higher income neighborhoods. (Byrd-Blake et al., 2010; Ingersoll, 2004; Johnson, 2006). Children in those schools are also more likely to be held back one or more grades and experience higher rates of suspension, school dropout, and teen pregnancy (Cauthen & Fass, 2008; Duncan & Brooks-Gunn, 2000; Hauser, Pager, & Simmons, 2004).

Parents are their children's first and primary guides through their schooling experiences, and therefore can serve to greatly buffer or compound risk factors for disengagement and low achievement. The achievement-related beliefs and behaviors of parents can have a profound influence on how children come to perceive their intellectual abilities and the value of learning and education (Eccles, Roeser, Vida, Fredricks, & Wigfield, 2006). Parents' educational socialization strategies operate at two levels that are inherently interconnected. Long before the start of formal schooling and throughout their children's schooling experiences, parents engage in cognitive socialization strategies to foster the development of intellectual skills children need to succeed in school. For example, when parents ask questions about an assigned reading or possible solutions to a math problem, they are helping their children develop critical thinking skills. Equally important, however, are the subtle ways in which parents engage motivational socialization strategies to foster the kinds of beliefs about learning that encourage persistence, diligence, and the ability to delay gratification. Thus, it is critically important to shed light on how parents, in collaboration with their children, their children's teachers, schools, and communities, can work to stem the tide of underachievement and disengagement.

In this chapter, we adopt a strength-based perspective to examine the multiple ways in which parents foster achievement motivation and student engagement. Our theoretical orientation is grounded in Bronfenbrenner's (1977) ecological systems theory in which the

---

[1] It is important to note that there is controversy around how the high school dropout rate is calculated. The commonly reported metric, based on a dataset (Common Core of Data or CCD) managed by the US Department of Education, is the averaged freshman graduation rate, which is said to reflect the percent of 9th graders who graduate on time, 4 years later. However, the CCD reports enrolled, but not entering, 9th graders. This means that the dropout rate can include, at any time, the number of students who were not promoted out of or are voluntarily repeating the 9th grade (Roy & Mishel, 2008).

child is situated at the center of increasingly distal and interconnected spheres of influence, from family and school to community and societal institutions. Given the increasingly diverse composition of our nation's schools, we place a premium on understanding how varied ethnic and cultural models of learning and socialization, particularly among low-income families, differentially influence parents' educational socialization strategies and how these come to affect children's developing achievement-related beliefs and behaviors. Clearly, not all economically disadvantaged and minority students are disengaged from school. There are many academically resilient students who beat the odds and demonstrate high levels of achievement and engagement in school.

In our own research, we are interested in understanding the more positive educational outcomes within these populations (Bempechat, 1998; Shernoff & Schmidt, 2008). We are interested in discovering: What are the learning beliefs and dispositions that characterize the motivational orientation of low-income and racial/ethnic minority students? What emotions and perceptions characterize such students' engagement with schoolwork when they are completing it? What are the influences on their motivation and engagement? Specifically, to what extent may parental involvement and other family-related variables influence such students' motivation and engagement with school learning and achievement? Finally, what is the role of culture in influencing educational socialization, and what differences in parental influences and socialization strategies exist within different cultures? We will here examine several theoretical models of engagement, motivation, and parental involvement and highlight some notable research efforts that seek to explain parents' roles in fostering motivation and engagement. We will then share several models of innovative programs that have experienced success in creating authentic partnerships between parents, children, schools, and communities.

Theoretical Perspective on Motivation and Engagement

Usually referring to students' involvement with schooling, academics, or learning (e.g., Finn, 1989, 1993; Marks, 2000; Skinner & Belmont, 1993), there is fairly broad agreement that student (or school) engagement involves both behaviors (e.g., completing assignments) and emotions (e.g., belongingness) and encompasses effort and persistence in schoolwork (Connell & Wellborn, 1991; Newmann, 1992; Skinner & Belmont, 1993; Smerdon, 1999). Engagement and motivation to learn (Stipek, 1993) are highly related and overlapping concepts, having many commonalities as measurable constructs (see Fig. 15.1). However, motivation has been traditionally viewed as a psychological construct, whereas engagement, even in its common definition, refers to an emotional involvement or

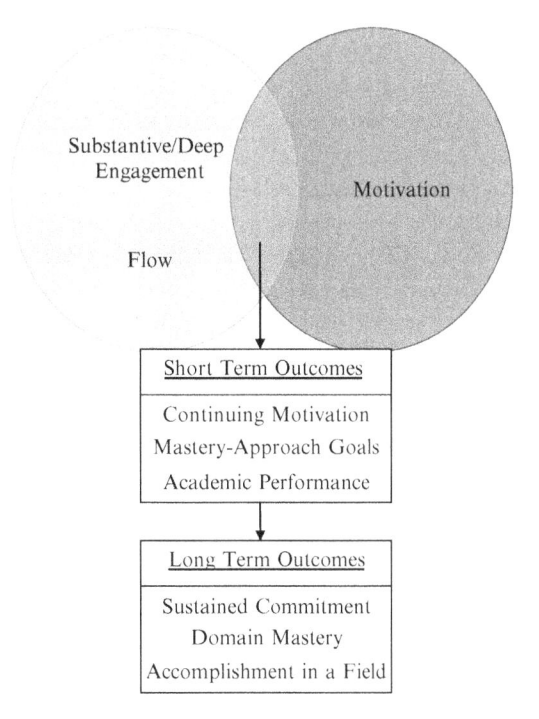

Fig. 15.1 Conceptual model of the interaction between deep engagement and motivation, with associated short-term and long-term outcomes

commitment to some object and describes the experiential intensity of a relationship or interaction. It can refer to a sustained relationship, as with engagement in the process of schooling or a domain of interest, and also to one's temporal involvement or interactions with activities and social partners in the immediate environments. An increasing amount of attention is directed to student engagement because it is presumed to be malleable and highly influenced by the learning environment, and thus considered a means to ameliorate downward student trajectories.

Engagement is increasingly recognized to be a complex, latent construct involving both observable (e.g., attending class) and unobservable (i.e., "investment" in learning) psychological events *and* positive emotions (e.g., enjoyment and interest) (Appleton, Christenson, & Furlong, 2008). It is presumed to encompass actions and behaviors, effort, as well as ambient emotional states. Fredricks, Blumenfeld, and Paris (2004) observed that a multitude of conceptualizations and measurements of engagement run throughout the literature and concluded that that student engagement should be conceptualized as a multidimensional metaconstruct made up of three distinct but related dimensions: cognitive engagement (i.e., investment in learning, self-regulation), behavioral engagement (i.e., positive conduct, demonstration of effort), and emotional engagement (e.g., interest and boredom). Behavioral engagement is based on observational and self-reported measures of on-task behavior, effort, participation, attendance, or other desirable behaviors typical of good students (Finn & Voelkl, 1993; Green, Rhodes, Hirsch, Suarez-Orozco, & Camic, 2008; Marks, 2000). Cognitive engagement is usually measured as students' investment or mastery in learning and depth of processing (Blumenfeld, 1992; Newmann, 1992; Newmann & Wehlage, 1993), students' intrinsic motivation to learn within a given learning environment (Brophy, 1987; Covington, 2000; Ryan & Deci, 2000; Sansone & Harackiewicz, 2000), and/or the use of self-regulated metacognitive strategies such as planning, monitoring, and evaluating one's understanding of a text (Zimmerman, 1990). Many of these conceptualizations and measurements of cognitive engagement have much in common with those used previously in the motivational literature. Emotional engagement refers to students' affect and emotions in schools, including interest, boredom, happiness, sadness, and anxiety (Finn, 1989; Shernoff, Csikszentmihalyi, Schneider, & Shernoff, 2003; Voelkl, 1997).

Both motivation and engagement have been conceptualized as a personal trait and context-varying psychological state (Fredricks et al., 2004; Schunk, Pintrich, & Meece, 2008). We find this to be a useful distinction, and to simplify, we generally think of *engagement* as the quality of temporal interactions with the learning activity, task, social companions, and other components of the proximal environment, not dissimilar from the concept of *situational interest* (Hidi & Anderson, 1992; Mitchell, 1993), whereas we characterize *motivation* as a more global set of personal orientations that influence how students approach schoolwork, learning, and achievement.

Conceptualizing Engagement

Many studies rely on observer ratings of engagement, but as both a latent and multidimensional construct, engagement may not always be an observable characteristic. In addition, behaviors rated high on engagement by observers may represent only compliance to authority figures or "going through the motions" characteristic of *procedural engagement*. This conceptualization of engagement contrasts with *substantive engagement* characterized by deep processing and intrinsic motivation (Brophy, 1983; Nystrand & Gamoran, 1991). For purposes of identifying students who are academically resilient, we are interested in identifying engagement that is more substantive and less procedural because substantive engagement is likely to be more strongly related to authentic motivational orientations and educational attitudes that are transferrable into higher levels of academic performance (see Fig. 15.1). We believe that when students are substantively and deeply engaged with learning, the psychological state is similar to that characterized as *flow experiences* (Csikszentmihalyi, 1990). Flow is a state of deep absorption in an activity that is intrinsically interesting and enjoyable, such as when athletes are focused on their play, dancers are immersed in their performance, or scientists are engrossed in solving a new problem (Csikszentmihalyi, 1990, 1997; Csikszentmihalyi & Csikszentmihalyi, 1988). The state of flow is all-encompassing, with no psychic energy left for distractions, including consciousness of time and self. During this state, individuals function at their fullest capacity, and the experience becomes its own reward (DeCharms, 1968; Deci, 1975). Notably, students with multiple risk factors have stated that concentrated experiences like dance can be therapeutic, providing a sort of sanctuary in which they can forget about their problems and allow their creative energies to "flow" (Csikszentmihalyi, 1990).

Based on flow theory, we have found it useful to define and operationalize engagement in educational contexts as the simultaneous experience of concentration, interest, and enjoyment in the task at hand (Shernoff & Schmidt, 2008; Shernoff & Vandell, 2007; Shernoff et al., 2003). Because all three components are strongly related to learning (Shernoff & Csikszentmihalyi, 2009), we argue that engagement defined in this way is very close to learning itself, or at least the *experience of learning*. It is of course unrealistic to conceptualize adolescent-aged students as routinely in flow during school; and indeed our research has demonstrated that this is not the case (Shernoff & Csikszentmihalyi). We concur with the observation of the National Research Council (2004) in writing, "We are not proposing that all high school students be in a constant state of flow, but we have seen youth deeply and enthusiastically engaged in schoolwork and we believe that this high standard should be our goal" (p. 32). In other words, deep problem-solving, authentic interest, and enjoyment in creating "works" encapsulated by the concept of flow are a way to conceptualize ideal engagement in learning and, indeed, the act of learning itself.

The type of experience that occurs as one becomes engrossed or entirely taken up with objects or activities of interest often results in a creative or scientific attitude toward the activity somewhat set apart from the ordinary range of experience (Henri, 1923/2007). These individual episodes may gradually accrue meaning, culminating in a strengthened, sustained, and persistent involvement in an area of interest (Nakamura, 2001). Thus, engagement may naturally progress and develop into a more stable, continuing motivational orientation that is directly related to academic performance (Maehr, 1976). For example, we found that student engagement reported at random moments in high school science classes was predictive of the choice of a college major in science 2 years later and that momentary interest and enjoyment in math and science classes were also predictive of academic performance in college (Shernoff, 2010; Shernoff & Hoogstra, 2001). These associations were statistically significant after controlling for grades in high school (which were not a significant predictor of a related college major or performance in college) as well as demographic characteristics. These findings are consistent with Hidi and Renninger's (2006) four-phase model of interest development, in which early interest is often situational, much like episodes of flow, but as value in the activity or topic deepens, interest becomes an enduring and sustained trait of the individual.

Conceptualizing Motivation

We, therefore, see substantive engagement with learning activities as having a cumulative progression toward more general motivational orientations and proclivities. We are particularly interested in motivational orientations that support learning and school achievement, or *achievement motivation*. Broadly speaking, achievement motivation consists of a constellation of beliefs influencing patterns of school achievement, including expectations and standards for performance, value placed on learning, and self-perceptions of ability (Deci & Ryan, 1985; Dweck, 2006; Eccles et al., 2006; Nicholls, 1989; Weiner, 2005). Research in achievement motivation today is located within a social-cognitive framework (Dweck & Leggett, 1988). That is, achievement-related beliefs are seen as influenced by the ways in which students interpret or make meaning from their educational experiences. Their school-related experiences may include feedback from parents and teachers, motivational and affective responses to success and failure, and their placement within school structures such as ability grouping. Importantly, children's achievement beliefs influence their achievement-related behavior. For example, children who believe that ability is fixed are more likely to avoid challenging tasks than those who view ability as malleable (Dweck, 2006).

Goal theory is one of the more prominent contemporary approaches to studying achievement motivation. Early research focused on two achievement goal orientations that students adopt about the nature and purpose of learning, beliefs about ability, and conceptions of school success, referred to as mastery and performance goals (Ames, 1992b; Elliott & Dweck, 1988; Maehr & Nicholls, 1980; Nicholls, 1978, 1989). Mastery goals are conceptualized as the desire to attain knowledge and understanding (a mastery-approach orientation), implying a positive form of motivation. As illustrated in Fig. 15.1, this motivational pattern is maintained over time both in the short term and in the long term (Weiner, 1979), underscoring the quality of involvement and a continued commitment to learning (Paris & Winograd, 1990; Pelletier et al., 1995; Pintrich & De Groot, 1990). Thus, we would expect cumulative episodes of substantive or flow-like engagement to progress into mastery-approach goals and dispositions.

Mastery goals can also include avoidance. Mastery-avoidance goals reflect a concern for maintaining one's skills that derives from the fear of losing them (Elliot, 1999). In contrast, performance goals represent a desire to appear competent (a performance-approach orientation), or at least to avoid appearing incompetent (a performance-avoidance orientation) (Ames, 1984; Dweck & Bempechat, 1983; Nicholls, 1984; Pintrich, 2000). An impressive body of experimental, survey, and, to a much lesser extent, qualitative research has demonstrated that individuals with mastery goals perform better, have more positive affect and self-efficacy beliefs, are more persistent in the face of difficulty, prefer challenging over easy tasks, and otherwise are better oriented toward learning (Ames, 1992a; Brophy, 1983; Meece, Blumenfeld, & Hoyle, 1988; Nicholls, 1983, 1984, 1989; see Kaplan & Maehr, 2007). Recent research also confirms that mastery goals are more likely to lead to subsequent, continuing interest including college course enrollment en route to early career development (Harackiewicz, Barron, Tauer, & Elliot, 2002; Hulleman, Durik, Schweigert, & Harackiewicz, 2008).

Motivational Orientations Among Low-Income Ethnic Minority Adolescents

In our recent research (e.g., Bempechat, Li, Wenk, & Holloway, submitted; Bempechat, Shernoff, Li, Holloway, & Arendtz, 2010), we conducted a series of in-depth interviews with an ethnically diverse sample of 92 ninth graders (approximately one third African American, one third European American, and one third Mexican American), all low-SES students (i.e., eligible for free/reduced-price lunch). We focused our analyses on the difference in achievement goals and educational attitudes between the higher and lower achievers, as determined by a median split. We asked the students about their perceptions of school and factors related to processes of learning and schooling in the context of their daily lives and routines.

To be sure, the high achievers expressed many more beliefs and attitudes expressive of a mastery orientation. However, our coding categories revealed that the predominant themes characterizing these students' educational attitudes and learning goals were more nuanced and varied than is typically reflected in the achievement goals literature. For example, high achievers were more likely to express three different types of mastery-related behaviors and habits: mastery-learning goals (e.g., the desire to learn new things; see Ames, 1992b), mastery behaviors (e.g., persistence, investment of effort, self-discipline), and mastery-emergent standards (e.g., high personal standards for performance or learning).

High achievers were also more likely to express a healthy conscientiousness for their future educational or career goals. The lower achievers also expressed mastery-related dispositions, but with the tendency to invest effort inconsistently, such as putting in more effort for some classes than others, seemingly perceiving their effort as more optional than high achievers. They were also more likely to avoid work altogether. Although on the surface, these motivational orientations appear similar to performance-approach and performance-avoidance goals, comparative performance did not seem to be a central concern; rather, lower achievers preferred activities perceived as more enjoyable until teachers or parents forced their attention to schoolwork—i.e., they had the need for external discipline in the absence of self-discipline.

We also sought to measure and compare individual levels of engagement in learning environments (mostly when in school) and while doing schoolwork in particular. To reach this goal, we utilized the Experience Sampling Method (or ESM; see Hektner, Schmidt, & Csikszentmihalyi, 2007). Students wore a watch programmed to beep randomly seven times per day, from 8:00 a.m. until 10:00 p.m. When signaled, students recorded their location, activity, preferred activity, companions, subjective experiences, and emotions (e.g., challenge, importance, etc.) into Experience Sampling Forms (ESFs). We then compared subjective experiences between the higher and lower achievers while completing schoolwork specifically. Results showed that higher achievers had significantly higher engagement (i.e., average of concentration, interest, and enjoyment) and consistently reported greater feelings of understanding and competence when completing their schoolwork than the lower achievers. However, they also reported significantly higher levels of negative affect such as feeling scared and confused. The magnitude of this difference was generally small (on average about 0.20 of a standard deviation, though this varied by the specific emotion examined), but the difference was greater (e.g., 0.60 of standard deviation in feeling confused) when the challenge of the school-related activity was perceived to be high. Higher achievers appeared to possess greater confidence in their academic competencies, but became more worried when higher levels of challenge threatened it. Consistent with their interview testimonies, lower achievers reported higher levels of choice and guilt when they were doing their schoolwork.

Overall, both the interview and ESM data converged on the central difference that higher achievers were more invested in schooling and seemed to take both their school learning and performance goals more seriously. On the whole, their educational values and future educational goals were decisively stronger. Although the goals literature may classify their goals to reach clearly defined future goals as performance-oriented (i.e., performance-approach goals), such goals, which guided the investment to learn and master material in a mature and purposeful way, may be better characterized as educational values for which the higher achievers demonstrated *identification* and *integration* in terms of Ryan and Deci's (2000) taxonomy of motivation.

Even though their educational goals and standards appeared to be internalized and integrated, this does not mean that this process of internalization was not highly influenced. On the contrary, we suspect that their values may be strongly influenced by a number of interacting contextual variables based on current theory and research. We turn to that theory and research next. An important question becomes: What are the salient contexts of influence on children's educational values? Are family factors, and parents in particular, especially salient influences?

Theoretical Background on Contextual Influences

In proposing his ecological model underscoring the primacy of context in child development, Bronfenbrenner (1977) observed that developmental psychology had become "…the science of the strange behavior of children in strange situations with strange adults for the briefest periods of time" (p. 513). His theory of nested and reciprocal spheres of influence in child development served to highlight a widely accepted organizing principle of development—individuals do not evolve in a vacuum, but rather are active participants in multiple social and historical contexts that shape their emerging beliefs about how the world around them functions. A great deal of research in parent involvement focuses on the two proximal systems. The microsystem consists of the immediate settings that contain the child—for example, what parents and families say and do in support of academic achievement. The mesosystem represents interactions between the environments that contain the child and thus theoretically situates the home-school connection in studies of how bonds between these settings can foster achievement and engagement. There may be many influences on student engagement within the microsystem and mesosystem alone. However, much of the research on flow in adolescents demonstrates that certain contexts in the microsystem (e.g., structured extracurriculars or organized sports) may exert a motivational pull so strong (i.e., to the point of complete absorption in the activity or context) that it can overcome the potentially distracting influence of other contexts within the microsystem or mesosystem (e.g., Csikszentmihalyi, 1975; Csikszentmihalyi & Larson, 1984; Schmidt, Shernoff, & Csikszentmihalyi, 2007).

No less important for the influence of parenting on developmental outcomes, however, are the two more distal circles of influence. Psychological anthropologists and cultural psychologists alike have argued that societal contexts (the exosystem) as well as cultural and historical contexts (the macrosystem) are critical in shaping thinking and the development of belief systems, including those that guide parental educational socialization practices (Cole, 1996; Harkness & Super, 1992; Rogoff, 2003; Vygotsky, 1978; Weisner, 2002). In her work, Rogoff (1990) has noted that cultural and historical contexts are key factors that drive the content and nature of meaning making.

Culture and context thus play central roles in helping us understand how parents foster their children's engagement with school. The child's role, however, is equally critical. Children actively co-construct their developing understanding of the nature and value of learning and education through their ongoing interactions with their caregivers, teachers, and mentors. Flow experiences are also considered to be the product of the quality of interaction between a person and the environment; thus, conceptualizing student engagement based on flow theory is consistent with bioecological views. Bronfenbrenner and Ceci's (Bronfenbrenner & Ceci, 1994) bioecological model of development provides a way of understanding the influences of an individual's background, personal attributes, peers, teachers, parents, the school, community, and macrolevel factors like society and culture through *proximal processes* described as "complex reciprocal interaction(s) between an active, evolving biophysical human organism and the persons, objects, and symbols in the immediate environment" (p. 572). Proximal processes vary as a function of the developing person and both distal and immediate environment. As we will discuss below, ecocultural theory and bioecological models of development are critical in understanding ethnic and cultural diversity in parental influences on student engagement.

Theoretical Approaches to Understanding Parent Involvement

Several decades of research have demonstrated that parental involvement in children's schooling is associated with a variety of positive academic and motivational outcomes. These include such indicators as higher GPA and achievement test scores, improved attendance in school, greater rates of high school graduation, and positive attitudes about schooling (Comer, 2005; Eccles & Gootman, 2002; Epstein, 1995; Mapp, Johnson, Strickland, & Meza, 2008). There is no universal pattern of parent involvement that results in higher achievement, nor do all forms of involvement enhance learning outcomes (Hill & Taylor, 2004; Jeynes, 2010; Pomerantz, Moorman, & Litwak, 2007). The overall benefits of parental involvement when taken as a whole, however, have been substantial enough to influence public policy. For example, under the mandate of the No Child Left Behind Act (NCLB), schools must enact policies and procedures that involve parents in their children's school lives (NCLB, 2002 Title I, Sec. 1001 [12]).

There exists a shared understanding that healthy academic and psychosocial development cannot occur if key constituents of the child's upbringing—parents, teachers, and community members—operate in a vacuum or, worse, are in conflict. While prominent models of parental involvement stress the co-construction of participation, they also place primary responsibility for engaging parents on schools and their agents—teachers, administrators, and support staff (Epstein, 1995; Reschly & Christenson, 2009). Epstein's influential theory of overlapping spheres of influence derives from Bronfenbrenner's ecological theory and, like it, places the child at the center of three contexts—home, school, and community—that need to work in concert to foster learning and development (Epstein, 1995). Epstein's typology of six types of family-school connections identifies family and school responsibilities that, when enacted, can create a seamless partnership between home and school. At the same time, schools are seen as bearing the responsibility for assisting parents to embrace beliefs (e.g., seeing their children as students) and engage in actions that support their children's learning. This is particularly so in high-poverty urban centers, where parents may not have the resources or social capital to maximize their own abilities to foster achievement.

Over time, conceptions of parent involvement have evolved from a focus on activities that schools can design to engage parents to the more recent realization that relationships are the foundation upon which successful partnerships are built (Reschly & Christenson, 2009). These relationships need to be perceived as warm, caring, and respectful in order to gain the trust and enduring participation of parents and family members. With Bronfenbrenner's mesosystem as its starting point, Reschly and Christenson have argued that family involvement represents a collaboration between homes and schools, one that is devoted to enhancing children's development across the domains of the self and not limited to only academic growth. This mesosystemic approach is at the core of the model of 4 A's—the school conditions necessary to establish strong partnerships (Christenson & Sheridan, 2001). These include an *approach* to families that communicates genuine respect for parents and the different ways they become involved; an *attitude* that respects parents' perspectives and views parental involvement as essential for student success; an *atmosphere* that supports interactions between home and school; and, with these three components in place, *actions* that can be adopted to support strong family-school relationships.

As we describe toward the end of this chapter, successful practitioners, such as James Comer and Geoffrey Canada, have embodied the 4 A's approach in their efforts to build meaningful connections between home, school, and communities.

The Influence of Parental Involvement on Well-Being and Engagement

Research evidence suggests at least two fundamental reasons that parental involvement influences engagement and motivation. The first is the strong association between parental relations with their children and overall psychological well-being, which positions parental involvement as a primary protective factor against disengagement. The second is the more direct influence of caring and supportive relationships with parents.

Parental Relations and Psychological Well-Being

Our conceptualization of engagement as defined by students' self-perceptions of their level of involvement in an activity places an emphasis on the relational and emotional well-being of the student. Such an outlook is based on the premise that engagement with learning environments is situated within the larger context of psychological and relational well-being emanating from effective adaptation to the environment (Griffiths, Sharkey, & Furlong, 2009). Within this larger perspective, meaningful engagement that leads to sustained motivation may be seen as a key driver of positive youth development (Larson, 2006), and fostering it is a primary goal of educational approaches that emphasize strengths and well-being of students rather than deficit-driven and reactive approaches (Gilman, Huebner, & Furlong, 2009).

Indeed, there appears to be a strong relationship between engagement and well-being. Students who are interested and involved in skill building and productive pursuits score higher on measures of psychological adjustment, including measures of self-esteem, responsibility, competence, and social relations (Steinberg, 1996), whereas students who report feeling alienated from school are more likely to have behavioral problems ranging from withdrawal to depression to aggression (Jessor & Jessor, 1977). Research has shown that the resources of families, schools, and communities may foster the positive development of youth through provisions of physical safety and security, developmentally appropriate structure, and expectations for behavior; emotional and moral support; and opportunities to make a contribution to one's community (Eccles & Gootman, 2002). In support of this ecological-adaptation view of engagement and positive development, Reschly, Huebner, Appleton, and Antaramian (2008) recently found that a significant relationship between positive emotions and student engagement was mediated by broadened cognitive capacities (i.e., problem-solving), behavioral coping strategies (i.e., social support seeking), and other proclivities toward healthy adaptation.

Because family life and parental relations are such powerful forces in overall adaptation and relational well-being, family cohesiveness and parental relations may be seen as a primary protective factor against behavioral and psychological problems including disengagement from school, while reciprocally serving as a salient influence on resiliency and positive psychological outcomes (Suldo, 2009). For example, spending time with one's family in grade five has been associated with positive affect (Larson & Richards, 1991). Not only have children's ratings of parents' warmth been related to life satisfaction (Chang, McBride-Chang, Stewart, & Au, 2003), but attesting to the long-ranging and formative influence of parental relations, a longitudinal study of 17,000 youth in Great Britain found that feeling close to one's mother at age 16 explained 5–11% of the variance in life satisfaction at age 42 (Flouri, 2004). Conversely, parental conflict has been associated with diminished life satisfaction both concurrently and 1 year later in a sample of 429 12–16-year-olds in Hong Kong (Shek, 1998).

The Influence of Parental Relationship Support

Caring and supportive relationships with peers and adults are an integral feature of settings promoting the motivation and development of youth (Eccles & Gootman, 2002). Developmentally speaking, adolescents are fully embedded in a world of interpersonal relationships (Kegan, 1982). As students enter middle school, their social networks have an increasingly important social-emotional influence on their attitudes toward school and motivation to succeed (Furlong et al., 2003). Due to the pervasive influence of relationships on multiple facets of student motivation, Martin and Dowson (2009) recently demonstrated that many of the most dominant motivational theories may be conceptualized in relational terms. A growing number of studies support this view. Typically, engagement research has examined the effect of connectedness with specific social partners: most commonly, teachers, peers, parents, and mentors. Research evidence has rapidly accumulated, demonstrating that relatedness in all of these categories has important and unique contributions to student engagement (e.g., Furrer & Skinner, 2003; Rhodes, 2002; Steinberg, 1996; See recent meta-analysis by Roorda et al. 2011). We here focus on the influence of parental relationship support.

The importance of parental relations for social competence and other positive developmental outcomes is rooted in the continuity view of relationships, which suggests that one's relationship style is relatively stable and strongly influenced by one's attachment to a primary caregiver as early as infancy, like relational "templates" carried forward into to adolescence and adulthood (Furrer & Skinner, 2003). During this time, the quality of parental relations may also operate in a great variety of ways to influence students' motivation. For example, many students are motivated by grades, but their interpretation of what the grades signify is often mediated though their relationship with their parents (Steinberg, 1996). The quality of parental relations has thus been linked not only to higher engagement (Chen, 2008), but also to academic performance (Furrer & Skinner, 2003; Sirin & Rogers-Sirin, 2004) and achievement (Hughes & Kwok, 2007). The quality of parent–child relations has also been associated with school satisfaction (Huebner & Diener, 2008). Findings like these suggest that supportive parental relations are important for students' engagement and attitudes about schooling beyond providing the child with templates for relating to others in the early years of life (Furrer & Skinner, 2003).

How Parents Influence Engagement and Foster Adaptive Achievement Beliefs

A considerable body of research has focused on what parents can do to foster their children's engagement and achievement in school and how schools can support parents in their efforts. While much attention is rightfully paid to particular activities (e.g., reading to children, assisting with homework) that positively contribute to school grades and achievement test scores, our understanding of the benefits of parent involvement has expanded to include the motivational factors involved. Research at the intersection of ecocultural theory and social cognitive theory has revealed that parents' own attitudes about learning, the value placed on education, achievement expectations, and approaches with the school and its agents have a profound influence on the development of their children's achievement-related beliefs and behaviors (Bempechat, 2004; Grolnick & Slowiaczek, 1994; Jeynes, 2010).

As we shall see, there is considerable variety in the ways in which, and circumstances under which, parents' participation in their children's learning enhances achievement and the development of adaptive motivational tendencies, such as mastery orientation toward learning. Research identifies at least three ways that parents and families can influence student engagement: through (a) parent involvement with homework, (b) parenting style, and (c) the transmission of educational values.

Parent Involvement in Homework

The literature on parent involvement in homework has been particularly illustrative of the profound influence that parents have to enhance as well as hinder the development of adaptive motivational beliefs and behaviors. This influence is not trivial, in light of the fact that students' subjective experiences while doing homework tend to be characterized by negative affect, including high apathy and low engagement (Leone & Richards, 1989; Shernoff & Vandell, 2007). Interestingly, this research suggests that the worst part of homework for children and adolescents may be that it is a solitary activity; affect improves considerably as a shared activity with parents or peers. Parents who provide assistance with homework play a critical role not only in fostering learning, but in scaffolding strategies for time management and problem-solving. Further, their interest in and assistance with homework predicts their children's self-perceptions of competence (Grolnick & Slowiaczek, 1994; Hoover-Dempsey et al., 2001; Pomerantz, Ng, & Wang, 2006). For example, Pomerantz and her colleagues examined mothers' mastery-oriented involvement with their children's homework as a function of children's perceptions of competence. Mothers who used mastery-oriented techniques to help their 8- to 12-year-old children with homework (e.g., helped them to understand their work, encouraged them to solve problems on their own) were particularly influential in enhancing mastery orientation in their children 6 months later. Importantly, these mothers' mastery-oriented practices predicted heightened self-perceptions of competence among children with initially low self-perceptions of ability (Pomerantz et al., 2006).

Parents also create environments for study that help students learn to deal with and manage their homework behavior (Epstein & Van Vooris, 2001; Hong & Lee, 1999; Xu & Corno, 1998, 2003). In their observation study of parents and their third grade children, Xu and Corno (1998) found that parents effectively arranged their children's homework environment by minimizing distractions, focusing their children on their assignments, and helping to make homework more interesting. Children of these parents actively engaged in strategies to help them complete their work, including preparing a place to work, keeping track of time, and self-monitoring their affect by praising themselves. These children, then, were able to model adaptive attitudes and behaviors that their parents had scaffolded for them.

This and other studies demonstrate the extent to which homework can be a social experience, in which children's subjective experience is coconstructed through interactions with parents. Indeed, parents' attitudes about homework have been found to have a direct and positive influence on their children's subsequent attitudes and academic outcomes (Cooper, Lindsay, Nye, & Greathouse, 1998; Else-Quest, Hyde, & Hejmadi, 2008; Leone & Richards, 1989). In a recent study, Else-Quest and her colleagues videotaped and coded mothers' and their 11-year-old children's affect during a teaching session. The authors invoke the notions of emotional contagion (unconscious copying of another's emotions) and emotional convergence (wherein members of a dyad express the same emotion) to suggest that mothers may in fact be able to shape their children's emotions during the homework experience by carefully monitoring the emotions they model (Else-Quest et al., 2008). These researchers documented a variety of positive (e.g., pride, positive interest, affection) and negative (e.g., frustration, distress, tension) emotions and found that these were associated with performance. For example, positive interest and pride were associated with higher achievement, while tension was linked to poorer performance.

The ongoing debate about the influence of homework on academic achievement has at times pitted parents against educators and educators against homework researchers (Bempechat, 2004). Mixed findings on the extent to which homework enhances achievement, especially at the elementary school level, have contributed to a popular view that its role should be very limited (Kohn, 2006; Kralovec & Buell, 2001). The above body of research makes clear that homework can be a powerful vehicle for fostering the development of adaptive motivational tendencies. When parent involvement with homework is warm and supportive, it serves to enhance both academic achievement and the development of adaptive beliefs about learning.

The Influence of Parenting Styles

Despite the variation that may exist in supportive parenting relations, Baumrind's (1971) typology of parenting styles has figured prominently in research on children's psychosocial outcomes. Research has found that authoritative parents—those who effectively set limits and enforce appropriate boundaries (i.e., a demandingness dimension, in which parents make age-appropriate demands for mature behavior) in the context of a caring and communicative relationship that supports children's independence (i.e., a responsiveness dimension, in which parents are sensitive to, but not indulgent of, children's requests)—promote social competence, especially in comparison with parents who provide only one or neither of the two dimensions (Baumrind, 1989). Various problem behaviors such as delinquency, drug and alcohol abuse, and conformity to antisocial peer pressure are lower among youth reared by authoritative parents (Lamborn, Brown, Mounts, & Steinberg, 1992; Steinberg, 1996). There is evidence that parenting that supports school success has similar authoritative characteristics—monitoring children's school activities, openly showing affection and becoming involved, and encouraging children to communicate their point of view. Actively participating in school activities and support for learning as an end in itself may instill intrinsic interest in learning and a tendency to persist in academic challenges (Lamborn et al., 1992). Thus, studies have found that children of authoritative parents are more engaged in school, spend more time in homework, have higher educational expectations and GPAs, and are less involved in school deviance than children of nonauthoritative parents (Lamborn et al., 1992).

More relevant to our own research, other studies have demonstrated that support and challenge experienced from the family is related to intrinsically motivated interest and flow experiences during work-related activities specifically, as measured by the Experience Sampling Method (ESM). The family challenge and support dimensions in Rathunde's (1996) study of 165 talented high school students (aged 14–15 years) somewhat expand on Baumrind's responsiveness and demandingness dimensions in the early years of life. Because developmental tasks during adolescence revolve around developing self-identity, managing unsupervised time, and directing one's pursuits, family challenge emanates from high expectations for doing one's best and behavioral control, and family support is provided by an authentic interest in the child, unconditional positive regard, acceptance/involvement, and autonomy granting. The study found that students' and parents' perceptions along both dimensions were corroborative. Moreover, students who reported their families to be high on both dimensions reported more flow experiences during productive activities.

Research suggests that authoritative parenting styles are associated with children's mastery goal motivational orientations as a potential mediator of positive school outcomes, whereas nonauthoritative styles are associated with performance goal orientations (Suldo, 2009). Some studies have suggested that the effect of parenting styles may not operate the same way for all ethnicities. For example, the use of physical discipline in childhood, generally associated with an authoritarian style, predicted more externalizing problems in adolescents for European Americans, but fewer among African Americans (Lansford, Deater-Deckard, Dodge, Bates, & Petit, 2004). However, this study did not examine parenting styles per se. Larger-scale research on parenting styles in adolescence, such as Steinberg, Mounts, Lamborn, and Dornbusch's (1991) study of 10,000 high school students, has found that positive correlates of authoritative parenting (i.e., higher grades and self-reliance, and less psychological stress and delinquency) transcended ethnicity, socioeconomic status, and family structure.

Mandara's research has shed some light on the inconsistent findings associated with ethnicity and parenting style (Mandara & Murray, 2002). In a recent study of African American parents and their 15-year-old children, he identified three styles of parenting that were similar to Baumrind's typology. Important differences set African American authoritative parents apart from their European American counterparts. For example, African American authoritative parents were found to be more exacting of their children and gave in less to their demands. From a European American perspective, this might be considered a sign of authoritarian parenting, yet this qualitatively different kind of authoritative parenting was associated with positive academic and social outcomes (Gorman-Smith, Tolan, Henry, & Florsheim, 2000; Taylor, Hinton, & Wilson, 1995).

Parenting styles are further influenced by social contexts. Recent research has demonstrated a positive association between residence in high-poverty neighborhoods and diminished parental warmth, increased control, and harsh discipline (Pinderhughes, Nix, Foster, & Jones, 2001; Tendulkar, Buka, Dunn, Subramanain, & Koenen, 2010; Zhang & Anderson, 2010). The stresses associated with living in communities characterized by violence, limited social resources, in addition to concerns for children's safety may undermine parents' ability to engage in more positive parenting (Pinderhughes et al., 2001). Together, these findings underscore the extent to which researchers need to understand parenting and educational socialization in cultural, ethnic, and social contexts.

The Transmission of Educational Values

As children progress through the school years, their interactions with schools and other contexts within the microsystem and mesosystem provide the basis for more stable, enduring educational attitudes and dispositions. While manifesting in a variety of ways, parents' own educational attitudes and beliefs may be the major influence on the educational attitudes that their children gradually adopt. Messages of educational values are often communicated more implicitly than explicitly. For example, if parents do not take advantage of opportunities to become involved with the child's schooling, even if they say that school is important, children may get the message that their parents do not have the time for school and conclude that they do not, either. Similarly, when parents support their children's opinions and encourage self-expression in an affirming and noncontingent manner, their children are more likely to express their beliefs and act in an autonomous and self-regulating manner important for success in school. Providing strong research evidence for this viewpoint, Jeynes (2010) conducted a series of meta-analyses of parent involvement research which showed that parent expectations, communicated through parental sacrifice, low stress communication, and a shared valuing of education, were more powerful in predicting academic outcomes than open communication, in which parents and children freely express themselves without fear of retribution.

Grolnick and her colleagues (Grolnick & Slowiaczek, 1994) also found evidence for the indirect influence of parent involvement on student achievement through motivational factors. Grolnick and Ryan (1989) found that youth whose parents were both autonomy supportive and involved in their schoolwork (i.e., talked with them about school and helped them with challenges) internalized the value of doing well in school, as demonstrated by regularly completing homework, enjoying their schoolwork, and doing their best to succeed. With greater internalization of their parents' educational values also came higher achievement and better psychological adjustment. Thus, parents who are present at school meetings or events may be communicating its importance to children and also modeling ways to deal with questions or concerns. As a result, children also come to view schooling as within their realm of control. Similarly, parents who are involved intellectually, by reading to their children or helping with homework, may foster beliefs that these are manageable and controllable tasks.

Studies of mentoring have likewise shown that a mentor's tacit values and practices leading toward high-quality work within a profession were found to become absorbed by multiple subsequent generations of mentees in the context of supportive relationships (Nakamura & Shernoff, 2009). Values that get transmitted from one generation to the next can be conceptualized as memes, the cultural units of intergenerational inheritance, as an analogue to genes. In the case of mentoring and apprenticeship within professions, the tacit transmission of values and practices appears to be one way in which professions are maintained and evolve. Similarly, cultural values transmitted from parents to children may be an important mechanism for the evolution and maintenance of culture itself, speaking to the potential interaction of parental influences with the macrosystem.

Social class in particular has been found to interact with parental involvement. In research with elementary school–aged children and their parents, Grolnick and Slowiaczek (1994) categorized types of parental involvement: overt behavior (going to parent-teacher and other school events), personal involvement (demonstrating that the parent enjoys the child's school and interactions with school personnel), and cognitive/intellectual involvement (providing intellectual resources and help with schoolwork). These dimensions of involvement were differentially associated with social class. Specifically, cognitive/intellectual involvement tended to be more characteristic of parents with higher levels of education. However, parent education was unrelated to behavioral involvement. This supports the notion that low-income, less educated parents are indeed involved in their children's education, albeit in different ways. This involvement is no less important in conveying to children that their parents care about their schooling and value their education.

Parental Involvement and the Building of Social Capital

The importance of parent involvement is well illustrated through the construct of social capital, the notion that individuals have at their disposal cultural resources they can access through their social networks (Bourdieu, 1985). Parent networks operate as a form of social capital in which individuals share tangible (books, educational videos) and intangible (knowledge about the college application process) resources to enhance their children's learning (Lareau, 2000). A body of ethnographic research has emerged to show that parents' means of creating and accessing social capital varies as a function of both social class and ethnicity (e.g., Delgado-Gaitan, 1994; Horvat, Weininger, & Lareau, 2003). Lareau's influential work underscores the power of social class in how parents build and use social networks to enhance their children's educational experiences (Lareau, 2002). Her early work on working- and middle-class European American parents of first graders showed how parental involvement practices are determined by social class, in spite of similarly active and supportive attempts on the part of teachers to enlist parental involvement, and the deep value that both working- and middle-class parents placed on education (Lareau, 1987).

Relative to their middle-class peers, working-class parents were less involved in fostering learning at home, less knowledgeable about their children's classroom and school lives, initiated less contact with teachers, and largely limited the content of their interactions to nonacademic issues such as the length of the lunch period. These parents believed that their own limited education rendered them less able to help their children with schoolwork, and therefore turned the responsibility of teaching to their children's teachers. In contrast, middle-class parents, often as well or better educated than the teachers, perceived their children's school progress as a partnership between themselves and their children's teachers. They initiated contact with teachers, participated in school events, were keenly aware of classroom dynamics and curricular issues, and felt empowered to voice concerns. Importantly, their social networks revolved around their children's friends' families, with the result that they benefited from a greater number of sources of information about their children's school and education. In contrast, working-class parents' social networks revolved around their extended families, resulting in less exposure to key information about school and schooling

In a later ethnography extended to include low-income, working-class, and middle-income African American families, social class was again the primary determinant of differences in educational socialization, whereas there was no effect of race/ethnicity (Lareau, 2002). Middle-class parents adopted efforts characterized by "concerted cultivation" to enhance their children's intellectual and social development (e.g., enrollment in extracurricular activities, use of reasoning as a means of socialization). By virtue of their parents' efforts, the middle-class children came to view themselves as both talented and entitled. Greater involvement in organized activities further extended middle-class parents' social networks by exposing them to similarly well-educated and connected adults while at the same time limiting their exposure to extended family.

In contrast, low-income parents of both European American and African American groups socialized their children toward the "accomplishment of natural growth" by structuring their children's lives around more spontaneous events, such as family gatherings. This pattern of kinship ties clearly had its own advantages, but resulted in a social network composed of few professionals and more limited in its understanding of how to negotiate the school system. This limitation was observed to hinder poor and working-class parents' attempts at school to intervene on behalf of their children. Middle-class parents were found to mobilize their social network in order to customize their children's curriculum (e.g., secure placement in special education or a gifted program), while low-income and working-class parents largely operated individually to try to bring about curricular change or contest a school policy (Horvat et al., 2003).

Ogbu's contribution to the discourse on social capital and race continues to be controversial but nonetheless important. Ogbu's (2003) study of the achievement gap at Shaker Heights High School revealed that the advantages associated with middle-class status did not serve to inoculate African American students from lower than average performance, as measured by GPA and

SAT scores. Ogbu's ethnographic study showed that many of the middle-class African American parents, professionals in most cases, embraced a model of learning more closely tied with the working-class parents. That is, while they all noted that effort is essential to school success, they believed it was largely the school's responsibility to ensure student success. These middle-class parents were minimally involved at school, attending few meetings or events, even when these were targeted toward improving their children's school performance. At home, parents did not effectively monitor homework, guide the development of organizational skills, or foster self-efficacy beliefs. From a social capital perspective, this finding is puzzling, since these parents' social networks included professionals like themselves. Yet as Mandara and colleagues (e.g., Mandara, Varner, Greene, & Richman, 2009) suggest, it is important to consider that many of the African American parents were first-generation professionals. They did not come from middle-class, high-achieving families whose parents would have understood what it takes to do well in school. Thus, the Shaker Heights parents may not have had the benefit of observing, experiencing, and learning from parenting practices that foster high achievement.

Research on parents' social networks has begun to consider how culture and ethnicity, in conjunction with social class, may explain students' academic achievement. This work presents a challenge, both to "deficit model" approaches to ethnic underachievement and to the premium placed on higher SES in social capital explanations of achievement. A variety of survey, ethnographic, and qualitative studies of Latino students and their families have converged to show that, contrary to popular stereotypes, Latino parents care deeply about their children's learning (Delgado-Gaitan, 1992; Gandara, 1995; Goldenberg & Gallimore, 1995; Valenzuela, 1999; Valenzuela & Dornbusch, 1994) and operate to socialize their children for learning within diverse cultural models. For example, parents within six Mexican American low-income immigrant families were found to support their children's schooling and conveyed the importance of education in a variety of ways (Delgado-Gaitan). At home, they provided a regular place for homework completion, rewarded good grades, and adhered to strict rules, such as those around homework completion and bedtime hour. For these families, the meaning of education—*educación*—went beyond individual achievement to include social behavior inherent to the concept of "buen educado," including respect and compliance (see also Reese, Balzano, Gallimore, & Goldenberg, 1995).

Similarly, researchers within the funds of knowledge framework (see Moll, Amanti, Neff, & Gonzalez, 1992) argue that culturally-based and historically accumulated resources and knowledge about education are powerful motivators of school achievement. An illustration of this comes from Espinoza-Herold's (2007) recent case study of a young Mexican American immigrant woman pursuing her doctorate. Her persistence in face of sometimes considerable odds, including a serious car accident, was made possible in large part by the support and encouragement of her mother, who communicated her value on education, belief in education, and the importance of future orientation through cultural folk tales and sayings.

Li and her colleagues recently demonstrated the primacy of culture in the creation and use of social networks among low-income Chinese American families (Li, Holloway, Bempechat, & Loh, 2008). Individual interviews with ninth graders revealed that their relatively high level of achievement (mean GPA of 3.27) was attained with little practical assistance from parents. Instead, students described parents as engaging in three strategies that supported their learning. First, they had identified and designated at least one person in the home or extended family (older sibling, relative)—an "*anchor helper*"—to be charged with guiding the student's school progress and providing tutoring. Second, according to students, their parents tried to motivate them by invoking *good learning models*—an exemplary individual(s) in the home or community whom they urged their children to emulate. Finally, students reported that their parents enlisted the *long reach of kin*—family members who were invited or obliged to be involved in their schooling, but who also willingly became involved by staying current about their progress in school.

Programs Modeling Parental Involvement and Home-School Partnerships

Perceptions of warmth, care, and support have emerged as critical factors in students' engagement in school. It should not be surprising, then, to find that these qualities are essential for the development of home-school partnerships that also draw on community resources. Prominent partnership models around the nation have demonstrated ways in which expressions of support for parents (and children) lead to more engaged parents, who are then able to successfully engage their children in learning. The importance of an atmosphere of warmth, care, and respect is evident in James Comer's School Development Program, Geoffrey Canada's Harlem Children's Zone project, and effective Catholic schools, three highly respected and successful initiatives modeling the importance of parental involvement and home-school partnerships. School-based family centers and quality after-school programs have also effectively modeled the building of social capital through networking with family, neighborhood, and community resources.

Comer's School Development Program and the Harlem Children's Zone Project

Comer's School Development Program (SDP, Comer, 2005) has been operating in the New Haven public schools since 1968 and has since been replicated around the nation. Through a mesosystemic approach, the SDP is a comprehensive home-school-community partnership that operates according to three guiding principles—"no fault" problem-solving, decision making through consensus, and collaboration across the school's constituencies. Schools are organized around three primary teams or structures. The School Planning and Management Team is composed of administrators, teachers, support staff, and parents charged with developing a vision for the school's academic and social goals for its students and is responsible for the overall operations of the school.

The Student and Staff Support Team is composed of the school's principal and staff members trained in mental health, charged with developing prevention programs and coordinating student services so that students' needs can be addressed in the most optimal ways. Finally, the Parent Team operates to support the school's social and academic goals and programs. Multimethod analyses have revealed a variety of positive short-term and long-term outcomes of SDP students as compared to non-SDP students attributable to the welcoming school climate, including improved self-concept, higher achievement, improved attendance, and higher high school graduation rates (Comer, 2005; Haynes, Emmons, Gebreyesus, & Ben-Avie, 1996).

More recently, the Harlem Children's Zone (HCZ) project, initiated in 1997 by educator Geoffrey Canada, has received increasing attention from educators and public policy makers. The HCZ is a community-based approach dedicated to reversing the negative effects of poverty on academic and psychosocial development. Its two guiding principles are that the participation of a critical mass of adults, trained in and oriented around healthy child development, can reverse the deleterious effects of poverty and that early and ongoing intervention is needed to ensure success. The initial success of this model based on the originally targeted 24-block area prompted a 10-year initiative to expand to 100 blocks starting in 2004. At its core, the HCZ is a comprehensive program of social services embedded within the community and oriented around serving the needs of families with children from in utero through 18 years of age and beyond. These community investment services include year-round after-school programs that include parent education components for expectant parents of infants, called Baby College; Promise Academy charter schools (with longer school days than the New York City public schools); college preparatory and employment centers; and a College Success Office to support college students' academic and psychosocial needs. Beyond the academic and intellectual activities, community members have access to a variety of family, community, and health programs, such as foster care prevention, obesity prevention, housing advocacy, and legal services.

The core of the Promise Academy schools, into which students gain access by lottery, is the Academic Case Management system (ACM), a holistic orientation toward youth development in which each student from middle school through college is assigned a student advocate. This individual is charged with working collaboratively with students and the adults in their lives (primarily parents and teachers) to develop goals and action plans that will enhance academic, social, and personal growth across the life span. These goals and plans are regularly reviewed, assessed, and modified as necessary in order to keep students on track toward success and provide support services, particularly at critical transition points, such as the move from high school to college.

A recent evaluation of the impact of the HCZ project revealed that students had made significant gains in math and English language arts, either eliminating or significantly reducing black-white achievement gap (Dobbie & Fryer, 2009). For example, after 3 years in the Promise Academy middle schools, students closed the black-white achievement gap in math, actually outperforming the average European American New York student. Relative to peers who did not win admittance to Promise Academy schools, enrolled students recorded lower absenteeism and higher rates of high school graduation. These gains were attributed to a combination of both high-quality schools and investments that had been made in the community. However, the latter alone could not account for the remarkable academic gains achieved by the students. The success of the HCZ project has garnered much public policy support, with President Obama having recently set aside $10 million to replicate the HCZ model in 20 high-poverty urban areas (Shulman, 2009).

School-Based Family Centers

In response to the challenge posed by decreased family involvement at the secondary level, Mapp et al. (2008) conducted an ethnographic investigation spotlighting eight family centers in several low-income urban communities. Each family center enjoyed a designated space in the high school, staffed by community insiders, and designed to engage family members in activities that foster student achievement. These included programs and workshops to build and sustain home-school bonds, programs for parents' own educational enhancement, and workshops to enhance parents' social capital by explaining, for example, how to negotiate the curriculum and understand the meaning, uses, and outcomes of standardized tests. Successful family centers witnessed improved attendance, academic performance, graduation rates, and college acceptance.

Mapp et al.'s observations and interviews with key stakeholders (students, parents and family members, teachers, administrators, staff members, and community members) revealed that these successful partnerships were maintained by a "joining process" in which schools were connected with families in different ways that welcomed, honored, and validated family members for their contributions to their children's learning. Successful family centers were characterized by three qualities: (1) a strong infrastructure, in which stakeholders shared a common vision and were supported by the principal; (2) skilled staff who could serve as "cultural brokers" connecting family and school; and (3) responsive programming, designed to meet parents' needs and enhance their parenting efficacy. These characteristics lead to a "zone of community" wherein parents perceived an atmosphere of mutual respect, allowing four positive outcomes to flourish: (1) stronger and more trusting relationships between adults, born of mutual respect; (2) parents' increased perceptions of themselves as active and effective participants in their children's learning; (3) the sense among students that teachers and administrators cared for them as individuals, resulting in a stronger trusting relationship; and (4) the development of greater confidence and self-efficacy on the part of students.

Embracing the Home-School Partnership: Catholic Schools

Academic achievement among low-income urban Catholic school students has been an enduring topic of interest and research since 1980s (Coleman, Hoffer, & Kilgore, 1982). Research has consistently demonstrated that, relative to their peers, poor and ethnic minority students in Catholic high schools attain greater levels of proficiency, as measured by an array of objective indicators, including participation in upper track courses, higher GPAs and SAT scores, greater rates of high school graduation and college attendance, and admittance to more selective colleges (Altonji, Elder, & Taber, 2005; Bryk, Lee, & Holland, 1993; Carbonaro, 2003; Eide, Goldhaber, & Showalter, 2004; Ellison & Hallinan, 2004; Morgan, 2001; Sander & Krautman, 1995). One exception to this pattern emerged in a recent analysis of National Assessment of Educational Progress (NAEP) data. This study confirmed that overall, Catholic school fourth and eighth graders outperformed their public school peers in mathematics (Lubienski, Lubienski, & Crane, 2008). However, unlike other research, this school-type advantage disappeared when the authors controlled for variables such as social class, teacher certification, and reform-driven instructional practices. Through complex statistical modeling, these researchers showed that public school students outperformed their Catholic school peers in math achievement. It is important to note that this study focused on one narrow outcome measure—math achievement—and relied on statistical assumptions (i.e., linearity) that may not have been met. In any case, these findings suggest that further research on a variety of achievement outcomes in different types of schools is warranted.

The generally higher achievement of Catholic high school students has been attributed in part to the perception of the school as a communal organization in which all stakeholders share a common vision—to prepare students for postsecondary education through high expectations and rigorous curricula. In their mixed methods study of urban Catholic high schools, Bryk and his colleagues (1993) described the relationship between parents and schools as fiducial, founded in an abiding sense of mutual trust. Many low-income parents, with low levels of education, trust the schools to operate in their children's best educational interests. In return, these schools expect parents to support their children's learning by seeing them, as Epstein (1995) would argue, as students. Because of this, Catholic schools are perceived to foster greater parent participation and more involvement at home (Bauch & Goldring, 1995). In the pursuit of their shared vision, parents, teachers, and administrators serve as a social network, which fosters greater cohesiveness between home and school. Indeed, norms for parent participation appear to be clearly communicated.

For example, research has found that parents in Catholic as compared to public schools are more likely to initiate contact with schools and adhere to rules at home. They are also more likely to perceive that they were on the receiving end of clearly communicated messages from their children's school, to feel more welcomed when they contact the school, and to perceive that the school is more responsive to their needs (Bauch & Goldring, 1995). Students similarly report an atmosphere of warmth and care in which teachers take a genuine interest not only in their students, but in their students' families as well. Indeed, students describe their schools as "feeling like a family," which ironically means that parents also trust teachers and administrators to see their children not only as students but also as children (Bempechat, Boulay, Piergross, & Wenk, 2008). Critics might argue that self-selection might be more implicated than other factors in the achievement of urban Catholic schools' students. Issues of self-selection aside (see Bempechat et al., 2008), research suggests that Catholic schools are emblematic of Christenson and Sheridan's (2001) mesosystemic 4 A's model of parent engagement.

Out-of-School Time Programs

Developmental psychologists have taken a keen interest in out-of-school time because structured and supervised after-school and extracurricular activities can help children and adolescents negotiate salient developmental tasks (Mahoney, Larson, & Eccles, 2005). Organized after-school programs, in particular, can be a unique context for supporting positive youth development (Lerner, Lerner, Phelps, & colleagues, 2008). Other than helping youth to develop talents in skill-building activities like sports, art, music, community projects, and special-interest academic pursuits, one reason programs are so developmentally supportive is that they can foster enhanced relations between peers and adults (Durlak & Weissberg, 2007; Eccles & Gootman, 2002) and improved social competence among participants (Mahoney, Parente, & Lord, 2007). For example, youths have reported learning cooperation and teamwork (Hansen, Larson, & Dworkin, 2003; Jarrett, 1998; Rogoff, Baker-Sennett, Lacasa, & Goldsmith, 1995) and experiencing increased empathy and understanding essential to perspective taking (Dworkin, Larson, & Hansen, 2003).

Some researchers have also cited social networking within the community and the building of social capital as a primary reason for the effectiveness of evidence-based programs. For example, in her studies of Los Angeles' BEST After School Enrichment Program (http://www.lasbest.org/), Huang and colleagues (Huang, Coordt, et al., 2009; Huang, Miyoshi, et al., 2009) not only found evidence for increased engagement with schooling and other educational outcomes among participants of the BEST programs, but described the overall effectiveness of the program in terms of building social, intellectual, and organizational capital among a network of participants and stakeholders. Parental involvement is a large part of the networking and building of social capital. Parents of the participants in the BEST program saw program staff not only as providing a caring and safe environment, but also as accessible liaisons between themselves and the school. Site coordinators and other staff became a bridge between parents and the school fostering trust and open communication. Los Angeles's BEST program has a high proportion of Latino and Spanish-speaking participants, many of whom live in low-income neighborhoods. The liaison or "cultural broker" role between families and the school is particularly important for such families because the staff help to translate Spanish and English, reducing the language barrier and thus providing families with increased social capital (i.e., access to school resources) and voice within the community. The programs not only provide a safe haven from violent crime and poverty in which valuable skills and resiliency are modeled, but also provide a broad network of partnerships with resources throughout the city such as museums and park districts. Because building collaborative, cooperative, and trusting relationships is the norm throughout the organization by virtue of its central philosophy, staff members understand implicitly the importance and value of involving families. The program's ability to leverage social and community capital and increase parental involvement was found to be a primary factor in its overall effectiveness.

Discussion

As we have seen, Bronfenbrenner's ecological systems theory is an especially useful lens, one that has enhanced our understanding of parents' roles in fostering student motivation and engagement. Several effective programs that we have presented demonstrate the extent to which interactions between the proximal (micro- and mesosystems) and distal (exo- and macrosystems) spheres of influences are dynamic and ever evolving in order to meet the varied and changing needs of children and families. This greater understanding has allowed researchers and practitioners to design family-centered and culturally sensitive programs that operate from a strength-based perspective.

The central message underlying the considerable body of research that we have reviewed is that affective and instrumental relational support across contexts is essential to student motivation and engagement. Perceptions of general acceptance, respect for and interest in students as individuals, and expressions of warmth and care are critical to well-being and essential in students' motivation to learn and expressions of engagement with schooling. This includes pragmatic assistance (e.g., shepherding students through the college application process) that adults such as teachers and mentors can provide to enable students to meet their goals. Importantly, research has demonstrated the extent to which relational support is vital as well to those individuals and entities that serve students. The programs initiated by Comer, Canada, and Mapp illustrate that respect for the various ways in which parents socialize their children for schooling creates a foundation of trust upon which strong parent-school connections can be forged. Systemically, administrative support for programs and individuals who work with students and their families (e.g., dedicated physical space) further signals the valuing of everyone's efforts—teachers, counselors, and mentors—in supporting student achievement. These elements of relational support serve as sources of guidance and represent protective factors that can help initiate, maintain, and reengage students' adaptive beliefs about learning and engagement in school.

Regrettably, public schooling in the USA is fraught with difficulties that challenge even the best teachers and administrators. The pressures inherent in high-stakes testing, pressures from the charter school movement, and ongoing school reform efforts may make it a great challenge for many educators to adopt and sustain partnerships with their students' families and communities. For one, it is difficult to create the ideal conditions and time for supportive relationships, engagement, and learning for students when they do not exist for teachers. Furthermore, teachers cannot be effective in providing support when they hold deficit-driven models of students, families, and communities (Ramirez, 2003). More generally, teachers, families, and schools as represented in Epstein's three circles cannot work together in a mutually supportive fashion if they do not understand each other. The research evidence and models of effective programming we have reviewed suggests that larger collaborative networks of schools, families, community organizations, and public institutions can provide for the nurturing and supportive socialization of youth, promoting engagement beyond what may be achieved by a single individual teacher or parent.

A variety of observers have concluded that school reform or transformation cannot be sustained in the long term without robust participation from the community (Schutz, 2006). However, educators and scholars often hold limited visions of school-community partnerships. This is especially the case for school-based models putting most of the responsibility for including the community on the school, because the efforts of even the best-intentioned schools to facilitate community involvement can be impeded by bureaucratic immobility and lack of resources. A review of some of the most influential efforts to foster engagement between inner city schools and low-income neighborhoods reveals that some of the most promising models, such as Comer's School Development Program and the Harlem Children's Zone project, have emerged from the community (Schutz, 2006). Models like these can also suggest to educators how parents become involved in partnerships when trust is not already in place as it is in the case of many Catholic schools—for example, by offering adult education classes and other resources that entice parents to become involved. Realistically, most schools and school districts are unlikely to be on the receiving end of the kinds of financial resources enjoyed by programs such as Comer's and Canada's. Yet as the research described above suggests, strong leadership and buy-in from teachers and other members of the school community can serve to launch and sustain strong home-school partnerships.

Implications and Future Directions for Research

Recently, and perhaps because our understanding of achievement goals has advanced so far, researchers have noted that an overreliance on experimental and survey methods may limit our understanding of the complex nature of achievement goals (Dowson & McInerney, 2001; Kaplan & Maehr, 2007). For example, experimental settings can bear little resemblance to the complex nature of classroom learning (Urdan & Turner, 2005). As Dowson and McInerney have also pointed out, the deductive approach to studying students' achievement goal orientations involves making a priori assumptions about the presence of certain achievement goals and then using quantitative, decontextualized measures to test these assumptions. Furthermore, there may be a variety of ways children construct meaning and form goals from their everyday educational experiences (Bempechat & Boulay, 2001). In particular, students who differ in social class, culture and ethnicity, and educational experiences may interpret survey or questionnaire items about their achievement goals differentially, further limiting our understanding.

Researchers in achievement motivation have therefore recognized the need to integrate qualitative methods in their investigations of students' and parents' learning beliefs. Indeed, we have seen the extent to which ethnographic research has enhanced our understanding of meaning making among ethnic and racial minority children and parents. The works of Gandara (1995), Goldenberg and colleagues (Goldenberg & Gallimore, 1995), Valenzuela (1999), and Delgado-Gaitan (1994) illustrate the value inherent in understanding the underlying cultural meanings of words and expressions that are meant to encourage and motivate students. For example, as mentioned earlier, Delgado-Gaitan's (1992) ethnographic study of six Mexican American low-income immigrant families found that parents supported their children's schooling and conveyed the importance of education in a variety of ways. In addition, their reliance on "consejos," culturally based nurturing advice, to help their children through difficult school-related issues, was itself a form of social capital, the sense that parents provided caring advice that allowed their children to successfully navigate the teacher's classroom rules (Delgado-Gaitan, 1994). For example, one mother responded to the teacher's concern about her child's inattentiveness by encouraging her child to view the teacher as a second mother, an individual to whom he had to pay attention.

Despite the knowledge gleaned from research that has examined differences between ethnic groups, researchers and educators must be wary about adopting stereotypic views of "Latino" or "African American" or "Chinese American" parents' educational socialization practices. While cultural beliefs may indeed guide parenting styles, it is important to recognize that within cultures and ethnicities, there exists variation in how individuals interpret cultural beliefs.

Engaging Students, Families, and Communities

In moving away from a deficit perspective to a strength-building approach, research and theory in achievement motivation and student engagement have expanded and deepened our understanding of how some low-income or minority children may succeed against the odds. Engagement and motivation appear to be strong mediators of resiliency to thrive in school as well as life in general. Superior engagement in skill-building tasks and an adaptive motivational orientation to succeed in school are often based in strong values for education and learning. Those values are neither created nor maintained in a vacuum, however. Parents, guardians, and teachers are perhaps the best poised to foster the motivation and engagement of children, with the potential to make a long-lasting influence, since they may have the most intimate understanding of their needs and potentialities. The most successful models converge to reveal that healthy patterns of engagement and motivation are fostered in supportive networks including students, teachers, parents, and community members who share a mutual interest and commitment in the future welfare of youth.

References

Alliance for Excellent Education. (2009). *Fact sheet: High school dropouts in America*. Retrieved September 28, 2009, from http://www.all4ed.org/files/GraduationRates_FactSheet.pdf.

Altonji, J. G., Elder, T. E., & Taber, C. R. (2005). Selection on observed and unobserved variables: Assessing the effectiveness of Catholic schools. *The Journal of Political Economy, 113*, 151–184.

Ames, C. (1984). Goal structures and motivation. *The Elementary School Journal, 85*, 39–52.

Ames, C. (1992a). Achievement goals and the classroom motivational climate. In D. H. Schunk (Ed.), *Student perceptions in the classroom*. Hillsdale, NJ: Erlbaum.

Ames, C. (1992b). Classrooms: Goals, structures, and student motivation. *Journal of Educational Psychology, 84*, 261–271.

Appleton, J. J., Christenson, S. L., & Furlong, M. J. (2008). Student engagement with school: Critical conceptual and methodological issues of the construct. *Psychology in the Schools, 45*, 369–386.

Bauch, P. A., & Goldring, E. B. (1995). Parent involvement and school responsiveness: Facilitating the home-school connection in schools of choice. *Educational Evaluation and Policy Analysis, 17*, 1–21.

Baumrind, D. (1971). *Current patterns of parental authority*. Washington, DC: American Psychological Association.

Baumrind, D. (1989). Rearing competent children. In W. Damon (Ed.), *Child development today and tomorrow*. San Francisco: Jossey-Bass.

Bempechat, J. (1998). *Against the odds: How 'at risk' students exceed expectations*. San Francisco: Jossey-Bass.

Bempechat, J. (2004). The motivational benefits of homework: A social-cognitive perspective. *Theory Into Practice, 43*, 189–196.

Bempechat, J., & Boulay, B. (2001). Beyond dichotomous characterizations: New directions in achievement motivation research. In D. McInerney & S. V. Etten (Eds.), *Research on sociocultural influences on motivation and learning* (Vol. 1, pp. 15–36). Greenwich, CT: Information Age Publishing.

Bempechat, J., Boulay, B. A., Piergross, S., & Wenk, K. (2008). Beyond the rhetoric: Understanding achievement and motivation in Catholic school students. *Education and Urban Society, 40*, 167–178.

Bempechat, J., Li, J., Wenk, K., & Holloway, S. D. Achievement goals of low income students: A qualitative study of adolescent meaning making. Manuscript submitted for publication.

Bempechat, J., Shernoff, D. J., Li, J., Holloway, S. D., & Arendtsz, A. L. (2010). *Achievement beliefs and school engagement in low income adolescents: A mixed-methods study*. Paper presented at the American Educational Research Association, Denver.

Blumenfeld, P. C. (1992). Classroom learning and motivation: Clarifying and expanding goal theory. *Journal of Educational Psychology, 84*, 272–281.

Bourdieu, P. (1985). The forms of capital. In J. G. Richardson (Ed.), *Handbook of theory and research for the sociology of education* (pp. 241–258). New York: Greenwood.

Bronfenbrenner, U. (1977). Toward an experimental ecology of human development. *American Psychologist, 32*, 513–531.

Bronfenbrenner, U., & Ceci, S. J. (1994). Nature-nurture reconceptualized in developmental perspective: A bioecological model. *Psychological Review, 101*, 568–586.

Brooks-Gunn, J., Linver, M. R., & Fauth, R. C. (2005). Children's competence and socioeconomic status in the family and neighborhood. In A. J. Elliot & C. S. Dweck (Eds.), *Handbook of competence and motivation* (pp. 414–435). New York: Guilford.

Brophy, J. E. (1983). Conceptualizing student motivation. *Educational Psychologist, 18*, 200–215.

Brophy, J. E. (1987). Synthesis of research on strategies for motivating students to learn. *Educational Leadership, 44*, 40–48.

Bryk, A., Lee, V., & Holland, P. (1993). *Catholic schools and the common good*. Cambridge, MA: Harvard University Press.

Byrd-Blake, M., Afolayan, M., Hunt, J. W., Fabunmi, M., Pryor, B. W., & Lender, R. (2010). Morale of teachers in high poverty schools: A post-NCLB mixed methods analysis. *Education and Urban Society, 42*, 450–472.

Carbonaro, W. J. (2003). Sector differences in student learning: Differences in achievement gains across school years and during the summer. *Catholic Education: A Journal of Inquiry and Practice, 7*, 219–245.

Cauthen, N. K., & Fass, S. (2008). *Measuring income and poverty in the United States*. New York: National Center for Children in Poverty, Columbia University, Mailman School of Public Health.

Chang, L., McBride-Chang, C., Stewart, S. M., & Au, E. (2003). Life satisfaction, self-concept, and family relations in Chinese adolescents and children. *International Journal of Behavioral Development, 27*, 82–189.

Chen, J. J.-L. (2008). Grade-level differences: Relations of parental, teacher and peer support to academic engagement and achievement among Hong Kong students. *School Psychology International, 29*, 183–198.

Christenson, S. L., & Sheridan, S. M. (2001). *School and families: Creating essential connections for learning*. New York: Guilford Press.

Cole, M. (1996). *Cultural psychology: A once and future discipline*. Cambridge, MA: Harvard University Press.

Coleman, J., Hoffer, T., & Kilgore, S. (1982). Cognitive outcomes in public and private schools. *Sociology of Education, 55*, 65–76.

Comer, J. P. (2005). The rewards of parent participation. *Educational Leadership, 62*, 38–42.

Connell, J. P., & Wellborn, J. G. (1991). Competence, autonomy, and relatedness: A motivational analysis of self-system processes. In M. R. Gunnar & L. A. Sroufe (Eds.), *Minnesota symposium on child psychology* (Vol. 23). Chicago, IL: University of Chicago Press.

Cooper, H., Lindsay, J. J., Nye, B., & Greathouse, S. (1998). Relationships among attitudes about homework, amount of homework assigned and completed, and student achievement. *Journal of Educational Psychology, 90*, 70–83.

Covington, M. V. (2000). Intrinsic versus extrinsic motivation in schools: A reconciliation. *Current Directions in Psychological Science, 9*, 22–25.

Csikszentmihalyi, M. (1975). Play and intrinsic rewards. *Journal of Humanistic Psychology, 15*(3), 41–63.

Csikszentmihalyi, M. (1990). *Flow: The psychology of optimal experience*. New York: Harper Perennial.

Csikszentmihalyi, M. (1997). *Finding flow: The psychology of engagement with everyday life*. New York: Basic Books.

Csikszentmihalyi, M., & Csikszentmihalyi, I. S. (Eds.). (1988). *Optimal experience: Psychological studies of flow in consciousness*. New York: Cambridge University Press.

Csikszentmihalyi, M., & Larson, R. (1984). *Being adolescent: Conflict and growth in the teenage years*. New York: Basic Books.

DeCharms, R. (1968). *Personal causation; the internal effective determinants of behavior*. New York: Academic.

Deci, E. L. (1975). *Intrinsic motivation*. New York: Plenum Press.

Deci, E. L., & Ryan, R. M. (1985). *Intrinsic motivation and self-determination in human behavior*. New York: Plenum.

Delgado-Gaitan, C. (1992). School matters in the Mexican-American home: Socializing children to education. *American Educational Research Journal, 29*, 495–513.

Delgado-Gaitan, C. (1994). Consejos: The power of cultural narratives. *Anthropology & Education Quarterly, 25*, 298–316.

Dobbie, W., & Fryer, R. G. (2009). *Are high-quality schools enough to close the achievement gap? Evidence from a bold social experiment in Harlem* (No. 15473). Cambridge, MA: NBER.

Dowson, M., & McInerney, D. M. (2001). Psychological parameters of students' social and work avoidance goals: A qualitative investigation. *Journal of Educational Psychology, 93*, 35–42.

Duncan, G. J., & Brooks-Gunn, J. (2000). Family poverty, welfare reform, and child development. *Child Development, 71*, 188–196.

Durlak, J. A., & Weissberg, R. P. (2007). *The impact of after-school programs that promote personal and social skills*. Chicago: Collaborative for Academic, Social, and Emotional Learning (CASEL).

Dweck, C. S. (2006). *Mindset: The new psychology of success*. New York: Random House.

Dweck, C. S., & Bempechat, J. (1983). Children's theories of intelligence: Consequences for learning. In S. G. Paris, G. M. Olson, & H. W. Stevenson (Eds.), *Learning and motivation in the classroom* (pp. 239–256). Hillsdale, NJ: Lawrence Erlbaum Associates.

Dweck, C. S., & Leggett, E. L. (1988). A social cognitive approach to motivation and personality. *Psychological Review, 95*, 256–273.

Dworkin, J. B., Larson, R., & Hansen, D. (2003). Adolescents' accounts of growth experiences in youth activities. *Journal of Youth and Adolescence, 32*, 17–26.

Eccles, J. S., & Gootman, J. A. (2002). *Community programs to promote youth development*. Washington, DC: National Academy Press.

Eccles, J. S., Roeser, R., Vida, M., Fredricks, J. A., & Wigfield, A. (2006). Motivational and achievement pathways through middle childhood. In L. Balter & C. S. Tamis-LeMonda (Eds.), *Child psychology: A handbook of contemporary issues* (2nd ed., pp. 325–355). New York: Psychology Press.

Eide, E. R., Goldhaber, D. D., & Showalter, M. H. (2004). Does Catholic high school attendance lead to attendance at a more selective college? *Social Science Quarterly, 85*, 1335–1352.

Elliot, A. J. (1999). Approach and avoidance motivation and achievement goals. *Educational Psychologist, 34*, 149–169.

Elliott, E. S., & Dweck, C. S. (1988). Goals: An approach to motivation and achievement. *Journal of Personality and Social Psychology, 54*, 5–12.

Ellison, B. J., & Hallinan, M. T. (2004). Ability grouping in catholic and public schools. *Catholic Education: A Journal of Inquiry and Practice, 8*, 107–129.

Else-Quest, N. M., Hyde, J. S., & Hejmadi, A. (2008). Mother and child emotions during mathematics homework. *Mathematical Thinking and Learning, 10*, 5–35.

Epstein, J. L. (1995). School/family/community partnerships: Caring for the children we share. *Phi Delta Kappan, 76*, 701–712.

Epstein, J. L., & Van Vooris, F. L. (2001). More than minutes: Teachers' roles in designing homework. *Educational Psychologist, 36*, 181–193.

Espinoza-Herold, M. (2007). Stepping beyond *Si Se Puede*: Dichos as a cultural resource in mother-daughter interaction in a Latino family. *Anthropology & Education Quarterly, 38*(3), 260–277.

Finn, J. D. (1989). Withdrawing from school. *Review of Educational Research, 59*, 117–142.

Finn, J. D. (1993). *School engagement and students at risk* (No. NCES-93–470). Washington, DC: National Center for Education Statistics.

Finn, J. D., & Voelkl, K. E. (1993). School characteristics related to student engagement. *The Journal of Negro Education, 62*, 249–268.

Flouri, E. (2004). Subjective well-being in midlife: The role of involvement of and closeness to parents in childhood. *Journal of Happiness Studies, 5*, 335–358.

Fredricks, J. A., Blumenfeld, P. C., & Paris, A. H. (2004). School engagement: Potential of the concept, state of the evidence. *Review of Educational Research, 74*, 59–109.

Furlong, M. J., Whipple, A. D., St. Jean, G., Simental, J., Soliz, A., & Punthuna, S. (2003). Multiple contexts of school engagement: Moving toward a unifying framework for educational research and practice. *The California School Psychologist, 9*, 99–114.

Furrer, C., & Skinner, E. (2003). Sense of relatedness as a factor in children's academic engagement and performance. *Journal of Educational Psychology, 95*, 148–162.

Gandara, P. C. (1995). *Over the ivy walls: The educational mobility of low income Chicanos*. Albany, NY: SUNY Press.

García Coll, C., & Marks, A. K. (2009). *Immigrant stories: Ethnicity and academics in middle childhood*. Oxford, UK: Oxford University Press.

Gilman, R., Huebner, E. S., & Furlong, M. J. (Eds.). (2009). *Handbook of positive psychology in schools*. New York: Routledge.

Goldenberg, C., & Gallimore, R. (1995). Immigrant Latino parents' values and beliefs about their children's education: Continuities and discontinuities across cultures and generations. In M. Maehr, P. R.

Pintrich, & D. E. Bartz (Eds.), *Advances in motivation and achievement: Culture, motivation, and achievement* (Vol. 9, pp. 183–228). San Francisco: JAI.

Gorman-Smith, D., Tolan, P. H., Henry, D. B., & Florsheim, P. (2000). Patterns of family functioning and adolescent outcomes among urban African American and Mexican American families. *Journal of Family Psychology, 14*, 436–457.

Green, G., Rhodes, J., Hirsch, A. H., Suarez-Orozco, C., & Camic, P. M. (2008). Supportive adult relationships and the academic engagement of Latin American immigrant youth. *Journal of School Psychology, 46*, 393–412.

Griffiths, A.-J., Sharkey, J. D., & Furlong, M. J. (2009). Student engagement and positive school adaption. In R. Gilman, E. S. Huebner, & M. J. Furlong (Eds.), *Handbook of positive psychology in schools*. New York: Routledge.

Grolnick, W. S., & Ryan, R. M. (1989). Parent styles associated with children's self-regulation and competence in school. *Journal of Educational Psychology, 81*, 143–154.

Grolnick, W. S., & Slowiaczek, M. L. (1994). Parents' involvement in children's schooling: A multidimensional conceptualization and motivational model. *Child Development, 65*, 237–252.

Hansen, D. M., Larson, R. W., & Dworkin, J. B. (2003). What adolescents learn in organized youth activities: A survey of self-reported developmental experiences. *Journal of Research on Adolescence, 13*, 25–56.

Harackiewicz, J. M., Barron, K. E., Tauer, J. M., & Elliot, A. J. (2002). Predicting success in college: A longitudinal study of achievement goals and ability measures as predictors of interest and performance from freshman year through graduation. *Journal of Educational Psychology, 94*, 562–575.

Harkness, S., & Super, C. (1992). Parental ethnotheories in action. In A. Sigel, J. McGillicuddy-DeLisi, & J. J. Goodnow (Eds.), *Parental belief systems: The psychological consequences for children* (2nd ed., pp. 373–391). Hillsdale, NJ: Erlbaum.

Hauser, R. M., Pager, D. I., & Simmons, S. J. (2004). Race-ethnicity, social background, and grade retention. In H. J. Walberg, A. J. Reynolds, & M. C. Wang (Eds.), *Can unlike students learn together?* (pp. 97–114). Greenwich, CT: IAP.

Haynes, N. M., Emmons, C. L., Gebreyesus, S., & Ben-Avie, M. (1996). The School Development Program evaluation process. In N. M. Haynes (Ed.), *Rallying the whole village: The Comer process for reforming education* (pp. 123–146). New York: Teachers College Press.

Hektner, J. M., Schmidt, J. A., & Csikszentmihalyi, M. (2007). *Experience sampling method: Measuring the quality of everyday life*. Thousand Oaks, CA: Sage.

Henri, R. (1923/2007). *The art spirit*. New York: Basic Books.

Hidi, S., & Anderson, V. (1992). Situational interest and its impact on reading and expository writing. In K. A. Renninger, S. Hidi, & A. Krapp (Eds.), *The role of interest in learning and development* (pp. 215–238). Hillsdale, NJ: Erlbaum.

Hidi, S., & Renninger, K. A. (2006). The four-phase model of interest development. *Educational Psychologist, 41*, 111–127.

Hill, N. E., & Taylor, L. C. (2004). Parental school involvement and children's academic achievement. *Current Directions in Psychological Science, 13*, 161–164.

Hong, E., & Lee, K. (1999, April). *Chinese parents' awareness of their children's homework style and homework behavior and its effects on achievement*. Paper presented at the American Educational Research Association, Montreal, Canada.

Hoover-Dempsey, K. V., Battiato, A. C., Walker, J. M., Reed, R. P., DeLong, J. M., & Jones, K. P. (2001). Parental involvement in homework. *Educational Psychologist, 36*, 195–209.

Horvat, E. M., Weininger, E. B., & Lareau, A. (2003). From social ties to social capital. *American Educational Research Journal, 40*, 319–351.

Huang, D., Coordt, A., La Torre, D., Leon, S., Miyoshi, J., Perez, P., et al. (2009). *The after-school hours: Examining the relationship between afterschool staff-based social capital and student engagement in LA's BEST*. Los Angeles, CA: National Center for Research on Evaluation, Standards, and Student Testing.

Huang, D., Miyoshi, J., La Torre, D., Marshall, A., Perez, P., & Peterson, C. (2009). *Exploring the intellectual, social, and organizational capitals at LA's BEST*. Los Angeles: National Center for Research on Evaluation, Standards, and Student Testing.

Huebner, E. S., & Diener, C. (2008). Research on life satisfaction of children and youth. In M. Eid & R. J. Larsen (Eds.), *The science of subjective well-being*. New York: The Guilford Press.

Hughes, J. N., & Kwok, O.-M. (2007). Influence of student-teacher and parent-teacher relationships on lower achieving readers' engagement and achievement in the primary grades. *Journal of Educational Psychology, 99*, 39–51.

Hulleman, C. S., Durik, A. M., Schweigert, S. B., & Harackiewicz, J. M. (2008). Task values, achievement goals, and interest: An integrative analysis. *Journal of Educational Psychology, 100*, 398–416.

Ingersoll, R. M. (2004). *Why do high-poverty schools have difficulty staffing their classrooms with qualified teachers?* Washington, DC: Center for American Progress.

Jarrett, R. L. (1998). African American children, families, and neighborhoods: Qualitative contributions to understanding developmental pathways. *Applied Developmental Science, 2*, 2–16.

Jessor, R., & Jessor, S. (1977). *Problem behavior and psychosocial development: A longitudinal study of youth*. New York: Academic.

Jeynes, W. H. (2010). The salience of the subtle aspects of parental involvement and encouraging that involvement: Implications for school based programs. *Teachers College Record, 112*, 747–774.

Johnson, S. M. (2006). *The workplace matters: Teacher quality, retention, and effectiveness.* Washington, DC: National Education Association.

Kaplan, A., & Maehr, M. (2007). The contributions and prospects of goal orientation theory. *Educational Psychology Review, 19*, 141–184.

Kegan, R. (1982). *The evolving self: Problem and process in human development.* Cambridge, MA: Harvard University Press.

Kohn, A. (2006). *The homework myth: Why our kids get too much of a bad thing.* Cambridge, MA: De Capo Lifelong Books.

Kralovec, E., & Buell, J. (2001). End homework now. *Educational Leadership, 58*(7), 39–42.

Lamborn, S. D., Brown, B. B., Mounts, N. S., & Steinberg, L. (1992). Putting school in perspective: The influence of family, peers, extracurricular participation, and part-time work on academic engagement. In F. M. Newmann (Ed.), *Student engagement and achievement in American secondary schools* (pp. 153–181). New York: Teachers College Press.

Lansford, J. E., Deater-Deckard, K., Dodge, K. A., Bates, J. E., & Petit, G. S. (2004). Ethnic differences in the link between physical discipline and later adolescent externalizing behaviors. *Journal of Child Psychology and Psychiatry, 45*, 801–812.

Lareau, A. (1987). Social class differences in family-school relationships: The importance of cultural capital. *Sociology of Education, 60*, 73–85.

Lareau, A. (2000). *Home advantage: Social class and parental intervention in elementary education.* Lanham, MD: Rowman & Littlefield Publishers, Inc.

Lareau, A. (2002). Invisible inequality: Social class and childrearing in black families and white families. *American Sociological Review, 67*, 747–776.

Larson, R. W. (2006). Positive youth development, willful adolescents, and mentoring. *Journal of Community Psychology, 34*, 677–689.

Larson, R. W., & Richards, M. H. (1991). Boredom in the middle school years: Blaming schools versus blaming students. *American Journal of Education, 99*, 418–443.

Leone, C. M., & Richards, M. H. (1989). Classwork and homework in early adolescence: The ecology of achievement. *Journal of Youth and Adolescence, 18*, 531–548.

Lerner, R. M., Lerner, J. V., Phelps, E., & Colleagues. (2008). *The positive development of youth: Report of the findings from the first four years of the 4-H study of positive youth development.* Retreived Dec. 4, 2011 from http://www.ase.tufts.edu/iaryd/documents/4HStudyFindings2008.pdf.

Leventhal, T., Fauth, R. C., & Brooks-Gunn, J. (2005). Neighborhood poverty and public policy: A 5-year follow-up of children's educational outcomes in the New York City moving to opportunity demonstration. *Developmental Psychology, 41*, 933–952.

Li, J., Holloway, S. D., Bempechat, J., & Loh, E. (2008). Building and using a social network: Nurture for low income Chinese American adolescents' learning. In Y. Hirokazu & N. Way (Eds.), *The social contexts of immigrant children and adolescents. New directions for child and adolescent development* (Vol. 121, pp. 9–25). San Francisco: Wiley.

Lubienski, S. L., Lubienski, C., & Crane, C. C. (2008). Achievement differences and school type: The role of school climate, teacher certification, and instruction. *American Journal of Education, 115*(1), 97–138.

Maehr, M. L. (1976). Continuing motivation: An analysis of a seldom considered educational outcome. *Review of Educational Research, 46*, 443–462.

Maehr, M. L., & Nicholls, J. G. (1980). Culture and achievement motivation: A second look. In N. Warren (Ed.), *Studies in cross cultural psychology.* San Diego, CA: Academic.

Mahoney, J. L., Larson, R. W., & Eccles, J. S. (Eds.). (2005). *Organized activities as contexts of development: Extracurricular activities, after-school and community programs.* Mahwah, NJ: Lawrence Erlbaum.

Mahoney, J. L., Parente, M. E., & Lord, H. (2007). After-school program engagement: Links to child competence and program quality and content. *The Elementary School Journal, 107*, 385–404.

Mandara, J., & Murray, C. B. (2002). Development of an empirical typology of African American family functioning. *Journal of Family Psychology, 16*, 318–337.

Mandara, J., Varner, F., Greene, N., & Richman, S. (2009). Intergenerational family predictors of the black–white achievement gap. *Journal of Educational Psychology, 101*, 867–878.

Mapp, K. L., Johnson, V. R., Strickland, C. S., & Meza, C. (2008). High school family centers: Transformative spaces linking schools and families in support of student learning. *Marriage and Family Review, 43*, 338–368.

Marks, H. M. (2000). Student engagement in instructional activity: Patterns in the elementary, middle and high school years. *American Educational Research Journal, 37*, 153–184.

Martin, A. J., & Dowson, M. (2009). Interpersonal relationships, motivation, engagement, and achievement: Yields for theory, current issues, and educational practice. *Review of Educational Research, 79*, 327–365.

Meece, J. L., Blumenfeld, P. C., & Hoyle, R. H. (1988). Students' goal orientations and cognitive engagement in classroom activities. *Journal of Educational Psychology, 80*, 514–523.

Mitchell, M. (1993). Situational interest: Its multifaceted structure in the secondary school mathematics classroom. *Journal of Educational Psychology, 85*, 424–436.

Moll, L. C., Amanti, C., Neff, D., & Gonzalez, N. (1992). Funds of knowledge for teaching: Using a qualitative approach to connect homes and classrooms. *Theory Into Practice, 31*(2), 132–141.

Morgan, S. L. (2001). Counterfactuals, causal effect heterogeneity, and the Catholic school effect on learning. *Sociology of Education, 74*, 341–374.

Nakamura, J. (2001). The nature of vital engagement in adulthood. In M. Michaelson & J. Nakamura (Eds.), *Supportive frameworks for youth engagement* (pp. 5–18). San Francisco: Jossey-Bass.

Nakamura, J., & Shernoff, D. J. (2009). *Good mentoring: Fostering excellent practice in higher education.* San Francisco: Jossey-Bass.

National Research Council, Institute of Medicine of the National Academies. (2004). *Engaging schools: Fostering high school students' motivation to learn*. Washington, DC: The National Academies Press.

Newmann, F. M. (Ed.). (1992). *Student engagement and achievement in American secondary schools*. New York: Teachers College Press.

Newmann, F. M., & Wehlage, G. G. (1993). Five standards of authentic instruction. *Educational Leadership, 50*, 8–12.

Nicholls, J. G. (1978). The development of the concepts of effort and ability, perception of academic attainment, and the understanding that difficult tasks require more ability. *Child Development, 49*, 800–814.

Nicholls, J. G. (1983). Conceptions of ability and achievement motivation: A theory and its implications for education. In S. G. Paris, G. M. Olson, & H. W. Stevenson (Eds.), *Learning and motivation in the classroom* (pp. 211–237). Hillsdale, NJ: Erlbaum.

Nicholls, J. G. (1984). Achievement motivation: Conceptions of ability, subjective experience, task choice, and performance. *Psychological Review, 91*, 328–346.

Nicholls, J. G. (1989). *The competitive ethos and democratic education*. Cambridge, MA: Harvard University Press.

No Child Left Behind (NCLB) Act of 2001, Pub. L. No. 107–110, § 115, Stat. 1425 (2002).

Nystrand, M., & Gamoran, A. (1991). Instructional discourse, student engagement, and literature achievement. *Research in the Teaching of English, 25*, 261–290.

Ogbu, J. U. (2003). *Black American students in an affluent suburb: A study of academic disengagement*. Mahwah, NJ: Erlbaum.

Paris, S. G., & Winograd, P. (1990). Promoting metacognition and motivation of exceptional children. *Rase: Remedial & Special Education, 11*, 7–15.

Pelletier, L. G., Fortier, M. S., Vallerand, R. J., Tuson, K. M., Briere, N. M., & Blais, M. R. (1995). Toward a new measure of intrinsic motivation, extrinsic motivation, and amotivation in sports: The sport motivation scale (SMS). *Journal of Sport & Exercise Psychology, 17*, 35–53.

Pinderhughes, E. E., Nix, R., Foster, E. M., & Jones, D. (2001). Parenting in context: Impact of neighborhood poverty, residential stability, public services, social network. *Journal of Marriage and Family, 63*, 941–953.

Pintrich, P. R. (2000). Multiple goals, multiple pathways: The role of goal orientation in learning and achievement. *Journal of Educational Psychology, 92*, 544–555.

Pintrich, P. R., & De Groot, E. V. (1990). Motivational and self-regulated learning components of classroom academic performance. *Journal of Educational Psychology, 82*, 33–40.

Pomerantz, E. M., Moorman, E. A., & Litwak, S. D. (2007). The how, whom, and why of parents' involvement in children's academic lives: More is not always better. *Review of Educational Research, 77*(3), 373–410.

Pomerantz, E. M., Ng, F. F., & Wang, Q. (2006). Mothers' mastery-oriented involvement in children's homework: Implications for the well-being of children with negative perceptions of competence. *Journal of Educational Psychology, 98*, 99–111.

Ramirez, A. Y. (2003). Dismay and disappointment: Parental involvement of Latino immigrant parents. *The Urban Review, 35*(2), 93–110.

Rathunde, K. (1996). Family context and talented adolescents' optimal experience in school-related activities. *Journal of Research on Adolescence, 6*, 605–628.

Reese, L., Balzano, S., Gallimore, R., & Goldenberg, C. (1995). The concept of "educaciòn": Latino family values and American schooling. *International Journal of Educational Research, 23*, 57–81.

Reschly, A. L., & Christenson, S. L. (2009). Parents as essential partners for fostering students' learning outcomes. In R. Gilman, E. S. Huebner, & M. J. Furlong (Eds.), *Handbook of positive psychology in schools* (pp. 257–272). New York: Routledge.

Reschly, A. L., Huebner, E. S., Appleton, J. J., & Antaramian, S. (2008). Engagement as flourishing: The contribution of positive emotions and coping to adolescents' engagement at school and with learning. *Psychology in the Schools, 45*, 419–431.

Rhodes, J. (2002). *Stand by me: The risks and rewards of mentoring today's youth*. Cambridge, MA: Harvard University Press.

Rogoff, B. (1990). *Apprenticeship in thinking: Cognitive development in a social context*. New York: Oxford University Press.

Rogoff, B. (2003). *The cultural nature of human development*. Oxford, UK: Oxford University Press.

Rogoff, B., Baker-Sennett, J., Lacasa, P., & Goldsmith, D. (1995). Development through participation in sociocultural activity. In J. J. Goodnow, P. J. Miller, & F. Kessel (Eds.), *Cultural practices as contexts for development* (Vol. 67, pp. 45–65). San Francisco: Jossey-Bass.

Roorda, D. L., Koomen, H. M. Y., Spilt, J. L., & Oort, F. J. (2011). The influence of affective teacher-student relationships on students' school engagement and achievement: A meta-analytic approach. *Review of Educational Research, 81*, 493–529.

Roy, J., & Mishel, L. (2008). Using administrative data to estimate graduation rates: Challenges, proposed solutions and their pitfalls. *Education Policy Analysis Archives, 16*(11), 2–27.

Ryan, R. M., & Deci, E. L. (2000). Intrinsic and extrinsic motivations: Classic definitions and new directions. *Contemporary Educational Psychology, 25*, 54–67.

Sander, W., & Krautman, A. C. (1995). Catholic schools, dropout rates and educational attainment. *Economic Inquiry, 33*, 217–233.

Sansone, C., & Harackiewicz, J. M. (2000). *Intrinsic and extrinsic motivation: The search for optimal motivation and performance*. San Diego, CA: Academic.

Schmidt, J. A., Shernoff, D. J., & Csikszentmihalyi, M. (2007). Individual and situational factors related to the experience of flow in adolescence: A multilevel approach. In A. D. Ong & Mv Dulmen (Eds.),

The handbook of methods in positive psychology (pp. 542–558). Oxford, UK: Oxford University Press.

Schunk, D. H., Pintrich, P. R., & Meece, J. L. (Eds.). (2008). *Motivation in education: Theory, research, and applications* (3rd ed.). Upper Saddle River, NJ: Merrill Prentice Hall.

Schutz, A. (2006). Home is a prison in the global city: The tragic failure of school-based community engagement strategies. *Review of Educational Research, 76*, 691–743.

Shek, D. T. L. (1998). A longitudinal study of the relations between parent-adolescent conflict and adolescent psychological well-being. *Journal of Genetic Psychology, 159*, 53–67.

Shernoff, D. J. (2010). *The experience of student engagement in high school classrooms: Influences and effects on long-term outcomes*. Saarbrucken, Germany: Lambert Academic Publishing.

Shernoff, D. J., & Csikszentmihalyi, M. (2009). Flow in schools: Cultivating engaged learners and optimal learning environments. In R. C. Gilman, E. S. Heubner, & M. J. Furlong (Eds.), *Handbook of positive psychology in schools* (pp. 131–145). New York: Routledge.

Shernoff, D. J., Csikszentmihalyi, M., Schneider, B., & Shernoff, E. S. (2003). Student engagement in high school classrooms from the perspective of flow theory. *School Psychology Quarterly, 18*, 158–176.

Shernoff, D. J., & Hoogstra, L. (2001). Continuing motivation beyond the high school classroom. *New Directions for Child and Adolescent Development, 93*, 73–87.

Shernoff, D. J., & Schmidt, J. A. (2008). Further evidence of an engagement-achievement paradox among U.S. high school students. *Journal of Youth and Adolescence, 36*, 891–903.

Shernoff, D. J., & Vandell, D. L. (2007). Engagement in after-school program activities: Quality of experience from the perspective of participants. *Journal of Youth and Adolescence, 36*, 891–903.

Shulman, R. (2009, August 2). Harlem program singled out as model. *Washington Post*.

Sirin, S. R., & Rogers-Sirin, L. (2004). Exploring school engagement of middle-class African American adolescents. *Youth & Society, 35*, 323–340.

Skinner, E. A., & Belmont, M. J. (1993). Motivation in the classroom: Reciprocal effects of teacher behavior and student engagement across the school year. *Journal of Educational Psychology, 85*, 571–581.

Smerdon, B. A. (1999). Engagement and achievement: Differences between African-American and white high school students. *Research in Sociology of Education and Socialization, 12*, 103–134.

Steinberg, L. (1996). *Beyond the classroom: Why school reform has failed and what parents need to do*. New York: Simon & Schuster.

Steinberg, L., Mounts, N. S., Lamborn, S. D., & Dornbusch, S. M. (1991). Authoritative parenting and adolescent adjustment across varied ecological niches. *Journal of Research on Adolescence, 1*, 19–36.

Stipek, D. J. (1993). *Motivation to learn: From theory to practice* (2nd ed.). Boston: Allyn & Bacon.

Suárez-Orozco, C., Suárez-Orozco, M., & Todorova, I. (2008). *Learning a new land: Immigrant students in American society*. Cambridge, MA: Belknap Press/Harvard University Press.

Suldo, S. M. (2009). Parent-child relationships. In R. Gilman, E. S. Huebner, & M. J. Furlong (Eds.), *Handbook of positive psychology in schools*. New York: Routledge.

Taylor, L. C., Hinton, I. D., & Wilson, G. J. (1995). Parental influences on academic performance in African American students. *Journal of Child and Family Studies, 4*, 293–302.

Tendulkar, S., Buka, S., Dunn, E. C., Subramanian, S. V., & Koenen, K. C. (2010). A multilevel investigation of neighborhood effects on parental warmth. *Journal of Community Psychology, 38*(5), 557–573.

Toppo, G. (2010). In Philadelphia, a bold move against "dropout factories." *USA Today*, 1A–2A.

Urdan, T., & Turner, J. C. (2005). Competence motivation in the classroom. In A. J. Elliot & C. S. Dweck (Eds.), *Handbook of competence and motivation* (pp. 297–317). New York: Guilford.

Valenzuela, A. (1999). *Subtractive schooling: US-Mexican youth and the politics of caring*. New York: SUNY Press.

Valenzuela, A., & Dornbusch, S. M. (1994). Familism and social capital in the academic achievement of Mexican origin and Anglo Americans. *Social Science Quarterly, 75*, 18–36.

Voelkl, K. E. (1997). Identification with school. *American Journal of Education, 105*, 294–318.

Vygotsky, L. S. (1978). *Mind in society: The development of higher psychological processes*. Cambridge, MA: Harvard University Press.

Weiner, B. (1979). A theory of motivation for some classroom experiences. *Journal of Educational Psychology, 71*, 3–25.

Weiner, B. (2005). Motivation from an attributional perspective and the social psychology of perceived competence. In A. J. Elliot & C. S. Dweck (Eds.), *Handbook of competence and motivation* (pp. 73–84). New York: Guilford Publications.

Weisner, T. (2002). Ecocultural understanding of children's developmental pathways. *Human Development, 45*, 275–281.

Xu, J., & Corno, L. (1998). Case studies of families doing third grade homework. *Teachers College Record, 100*, 402–436.

Xu, J., & Corno, L. (2003). Family help and homework management reported by middle school students. *The Elementary School Journal, 103*, 503–519.

Zhang, S., & Anderson, S. G. (2010). Low-income single mothers' community violence exposure and aggressive parenting practices. *Children and Youth Services Review, 32*, 889–895.

Zimmerman, B. J. (1990). Self-regulated learning and academic achievement: An overview. *Educational Psychologist, 25*, 3–17.

Families as Facilitators of Student Engagement: Toward a Home-School Partnership Model

16

Jacquelyn N. Raftery, Wendy S. Grolnick, and Elizabeth S. Flamm

Abstract

Homes make key contributions to children's achievement. Parents are salient facilitators of engagement, and schools, through their active collaboration with families, can help caregivers create home environments that promote academic success. Engagement, from a Self-determination Theory (SDT) framework, is the outward manifestation of motivation and occurs most readily in contexts that satisfy children's needs for relatedness, autonomy, and competence. We review the substantial literature pointing to three corresponding parent variables, involvement, autonomy support, and structure that contribute to motivation and thereby engagement. We then consider the role of schools in promoting facilitative parenting. Research identifies barriers to involving families as well as sociodemographic and school structural variables that predict parent participation in children's learning. Emerging work also highlights the efficacy of system-wide interventions to develop school-family partnerships wherein educators and parents work together toward enhancing student success. Suggestions for future directions include developing interventions that target parent autonomy support and structure and conducting research that embraces the bidirectional and transactional nature of home and school influences on student engagement.

J.N. Raftery (✉)
Frances L. Hiatt School of Psychology,
Clark University, Worcester, MA, USA
e-mail: jraftery@clarku.edu

W.S. Grolnick, Ph.D.
Frances L. Hiatt School of Psychology, Clark University,
Worcester, MA, USA
e-mail: wgrolnick@clarku.edu

E.S. Flamm
Frances L. Hiatt School of Psychology,
Clark University, Worcester, MA, USA
e-mail: eflamm@clarku.edu

It is Multicultural Night at Center School, and students are presenting to teachers, parents, and classmates the creative projects they have completed that celebrate their own cultural backgrounds. In Ms. Jones' 6th grade class, it is Maria's turn to present her project. Maria, whose family is from Ecuador, has spent weeks working on her presentation. She begins by talking about the upcoming holiday, El Día de los Muertos. "On this day," she says "we gather and pray for and remember friends and family members who have passed away." Maria glances over at her mother who is sitting in the back of the classroom, smiling, as Maria talks about the deep-rooted traditions and meaning behind the holiday. Maria gives her mother a nod and continues, "And on El Día de los Muertos, we eat colada morado, a spiced fruit porridge that is purple! My mother and I made some last night and she will pass out samples for you all to try." Maria's classmates giggle with anticipation to try the bright purple porridge. After passing out all the samples, Maria's mother joins Maria at the front of the classroom. Together, they look out onto the audience of teachers, parents and students, and can only laugh as a chorus of "yum!" fills the room. "How did you get this to be such a deep purple?" Maria's teacher eagerly asks. Maria looks at her mother and whispers, "Should we tell them our secret family recipe?" Maria's mother smiles and gives an approving nod, and together, they take turns sharing the recipe that has been in their family for more than six generations. And when they are done, the audience roars in applause and Maria feels a sense of satisfaction and pleasure that she has shared a piece of her culture with others.

There are a number of things going on in Ms. Jones' classroom on Multicultural Night. First, the students are engaged in the presentations— they are enthusiastically asking and answering questions of one another, intensely and attentively listening to their peers, and expressing a genuine desire to understand differences in the world. They seem to be enjoying one another's projects and are having fun learning about other cultures.

And if we take a step back, we can see that there is even more going on in this classroom. There are parents who, too, are involved in the presentations. They are not only members of the audience, but active participants, presenting right alongside their children. Further, it is the parents who envisioned this night from the start. They recognized that there was immense diversity in their school community that should be celebrated. And so, these parents created and organized this night devoted to honoring and appreciating difference. And then there are the teachers. Sitting among the students and parents, these educators are teaching, yet are also learning from the families about the diversity of experience.

This night, as successful as it has been, did not happen by accident. Instead, it was an active effort by the school and its families to work together, based on a mutual interest and shared responsibility for children's learning. Involving families in this event recognizes the importance of parents in children developing the attitudes and motives necessary for success in school. Further, it illustrates how schools can play a key role in facilitating parent involvement.

In this chapter, we explore the roles of homes in facilitating student success and, in addition, how schools and families can interact in ways that will positively affect students. While educational success can encompass a number of outcomes, we will focus on student engagement. Most psychologists and educators agree that facilitating students' active engagement in learning—like the engagement Center School's students displayed on Multicultural Night—is a key goal for education. Researchers are beginning to recognize that enhancing student engagement is a complex process involving a number of factors and institutions including those within students, schools, families, and communities (Southwest Educational Developmental Laboratory, 2002). In this chapter, we will explore the role of families in student engagement, taking into account interactions with student and school characteristics. Most notably, we look at these interactions in bidirectional and transactional frameworks as dynamic processes ultimately affecting student engagement.

Engagement

We begin by defining engagement and then move to a motivational perspective that considers engagement as the quality of children's interactions with academic activities (Skinner, Kindermann, Connell, & Wellborn, 2009). There have been a variety of definitions of engagement as well as some controversy over the nature of engagement and its boundaries (Appleton, Christenson, & Furlong, 2008). Some perspectives on academic engagement have focused on behavior, especially participation in the school process (e.g., Natriello, 1984). Many perspectives also include a second affective or emotional component concerning students' positive attitudes, interest, and sense of belonging (e.g., Finn, 1989). Recent views have added a cognitive component involving the types of goals or values students have with regard to learning (e.g., Fredricks, Blumenfeld, & Paris, 2004) and thus include three components. In this chapter, we adopt Skinner et al.'s (2009) definition of engagement and three-component conceptualization. According to Skinner et al., engagement is the "outward manifestation of motivation-namely energized, directed, and sustained action" (p. 225). Their model includes the three components of behavior, cognition, and affect. The behavioral component concerns a child's determination, effort, intensity, persistence, and perseverance in response to challenges. The emotional dimension includes an enthusiasm about learning, enjoyment and pleasure in activities, and a sense of satisfaction when completing challenges. Finally, cognitive engagement encompasses a student's attention, participation, focus, and propensity to set goals beyond what is minimally expected.

Researchers suggest that engagement in school may contribute to important academic outcomes because it is through active participation that children learn best (Klem & Connell, 2004). Research has found that engagement in academic activities predicts critical school outcomes, such as academic resilience (Finn & Rock, 1997), attendance and retention in school (Connell, Halpern-Felsher, Clifford, Crichlow, & Usinger, 1995; Connell, Spencer, & Aber, 1994; Goodenow, 1993; Sinclair, Christenson, Lehr, & Anderson, 2003), as well as grades and achievement test scores (Connell et al., 1995; Skinner, Zimmer-Gembeck, & Connell, 1998). Given its critical role in students' learning and school success, it is crucial to understand the factors that influence engagement.

In addressing ways in which families, in interaction with schools, influence student engagement, it is important to use a framework specifying what children need to fully engage with their environments. In this chapter, we take a motivational perspective on this issue. Motivational perspectives focus on the energy and direction of behavior, for example, what makes children engaged in particular activities, rather than behavior alone. Thus, we focus on the processes that underlie behavior and how the active individual constructs self-related beliefs and affects relevant to him or herself and his or her learning that fuel engagement. Our chapter utilizes the motivational perspective of Self-determination Theory (SDT; Deci & Ryan, 1985).

A Motivational Perspective on Engagement

Self-determination Theory (Deci & Ryan, 1985) posits that individuals have psychological needs for autonomy, competence, and relatedness which they attempt to satisfy in their interactions with their environments. The need for autonomy concerns a need to feel volitional regarding one's actions and to feel that behaviors are self-initiated, rather than externally regulated (Ryan & Connell, 1989; Ryan, Connell, & Grolnick, 1992). The need for competence concerns individuals' need to feel effective in interactions with the environment, that is, to feel like they can produce positive or prevent negative outcomes and that they have the capacity to master challenges (Harter, 1982; Skinner, Wellborn, & Connell, 1990). Lastly, the need for relatedness is a need to feel related or connected to others and loved and valued by them.

Based on their experiences with contexts that support or neglect their needs, children will construct and revise self-system processes, which are their attitudes, beliefs, and motivational propensities with regard to themselves and the world. These self-system processes can be organized around the psychological needs of autonomy, competence, and relatedness and filter children's experiences of the environment and future social interactions (Connell & Wellborn, 1991). The experience of autonomy can be seen in the degree to which individuals initiate and sustain their behavior volitionally versus doing so out of a sense of pressure or coercion. This manifests in children engaging in inherently interesting activities out of a sense of pleasure and enjoyment—that is, displaying intrinsic motivation to learn and master materials. In addition, autonomy can be seen in children increasingly taking on or internalizing the regulation of activities that may not be inherently interesting and doing them out of a sense of importance or value. Ryan and Connell (1989) thus described children's self-regulation of learning activities as varying along a continuum of autonomy from external regulation, in which children engage in activities because of externally imposed contingencies (e.g., I do my homework because I'd get in trouble if I didn't), to identified regulation where students engage in activities because of a sense of their value or importance (e.g., I do my homework because it is important for my learning). The motivational resources centering around competence concern whether children believe that they have control over outcomes and whether they see themselves as capable or as incompetent in their world (Bandura, 1977; Dweck, 1991; Skinner, 1996; Weisz, 1986). Thus, perceived control and perceived competence are motivational resources connected to the satisfaction of the need for competence (Skinner et al., 1990). Finally, experiences of relatedness involve individuals feeling secure in their relationships and feeling worthy of love and positive regard (Bretherton, 1985; Crittenden, 1990). Thus, the experience of relatedness can be seen in children's sense of worth and security with themselves and others.

Children's motivational resources will then relate to their engagement in learning. For example, if children's school behavior is autonomously regulated, they will prefer a challenge and will set goals for themselves beyond what is required (Deci & Ryan, 1985). When students have a sense of who or what controls outcomes and are convinced of their own efficacy, they will persevere in the face of setbacks. They will be enthusiastic, even when confronted with obstacles, concentrate on learning activities, and expend effort beyond what is minimally expected (Skinner et al., 2009). When children feel connected to others and feel that they are lovable and important, they will show effortful participation and persistence in the classroom (Murdock, 1999). In these ways, motivational resources result in patterns of action involving affect, attention, and behavior that encompass engagement—enthusiastic, focused, and purposeful participation in learning.

Linked to the needs are three aspects of the environment: autonomy support, structure, and involvement, which should facilitate satisfaction of the needs. Autonomy-supportive environments support children's autonomous problem-solving, action, and decision-making and take children's perspectives and points of view (Grolnick & Ryan, 1989). In addition to autonomy-supportive contexts which support autonomy, structured environments meet the need for competence by providing clear and consistent expectations, predictable consequences for not meeting expectations, and feedback about how to better meet expectations in the future. Lastly, involved contexts that meet children's need for relatedness are those that provide tangible resources, such as attention and time, and psychological resources such as emotional support and warmth (Grolnick & Ryan, 1989). With regard to academics, these contexts are communicating to children that learning is connected, important, and relevant to their personal goals, that they have the capacity to succeed in school, and that they belong and are valued by others.

Taking this perspective on engagement (see Fig. 16.1 for a summary of the model), we explore contexts that are likely to satisfy students' psychological needs and thus increase their engagement. We first turn to work that focuses on the role of parents. Notably, families provide environments higher or lower on dimensions of involvement, autonomy support, and structure, and these resources can affect student motivation and engagement. Yet, whether families provide these resources is not solely a function of qualities of the families themselves—the larger social context and schools can play an active role in whether families are involved and how they see themselves in terms of their roles in student learning.

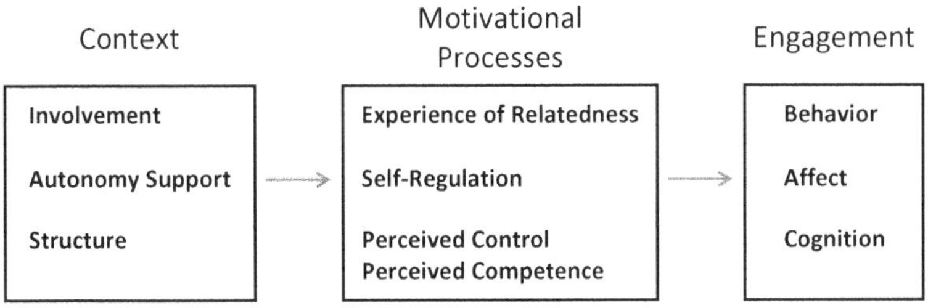

Fig. 16.1 A motivational model of the effects of context and motivational processes on children's engagement (From Connell & Wellborn, 1991, p. 51, Copyright 1991 by Erlbaum. Adapted with permission)

Further, schools' attitudes about families are in part a function of the backgrounds of families. Thus, we will then turn to a discussion of families and schools as overlapping spheres of influence (in the tradition of Epstein). We will focus on how schools and families can move beyond one-way and traditional interactions to more effective and dynamic interactions that can have important implications for student engagement.

Parent Involvement

Parent involvement in children's schooling has been a frequent target of research and intervention in the past two decades. Importantly, parent involvement has been identified as a way to close gaps in achievement between more and less disadvantaged children and minority and majority youth (e.g., Dearing, Kreider, Simpkins, & Weiss, 2006; Hara, 1998). There have been a number of definitions of parent involvement. Grolnick and Slowiaczek (1994) defined involvement as the dedication of resources by the parent to the child in a given domain. Gonzalez-DeHass, Willems, and Holbein (2005) defined parent involvement as "parenting behaviors directed toward children's education" (p. 101). Hill and Taylor (2004) suggested that involvement is "parents' interaction with schools and with their children to promote academic success" (p. 1491). All these definitions are purposefully broad and ultimately include multiple components to account for the myriad ways in which parents are involved and in which involvement can affect children.

A growing and consistent literature supports the importance of parent involvement in children's school achievement across school level and various ethnic and racial groups. For example, a recent meta-analysis of 41 studies addressing the relations between parent involvement and the academic achievement of elementary students (Jeynes, 2005) revealed an overall effect size of .74. Such a strong effect size was seen in studies including white and African American families and boys and girls. Nye, Turner, and Schwartz (2006) reported results of a review of 19 studies of parent involvement programs involving elementary age children. These studies resulted in an average effect size of .43, suggesting that children of parents receiving an intervention achieved at a level a half standard deviation higher than those of controls. Hill and Tyson (2009) reviewed 50 studies involving middle school students. The average correlation between parent involvement and achievement in middle school was .18, a highly significant, though low to moderate, effect. Finally, a second meta-analysis by Jeynes examining 52 studies of secondary school students demonstrated positive effects of parent involvement on academic achievement, with an overall effect size of .53 and an effect size for parent involvement programs of .36 again across white and minority children (Jeynes, 2007). Thus, although somewhat stronger for younger children, across a wide range of ages and in studies of various types, parent involvement appears to have a robust effect on children's achievement.

One key question researchers have addressed is how parent involvement impacts children's achievement. Grolnick and Slowiaczek (1994) suggested two models for understanding the effects of parent involvement—a direct effects model and an indirect or motivational model.

The direct effects model would suggest that parent involvement in children's schooling helps children by teaching them the academic skills they require to do well in school. Thus, parents, for example, would be increasing children's math and reading skills through their interactions with them, particularly at home. Another model suggests that parent involvement impacts children by facilitating their motivation to engage in and do well in school. According to this model, when parents place importance on school by discussing school with students, going to the school, and linking school topics with outside activities, children themselves come to value school and develop the sense of competence that would enable them to put forth effort in learning activities. In short, the motivational model suggests that parent involvement facilitates the motivational resources that would enhance children's engagement in school. What is the evidence for this proposition?

While studies have generally supported the overall relations between parent involvement and children's achievement, most have also found different effects of various types of involvement, and the results may well speak to the question of how involvement is related to school success. McWayne, Hampton, Fantuzzo, Cohen, and Sekino (2004) divided parent involvement into supportive home learning environments, including behaviors such as talking about school and structuring the home environment to support learning; direct involvement, including involvement in school activities and direct communication between parents and school personnel; and inhibited involvement, which included barriers to involvement such as time constraints and competing responsibilities. In 307 urban ethnic minority kindergarteners, the supportive environment type of involvement was positively and the inhibited type negatively associated with children's reading and math achievement. There were no significant relations for direct involvement. The strongest findings were for the supportive home learning environment type of involvement. Hill and Tyson (2009) divided parent involvement in the studies they reviewed into three types. School-based involvement strategies included activities such as volunteering at school, communication between parents and teachers, and involvement in school governance. Home-based strategies included helping with homework and providing children experience with cultural activities. Finally, academic socialization involved activities such as communicating expectations for the value of education, linking schoolwork to current events, and fostering children's educational and occupational aspirations. The researchers' analyses for middle school students showed no significant effects of home-based involvement and a significant relation for school-based involvement. However, the strongest effects on achievement were for academic socialization. Jeynes (2005) showed a similar finding with parent expectations, the degree to which parents held high expectations of students' potential to achieve at high levels, yielding larger effect sizes than parental reading, checking homework, parental styles, and specific types of parent involvement such as participation at school. It should be noted, however, that parents may have higher expectations for their higher-performing students, and thus the finding for parental expectations may represent a bidirectional effect. Overall though the findings from these studies suggest that parent involvement may likely have its largest effects by facilitating the attitudes and values children need to put forth effort in school, especially for older students.

Interestingly, there is some evidence that the effects of various types of involvement may differ somewhat for families from different backgrounds. Hong and Ho (2005), using data from the National Education Longitudinal Survey, examined four types of involvement in parents of eighth graders: communication, which included students discussing their school activities and plans with their parents; parent educational aspirations for their children; participation in school activities; and supervision. Results showed that for white and Asian American families, communication and educational aspirations were most predictive of initial achievement and growth in achievement. For Asian American families, participation was also predictive. For African American families, supervision predicted achievement outcomes, while for Hispanic families, communication was key. The results underscore the importance of considering family background in understanding which involvement strategies may work best (Bempechat, Graham, & Jimenez, 1999).

Fewer studies have specifically examined motivational outcomes of parent involvement for students. Sanders (1998) examined 12–17-year-old students' perceptions of parents' encouragement of academic endeavors and achievement. She found positive relations, over and above background variables such as single-parent status and poverty, with academic self-concept, school behavior, and achievement ideology, which was the students' perceptions of the importance of academic achievement for future success.

Fan and Williams (2010) examined whether various dimensions of parent involvement predicted tenth graders' academic self-efficacy, school engagement, and intrinsic motivation. Results showed that both parents' educational aspirations for their children and school-based involvement had strong effects on these outcomes. Similarly, Hong and Ho (2005) showed the importance of parents' educational aspirations for children's educational aspirations, a finding that did not differ across ethnic groups. Marchant, Paulson, and Rothlisberg (2001) examined fifth and sixth grade students' perceptions of their parents' value for school and academics as well as involvement in school activities and events in relation to the importance students place on effort, ability, and grades—a composite that is highly related to engagement. Interestingly, while parent participation in school was not related to motivational outcomes, children who reported that their parents valued academics had higher perceived competence and placed a higher priority on academic ability, effort, and grades. Consistent with the results of these studies, Gonzalez-DeHass et al. (2005) synthesized multiple studies of relations between parent involvement and children's motivation and concluded that parent involvement boosts students' perceived control and competence and helps them to internalize educational values.

Cooper and Crosnoe (2007) conducted an interesting study showing that the effects of involvement on engagement may differ for families differing in economic advantage. This study examined the effects of parent involvement on children's academic orientations in 489 11–15-year-old children and mothers. Academic orientations were defined as the degree to which students are committed to school and education and to doing well. To assess this construct, students responded to questionnaire items such as, "In general, you like school a lot," and "You usually finish your homework"—items that indicate greater student engagement. Parent involvement (a mix of involvement at school and home and socialization of positive attitudes toward school) was associated with children's greater endorsement of an academic orientation in disadvantaged families. However, for nondisadvantaged families, the results were in the opposite direction: greater involvement was associated with lower academic orientation. The authors suggested that academic orientation and school performance are more tightly coupled in more advantaged children; in other words, academic orientation may become more actualized. Thus, parents of advantaged children may become less involved when their children are high in academic orientation because the children are doing well and do not need these resources. On the other hand, parents of disadvantaged children may keep their involvement levels consistent regardless of orientation as these resources are still necessary.

Grolnick and Slowiaczek (1994) directly addressed the motivational model suggesting that parent involvement has its impact on student school success by facilitating motivation. These authors examined three types of involvement—behavioral (involvement in school activities and events), cognitive-intellectual (exposing children to educationally stimulating activities and experiences), and personal (interest in the school, asking about the school day)—on children's motivational resources of self-regulation, perceived control, and perceived competence. Results showed modest relations between mothers' behavioral and cognitive-intellectual involvement and students' perceived competence and control understanding (correlations .18–.28). For fathers, there were relations between behavior and cognitive intellectual involvement and students' perceived competence (correlations .15–.23) Further, regression analyses supported a mediational model in which parent involvement affects children's grades by facilitating children's perceived competence and their understanding of the sources of control of their success and failure outcomes, crucial motivational resources that have been found to be associated with student engagement. Marchant et al. (2001) also demonstrated support for a mediational model in which parent values affect student achievement by facilitating students' motivation and perceptions of competence.

Overall, the research on parent involvement supports its importance for students' engagement in school. The consistently positive effects of parent expectations, value for education, and knowledge of what goes on for the child in school suggest that such attitudes and behaviors help children to internalize the attitudes and motivation necessary to truly engage in the school enterprise. While the level of involvement parents provide is clearly important, we now turn to another parental resource addressing the way parents engage with their children around school—autonomy support versus control.

Autonomy Support Versus Control

Parents impact student engagement not only in terms of the extent of their involvement, but through the style with which they engage with their children around school (Grolnick, Deci, & Ryan, 1997b; Pomerantz, Moorman, & Litwack, 2007). A second parenting dimension, autonomy support versus control, addresses qualities of parents' communications and interactions that can have meaningful consequences for children's motivation, engagement, and academic performance.

When children experience themselves as agents and their actions as volitionally initiated, they have a sense of autonomy. Parents foster this experience by encouraging their children's initiations and autonomous problem-solving and taking their perspectives. At the opposite end of this spectrum lie parenting practices that pressure children toward specific ends, deny them a chance to solve problems for themselves, and ignore their points of view. These behaviors characterize parental control; they hinder children's autonomy and instead cause them to feel coerced and externally regulated (Grolnick & Ryan, 1989).

From an SDT perspective, a sense of autonomy and a lack of feeling controlled are crucial to children's engagement in learning. This section outlines evidence that parents enhance motivation, and thereby engagement, by meeting their children's need for autonomy.

Research demonstrates a clear link between parental autonomy support and a variety of outcomes relevant to children's success in school. Studies support the positive relation between parental autonomy support and children's behavior regulation (Grolnick et al., 1997b), emotion regulation (Ryan, Deci, Grolnick, & La Guardia, 2006), and social competence (Soenens & Vansteenkiste, 2005). Parental control, on the other hand, relates to greater internalizing and externalizing symptomatology (Barber, Olsen, & Shagle, 1994; Barber, Stolz & Olsen, 2005; Soenens et al., 2005) and stronger propensities to engage in risky social (Goldstein, Davis-Kean, & Eccles, 2005) and health-related behaviors (Turner, Irwin, Tschann, & Millstein, 1993). Largely, these patterns exist across demographically (Barber, 1996; Goldstein et al., 2005) and ethnically (Barber et al., 2005; Hill & Bush, 2001; Hill, Bush, & Roosa, 2003) diverse samples.

Of particular importance here is the growing body of work highlighting the significance of parental autonomy support for academic motivation, which then fuels engagement and achievement in children. We present some particularly illustrative studies below. Grolnick and Ryan (1989) assessed parents' support for autonomy in elementary school-age children with a structured interview. Parenting that favored autonomous problem-solving, choice, and joint decision-making over pressure, punishment, and controlling rewards was moderately associated with children's reports of more autonomous self-regulation—that is, more autonomously initiated and managed learning and achievement behaviors. Autonomy-supportive parenting was further strongly related to teachers' ratings of children's competence and moderately related to classroom behavior, as well as two measures of school performance: grades and achievement test scores.

Ginsburg and Bronstein (1993) also showed that fifth graders from more autonomy-supportive family contexts were more likely to have an intrinsic orientation toward learning—they engaged in mastery processes with curiosity and interest, had internal standards for success, and initiated schoolwork without direction. In contrast, controlling parenting behaviors, such as intrusively monitoring homework and responding to grades with punishment, criticism, or external rewards, were associated with children's lower intrinsic orientation and lower academic performance. The strength of associations in this study was moderate to low.

Research suggests that the relations between parent autonomy support and student engagement hold in diverse populations (d'Ailly, 2003; Soenens et al., 2007; Vansteenkiste, Zhou, Lens, & Soenens, 2005; Wang, Pomerantz, & Chen, 2007). Most of the studies on this topic have taken place in East Asia, within cultures characterized by communalism and interdependence. In their review of this work, Pomerantz and Wang (2009) conclude that, despite the notion that aspects of East Asian culture may make children more accepting of parental control, the effects of a controlling parenting style on children's academic and psychological functioning are negative across both United States and East Asian cultures, though the effects sometimes appear stronger in the United States.

These and other studies establish a consistent picture of three related variables: autonomy support, motivation, and achievement; but what is the nature of these relations? Motivation scholars have employed longitudinal designs and structural equation modeling to address this question.

Joussemet, Koestner, Lekes, and Landry (2005) coded interviews for the style with which mothers communicated standards for their 5-year-old children's behavior. A more autonomy-supportive style was associated with children's academic adjustment and reading performance 3 years later, even after controlling for initial adjustment, IQ, and SES. Specifically, children from more autonomy-supportive homes listened more attentively, set higher standards for their work, and used downtime more productively. This focus and preference for challenge exemplify engaged learning. In older children, parental autonomy support has been shown to serve as a protective factor, buffering against the increased risk for academic and behavior problems associated with the transition to middle school (Grolnick, Kurowski, Dunlap, & Hevey, 2000).

Grolnick, Ryan, and Deci (1991) hypothesized a motivational link between elementary school students' perceptions of their parents' autonomy support and their achievement. Specifically, the authors examined the mediating role of children's inner motivational resources, namely, their sense of autonomy, perceptions of control (Connell, 1985), and perceptions of competence (Harter, 1982) in school activities. Perceived autonomy support evidenced a low but significant correlation with the three motivational resources, and these resources accounted for 13% of the variance in children's grades, 17% of the variance in achievement test scores, and 16% of the variance in teacher-rated competence. In addition, structural equation results supported the process model: perceived autonomy support predicted enhanced motivational resources, which in turn predicted achievement.

Mothers' self-reported emphasis on the pleasure inherent in academic tasks and the value of learning, rather than their implementation of task-extrinsic contingencies, initiates an analogous process. Such "task endogeny" was associated with enhanced intrinsic motivation in 9-year-olds (Gottfried, Fleming, & Gottfried, 1994). Further, it was through this enhanced intrinsic motivation that mothers' motivational practices ultimately predicted their children's math and reading achievement 1 year later. This longitudinal path model explained 8% of the variance in 10-year-olds' reading achievement and 32% of the variance in math achievement.

There is also other research addressing the pathways through which parental autonomy support predicts children's motivation and achievement. Bronstein, Ginsburg, and Herrera (2005) demonstrated that mothers' autonomy-supportive behaviors were associated with higher concurrent achievement in fifth graders. In turn, higher achievement led to greater perceived competence and greater intrinsic motivation 2 years later. The model yielded a squared multiple correlation of .60.

The compelling evidence for the positive impact of autonomy support likely also represents a bidirectional transaction, whereby a parent's autonomy-supportive or controlling style is partly a response to her child's level of self-regulation and competence (Grolnick & Ryan, 1989). In Bronstein et al.'s (2005) longitudinal study, autonomy support led to higher achievement, which in turn brought about greater autonomy support. Similarly, Pomerantz and Eaton (2001) found that fourth through sixth graders' poor academic performance elicited heightened intrusive homework checking and helping from their mothers 6 months later. Two mechanisms mediated this relation: mothers' worry over children's low achievement and children's uncertainty about how to meet academic standards, which apparently manifested in behaviors that cued parental assistance.

Importantly, children with more negative competence experiences may be particularly sensitive to autonomy-supportive versus controlling parenting practices (Pomerantz, Wang, & Ng, 2005). In Ng, Kenney-Benson, and Pomerantz's (2004) laboratory study, mothers' autonomy-supportive behaviors during a challenging, homework-like task predicted enhanced achievement, whereas control predicted diminished engagement, more for low-achieving than for high-achieving elementary school students.

Certainly, autonomy support is crucial to child engagement. But just how important is it for children to experience autonomy-supportive interactions in the context of the family, as compared to the other environments in which they grow and learn? Soenens and Vansteenkiste (2005) found that, above and beyond teacher autonomy support, parent autonomy support predicted adolescents' self-determination and adjustment in school. Vallerand, Fortier, and Guay (1997) also showed that parental autonomy support predicted adolescents' subsequent academic outcomes above and beyond the autonomy support they perceived from teachers and the school administration. In this study, parental control led ultimately to an increased likelihood of deciding to drop out of high school.

In sum, clearly parent autonomy support contributes to children's motivation. It is a critical element in the bidirectional process whereby autonomy support affects motivation, motivation results in engagement, and engagement feeds back to motivational processes and parenting. Given this ongoing transaction, facilitating parents' autonomy support is a worthy goal for educators as doing so can likely have long-lasting and broad effects.

Parental Structure

Self-determination Theory (Deci & Ryan, 1985) posits that in addition to providing autonomy support and involvement, environments need to provide resources that facilitate children's competence. According to this theory, social contexts facilitate competence by providing structure. From an SDT framework, environments that are structured include clear guidelines, expectations, and rules as well as predictable consequences and clear feedback (Farkas & Grolnick, 2010). Such structure allows individuals to anticipate outcomes and plan their behavior accordingly. Thus, homes that provide structure should give children a clear sense of how their actions are connected to important outcomes. When this is the case, children should feel more in control of their successes and failures, in other words, have a sense of perceived control (Skinner et al., 1990). By contrast, when expectations, consequences for action, and feedback are unclear or left unspecified, children may experience themselves as unable to make outcomes happen. Feelings of incompetence and lack of control may undermine effective engagement.

Relative to involvement and autonomy support, there is much less work addressing the structure dimension and school outcomes. Grolnick and Ryan (1989) interviewed parents and coded them for level of structure, which included two components: the degree to which there were clear rules, expectations, and guidelines in the home and the degree to which rules and expectations were consistently enforced. Higher levels of parental structure were associated with children's greater understanding of how to attain successes and avoid failures. Grolnick and Wellborn (1988) developed a questionnaire to assess parental structure including the predictability of consequences for children's actions and clarity of expectations. Children who described their parents as higher in structure also reported lower levels of maladaptive control beliefs (i.e., believing they succeeded in school because of luck or powerful others) and higher perceived competence. Skinner, Johnson, and Snyder (2005) developed parent and child reports of parental structure and its obverse, chaos. High parental structure and low parental chaos were associated with higher levels of perceived control, engagement in school, and self-worth.

In our recent work, we have been attempting to specify the particular components of structure and how they relate to motivational outcomes. Farkas and Grolnick (2010), in particular, specified six components of structure: (1) clear and consistent guidelines, rules, and expectations; (2) predictability of consequences for action; (3) information feedback; (4) opportunities to meet expectations; (5) provision of rationales for rules and expectations; and (6) parental authority (i.e., parents taking a leadership role in the home). In a first study of these components, 75 seventh and eighth grade students from two large middle schools were interviewed about their homes with regard to homework and grades. From the interviews, parents were rated on the six components of structure. Children completed questionnaires about their perceptions of control and competence and academic engagement. Schools provided children's grades. Structure components correlated with these outcomes—clear and consistent guidelines and expectations were associated with children feeling more in control of outcomes and with perceived competence, engagement in school, and grades. Further, relations between structure and outcomes were apparent above and beyond the effects of parental autonomy support and involvement.

In a second study of over 160 sixth grade children from nine schools within an urban school district, our lab group identified three key components of parental structure: clear and consistent guidelines and expectations, predictability of consequences, and authority. Similar to the above study, children were interviewed about rules and expectations in the home with regard to homework and studying, and interviews were rated for these aspects of structure. However, in addition to examining the effects of the components of structure on children's motivation and engagement, we also looked at the manner in which parents implemented structure on the autonomy support to control continuum. In contrast to views that conceptualize structure as at odds with autonomy support, our framework specifies that these dimensions are separable: parents can provide structure in a manner that supports children's autonomy (e.g., by allowing children input about the rules and expectations, being open to discussing the rules, and being empathic about children not wanting to follow the rules) or in a way that controls children (e.g., by dictating rules and expectations, prohibiting dissension and discussion, and providing parent-oriented rationales for rules) (Grolnick & Pomerantz, 2009). Thus, raters also coded the degree to which rules and expectations were implemented in an autonomy-supportive or controlling manner. Autonomy-supportive versus controlling implementation of rules and expectations was coded for five components: (1) whether rules and expectations were jointly established with children (or parent dictated), (2) whether there was open exchange around rules and expectations, (3) parent empathy, (4) provision of choice, and (5) provision of rationales that would be meaningful for children's goals.

Consistent with the previous study, structure, including more clear and consistent rules and expectations and higher parental authority, was associated with children's lower endorsement of maladaptive control beliefs. Lower levels of maladaptive control beliefs then led to less use of maladaptive coping strategies for dealing with academic failure including less avoidance, rumination, and blaming the teacher (Raftery & Grolnick, 2010). The degree to which parents implemented structure in an autonomy-supportive manner was also associated with children's competence. In particular, greater use of empathy, provision of choice, and provision of meaningful rationales were associated with lower endorsement of maladaptive control. Further, when parents implemented structure in a more autonomy-supportive manner, children reported feeling more competent in school, were more engaged in the classroom, and attained better grades. Though these correlations were low to moderate, generally, in the .2 range, given the myriad of factors that can effect children's motivation, engagement, and achievement, the results are worthy of attention, particularly since they are so focused on concrete behaviors parents can engage in to facilitate their children's motivation and engagement.

The results of studies of structure indicate the importance of parents providing rules and expectations for children. Such rules and expectations help children to develop the competence and confidence they need to channel their efforts in school. However, it is also important for parents to institute and enforce rules and expectations in a way that supports children's agency and respects their roles as active participants in their school activities.

Supporting Families to Facilitate Student Engagement

Substantial research points to parental involvement, autonomy support, and structure as key elements in facilitating student engagement. Yet, most research on parenting has treated parents as an influence separate from that of schools. However, researchers are recognizing that whether families provide facilitative resources is not solely a function of qualities of the families themselves; schools play an active role in whether and how families are involved in student learning. Thus, a key direction in research is understanding what schools can do to help families influence student engagement.

The idea of lack of separation between families and schools is consistent with the new work on family-school partnerships. This model moves beyond families and schools as separate influences to see them as partners with shared responsibility for ensuring the success of students. Christenson and Sheridan (2001) defined school-family partnerships as "[developing an] intentional and ongoing relationship between school and family designed to directly or indirectly enhance children's learning and development, and/or to address the obstacles that impede it" (p. 38). They further suggested that family-school partnerships are characterized by: (1) a student focus, (2) a belief that families and schools share responsibility for student success and are both essential to it, (3) an emphasis on families and schools working together, and (4) a preventive solution-focused approach where families and schools strive to create conditions that will facilitate learning. This theory of partnership entails a deeper understanding of families and the potential barriers that some families, including those of low income and minority status, may face in initiating or maintaining this school-home connection. In addition, true partnerships not only recognize these potential barriers but address them. In particular, there are many ways that schools can work to help families remain involved in light of barriers by using an ecological approach, taking into consideration the needs and resources of the community, and by seeking to understand parents' unique needs and views of the education system (Rafaele & Knoff, 1999).

This way of thinking about connections among families and schools is best exemplified in Epstein's (1990) work in which she identified six types of parent involvement that should be included in any comprehensive family-school partnership program. The first type of involvement refers to basic responsibilities of families. This includes obligations such as providing adequate housing; ensuring the child's health, safety, and general well-being; and providing a home environment that supports children's learning across grade levels. A second type of involvement refers to home-school communication. Epstein suggested that it is important for parents and schools to communicate about children's progress and school programs through the use of conferences, notices, memos, or report cards. A third type, parent involvement at the school, includes parent volunteering in the classroom or for other in-school activities. Parent involvement at the school also includes parent attendance at school-wide events such as student sports games or performances. Epstein labeled the fourth type involvement in learning activities at home. This refers to parents' role in monitoring or helping children complete homework assignments or other take-home learning activities. Fifth, parents can also take on roles in advocacy, governance, and decision-making. This type of involvement includes parents' participation on committees at the school, district, or even state level such as the PTA/PTO, Advisory Councils, or Advocacy Groups. Lastly, the sixth type of involvement refers to family collaboration with community stakeholders, such as agencies, businesses, or other groups in the community.

Epstein (1990) suggested that these six parent involvement practices are not responsibilities of parents alone but that there are many things that schools can do to help parents take a more active role in their children's education. Before providing more detail about what explicitly schools can do to help families provide these facilitative resources to their children, it is important to identify some of the challenges of involving families. In the true spirit of partnerships, schools will be most effective in involving families if they address realistic barriers that many families face in becoming and remaining involved.

Challenges to Involving Families

Low-income and less educated parents have been found to be less involved in their children's schooling than parents with a higher education level and income (Grolnick, Benjet, Kurowski, & Apostoleris, 1997a; Horvat, Weininger, & Lareau, 2003; Lareau, 1987). Other research suggests that language may be a barrier to involvement as minority families are less involved in school activities (Epstein, 1990; Pena, 2000). Without a common language in which to communicate and discuss issues, these families may feel isolated from the school system or may not be aware of their important role in their children's learning.

To help parents be involved, it is important for schools to understand what it is that makes lower class and minority families less involved. In her work on social class and parent-school relationships, for example, Lareau (1987) suggested that there are differences between working-class and middle-class families in cultural, economic, and social resources that influence parent involvement. For example, during qualitative interviews, many working-class parents reported doubting their ability to help their children in academic activities because of their limited formal education. Further, many working-class parents viewed educators as possessing superior education skills and prestige and thus felt they should defer to these professionals the responsibility of educating their children. Lareau also addressed how differences in financial resources have implications for school involvement. Many working-class families have limited time and disposable income, making parent involvement a challenge. For example, many working-class parents reported difficulty in even attending school events because they lacked transportation, childcare arrangements, flexible work hours, and other resources more readily available to middle-class families.

In more recent work, Horvat et al. (2003) have focused on parental networks as one type of social capital that influences the relationship between families and schools. The researchers found that whereas social networks of working-class and poor families are bounded by kinship, middle-class families form social networks that include parents of their children's peers and are much more likely to include a variety of professionals. These network differences were found to parallel class differences in how parents interact with schools. In particular, middle-class families were more likely to rely on their social networks when problems arose with their child in school or to customize their children's learning and educational experience. For instance, these families used their networks to obtain additional resources for a child with a learning disability or to challenge a child's placement decision. In contrast, working-class and poor parents were less likely to use their social networks and often responded to school problems in an individualized fashion. These families were also less likely to dispute school decisions and the authority they perceived the school to have.

In a comprehensive study identifying challenges to parent involvement, Grolnick et al. (1997a) examined individual, contextual, and institutional factors that might affect parent involvement. At the individual level, the authors examined parent characteristics (i.e., thoughts and beliefs about their role in their children's learning and perceived efficacy) and child characteristics (i.e., temperament). At the contextual level, they assessed stressful life events and support for the family. The institutional context, that is, teachers' attitudes and practices toward parents, will be discussed in the next section. In a sample of 209 mothers and their third to fifth grade children, the authors found that factors from both individual and contextual levels were important. In particular, parents who believed more strongly that their role was to be a teacher and those who felt efficacious were more involved. Further, mothers who rated their children as more difficult were less involved in personal and cognitive activities. In addition, mothers who experienced a more difficult context including frequent stressful life events and stretched economic resources and those who reported little social support tended to be less involved personally and in cognitive activities. Interestingly, the effects of a difficult context were stronger for mothers of boys than mothers of girls. Grolnick and her colleagues (1997a) suggested that mothers may perceive their sons as more independent than daughters. Thus, in difficult contexts, mothers may be more likely to withdraw resources from their sons, whereas they may be more likely to remain involved for daughters who they perceive as more needy of support.

When thinking about what schools can do to help parents influence student engagement, it will be important to consider these challenges in involving families. In particular, schools' efforts to involve families must take into account the barriers that families may experience in becoming involved or sustaining involvement and consider innovative ways to overcome such barriers. We now turn to research addressing the ways in which schools can affect parents' provision of facilitative resources, with a particular focus on how to address some of the logistical, structural, and interpersonal barriers preventing caregiver involvement.

What Can Schools Do?

There has been an abundance of research that suggests that schools are salient contexts that influence the kinds of support parents may provide for their children's academic engagement. Much of the research in this area has focused on how exogenous characteristics of schools and teachers (e.g., sociodemographic variables, school compositional and structural characteristics, and school resources; Stone, 2006) influence parents' involvement in their children's schooling. Researchers have found that teachers from schools with high proportions of low-income and minority students reported poorer relationships with parents than those from schools with few minority students (Metropolitan Life Survey of the American Teacher, 2001). Likewise, Gardner, Riblatt, and Beatty (2000) found that small high schools had higher parent involvement than larger schools. Others have recognized grade level as an important factor, finding decreases in parent involvement with increases in grade level, perhaps due to the greater bureaucracy of secondary schools (Grolnick et al., 2000; Stevenson & Baker, 1987). However, research that moves beyond these exogenous factors and focuses on what teachers and schools can actually do to facilitate more involvement may be more crucial in understanding how to facilitate student engagement.

Teacher Beliefs and Practices

There is some evidence that teachers' attitudes and practices impact parent involvement. Epstein and Becker (1982) found that teachers widely vary in their beliefs about the utility of involving parents in their student's education. Some teachers were positive about parent involvement and believed that efforts to involve parents are essential. In particular, these teachers reported that parents are interested and willing to be involved in their children's education and can be helpful resources to educators if they are shown how to help their children. Epstein (1986) also found that many teachers see the value of school-family cooperation and believe the two contexts should share responsibilities, particularly given their shared goals and investment in students.

Other teachers, discouraged by unsuccessful attempts to involve parents, reported concerns about the likely success of parent involvement practices. In particular, these teachers expressed concern that involving parents may cause undue stress on parents and their children. These teachers also reported that some parents are less willing or able to be involved in their children's education, identifying parents of older students, parents with little formal education, working parents, and single parents as having unique barriers that challenge the utility and effectiveness of parent involvement practices. Namely, these teachers saw efforts to involve parents as being overwhelmingly time-consuming and "not worth the trouble" (p. 104). Further, Epstein (1986) suggests that some teachers believe that there is competition, conflict, and incompatibility between families and schools and that parents and teachers should fulfill their roles independently. Some teachers may in fact believe that their professional status may be undermined if parents become involved in academic activities generally considered to be responsibilities of educators.

Researchers have found that teachers' attitudes, beliefs, and practices toward parent involvement impact parental behavior and thus the extent to which they provide facilitative resources for their children. For instance, Epstein (1986) identified teachers who strongly supported parent involvement and were considered "leaders" in using parent involvement practices. Parents whose children's teachers were "leaders" reported that they received the most ideas for home learning activities from the teacher, believed they should help their children more at home, felt that they had an increased understanding about what their child was learning in school, and judged their children's teacher higher in overall teaching ability and interpersonal skills. These results suggest that teachers' attitudes are important in influencing parents' self-efficacy around school involvement and ultimately parental behaviors that have been found most crucial to facilitating academic motivation and engagement.

Patrikakou and Weissberg (2000) explored the relationship between teacher outreach practices and parent involvement at home and school to understand ways in which schools can help parents support their children's academic efforts. The researchers found that parents' perceptions of teacher outreach were the strongest predictor of parent involvement, even after controlling for background characteristics (e.g., parental education level, parent employment status, child age, gender, or race). For example, the more parents reported that teachers encouraged them to visit the school (Epstein's third type of parent involvement; Epstein, 1990), the more likely they were to participate in a variety of school activities. Similarly, when parents perceived that teachers were keeping them informed about their child's progress and school programs through the use of phone calls, notes, home-school journals, etc. (Epstein's second type of involvement; Epstein, 1990), they were more involved in their children's schooling. In another study on teachers' efforts to initiate and maintain contact with parents, Ames (1993) found that teacher communication to parents about student progress, in-school learning activities, and feedback to parents on how to best help their children with learning activities at home influenced parents' feelings of comfort with the school. Further, such feelings of comfort were found to be associated with parental involvement.

In the previously described study, Grolnick and colleagues (1997a) also examined teacher attitudes and practices to understand how schools may facilitate or undermine parent involvement efforts. In particular, teachers reported on the extent to which they believed parent involvement was important and the frequency with which they used various practices to involve parents. Teachers' practices to solicit involvement were found to predict parent involvement, but only when other contexts (e.g., parental attitudes and social context) were optimal. For example, parents who experienced more optimal contexts, felt efficacious, and viewed their role as that of a teacher became more involved when teachers used more parent involvement practices. However, parents who reported experiencing more difficult contexts, did not feel efficacious, and did not believe they had a role in the teaching-learning process were less affected by teacher beliefs or practices. Grolnick et al. (1997a) speculated that parents in the most difficult contexts or those whose beliefs clash with the attitudes and values of the teachers may not receive the teachers' messages or be able to benefit from them, even with active attempts to involve families. Given these findings, it seems important for schools to think creatively, beyond traditional classroom-based individual teacher efforts to involve parents, to be most successful in targeting these harder to reach families.

School Interventions to Increase Family Involvement

Certainly there is a need for schools to think creatively about how to involve traditionally hard to reach families, and we present some examples of systematic approaches below. Less work has specifically examined ways in which schools systematically organize and implement programs to increase connection and collaboration with families. However, one approach to developing, maintaining, and improving school-family relationships that has received some attention is the National Network of Partnership Schools (NNPS; Sanders & Epstein, 2000). Schools that are members of the NNPS receive materials, tools, and training on how to foster family-school relationships and create "action teams," (p.128) made up of school, family, and community stakeholders. These "action teams" generate specific goals for implementing more effective family-school partnerships and assess progress toward meeting these goals. Encouraging parents to join these "action teams" is one way in which schools may help increase parent involvement in governance and advocacy as in Epstein's (1990) fifth type of parent involvement. In a longitudinal study of schools in the NNPS, Sheldon and Van Voorhis (2004) examined whether the quality of schools' partnership programs predicted family involvement. They found that in schools with higher quality partnership programs, higher percentages of parents volunteered in school, were involved on school councils and committees, and were involved in school-assigned homework. Epstein (2005) found further support for the importance of school-family partnerships in increasing parental involvement. In one partnership school, school climate changed from one in which teachers worked alone to an environment in which educators and parents collaborated to reach agreed-upon goals. During this transition, the school implemented activities that encouraged communication and exchange of information between parents and teachers, which increased family involvement. These results suggest that when schools devote attention and resources to family-school relationships, parents are likely to be better able to support their children's academic endeavors.

Epstein and Van Voorhis (2001) also found that system-wide efforts to improve family-school relationships may impact parenting behavior. In particular, these researchers reviewed the Teachers Involve Parents in Schoolwork (TIPS) program, an innovative approach to homework in which teachers assign homework that requires students to interact with family members. Epstein and Van Voorhis found that in classrooms using the TIPS program, more families were involved in their children's education, even during middle school when parents are traditionally less involved in school activities (Grolnick et al., 2000; Stevenson & Baker, 1987). The researchers also found that family socioeconomic status did not predict whether the TIPS design was effective in involving parents. Thus, the TIPS design may be one creative and effective way to support Epstein's (1990) fourth type of involvement, parent involvement in learning activities at home. In addition, this program may be particularly useful for reaching families who are often less involved in learning activities given limited social, cultural, and economic resources. Other more systemic school practices may include organizing workshops for families to help them fulfill their basic home obligations, as in Epstein's first type of involvement, and future research should address the effectiveness of this and other school efforts to increase parent involvement.

Schools and Parent Autonomy Support

Research suggests that parental autonomy support is crucial for engagement and is associated with children's self-regulation, motivation, and achievement in the classroom. Thus, it is important to consider whether there are things schools can do to help parents provide more autonomy support. Though there is no specific research on this question, work on why parents provide more control can identify areas of possible intervention.

There has been some work suggesting that the pressure parents experience may predict their autonomy-supportive and controlling practices. For example, Grolnick, Gurland, DeCourcey, and Jacob (2002) examined the role of evaluative pressure in influencing mothers' behavior while they worked on tasks in the laboratory with their children. Mother-child dyads were asked to complete two homework-like tasks, a map task and a poem task. Dyads were assigned to either a high-pressure condition, in which the experimenter told them their child would be evaluated and that there were performance standards, or a low-pressure condition in which there was no mention of performance standards. Children also completed a questionnaire which assessed the extent to which they perceived their mother as being autonomy-supportive or controlling. On the poem task, mothers in the high-pressure condition used more controlling practices with their children, whether or not their style was more autonomy-supportive or controlling. On the map task, observers rated controlling mothers in the high-pressure condition as more controlling in their nonverbal behavior and in their practices than controlling mothers in the low-pressure condition or autonomy-supportive mothers in either of the two manipulation groups. Autonomy-supportive mothers, however, did not appear influenced by the pressure manipulation. The findings underscore the importance of individual differences and situational factors, such as pressure, in predicting autonomy-supportive versus controlling parental practices.

While Grolnick et al. (2002) looked at in-the-moment pressure that parents experienced in the laboratory, another type of pressure that may be particularly salient for parents is their perception of threat in society. Gurland and Grolnick (2003) found that mothers who perceived the world as threatening (a world in which there is little predictability, a lack of security, and limited resources) endorsed more controlling attitudes and values and used more controlling behaviors with their children compared to mothers who perceived less threat in their child's current and future environment. The researchers interpreted these findings as suggesting that mothers who perceive threat in the world may try to ensure outcomes by over-directing their children's behavior and problem-solving for them. Although well intentioned, this may actually undermine children's own autonomous self-regulation and motivation.

Findings that pressure influences parents' provision of autonomy support have important implications for ways in which school-home partnerships are designed. For example, several programs have been developed that encourage parents to be involved in their children's homework. It seems particularly necessary for schools and teachers to clarify this role for parents, stressing that these homework assignments are not evaluative, but instead are used to provide information to the teacher about children's progress. In this way, parents will not feel pressured for their child to meet performance standards or feel compelled to "take over" when their child is struggling to ensure achievement. This seems particularly important in light of Pomerantz and Eaton's (2001) finding that mothers of low-achieving children were more likely to use intrusive practices such as checking or helping their child with homework without the child's request.

Summary and Future Directions

Student engagement is a key outcome for students as it is through active participation that students best learn. The description of Mr. Jones' sixth grade class at the beginning of the chapter illustrates what this engagement can look like, particularly in the context of family involvement. Our examination of families, students, and schools suggests the important role that families play in facilitating student engagement. In particular, our chapter focuses on the important contributions of parental autonomy support, involvement, and structure to student engagement. It also illustrates the challenges families face in providing resources to children and the crucial role that schools can play in fostering parent engagement. Through their attitudes and practices, schools can help families provide facilitative contexts for children. At the same time, parent involvement, autonomy support, and structure at home can boost schools' missions to develop engaged, committed learners. Clearly, it is only through an active partnership that the optimal context for student engagement is possible.

We end with some future directions for research:

1. While there has been work, much of which we have reviewed in this chapter, that has explored how schools can help caregivers provide facilitative resources to their children, future research needs to address the bidirectionality of these home-school relations. There has been some evidence suggesting that while schools affect parent behavior, parents can also have a powerful influence on teacher behaviors and school climate. For instance, Epstein and Dauber (1991) found that teachers who believed parents shared their beliefs about the importance of a strong home-school connection had more positive attitudes about involving parents and made more active efforts to make contact and interact with families. Hoover-Dempsey, Bassler, and Brissie (1992) suggested that the correlation they uncovered between parent involvement and teacher self-efficacy could indicate that teachers with higher self-efficacy are more likely to involve parents *or* that when parents are involved in the classroom, teachers actually develop higher levels of teaching self-efficacy. Certainly more research is needed that considers family-school relationships in more bidirectional and transactional frameworks.

2. Just as the investigation into environmental influences on parent involvement has proven immensely productive, research on the school and community factors that promote parent autonomy support and structure would likely make valuable contributions to our understanding of student engagement in context. What demographic characteristics, teacher attitudes, and school programming affect autonomy support and structure? And how do these factors translate into student engagement and achievement outcomes? Grolnick and colleagues provide some preliminary answers with their work on evaluative pressure and threat; however, there is much more to learn. Further research can inform our development of home-school partnerships such that they promote more optimally facilitative family contexts for children.

3. Another key direction for future research is to focus on the needs and circumstances of traditionally hard to reach families. As was seen in the Grolnick et al. (1997a) study, teacher efforts to involve families may not reach stressed families or those with limited resources, as barriers such as time, transportation, and language may interfere. Further, teachers' and parents' assumptions and attitudes about parents' roles in student learning may not coincide (Christenson, 2004). Finally, research on social capital (Horvat et al., 2003) suggests that families with limited economic resources may not have the same interpersonal resources, such as network ties connecting parents of school peers, which are key in helping parents effectively intervene in school issues.

Such findings point to the need for schools to identify and overcome these logistical, structural, and interpersonal barriers through active communication between families and schools and innovative approaches such as flexible meeting times (e.g., alternating evening and morning activities) and provision of transportation, babysitting, and translation services.

4. Finally, our review suggests the need for more research on interventions targeting families. More information is needed on the kinds of programs that are most effective in increasing positive interactions between families and schools. Further, as suggested by Christenson and Carlson (2005), when successful programs are identified, research addressing the key features responsible for such success and the processes through which they ultimately affect student engagement is crucial. Isolating the active ingredients of effective approaches can provide crucial information to schools attempting to create active partnerships.

The engagement literature to date covers tremendous ground in illuminating the complex relations among families, schools, and children, but there is still much more to learn. Fascinating research questions abound regarding how these transactions ultimately impact students and how to apply this knowledge toward a worthy goal of parents, educators, and community members alike, fostering motivation, engagement, and love of learning in future generations.

References

Ames, C. (1993). How school-to-home communications influence parent beliefs and perceptions. *Equity and Choice, 9*(3), 44–49.

Appleton, J., Christenson, S., & Furlong, M. (2008). Student engagement with school: Critical conceptual and methodological issues of the construct. *Psychology in the Schools, 45*(5), 369–386.

Bandura, A. (1977). Self efficacy: Toward a unified theory of behavioral change. *Psychological Review, 84*, 191–215.

Barber, B. K. (1996). Parental psychological control: Revisiting a neglected construct. *Child Development, 67*, 3296–3319.

Barber, B. K., Olsen, J. E., & Shagle, S. C. (1994). Associations between parental psychological and behavioral control and youth internalized and externalized behaviors. *Child Development, 65*, 1120–1136.

Barber, B. K., Stolz, H. E., & Olsen, J. E. (2005). Parental support, psychological control, and behavioral control: Assessing the relevance across time, method, and culture. *Monographs of the Society for Research in Child Development, 70*(70), 1–137.

Bempechat, J., Graham, S. E., & Jimenez, N. V. (1999). The socialization of achievement in poor and minority students: A comparative study. *Journal of Cross-Cultural Psychology, 30*, 139–158.

Bretherton, I. (1985). Attachment theory: Retrospect and prospect. *Monographs of the Society for Research in Child Development, 50*, 3–35.

Bronstein, P., Ginsburg, G. S., & Herrera, I. S. (2005). Parental predictors of motivational orientation in early adolescence: A longitudinal study. *Journal of Youth and Adolescence, 34*, 559–575.

Christenson, S. L. (2004). The family-school partnership: An opportunity to promote the learning competence of all students. *School Psychology Review, 33*, 83–104.

Christenson, S. L., & Sheridan, S. M. (2001). *Schools and families: Creating essential connections for learning.* New York: Guilford Press.

Connell, J. P. (1985). A new multidimensional measure of children's perceptions of control. *Child Development, 56*, 1018–1041.

Connell, J. P., Halpern-Felsher, B. L., Clifford, E., Crichlow, W., & Usinger, P. (1995). Hanging in there: Behavioral, psychological, and contextual factors affecting whether African-American adolescents stay in high school. *Journal of Adolescent Research, 10*, 41–63.

Connell, J. P., Spencer, M. B., & Aber, J. L. (1994). Educational risk and resilience in African-American youth: Context, self-action, and outcomes in school. *Child Development, 65*, 493–506.

Connell, J. P., & Wellborn, J. G. (1991). Competence, autonomy and relatedness: A motivational analysis of self-system processes. In M. Gunnar & L. A. Sroufe (Eds.), *Minnesota symposium on child psychology: Vol. 23. Self processes in development* (pp. 43–77). Chicago: University of Chicago Press.

Cooper, C. E., & Crosnoe, R. (2007). The engagement in schooling of economically disadvantaged parents and children. *Youth and Society, 38*, 372–391.

Christenson, S.L., & Carlson, C. (2005). Evidence-based parent and family interventions in school psychology: State of scientifically based practice. *School Psychology Quarterly, 20*, 525–528.

Crittenden, P. M. (1990). Internal representational models of attachment relationships. *Infant Mental Health Journal, 11*, 259–277.

d'Ailly, H. (2003). Children's autonomy and perceived control in learning: A model of motivation and achievement in Taiwan. *Journal of Educational Psychology, 95*, 84–96.

Dearing, E., Kreider, H., Simpkins, S., & Weiss, H. B. (2006). Family involvement in school and low-income children's literacy: Longitudinal association between and within families. *Journal of Educational Psychology, 98*, 653–664.

Deci, E. L., & Ryan, R. M. (1985). *Intrinsic motivation and self-determination in human behavior.* New York: Plenum Press.

Dweck, C. S. (1991). Self theories and goals: Their role in motivation, personality, and development. In R. Dienstbier (Ed.), *Nebraska symposium on motivation.* Lincoln, NE: University of Nebraska Press.

Epstein, J. L. (1986). Parents' reactions to teacher practices of parent involvement. *The Elementary School Journal, 86*, 277–294.

Epstein, J. L. (1990). School and family connections: Theory, research, and implications for integrating sociologies of education and family. *Marriage and Family Review, 15*, 99–126.

Epstein, J. L. (2005). A case study of the partnership schools comprehensive school reform (CSR) model. *The Elementary School Journal, 106*, 151–170.

Epstein, J. L., & Becker, H. J. (1982). Teachers' reported practices of parent involvement: Problems and possibilities. *The Elementary School Journal, 83*, 103–113.

Epstein, J. L., & Dauber, S. L. (1991). School programs and teacher practices of parent involvement in inner city elementary and middle schools. *The Elementary School Journal, 91*, 289–303.

Epstein, J. L., & Van Voorhis, F. L. (2001). More than minutes: Teachers' roles in designing homework. *Educational Psychologist, 36*, 181–193.

Fan, W., & Williams, C. M. (2010). The effects of parental involvement on students' academic self-efficacy, engagement and intrinsic motivation. *Educational Psychology, 30*, 53–74.

Farkas, M. S., & Grolnick, W. S. (2010). Examining the components and concomitants of parental structure in the academic domain. *Motivation and Emotion, 34*, 266–279.

Finn, J. D. (1989). Withdrawing from school. *Review of Educational Research, 59*, 117–142.

Finn, J. D., & Rock, D. A. (1997). Academic success among students at risk for school failure. *Journal of Applied Psychology, 82*, 221–234.

Fredricks, J. A., Blumenfeld, P. C., & Paris, A. H. (2004). School engagement: Potential of the concept, state of the evidence. *Review of Educational Research, 74*, 59–109.

Gardner, P., Riblatt, S., & Beatty, N. (2000). Academic achievement and parental involvement as a function of school size. *High School Journal, 83*, 21–27.

Ginsburg, G. S., & Bronstein, P. (1993). Family factors related to children's intrinsic/extrinsic motivational orientation and academic performance. *Child Development, 64*, 1461–1474.

Goldstein, S. E., Davis-Kean, P. E., & Eccles, J. S. (2005). Parents, peers, and problem behavior: A longitudinal investigation of the impact of relationship perceptions and characteristics on the development of adolescent problem behavior. *Developmental Psychology, 41*, 401–413.

Gonzalez-DeHass, A., Willems, P., & Holbein, M. (2005). Examining the relationship between parental involvement and student motivation. *Educational Psychology Review, 17*(2), 99–123.

Goodenow, C. (1993). The psychological sense of school membership among adolescents: Scale development and educational correlates. *Psychology in the Schools, 30*, 79–90.

Gottfried, A. E., Fleming, J. S., & Gottfried, A. W. (1994). Role of parental motivational practices in children's academic intrinsic motivation and achievement. *Journal of Educational Psychology, 86*, 104–113.

Grolnick, W. S., Benjet, C., Kurowski, C. O., & Apostoleris, N. (1997a). Predictors of parent involvement in children's schooling. *Journal of Educational Psychology, 89*, 538–548.

Grolnick, W. S., Deci, E. L., & Ryan, R. M. (1997b). Internalization within the family: The self-determination theory perspective. In J. Grusec & L. Kuczynski (Eds.), *Parenting and children's internalization of values: A handbook of contemporary theory* (pp. 135–161). New York: Wiley.

Grolnick, W. S., Gurland, S., DeCourcey, W., & Jacob, K. (2002). Antecedents and consequences of mothers' autonomy support. An empirical investigation. *Developmental Psychology, 38*, 143–155.

Grolnick, W. S., Kurowski, C. O., Dunlap, K. G., & Hevey, C. (2000). Parental resources and the transition to junior high. *Journal of Research on Adolescence, 10*, 465–488.

Grolnick, W., & Pomerantz, E. (2009). Issues and challenges in studying parental control: Toward a new conceptualization. *Child Development Perspectives, 3*, 165–170.

Grolnick, W. S., & Ryan, R. M. (1989). Parent styles associated with children's self-regulation and competence in school. *Journal of Educational Psychology, 81*, 143–154.

Grolnick, W. S., Ryan, R. M., & Deci, E. L. (1991). Inner resources for school achievement: Motivational mediators of children's perceptions of their parents. *Journal of Educational Psychology, 83*, 508–517.

Grolnick, W. S., & Slowiaczek, M. L. (1994). Parents' involvement in children's schooling: A multidimensional conceptualization and motivational model. *Child Development, 65*, 237–252.

Grolnick, W. S, & Wellborn, J. (1988). *Parent influences on children's school-related self-system process.* Paper presented at the annual meeting of the American Educational Research Association, New Orleans, LA.

Gurland, S. T., & Grolnick, W. S. (2003). Perceived threat, controlling parenting, and children's achievement orientations. *Motivation and Emotion, 29*, 103–121.

Hara, S. R. (1998). Parent involvement: The key to improved student achievement. *School Community Journal, 8*(2), 9–19.

Harter, S. (1982). The perceived competence scale for children. *Child Development, 53*, 87–97.

Hill, N. E., & Bush, K. R. (2001). Relationships between parenting environment and children's mental health among African American and European American mothers and children. *Journal of Marriage and Family, 63*, 954–966.

Hill, N. E., Bush, K. R., & Roosa, M. W. (2003). Parenting and family socialization strategies and children's mental health: Low-income Mexican-American and Euro-American mothers and children. *Child Development, 74*, 189–204.

Hill, N. E., & Taylor, L. C. (2004). Parental school involvement and children's academic achievement: Pragmatics and issues. *Current Directions in Psychological Science, 13*, 161–164.

Hill, N. E., & Tyson, D. F. (2009). Parental involvement in middle school: A meta-analytic assessment of the strategies that promote achievement. *Developmental Psychology, 45*(3), 740–763.

Hong, S., & Ho, H. (2005). Direct and indirect longitudinal effects of parental involvement on student achievement: Second order latent growth modeling across ethnic groups. *Journal of Educational Psychology, 97*, 32–42.

Hoover-Dempsey, K. V., Bassler, O. C., & Brissie, J. S. (1992). Explorations in parent-school relations. *The Journal of Educational Research, 85*, 287–294.

Horvat, E. M., Weininger, E. B., & Lareau, A. (2003). From social ties to social capital: Class differences in the relations between schools and parent networks. *American Educational Research Journal, 40*, 319–351.

Jeynes, W. H. (2005). A meta-analysis of the relation of parental involvement to urban elementary school student academic achievement. *Urban Education, 40*, 237–269.

Jeynes, W. H. (2007). The relationship between parental involvement and urban secondary school student academic achievement: A meta-analysis. *Urban Education, 42*, 82–110.

Joussemet, M., Koestner, R., Lekes, N., & Landry, R. (2005). A longitudinal study of the relationship of maternal autonomy support to children's adjustment and achievement in school. *Journal of Personality, 73*, 1216–1235.

Klem, A. M., & Connell, J. P. (2004). Relationships matter: Linking teacher support to student engagement and achievement. *Journal of School Health, 74*, 262–273.

Lareau, A. (1987). Social class differences in family – School relationships: The importance of cultural capital. *Sociology of Education, 60*, 73–85.

Marchant, G. J., Paulson, S. E., & Rothlisberg, B. A. (2001). Relations of middle school students' perceptions of family and school contexts with academic achievement. *Psychology in the Schools, 38*, 505–519.

McWayne, C., Hampton, V., Fantuzzo, J., Cohen, H. L., & Sekino, Y. (2004). A multivariate examination of parent involvement and the social and academic competencies of urban kindergarten. *Psychology in the Schools, 41*, 363–377.

Metropolitan Life Survey of the American Teacher. (2001). *Key elements of quality schools.* http://www.metlife.com/Companyinfo/Community/Found/Docs/2001ats.pdf

Murdock, T. B. (1999). The social context of risk: Status and motivational predictors of alienation in middle school. *Journal of Educational Psychology, 91*, 62–76.

Natriello, G. (1984). Problems in the evaluation of students and student from secondary schools. *Journal of Research and Development in Education, 17*, 14–24.

Ng, F. F., Kenney-Benson, G. A., & Pomerantz, E. M. (2004). Children's achievement moderates the effects of mothers' use of control and autonomy support. *Child Development, 75*, 764–780.

Nye, C., Turner, H., & Schwartz, J. (2006). *Approaches to parent involvement for improving the academic performance of elementary school age children.* Oslo, Norway: The Campbell Collaboration, Campbell Systematic Reviews.

Patrikakou, E. N., & Weissberg, R. P. (2000). Parents' perceptions of teacher outreach and parent involvement in children's education. *Journal of Prevention & Intervention in the Community, 20*, 103–119.

Pena, D. C. (2000). Parent involvement: Influencing factors and implications. *The Journal of Educational Research, 94*, 42–54.

Pomerantz, E. M., & Eaton, M. M. (2001). Maternal intrusive support in the academic context: Transactional socialization processes. *Developmental Psychology, 37*, 174–186.

Pomerantz, E. M., Moorman, E. A., & Litwack, S. D. (2007). The how, whom and why of parents' involvement in children's academic lives: More is not always better. *Review of Educational Research, 77*, 373–410.

Pomerantz, E. M., & Wang, Q. (2009). The role of parental control in children's development in Western and East Asian countries. *Current Directions in Psychological Science, 18*, 285–289.

Pomerantz, E. M., Wang, Q., & Ng, F. F. (2005). The role of children's competence experiences in the socialization process: A dynamic process framework for the academic arena. In R. Kail (Ed.), *Advances in child development and behavior* (Vol. 33, pp. 193–227). San Diego, CA: Academic.

Rafaele, L. M., & Knoff, H. M. (1999). Improving home-school collaboration with disadvantaged families: Organizational principles, perspectives, and approaches. *School Psychology Review, 28*, 448–466.

Raftery, J. R., & Grolnick, W. S. (2010, May). *Coping with academic failure: Effects of structure and perceived control.* Fourth International Conference on Self-Determination Theory, Gent, Belgium.

Ryan, R. M., & Connell, J. P. (1989). Perceived locus of causality and internalization: Examining reasons for acting in two domains. *Journal of Personality and Social Psychology, 57*, 749–761.

Ryan, R. M., Connell, J. P., & Grolnick, W. S. (1992). When achievement is not intrinsically motivated: A theory and assessment of self-regulation in school. In

A. K. Boggiano & T. S. Pittman (Eds.), *Achievement and motivation: A social-developmental perspective* (pp. 167–188). New York: Cambridge University Press.

Ryan, R. M., Deci, E. L., Grolnick, W. S., & La Guardia, J. G. (2006). The significance of autonomy and autonomy support in psychological development and psychopathology. In D. Cicchetti & D. J. Cohen (Eds.), *Developmental psychopathology: Theory and method* (2nd ed., pp. 795–849). Hoboken, NJ: Wiley.

Sanders, M. G. (1998). The effects of school, family, and community support on the academic achievement of African American adolescents. *Urban Education, 33*, 385–409.

Sanders, M. G., & Epstein, J. L. (2000). The National Network of Partnership Schools: How research influences educational practice. *Journal of Education for Students Placed at Risk, 5*, 61–76.

Sheldon, S. B., & Van Voorhis, F. L. (2004). Partnership programs in U.S. schools: Their development and relationship to family involvement outcomes. *School Effectiveness and School Improvement, 15*, 125–148.

Sinclair, M. F., Christenson, S. L., Lehr, C. A., & Anderson, A. R. (2003). Facilitating student learning and engagement: Lessons learned from Check and Connect longitudinal studies. *The California School Psychologist, 8*, 29–41.

Skinner, E. A. (1996). A guide to constructs of control. *Journal of Personality and Social Psychology, 71*, 549–570.

Skinner, E. A., Johnson, S., & Snyder, T. (2005). Six dimensions of parenting: A motivational model. *Parenting: Science and Practice, 5*(2), 175–235.

Skinner, E. A., Kindermann, T. A., Connell, J. P., & Wellborn, J. G. (2009). Engagement as an organizational construct in the dynamics of motivational development. In K. Wentzel & A. Wigfield (Eds.), *Handbook of motivation in school* (pp. 223–245). Mahwah, NJ: Erlbaum.

Skinner, E. A., Wellborn, J. G., & Connell, J. P. (1990). What it takes to do well in school and whether I've got it: The role of perceived control in children's engagement and school achievement. *Journal of Educational Psychology, 82*, 22–32.

Skinner, E. A., Zimmer-Gembeck, M. J., & Connell, J. P. (1998). Individual differences and the development of perceived control. *Monographs of the Society for Research in Child Development, 63* (nos 2 and 3) whole no. 254 pp. v-220.

Soenens, B., Elliot, A. J., Goossens, L., Vansteenkiste, M., Luyten, P., & Duriez, B. (2005). The intergenerational transmission of perfectionism: Parents' psychological control as an intervening variable. *Journal of Family Psychology, 19*, 358–366.

Soenens, B., & Vansteenkiste, M. (2005). Antecedents and outcomes of self-determination in three life domains: The role of parents' and teachers' autonomy support. *Journal of Youth and Adolescence, 34*, 589–604.

Soenens, B., Vansteenkiste, M., Lens, W., Luyckx, K., Goossens, L., Beyers, W., et al. (2007). Conceptualizing parental autonomy support: Adolescent perceptions of promotion of independence versus promotion of volitional functioning. *Developmental Psychology, 43*, 633–646.

Southwest Educational Developmental Laboratory. (2002). *A new wave of evidence: The impact of school, family, and community connections on student achievement* (Annual Synthesis 2002). www.sedl.org/connections/

Stevenson, D., & Baker, D. (1987). The family-school relation and the child's school performance. *Child Development, 58*, 1348–1357.

Stone, S. (2006). Correlates of change in student reported parent involvement in schooling: A new look at the National Longitudinal Study of 1988. *Journal of Orthopsychiatry, 76*, 518–530.

Turner, R. A., Irwin, C. E., Jr., Tschann, J. M., & Millstein, S. G. (1993). Autonomy, relatedness, and the initiation of health risk behaviors in early adolescence. *Health Psychology, 12*, 200–208.

Vallerand, R. J., Fortier, M. S., & Guay, F. (1997). Self-determination and persistence in a real-life setting: Toward a motivational model of high school dropout. *Journal of Personality and Social Psychology, 72*, 1161–1176.

Vansteenkiste, M., Zhou, M., Lens, W., & Soenens, B. (2005). Experiences of autonomy and control among Chinese learners: Vitalizing or immobilizing? *Journal of Educational Psychology, 97*, 468–483.

Wang, Q., Pomerantz, E. M., & Chen, H. (2007). The role of parents' control in early adolescents' psychological functioning: A longitudinal investigation in the United States and China. *Child Development, 78*, 1592–1610.

Weisz, J. R. (1986). Contingency and control beliefs as predictors of psychotherapy outcomes among children and adolescence. *Journal of Consulting and Clinical Psychology, 54*, 789–795.

17. Teacher-Student Relationships and Engagement: Conceptualizing, Measuring, and Improving the Capacity of Classroom Interactions

Robert C. Pianta, Bridget K. Hamre, and Joseph P. Allen

Abstract

Classrooms are complex social systems, and student-teacher relationships and interactions are also complex, multicomponent systems. We posit that the nature and quality of relationship interactions between teachers and students are fundamental to understanding student engagement, can be assessed through standardized observation methods, and can be changed by providing teachers knowledge about developmental processes relevant for classroom interactions and personalized feedback/support about their interactive behaviors and cues. When these supports are provided to teachers' interactions, student engagement increases. In this chapter, we focus on the theoretical and empirical links between interactions and engagement and present an approach to intervention designed to increase the quality of such interactions and, in turn, increase student engagement and, ultimately, learning and development. Recognizing general principles of development in complex systems, a theory of the classroom as a setting for development, and a theory of change specific to this social setting are the ultimate goals of this work. Engagement, in this context, is both an outcome in its own

---

*Preparation of this chapter was supported in part by the Wm. T. Grant Foundation, the Foundation for Child Development, and the Institute of Education Sciences.

R.C. Pianta, Ph.D. (✉)
Curry School of Education, University of Virginia,
PO Box 400260, Charlottesville, VA 22904-4260, USA
e-mail: rcp4p@virginia.edu

B.K. Hamre, Ph.D.
Center for Advanced Study of Teaching and Learning,
University of Virginia, Charlottesville, VA, USA
e-mail: bkh3d@virginia.edu

J.P. Allen, Ph.D.
Department of Psychology, University of Virginia,
Charlottesville, VA, USA
e-mail: allen@virginia.edu

right and a mediator of impacts that teachers have on student outcomes through their interactions with children and youth. In light of this discussion, we offer suggestions or directions for further research in this area.

Introduction

Students spend at least one-quarter of their waking hours in schools, most of it in classrooms, one of the most proximal and potentially powerful settings for influencing children and youth. Students' relationships and interactions with teachers either produce or inhibit developmental change to the extent that they engage, meaningfully challenge, and provide social and relational supports. In this sense, relationships between teachers and students reflect a classroom's capacity to promote development, and it is precisely in this way that relationships and interactions are the key to understanding engagement. As just one example of this connection between engagement and relationships, the National Research Council (NRC, 2004) published a groundbreaking recasting of settings in terms of features that engage developmental mechanisms in adolescence in positive, promotive ways. Notably, the NRC report shifted discussions from how various contexts (e.g., classrooms, clubs) and programs should focus on reducing the rate of problems in child and adolescent development to one that recognizes that perhaps the best way for these contexts to benefit youth is to emphasize the positive ways that relational experiences in these settings provide children and youth experiences that draw them in—that engage with their desires and needs for feeling competent and connected to others. From the perspective of the NRC report, relationships are a mechanism or medium through which settings engage developmental processes.

Building on extensive observational work that had been underway in early childhood settings for the past two decades, as well as a very compelling literature demonstrating the value of adult-child relationships for promoting competence in the birth to 8 years period (see Pianta, Hamre, & Stuhlman, 2003), we embarked on a program of study to conceptualize, measure, and ultimately improve the quality of teacher-child relationships through a focus on their interactions, starting in the preschool and early elementary period. This work resulted in an observational tool for assessing interactions in early childhood and elementary classrooms, the Classroom Assessment Scoring System (CLASS; Pianta, La Paro, & Hamre, 2004); an accompanying conceptualization of classrooms, the CLASS framework (Hamre, Pianta, Mashburn, & Downer, 2010); and an approach to enhancing the quality of teacher-child interactions that we call MyTeachingPartner. Recently, we extended this approach to measuring and improving relationships to middle and high school classrooms (Pianta, Hamre, & Mintz, 2010). As we have deepened this work in the early grades and extended these ideas toward classrooms serving older children, evidence has been revealed not only for the NRC report but also for the recasting of classrooms as contexts in which perhaps the key mechanism through which classroom experiences add value for development is through the pivotal role of student-teacher relationships in the very process of engagement.

In our view, and reflected throughout this chapter, engagement is a relational process. It reflects students' cognitive, emotional, behavioral, and motivational states and capacities but is conditioned in part on interpersonal relationships as activators and organizers of these states and capacities in the service of some larger developmental task or aim (Allen & Allen, 2009; Crosnoe, 2000; Dornbusch, Glasgow, & Lin, 1996; Eccles, Lord, & Midgley, 1991). From this perspective, engagement is best understood by understanding relationships and their behavioral expression in interpersonal interactions in the classroom—through observation of exchanges and interpretation of their value and meaning with regard to fostering opportunity to learn and develop.

Engagement reflects relationally mediated participation in opportunity.

In this chapter, we describe this and related work in an effort to frame conceptually the discussion of student engagement not as a property of a child but rather as embedded in interactions and relationships. We organize our discussion in three main sections: the first provides a depiction of classrooms as a relational setting for development, the second describes efforts to conceptualize and measure teacher-student classroom interactions, and the third reports early results from efforts to enhance engagement in classrooms as a function of improving the quality of teacher-student interactions.

Underperformance of the Classroom Setting as a Context for Youth Development

There is little question that academic achievement, personal well-being, and civic-related outcomes for children and adolescents are in dire need of improvement and enhancement (Carbonaro & Gamoran, 2002; National Center for Education Statistics [NCES], 2003). For all of the resources devoted to schooling, the capacity of classrooms as settings that promote and enhance development is sorely lacking. For example, adolescents report that social and task-related disengagement and alienation are directly tied to classroom experiences that are disconnected from youths' developmental needs and motivations (Crosnoe, 2000; Dornbusch et al., 1996; Eccles et al., 1991). Youth describe school experiences as irrelevant and lacking appropriate and meaningful challenges. These patterns are exacerbated dramatically for youth attending schools in low-income communities, rural communities, large schools, and for those with histories of poor achievement or problem behavior (e.g., Crosnoe, 2001; Eccles, Lord, Roeser, Barber, & Jozefowicz, 1997).

Even more disconcerting is recent evidence from observational studies of large samples of fifth grade classrooms that the nature and quality of the instructional and social supports actually offered to early adolescents in classrooms is generally low and even lower for the groups noted above. Moreover, findings from studies of large and diverse samples of middle schools demonstrate quite clearly that competitive, standards-driven instruction in decontextualized skills and knowledge contributes directly to this sense of alienation and disengagement (Eccles et al., 1997; Shouse, 1996). Engagement in school begins to decline early in adolescence, and by entry into high school this decline is pronounced to the point where more than half of high school students from all types of schools report that they do not take their school or their studies seriously (Marks, 2000; Steinberg, Brown, & Dornbusch, 1996). Further, adolescents bring their peers along with them: doing well in school switches from being a positively valued behavior among peers in childhood to a somewhat negatively valued behavior by mid-adolescence. Yet, engagement and intrinsic motivation become pivotal in adolescence, as students at this age have the means to not only withdraw energy from educational pursuits but also the ability to drop out altogether (NRC, 2004).

With regard to achievement outcomes, there is recent evidence that middle and high school youth are underperforming in relation to expectations set by state standards tests and in international competitions. Moreover, performance gaps related to culture, race, and income are not closing despite years of rhetoric and attention (NCES, 2003). For example, after years of standards-based educational reform under No Child Left Behind (NCLB), roughly 40% of poor or African-American eighth graders in Virginia perform below standards for reading achievement, and the corresponding rates of failure for youth in the District of Columbia are close to 80% (Aratani, 2006). These rates of failure in reading, which was one of the spurs for NCLB, reflect a fundamental misunderstanding of the mechanisms by which students are engaged through relationships and the need to reconceptualize and redesign how we support teachers to build upon and foster relationships with students.

Consider a second target of school reform, the dropout rate. Fewer than 60% of ninth graders in certain demographic groups (NCES, 2003) actually graduate 4 years later. Yet for 10 years, decreasing the dropout rate has been a singular focus of most secondary schools, and the average *annual* dropout rate remains near 10% and ranges up for some groups. These figures make strikingly clear that the high school classroom as a setting for youth development is fundamentally flawed. Put another way, it does not appear to us that the central problem in school reform is curriculum, school/class size, or outcomes assessment but rather the extent to which teachers are supported to interact with students and form relationships with them that engage them in opportunities to learn and develop.

Youth report that they are highly concerned with the actual experiences they have in classroom settings, which they find lacking in terms of supportive relationships that draw them into meaningful challenges and competence-building experiences (Crosnoe, 2001; Csikszentmihalyi & Schneider, 2000; Marks, 2000; NRC, 2004; Roeser, Eccles, & Sameroff, 2000). Perhaps they are right, and the capacity of schools to support youth development, particularly for "high risk" youth, depends on whether the relationships and interactions among students and teachers within a classroom offer a developmentally meaningful and challenging experience (NRC). Because teacher-student interactions embody the relational capacity of the classroom to promote positive development, our focus is on improving and changing these relationships and interactions and involves working with teachers. Thus, our theory and method of change is centered on teachers' relationships and interactions with students.

A Theory of Engagement Within Classroom Settings

We start with a brief description of a typical classroom experience in a school in the United States, public or private, regardless of grade or content area. Whether based on observations of teacher-student interactions or youth reports, experiences in classrooms too often fail to capitalize on student interests, goals, and motivation and rather promote disengagement and alienation. One cannot read these accounts and escape the sense that school and classroom settings and the adults responsible for their quality are simply not involved relationally (Crosnoe, 2000; Dornbusch et al., 1996; Eccles et al., 1991). Yet, despite this generally dismal picture of classrooms, it is also true that nearly every student can describe, with enthusiasm and passion, a relationship with a teacher that they felt was meaningful and important to them, often with considerable evidence to back up those claims (Resnick et al., 1997).

The impressions gleaned from youth reports are confirmed in observations, some of which are ethnographic in nature while others rely on large-scale assessments of hundreds of classrooms. For example, evidence gleaned from observing large numbers of typical American classrooms in first, third, and fifth grades shows clearly that the nature and quality of adult-student interactions in classrooms are lacking in the kind of assets outlined in the NRC report. For example, in the NICHD Study of Early Child Care and Youth Development observations in more than 2,500 elementary classrooms, of the opportunities for academic activities and learning to which a typical student is exposed, more than 85% of those opportunities take place in the context of teacher-directed whole group instruction or individual seatwork, in contrast to small-group work that might capitalize on teacher-student relationships as key mediators of engagement. The typical student interacted with their teacher (individually or in a small group) fewer than four times in an hour, and in most cases, these exchanges were perfunctory and compliance-directed. Furthermore, most instructional exchanges had a pronounced and almost singular focus on performing basic skills, tasks that require a discrete answer that is correct or not rather than eliciting analysis, reasoning, or problem-solving around a more ambiguous challenge. From a relational standpoint, these exchanges were devoid of personal, emotional, motivational properties that would engage the student in the task at hand. Recalling the NRC report's emphasis on meaningful challenges for cognitive development (as well as recent calls for raising standards for "twenty-first century skills"), this focus on basic skills neglects the ways in which reasoning, problem-solving, and more advanced cognition can be a force for engaging students in activities that are highly salient developmentally but which also require relational supports to sustain students' participation. Despite rhetoric that paints a picture of middle and high school as challenging and interesting, the actual experiences youth have in classroom settings (observed or reported) are often lacking in terms of meaningful challenges, supportive relationships, and competence-building opportunities (Crosnoe, 2001; Csikszentmihalyi & Schneider, 2000; Marks, 2000; NRC, 2002; Roeser et al., 2000).

Schools all fundamentally rise or fall on the success of what occurs within the classroom (e.g., Crosnoe, 2001; Nye, Konstantopoulos, & Hedges, 2004; Resnick et al., 1997) Ironically, close observation of most any secondary school in America reveals that adolescents—both at risk and high functioning—often display remarkably high degrees of motivation and engagement within the school setting. Rarely, however, does this occur *within* the classroom. High school hallways, playing fields, and lunchrooms literally brim over with youthful energy, excitement, and enthusiasm. Intense interactions occur in sports and extracurricular activities, and interactions with peers dominate students' perception of the social ecology of school. It is only when these students enter their classroom that energy levels decline precipitously, and it is rare that a given student will "connect" with a teacher or material in classroom or subject area in such a way that they perform at high levels of capacity or "flow" (Csikszentmihalyi & Schneider, 2000). The classroom setting looks equally bleak from the perspective of teachers, who are also dropping out and becoming more disengaged. Fifteen percent of the entire teaching workforce turns over every year. Rates of teachers leaving the profession are increasing. And those who stay report a sense of malaise and frustration—they feel their job is getting harder and they have fewer tools with which to work and feel effective (Hart, Stroot, Yinger, & Smith, 2005).

A fundamental principle in addressing the chronically resource-starved classroom is that modifying the classroom as a relational setting to engage children and youth more fully may be the single best way to unleash and expand the level of *human resources* (e.g., relationships and interpersonal interactions) available to the educational process (Sarason, 1982). Below, we discuss three features of classrooms likely to influence levels of behavioral/psychological engagement—relational supports, competence supports, and relevance. These features form the core theoretical foundation of our subsequent efforts to assess and improve the relational properties of classrooms and, thereby, engagement.

Understanding the primary role of interactions and relationships in creating the capacity for children and youth to engage the classroom as a setting for development is a fundamental precursor to understanding our approach to measuring interactions and to *changing* classroom settings' capacity for engagement. Readers will recognize applications and extensions of Vygotsky's (1978, 1991) ideas about the contextualized nature of learning and development and close, interdependent connection among relational supports, task-related challenges, and learning. Pianta (1999) also has discussed the connection between classroom contexts and learning in terms of the relational, structural, and motivational affordances available in classrooms. Central to each of these perspectives, and elaborated below, is an appreciation of engagement as a contextualized process mediated by relationships and interpersonal interactions.

Relational Supports

As a behavior setting, the classroom runs on interactions between and among participants: the relationship between the student and the teacher and the relationships of students with one another. These relationships and their value emotionally, instrumentally, and psychologically are fundamental supports to the value of their experience in the classroom setting for furthering development. It is not an overstatement to suggest that most children and adolescents *live* for their social relationships (Collins & Repinski, 1994), and for many young people, relationships with teachers are core organizers of experience; they are fundamental to core developmental functions. Yet, the qualities of teacher-student relationships are frequently afterthoughts in battles over curricula, testing, school structure, and funding. Positive relationships with adults are perhaps the single most important ingredient in promoting positive student development. For example, when teachers learn to make modest efforts to form a personal connection with their adolescent students—such that the students feel known—they can dramatically enhance student motivation in school and emotional functioning outside of school (Roeser, Eccles, & Sameroff, 1998; Skinner, Zimmer-Gembeck, & Connell, 1998). In the early grades, when teachers spend nondirective individual time with children who they find challenging, the disruptive behavior of these students drops, and teachers report more harmonious and learning-oriented interactions (Mashburn et al., 2008).

Adolescents report both that they would learn more if their teachers cared about them personally and that such personal connections are rare (Public Agenda, 1997). A close, supportive relationship with a teacher is a key feature distinguishing at-risk children and adolescents who succeed in school from those who do not (Pianta, Steinberg, & Rollins, 1995; Resnick et al., 1997), and youths' sense of social connection within settings predicts outcomes ranging from higher achievement scores to greater student engagement and more positive academic attitudes (Bryk & Driscoll, 1988; Bryk, Lee, & Holland, 1993; Connell & Wellborn, 1991; Crosnoe, Johnson, & Elder, 2004; Ryan & Deci, 2000; see also, NRC, 2004, for extended review of other similar findings). Notably, even for relatively highly motivated late adolescents in college, recent experimental work has shown that a sense of isolation can significantly reduce energy for intellectual pursuits and that this reduction is powerful enough to temporarily depress results on IQ tests (Baumeister, Twenge, & Nuss, 2002), while increasing irrational and risk-taking behavior (Twenge, Catanese, & Baumeister, 2002). Thus, regardless of age or grade, interpersonal relational supports provided through teachers' interactions with students are a fundamental facet of classrooms' capacity to support development.

Autonomy/Competence Supports

Children and youth are engaged by challenges that are within reach and that provide a sense of self-efficacy and control: experiences that offer challenges viewed as "older" or adultlike but for which appropriate scaffolding and support are provided (Bandura, Barbaranelli, Caprara, & Pastorelli, 1996; Eccles et al., 1993). Any setting that intends to advance development and learning outcomes for children or youth must carefully craft the nature of experience it provides in order to give participants a developmentally calibrated sense of control, autonomy, choice, and mastery. Absent these considerations or in settings that rely on approaches characterized as overly top-down or passive, in which teachers are over- or underinvolved, classrooms are doomed to be places lacking in engaged participants. For example, one of the most tragically avoidable errors that some secondary school teachers make is to assume that youth strivings for autonomy and self-expression represent negative forces to be countered rather than positive energy to be harnessed. This basic misunderstanding of adolescent development (one often promoted in teacher education courses and reinforced by school policies) then takes form in highly controlling and punitive classroom and school settings and in instruction that is highly teacher-driven and discouraging of exploration and curiosity. At the other end of the age spectrum, all too often, teachers espouse a "child-centered" or "play-based" philosophy around learning and development that all too often expresses itself in children wandering around activity centers while teachers are not involved in actively scaffolding learning (Pianta, Mashburn, Downer, Hamre, & Justice, 2008). In both instances, overcontrolled responses to adolescents and underinvolved responses to young children, adult-child relationships, and interactions are not calibrated to developmental tendencies of students. This mismatch of classroom and development results in schools narrowing, rather than expanding, the "space" in which zones of proximal development can be created.

Relevance

For children and youth, the connection of academic skills and knowledge to their real-life experience is a near-universal property of classrooms that foster engagement. Adolescents, like adults, deploy a considerable amount of effort in attempts to make meaning in their lives. For many, adolescence is a period in which this becomes a focus for the first time. This process ultimately leads to a bias in adolescents' evaluation of experience (particularly those experiences offered by adults) toward choices they view as relevant, or connected to their emerging views on what is meaningful and what is not. Too often, the high school curriculum and the rationales behind it are taken as a "given" without recognition that these rationales need to be made clear to each new cohort of students. Drawing even very distal connections between what occurs within high school and the larger "real world" can alter student behavior. For example, involving students in significant, real-world, voluntary community service and then discussing it within the classroom in an ongoing way has been found to reduce disruptive behavior by 50% in randomly controlled trials, with similar effects upon other outcomes in youths' lives as well (Allen, Philliber, Herrling, & Kuperminc, 1997). Centuries ago, late adolescents were commanding armies and running countries (Barzun, 2000). Today, a generation of children and adolescents who grew up with the internet, social networks, and sophisticated video games is confined to a classroom for hours a day with little vision of how what occurs within that classroom relates to the larger world.

In the early grades, as we recounted previously, virtually no instruction occurs that does not have a "correct/incorrect" focus. Thinking, problem-solving, and reasoning with real-world information is conspicuously absent in the vast majority of classrooms (see Pianta, Belsky, Houts, Morrison, & NICHD ECCRN, 2007). When academic learning is almost completely organized and focused in this way, there is virtually no way in which teachers can make the content or activity relevant. Rather than drawing on relationships and interpersonal interactions with students as a front-end asset to draw them into solving a somewhat ambiguous and perhaps uncertain real-life problem, teachers end up relying on relationships and interactions to cajole or to address behavioral disruptions and inattention (i.e., disengagement) that are the inevitable by-product of miscalibration.

Consciously addressing the relevance of what occurs within the classroom to the larger world is critical to engaging otherwise restless young minds. On a smaller scale, teachers may increase the relevance of the classroom by making repeated, explicit ties between curricular material and real-world applications and engaging relational processes that scaffold participation in learning that is somewhat less constricted. The key factor here is that the real-world connections must be made in ways that are meaningful *as perceived by the student*. For some, it may be through a very close and comforting emotional connection to a teacher, while for others it will be through a teacher providing challenging problems.

These ideas about the central role of teacher-student interactions and relationships as the primary mechanism by which student engagement is fostered form the basis for our developmentally informed analysis of classroom effects on student outcomes. In our view, the capacity of classroom settings to engage children and youth is the core "criterion" by which they should be judged, and the features of relational supports, autonomy/competence supports, and relevance are how classrooms, through relationships and interactions, accomplish that goal.

These supports, enacted in teacher-student interactions, produce cycles of student engagement, teacher efficacy, and student performance. We suggest that in the best classrooms, these supports operate in concert to initiate self-reinforcing linkages among engaged students, effective teachers, and growth in student performance. Relationships and interactions in the classroom are the media through which relational, competence, and relevance supports are made available to students. In the next section, we present our conceptualization and technical approach to interactions and relationships between teachers and students as the focus of measurement and change.

Conceptualizing and Measuring Teacher-Student Classroom Interactions

To help organize the diverse literatures that inform conceptualization and assessment of classroom processes, Hamre and Pianta (2007) presented the Teaching Through Interactions (TTI) framework, a theoretically driven and empirically supported system for conceptualizing, organizing, and measuring classroom interactions between teachers and students into three major domains—emotional supports, classroom organization, and instructional supports. This framework recognizes that the starting point for understanding contextual influences on development is to recognize that development occurs through interactions between the capacities and skills of the person and the resources available to them in various settings, and that this process is very dynamic (Bronfenbrenner & Morris, 1998; Magnusson & Stattin, 1998).

A feature of the TTI framework is that the latent structure of teacher-child interactions applies consistently across grades from preschool through to secondary grades; thus, the three-domain TTI latent structure is hypothesized as grade invariant. Critically, although latent structure is hypothesized as *invariant*, the TTI framework reflects the developmentally relevant construct of *heterotypic continuity* and allows for variation across grades in the specific behavioral indicators that reflect positive and negative features of interactions.

In the section that follows, we briefly review the three major domains of teacher-student interactions described in the TTI framework (emotional, organizational, and instructional), including a summary of the developmental theories and empirical studies on which they are based. Within each of these three broad domains of interaction, we then describe in subsections a number of specific dimensions that form the basis of behavioral interactions and observations of interactions. Thus, we present two levels of the TTI framework—three broad domains and the dimensions of behavioral interactions between teachers and students that more specifically define these domains. Much of what we present below is based on work in elementary classrooms;

however, as is evident in the discussion above and in reports such as that of the NRC (2004), these concepts of the TTI framework and their relevance for understanding engagement are applicable to adolescents as well.

Emotional Interaction Domain

Teacher efforts to support students' social and emotional functioning in the classroom, through positive facilitation of teacher-student and student-student interactions, are key elements of effective classroom practice. Two broad areas of developmental theory guide much of the work on emotional support in classrooms—attachment (Ainsworth, Blehar, Waters, & Wall, 1978; Bowlby, 1969; Pianta, 1999) and self-determination theory (Connell & Wellborn, 1991; Ryan & Deci, 2000; Skinner & Belmont, 1993). Attachment theorists posit that when parents provide emotional support, and a predictable, consistent, and safe environment, children become more self-reliant and are able to take risks as they explore the world because they know that an adult will be there to help them if they need it (Ainsworth et al., 1978; Bowlby, 1969). This theory has been broadly applied to and validated in school environments (Birch & Ladd, 1998; Hamre & Pianta, 2001; Howes, Hamilton, & Matheson, 1994; Lynch & Cicchetti, 1992; Pianta, 1999). Self-determination (or self-systems) theory (Connell & Wellborn, 1991; Ryan & Deci, 2000; Skinner & Belmont, 1993) suggests that children and youth are most motivated to learn when adults support their need to feel competent, positively related to others, and autonomous. Throughout schooling, students who are more emotionally connected to teachers and peers demonstrate positive trajectories of development in both social and academic domains (Hamre & Pianta, 2001; Harter, 1996; Ladd, Birch, & Buhs, 1999; Pianta et al., 1995; Roeser et al., 2000; Ryan, Stiller, & Lynch, 1994; Silver, Measelle, Essex, & Armstrong, 2005; Wentzel, 1998). Within this domain, we focus on behavioral interactions related to emotional climate, teacher sensitivity, and regard for student perspectives.

Emotional Climate

Classrooms are, by their very nature, social places. Teachers and children laugh and play together, share stories about their lives outside of the classroom, and work together to create an environment in which all learning occurs. The classroom climate can be described along positive and negative dimensions. Positive climate encompasses the degree to which students experience warm caring relationships with adults and peers and enjoy the time they spend in the classroom. Negative climates are those in which students experience frequent yelling, humiliation, or irritation in interactions with teachers and peers.

The aspect of climate that has been studied most extensively in the past 10 years is the nature and quality of teachers' relationships with students. There is strong evidence for the salience of student-teacher relationships as an important context for children's development (see Pianta et al., 2003); student-teacher relationships are associated with children's peer competencies (e.g., Birch & Ladd, 1998; Howes, 2000; Howes et al., 1994) and trajectories toward academic success or failure (Birch & Ladd, 1996, 1998; Hamre & Pianta, 2001; Ladd et al., 1999; Pianta et al., 1995; Silver et al., 2005; van Ijzendoorn, Sagi, & Lambermon, 1992). There is evidence that certain teachers have tendencies to develop more positive relationships, across multiple students in their classroom, than do others (Hamre, Pianta, Downer, & Mashburn, 2005; Mashburn, Hamre, Downer, & Pianta, 2007). Children and youth in classrooms with higher levels of teacher support have higher levels of peer acceptance and classroom engagement than do their peers in less supportive classrooms, even after controlling for individual levels of teacher-support (Hughes, Zhang, & Hill, 2006).

Teacher Sensitivity

Teachers provide more than a warm and caring social environment. They must be attuned and responsive to the individual cues and needs of students in their classrooms, a dimension of teaching referred to here as teacher sensitivity. Highly sensitive teachers, through their consistent, timely, and responsive interactions, help students see adults as a resource and create environments in which students feel safe and free to explore and learn (Pianta et al., 2004). Highly sensitive teaching requires teachers to attend to, process, and respond to a lot of information simultaneously. For example, during whole group instruction, a sensitive teacher may, within quick succession, notice some children not paying attention, see that one child is frustrated because he does not understand her questions, and observe a sad look on a child she knows is generally very happy and engaged. The sensitive teacher not only notices these subtle cues from students, but knows her students well enough to respond in ways that help alleviate their problems. She may, for example, change the tone of her voice to reengage those students not participating, take a quick moment to restate her question in simpler language, and make a mental note to check in with the sad student at recess. In contrast, an insensitive teacher may completely miss these subtle cues or respond in ways that aggravate, rather than alleviate, students' problems.

Students in classrooms with sensitive teachers are more engaged and self-reliant in the classroom and have lower levels of mother-reported internalizing problems than do those with less sensitive teachers (NICHD ECCRN, 2003; Rimm-Kaufman, Early, & Cox, 2002). Sensitive teaching is important to not only social outcomes, but also to academic outcomes. For example, among a group of preschoolers, those who experienced more responsive teacher interactions in preschool displayed stronger vocabulary and decoding skills at the end of first grade (Connor, Son, & Hindman, 2005). Sensitivity—timing and responsiveness to student cues—is perhaps one of the single most important features of interaction in relation to engagement as these behaviors on the part of the teacher literally denote the extent of calibration in drawing the student toward an opportunity.

Regard for Students' Perspectives

The final dimension of emotional support is the degree to which classrooms and interactions are structured around the interests and motivations of the teacher, versus those of the students.

In some classrooms, teachers frequently ask for students' ideas and thoughts, follow students' lead, and provide opportunities for students to have a *formative* role in the classroom. In these classrooms, students are not just allowed to talk but are actively encouraged to talk to one another (Pianta et al., 2004). At the other end of the continuum are classrooms in which teachers follow very scripted plans for how the day should run, show little flexibility or response to students' interests and motivations, and provide few opportunities for students to express their thoughts or to assume responsibility for activities in the classroom. Teachers in these classrooms may also be very controlling of student movement, requiring, for example, young children to sit quietly on the rug with their legs crossed and hands in their laps for long periods of time, or for older children, requiring long stretches of drill.

Children and adolescents report more positive feelings about school, display more motivation, and are more engaged when they experience more student-focused and autonomy-supportive instruction (deKruif, McWilliam, Ridley, & Wakely, 2000; Gutman & Sulzby, 2000; Pianta, La Paro, Payne, Cox, & Bradley, 2002; Valeski & Stipek, 2001). Students in more teacher-directed classrooms have higher levels of internalizing problems (NICHD ECCRN, 2003). There are some findings, however, suggesting that the optimal level of teacher control may vary depending on factors such as learning objectives (Brophy & Good, 1986; Soar & Soar, 1979) and grade (Valeski & Stipek, 2001). Interestingly, there is ample support that adolescents also thrive when given some degree of control and choice over their learning (NRC, 2004).

Classroom Organization Domain

Educational research and practice place tremendous emphasis on the role of organization and management in creating a well-functioning classroom. In the TTI framework, classroom organization is the domain of teacher-student interactions through which teachers organize *behavior*, *time*, and *attention* (Emmer & Stough, 2001). Teachers using more effective behavior management strategies (Arnold, McWilliams, & Arnold, 1998; Emmer & Strough, 2001; Evertson, Emmer, Sanford, & Clements, 1983; Evertson & Harris, 1999), having more organized and routine management structures (Bohn, Roehrig, & Pressley, 2004; Cameron, Connor, & Morrison, 2005), and implementing strategies that make students active participants in classroom activities (Bowman & Stott, 1994; Bruner, 1996; Rogoff, 1990; Vygotsky, 1978) have less oppositional behavior, higher levels of engagement in learning, and ultimately, students who learn more. Thus, the dimensions of teacher-student interaction that are reflected in the classroom organization domain include effective behavior management, productivity, and learning formats.

Effective Behavior Management

Behavior management is a term that is often applied to a broad spectrum of classroom management strategies, including teachers' abilities to engage students and make constructive use of time. Within the TTI framework, behavior management is defined more narrowly as teacher-student interactions intended to *promote positive behavior* and *prevent or terminate misbehavior* in the classroom. There is general consensus around a set of practices associated with more positive student behavior including: (a) providing clear and consistent behavioral expectations; (b) monitoring the classroom for potential problems and proactively preventing problems rather than being reactive; (c) efficiently redirecting minor misbehavior before it escalates; (d) using positive, proactive strategies such as praising positive behavior rather than calling attention to misbehavior; and (e) spending a minimal amount of time on behavior management issues (Emmer & Stough, 2001; Pianta et al., 2004). At the low end of this dimension, classrooms are chaotic with very few consistently enforced rules and a great deal of student misbehavior.

Most of the research on behavior management was conducted by process-product researchers in the 1970s and 1980s with studies consistently showing that classrooms with positive behavior management tend to have students who make greater academic progress (Good & Grouws, 1977; Soar & Soar, 1979). Intervention studies suggest that teachers who adopt these types of practices after training are more likely than teachers in control groups to have students who are engaged and learning (Emmer & Strough, 2001; Evertson & Harris, 1999; Evertson et al., 1983). Surprisingly, researchers have yet to examine the extent to which these specific behavioral strategies are associated with the more recent concept of self-regulated learning behaviors, though prior work would suggest clear linkages.

Productivity

In productive classrooms, teachers are not only effective managers of behavior, but are well organized, spend a minimal amount of time on basic management activities such as taking attendance or passing out and collecting homework, and are prepared for instructional activities so that little time is lost in transition. Highly productive classrooms may resemble a "well-oiled machine" in which everyone in the classroom seems to know what is expected of them and how to go about doing it (Pianta et al., 2004). In contrast, when teachers do not manage time efficiently, students may spend extraordinary amounts of time looking for materials, waiting for the next activity, or simply sitting around.

Early work by process-product researchers focused attention on the importance of time management, providing consistent evidence that students are most engaged in productive classrooms, and that this engagement is, in turn, directly associated with student learning (Brophy & Evertson, 1976; Coker, Medley, & Soar, 1980; Good & Grouws, 1979; Stallings, 1975; Stallings, Cory, Fairweather, & Needels, 1978). Several more recent studies suggest that teachers observed to foster productive classrooms spend more time creating efficient routines at the beginning of the school year and that this early investment pays off for students and teachers by enabling them to spend less time in transition and more time in child-managed activities later in the school year (Bohn et al., 2004; Cameron et al., 2005).

Instructional Learning Formats

The instructional learning formats dimension of interaction focuses directly on the extent to which teachers provide interesting activities, instruction, centers/projects, and materials and facilitate those activities so that students are actively engaged through various modalities. Consistent with constructivist theories as well as information-processing views of learning and cognition (Bowman & Stott, 1994; Bruner, 1996; Rogoff, 1990; Vygotsky, 1978), formats for instruction should foster *active* participation in a specific learning opportunity such that the students are not only participating behaviorally but they are engaged cognitively as well. In classrooms low on this dimension, teachers may rely on one format, typically lecture, and fail to format instruction or provide opportunity for interaction that foster students' engagement. Again, formatting instruction developmentally is not solely contingent on the *type* of instruction or number of materials a teacher uses but rather how effectively the teacher interacts to use instruction and materials to engage students (Rimm-Kaufman, La Paro, Downer, & Pianta, 2005).

Instructional Interaction Domain

Instructional methods have been put in the spotlight in recent years, as more emphasis has been placed on the translation of cognitive science, learning, and developmental research to educational environments (Carver & Klahr, 2001). The theoretical foundation for the conceptualization of instructional supports in the TTI framework comes primarily from research on cognitive and language development (e.g., Carver & Klahr, 2001; Catts, Fey, Zhang, & Tomblin, 2001; Fujiki, Brinton, & Clarke, 2002; Romberg, Carpenter, & Dremock, 2005; Taylor, Pearson, Peterson, & Rodriguez, 2003; Vygotsky, 1991; Wharton-McDonald, Pressley, & Hampston, 1998). This literature highlights the distinction between simply learning facts and gaining "usable knowledge," which is built upon learning how facts are interconnected, organized, and conditioned upon one another (Bransford, Brown, & Cocking,

1999; Mayer, 2002). A student's cognitive and language development is contingent on the opportunities adults provide to express existing skills and scaffold more complex ones (Davis & Miyake, 2004; Skibbe, Behnke, & Justice, 2004; Vygotsky, 1991). The development of "metacognitive" skills, or the awareness and understanding of one's thinking processes, is also critical (Veenman, Kok, & Blöte, 2005; Williams, Blythe, & White, 2002). The exemplary work of the National Research Council's series, *How Students Learn* (Donovan & Bransford, 2005), summarizes research across disciplines to emphasize how specific teaching strategies can enhance students' development and application of these core thinking skills (Bransford et al., 1999). Within this broad, cognitively focused definition of instruction, we describe below three aspects of teachers' interactions with students that not only promote engagement but student learning outcomes as well.

Concept Development

Through instructional behaviors, conversations, and activities, teachers foster students' development of *concepts and higher-order thinking skills* (Pianta et al., 2004). In an extension of Bloom's Taxonomy (Bloom, Engelhart, Furst, Hill, & Krathwohl, 1956), Mayer (2002) offers a helpful description of the teaching and learning practices associated with the development of these cognitive skills. According to Mayer, learning requires not only the acquisition of knowledge (retention), but the ability to access and apply this knowledge in new situations (transfer). Teachers can facilitate this transfer process by providing students with opportunities to: *understand*—build connections between new and previous knowledge; *apply*—use procedures and knowledge to help solve new problems; *analyze*—divide information into meaningful parts; *evaluate*—make conclusions based on criteria or standards; and *create*—put pieces of knowledge together to produce new ideas. These features of students' cognitive engagement are directly promoted through teacher-student interactions. At the high end of this dimension, teachers are opportunists who not only plan activities in ways that will stimulate higher-order thinking, but they take advantage of the moment-to-moment opportunities *within* their daily interactions to push students toward deeper thinking. In contrast, in classrooms low on concept development, interactions between teachers and students focus on *remembering* facts, or simple tasks in which they must *recognize* or *recall* information.

Interactions that stimulate concept development predict greater achievement gains for students (Romberg et al., 2005; Taylor et al., 2003; Wharton-McDonald et al., 1998). As noted by Brophy (1986), this does not require that all of a teacher's questions are "higher level" questions, but that there is a balance in which teachers use higher level questions to help focus student attention on the process of learning rather than solely on the product. In one recent study, Taylor and colleagues (2003) examined the role of these teacher practices in reading development among children in 88 high-poverty classrooms (first to fifth grade) across the United States. They observed in classrooms three times over the course of the year and examined growth in a randomly selected nine students per classroom. Their observations consisted of mixed methods in which they collected quantitative information on the types and frequency of questions used by teachers, as well as detailed qualitative information on teacher practices. Results suggested that children in classrooms in which teachers emphasized higher-order thinking skills, through questioning and activities, displayed more reading growth over the course of the year.

Feedback

In order to get the most benefit from the instructional opportunities described above, students need feedback about their learning. Feedback refers to a broad range of teachers' interactions with students in which the teacher provides some information back to the student about their performance or effort. Research on feedback has typically focused on praise (Brophy & Evertson, 1976; Stallings, 1975), behavioral feedback, or attributional feedback, in which teachers make statements to students attributing their performance to either ability (e.g., "you did this well because you are a good reader") or effort (e.g., "you did this well because you worked hard") (Burnett, 2003; Dohrn & Bryan, 1994; Mueller & Dweck, 1998). Although the TTI definition includes these forms of feedback, the focus is on feedback that provides students with specific information about the content or process of learning. High-quality feedback is described as communication from teachers that provides students with specific information about not only whether or not they are correct (Brophy, 1986), but about how they might get to the correct answer, how they might perform at a higher level, or how their performance meshes with larger goals. Teachers providing high-quality feedback provide frequent feedback loops or back-and-forth exchanges in which a teacher responds to an initial student comment by engaging with the student, or group of students, in a sustained effort to reach deeper understanding (Pianta et al., 2004).

Most research on feedback has focused on quantity rather than the quality. For example, within a group of elementary, middle, and secondary Kentucky schools, those identified as successful in reducing the achievement gap between White and African-American students had teachers who were more likely to provide frequent corrective and immediate feedback to students (Meehan, Hughes, & Cavell, 2003); in this regard, timing was clearly important. In studies in which quality of feedback was observed, these interactions were associated with gains in literacy and language across the preschool and kindergarten years (Howes et al., 2008) and a closing of the achievement gap among first grade students coming from disadvantaged backgrounds (Hamre & Pianta, 2005).

Language and Instructional Discourse

Children's ability to navigate the instructional and social opportunities in classrooms is dependent in large part on their language skills (Catts, Fey, Zhang, & Tomblin, 1999; Fujiki et al., 2002) and in turn requires that teachers engage students in conversations that promote the development of specific language skills such as social language and pragmatics (Ninio & Snow, 1999; Whitehurst et al., 1988), vocabulary (Justice, 2002; Penno, Wilkinson, & Moore, 2002), and narrative skills (Catts et al., 1999; Zevenbergen, Whitehurst, & Zevenbergen, 2003). In classrooms offering high levels of language modeling, teachers often converse with students, ask many open-ended questions, repeat or extend children's responses, and use a variety of words, including more advanced language which is explicitly linked to words the students already know. Although there is a mix of teacher and student talk in these classrooms, there is a clear and intentional effort by teachers to promote students' language use, including explicit attempts to facilitate peer conversations (Justice, Mashburn, Hamre, & Pianta, 2008; Pianta et al., 2004). At the low end, classrooms are dominated by teacher talk, and student utterances are rarely attended or responded to in any meaningful way.

Young children exposed to high-quality language modeling, at home and at school, display more positive language development (Catts et al., 1999; Justice, 2002; Ninio & Snow, 1999; Penno et al., 2002; Reese & Cox, 1999; Schuele, Rice & Wilcox, 1995; Whitehurst et al., 1988; Zevenbergen et al., 2003) which, in turn, is associated with more positive social adjustment (Hemphill & Siperstein, 1990; Pianta & Nimetz, 1991) and greater reading abilities (Catts et al., 1999). In one example, Justice, Meier, and Walpole (2005) tested the degree to which teacher-child interactions influenced kindergarten children's increases in vocabulary. Results suggest that when children are explicitly introduced to new words through providing a definition (e.g., a *marsh* is a very wet place where there are wetlands covered with grasses) and using the new word in a supportive context (e.g., like, we took a boat through the *marsh* and we saw lots of birds and alligators), they show greater vocabulary development relative to a comparison group (Justice et al., 2005). In contrast, simple exposure to new words through book reading was not associated with significant vocabulary gains.

In the upper grades, language-related interactions between teachers and students can be characterized in terms of instructional discourse in the classroom. Teachers promoting rich instructional discourse do so through verbal interactions that foster exchanges of ideas, concepts, and perspectives as well as student control over discourse. Because of the fundamental importance of language as both a social medium and a medium for conveying information, teachers' language and their interactions around language with and among students are fundamental to the ways in which teacher-student interactions are a medium for student engagement.

Measuring Teacher-Student Interactions

When approaching the task of translating the Teaching Through Interactions framework into a measurement tool for observing teacher-student relationships and interactions, we proposed a model (Hamre & Pianta, 2007) that organizes teacher-student interactions at four levels, from broad to micro in nature. As described earlier, the broad *domain* of emotional supports is defined in terms of three *dimensions*: classroom climate, teacher sensitivity, and regard for student perspectives. Each dimension is operationalized at more granular levels of analysis in terms of a set of specific *behavioral indicators* that are then defined in terms of observable *behavioral interactions*. Classroom climate includes observable behavioral indicators such as the frequency and quality of teachers' affective communications with students (further specified in terms of smiles, positive verbal feedback) as well as the degree to which students appear to enjoy spending time with one another. This multilevel conceptualization of the interactions between a student and teacher can be observed in actual classroom environments, moving from broad theoretically based domains (as described above in the TTI framework) to very specific behaviors. The resulting articulation of the TTI framework into the four levels of description and accompanying scaling into examples of interaction from "low" to "high" quality along a seven-point rating scale is described in the Classroom Assessment Scoring System, or CLASS (Pianta, Mashburn, et al., 2008). The CLASS is the measurement tool for observing and evaluating teacher-student interactions derived from the TTI theoretical framework.

In an attempt to test the validity of the three-domain organization of the TTI across multiple grade levels, Hamre and colleagues (2010) drew from a sample of over just under 4,000 preschool to fifth grade classrooms that were a part of several large national and regional studies. Results of a confirmatory factor analysis suggested adequate fit of the three-factor model, and that the fit of this model was superior to a one- or two-factor model. This means that all three of the domains of teacher-child interactions described in the TTI framework and assessed by CLASS are important for describing teacher-child interactions and understanding the impacts that classrooms have on students; no single domain on its own may be enough. That is, interactions and relationships between teachers and students reflect a number of facets and features, common across grades and ages, but nonetheless multidimensional.

We also were interested in the extent to which classroom processes at different levels (behavior, indicator, dimension, domain) predict differentially to outcomes (gains). Put another way, do teacher-child interactions encoded at the level of dimension based on global 1–7 ratings of teacher-interaction across a 15–20-min period predict to student achievement gains better or worse than teacher-student behavior encoded as counts or checklists of discrete teacher interactions toward a student? This question concerning level of analysis reflects major conceptual issues regarding the actual level at which developmentally meaningful or salient connections between the child and classroom context occur. Drawing on Sroufe's (1996) work and a developmentally informed theory of teacher-child interactions as embedded in a relationship (Pianta, 1999), the TTI framework posits that the level at which interactions with adults predicts development is best captured at the level of *dimensions* of interaction that take place over time. In the case of the CLASS as a measure, this is operationalized by ratings on a seven-point dimension made after 20 min of observation. In preliminary analyses, we find fairly consistent support for prediction of achievement and social gains at the level of dimensions of teacher-student interaction (i.e., seven-point ratings) rather than for counts or time samplings of discrete teacher behaviors.

Moreover, we find that discrete teacher behaviors are highly unstable from moment to moment across time, and the frequency of their display is highly contingent on the nature of the activity. In terms of a theory of relationships and engagement, these results suggest that to capture the qualities of interactions and relationships that foster and reflect engagement, it may be important to conceptualize and assess those interactions over episodes and patterns of behavior rather than discrete instances. In other words, the whole may be greater than the sum of the parts.

Conceptually, the reason for expecting that discrete teacher behaviors would be less strongly related to student growth is that measures of isolated behaviors, by definition, do not capture aspects of the teacher's behavior that reflects either a *response to the child* or a *calibrated intent to stimulate development* that are both stable across moment-to-moment fluctuations and reflect reliable differences between individual teachers in their approach (Magnusson & Stattin, 1998). This ongoing process of calibration is where we believe the focus on interactions maps well onto the discussion of student engagement and its importance. Not surprisingly, we find that indeed, dimensions of teacher-student interactions are rather stable across time and reflect variance that is reliably located between teachers (Mashburn et al., 2007).

The dimensions of interaction assessed by the CLASS elementary version predict growth in literacy and math as well as reduced teacher-child conflict and problem behavior from pre-K through fifth grade (Hamre & Pianta, 2005; Howes et al., 2008; NICHD ECCRN, 2004). The CLASS is one of the most current and widely used standardized assessments of social and instructional interactions in classrooms (Hart et al., 2005; NICHD ECCRN, 2002, 2005; McCaslin, Burross, & Good, 2005). The CLASS-Secondary version, or CLASS-S, is explicitly designed to capture precisely those aspects of classroom interactions that we hypothesize above to be resources for adolescent engagement. As such, it builds on and incorporates all of the strengths of the CLASS system at elementary levels, while adding specific dimensions conceptualized and operationalized to maximize adolescent engagement.

Changing Interactions Between Teachers and Students in Classrooms

In this section, we briefly outline results from descriptive research using CLASS that forms the basis and rationale for the steps we have taken to improve teacher-student interactions. It then summarizes our approach to professional development, which we call MyTeachingPartner, which is designed explicitly around the CLASS as a focus for changing interactions.

Improving Teacher-Student Interactions

We posit four levers producing developmental change for teacher-student relationships and interactions: (1) *teachers' knowledge and cognitions* related to their interactions with students, (2) availability of ongoing *relational supports for teachers* themselves, (3) teachers' regular *exposure to individualized feedback* about their actual interactions with students, and (4) *a standard and valid "target" around which to focus* efforts to change interactions. The hypothesis we are testing in our ongoing work is that intervention packages that activate these levers in a coordinated way are most likely to induce and maintain change, given the systemic nature of teacher-student relationships and interactions in classrooms. Here we describe the theoretical and technical features of MyTeachingPartner (MTP), an innovative professional development approach that by design incorporates these four levers for changing teacher-student interactions and relationships. MTP utilizes a collaborative consultation process and web-based resources to provide ongoing, classroom-focused in-service training across a distance.

MTP is an ongoing, systematic professional development program for teachers, one feature of which centers on a supportive consultation relationship, which is sustained via web-based interactions in which teachers have the opportunity to view video of their own and others' interactions with students, annotated using the CLASS framework in language that is both at the level of specific behaviors and indicators but also connects to the level of dimensions.

These opportunities are provided in the context of a college course (Hamre et al., 2010), a library of annotated video clips that are exemplars of highly rated interaction, and a web-mediated process of ongoing individualized consultation (Pianta, Mashburn, et al., 2008).

The web-based consultation revolves around observation-based reflection, and feedback is enacted through a regular cycle of interactions between a teacher and consultant. Every 2 weeks, teachers videotape their practices in the classroom and share this footage with consultants. Together, they then use the CLASS (Pianta et al., 2007) as a common lens with which to observe and reflect upon aspects of teaching and teacher-child interactions that have known links to children's skill development and start by choosing a dimension of the CLASS that will serve as the basis for consultation and feedback.

MTP consultants provide direct, individualized, regular, and systematic feedback to teachers based on validated, observational assessment of the classroom environment. The MTP consultancy process functions by increasing teachers' knowledge and skills to observe the qualities of their interactions with students and the contingencies involved, and their awareness of the meanings of these interactions in terms of their contributions to motivational, relational, and competence-enhancing processes. The process also encourages reflection on the teachers' own personal motivations and tendencies in these interactions and their impact on interactive behaviors in an effort to internalize change and sustain it.

Recent controlled evaluations of these professional development assets demonstrate several benefits for improving the quality of teachers' interactions with children (Pianta, Belsky, et al., 2008), children's attentiveness and literacy outcomes in pre-K (Mashburn et al., 2008), as well as student reports and observation of engagement in secondary classrooms, and student test scores (Allen et al., 2010). Preliminary evaluations of a course that focuses on teachers' learning of CLASS dimensions and indicators show positive effects on teachers' knowledge and beliefs about teaching and significant effects on their interactive behaviors in the classroom. Opportunities for observing annotated video exemplars of other teachers' effective interactions with students shows positive effects for improvements in teacher-child interactions (assessed by the CLASS) for teachers with low levels of experience, and consultation involving ongoing observation, analysis, and feedback regarding one's own behavior shows clear positive impacts on teacher-child interactions, with particular benefits for teachers in high-need classrooms.

Interestingly, as we further interpret these results, particularly in light of focus group interviews with teachers, we have started to hypothesize that the process of changing teacher-child relationships and interactions involves entering the systems (behavioral, psychological, emotional) that teachers use to self-regulate around their interactions with students. In terms of the psychological processes involved, we find that teachers routinely report the value of the CLASS as a "roadmap" for how to improve their teaching, or that CLASS validates and provides a structure for their own explanations, interpretations, and analysis of their practice. Teachers regularly note that having a common language and lens for their interactions with students that is directly, overtly, and explicitly articulated in a set of professional development resources is of great benefit to them as it grounds those resources in the realities of their practice and experience. Although teachers describe their interactions with reference to the more molar dimensions of the CLASS framework, what is of most use to them is the very detailed and explicit descriptions of interaction at the levels of behavioral indicators and behavioral interactions. Our hypothesis is that this more granular level of analysis meshes well with the psychological and behavioral systems that teachers and students use to calibrate their engagement with one another and with the focus of classroom activities. We plan further tests of this idea in subsequent studies.

Conclusions and Future Directions

Although classrooms are complex social systems and student-teacher relationships and interactions are also complex, multicomponent systems, we posit that the nature and quality of interactions between teachers and children are fundamental to understanding student engagement, can be assessed through standardized observation methods, and can be changed by providing teachers knowledge about developmental processes relevant for classroom interactions and personalized feedback/support about their interactive behaviors and cues.

A theory of classroom settings must be premised on an understanding of the developmental significance of those settings' influence on children and youth and the mechanisms of these effects. Once that knowledge base is established, then theory can move to how those mechanisms (in this case, student-teacher interactions) themselves can be changed. In this chapter, we focused on the theoretical and empirical links between interactions and engagement and presented an approach to intervention designed to increase the quality of such interactions and in turn increase student engagement and, ultimately, learning and development. Recognizing general principles of development in complex systems, a theory of the classroom as a setting for development and a theory of change specific to this social setting are the ultimate goals of this work. Engagement, in this context, is both an outcome in its own right and a mediator of impacts that teachers have on student outcomes through their interactions with children and youth. In light of this discussion, we offer the following suggestions or directions for further research in this area.

First, it is apparent that researchers must distinguish, in their conceptual models and empirical work, the positioning of engagement in the causal chain—as an input to learning, a mediator situated between experience and outcomes, or as an outcome in its own right. Failure to specify this role can easily lead to confusion and misinterpretation. In the context of a focus on interactions and relationships, we have focused on engagement as a mediator and potential outcome. By specifying the role of engagement in a putative causal chain, investigators can then more strategically and systematically confirm or disconfirm hypotheses rather than report assortments of correlations.

Relatedly, a molar, pattern-oriented view of relationships and interactions appears most helpful when using assessments to capture classroom inputs related to engagement. Approaches that are highly focused on occurrences of granular, discrete behaviors captured in isolation or extracted from the ongoing behavioral stream are less likely to yield interpretable or meaningful findings. This does not mean that a focus on specific teacher behaviors is not of use; in fact, in our professional development work, we are highly focused on analysis of teachers' specific behaviors but always in reference to broader dimensions and patterns of interaction. It appears important to us that programs of research conceptualize and assess relationships and interactions in coherent systems that reflect multiple levels of analysis.

Finally, we believe it is critical to subject hypotheses to experimental tests in research on classroom processes. Classrooms are indeed complex, and there is no shortage of description and theoretical narrative available. In too many cases, descriptive studies simply confirm the narrative and theory and do not provide tests that could actually disconfirm hypotheses and helps simplify complexity into actionable models. In a literature focused so heavily on processes—engagement, relationships, and interaction—it might be even more important for research designs to have the capacity to disconfirm hypotheses or speculation. Thus, we posit that advances in both theory and intervention concerning engagement and relational processes can benefit from a dialectical balance in research design—experiments and rich description of processes.

References

Ainsworth, M. D., Blehar, M. C., Waters, E., & Wall, D. (1978). *Patterns of attachment: A psychological study of the strange situation*. Hillsdale, NJ: Erlbaum.

Allen, J. P., & Allen, C. W. (2009). *Escaping the endless adolescence: How we can help our teenagers grow up before they grow old*. New York: Random House.

Allen, J. P., Gregory, A., Mikami, A., Lun, J., Hamre, B. K., & Pianta, R. C. (2010). *Observations of effective secondary school teaching: Predicting student achievement with the CLASS-S*. Manuscript in preparation, University of Virginia, Charlottesville, VA.

Allen, J. P., Philliber, S., Herrling, S., & Kuperminc, G. P. (1997). Preventing teen pregnancy and academic failure: Experimental evaluation of a developmentally based approach. *Child Development, 68*(4), 729–742.

Aratani, L. (2006, July 13). Upper grades, lower reading skills. *The Washington Post*, B1.

Arnold, D. H., McWilliams, L., & Arnold, E. H. (1998). Teacher discipline and child misbehavior in day care: Untangling causality with correlational data. *Developmental Psychology, 34*, 276–287.

Bandura, A., Barbaranelli, C., Caprara, G. V., & Pastorelli, C. (1996). Multifaceted impact of self-efficacy beliefs on academic functioning. *Child Development, 67*(3), 1206–1222.

Barzun, J. (2000). *From dawn to decadence: 500 years of western cultural life 1500 to the present*. London: Harper Collins.

Baumeister, R. F., Twenge, J. M., & Nuss, C. K. (2002). Effects of social exclusion on cognitive processes: Anticipated aloneness reduces intelligent thought. *Journal of Personality and Social Psychology, 83*, 817–827.

Birch, S. H., & Ladd, G. W. (1996). Interpersonal relationships in the school environment and children's early school adjustment: The role of teachers and peers. In K. Wentzel & J. H. Juvonen (Eds.), *Social motivation: Understanding children's school adjustment*. New York: Cambridge University Press.

Birch, S. H., & Ladd, G. W. (1998). Children's interpersonal behaviors and the teacher-child relationship. *Developmental Psychology, 34*, 934–946.

Bloom, B. S., Engelhart, M. D., Furst, E. J., Hill, W. H., & Krathwohl, D. R. (1956). *Taxonomy of educational objectives: The cognitive domain*. New York: Longman.

Bohn, C. M., Roehrig, A. D., & Pressley, M. (2004). The first days of school in the classrooms of two more effective and four less effective primary-grades teachers. *The Elementary School Journal, 104*(4), 269–287.

Bowlby, J. (1969). *Attachment and loss* (Attachment, Vol. 1). New York: Basic Books.

Bowman, B., & Stott, F. (1994). Understanding development in a cultural context: The challenge for teachers. In B. Mallory & R. New (Eds.), *Diversity and developmentally appropriate practices: Challenges for early childhood education* (pp. 19–34). New York: Teachers College Press.

Bransford, J., Brown, A. L., & Cocking, R. R. (Eds.). (1999). *How people learn: Brain, mind, experience, and school*. Washington, DC: National Academy Press.

Bronfenbrenner, U., & Morris, P. A. (1998). The ecology of developmental processes. In W. Damon & R. M. Lerner (Eds.), *Handbook of child psychology* (Theoretical models of human development 5th ed., Vol. 1, pp. 993–1029). New York: Wiley.

Brophy, J. (1986). Teacher influences on student achievement. *American Psychologist, 41*(10), 1069–1077.

Brophy, J., & Evertson, C. (1976). *Learning from teaching: A developmental perspective*. Boston: Allyn & Bacon.

Brophy, J. E., & Good, T. L. (1986). Teacher behavior and student achievement. In M. C. Wittrock (Ed.), *Handbook of research on teaching* (3rd ed., pp. 328–375). New York: Macmillan.

Bruner, J. (1996). *The culture of education*. Cambridge, MA: Harvard University Press.

Bryk, A. S., & Driscoll, M. (1988). *The high school as a community: Contextual influences and consequences for teachers*. Madison, WI: University of Wisconsin, National Center on Effective Secondary Schools.

Bryk, A. S., Lee, V. E., & Holland, P. B. (1993). *Catholic schools and the common good*. Cambridge, MA: Harvard University Press.

Burnett, P. C. (2003). The impact of teacher feedback on student self-talk and self-concept in reaching and mathematics. *Journal of Classroom Interaction, 38*(1), 11–16.

Cameron, C. E., Connor, C. M., & Morrison, F. J. (2005). Effects of variation in teacher organization on classroom functioning. *Journal of School Psychology, 43*(1), 61–85.

Carbonaro, W. J., & Gamoran, A. (2002). The production of achievement inequality in high school English. *American Educational Research Journal, 39*, 801–827.

Carver, S. M., & Klahr, D. (Eds.). (2001). *Cognition and instruction: 25 years of progress*. Mahwah, NJ: Erlbaum.

Catts, H. W., Fey, M. E., Zhang, X., & Tomblin, J. B. (1999). Language basis of reading and reading disabilities: Evidence from a longitudinal investigation. *Scientific Studies of Reading, 3*(4), 331–361.

Coker, H., Medley, D. M., & Soar, R. S. (1980). How valid are expert opinions about effective teaching? *The Phi Delta Kappan, 62*, 131–134.

Collins, W. A., & Repinski, D. J. (1994). Relationships during adolescence: Continuity and change in interpersonal perspective. In R. Montemayor, G. Adams, & T. P. Gullotta (Eds.), *Personal relationships during adolescence* (pp. 7–36). San Francisco: Sage Publications.

Connell, J. P., & Wellborn, J. G. (1991). Competence, autonomy, and relatedness: A motivational analysis of self-system processes. In M. Gunnar & L. A. Sroufe (Eds.), *Self processes in development: Minnesota symposium on child psychology* (Vol. 23, pp. 43–77). Hillsdale, NJ: Erlbaum.

Connor, C. M., Son, S., & Hindman, A. H. (2005). Teacher qualifications, classroom practices, family characteristics, and preschool experience: Complex effects on first graders' vocabulary and early reading outcomes. *Journal of School Psychology, 43*, 343–375.

Crosnoe, R. (2000). Friendships in childhood and adolescence: The life course and new directions. *Social Psychology Quarterly, 63*, 377–391.

Crosnoe, R. (2001). Academic orientation and parental involvement in education during high school. *Sociology of Education, 74*, 210–230.

Crosnoe, R., Johnson, M. K., & Elder, G. H., Jr. (2004). Intergenerational bonding in school: The behavioral and contextual correlates of student-teacher relationships. *Sociology of Education, 77*(1), 60–81.

Csikszentmihalyi, M., & Schneider, B. (2000). *Becoming adult: How teenagers prepare for the world of work.* New York: Basic Books.

Davis, E. A., & Miyake, N. (2004). Explorations of scaffolding in complex classroom systems. *The Journal of the Learning Sciences, 13*(3), 265–272.

de Kruif, R. E. L., McWilliam, R. A., Ridley, S. M., & Wakely, M. B. (2000). Classification of teachers' interaction behaviors in early childhood classrooms. *Early Childhood Research Quarterly, 15*, 247–268.

Dohrn, E., & Bryan, T. (1994). Attributional instruction. *Teaching Exceptional Children, 26*, 61–63.

Donovan, M. S., & Bransford, J. D. (2005). *How students learn: History, mathematics, and science in the classroom.* Washington, DC: National Academies Press.

Dornbusch, S. M., Glasgow, K. L., & Lin, I.-C. (1996). The social structure of schooling. *Annual Review of Psychology, 47*, 401–429.

Eccles, J., Lord, S., & Midgley, C. (1991). What are we doing to early adolescents? The impacts of educational contexts on early adolescents. *American Educational Journal, 99*, 521–542.

Eccles, J. S., Lord, S. E., Roeser, R. W., Barber, B. L., & Jozefowicz, D. M. H. (1997). The association of school transitions in early adolescence with developmental trajectories during high school. In J. Schulenberg, J. L. Maggs, & K. Hurrelmann (Eds.), *Health risks and developmental transitions during adolescence* (pp. 283–321). New York: Cambridge University Press.

Eccles, J. S., Midgley, C., Wigfield, A., Buchanan, C. M., Reuman, D., Flanagan, C., et al. (1993). Development during adolescence: The impact of stage-environment fit on young adolescents' experiences in schools and in families. *American Psychologist, 48*(2), 90–101.

Emmer, E. T., & Stough, L. (2001). Classroom management: A critical part of educational psychology, with implications for teacher education. *Educational Psychologist, 36*(2), 103–112.

Evertson, C., Emmer, E., Sanford, J., & Clements, B. (1983). Improving classroom management: An experiment in elementary classrooms. *The Elementary School Journal, 84*, 173–188.

Evertson, C., & Harris, A. (1999). Support for managing learning-centered classrooms: The Classroom Organization and Management Program. In H. J. Freiberg (Ed.), *Beyond behaviorism: Changing the classroom management paradigm* (pp. 59–74). Boston: Allyn & Bacon.

Fujiki, M., Brinton, B., & Clarke, D. (2002). Emotion regulation in children with specific language impairment. *Language, Speech, and Hearing Services in Schools, 33*, 102–111.

Good, T. L., & Grouws, D. A. (1977). A process-product study in fourth-grade mathematics classrooms. *Journal of Teacher Education, 28*(3), 49–54.

Good, T. L., & Grouws, D. A. (1979). The Missouri mathematics effectiveness project in fourth-grade classrooms. *Journal of Educational Psychology, 71*, 355–362.

Gutman, L. M., & Sulzby, E. (2000). The role of autonomy-support versus control in the emergent writing behaviors of African American kindergarten children. *Reading Research and Instruction, 39*, 170–184.

Hamre, B. K., & Pianta, R. C. (2001). Early teacher-child relationships and the trajectory of children's school outcomes through eighth grade. *Child Development, 72*(2), 625–638.

Hamre, B. K., & Pianta, R. C. (2005). Can instructional and emotional support in the first grade classroom make a difference for children at risk of school failure? *Child Development, 76*(5), 949–967.

Hamre, B. K., & Pianta, R. C. (2007). Learning opportunities in preschool and early elementary classrooms. In R. C. Pianta, M. J. Cox, & K. L. Snow (Eds.), *School readiness and the transition to kindergarten in the era of accountability* (pp. 49–84). Baltimore: Brookes.

Hamre, B. K., Pianta, R. C., Burchinal, M., & Downer, J. T. (2010, March). *A course on supporting early language and literacy development through effective teacher-child interactions: Effects on teacher beliefs, knowledge and practice.* Paper presented at the annual meeting of the Society for Research on Educational Effectiveness, Washington, DC.

Hamre, B. K., Pianta, R. C., Downer, J. T., & Mashburn, A. J. (2005). Teachers' perceptions of conflict with young students: Looking beyond problem behaviors. *Social Development, 17*(1), 115–136.

Hamre, B. K., Pianta, R. C., Mashburn, A. J., & Downer, J. T. (2010). *Building a science of classrooms: Application of the CLASS framework in over 4,000 U.S. early childhood and elementary classrooms.* Manuscript submitted for publication.

Hart, P., Stroot, S., Yinger, R., & Smith, S. (2005). *Meeting the teacher education accountability challenge: A focus on novice and experienced teacher studies.* Mount Vernon, OH: Teacher Quality Partnership.

Harter, S. (1996). Teacher and classmate influences on scholastic motivation, self-esteem, and level of voice in adolescents. In J. Juvonen & K. Wentzel (Eds.), *Social motivation: Understanding children's school adjustment* (pp. 11–42). New York: Cambridge University Press.

Hemphill, L., & Siperstein, G. M. (1990). Conversational competence and peer response to mildly retarded children. *Journal of Educational Psychology, 82*(1), 1–7.

Howes, C. (2000). Socio-emotional classroom climate in child care, child–teacher relationships and children's second grade peer relations. *Social Development, 9*, 191–204.

Howes, C., Burchinal, M., Pianta, R., Bryant, D., Early, D., Clifford, R., & Barbarin, O. (2008). Ready to learn? Children's pre-academic achievement in pre-kindergarten programs. *Early Childhood Research Quarterly, 23,* 27–50.

Howes, C., Hamilton, C. E., & Matheson, C. C. (1994). Children's relationships with peers: Differential associations with aspects of the teacher-child relationship. *Child Development, 65,* 253–263.

Hughes, J. W., Zhang, D., & Hill, C. R. (2006). Peer assessment of normative and individual teacher-student support predict social acceptance and engagement among low-achieving children. *Journal of School Psychology, 43,* 447–463.

Justice, J. M. (2002). Word exposure conditions and preschoolers' novel word learning during shared storybook reading. *Reading Psychology, 23*(2), 87–106.

Justice, L. M., Mashburn, A. J., Hamre, B. K., & Pianta, R. C. (2008). Quality of language and literacy instruction in preschool classrooms serving at-risk pupils. *Early Childhood Research Quarterly, 23,* 51–68.

Justice, L., Meier, J., & Walpole, S. (2005). Learning new words from storybooks: An efficacy study with at-risk kindergartners. *Language, Speech, and Hearing Services in Schools, 36,* 17–32.

Ladd, G. W., Birch, S. H., & Buhs, E. S. (1999). Children's social and scholastic lives in kindergarten: Related spheres of influence? *Child Development, 70,* 1373–1400.

Lynch, M., & Cicchetti, D. (1992). Maltreated children's reports of relatedness to their teachers. In R. C. Pianta (Ed.), *Relationships between children and non-parental adults: New directions in child development* (pp. 81–108). San Francisco: Jossey-Bass.

Magnusson, D., & Stattin, H. (1998). Person-context interaction theory. In W. Damon & R. M. Learner (Eds.), *Handbook of child psychology* (Theoretical models of human development 5th ed., Vol. 1, pp. 685–760). New York: Wiley.

Marks, H. M. (2000). Student engagement in instructional activity: Patterns in the elementary, middle, and high school years. *American Educational Research Journal, 37*(1), 153–184.

Mashburn, A. J., Hamre, B. K., Downer, J. T., & Pianta, R. C. (2007). Teacher and classroom characteristics associated with teachers' ratings of pre-kindergartners' relationships and behavior. *Journal of Pyschoeducational Assessment, 24,* 367–380.

Mashburn, A. J., Pianta, R. C., Hamre, B. K., Downer, J. T., Barbarin, O., Bryant, D., Burchinal, M., Early, D., & Howes, C. (2008). Pre-k program standards and children's development of academic, language, and social skills. *Child Development, 79,* 732–749.

Mayer, R. E. (2002). Rote versus meaningful learning. *Theory into Practice, 41,* 226–233.

McCaslin, M., Burross, H. L., & Good, T. L. (2005, January 2). Change and continuity in student achievement from grades 3 to 5: A policy dilemma. *Education Policy Analysis Archives, 13*(1). Retrieved February 2, 2006, from http://epaa.asu.edu/epaa/v13n1/.

Meehan, B. T., Hughes, J. N., & Cavell, T. A. (2003). Teacher-student relationships as compensatory resources for aggressive children. *Child Development, 74,* 1145–1157.

Mueller, C., & Dweck, C. (1998). Praise for intelligence can undermine children's motivation and performance. *Journal of Personality and Social Psychology, 75*(1), 33–52.

National Center for Education Statistics. (2003). *The condition of education 2003.* Washington, DC: U.S. Department of Education, Institute of Education Sciences.

National Research Council. (2002). *Achieving high educational standards for all.* Washington, DC: National Academy Press.

National Research Council. (2004). *Engaging schools: Fostering high school students' motivation to learn.* Washington, DC: National Academies Press.

NICHD Early Child Care Research Network [ECCRN]. (2002). The relation of global first-grade classroom environment to structural classroom features and teacher and student behaviors. *The Elementary School Journal, 102*(5), 367–387.

NICHD Early Child Care Research Network. (2003). Social functioning in first grade: Prediction from home, child care and concurrent school experience. *Child Development, 74,* 1639–1662.

NICHD Early Child Care Research Network. (2004). Social functioning in first grade: Associations with earlier home and child care predictors and with current classroom experiences. *Child Development, 75,* 1639–1662.

NICHD Early Child Care Research Network. (2005). A day in third grade: A large-scale study of classroom quality and teacher and student behavior. *The Elementary School Journal, 105,* 305–323.

Ninio, A., & Snow, C. E. (1999). The development of pragmatics: Learning to use language appropriately. In W. C. Ritchie & T. K. Bhatia (Eds.), *Handbook of child language acquisition* (pp. 347–383). San Diego, CA: Academic.

Nye, B., Konstantopoulos, S., & Hedges, L. (2004). How large are teacher effects? *Educational Evaluation and Policy Analysis, 26,* 237–257.

Penno, J. F., Wilkinson, A. G., & Moore, D. W. (2002). Vocabulary acquisition from teacher explanation and repeated listening to stories: Do they overcome the Matthew effect? *Journal of Educational Psychology, 94,* 23–33.

Pianta, R. C. (1999). *Enhancing relationships between children and teachers.* Washington, DC: American Psychological Association.

Pianta, R. C., Belsky, J., Houts, R., Morrison, F., & The NICHD Early Child Care Research Network. (2007). Opportunities to learn in America's elementary classrooms. *Science, 315,* 1795–1796.

Pianta, R. C., Belsky, J., Vandergrift, N., Houts, R., Morrison, F., & The NICHD Early Child Care Research Network. (2008). Classroom effects on children's achievement trajectories in elementary school. *American Educational Research Journal, 45*(2), 365–397.

Pianta, R. C., Hamre, B. K., & Mintz, S. L. (2010). *The CLASS-secondary manual*. Unpublished measure, University of Virginia, Charlottesville, VA.

Pianta, R. C., Hamre, B. K., & Stuhlman, M. (2003). Relationships between teachers and children. In W. Reynolds & G. Miller (Eds.), *Comprehensive handbook of psychology* (Educational psychology, Vol. 7, pp. 199–234). Hoboken, NJ: Wiley.

Pianta, R. C., La Paro, K. M., & Hamre, B. K. (2004). *Classroom assessment scoring system [CLASS]*. Unpublished measure, University of Virginia, Charlottesville, VA.

Pianta, R. C., La Paro, K. M., Payne, C., Cox, M., & Bradley, R. (2002). The relation of kindergarten classroom environment to teacher, family, and school characteristics and child outcomes. *The Elementary School Journal, 102*(3), 225–238.

Pianta, R. C., Mashburn, A. J., Downer, J. T., Hamre, B. K., & Justice, L. (2008). Effects of web-mediated professional development resources on teacher-child interactions in pre-kindergarten classrooms. *Early Childhood Research Quarterly, 23*(4), 431–451.

Pianta, R. C., & Nimetz, S. (1991). Relationships between children and teachers: Associations with classroom and home behavior. *Journal of Applied Developmental Psychology, 12*, 379–393.

Pianta, R. C., Steinberg, M. S., & Rollins, K. B. (1995). The first two years of school: Teacher-child relationships and deflections in children's classroom adjustment. *Development and Psychopathology, 7*, 295–312.

Public Agenda. (1997). *Getting by: What American teenagers really think about their schools*. New York: Public Agenda.

Reese, E., & Cox, A. (1999). Quality of adult book-reading style affects children's emergent literacy. *Developmental Psychology, 35*, 20–28.

Resnick, M. D., Bearman, P. S., Blum, R. W., Bauman, K., Harris, K. M., Jones, J., Tabor, J., et al. (1997). Protecting adolescents from harm: Findings from the National Longitudinal Study of Adolescent Health. *Journal of the American Medical Association, 278*, 823–832.

Rimm-Kaufman, S. E., Early, D. M., & Cox, M. J. (2002). Early behavioral attributes and teachers' sensitivity as predictors of competent behavior in the kindergarten classroom. *Journal of Applied Developmental Psychology, 23*(4), 451–470.

Rimm-Kaufman, S. E., La Paro, K. M., Downer, J. T., & Pianta, R. C. (2005). The contribution of classroom setting and quality of instruction to children's behavior in the kindergarten classroom. *The Elementary School Journal, 105*(4), 377–394.

Roeser, R. W., Eccles, J. S., & Sameroff, A. J. (1998). Academic and emotional functioning in early adolescence: Longitudinal relations, patterns, and prediction by experience in middle school. *Development and Psychopathology, 10*(2), 321–352.

Roeser, R. W., Eccles, J. S., & Sameroff, A. J. (2000). School as a context of early adolescents' academic and social-emotional development: A summary of research findings. *The Elementary School Journal, 100*, 443–471.

Rogoff, B. (1990). *Apprenticeship in thinking: Cognitive development in social context*. New York: Oxford University Press.

Romberg, T. A., Carpenter, T. P., & Dremock, F. (2005). *Understanding mathematics and science matters*. Mahwah, NJ: Lawrence Erlbaum Associates.

Ryan, R. M., & Deci, E. L. (2000). Self-determination theory and the facilitation of intrinsic motivation, social development, and well-being. *American Psychologist, 55*(1), 68–78.

Ryan, R. M., Stiller, J. D., & Lynch, J. H. (1994). Representations of relationships to teachers, parents, and friends as predictors of academic motivation and self-esteem. *Journal of Early Adolescence, 14*(2), 226–249.

Sarason, S. B. (1982). *The culture of the school and the problem of change* (2nd ed.). Boston: Allyn & Bacon.

Schuele, C. M., Rice, M. L., & Wilcox, K. A. (1995). Redirects: A strategy to increase peer interactions. *Journal of Speech and Hearing Research, 28*, 1319–1333.

Shouse, R. C. (1996). Academic press and sense of community: Conflict, congruence, and implications for student achievement. *Social Psychology of Education, 1*(1), 47–68.

Silver, R. B., Measelle, J., Essex, M., & Armstrong, J. M. (2005). Trajectories of externalizing behavior problems in the classroom: Contributions of child characteristics, family characteristics, and the teacher-child relationship during the school transition. *Journal of School Psychology, 43*, 39–60.

Skibbe, L., Behnke, M., & Justice, L. M. (2004). Parental scaffolding of children's phonological awareness skills: Interactions between mothers and their preschoolers with language difficulties. *Communication Disorders Quarterly, 25*(4), 189–203.

Skinner, E. A., & Belmont, M. J. (1993). Motivation in the classroom: Reciprocal effects of teacher behavior and student engagement across the school year. *Journal of Educational Psychology, 85*, 571–581.

Skinner, E. A., Zimmer-Gembeck, M. J., & Connell, J. P. (1998). Individual differences and the development of perceived control. *Monographs of the Society for Research in Child Development, 63*(2–3).

Soar, R., & Soar, R. (1979). Emotional climate and management. In P. Peterson & H. Walberg (Eds.), *Research on teaching: Concepts, findings, and implications* (pp. 97–119). Berkeley, CA: McCutchan.

Sroufe, L. A. (1996). *Emotional development: The organization of emotional life in the early years*. Cambridge, UK: Cambridge University Press.

Stallings, J. (1975). Implementation and child effects of teaching practices in follow through classrooms. *Monographs of the Society for Research in Child Development, 40*(7–8), Serial No. 163.

Steinberg, L., Brown, B. B., & Dornbusch, S. M. (1996). *Beyond the classroom: Why school reform has failed and what parents need to do*. New York: Simon and Schuster.

Taylor, B. M., Pearson, P. D., Peterson, D. S., & Rodriguez, M. C. (2003). Reading growth in high-poverty classrooms: The influence of teacher practices that encourage cognitive engagement in literacy learning. *The Elementary School Journal, 104*, 3–28.

Twenge, J. M., Catanese, K. R., & Baumeister, R. F. (2002). Social exclusion causes self-defeating behavior. *Journal of Personality and Social Psychology, 83*(3), 606–615.

Valeski, T., & Stipek, D. (2001). Young children's feelings about school. *Child Development, 72*, 1198–1213.

van Ijzendoorn, M. H., Sagi, A., & Lambermon, M. W. E. (1992). The multiple caretaker paradox: Data from Holland and Israel. In R. C. Pianta (Ed.), *Beyond the parent: The role of other adults in children's live* (New directions for child development, Vol. 57, pp. 5–24). San Francisco: Jossey-Bass.

Veenman, M. V. J., Kok, R., & Blöte, A. W. (2005). The relation between intellectual and metacognitive skills in early adolescence. *Instructional Science, 33*(3), 193–211.

Vygotsky, L. S. (1978). *Mind and society: The development of higher mental processes*. Cambridge, MA: Harvard University Press.

Vygotsky, L. S. (1991). Genesis of the higher mental functions. In P. Light, S. Sheldon, & M. Woodhead (Eds.), *Learning to think* (pp. 32–41). Florence, KY: Taylor & Frances/Routledge.

Wentzel, K. (1998). Social relationships and motivation in middle school: The role of parents, teachers, and peers. *Journal of Educational Psychology, 90*(2), 202–209.

Wharton-McDonald, R., Pressley, M., & Hampston, J. M. (1998). Literacy instruction in nine first-grade classrooms: Teacher characteristics and student achievement. *The Elementary School Journal, 99*(2), 101–128.

Whitehurst, G. J., Falco, F. L., Lonigan, C. J., Fischel, J. E., DeBaryshe, B. D., Valdez-Menchaca, M. C., & Caulfield, M. (1988). Accelerating language development through picture book reading. *Developmental Psychology, 24*, 552–559.

Williams, W. M., Blythe, T., & White, N. (2002). Practical intelligence for school: Developing metacognitive sources of achievement in adolescence. *Developmental Review, 22*(2), 162–210.

Zevenbergen, A. A., Whitehurst, G. J., & Zevenbergen, J. A. (2003). Effects of a shared-reading intervention on the inclusion of evaluative devices in narratives of children from low-income families. *Journal of Applied Developmental Psychology, 24*, 1–15.

The Role of Peer Relationships in Student Academic and Extracurricular Engagement

Jaana Juvonen, Guadalupe Espinoza, and Casey Knifsend

Abstract

Friends and other peer relationships can motivate students to engage in school work as well as in extracurricular activities. To understand when and how peers matter, research on the positive and negative engagement "effects" of friends, peer support, and socially marginalizing experiences, such as peer rejection and bullying, is reviewed. The chapter starts with a brief summary of research demonstrating the links between school belonging and academic engagement and extracurricular involvement. The ways in which selection of friends and the influence of friends, quality of friendships, and type of friendship support (academic or emotional) are related to academic engagement and extracurricular involvement in school are then discussed. Studies examining whether the number of friends or the size of peer network is related to school engagement are also included. The chapter ends with a discussion about future research needs in relation to the role of peer relationships and student engagement, and implications for school policies (e.g., academic tracking, grade retention, and extracurricular practices).

Peers are a major part of schooling. Given the amount of time students spend with their classmates and friends in school, they are likely to be influenced by them. Moreover, when students have friends and feel socially connected and supported at school, one would expect these factors to predispose them to feel positively toward academic work and other school activities. The assumptions guiding this review are first, that friends and other peer relationships can motivate students to engage in school work as well as in extracurricular activities. However, we recognize that some peers and social experiences in school can also discourage engagement. To be able to understand when and how peers matter, we review research on the positive and negative "effects" of friendships and peer support, and

J. Juvonen, Ph.D.(✉)
Department of Psychology, University of California,
Los Angeles, CA, USA
e-mail: j_juvonen@yahoo.com

G. Espinoza, M.A. • C. Knifsend, M.A.
Department of Psychology, University of California,
Los Angeles, CA, USA
e-mail: g.espinoza@ucla.edu; cknifsend@ucla.edu

Peer relationships → Sense of belonging → Student engagement

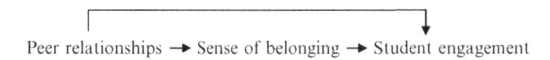

Fig. 18.1 Conceptual framework guiding this review

socially marginalizing experiences, such as peer rejection and bullying, on student engagement. Our second guiding assumption is that positive relationships with schoolmates facilitate a sense of belonging to school. We presume that both peer relationships and belonging to school are related to student engagement, with peer relationships contributing to both the sense of belonging and student engagement, as indicated in Fig. 18.1.

In our review, terms referring to school belonging (i.e., sense of connection) and peer relationships are used broadly. For example, we use "belongingness" and "connectedness" interchangeably. The term "peer relationships" is used as a superordinate construct to refer to close friendships (i.e., relationships characterized by mutual liking) as well as to peer group affiliations (i.e., less tight relationships united by common interests and activities).

We also use a broad definition of student engagement, focusing primarily on observable indicators, such as attendance and classroom participation. Although we primarily focus on engagement behaviors as a means to achieve good grades, we also refer to findings regarding academic performance as an indication of student engagement. School-based extracurricular involvement in sports, arts, and other activities is included in this review for two reasons. First, by assessing engagement in both academic and non-academic activities, we are able to determine whether peer relationships operate in similar ways across these two domains. Second, although extracurricular participation mostly involves nonacademic activities, such involvement is related to student engagement in academic activities, including school attendance (e.g., Mahoney, 2000). Thus, we review how peer relationships affect and are affected by extracurricular involvement in ways that can facilitate academic engagement.

We start the chapter with a brief summary of research demonstrating the links between school belonging and academic engagement and extracurricular involvement. We then proceed to review the ways in which selection of friends and the influence of friends is related to students' school engagement. Quality of friendships and type of friendship support (academic or emotional) are discussed. Studies examining the relationships between number of friends and the size of peer networks and student engagement are also reviewed. Research on students who are rejected or bullied by their peers shows, in turn, the ways in which negative social experiences may alienate students from school and possibly increase the chances of their dropping out. The chapter ends with a discussion about future research needs in relation to the role of peer relationships and student engagement, and implications from the work already done on this topic for school policies (e.g., academic tracking, grade retention, and extracurricular practices).

School Belonging

Research on school belonging is based on the assumption that environments characterized by caring and supportive relationships facilitate student engagement (e.g., Brand, Felner, Shim, Seitsinger, & Dumas, 2003; Felner & Felner, 1989; Goodenow & Grady, 1993; Voelkl, 1997). Consequently, motivation and achievement are presumed to be undermined when students feel unsupported and disconnected from others (e.g., Becker & Luthar, 2002; Finn, 1989, 1993). A particularly strong association between peer acceptance and school belonging (Adelabu, 2007) suggests that school-based relationships are critical. Although both relationships with teachers and peers are likely to matter (Furrer & Skinner, 2003), the need to "fit in" with one's peers is especially pronounced during adolescence (LaFontana & Cillessen, 2010). Hence, it is not surprising that much of the existing research on school belonging has focused on middle and high school students. Yet, school belonging matters as early as elementary school.

Does School Belonging Promote Academic Engagement?

Capitalizing on a large sample of over 4,000 students across 24 elementary schools, Battistich, Solomon, Kim, Watson, and Schaps (1995) investigated the association between students' sense of school community (e.g., perceptions of caring and supportive school-based relationships) and a range of measures tapping attitudes, motivation, and achievement. Using hierarchical linear modeling techniques that allow examination of students nested within schools, the findings revealed that a greater sense of school community was associated with higher levels of class enjoyment, lower levels of work avoidance, and higher mathematics scores. Generally, stronger associations were documented in schools serving the most economically disadvantaged families, suggesting that school belonging might be particularly important for students from educationally and financially disadvantaged homes.

In one of the earliest studies on school belonging in middle school, Goodenow and Grady (1993) demonstrated that a strong sense of school belonging was associated with increased academic engagement among an ethnically diverse sample of students. Based on self-report measures, a positive association between school belonging, the importance of schoolwork, and persistence with schoolwork was observed. Sampling middle schools serving predominantly White youth from working class families, Roeser, Midgley, and Urdan (1996), in turn, showed that school belonging was associated with higher levels of academic performance. The association was robust inasmuch as other relevant motivational constructs (e.g., goal structures fostered by the school, personal achievement goal orientations) were taken into account in the analyses.

The link between school belonging and student engagement has been studied most extensively among high school students. Focusing on a predominantly Latino sample of urban high school seniors, Sánchez, Colón, and Esparza (2005) documented that school belonging was associated with more frequent classroom participation, homework completion, exam preparation, and better school attendance. Consistent with these findings, analyses of the National Longitudinal Study of Adolescent Health (Add Health) of 20,000 ethnically diverse students from 132 secondary schools showed that higher levels of school belonging were associated with fewer school absences (Anderman, 2002). A large-scale longitudinal study of Australian secondary school students, in turn, demonstrated that low school connectedness decreased the likelihood of students finishing school (Bond et al., 2007).

In sum, these findings suggest that students' school belonging, which we presume to be integrally linked with school-based peer relationships (although student school belonging also encompasses relationships with adults in the school) (e.g., Hamm & Faircloth, 2005), is an important factor associated with engagement in academic work especially in secondary school. However, we are not in the position to conclude that school belonging causes students to engage. The association between school belonging and engagement may operate in both directions, possibly in a mutually reinforcing manner. That is, the more engaged students are, the stronger their sense of belonging; and the more strongly they feel they belong, the more actively they engage academically. In the next section, we turn to extracurricular engagement to review research on sense of belonging and participation in voluntary activities in school.

Is Extracurricular Participation a Way to Strengthen School Belonging?

A handful of survey and qualitative studies have examined the association between school belonging and students' engagement in extracurricular activities. Students with a stronger sense of school belonging are more likely to engage in activities, such as after-school sports or extracurricular academic programs. Sampling an ethnically diverse group of seventh through twelfth grade students, Brown and Evans (2002) showed that extracurricular activity participation was significantly associated with greater school connection, which was measured with school belonging as one of its main dimensions. Although the authors only tested a direct path from extracurricular activities to school connection, they posited that participation in extracurricular activities facilitates positive school-related experiences, which in turn, facilitate school belonging and commitment to school. In a study using daily phone interviews of African-American students in sixth to ninth grade, Dotterer, McHale, and Crouter (2007) found that the more time students spent on extracurricular activities, the more strongly they bonded with school. Such a positive association may, however, merely indicate that youth who are school-oriented and who feel that they belong and fit in at school spend time in school with peers sharing similar interests.

Research utilizing mixed methods provides some insights into whether extracurricular involvement in fact affects school belonging or whether those who feel they belong are more likely to participate in activities provided by school. Barnett (2006) surveyed female high school students before, and interviewed them after, they received notification of whether they had been selected to the cheer or dance team following competitive tryouts. In the initial surveys, all applicants reported liking school and wanting to be at school, which is partly tapping into the sense of school belonging. The girls who made the team maintained their high levels of school liking, whereas school liking significantly decreased among the unsuccessful aspirants not only the day after the decision was made, but also 2 months after the decision. When interviewed, one of the nonselected girls explained that one of the main reasons why she wanted to be on the dance team was "to find a way to be connected with my school." Thus, individuals may have different reasons to pursue extracurricular activities.

Research shows positive links between school belonging and academic engagement, such as classroom participation and school attendance, and involvement in extracurricular activities. Although the rest of our review is based on the premise that positive peer relationships are important in facilitating a sense of school belonging, it becomes evident that not all peer relationships are related with increased levels of engagement.

Peer Selection and Socialization

Children tend to have relationships and affiliate with similar others (Hallinan, 1983). That is, students engaged in classwork form friendships with engaged classmates, whereas students who are not so engaged are friends with similarly disengaged peers. Given the similarities between friends, it is not surprising that friendships amplify students' school-related behaviors (Dishion, Spracklen, Andrews, & Patterson, 1996; Mounts & Steinberg, 1995). In other words, engaged students get more involved in academic work, whereas disengaged students become alienated from school-related activities. Whether these peer "effects" are due to selection of friends, or their influence – or both – is less clear (Kandel, 1996).

Characteristics of Friends and the Relation with Academic Engagement

Perhaps the best evidence for peer influence on academic engagement comes from studies on peer networks (Cairns, Cairns, & Neckerman, 1989; Kindermann, 1993; Kindermann, McCollam, & Gibson, 1996). Kindermann et al. (1996) found that when students were members of groups with high average academic engagement, their own individual academic engagement improved over time. The opposite effect was obtained for members of groups with low academic engagement profiles. In spite of relatively high turnover of specific members across the school year, the groups' engagement "profiles," or overall orientation toward school work, remained stable. This finding highlights that students select peer groups, and groups accept members based on similarities.

Besides academic orientation, a wide range of characteristics of friends is related to academic engagement. A survey study of almost 1,000 adolescents examined how a set of academic, social, and mental health attributes of friends was related to students' academic engagement and performance from seventh to eighth grade

(Cook, Deng, & Morgano, 2007). Cook and colleagues discovered that students with all-around adjusted friends spent more time doing homework and in extracurricular activities, and were absent less frequently, than were students with friends who obtained lower grades and engaged in drug use or other misbehaviors. Students with all-around adjusted friends also improved their grade point average from seventh to eighth grade. Thus, friends' academic behaviors and socioemotional well-being were each related to student engagement in academic work and extracurricular activities.

The studies described above relied on independent assessments of friends' behaviors and other attributes (i.e., friends were identified and they provided self-reports). Methodologically less strong research relies on subjective perceptions of friends' behaviors or values, perceptions which may be biased by the student's own values and behavior. However, the same patterns are evident. In cross-sectional studies, student perceptions of their friends' behaviors and values are consistently related to students' own engagement and conduct. For example, in a survey study of seventh and ninth grade students, Nelson and DeBacker (2008) showed that perceptions of one's best friend having high academic values (e.g., "My best friend believes that school is more important than most people think") were related to self-reports of a greater desire for mastery of school work (e.g., "I do the work in this class because I like to understand what I am learning").

Perceptions of friends' behavior also predict changes in engagement over time. Berndt and Keefe (1995) found that seventh and eighth graders became more involved in classroom activities over the course of the school year, as indicated by self-reports, when they perceived that their three closest friends were highly involved in classroom activities at the beginning of the school year. Conversely, students who perceived their friends to disrupt class in the beginning of the year become more disruptive themselves across the year. With a sample of about 2,500 students, Simons-Morton and Chen (2009) showed that students who perceived a higher proportion of their five closest friends engaging in negative behaviors (e.g., being disrespectful of teachers) reported making less effort in class and lower motivation to do well in school over the course of sixth to ninth grade. These findings are particularly troublesome because decreases in academic engagement levels appear to be a precursor of dropping out of school (Janosz, Archambault, Morizot, & Pagani, 2008), indicating that friends may indirectly influence school dropout (a topic that we will return to later in the chapter).

Extracurricular Engagement: Are Friends a Reason to Get and Stay Involved?

Consistent with findings regarding academic engagement, students with friends who are highly involved in extracurricular activities are more likely to participate in activities themselves. An interview study with highly involved high school students explored the factors that motivate students to become involved and maintain their involvement in extracurricular activities (Fredricks et al., 2002). Students discussed their friends' involvement in the activities as a reason to continue their own participation. The role of friends seems to be especially important in encouraging continued involvement, potentially even when individual interest in the activity itself has waned.

Beyond the influence of existing friendships, Fredricks et al. (2002) found that high school students were motivated to join extracurricular activities in order to acquire new friendships. Moreover, through extracurricular participation, students are likely to be exposed to peers they may not normally associate with over the course of the school day. Dworkin, Larson, and Hansen (2003) used focus group methodology to examine the ways in which extracurricular involvement is related to friendships among high school students. Students specifically commented on the opportunities that extracurricular activities provided to socialize with peers outside of their typical friendship groups, including students of different racial backgrounds. This research suggests that extracurricular activities can play an important role in helping students form new relationships with peers with whom they might otherwise not interact.

In sum, friends' behaviors and engagement are related to student academic and extracurricular engagement. Although the mechanisms of peer influence and selection are not necessarily investigated in most studies, research suggests that students with more academically engaged friends perform better academically than those whose friends are disengaged. Similarly, those with friends involved in extracurricular activities are more likely to start and stay engaged in the activity. Thus, friends seem to amplify students' initial level of involvement. What is not clear from these studies is whether the quality of friendships and the type of peer support might matter also in terms of student engagement.

Quality of Friendships and Type of Peer Support

High-quality friendships typically involve positive features such as support, companionship, and commitment, as well as low levels of conflict (Berndt, 2002). A number of studies have shown direct effects of high-quality friendships on student engagement behaviors. For example, Berndt and Keefe (1995) examined the importance of friendship quality in addition to friends' school-related behaviors (class involvement and disruptiveness) in a study of seventh and eighth graders. The perceived quality of the friendship predicted changes in self-reported behaviors across the school year. Students with a supportive, intimate, and validating closest friend became more involved in class across the school year. In contrast, students whose closest friendship involved frequent conflict and rivalry or competition increased in disruptive behavior during the school year. These results highlight that it is not only the behaviors of friends, but also the relationship qualities of friendships, that matter.

The quality of friendships also matters because stable, supportive relationships with classmates encourage student engagement through consistent reinforcement. In the same investigation described above, Berndt and Keefe (1995) discovered that students who retained stable friendships over the course of the academic year reported less disruptive behavior, were rated by their teachers as involved in class, and also received higher grades than peers with unstable friendships. Because stable friendships with specific qualities might encourage student engagement, it is also possible that students with good grades select friends with whom they can study together. In a longitudinal survey study of seventh through ninth grade students examined at two time points, an earlier high grade point average indeed correlated with subsequent social support obtained from friends (DuBois, Felner, Brand, Adan, & Evans, 1992). Thus, the association between supportive friends and academic engagement is likely to work both ways.

The *type* of peer support received might also matter. That is, while academic support might be particularly critical in allowing students to work together on homework or projects, emotional or social support might be especially critical at times of heightened distress. In concurrent and short-term longitudinal analyses (i.e., start and end of kindergarten), Ladd, Kochenderfer, and Coleman (1996) found that when young elementary school students considered their friends as sources of aid and validation, they were particularly likely to develop positive attitudes toward school as the year progressed.

Wentzel (1994) examined whether social support, defined as peers' concerns about an individual's emotions (e.g., "My classmates care about my feelings"), and academic support, defined as peers' concern for an individual's learning (e.g., "My classmates care about how much I learn"), were related to students' pursuit of socially valued outcomes in middle school. The results revealed that sixth and seventh grade students' perceptions of both social and academic support were associated with willingness to follow classroom rules. Peers' academic support was additionally related to what Wentzel described as students' academic social responsibility goals, such as the desire to comply with teacher requests.

Most importantly, perceived academic support from peers is related to active class participation.

Focusing on seventh grade students, Murdock (1999) demonstrated that students who reported high levels of academic support from peers were rated by their teachers as attending classes, participating in class, and completing assignments more frequently than those who did not feel academically supported by their peers. Perceived academic support from peers was also related to lower rates of discipline problems (e.g., detention, in-school suspension).

While relatively little is known about the relation between extracurricular involvement and peer support, it is possible that at least some types of extracurricular activities foster skills that allow students to be more supportive of one another. In a focus group study of high school students who took part in extracurricular and community-based activities, students reported that their involvement in the activities helped them develop a stronger sense of empathy and ability to handle stress and anxiety (Dworkin et al., 2003). This may mean that the effects of extracurricular activities on academic engagement are indirect. Personal skills and competencies to understand and support peers in distress gained in the context of extracurricular activities may help students to provide academic support.

In sum, the research available suggests that the quality of student friendships and peer support are each related to academic engagement. Students with stable, nonconflictive friendships are likely to engage in academic tasks. While close friends can encourage student engagement, students are also likely to seek friends who can help them with academic work. Although friends are in the position to provide various types of support, not surprisingly, academic support is consistently related to academic engagement. Extracurricular involvement, in turn, may aid the ability to support others.

Does the Number of Friends and Ability to Make Friends Matter?

As shown above, school-based friendships often serve as sources of instrumental and social support. Does this mean then that students with larger friendship networks are more engaged in school? Focusing on initial school entry and the year of kindergarten, Ladd (1990) found that children with multiple existing friendships during school entrance developed more favorable school attitudes during the first 2 months of kindergarten. Those maintaining these friendships also liked school more over time. These findings are particularly robust because students' preschool experience, mental age, and gender were taken into account in the analyses. Ladd (1990) also found that children who formed new friendships during kindergarten performed better academically (as measured by teacher reports and student performance on school readiness and achievement tests) than children who did not establish friendships. New friendships accounted for a significant proportion of the variance in academic performance even when controlling for existing friendships.

In a study of students transitioning from fifth to sixth grade, Kingery and Erdley (2007) relied on both student self-reports and peer nominations to examine the role of schoolmates as students acclimate to their new middle school. Correlation analysis showed that greater peer acceptance and number of friends prior to the transition to middle school was related to greater involvement (e.g., participating in class and other school activities) at the start of the sixth grade. Hence, having more friends even before the transition seems to help students when transitioning to a new school. However, larger friendship networks may simply reflect the social skills of students. That is, the most socially skillful students (who are likely to have lots of friends) may have the easiest time navigating in a new environment, and therefore they remain highly engaged.

Although a greater number of friends might help, having one friend may be sufficient to help adjust to a new school environment. The power of one friend is highlighted in research on school transitions, when students frequently experience a disruption in peer networks and loss of friends (Kenny, 1987). Linking early middle school friendships with school outcomes in a longitudinal survey study over the course of middle school, Wentzel, Barry, and Caldwell (2004) found that students with no friends in the first year of middle school were initially more distressed and received lower grades in their school record than students with at least one friend. Although a lack of friends may have caused distress which interfered with achievement, it is also possible that stress caused by low grades from elementary school made it hard for students to make friends. Nevertheless, this study demonstrates that an absence of even just one friend is related with compromised academic performance.

Research on extracurricular activities also suggests that one friend may be sufficient to get students engaged in nonacademic activities. Huebner and Mancini (2003) showed that high school students with just one friend whom they could "count on" were more likely to report that they participated in after-school extracurricular activities (e.g., sports, clubs), regardless of whether that friend participated in that activity or not. Thus, it is possible that a close friendship provides enough support and confidence for students to explore and become involved in school, much like secure attachment to a caregiver is related to exploration early in life.

While one good friendship may be enough to get students more engaged in school, friends are not the only way to improve academic outcomes. Wentzel et al. (2004) also found that the students with no friends in the first year of middle school did improve their academic performance over the course of middle school, despite initially having lower grades in sixth grade than those with friendships. It is possible that friendless students obtain support for academic engagement from other sources (e.g., adults at school, parents).

In sum, the existing research shows that lack of close friendships is associated with lower student engagement (especially at times of school transitions), while the ability to develop and maintain friendships is related with academic engagement. Although a larger number of friends might increase the probability of receiving positive support for academic performance, the size of the peer network may simply reflect social skills that are particularly helpful to students during school transitions. Yet, having just one friend is enough to help students become involved in both academic and extracurricular activities. One study also suggests that academic progress is possible without friends. But what happens when a student is rejected or bullied in school? We now turn to research on negative social experiences with peers.

Negative Social Experiences: Rejected and Bullied Students

Given the literature covered thus far, it appears that having high-quality, supportive friendships can promote school engagement behaviors possibly because such relationships facilitate school belonging. Conversely, students who are friendless are less engaged, perhaps because they feel they do not belong in school. In this section, we go beyond the lack of friends to examine how negative peer experiences (rejection and bullying) are related to academic disengagement, and potentially to alienation from school.

Peer rejection is commonly defined as peers' social avoidance of, dislike of, or reluctance to affiliate with a student. Therefore, rejection by classmates may threaten school belonging even more than lack of friends, inasmuch as rejection affects group membership at the classroom level (Furman & Robbins, 1985). Indeed, peer rejection is associated with avoidance of school, less positive perceptions about school, and lower academic performance in kindergarten (Ladd, 1990), as well as lower grades in the first and second grade (O'Neil, Welsh, Parke, Wang, & Strand, 1997). In secondary school, peer rejection is associated with increased absenteeism and truancy (DeRosier, Kupersmidt, & Patterson, 1994; Kupersmidt & Coie, 1990) as well as subsequent grade retention (Coie, Lochman, Terry, & Hyman, 1992).

Even temporary rejection is associated with negative academic outcomes. Examining peer rejection across time among elementary school students, Greenman, Schneider and Tomada (2009) showed that students rejected at even just one time point performed worse academically than children who had never been rejected. Moreover, Buhs, Ladd, and Herald (2006) demonstrated that students who were excluded and victimized in elementary school became increasingly less engaged over time. Thus, negative experiences with schoolmates can also be associated with lasting disengagement.

Given that aggressive students are at high risk for being rejected by classmates at least in elementary school (Asher & Coie, 1990), it is important to understand whether peer rejection independently contributes to subsequent problems or whether it functions merely as a marker of problem behaviors (Parker & Asher, 1987). Following a large sample of African-American children from elementary school to middle school, Coie et al. (1992) demonstrated that childhood peer rejection contributed to behavior problems 3 years later, over and above earlier levels of aggression. Subsequent analyses of data from the same sample revealed that the combination of childhood aggression and peer rejection significantly increased the risk of committing assaults by the second year in high school (Coie, Terry, Lenox, & Lochman, 1995). Because aggression is associated with school disengagement, independent of rejection (e.g., Lessard et al., 2008; Schwartz, Gorman, Nakamoto, & Toblin, 2005), it is therefore likely that rejection amplifies the risk for subsequent school disengagement.

In the studies described above, peer rejection is assessed via peer nominations by asking students to name classmates they do not like to sit next to or spend time with. But self-reports also show associations between feeling rejected by peers and student, disengagement. Buhs (2005) found that fifth grade students who reported that they were excluded by their peers, were less likely to participate in class. In a cross-sectional study of sixth and seventh graders, Lopez and DuBois (2005) showed that students who felt disapproved of by their peers had lower grade point averages and were absent from school on more days than students who felt accepted. The authors suggested that both perceived rejection and the low self-esteem associated with such perceptions make it difficult for students to concentrate on schoolwork and engage in productive, collaborative work with peers.

Consistent with the findings of research on rejected students, victims of bullying in elementary school are less likely to feel that they belong in school and are more likely to disengage. Kochenderfer and Ladd (1996) showed that bullied kindergartners displayed increased loneliness and school avoidance by the end of the school year. Examining the association between bullying experiences and teacher-rated academic engagement as well as grade point average in middle school, Juvonen, Wang, and Espinoza (2011) discovered that bullied students were less engaged and obtained lower academic grades across 3 years of middle school. Although the study did not test the directionality of the associations (i.e., whether bullying experiences preceded disengagement or vice versa), the robust association between bullying experiences (regardless of being based on self-reports or peer nominations) and the academic indicators among an ethnically diverse sample of about 1,500 students suggest that bullying cannot be ignored when trying to improve academic engagement and performance.

Nishina, Juvonen, and Witkow (2005) reported evidence for both direct and mediated effects of bullying on middle school functioning. Among close to 2,000 students of diverse ethnic backgrounds, bullying experiences at the start of the sixth grade were linked with subsequent psychological maladjustment as well as health complaints, which were related to end-of-the-year absences and grades. At the same time, symptoms of psychological distress at the start of the sixth grade also increased the chances of students being bullied by the end of the year, which was associated with higher absences and lower grades. Hence, negative peer experiences and distress are interrelated in a cyclical manner (see also Egan & Perry, 1998) and therefore especially likely to compromise academic engagement (see also Juvonen, Nishina, & Graham, 2000).

Bullying research suggests that emotional distress associated with hostile peer interactions contributes also to negative school attitudes and a desire to withdraw from or avoid school. The mere prospect of potential rejection may discourage academic success, at least among older students. Ishiyama and Chabassol (1985) surveyed seventh to twelfth graders about their concerns of the social implications of high academic achievement (e.g., peer rejection and/or criticism, pressure to continue success). Seventh to ninth grade students (particularly girls) expressed more concern about the social repercussions of performing well than older participants. Hence, students' concern about rejection may temper their classroom participation. Given that earlier academic performance sets the stage for subsequent performance, it is particularly troublesome if young teens downplay their academic success and engagement.

In sum, both peer rejection and bullying experiences are associated with lower levels of academic engagement and academic performance. It is likely that negative social experiences cause students to disengage. However, it is also possible that low-performing students are bullied and rejected by their classmates. In the latter case, the odds against these students accumulate. Their distress and concerns about being ridiculed or excluded can propel students into avoiding school altogether. Thus, the associations are likely to be cyclical. Moreover, even mere concerns about rejection are related to decreased academic engagement in middle and high school. Although additional longitudinal research on this topic is warranted, there is important evidence illustrating that a sense of social alienation precedes an ultimate form of disengagement, namely dropping out of school, as summarized below.

Social Alienation and Dropping Out

When interviewed about reasons for dropping out, one out of four youth reported that they did not belong at school (U.S. Department of Education, Center for Education Statistics, 1993). Finn (1989, 1993) proposed that the relationship between students not participating in school and dropping out is explained by a lack of sense of belonging and identification with school. Consistent with this idea, an early study (Dillon & Grout, 1976) reported that students become alienated from school when they feel they are denied meaningful participation in both classroom and other school activities.

Extracurricular involvement may serve as a meaningful activity, and thereby protect youth from dropping out of school. Focusing on Mexican-American and White non-Hispanic high school–aged students who were either in good academic standing or had dropped out of school, Davalos, Chavez, and Guardiola (1999) found that students who had been involved in any extracurricular activity were more than twice as likely to be enrolled in school. In a prospective longitudinal study, Mahoney and Cairns (1997) demonstrated that students who participated in extracurricular activities in middle or high school were less likely to drop out of school. This effect was particularly strong for those considered at high risk of dropping out who participated in extracurricular activities early in high school (Mahoney & Cairns, 1997). In a subsequent study, Mahoney (2000) showed that participation in extracurricular activities before 11th grade decreased the chance of leaving school early or engaging in criminal behavior as an adult among students considered at high risk. Moreover, the likelihood of dropping out was reduced further when the students' friends also participated in school extracurricular activities. These findings suggest that opportunities to engage in school-related activities together with peers are critical, especially for youth who might otherwise be at risk of leaving school prematurely (Hymel, Comfort, Schonert-Reichl, & McDougall, 1996).

Consistent with the importance of the sense of school belonging, Kaplan, Peck, and Kaplan (1997) showed that in addition to low grades and lack of motivation, social alienation from school-based peer networks and relationships with deviant schoolmates during eighth and ninth grade independently contributed to the risk of dropping out. Also, students who were held back during middle school were seven times more likely to drop out of school than their peers with similar academic performance who were not held back (Alexander, Entwisle, & Kabbani, 2001). The authors concluded that this independent effect of grade retention partly reflects a lack of social integration. Hence, feeling that one does not socially fit in or belong is an important risk factor for dropping out.

In sum, socially alienated youth who feel that they do not fit in and are not engaged in school are at risk of dropping out of school. Although both grade retention and behavior problems may in part alienate youth from their peers as well as their teachers, negative peer experiences may also increase sense of alienation. In addition to not retaining students, encouraging socially vulnerable youth to participate in extracurricular activities might help keep these students engaged in the schooling process.

Conclusion

One of the main reasons given by high school students for attending school is that they get to see their friends (Brown & Theobald, 1998). Students select to affiliate with certain types of peers, and the way they feel about fitting in with their schoolmates is associated with their level of engagement in school. We now briefly summarize some of the positive and negative effects of peers, as well as point out questions that need to be further examined.

Summary of Positive Peer "Effects"

Relationships with friends who are academically engaged in school are associated with higher academic motivation and achievement. Friends' overall social adjustment (e.g., lack of behavior problems) is also associated with academic engagement and involvement in extracurricular activities. Although having a greater number of friends may help students get engaged in school, having just one friend helps alleviate the stress related with transitioning to a new school. Friends are typically good sources of emotional and social support; however, it is academic support that is most clearly associated with increased achievement motivation and classroom participation. Extracurricular activities, in turn, provide students with opportunities to form new friendships, just as those with friends are more likely to explore new extracurricular options and stay involved. Based on the research reviewed, we conclude that friendships and peer affiliations with engaged classmates generally facilitate a sense of belonging in school that in turn promotes engagement, as suggested by the pathway depicted in the beginning of the chapter.

Summary of Negative Peer "Effects"

Not all friendships are beneficial, however. Not only do critical qualities (e.g., supportiveness, validation) of friendships vary, but also the level of support and collaboration on school assignments varies depending on the abilities and aspirations of friends (e.g., Berndt, 1989, 2002). Students who have disengaged friends are unlikely to excel academically. Additionally, negative social experiences with classmates may make rejected youth seek the company of other students who misbehave and encourage bullied students to avoid school. Feelings of social alienation from the institution and repeated absences, in turn, increase the risk of dropping out of school. Thus, particular types of friendships, lack of any friendships, as well as bullying and rejection experiences are all related to school disengagement.

Are Peers Necessary to Maintain School Engagement?

Although many students are motivated to attend school to spend time with their friends, it should be clear from the research reviewed that peers are not always essential for student engagement and achievement. There is evidence suggesting that parent support and teacher support may be more important than peer support for student engagement (Chen, 2005; Garcia-Reid, 2007; Wentzel, 1998). When and if these other sources of support can compensate for the support that friends provide in relation to engagement in academic work is a critical question to further investigate. This issue may be best studied with students who lack friendships. It would be equally important to know whether other sources of support, besides support from peers, can alleviate the distress associated with negative social experiences (such as bullying).

The studies reviewed in this chapter also convey that not all peer relationships promote academic engagement. Clearly, there are peer groups of disengaged students whose effects are more harmful than productive. Also, while a lack of friends might be a sign of social isolation or alienation, there are students with no friends in school who do well. For some, it may be to their benefit not to form close ties with classmates who are not engaged. Moreover, youth can form valuable peer relationships outside of school. That is, neighborhood friends or friends from out-of-school activities may compensate for the lack of close ties in school. These are questions that remain to be investigated.

Implications for Future Research and School Policies

A few key longitudinal studies suggest that both selection of friends and their influence play a part in whether students engage in class or get involved in extracurricular activities. It is therefore important to consider the opportunities that schools provide for students to seek and find friends who are in the position to provide support. This is particularly critical when considering how certain educational policies and practices may restrict students' opportunities to establish and maintain positive peer relationships. Based on the current review, it seems that academic tracking is particularly problematic. In low-track classrooms that often have an overrepresentation of disengaged students, youth lack opportunities to form positive peer relationships supporting academic involvement. Similar problems can arise in classrooms that segregate students with disabilities. That is, the range of potential friends is limited.

For extracurricular activities, in turn, selection procedures are problematic. Exclusion based on tryouts can disengage and alienate students from school. When nonselected students are the ones who need most support, an opportunity to make them feel part of the school is lost. Therefore, schools should consider offering meaningful alternative activities for students who are not among the top performers within their extracurricular activities.

The benefits of having at least one friend through the transition to a new school are consistent across studies of kindergartners to middle school students. Similarly, research on bullying suggests that one friend is enough to both decrease the risk of getting bullied as well as to buffer the emotional distress associated with peer harassment (Hodges, Boivin, Vitaro, & Bukowski, 1999; Hodges, Malone, & Perry, 1997). Whether one friend or *any* friend is enough in other stressful situations as well is less clear. It is therefore important to examine the potential power of one friend when youth experience academic difficulties or when they get cut from a team. Equally important is research examining the ways in which some extracurricular involvement (e.g., team sports) might help students provide support to one another. Unless group work and other cooperative methods are used in classrooms, certain extracurricular activities may be one of the only ways to learn support giving.

Because the bodies of research on academic and extracurricular activities are largely separate, it is valuable to compare the two domains of engagement. It is interesting not only to note differences in assumptions and research traditions for each but also to learn about the generalizability of the findings across the two domains. For example, it appears that rejection by peers and exclusion from a sports team may have similarly alienating effects that are related to disengagement. Whether course selections, much like extracurricular choices, might be influenced in part by whether friends or high-status (i.e., popular) peers are involved in the class is also needed. Particularly intriguing is the idea that extracurricular activities or peer relations fostered by those activities might help academic engagement.

References

Adelabu, D. H. (2007). Time perspective and school membership as correlates to academic achievement among African American adolescents. *Adolescence, 42*, 525–538.

Alexander, K. L., Entwisle, D. R., & Kabbani, N. (2001). The dropout process in life course perspective: Early risk factors at home and school. *Teachers College Record, 103*, 760–822.

Anderman, E. M. (2002). School effects on psychological outcomes during adolescence. *Journal of Educational Psychology, 94*, 795–809.

Asher, S. R., & Coie, J. D. (1990). *Peer rejection in childhood* (Cambridge studies in social and emotional development). New York: Cambridge University Press.

Barnett, L. A. (2006). Flying high or crashing down: Girls' accounts of trying out for cheerleading and dance. *Journal of Adolescent Research, 21*, 514–541.

Battistich, V., Solomon, D., Kim, D., Watson, M., & Schaps, E. (1995). Schools as communities, poverty levels of student populations, and students' attitudes, motives and performance: A multilevel analysis. *American Educational Research Journal, 32*, 627–658.

Becker, B. E., & Luthar, S. S. (2002). Social-emotional factors affecting achievement outcomes among disadvantaged students: Closing the achievement gap. *Educational Psychologist, 37*(4), 197–214.

Berndt, T. J. (1989). Obtaining support from friends during childhood and adolescence. In D. Belle (Ed.), *Children's social networks and social supports* (pp. 308–331). Oxford, UK: Wiley.

Berndt, T. J. (2002). Friendship quality and social development. *Current Directions in Psychological Science, 11*, 7–10.

Berndt, T. J., & Keefe, K. (1995). Friends' influence on adolescents' adjustment to school. *Child Development, 66*, 1312–1329.

Bond, L., Butler, H., Thomas, L., Carlin, J., Glover, S., Bowes, G., & Patton, G. (2007). Social and school connectedness in early secondary school as predictors of late teenage substance use, mental health and academic outcomes. *Journal of Adolescent Health, 40*, 357.e9–357.e18.

Brand, S., Felner, R., Shim, M., Seitsinger, A., & Dumas, T. (2003). Middle school improvement and reform: Development and validation of a school-level assessment of climate, cultural pluralism, and school safety. *Journal of Educational Psychology, 95*(3), 570–588.

Brown, R., & Evans, W. P. (2002). Extracurricular activity and ethnicity: Creating greater school connection among diverse student populations. *Urban Education, 37*, 41–58.

Brown, B. B., & Theobald, W. (1998). Learning contexts beyond the classroom: Extracurricular activities, community organizations, and peer groups. In K. Borman & B. Schneider (Eds.), *The adolescent years: Social influences and educational challenges* (The 97th yearbook of the National Society for the Study of Education. Part I, pp. 109–141). Chicago: National Society for the Study of Education.

Buhs, E. S. (2005). Peer rejection, negative peer treatment, and school adjustment: Self-concept and classroom engagement as mediating processes. *Journal of School Psychology, 43*, 407–424.

Buhs, E. S., Ladd, G. W., & Herald, S. L. (2006). Peer exclusion and victimization: Processes that mediate the relation between peer group rejection and children's classroom engagement and achievement? *Journal of Educational Psychology, 98*, 1–13.

Cairns, R. B., Cairns, B. D., & Neckerman, H. J. (1989). Early school dropout: Configurations and determinants. *Child Development, 60*, 1437–1452.

Chen, J. J. (2005). Relation of academic support from parents, teaches, and peers to Hong Kong adolescents' academic achievement: The mediating role of academic engagement. *Genetic, Social, and General Psychology Monographs, 131*(2), 77–127.

Coie, J. D., Lochman, J., Terry, R., & Hyman, C. (1992). Predicting early adolescent disorder from childhood aggression and peer rejection. *Journal of Consulting and Clinical Psychology, 60*, 783–792.

Coie, J. D., Terry, R., Lenox, K., & Lochman, J. (1995). Childhood peer rejection and aggression as predictors of stable patterns of adolescent disorder. *Development and Psychopathology, 7*, 697–713.

Cook, T. D., Deng, Y., & Morgano, E. (2007). Friendship influences during early adolescence: The special role of friends' grade point average. *Journal of Research on Adolescence, 17*, 325–356.

Davalos, D. B., Chavez, E. L., & Guardiola, R. J. (1999). The effects of extracurricular activity, ethnic identification, and perception of school on student dropout rates. *Hispanic Journal of Behavioral Sciences, 21*, 61–77.

DeRosier, M. E., Kupersmidt, J. B., & Patterson, C. P. (1994). Children's academic and behavioral adjustment as a function of the chronicity and proximity of peer rejection. *Child Development, 65*, 1799–1813.

Dillon, S. V., & Grout, J. A. (1976). Schools and alienation. *The Elementary School Journal, 76*, 481–489.

Dishion, T. J., Spracklen, K. M., Andrews, D. W., & Patterson, G. R. (1996). Deviancy training in male adolescent friendships. *Behavior Therapy, 27*, 373–390.

Dotterer, A. M., McHale, S. M., & Crouter, A. C. (2007). Implications of out-of-school activities for school engagement in African American adolescents. *Journal of Youth and Adolescence, 36*, 391–401.

DuBois, D. L., Felner, R. D., Brand, S., Adan, A. M., & Evans, E. G. (1992). A prospective study of life stress, social support, and adaptation in early adolescence. *Child Development, 63*, 542–557.

Dworkin, J. B., Larson, R., & Hansen, D. (2003). Adolescents' accounts of growth experiences in youth activities. *Journal of Youth and Adolescence, 32*, 17–26.

Egan, S. K., & Perry, D. G. (1998). Does low self-regard invite peer victimization? *Developmental Psychology, 34*, 299–309.

Felner, R. D., & Felner, T. Y. (1989). Primary prevention programs in the educational context: A transactional-ecological framework and analysis. In L. A. Bond & B. E. Compas (Eds.), *Primary prevention and promotion in the schools* (pp. 13–49). Thousand Oaks, CA: Sage.

Finn, J. D. (1989). Withdrawing from school. *Review of Educational Research, 59*, 117–142.

Finn, J. D. (1993). *School engagement and students at risk* (National Center for Education Statistics Research and Development Reports). Washington, DC: U.S. Department of Education, National Center for Education Statistics.

Fredricks, J. A., Alfeld-Liro, C. J., Hruda, L. Z., Eccles, J. S., Patrick, H., & Ryan, A. M. (2002). A qualitative exploration of adolescents' commitment to athletics and the arts. *Journal of Adolescent Research, 17*, 68–97.

Furman, W., & Robbins, P. (1985). What's the point?: Selection of treatment objectives. In B. Schneider, K. H. Rubin, & J. E. Ledingham (Eds.), *Children's peer relations: Issues in assessment and intervention* (pp. 41–54). New York: Springer.

Furrer, C., & Skinner, E. (2003). Sense of relatedness as a factor in children's academic engagement and performance. *Journal of Educational Psychology, 95*, 148–163.

Garcia-Reid, P. (2007). Examining social capital as a mechanism for improving school engagement among low income Hispanic girls. *Youth and Society, 39*(2), 164–181.

Goodenow, C., & Grady, K. E. (1993). The relationship of school belonging and friends' values to academic motivation among urban adolescent students. *The Journal of Experimental Education, 62*, 60–71.

Greenman, P. S., Schneider, B. H., & Tomada, G. (2009). Stability and change in patterns of peer rejection: Implications for children's academic performance over time. *School Psychology International, 30*, 163–183.

Hallinan, M. R. (1983). Commentary: New directions for research on peer influence. In J. L. Epstein & N. Karweit (Eds.), *Friends in school: Patterns of selection and influence in secondary schools* (pp. 219–231). New York: Academic.

Hamm, J. V., & Faircloth, B. S. (2005). The role of friendship in adolescents' sense of school belonging. *New Directions for Child and Adolescent Development, 107*, 61–78.

Hodges, E. V. E., Boivin, M., Vitaro, F., & Bukowski, W. M. (1999). The power of friendship: Protection against an escalating cycle of peer victimization. *Developmental Psychology, 25*, 94–101.

Hodges, E. V. E., Malone, M. J., & Perry, D. G. (1997). Individual risk and social risk as interacting determinants of victimization in the peer group. *Developmental Psychology, 33*, 1032–1039.

Huebner, A. J., & Mancini, J. A. (2003). Shaping structured out-of-school time use among youth: The effects of self, family, and friend systems. *Journal of Youth and Adolescence, 32*, 453–463.

Hymel, S., Comfort, C., Schonert-Reichl, K., & McDougall, P. (1996). Academic failure and school dropout: The influence of peers. In K. Wentzel & J. Juvonen (Eds.), *Social motivation: Understanding children's school adjustment* (pp. 313–345). New York: Cambridge University Press.

Ishiyama, F. I., & Chabassol, D. J. (1985). Adolescents' fear of social consequences of academic success as a function of age and sex. *Journal of Youth and Adolescence, 14*, 37–46.

Janosz, M., Archambault, I., Morizot, J., & Pagani, L. S. (2008). School engagement trajectories and their differential predictive relations to dropout. *Journal of Social Issues, 64*, 21–40.

Juvonen, J., Nishina, A., & Graham, S. (2000). Peer harassment, psychological adjustment, and school functioning in early adolescence. *Journal of Educational Psychology, 92*, 349–359.

Juvonen, J., Wang, Y., & Espinoza, G. (2011). Bullying experiences and compromised academic performance across middle school grade. *Journal of Early Adolescence, 31*, 152–173.

Kandel, D. B. (1996). The parental and peer contexts of adolescent deviance: An algebra of interpersonal influences. *Journal of Drug Issues, 26*, 289–315.

Kaplan, D. S., Peck, B. M., & Kaplan, H. B. (1997). Decomposing the academic failure-dropout relationship: A longitudinal analysis. *The Journal of Educational Research, 90*, 331–343.

Kenny, M. (1987). Family ties and leaving home for college: Recent findings and implications. *Journal of College Student Personnel, 28*, 438–442.

Kindermann, T. A. (1993). Natural peer groups as contexts for individual development: The case of children's motivation in school. *Developmental Psychology, 29*, 970–977.

Kindermann, T. A., McCollam, T., & Gibson, E. (1996). Peer networks and student's classroom engagement during childhood and adolescence. In J. Juvonen & K. Wentzel (Eds.), *Social motivation: Understanding children's school adjustment* (pp. 279–312). Cambridge, UK: Cambridge University Press.

Kingery, J. N., & Erdley, C. A. (2007). Peer experiences as predictors of adjustment across the middle school transition. *Education and Treatment of Children, 30*, 73–88.

Kochenderfer, B. J., & Ladd, G. W. (1996). Peer victimization: Cause or consequence of school maladjustment? *Child Development, 67*, 1305–1317.

Kupersmidt, J. B., & Coie, J. D. (1990). Preadolescent peer status, aggression, and school adjustment as predictors of externalizing problems in adolescence. *Child Development, 61*, 1350–1362.

Ladd, G. W. (1990). Having friends, keeping friends, and being liked by peers in the classroom: Predictors of children's early school adjustment? *Child Development, 61*, 1081–1100.

Ladd, G. W., Kochenderfer, B. J., & Coleman, C. C. (1996). Friendship quality as a predictor of young children's early school adjustment. *Child Development, 67*(1103), 1118.

LaFontana, K. M., & Cillessen, A. H. N. (2010). Developmental changes in the priority of perceived status in childhood and adolescence. *Social Development, 19*(1), 130–147.

Lessard, A., Butler-Kisber, L., Fortin, L., Marcotte, D., Potvin, P., & Royer, E. (2008). Shades of disengagement: High school dropouts speak out. *Social Psychology of Education, 11*(1), 25–42.

Lopez, C., & DuBois, D. L. (2005). Peer victimization and rejection: Investigation of an integrative model of effects on emotional, behavioral, and academic adjustment in early adolescence. *Journal of Clinical Child and Adolescent Psychology, 34*, 25–36.

Mahoney, J. L. (2000). School extracurricular activity participation as a moderator in the development of antisocial patterns. *Child Development, 71*, 502–516.

Mahoney, J. L., & Cairns, R. B. (1997). Do extracurricular activities protect against early school dropout? *Developmental Psychology, 33*, 241–253.

Mounts, N. S., & Steinberg, L. (1995). An ecological analysis of peer influence on adolescent grade point average and drug use. *Developmental Psychology, 31*, 915–922.

Murdock, T. B. (1999). The social context of risk: Status and motivational predictors of alienation in middle school. *Journal of Educational Psychology, 91*, 62–75.

Nelson, R. M., & DeBacker, T. K. (2008). Achievement motivation in adolescents: The role of peer climate and best friends. *The Journal of Experimental Education, 76*, 170–189.

Nishina, A., Juvonen, J., & Witkow, M. R. (2005). Sticks and stones may break my bones, but names will make me feel sick: The psychosocial, somatic and scholastic consequences of peer harassment. *Journal of Clinical Child and Adolescent Psychology, 34*, 37–48.

O'Neil, R., Welsh, M., Parke, R. D., Wang, S., & Strand, C. (1997). A longitudinal assessment of the academic correlates of early peer acceptance and rejection. *Journal of Clinical Child Psychology, 26*, 290–303.

Parker, J. G., & Asher, S. R. (1987). Peer relations and later personal adjustment: Are low-accepted children at risk? *Psychological Bulletin, 102*, 357–389.

Roeser, R. W., Midgley, C., & Urdan, T. C. (1996). Perceptions of the school psychological environment and early adolescents' psychological and behavioral functioning in school: The mediating role of goals and belonging. *Journal of Educational Psychology, 88*, 408–422.

Sánchez, B., Colón, Y., & Esparza, P. (2005). The role of sense of school belonging and gender in the academic adjustment of Latino adolescents. *Journal of Youth and Adolescence, 34*, 619–628.

Schwartz, D., Gorman, A. H., Nakamoto, J., & Toblin, R. L. (2005). Victimization in the peer group and children's academic functioning. *Journal of Educational Psychology, 97*, 425–435.

Simons-Morton, B., & Chen, R. (2009). Peer and parent influences on school engagement among early adolescents. *Youth and Society, 41*, 3–25.

U.S. Department of Education. (1993). *Dropout Rates in the United States*: 1992 (NCES 93–901). Washington, DC: National Center for Education Statistics.

Voelkl, K. E. (1997). Identification with school. *American Journal of Education, 105*, 294–318.

Wentzel, K. R. (1994). Relations of social goal pursuit to social acceptance, classroom behavior and perceived social support. *Journal of Educational Psychology, 86*, 173–182.

Wentzel, K. R. (1998). Social relationships and motivation in middle school: The role of parents teachers and peers. *Journal of Educational Psychology, 90*, 202–209.

Wentzel, K. R., Barry, C. M., & Caldwell, K. A. (2004). Friendships in middle school: Influences on motivation and school adjustment. *Journal of Educational Psychology, 96*, 195–203.

Understanding Student Engagement with a Contextual Model*

Shui-fong Lam, Bernard P.H. Wong, Hongfei Yang, and Yi Liu

Abstract

In the present study, student engagement was conceptualized as a meta-construct with affective, behavioral, and cognitive dimensions. As the indicators in each of the three dimensions were unpacked from facilitators and outcomes, we were able to investigate how student engagement was associated with its antecedents and outcomes in a sample of Chinese junior secondary school students ($N=822$). The results supported a contextual model for understanding student engagement. They revealed that students were engaged in school when they felt that their teachers adopted motivating instructional practices and they had social-emotional support from their teachers, parents, and peers. Their engagement was high when they had high self-efficacy, endorsed learning goals, and effort attribution. Most importantly, when students were engaged in schools, they experienced positive emotions frequently and their teachers rated them high on academic performance and conduct. The findings have implications for interventions for the enhancement of student engagement in school.

In recent years, the concept of student engagement has attracted much attention from educators and researchers (Fredricks, Blumenfeld, & Paris, 2004). Many studies have indicated that student engagement has both short-term and long-term impacts on students. In the short term, it is predictive of students' learning, grades, and conduct in school (Connell, Spencer, & Aber, 1994; Hill & Werner, 2006; Marks, 2000; Skinner & Belmont, 1993; Voelkl, 1997). Over the long term, it is linked to a variety of life outcomes, such as academic achievement, self-esteem, and socially appropriate behaviors (Finn & Rock, 1997; Hawkins, Gou, Hill, Battin-Pearson, & Abbott, 2001; Maddox & Prinz, 2003). It is considered

---

*The study reported in this chapter is part of an international research project initiated by the International School Psychology Association (Lam et al., 2009).

S.-f. Lam, Ph.D. (✉) • B.P.H. Wong, Ph.D.
Department of Psychology, University of Hong Kong, Pokfulam, Hong Kong
e-mail: lamsf@hku.hk

H. Yang, Ph.D.
Department of Psychology and Behavioral Sciences, University of Zhejiang, Hangzhou, Zhejiang, China

Y. Liu, M.A.
Urban Community and Mental Health Education Office, Yunnan Health Education Institute, Kunming, Yunnan, China

as a protective factor against school dropout, substance abuse, delinquency, and antisocial behaviors (Appleton, Christenson, & Furlong, 2008; Chung, Hill, Hawkins, Gilchrist, & Nagin, 2002; O'Farrell & Morrison, 2003). Given the abundant evidence that student engagement is related not only to an adaptive orientation toward school but also to a wide range of developmental and adjustment outcomes, no wonder it has emerged in recent decades as an important concept in the field of education.

Conceptualization and Measurement of Student Engagement

While there is a consensus about the importance of student engagement and the necessity to investigate how to enhance it, there is little consensus about its conceptualization and measurement. Most researchers agree that it is a metaconstruct encompassing multiple dimensions of involvement in school or commitment in learning (Appleton et al., 2008; Fredricks et al., 2004; Jimerson, Campos, & Greif, 2003). However, the number and nature of dimensions within this metaconstruct remain confusing and require clarification. Some researchers use a three-part typology and conceptualize it as comprising affective, behavioral, and cognitive dimensions (Fredricks et al., 2004; Jimerson et al., 2003; Lam et al., 2009), whereas some researchers use a four-part typology, adding an academic dimension to this metaconstruct (Appleton, Christenson, Kim, & Reschly, 2006). Some researchers include antecedents of student engagement, such as teacher support and peer relationships, in the measurement of student engagement (e.g., Appleton et al., 2006), whereas others include outcomes, such as grades and discipline, in the measurement (e.g., Archambault, Janosz, Fallu, & Pagani, 2009).

The fusion of several dimensions under the idea of student engagement is valuable because it may provide a richer characterization of students than is possible in research on a single dimension (Fredricks et al., 2004). However, to capitalize on the merits of this metaconstruct, clarification must be made regarding the number and nature of its dimensions. Otherwise, a comprehensive but elusive metaconstruct may cause more confusion than understanding. Three concerns regarding the conceptualization and measurement of this metaconstruct need to be addressed. The first relates to the distinction between indicators versus facilitators of student engagement. Indicators refer to the features that define student engagement, while facilitators are contextual factors that influence student engagement (Sinclair, Christenson, Lehr, & Anderson, 2003; Skinner, Furrer, Marchand, & Kindermann, 2008). Indicators are the characteristics that belong inside the construct of student engagement proper, e.g., students' effort and enthusiasm in school work. By contrast, facilitators are the causal factors outside the construct, e.g., teacher support that contributes to student engagement. We agree with Skinner et al. (2008) that a clear demarcation between these two is needed. If facilitators are defined as part of student engagement itself, researchers cannot explore how contextual factors, such as teacher support, influence student engagement. Therefore, facilitators should not be included in the conceptualization and measurement of student engagement.

The second concern relates to the distinction between indicators versus outcomes of student engagement. This concern is parallel with the first one. Similarly, outcomes such as grades, discipline, and number of credits the student has accrued should not be defined as part of student engagement itself. Otherwise, researchers cannot explore the consequences of student engagement. Therefore, there is also a need for a clear demarcation between indicators and outcomes of student engagement. Outcomes should not be included in the conceptualization and measurement of student engagement.

The third concern relates to the uniqueness and redundancy of the dimensions in student engagement. Although the dimensions in this metaconstruct are not isolated processes and should be interrelated dynamically within individual students, their features should not be overlapping with one another across the dimensions. Otherwise, the justification for the proposed dimensions is in question. For example, in a four-part typology (Appleton et al., 2006), the amount of time spent on schoolwork and the amount of homework completed are considered as academic engagement. However, involvement in academic activities and on-task behavior can also be considered as behavioral engagement (Skinner & Belmont, 1993). The overlapping between the academic and behavior engagement may result in redundancy and confusion. Parsimony is important in the development of theoretical models (Gauch, 2003). There is a need to streamline the dimensions in the metaconstruct of student engagement and to avoid redundancy.

To address the above concerns, we have adopted a three-part typology and conceptualized student engagement as a metaconstruct that comprises affective, behavioral, and cognitive dimensions. They are the most critical dimensions of student involvement in school (Fredricks et al., 2004; Jimerson et al., 2003). Affective engagement refers to students' feelings about learning (Connell & Wellborn, 1991; Skinner & Belmont, 1993) and the school they attend (Finn, 1989; Voelkl, 1997). The feelings about learning activities are reflections of intrinsic motivation, while the feelings about the school are a manifestation of school bonding. Students with high affective engagement enjoy learning and love going to school. Behavioral engagement refers to student participation in learning (Birch & Ladd, 1997; Skinner & Belmont, 1993) and extracurricular activities in school (Finn, Pannozzo, & Voelkl, 1995). Students with high behavioral engagement are diligent in learning activities and active in extracurricular activities. Cognitive engagement refers to the amount and types of cognitive strategies that students employ (Walker, Greene, & Mansell, 2006). Students may employ deep or shallow processing strategies. Deep processing is associated with cognitive elaboration of the to-be-learned material, whereas shallow processing involves rote memorization, basic rehearsal, and other types of superficial engagement with the new material. Students who engage in deep cognitive processing have better understanding and retention of meaningful learning materials.

In this three-part typology, the three dimensions of student engagement have clear and distinctive features that do not overlap with one another. The components in each of the dimensions are actually well-established constructs in the literature. They have been addressed by robust bodies of work separately. For example, enjoyment in learning, a component of affective engagement, is intrinsic motivation, the eagerness that comes from the pleasure in learning itself. This component is a well-researched construct in the field of motivation (Ryan & Deci, 2000). To build a metaconstruct on well-defined and well-researched constructs enables researchers to tap into their existing body of knowledge and examine their additive and interactive effects simultaneously and dynamically. Compared to the research that focuses on only one construct, the study of student engagement as metaconstruct provides a new and comprehensive perspective.

In this three-part typology of student engagement, indicators are conceptually unpacked from facilitators and outcomes. The clear demarcation among the three enables researchers to examine the consequences of student engagement in both the short and the long run. Most importantly, it also enables researchers to examine how and what contextual factors contribute to the development of student engagement. As Furlong and Christenson (2008) pointed out, student engagement is "a state of being that is highly influenced by contextual factors – home, school, and peers – in relation to the capacity of each to provide consistent support for student learning" (p. 366). It is not a nonmalleable trait of the student. The conceptualization of student engagement as a state instead of a trait is very important because it makes intervention possible and legitimate. If student engagement is a nonmalleable trait, there is no point to do any intervention. By contrast, if student engagement is influenced highly by contextual factors, intervention with these factors will bring changes to student engagement.

Contextual Factors

Given the important impact of student engagement on the wide range of developmental and adjustment outcomes, researchers and educators need to know how and what contextual factors can enhance it. The contextual factors of student engagement are best conceptualized from the

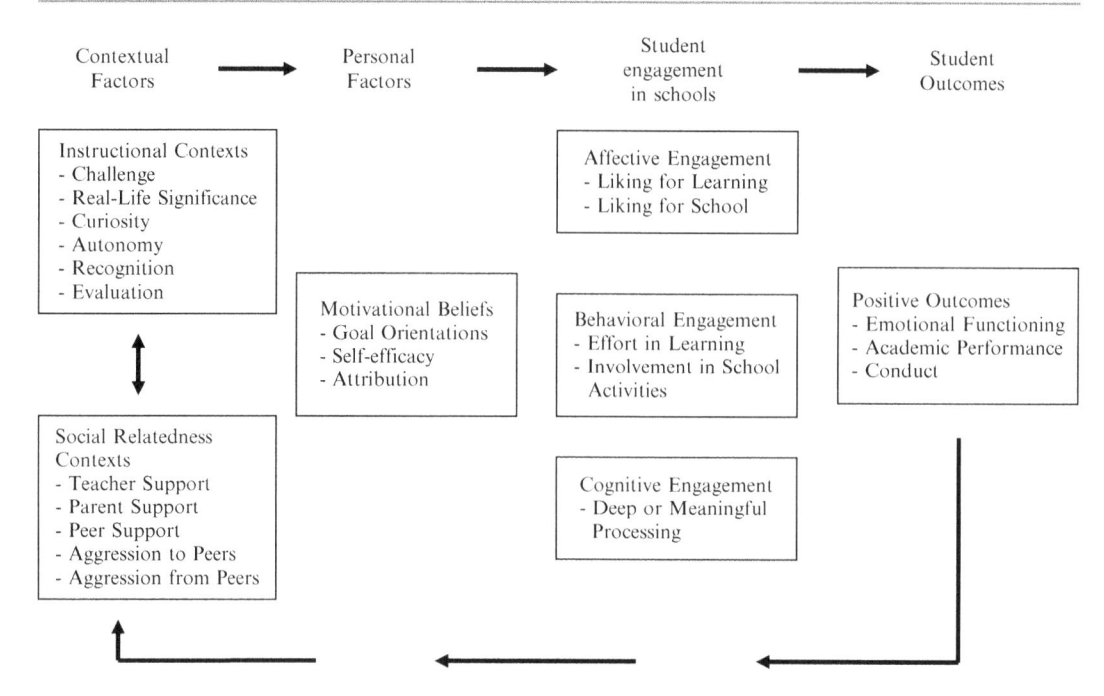

Fig. 19.1 A contextual model for student engagement

ecological system theory (Bronfenbrenner, 1986). According to this theory, human development occurs in a nested arrangement of systems, each contained within the next. The most immediate systems in which a human organism develops are the microsystems (e.g., school, family, workplace). The dynamics and relationships in these microsystems have a significant impact on human development. To learn about how student engagement develops in an intricate web of mutually influencing contexts, it is important to explore its antecedents in the school and family.

Figure 19.1 presents a contextual model of the antecedents and outcomes of student engagement. In the school, at least two sets of contextual factors are likely to influence students' personal motivational beliefs and their engagement in school. The first set pertains to instructional contexts, and the second pertains to social-relatedness contexts. How teachers teach in classrooms has tremendous impact on student motivation (Perry, Turner, & Meyer, 2006). On the basis of social-cognitive theories and empirical research findings in motivation and instructional strategies, Lam, Pak, and Ma (2007) have identified six important components of motivating instructional contexts: (1) challenge, (2) real-life significance, (3) curiosity, (4) autonomy, (5) recognition, and (6) evaluation. The more the students reported that their teachers assigned challenging work, integrated real-life significance to learning tasks, aroused their curiosity, supported their autonomy, recognized their effort or improvement, and used formative evaluation, the stronger was the intrinsic motivation they reported in learning.

Social-relatedness factors can also affect student engagement. Children who report a higher sense of relatedness with teachers and peers show greater affective and behavioral engagement (Connell & Wellborn, 1991; Eccles et al., 1993; Furrer & Skinner, 2003; Gest, Welsh, & Domitrovich, 2005; Murray & Greenberg, 2000; Wentzel, 1998). Research on school bullying and victimization has also revealed that children with larger circles of friends, higher levels of peer acceptance, and lower levels of peer victimization tend to like school more (Ladd, Kochenderfer, & Coleman, 1997). Students' enthusiasm, interest, happiness, and comfort in school, then, seem to be shaped by their sense of relatedness to others.

By contrast, feelings of boredom, frustration, sadness, and anxiety in the school are exacerbated when children feel alienated from others.

Other than social relatedness in school, social relatedness at home is also influential to student engagement in school. Family is one of the most immediate microsystems for human development. Parent support is expected to play an important role in student engagement in school. It is well documented that parenting styles (e.g., Donrbush, Ritter, Leiderman, Roberts, & Fraleigh, 1987) and parental involvement (e.g., Hoover-Dempsey & Sandler, 1995) contribute to children's academic performance in school. Students will be engaged in school when they perceive that their parents have high expectation on them and provide them with encouragement and assistance.

Personal Factors

Some personal factors may have direct impact on student engagement. They may mediate the effect of contextual factors on student engagement. It is well documented that some motivational beliefs are essential to students' intrinsic interest and may be important proximal determinants of student engagement (see Schunk & Zimmerman, 2006 for a review). These beliefs include goal orientations (Dweck, 2006), attribution (Weiner, 1985), and self-efficacy (Bandura, 1977). Students with learning goals are more persistent after failure than students with performance goals (Lam, Yim, Law, & Cheung, 2004). They focus on gaining new skills and knowledge even if failures occur during the process. On the contrary, students with performance goals focus on gaining positive evaluation of their ability. They tend to avoid challenges when they are not sure that they can gain positive feedback from others. Goal orientations affect not only students' persistence and effort in learning but also their cognitive engagement (Elliot, McGregor, & Gable, 1999; Graham & Golan, 1991; Meece, Blumenfeld, & Hoyle, 1988; Nolen, 1988). Learning goals are positive predictors of deep processing, whereas performance goals are positive predictors of surface processing.

Attribution can also be an important antecedent of student engagement. Weiner (1985) postulated that differences in effort expenditure by students can be explained by differences in how they explain their successes and failures. When students attribute success and failure to effort, they are more likely to invest effort in future tasks. Another potential determinant of students' effort expenditure is self-efficacy (Bandura, 1977). Students with high self-efficacy believe that they are capable of successfully performing the course of action that will lead to success. They attempt challenging tasks and do not give up easily. It is reasonable to expect that students with high self-efficacy tend to be engaged in school.

Overview of the Study

The study reported in this chapter is a part of a multicountry project initiated by the International School Psychology Association (Lam et al., 2009). Twelve countries (Austria, Canada, China, Cyprus, Estonia, Greece, Korea, Malta, Portugal, Romania, United Kingdom, and United States) participated in this project with the purpose of investigating both the personal and contextual antecedents of student engagement in schools across different countries. This was a large-scale international project that involved many themes of investigation. In this chapter, the focus is on the validation of the contextual model presented in Fig. 19.1. With the data from China, we examined how student engagement was associated with contextual factors, personal factors, and student outcomes. It is noteworthy that the relations among these constructs may be bidirectional. Better student outcomes may reinforce student engagement, which in turn may have positive impact on personal and contextual factors. Reciprocal relationships between contextual factors and student engagement were found in previous research (Skinner & Belmont, 1993).

Method

Participants

The participants were 822 junior secondary school students from three cities in China, namely, Hangzhou, Hong Kong, and Kunming. The three cities are located in different regions of the country and are considered as big cities in their regions. The population of these three cities ranged from 6.25 million to 7 million. The sample consisted of 280 seventh graders, 236 eighth graders, and 306 ninth graders from the three cities. About 34% of the students came from Hangzhou, 29% from Hong Kong, and 37% from Kunming. Parental consent was obtained in Hong Kong and approval was sought from local education authorities in Hangzhou and Kunming. All the students gave assent to the participation. Their mean age was 14.14, with a range of 12–19 and a standard deviation of 1.21. The percentages of boys and girls were 54.8% and 45.2%, respectively. To make sure that the sample was representative of the average urban Chinese students, the students were recruited from an ordinary school with an average academic performance in each city. Elite schools or special schools were not included in the present study.

Procedures

The participants were asked to complete a questionnaire in their schools. The questionnaire included questions about their engagement in school and antecedent factors of their engagement. The questionnaire was either administered by project research assistants or the teachers in their respective schools. The survey was administered at the end of a semester, and the students were asked to answer the questions with reference to their experience in that semester. At about the same time, their teachers completed a rating form to report each student's academic performance and conduct in that semester.

Measures

Student Engagement

Student engagement in school was measured by a scale that consisted of three subscales, namely, affective engagement, behavioral engagement, and cognitive engagement Subscales. The affective engagement subscale consisted of nine items that measured the student's liking for learning and school (e.g., "I like what I am learning in school."). The behavioral engagement subscale consisted of 12 items that measure students' persistence and effort in learning (e.g., "I try hard to do well in school."). The cognitive engagement subscale consisted of 12 items that measured students' use of meaningful information processing strategies in learning (e.g., "When I study, I try to connect what I am learning with my own experiences."). The students were asked to indicate their agreement to the items in the affective and behavioral subscales on a 5-point Likert scale with 1 for *strongly disagree* and 5 for *strongly agree*. As for the cognitive subscale, responses were made on a 5-point Likert scale with 1 for *never* and 5 for *always*. We used the average of the three subscale scores to indicate student engagement. A high score indicated high engagement and a low score indicated otherwise. The Cronbach's α of the three subscale-scores was .78 for this sample.

Motivating Instructional Contexts

Students' perceptions of their teachers' instructional practices were measured by the Motivating Instructional Contexts Inventory (MICI) (Lam et al., 2007). The MICI consisted of 24 items with four items in each of the six subscales: challenge (e.g., "Teachers give assignments at the right level, neither too difficult nor too easy."), real-life significance (e.g., "Teachers point out the relation between the subject and our everyday life."), curiosity (e.g., "During the course of teaching, teachers will pinpoint the intriguing part and demand us to think it over and sort it out."), autonomy (e.g., "Teachers let us choose exercises that match our individual interests."), recognition (e.g., "Teachers give recognition to our self-improvement and care not so much if we can win over others."), and evaluation (e.g., "When giving comments on our work, teachers specifically point out those areas for improvement instead of just grading it good or bad."). These six subscales, respectively, measured students' perceptions of the proportion of their teachers who had provided them with challenging tasks, ensured real-life significance in their learning activities, stimulated their curiosity, granted them autonomy, recognized their efforts, and provided useful feedback for their improvement. The students were asked to indicate the proportions on a 5-point Likert scale with 1 for *none of them* and 5 for *all of them*. We used the average of the six subscale-scores as an indicator of the students' perceptions of their teachers' instructional practices. A high score indicated that the students perceived that most of their teachers adopted instructional practices that were motivating. A low score indicated otherwise. The Cronbach's α of these six subscale-scores was .92 for this sample.

Teacher Support

Student perception of teacher support was measured by the Caring Adult Relationships in School Scale of the California Healthy Kids Survey (WestEd, 2000). The scale consisted of three items: (1) "At my school, there is a teacher who cares about me"; (2) "At my school, there is a teacher who is kind to me"; and (3) "At my school, there is a teacher who listens to me when I have something to say." Students were asked to indicate how much they agreed to these three statements on a 5-point Likert scale with 1 for *strongly disagree* and 5 for *strongly agree*. A high score indicated perception of high teacher support and a low score indicated otherwise. The Cronbach's α of the three item-scores was .79 for this sample.

Parent Support

Student perception of parent support was measured by eight items adapted from the components of home support for learning in the Functional Assessment of Academic Behavior (Ysseldyke & Christenson, 2003). These items described parent involvement in their children's learning, such as asking their children about school, monitoring their children's academic progress, and discussing schoolwork with their children at home. The students indicated the frequency of their parent support as stated in these items on a 5-point Likert scale with 1 for *never* and 5 for *always*. A high score indicated perceptions of high parent support and a low score indicated otherwise. The Cronbach's α of the eight item-scores was .85 for this sample.

Peer Support

It was measured by the Caring Peer Relationships in School Scale of the California Healthy Kids Survey (WestEd, 2000). The scale consisted of three items: (1) "At my school, I have a friend who really cares about me"; (2) "At my school, I have a friend who talks with me about my problems"; and (3) "At my school, I have a friend who helps me when I'm having a hard time." The students were asked to indicate how much they agreed to these three statements on a 5-point Likert scale with 1 for *strongly disagree* and 5 for *strongly agree*. A high score indicated perceptions of high peer support and a low score indicated otherwise. The Cronbach's α of the three item-scores was .79 for this sample.

Aggression to Peers

This was measured by a 7-item scale of peer aggression (Hill & Werner, 2006). The students indicated how often over the semester they had engaged in aggressive behaviors toward their peers (e.g., "hit someone because you didn't like what that person said or did."). Responses were made on a 5-point scale with 1 for *never* and 5 for *at least once every day*. A high score indicated high aggression to peers in the school and a low score indicated otherwise. The Cronbach's α of the seven item-scores was .76 for this sample.

Aggression from Peers

This was measured by a scale modified from the scale that measured aggression to peers (Hill & Werner, 2006). The students indicated how often over the semester someone was aggressive to them (e.g., "Someone who didn't like you hit you."). Responses were made on a 5-point scale with 1 for *never* and 5 for *at least once every day*. A high score indicated high aggression from peers in the school and a low score indicated otherwise. The Cronbach's α of the seven item-scores was .86 for this sample.

Self-Efficacy

This was measured by a 7-item scale adapted from the self-efficacy scale used by Pintrich and de Groot (1990). The students indicated the extent to which they agreed with the statement about their self-efficacy in learning (e.g., "I can do very well in this class if I work hard."). Responses were made on a 5-point scale with 1 for *strongly disagree* and 5 for *strongly agree*. We used the average of the five item-scores to indicate students' self-efficacy. A high score indicated that students believed strongly that they were capable of successfully performing the course of action that would lead to success and a low score indicated otherwise. The Cronbach's α of the five item-scores was .74 for this sample.

Learning Goals

A 3-item scale, adapted from the Scales of Achievement Goal Orientations (Midgley et al., 1998), was used to measure learning goals. These three items were (1) "I like school work best when it really makes me think," (2) "An important reason I do my school work is because I want to get better at it," and (3) "I do my school work because I am interested in it." The students were asked to indicate their agreement to these items on a 5-point scale with 1 for *strongly disagree* and 5 for *strongly agree*. The average of the three item-scores reflected the extent to which the students endorsed the goals to develop their ability or master the task. A high score indicated high endorsement of learning goals and a low score indicated otherwise. The Cronbach's α of the three item-scores was .68 for this sample.

Performance Approach Goals

These were also measured by a three-item scale adapted from the Scales of Achievement Goal Orientations (Midgley et al., 1998). These three items were (1) "It's important to me that the other students in my classes think that I am good at my work," (2) "I'd like to show my teachers that I'm smarter than the other students in my classes," and (3) "Doing better than other students in school is important to me." The students were asked to indicate their agreement to these items on a 5-point scale with 1 for *strongly disagree* and 5 for *strongly agree*. The average of the three item-scores reflected the extent to which the students endorsed the goals to seek positive evaluation of their performances or abilities. High scores indicated high endorsement of performance approach goals and low scores indicated otherwise. The Cronbach's α of the three item-scores was .60 for this sample.

Performance Avoidance Goals

These were also measured by a 3-item scale adapted from the Scales of Achievement Goal Orientations (Midgley et al., 1998). These three items were (1) "It's very important to me that I don't look stupid in my classes," (2) "An important reason I do my school work is so that I don't embarrass myself," and (3) "The reason I do my work is so others won't think I'm dumb." The students were asked to indicate their agreement to these items on a 5-point scale with 1 for *strongly disagree* and 5 for *strongly agree*. The average of the three item-scores reflected the extent to which the students endorsed the goals to avoid negative evaluation of their performance or ability. A high score indicated high endorsement of performance avoidance goals and a low score indicated otherwise. The Cronbach's α of the three item-scores was .59 for this sample.

Attribution

To measure students' beliefs in attribution, we asked them to indicate how much their academic performances in that semester were influenced by their abilities, efforts, luck (e.g., boring learning materials), and situations (e.g., being sick). They were asked to write down the percentage of each factor's contribution and the total was required to add up to 100%. The higher the percentage that a student assigned to a factor indicated the more that the student attributed his/her academic performance to that factor.

Emotional Functioning

This was measured by a scale adapted from the Emotional Functioning Scale (Diener, Smith, & Fujita, 1995). The item with the highest factor loading in each of the six clusters of emotion in this scale was selected. The students were asked to indicate how often they had felt happiness, anxiety, anger, shame, sadness, or caring in that semester. Their responses were made on a 5-point scale with 1 for *never* and 5 for *always*. The scores for happiness and caring were averaged to indicate positive emotion. The scores for anxiety, anger, shame, and sadness were averaged to indicate negative emotion. The Cronbach's α of the positive emotion scores and negative emotion scores were .50 and .70, respectively, for this sample.

Academic Performance

The students' academic performances were reported by their teachers. The teachers reported how much each of the students in their class was "good at school work," had "good performance on tests," and did "well on assignments." They were asked to indicate their agreement to the above three statements on a 5-point Likert scale with 1 for *strongly disagree* and 5 for *strongly agree*. The average of these three item-scores was used as an indicator of the students' academic performances in school. A high score indicated good academic performances and a low score indicated otherwise. The Cronbach's α of the six item-scores was .89 for this sample.

Conduct

The students' conduct was also reported by their teachers. The teachers reported how much each of the students in their class was "well behaved in class," "followed all of the rules," and "never got in trouble in class." They were asked to indicate their agreement to the above three statements on a 5-point Likert scale with 1 for *strongly disagree* and 5 for *strongly agree*. The average of these three item-scores was used as an indicator of the students' conduct in school. A high score indicated good conduct and a low score indicated otherwise. The Cronbach's α of the six item-scores was .92 for this sample.

Results

Intraclass Correlations

Before completing the main analyses to examine how student engagement was related to the antecedent factors and outcomes, it was essential to determine the proportion of total variance that occurred systematically between the three cities, i.e., the intraclass correlation (ICC). In the current study, the students were nested within cities. If the ICC was high, one could not treat the students as independent subjects and do the analyses as if they were not nested within cities. Ignoring their cities would have resulted in an overestimation of the correlation among the variables. Lee (2000) argued that researchers should consider a multilevel analytic method when the ICC is more than trivial (i.e., greater than 10% of the total variance in the outcome). To determine the ICC, we conducted analyses of unconditional models for the three subscales and the full scale of student engagement using Hierarchical Linear Modeling (Raudenbush & Bryk, 2002). The between-city ICCs of affective engagement, behavioral engagement, cognitive engagement, and the full scale were .07, .05, .04, and .04, respectively. All the ICC indicated that less than 10% of the total variance in these variables occurred systematically between cities. Thus, it was justifiable to pool the data from the three cities and to run the analyses with the students as independent subjects.

Student Engagement and Instructional Contexts

The means for the subscale scores of affective engagement, behavioral engagement, cognitive engagement, and the full-scale score of student engagement were 3.32, 3.56, 3.18, and 3.36, respectively. The correlation coefficients of these scores with the subscale and full-scale scores of the Motivating Instructional Contexts Inventory are presented in Table 19.1. Given the many correlation tests and large sample size, attention

Table 19.1 Means of the subscale and full-scale scores of the Motivating Instructional Contexts Inventory (MICI) and their correlations with student engagement

	Mean (SD)	Affective engagement	Behavioral engagement	Cognitive engagement	Student engagement
Challenge	2.80 (.86)	.30**	.24**	.31**	.34**
Curiosity	3.50 (.86)	.39**	.35**	.31**	.42**
Real-life significance	3.29 (.92)	.47**	.38**	.35**	.48**
Autonomy	2.77 (1.02)	.35**	.25**	.30**	.36**
Recognition	3.41 (.96)	.32**	.31**	.26**	.35**
Evaluation	3.11 (.86)	.40**	.34**	.31**	.42**
Full-scale score	3.15 (.78)	.43**	.36**	.36**	.46**

Note: **$p<.01$

Table 19.2 Means of the factors in the social-relatedness contexts and their correlations with student engagement

	Mean (SD)	Affective engagement	Behavioral engagement	Cognitive engagement	Student engagement
Teacher support	3.80 (.84)	.46**	.42**	.32**	.48**
Parent support	3.62 (.84)	.32**	.34**	.30**	.38**
Peer support	4.07 (.78)	.25**	.29**	.25**	.31**
Aggression toward peers	1.46 (.57)	−.26**	−.27**	−.16**	−.27**
Aggression from peers	1.50 (.72)	−.10**	−.09*	−.01	−.08*

Note: **$p<.01$, *$p<.05$

should be focused on the effect size of the correlation instead of the p value. As suggested by Cohen (1992), $r=.1-.23$ is considered as small; $r=.24-.36$ is considered medium; and $r>0.37$ is considered as large. The correlations in Table 19.1 were mostly medium and large. Student engagement was associated significantly with instructional contexts. The more the students perceived that their teachers assigned challenging work, integrated real-life significance to learning tasks, aroused their curiosity, supported their autonomy, recognized their effort or improvement, and used formative evaluation, the more they reported that they were engaged affectively, behaviorally, and cognitively in school. It is noteworthy that among the six instructional practices, the practice to integrate real-life significance with learning tasks had the highest correlation with student engagement. We regressed student engagement on the six instructional practices and obtained similar results. Real-life significance had the highest predictive power of student engagement ($\beta=.33, p<.001$). It is also noteworthy that, among the three subscales of student engagement, affective engagement had the highest correlation with all the six motivating instructional practices. It seemed that liking for learning and for school was most sensitive to motivating instructional contexts.

Student Engagement and Social-Relatedness Contexts

The correlation coefficients between the factors in social-related contexts and the subscales and full scale of student engagement are presented in Table 19.2. All the correlation coefficients were significant except the one between aggression from peers and cognitive engagement. The results indicated that student engagement was related closely to teacher support, parent support, peer support, aggression to peers, and aggression from peers. It is interesting to note that teacher support had a stronger association with student engagement than parent support and peer support. We regressed student engagement on all the five contextual variables and found that teacher support had the highest predictive power of student

Table 19.3 Means of motivational beliefs and their correlations with student engagement

	Mean (SD)	Affective engagement	Behavioral engagement	Cognitive engagement	Student engagement
Self-efficacy	3.83 (.61)	.41**	.55**	.46**	.56**
Learning goals	3.36 (.83)	.58**	.52**	.45**	.62**
Performance approach goals	3.20 (.78)	.22**	.17**	.25**	.26**
Performance avoidance goals	2.80 (.84)	−.06	−.11**	.04	−.05
Effort attribution	37.50 (19.20)	.20**	.17**	.14**	20**
Ability attribution	29.46 (17.21)	−.03	.03	.01	.00
Luck attribution	12.25 (11.75)	−.06	−.06	−.07*	−.08*
Situation attribution	21.59 (14.98)	−.20**	−.29**	−.14**	−.21**

Note: **$p < .01$, *$p < .05$

engagement ($\beta = .35$, $p < .001$). In addition, Table 19.2 shows that aggression to peers had a stronger association with student engagement than aggression from peers. The results of the multiple regression analysis also corroborated with this finding. Aggression to peers had higher predictive power of student engagement ($\beta = -.26$, $p < .001$) than aggression from peers ($\beta = -.14$, $p < .001$). In other words, the chances for the bullies to be disengaged from school were higher than those of the victims who got bullied.

Student Engagement and Motivational Beliefs

The correlation coefficients between the motivational beliefs and the subscales and full scale of student engagement are presented in Table 19.3. Self-efficacy had a strong association with student engagement. The more the students believed that they were capable of successfully performing the course of action that would lead to success, the more they were engaged affectively, behaviorally, and cognitively in school. Among the three goal orientations, learning goals had the strongest association with student engagement. It is noteworthy that performance approach goals were also associated positively with student engagement although the effect size was not as big as that of learning goals. Performance avoidance goals did not have much association with student engagement although it had a small negative association with behavioral engagement ($r = -.11$, $p < .01$). Among the four types of attribution, effort attribution and situation attribution had the strongest association with student engagement. The more the students attributed their academic performances to their efforts, the more they would be engaged in school. By contrast, the more the students attributed their academic performances to situations, such as teachers' teaching strategies or boring learning materials, the less they would be engaged. In addition, the associations of ability attribution and luck attribution with student engagement were not obvious.

Given the strong association between self-efficacy and student engagement, self-efficacy was very likely a mediator in the relationship between instructional contexts and student engagement. To verify this mediation model, we examined the mediation effect of self-efficacy in the relationship between instructional contexts and student engagement. The Sobel Test indicated that the effect of instructional contexts on student engagement was mediated partially by self-efficacy, $z = 6.63$, $p < .01$. The indirect and direct effects of instructional contexts on student engagement were .12, $p < .01$, and .35, $p < .01$, respectively.

Student Engagement and Student Outcomes

The correlation coefficients between the four outcome variables and the subscales and full scale of student engagement are presented in Table 19.4.

Table 19.4 Means of the student outcomes and their correlations with student engagement

	Mean (SD)	Affective engagement	Behavioral engagement	Cognitive engagement	Student engagement
Positive emotion	3.63 (.92)	.38**	.32**	.26**	.38**
Negative emotions	2.55 (.76)	−.06	−.03	.02	−.03
Academic performance	3.72 (1.05)	.18**	.24**	.15**	.22**
Conduct	3.99 (.98)	.16**	.18**	.07*	.16**

Note: **$p<.01$, *$p<.05$

As predicted, student engagement was correlated significantly with positive emotions. The more the students reported that they were engaged affectively, behaviorally, and cognitively in school, the more they would report that they often had positive emotions. However, there was little association between negative emotions and student engagement. Both academic performances and conduct had significant correlations with student engagement. The more the students reported that they were engaged in school, the more their teachers would report that they had good academic performance and conduct.

Discussion

With the conceptualization and measurement of student engagement with indicators in three dimensions that were unpacked from facilitators and outcomes, we were able to investigate how student engagement was associated with its antecedents and outcomes. The results indicated that student engagement was associated significantly with the contextual factors, motivational beliefs, and student outcomes. They provided empirical support to the contextual model proposed in Fig. 19.1. Students were engaged affectively, behaviorally, and cognitively in school when they felt that their teachers adopted motivating instructional practices and they had social-emotional support from their teachers, parents, and peers. Their engagement in school was also high when they had high self-efficacy, endorsed learning goals, and attributed their academic performances to how much effort they had made. Most importantly, when students were engaged in schools, they experienced positive emotions frequently and their teachers rated them high on academic performance and conduct.

The data of the present study were collected from junior secondary students in China, a developing country where a collectivistic culture prevails. One may query the generalizability of the results to other countries with different cultures. As this is a subproject of an international research project that involved 12 countries (Lam et al., 2009), cross-country comparisons could be made. Lam et al. found that the proposed contextual model was consistent across the 12 countries. They found that how student engagement was related to the contextual factors and student outcomes did not vary between countries according to gross domestic product (GDP) per capita, an important indicator of economic development. Neither did the relationships vary between countries according to Hofstede's Individualism Index (2009), an indicator of cultural value that distinguished individualistic cultures from collectivistic cultures. The contextual model in Fig. 19.1 is valid for the 12 countries although they are very different in economic development and cultures. There are more cultural similarities than differences when it comes to matters about how student engagement is related to its contexts, antecedents, and outcomes.

Instructional and Social-Relatedness Contexts

The results of the present study indicated that instructional contexts were related closely to student engagement. A close examination of the correlations between student engagement and the subscales of the Motivating Instructional Contexts Inventory revealed an interesting pattern. Real-life significance stood out to be the subscale that had the highest correlation with student engagement. The more the students perceived that many of their teachers integrated real-life significance into their learning tasks, the more they reported that they were engaged affectively, behaviorally, and cognitively in school. According to expectancy x value theory, the amount of effort invested in a task is a product of expectation of success and the values of the task (Wigfield & Eccles, 2000). To increase the value of a task, one strategy is to incorporate real-life significance into the task. Students are more likely to be interested in a task and to think highly of its successful completion if it is relevant to their lives. The results of the present study support the claims of the expectancy x value theory and have important implications for instructional practices. To enhance student engagement, teachers need to provide learning materials and activities relevant to their students' real-life experiences. Instructional strategies specific to the promotion of real-life significance include explaining the text with reference to daily life examples and pointing out the practical use of the learning activities.

Among the three dimensions of student engagement, affective engagement had the highest positive association with instructional contexts. This seemed to be the most responsive and sensitive dimension to motivating instructional strategies. Affective engagement refers to the intrinsic motivation (liking for learning) and school bonding (liking for school). It is the direct feeling toward learning and school. Compared to behavioral and cognitive engagement, the response of affective engagement to instructional contexts may be more direct and intuitive. In a longitudinal study of the internal dynamics of student engagement, Skinner et al. (2008) found that emotional components of engagement contributed significantly to changes in their behavioral counterparts. The affective dimension may be the engine that drives the other dimensions of student engagement. Interventions that target affective dimension are particularly important because they may provide leverage to uplift student engagement as a whole.

In the present study, most of the factors in social-relatedness contexts were associated with student engagement. The most outstanding one was teacher support. Its correlation with the full-scale score of student engagement ($r=.48, p<.01$) was much higher than those of parent support ($r=.38, p<.01$) and student support ($r=.32, p<.01$). The findings that peer support ranked the last does not seem to be consistent with the common belief that peers are influential to adolescents. However, these findings are understandable when the support from teachers, parents, and teachers is compared across various outcomes of children. In a study with sixth grade students, Wentzel (1998) found that peer support was a positive predictor of prosocial goal pursuit, teacher support was a positive predictor of class-related and school-related interest, and parent support was a positive predictor of school-related interest and goal orientations. Different outcomes were associated with support from different socializing agents. Peer support was still important; however, it was not as important as teacher and parent support when the matter of concern was school-related interest. The findings of the present study supported the importance of teacher support in student engagement. Students will be engaged in school when they feel that their teachers provide them with social-emotional support. Teacher support can be a pivotal factor in the enhancement of student engagement.

In the present study, aggression to peers was found to have negative association with student engagement ($r=-.27, p<.01$). This association was much higher than that of aggression to peers ($r=-.08, p<.05$) with student engagement. The findings suggest that the chances for the bullies to be disengaged from school are higher than those of the victims who get bullied. The vulnerable victims are usually the center of attention for the research in peer aggression (Juvonen & Graham, 2001; Ladd et al., 1997). However, the findings of the present study remind us that the bullies may be more susceptible to disengagement from school. They are also a group of students who need attention from researchers and educators.

Motivational Beliefs

As presented in Table 19.3, self-efficacy was associated positively with student engagement. The more the students believed that they were capable of successfully performing the course of action that would lead to success, the more they were engaged in schools. It was found in the present study that self-efficacy was a mediator in the relationship between instructional contexts and student engagement. The instructional contexts had impact on students' self-efficacy, which in turn had impact student engagement. This mediation model can be explained by expectancy x value theory (Wigfield & Eccles, 2000). According to this theory, the amount of effort invested in a task is a product of expectation of success and the values of the task, the increase in the expectation of success would be motivational. When teachers adopt instructional practices that enable students to master challenging tasks successfully, they will increase their students' self-efficacy. As indicated in the challenge subscale of the Motivating Instructional Contexts Inventory, these instructional practices include providing scaffolding and assigning a task at the appropriate difficulty level. The results of the mediation analysis showed that the more the teachers adopted these practices, the more the students would feel efficacious. When the students felt more efficacious, they would be more engaged in school. These results illustrate the mechanism by which instructional contexts affect student engagement. They help teachers understand how they can enhance student engagement by promoting self-efficacy.

Among the three goal orientations, learning goals had the strongest correlation with student engagement. Nevertheless, performance approach goals also had a positive association with student engagement. The role of performance approach goals in learning and achievement has been controversial (Midgley, Kaplan, & Middleton, 2001). Experimental studies with manipulation (e.g., Lam et al., 2004) have usually shown that performance goals have detrimental effects on learning and achievement, but correlational studies with observed data (e.g., Pintrich, 2000) showed otherwise. As the present study was also a correlational study, its results were consistent with those of the previous correlational studies and showed that performance approach goals had a positive association with student engagement. It was only the performance avoidance goals that had any negative association with behavioral engagement. The discrepancy between the findings of experimental and correlational studies may be due to the differences in methodology. Studies with experimental design usually manipulate performance goals and look into how students with these goals respond to setbacks. As Dweck described clearly in a seminal paper (1986), performance goals with high self-confidence are as motivating as learning goals. It is only in the condition of low self-confidence that performance goals will elicit avoidance and self-handicapping behaviors. Performance goals with high self-confidence are similar to performance approach goals, whereas performance goals with low self-confidence are similar to performance avoidance goals. It is understandable that correlational studies, without controlling the level of self-confidence, will find that performance approach goals are associated with positive outcomes. The positive role of performance approach goals in learning and achievement is unstable because it may turn negative once self-confidence is low. Educators must be cautious in promoting performance approach goals because it may backfire when learning becomes difficult and challenging.

The results of the present study indicated that, among the four types of attribution, effort attribution had the highest correlation with student engagement. The more the students attributed their academic performances to their efforts, the more they reported that they were engaged affectively, behaviorally, and cognitively in school. Effort is an internal, controllable, and changeable factor (Weiner, 1985). Students will believe that they can control and change their academic performance if they endorse effort attribution. By contrast, attribution to external and uncontrollable factors, such as luck and situation, does not help them think that they can control and change their academic performance. It is interesting to note that ability attribution did not have any association with student engagement. Ability is an internal factor, but whether it is controllable and changeable depends on one's implicit theory of intelligence (Dweck, 1986). If students believe that ability is inherited and nonmalleable, ability attribution does not help them much. This is particularly so in the face of setback. Out of good intention, many teachers may praise their students' abilities for good academic performance. This practice may also backfire if their students believe that ability is inherited and nonmalleable (Mueller & Dweck, 1998).

Limitations and Future Directions

The present study has provided support to a contextual model for understanding student engagement. With the conceptualization and measurement of student engagement with indicators in three dimensions that were unpacked from facilitators and outcomes, the present study showed how student engagement was associated with its antecedents and outcomes. The findings have significant implications for strategies for the enhancement of student engagement.

Despite its contributions, the present study also has some obvious limitations. This is a correlational study with observed data, so causal relations between variables cannot be ascertained. To address this limitation, future studies may consider field experiments on the effects of intervention (e.g., motivating instructional practices) on student engagement. Another possibility is to employ longitudinal designs that allow time series analyses in field studies. With longitudinal data, one can justify the temporal ordering of variables and possible causal effects according to the time of measurement.

Another limitation of the present study is its dependence on self-report measures from students. Almost all of the measures were reported by students. The exceptions were the measures of academic performance and conduct, which were reported by teachers. There is a possibility of inflation of correlations when variables are measured at the same time from the same participants. Although self-reports are valid measures of subjective psychological constructs, such as liking for learning and for school, the results of the present study would be much stronger if measures other than self-reports were included. For example, instructional contexts can be measured with a third party's observation. This objective measure might provide stronger evidence for the current contextual model.

The findings of the present study have only presented a general picture or overview about how student engagement is related to its antecedents and outcomes in a contextual model. It provides understanding in a broad stroke. Details about the mechanisms among the variables in this contextual model still need further investigation. For example, we only did one mediation analysis to see the relationship among instructional contexts, self-efficacy, and student engagement. Actually, there may be more mediation relations among other variables in this contextual model. In addition, the internal dynamics among the three dimensions of student engagement should also be studied. Further investigation into the details of this contextual model will definitely enhance our understanding of student engagement and its facilitators.

References

Appleton, J. J., Christenson, S. L., & Furlong, M. J. (2008). Student engagement with school: Critical conceptual and methodological issues of the construct. *Psychology in the Schools, 45*, 369–386.

Appleton, J. J., Christenson, S. L., Kim, D., & Reschly, A. L. (2006). Measuring cognitive and psychological engagement: Validation of the student engagement instrument. *Journal of School Psychology, 44*, 427–445.

Archambault, I., Janosz, M., Fallu, J.-S., & Pagani, L. S. (2009). Student engagement and its relationship with early high school dropout. *Journal of Adolescence, 32*, 651–670.

Bandura, A. (1977). Self-efficacy: Toward a unifying theory of behavioral change. *Psychological Review, 84*, 191–215.

Birch, S. H., & Ladd, G. W. (1997). The teacher-child relationship and children's early school adjustment. *Journal of School Psychology, 35*, 61–79.

Bronfenbrenner, U. (1986). Ecology of the family as a context for human development: Research perspectives. *Developmental Psychology, 22*, 723–742.

Chung, I. J., Hill, K. G., Hawkins, J. D., Gilchrist, L. D., & Nagin, D. S. (2002). Childhood predictors of offense trajectories. *Journal of Research in Crime and Delinquency, 39*, 60–90.

Cohen, J. (1992). A power primer. *Psychological Bulletin, 112*, 155–159.

Connell, J. P., Spencer, M. B., & Aber, J. L. (1994). Educational risk and resilience in African-American youth: Context, self, action, and outcomes in school. *Child Development 65*, 493–506.

Connell, M. P., & Wellborn, J. G. (1991). Competence, autonomy and relatedness: A motivational analysis of self-system processes. In M. R. Gunnar & L. A. Sroufe (Eds.), *Self processes and development: The Minnesota symposia on child psychology* (pp. 43–78). Hillsdale, NJ: Erlbaum.

Diener, E., Smith, H., & Fujita, F. (1995). The personality structure of affect. *Journal of Personality and Social Psychology, 69*, 130–141.

Donrbush, S. M., Ritter, P. L., Leiderman, P. H., Roberts, D. F., & Fraleigh, M. J. (1987). The relation of parenting style to adolescent school performance. *Child Development, 58*, 1244–1257.

Dweck, C. S. (1986). Motivational processes affecting learning. *American Psychologist, 41*, 1040–1048.

Dweck, C. S. (2006). *Mindset: The new psychology of success*. New York: Random House.

Eccles, J. S., Midgley, C., Wigfield, A., Buchanan, C. M., Reuman, D., Flanagan, C., et al. (1993). Development during adolescence: The impact of stage-environment fit on young adolescents' experiences in schools and in families. *American Psychologist, 48*, 90–101.

Elliot, A. J., McGregor, H. A., & Gable, S. (1999). Achievement goals, study strategies, and exam performance: A mediational analysis. *Journal of Educational Psychology, 91*(3), 549–563.

Finn, J. D. (1989). Withdrawing from school. *Review of Educational Research, 59*, 117–142.

Finn, J. D., Pannozzo, G. M., & Voelkl, K. E. (1995). Disruptive and inattentive withdrawn behavior and achievement among fourth graders. *The Elementary School Journal, 95*, 421–454.

Finn, J. D., & Rock, D. A. (1997). Academic success among students at risk for school failure. *Journal of Applied Psychology, 82*, 221–234.

Fredricks, J. A., Blumenfeld, P. C., & Paris, A. H. (2004). School engagement: Potential of the concept, state of the evidence. *Review of Educational Research, 74*, 59–109.

Furlong, M. J., & Christenson, S. L. (2008). Engaging students at school and with learning: A relevant construct for ALL students. *Psychology in the Schools, 45*, 365–368.

Furrer, C., & Skinner, E. (2003). Sense of relatedness as a factor in children's academic engagement and performance. *Journal of Educational Psychology, 95*, 148–162.

Gauch, H. G. (2003). *Scientific method in practice*. Cambridge, MA: Cambridge University Press.

Gest, S. D., Welsh, J. A., & Domitrovich, C. E. (2005). Behavioral predictors of changes in social relatedness and liking school in elementary school. *Journal of School Psychology, 43*, 281–301.

Graham, S., & Golan, S. (1991). Motivational influences on cognition: Task involvement, ego involvement, and depth of information processing. *Journal of Educational Psychology, 83*, 187–194.

Hawkins, J. D., Gou, J. G., Hill, K. G., Battin-Pearson, S., & Abbott, R. D. (2001). Long term effects of the Seattle social development intervention on school bonding trajectories. *Applied Developmental Science, 5*, 225–236.

Hill, L. G., & Werner, N. E. (2006). Affiliative motivation, school attachment, and aggression in school. *Psychology in the Schools, 43*, 231–246.

Hofstede, G.. (2009). *Geert HosfstedeTM cultural dimensions*. Retrieved from http://www.geert-hofstede.com/hofstede_dimensions.php.

Hoover-Dempsey, K. V., & Sandler, H. M. (1995). Parental involvement in children's education: Why does it make a difference? *Teachers College Record, 97*, 310–331.

Jimerson, S., Campos, E., & Greif, J. (2003). Towards an understanding of definitions and measures of school engagement and related terms. *The California School Psychologist, 8*, 7–28.

Juvonen, J., & Graham, S. (Eds.). (2001). *Peer harassment in school: The plight of the vulnerable and victimized*. New York: Guilford Press.

Ladd, G. W., Kochenderfer, B. J., & Coleman, C. C. (1997). Classroom peer acceptance, friendship, and victimization: Distinct relational systems that contribute uniquely to children's school adjustment? *Child Development, 68*, 1181–1197.

Lam, S.-f., Jimerson, S., Basnett, J., Cefai, C., Duck, R., Farrell, P., et al. (2009, July). *Exploring student engagement in schools internationally: A collaborative international study yields further insights*. A symposium at the 31st annual International School Psychology Association Colloquium, Malta.

Lam, S.-f., Pak, T. S., & Ma, W. Y. K. (2007). Motivating Instructional Contexts Inventory. In P. R. Zelick (Ed.), *Issues in the psychology of motivation* (pp. 119–136). Huppauge, NJ: Nova Science.

Lam, S.-f., Yim, P.-s., Law, J. S. F., & Cheung, R. W. Y. (2004). The Effects of competition on achievement motivation in Chinese classrooms. *British Journal of Educational Psychology, 74*, 281–296.

Lee, V. (2000). Using hierarchical linear modeling to study social contexts: The case of school effects. *Educational Psychologist, 35*, 125–141.

Maddox, S. J., & Prinz, R. J. (2003). School bonding in children and adolescents: Conceptualization, assessment, and associated variables. *Clinical Child and Family Psychology Review, 6*, 31–49.

Marks, H. M. (2000). Student engagement in instructional activity: Patterns in the elementary, middle, and high school years. *American Educational Research Journal, 37*, 153–184.

Meece, J. L., Blumenfeld, P. C., & Hoyle, R. H. (1988). Student's goal orientations and cognitive engagement in classroom activities. *Journal of Educational Psychology, 80,* 514–523.

Midgley, C., Kaplan, A., & Middleton, M. (2001). Performance-approach goals: Good for what, for whom, under what circumstances, and at what cost? *Journal of Educational Psychology, 93,* 77–86.

Midgley, C., Kaplan, A., Middleton, M., Maehr, M. L., Urdan, T., Anderman, L. H., et al. (1998). The development and validation of scales assessing students' achievement goal orientations. *Contemporary Educational Psychology, 23*(2), 113–131.

Mueller, C. M., & Dweck, C. S. (1998). Praise for intelligence can undermine children's motivation and performance. *Journal of Personality and Social Psychology, 75,* 33–52.

Murray, C., & Greenberg, M. T. (2000). Children's relationships with teachers and bonds with school: An investigation of patterns and correlates in middle childhood. *Journal of School Psychology, 38,* 423–445.

Nolen, S. B. (1988). Reasons for studying: Motivational orientations and study strategies. *Cognition and Instruction, 5,* 269–287.

O'Farrell, S. L., & Morrison, G. M. (2003). A factor analysis exploring school bonding and related constructs among upper elementary students. *The California School Psychologist, 8,* 53–72.

Perry, N. E., Turner, J. C., & Meyer, D. K. (2006). Classrooms as contexts for motivating learning. In P. A. Alexander & P. H. Winnie (Eds.), *Handbook of educational psychology* (Vol. 2). Mahwah, NJ: Lawrence Erlbaum.

Pintrich, P. R. (2000). Multiple goals, multiple pathways: The role of goal orientation in learning and achievement. *Journal of Educational Psychology, 92,* 544–555.

Pintrich, P. R., & de Groot, E. V. (1990). Motivational and self-regulated learning components of classroom academic performance. *Journal of Educational Psychology, 82*(1), 33–40.

Raudenbush, S. W., & Bryk, A. S. (2002). *Hierarchical linear models: Applications and data analysis methods* (2nd ed.). Thousand Oaks, CA: Sage Publications.

Ryan, R. M., & Deci, E. L. (2000). Intrinsic and extrinsic motivations: Classic definitions and new directions. *Contemporary Educational Psychology, 25,* 54–67.

Schunk, D. H., & Zimmerman, B. J. (2006). Competence and control beliefs: Distinguish the means and ends. In P. A. Alexander & P. H. Winnie (Eds.), *Handbook of educational psychology* (Vol. 2, pp. 349–367). Manhwah, NJ: Lawrence Erlbaum.

Sinclair, M. F., Christenson, S. L., Lehr, C. A., & Anderson, A. R. (2003). Facilitating school engagement: Lessons learned from Check & Connect longitudinal studies. *The California School Psychologists, 8,* 29–41.

Skinner, E., & Belmont, M. J. (1993). Motivation in the classroom: Reciprocal effects of teacher behavior and student engagement across the school year. *Journal of Educational Psychology, 85,* 571–581.

Skinner, E., Furrer, C., Marchand, G., & Kindermann, T. (2008). Engagement and disaffection in the classroom: Part of a larger motivational dynamic? *Journal of Educational Psychology, 100,* 765–781.

Voelkl, K. E. (1997). Identification with school. *American Journal of Education, 105,* 204–319.

Walker, C. O., Greene, B. A., & Mansell, R. A. (2006). Identification with academics, intrinsic/extrinsic motivation, and self-efficacy as predictors of cognitive engagement. *Learning and Individual Differences, 16,* 1–12.

Weiner, B. (1985). An attributional theory of achievement motivation and emotion. *Psychological Review, 92,* 548–573.

Wentzel, K. R. (1998). Social relationships and motivation in middle school: The role of parents, teachers and peers. *Journal of Educational Psychology, 90,* 202–209.

WestEd. (2000). *California healthy kids survey.* Los Alamitos, CA: WestEd.

Wigfield, A., & Eccles, J. S. (2000). Expectancy-value theory of achievement motivation. *Contemporary Educational Psychology, 25,* 68–81.

Ysseldyke, J., & Christenson, S. (2003). *Functional assessment of academic behavior: Creating successful learning environments.* Longmont, CO: Sopris West.

Allowing Choice and Nurturing an Inner Compass: Educational Practices Supporting Students' Need for Autonomy*

Avi Assor

Abstract

This chapter focuses on seven practices of autonomy support which are likely to promote two major components of the need for autonomy: (a) lack of coercion and optional choice and (b) formation and realization of an inner compass: authentic, direction-giving values, goals, and interests. A special emphasis is put on research pertaining to three autonomy supportive practices which are assumed to support formation and realization of authentic, direction-giving values, goals, and interests, whose impact on perceived autonomy was not sufficiently examined so far: (a) IVD – intrinsic value demonstration, (b) SVE – support for value/goal/interest examination, and (c) FIV – fostering inner-directed valuing processes. The autonomy supportive practices that foster the development of stable authentic values and goals might be especially important in western countries, in which postmodern moral relativism and the abundance of information and options make it particularly difficult for youth to form stable and authentic values and goals.

The hope to see students motivated and engaged in activities that contribute to their intellectual, socioemotional, and moral growth is widely shared. However, students often appear less and less engaged in learning as they grow older (e.g., Gottfried, Marcoulides, Gottfried, Oliver, & Guerin, 2007). According to self-determination theory (SDT, Ryan & Deci, 2000), one major factor which may explain why students are often poorly motivated and poorly engaged is that they do not feel that school-related activities support their need for autonomy.

The need for autonomy is conceptualized in this chapter as involving two major components: (a) the striving to avoid coercion and have optional choice and (b) the striving to form and realize authentic and direction-giving values, goals, and interests (i.e., the striving for an inner compass). In this chapter, I describe various practices of teachers, parents, and schools that can support students' need for autonomy and therefore promote engagement. In particular, I describe

---

*The research reported in this chapter was supported by grants from the Israel Science Foundation, the US-Israel Binational Science Foundation, and the chief scientist of the Israel education ministry.

A. Assor (✉)
Educational and School Psychology Program,
Ben Gurion University, Be'er-Sheva, Israel
e-mail: assor@bgu.ac.il

three practices that promote the examination (and consequent formation) of authentic goals and values and are relatively underemphasized in extant work on autonomy support:

(a) Intrinsic value demonstration (IVD)
(b) Support for value/goal/interest examination (SVE)
(c) Fostering inner-directed valuing processes (FIV)

These practices are especially important in the postmodern era in which many face considerable value confusion.

Motivation

I view the concept of motivation as referring to people's intentions to perform actions. These inclinations or intentions (i.e., motives) have two important attributes: intensity (strength) and phenomenological quality. The intensity dimension refers to the amount of effort which people intend to put in an attempt to reach a certain goal, often in the face of difficulties. The quality dimension refers to people's perception and experience of the reasons or sources of their intentions or motives. Specifically, when people perceive their intentions as emanating from their authentic self, the phenomenological quality of the motivation is high because the intentions are experienced as autonomous, whereas intentions that are perceived as unauthentic are experienced as controlling and unpleasant (e.g., Roth, Assor, Niemiec, Ryan, & Deci, 2009; Ryan & Deci, 2000). For example, two students may intend to invest a great deal of effort in a school assignment, so the intensity of their motivation is similar (both are high on intensity). However, the quality of the motivation may be high for the student who perceives the assignment as something that she/he would authentically want to do. In contrast, the quality of the motivation to do the assignment would be low for the person who feels that the assignment is a task that is completely unconnected to her/his authentic values and interests.

Based on SDT, then, I differentiate between: (1) Motives or intentions that are experienced as controlling, nonautonomous and therefore stressful and nonoptimal, and (2) Motives or intentions that are experienced as autonomous, emanating from one's true self, highly volitional, and therefore leading to full engagement and well-being (e.g., Ryan & Deci, 2000). Specifically, controlled motives can be driven by (1) the desire to avoid external punishments and threats and/or the hope to attain rewards (e.g., doing your homework in order to avoid being grounded or in order to win a desired gadget) and/or (2) the desire to avoid internal feelings of guilt and shame and/or the hope to feel grand and unique (e.g., Assor, Vansteenkiste, & Kaplan, 2009). Autonomous motives can be guided by (1) the perception of the task as valuable, perhaps even central to the realization of one's central values (but not necessarily pleasant), and/or (2) the perception of the task as interesting and enjoyable.

The concept of engagement refers to the amount and quality of *actual* efforts and actions aimed at reaching a certain goal. While motives refer to *intentions or inclinations* to do something in order to reach a certain goal, engagement refers to *actual actions* that are performed as one attempts to reach a certain goal. Simply put, the difference between motives and engagement is the difference between goal-oriented intention and action. If the goal is learning new concepts or skills, then people can differ in the amount of effort they invest (i.e., persistence, determination), as well as the effectiveness, flexibility, or creativity that characterize their efforts. Research guided by SDT indicates that while controlling motives can lead to a great deal of effort, *autonomous motives are much more likely to promote flexible and creative engagement in learning* (e.g., Deci & Ryan, 1985; Roth et al., 2009).

Given the pleasant emotional experience associated with autonomous motives and the role of such motives in facilitating flexible and creative engagement in learning, it is important to discover factors which may contribute to autonomous motivation. SDT posits that there are at least three basic human needs whose satisfaction promotes autonomous motivation and therefore high-quality engagement: the need for relatedness, competence, and autonomy (e.g., Ryan & Deci, 2000).

While the needs for competence and relatedness have received considerable attention from other theorists (e.g., Baumeister & Leary, 1995; Elliot & Dweck, 2005; White, 1959), SDT is unique in its emphasis on the need for autonomy.

Freedom from Coercion and Optional Choice

The first striving within the need for autonomy, to be free from coercion and have the possibility to choose one's actions, is similar to Fromm's (1941) notion of "Freedom From," as well as Berlin's (1969) notion of negatively defined autonomy (see also Aviram & Assor, 2010, on this issue). Research anchored mainly in SDT has shown that when people are pressured and coerced (from outside or from within) to behave in specific ways, they experience frustration. This frustration has been shown to undermine engagement, well-being, and vitality (e.g., Assor, Kaplan, Kanat-Maymon, & Roth, 2005; Assor, Kaplan, & Roth, 2002; Reeve, 2006; Reeve & Jang, 2006).

As for choice, there is ample research showing that people, in general, prefer to have the option to choose (see Patall, Cooper & Robinson, 2008), although they do not always need to be the ones who make the choice, especially when someone else chooses for them what they anyway want (e.g., Katz & Assor, 2007). For example, Katz and Assor showed that when parents choose for children learning and leisure activities that children have a sustained interest in, children willingly engage in these activities. In contrast, when parents choose activities that are inconsistent with the child's interests, children do feel controlled and nonautonomous. Thus, it appears that while people do not always have to choose things by themselves, they do want to have the *option* to choose so that if they lose trust in a person who does the choice for them, they could determine their choices and actions themselves.

Inner Compass

The striving to develop and realize direction-giving and authentic values, goals, and interests (an inner compass) is similar to Fromm's (1941) notion of "Freedom For," as well as Berlin's (1969) notion of positively defined autonomy (see also Aviram & Assor, 2010). The formation of this inner compass is very important because it *provides inner criteria for making important decisions*. When people do not have clear and authentic values, goals, and interests, the availability of choices might be a threat or a burden, as indicated in Fromm's writings on the phenomena of escape from freedom. *It is only when one has clear and authentic inner compass that one welcomes choice* (if this choice is meaningful; see Katz & Assor, 2007). Thus, it is possible that the finding that people feel burdened by too much consumerist choice (e.g., Iyengar & Lepper, 2000) may at least, in part, be a product of lack of clear and authentic values which enable people to quickly discard many of the choices offered to them as irrelevant and harmful.

Authentic, direction-giving goals, values, and interests also provide people with internal criteria for evaluating others and themselves and a foundation a for feeling that their actions are coherent and meaningful, and they also make people less dependent on others' evaluations (Assor, 2010, 2011; Reeve & Assor, 2011). Highly developed and authentic value systems which guide decisions and actions function as elaborate, multilevel, categories which are anchored in a more general self and world view, embedded in a historical perspective (e.g., Assor, 1999, 2011; Assor, Cohen-Melayev, Kaplan, & Friedman, 2005).

Teacher, Parent, and School Practices That Support the Need for Autonomy

In this section, I will describe seven practices of teachers, parents, and schools that are likely to support the two components of the need for autonomy. Research demonstrating the contributions of these practices to students' perceived autonomy, engagement, achievement, high-quality learning, and/or well-being will be briefly described. I will start with practices that support the striving for no coercion and optional choice and then move to practices supporting the formation of authentic values, goals, and interests (Fig. 20.1).

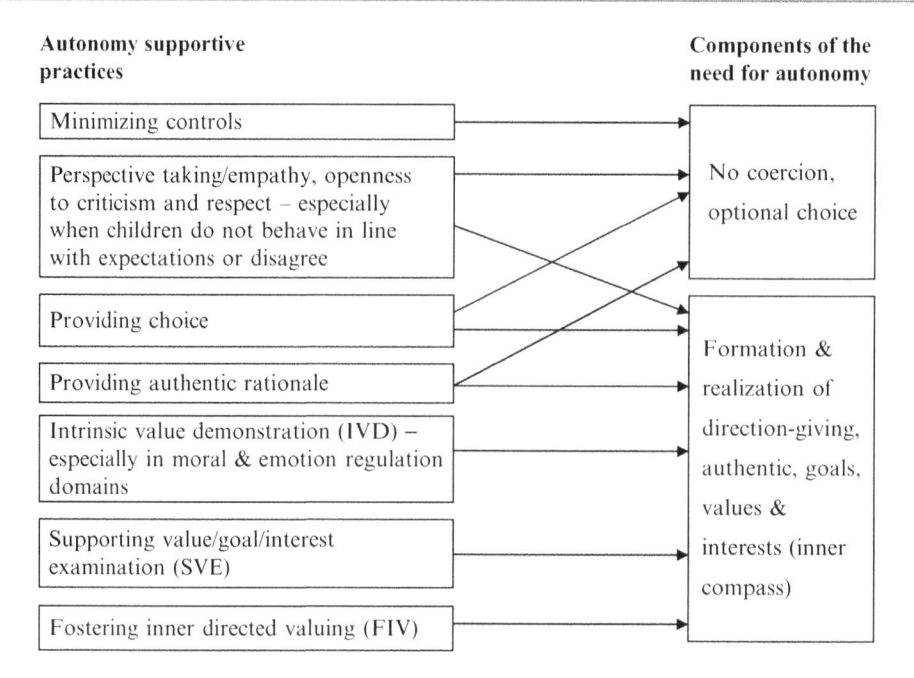

```
Autonomy supportive                              Components of the
practices                                        need for autonomy

┌─────────────────────────────────┐
│ Minimizing controls             │──────────┐
└─────────────────────────────────┘          │
┌─────────────────────────────────┐          │    ┌──────────────────┐
│ Perspective taking/empathy,     │──────────┼───▶│ No coercion,     │
│ openness to criticism and       │          │    │ optional choice  │
│ respect – especially when       │          │    └──────────────────┘
│ children do not behave in line  │          │
│ with expectations or disagree   │          │
└─────────────────────────────────┘          │
┌─────────────────────────────────┐          │
│ Providing choice                │──────────┤
└─────────────────────────────────┘          │
┌─────────────────────────────────┐          │    ┌──────────────────┐
│ Providing authentic rationale   │──────────┼───▶│ Formation &      │
└─────────────────────────────────┘          │    │ realization of   │
┌─────────────────────────────────┐          │    │ direction-giving,│
│ Intrinsic value demonstration   │──────────┤    │ authentic, goals,│
│ (IVD) – especially in moral &   │          │    │ values &         │
│ emotion regulation domains      │          │    │ interests (inner │
└─────────────────────────────────┘          │    │ compass)         │
┌─────────────────────────────────┐          │    └──────────────────┘
│ Supporting value/goal/interest  │──────────┤
│ examination (SVE)               │          │
└─────────────────────────────────┘          │
┌─────────────────────────────────┐          │
│ Fostering inner directed        │──────────┘
│ valuing (FIV)                   │
└─────────────────────────────────┘
```

Fig. 20.1 Practices supporting the need for autonomy

Minimizing Controls

This practice refers to behaviors of other people or features of the educational context which cause students to feel controlled. Minimizing controls may be a necessary but not sufficient condition for supporting the need for autonomy. That is, while the presence of controls can undermine the need for autonomy, its absence may not be enough to make people feel that they can choose and organize their actions or formulate and realize direction-giving values, goals, and interests.

Soenens and Vansteenkiste (2010) describe two forms of control: (a) behaviors that pressure one to behave in a specific way in order to avoid unpleasant bodily experiences, loss of material benefits and privileges, as well as in order to gain various material benefits and privileges (external control), and (b) behaviors that pressure one to behave in a specific way in order to feel worthy of love and esteem (internal control; see also Assor, Roth & Deci, 2004).

External control includes behaviors such as physical punishment, withdrawing privileges, physical threats, and power assertion, as well as bribes or material rewards that are not informative in terms of level or quality of one's performance. Research surveyed by Deci, Koestner, and Ryan (1999) indicated that when people are already intrinsically motivated to perform certain tasks (including learning), the offering of material rewards, in general, tends to undermine intrinsic motivation, perceived autonomy, and performance quality. Other external controls involve direct commands and surveillance, imposing of deadlines, intruding and interfering with the child's natural rhythm of work, and suppressing the expression of disagreement or critical opinions.

One study that examined the impact of the teachers' use of external controls on children was conducted by Assor, Kaplan, Kanat-Maymon and Roth (2005). Israeli fourth and fifth graders completed questionnaires assessing teachers' tendency to intrude and interfere as children worked on their assignments, as well as to discourage any answer that diverts from teachers' opinion. Children's academic engagement was assessed by their primary teachers. Path analyses supported the hypothesis that children's perceptions of their teachers as using external controls arouse children's anger and anxiety, and these emotions then undermine academic engagement. Similarly, Assor et al. (2002), in a study conducted with Israeli students in grades 3–8, also showed that interfering with children's or early adolescents' preferred pace of learning and not allowing critical and independent opinions predicted negative emotions during learning and poor academic engagement. Importantly, these findings were obtained also when the effects of autonomy supportive behaviors such as providing choice were held constant via regression analyses.

Research by Assor, Roth, and their colleagues (Assor & Roth, 2005; Assor, Roth, & Deci, 2004; Roth et al., 2009) has identified one type of control that undermines students' need of autonomy by linking their sense of love-worthiness and self-worth to the enactment of expected behaviors. This type of controlling behavior was termed "using *conditional regard* as a socializing practice." In this practice, educators provide more affection or esteem when children enact behaviors or attain outcomes that are valued by educators; similarly, children lose affection or esteem when they do not comply with expectations (see Assor et al., 2004). Research with ninth-grade Israeli adolescents has shown that when parents were perceived by their children as using conditional regard to promote academic achievement and investment, children felt a sense of internal compulsion, as well as anger and resentment in relation to parents. Importantly, research by Roth et al. (2009) has shown that even the seemingly benign practice of using conditional *positive* regard (i.e., providing more affection and esteem when the child invests and achieves in school) is also associated with feelings of internal compulsion and a rather rigid, grade-focused mode of engagement in school.

Assor, Roth, Israeli, and Freed (2007) conducted a follow-up study to examine whether the Roth et al. (2009) findings concerning conditional regard predicting adolescents' sense of internal compulsion would emerge also when conditional regard was assessed via parents' reports. Results obtained with ninth-grade Israeli adolescents clearly replicated the pattern obtained by Roth et al., thus indicating that the negative emotional effects of parental conditional regard are not simply an artifact of adolescents' self-reports.

Indirect evidence for the autonomy suppressive nature of conditional regard comes also from research on the construct of psychological control. The concept and measure of psychological control (Barber, 1996; Barber, Stolz, & Olsen, 2005) is essentially similar to that of conditional *negative* regard, as both concepts include clear elements of love withdrawal when children do not comply with parents' expectations. Research on this widely used concept has shown that parents' use of psychological control in the domain of achievement predicts a variety of maladaptive child outcomes such as depressive feelings, poor self esteem, and maladaptive perfectionism (e.g., Barber et al., 2005; Soenens & Vansteenkiste, 2010; Soenens et al., 2005). The offspring participating in these studies ranged in age from 11 to 24 years and came from ethnic groups characterized by widely different religions and cultural values in Europe, North and South America, Africa, and Asia. The major negative effects of psychological control were observed in all the ethnic groups examined.

Perspective Taking, Empathy, Openness to Criticism, and Respect When Children Disagree or Display Negative Feelings

This practice refers to the ability and inclination to try to understand and respect the other's perspective, including perspectives that are inconsistent with one's own views or seem unreasonable or wrong. Perspective taking and respect in the case of disagreements can take different forms depending on the content of the disagreement. For example, when children do not want to engage in studying a certain topic, the teacher can first ask them why they do not invest much in this topic. If the students say that they are bored or that they feel that no matter what they would do, they would never succeed, the empathic teacher acknowledges those feelings and respects them, and then relies on additional autonomy supportive practices such as offering a rationale and some choice to try to promote autonomous internalization of the value of learning the task at hand.

The task of being empathic, taking others' perspective, and respecting their feelings and opinions is relatively easy when others feel incompetent, confused, or distressed and therefore need someone to help them. In such cases, our interest and respect may only mean that we care and are not threatened by the distress or the other person. Moreover, such cases usually do not pose a threat to our beliefs, values, power, or self-esteem (as people who know what is right or wrong).

In contrast, being empathic and respectful is much more challenging when others do not necessarily feel incompetent and/or in need of help but simply hold *opposite* views and beliefs. Let us consider, for example, a high school student who is interested in arts and literature and therefore wants to take a minimal load of studies in the natural sciences. For parents who admire the natural sciences and want their child to study these subjects because they know she/he is very intelligent (and/or think these subjects can secure a high income), it might be extremely difficult to show respect for the child's different opinions, plans, and feelings on this issue. The difficulties in respecting the child's view may arise not only from our concern about the child's well-being and future opportunities but also from the feeling that respecting opposite opinions may indicate that our view is not so valid or even that we have no authority or are unsure of our views.

Because children and adolescents have at least some understanding of the challenge involved in respecting their opinions and feelings *because they have already have at least some capacity for perspective taking* (e.g., Epley, Morewedge, & Keysar, 2004), they really value the capacity of significant others to respect their differing opinions and negative feelings. Consequently, *empathy and respect for oppositional opinions and feelings may provide particularly strong support for the child's need for autonomy*. Consistent with this view, reports by Assor et al. (2002) and Assor and Kaplan (2001) on research with elementary and high school students in Israel showed that their perceptions of their teachers as suppressing the expression of different and sometime critical opinions were negatively associated with their engagement in studying and positive feelings during studying. Importantly, this effect was also detected when the effects of other aspects of teacher behavior (as perceived by students) were statistically controlled for. The aspects of teacher behavior that were held constant were teachers' provision of choices, clarification of the relevance of the subject matter to students' goals, competence supporting feedback, and a warm behavior toward the student. While in these studies acceptance of differing opinions or negative feelings was not found to have positive correlates when entered with other variables in the regression analyses, it should be noted that openness to differing opinions was found to have positive and significant Pearson correlations with engagement.

The importance of perspective taking and empathy when teachers or parents disagree with children was also demonstrated in several studies conducted by Assor, Roth, and their colleagues, as in these studies, one major component of the autonomy support measure reflects the capacity to take children's perspective when they disagree with adults regarding school issues (e.g., Assor et al., 2007; Roth et al., 2009). The Roth et al. (2009) study is described in some detail in the section focusing on intrinsic value demonstration.

Providing Rationale

This attribute refers to teachers' inclination and ability to provide a coherent, age-appropriate rationale for their expectations. When students are provided with clear and convincing rationale for actions they do not find particularly interesting or valuable, they tend to feel less coerced (Assor, 2011; Grolnick, Deci, & Ryan, 1997). Moreover, when students understand and identify with the rationale for their school-related activities, they feel that the act of studying supports their need for autonomy because studying allows them to express and promote their values and goals. For example, when a high school teacher shows students how good writing ability has allowed many past graduates to attain jobs they find interesting and socially valuable, this rationale enables many students to believe that by improving their writing abilities, they would be able to realize their authentic goals and values and therefore feel autonomous. Consistent with this view, Assor et al. (2002) and Assor and Kaplan (2001) have shown that the provision of a sound rationale to students in elementary school, middle school, or high school was a particularly good predictor of engagement and positive feelings regarding studying. Other research, conducted with adolescents and young adults in Israel and the USA, also supports the benefits of providing a rationale for actions expected from children (e.g., Deci, Eghrari, Patrick, & Leone, 1994; Koestner, Ryan, Bernieri, & Holt, 1984; Roth et al., 2009). In all these studies, it was found that children showed more autonomous motivation to act in accordance with adults' requests when adults provided a rationale for their requests.

Supporting Choice and Initiation

This attribute directly supports the striving for optional choice. Studies examining the impact of choice provision on the motivation to perform a relatively uninteresting task or on effort investment in class have shown that choice provision often enhances autonomous motivation and positive feelings while working on the task at hand (e.g., Assor et al., 2002; Cordova & Lepper, 1996; Deci et al., 1994; Katz & Assor, 2007; Reynolds & Symons, 2001; Zuckerman, Porac, Lathin, Smith, & Deci, 1978).

However, Katz and Assor (2007) noted that choice may be unimportant or even frustrating when students do not have clear goals or values or when the options available do not allow realization of students' goals and values. For example, Katz and Assor described research showing that when students can work on a task that they are highly interested in, the choice factor makes no difference. That is, students show similar (high) level of autonomous motivation irrespective of whether they were given choice on not given choice. Thus, it appears that if one is able to do what one values as important or interesting, the provision of choice becomes insignificant. Thus, choice appears to be important mainly when it allows student to better realize their interests and values, or at least avoid activities that undermine their interests or values.

Intrinsic Value Demonstration

This attribute refers to the demonstration of valued attributes and behaviors by parents and teachers. It is important that the people demonstrating the valued behavior would not only enact it often but would also fully identify with it and perhaps would also appear to enjoy it. These feelings indicate that the behavior is worth engaging in, and as a result, children may feel that they really want to adopt these behaviors and they do not have to be forced to do them. IVD differs from modeling in that in IVD, it is important not only that the behavior is demonstrated often but also that the modeled behavior appears intrinsically worthy (valuable and/or enjoyable). IVD might be even more convincing than the provision of rationale because rather than talking about the importance of the valued behavior, you demonstrate its value in your own life and ongoing actions.

The identification with the demonstrated valued behaviors helps children to internalize values and goals around which their identity is formed and then renegotiated as they grow older (Erikson, 1950, 1968). As such, IVD by significant others may be necessary to support one key striving constituting the need for autonomy, namely, the striving for the formation of authentic direction-giving values and goals. One implication of the important role of IVD in the formation of values and goals is that when parents and educators do not provide IVD, youth may find it very difficult to feel that they have authentic values and goals that they really identify with and experience as a source of perceived autonomy and vitality. Thus, lack of IVD by significant others, especially in the moral, religious, and character domain, may lead to a state of identity diffusion that is characterized by the feeling and the belief that nothing is really valuable and worthy to put effort into (e.g., Assor, 2011; Marcia, Waterman, Matteson, Archer, & Orlofsky, 1993). And indeed, research carried by Cohen-Malayev (2009) (see also Assor, Cohen-Malayev et al., 2005; Cohen-Malayev, Assor, & Kaplan, 2009) indicates that young adults raised in modern Orthodox Jewish families had significant difficulties developing a firm and satisfying religious identity and experienced many of the features characterizing identity diffusion when their parents were low on IVD of religious behavior.

The first study demonstrating the value of IVD from an SDT perspective was conducted by Roth and Assor (2000). They found that Israeli college students' perceptions of their parents as demonstrating the intrinsic value of prosocial actions predicted autonomous prosocial motivation, which in turn predicted students' engagement in prosocial behavior. All variables in this research were assessed via students' self-reports, and therefore the findings may, in part, reflect self-report bias.

A second, and more comprehensive, study of the correlates of IVD was conducted by Roth et al. (2009) with ninth-grade Israeli adolescents. IVD was assessed via items such as "My mom enjoys studying and expanding her knowledge." In addition, the study also assessed parents' perspective taking and rationale provision when the parent and child disagreed about how much studying the child should do. Results showed that adolescents' perceptions of their parents as using the practices of IVD, perspective taking, and rationale provision in the academic domain predicted adolescents' sense of choice with regard to studying, which in turn predicted teacher ratings of adolescents as showing interest-focused engagement in learning. The participants in the study came from diverse socioeconomic backgrounds, but there was no information available on the socioeconomic status of each participant; consequently potential effects of SES on the relations detected were not examined.

Another interesting finding in that research pertained to adolescents' perception of their parents as using the practice of conditional positive regard. Conditional Positive Regard (CPR) in the academic domain involves the provision of more affection and esteem when the child studies and achieves more. It was found that CPR, unlike the autonomy supportive practices, predicted feelings of internal compulsion with regard to studying, which in turn predicted teacher ratings of adolescents' engagement as grade-focused rather than interest-focused. (see Roth et al., 2009). It should be noted that the correlation between CPR and IVD was very low and not significant.

The importance of modeling, a construct somewhat similar to IVD, for engagement in prosocial acts has long been demonstrated by empirical research (see Eisenberg, Fabes, & Spinrad, 2006). However, so far there is almost no research comparing IVD and modeling in the domain of prosocial behavior.

Intrinsic value demonstration obviously does not apply to domains which students may find interesting and educators may value yet have no expertise or interest in. For example, adolescents may develop a serious individual interest in a musical instrument or a certain kind of art or sports domain which the parents know little about. In such cases, of course, parents cannot engage in IVD. However, if they value the development of intrinsic interests, engagement, and competence in their children and/or value the domain, they can rely on other autonomy supportive practices to foster the continual engagement and growth of their child within the relevant domain. For example, they can minimize controls and provide choice and, in addition, also support their child's need for competence by helping them find a teacher who presents optimal challenges and feedback (for applied implications of this point, see Madjar & Assor, in press).

Moreover, although parents may not be able to engage in IVD in the specific domain the child is interested in, they can demonstrate the value of general attitudes and skills that can help their children to persist and overcome difficulties in the domain they have chosen. For example, parents can show persistence and task-oriented coping skills in their personal hobby or some volunteer work, and their children can then adopt this orientation and skills in their specific interest domain.

While IVD may not be crucial to the development of individual interests, it is likely to be especially important in the moral, prosocial, and emotion regulation domains (Assor, 2011), and to some extent also in the academic domain. In these domains, the great majority of parents and teachers believe that it is important that their children adopt certain values and attitudes, for example, being honest, responsible, and considerate; regulating one's anger and aggressive reactions in order to avoid inflicting extreme pain on others or avoid undermining one's own future chances; and being able to persist in the face of difficulties in the pursuit of important self-determined goals. In all these domains, parents are likely to face significant difficulties in transmitting their values to their children if they do not demonstrate these valued behaviors in their every day conduct.

Importantly, if parents demonstrate behaviors and use additional autonomy supportive methods (such as minimizing controls, perspective taking, rationale, and choice), the demonstrated behaviors can serve as a potential foundation for offspring's sense of authentic self and identity. In particular, deep internalization of parents' values is more likely to occur if parents support adolescents' inclination to seriously examine the values endorsed and demonstrated by them. Research supporting this idea is presented in the next section which focuses on the practice of supporting value and goal examination.

The role of IVD in supporting the construction of direction-giving values and goals might be especially important in postmodern western societies and perhaps also to other societies in a globalized world (e.g., Aviram & Assor, 2010). In these societies, clear guidelines regarding the worthy and unworthy do not exist anymore due to increasing moral relativism, and the collapse of traditional moral and ideological authorities and norms. As in postmodern societies it is less possible to rely on recognized societal authorities and traditions, IVD by parents and teachers can fill an important social gap and become a particularly important source of authentic direction-giving values and goals, which then provide a relatively solid basis for youth emerging identity and future goals.

It appears then that the accumulating experience of being exposed to adults who have again and again demonstrated the value of certain values and virtues, and at the same time were careful not to force these values on their children, is likely to create a deep appreciation for the importance of these values and virtues even in a cynical and morally relativistic world. Consistent with the above view, it is probable that students would be much more engaged in various school-related activities if the intrinsic value of persistence, trying to understand things in depth, high-quality performance, and learning were often demonstrated by their parents and teachers in their own behavior. However, among adolescents in postmodern western cultures, IVD may not be sufficient to promote persistent engagement in learning (or other parentally valued activities) and might have to be complemented by educators' willingness to support youth inclination to examine parentally valued behaviors in terms of their own personal judgements, goals and values. The next section focuses on the practice of support for value examination and its potential contribution to youth engagement in various tasks.

Supporting Value/Goal/Interest Examination

This practice refers to acts that encourage youth to engage in activities, experiences, and discussions that allow them to examine and reflect seriously and critically on their goals, values, and interests. The notion of support for value examination (SVE) is illustrated in Table 20.1 via items of a scale assessing school-based support for value examination (Assor, 2010, 2011; Kanat-Maymon & Assor, 2011). As the concept of SVE is fairly new, research demonstrating the utility of this scale is only now emerging and is described in the following sections.

While SVE shares some similarities with perspective taking, it also differs from the latter in that in a typical perspective-taking act, the child already has relatively clear feelings or desires, which the educator tries to understand. In contrast, in the case of SVE, the youngster does not

Table 20.1 A scale assessing school support for value examination (SVE)

1. The activities/studies in school sometimes cause me to think about important things I would like to do in my life
2. The activities/studies in school help me to find out what are the things I value in people
3. School studies/activities enable me to examine my attitude to important issues in life
4. School studies/activities do *not* provide me with opportunities to examine important questions that I am concerned with (Reverse coded)
5. School studies/activities cause me to think of traits (attributes) I would like to have
6. School studies/activities help me to think about just and desirable ways of acting in complex situations
7. School studies/activities help me to think about what is more important and what is less important in life

Students respond to the above items on a 5-point Likert scale

know what she/he feels or wants, and it is the role of the educator to support an active, reflective, open-ended search of what one truly values, wants and feels. SVE also shares some similarities with choice provision. However, here too, the options may not be clear or they do not even exist at the present. But, as part of the exploration process they can be discovered or created.

As depicted in Fig. 20.2, the examination and reflection process is assumed to be part of a larger integration process, in which youth construct direction-giving, authentic goals, values, and interests (i.e., an inner compass). In Fig. 20.2, the process is depicted as a linear one. However, in reality, the process may often be spiral; for example, sense of autonomy may support deeper reflection and examination of one's goals and values. However, there is a general progress in the direction depicted in Fig. 20.2.

Following Ryan and Deci (2000), I view the integration process as a gradual attempt to resolve intra- and interpersonal inconsistencies between important goals and values (including conflicts between parents' and teachers' values and new ideas the adolescent develops). This can be accomplished by prioritizing goals and modifying practices so they fit together and, most importantly, so they reflect one's authentic inclinations, values, and goals. However, before goals and values can be prioritized, they have to be seriously examined. The exploration process allows such an examination.

As shown in Fig. 20.2, an open and reflective examination process is assumed to advance a deep integration process, one in which values and goals are experienced as authentic, fit each other, and are embedded in a rich world view. As cognitive-emotional structures, these values constitute elaborate, multilevel categories. Consequently, when youth hold a certain value, they not only endorse abstract categories such as social justice or self-direction (as is typically the case in value questionnaires), but they also have representations of specific attitudes and actions reflecting these values, as well cultural and historical narratives, symbols, and memories associated with these values. The formation of such integrated schemas is assumed to support youth sense of autonomy and also contributes directly to the enactment of demanding actions (e.g., Assor, 1999). Sense of autonomy is then assumed to enhance vitality and positive affect, as well as engagement in demanding actions. Empirical evidence for the processes depicted above is presented below.

As was already noted, the formation of integrated, direction-giving values and goals might be especially important in postmodern western societies in which clear guidelines regarding the worthy and unworthy do not exist anymore (see Aviram & Assor, 2010). Under these conditions, reflection-based integrated values and goals may be a crucial source of sense of autonomy and therefore vitality. These integrated values and goals can then provide a solid foundation for an identity that can resist the pressures and pulls of passing fads and contradictory cultural beliefs.

The above model was supported by two research projects. The first set of studies (Assor, 2010, 2011; Kanat-Maymon & Assor, 2011) focused on adolescents' perceptions of the extent to which their schools or their youth movement contexts support value and goal examination. The second project focused on parents' support for value examination in the religious domain.

Inspection of the model in Fig. 20.3 indicates that the first research project focused on two components of the comprehensive model presented

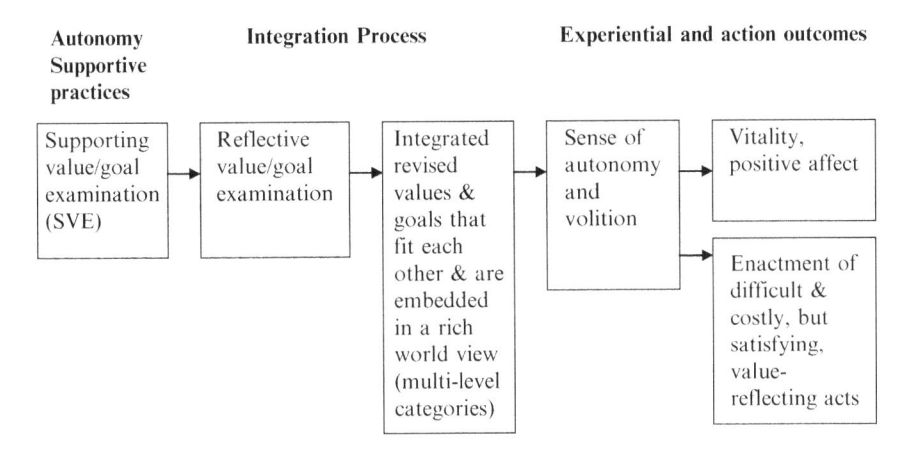

Fig. 20.2 The process by which support for value examination (*SVE*) is assumed to promote the formation of integrated and authentic values/goals and consequent positive outcomes

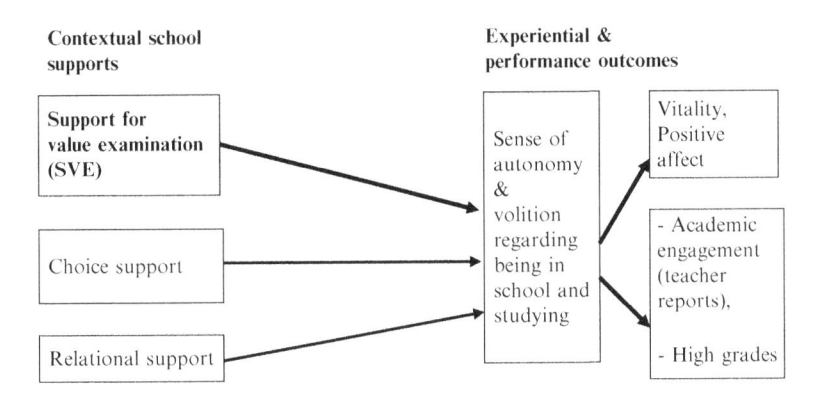

Fig. 20.3 The model examined in research project 1: SVE as a predictor of perceived autonomy and consequent affective and behavioral outcomes in educational contexts

in Fig. 20.2. Specifically, this project focused on SVE as a predictor of perceived autonomy and consequent positive outcomes. As can be seen from Fig. 20.3, this research did not examine the hypothesis that SVE promotes an integrative value examination process which then leads to the formation of authentic and elaborate value and goal schemas. This aspect of the comprehensive model is examined in the second project to be described later.

The first test of the model described in Fig. 20.3 was conducted with adolescents (11th grade) who completed a self-report questionnaire assessing the variable of interest with regard to their schools (Assor, 2010). Adolescents came from four schools serving students coming mostly from middle class neighborhoods. Factor analysis indicated that students clearly distinguished between school supports for value examination, choice, and relatedness. The construct validity of the SVE scale (presented in Table 20.1) was supported by the finding that this scale was unrelated to social desirability or neuroticism measures. Moreover, as expected, perceptions of the school context as high on SVE were positively and significantly associated with reporting that studying and participating in school activities increased the importance of the intrinsic values of community contribution, self-understanding, and health, and at the same time reduced the importance of the extrinsic values of wealth and power and prestige (see Kasser & Ryan, 1996 on intrinsic versus extrinsic values).

The degree to which participating in school activities increased or decreased the importance of intrinsic or extrinsic values was assessed via a questionnaire which included a list of 15 items reflecting the three intrinsic values noted above and 10 items reflecting the two extrinsic values. In relation to each item, participants were asked to indicate: "To what extent did the activities, studies and discussions in school strengthen or weaken your belief in the following values, goals and aspirations?" The response scale ranged from 1(weakened the importance of this value for me) to 5 (strengthened the importance of this value for me). An example of an extrinsic value is "being wealthy," and an example of intrinsic value is "work for the improvement of society." Each value was assessed via five items.

According to SDT, authentic value examination should connect people with their basic needs and the intrinsic values associated with them. Therefore, the positive correlations between SVE and enhanced intrinsic values and the negative correlation between SVE and enhanced extrinsic values suggested that the process assessed by our measure of SVE indeed promoted a relatively authentic, intrinsically oriented value examination.

Results of structural equation modeling and mediation analyses confirmed that perceptions of the school as supporting value examination predicted perceived autonomy regarding studying in the school, which in turn predicted engagement in studying and feelings of vitality while in school. Interestingly, choice support did not have a unique effect on the outcomes examined (i.e., choice provision was not significantly associated with engagement and vitality when the effects of SVE were also considered). Importantly, the effects of SVE were detected also when the effects of choice support were statistically controlled for. Together, these findings indicate that SVE may be a more important determinant of student engagement and vitality in high school.

The second test of the model was conducted with many of the adolescents who completed questionnaires on their school context. However, in this part of the study, the context and the investment referred to youth movement activities (Assor, 2010; Kanat-Maymon & Assor, 2011). The term "youth movement" refers to informal education set ups like the scouts or other frameworks. Specifically, the youth movement studied was the Israeli Scouts, which is an organization that tries to promote youth activities that contribute to society, as well as conduct social activities and nature trips. The instructors in this setup are typically only several years older than the members of the group, and the relation between instructors and members is rather informal.

Results again highlighted the importance of SVE as a predictor of perceived autonomy and consequent positive outcomes. Choice support again had no unique effect. The fact that choice support did not have a unique effect suggests that perhaps the choices offered to students were not sufficiently meaningful to students, and consequently, the provision of choice did not have positive effects.

One limitation of the first two studies was their complete reliance on students' self-report measures. This problem was addressed by the second study (Assor, 2010; Kanat-Maymon & Assor, 2011), in which students' engagement in studying was assessed by teacher ratings. In addition, students' grades and student-rated positive affect were also assessed. Results were consistent with the results of the first two studies. The third study (Assor, 2010; Kanat-Maymon & Assor, 2011) used the same measures employed in the third study but, in addition, also included two additional scales: social desirability and students' perception of teacher as providing warmth and caring (relational support). Results again replicated the findings of previous studies, showing that SVE had unique positive effects on teacher-rated student engagement, student grades, and student-rated positive affect.

In sum, the studies described in this section suggest that when adolescents and children feel that being in their school (or in the youth movement) helps them to form personal goals and values, this promotes a sense of autonomy and volition regarding being in the school (or the youth movement), which in turn leads to increased engagement, vitality, and positive affect. Importantly, in all these studies, perceived support for value examination (SVE) had unique positive effects on perceived autonomy, investment, and well-being also when perceived choice and perceived teacher warmth and caring were statistically controlled for. In fact, SVE consistently had considerably stronger effects on perceived autonomy, investment, and well-being than did choice support. This is not surprising in view of other studies showing that choice provision is useful only when the choices are meaningful or when choice recipients have clear interests and goals (e.g., Assor et al., 2002; Katz & Assor, 2007). The detection of unique effects of SVE is of special interest because it indicates that SVE is a unique component of autonomy support and consequent engagement and well-being. Thus, provision of choice and relational support may not be enough to promote desired student processes and outcomes. Moreover, the fact the SVE had unique effects beyond two other positive teacher supports indicates that the positive effects of SVE cannot be ascribed to a general positive perception of the teacher or the youth movement instructor. However, one limitation of the above studies is their reliance on correlations, which precludes conclusions regarding causal inferences.

The second research project examined the complete model depicted in Fig. 20.1, referring to the process by which SVE is assumed to promote the construction of integrated, direction-giving goals and values and consequent positive outcomes. This research project was conducted by Cohen-Malayev and her colleagues (Assor, Cohen-Melayev et al., 2005; Cohen-Malayev, 2009; Cohen-Malayev et al., 2009). Participants were modern Orthodox Jewish students in Israel, coming from religious homes who also embraced modern technology and ways of life, and were therefore exposed to views and materials disseminated by the secular mass media. Moreover, these students also studied in a nonreligious and fairly secular institution. Because the norms and values of the secular contexts and of Orthodox Judaism often differ widely, modern Orthodox Jewish students face a rather demanding task of forming values and goals that integrate contradictory religious and secular viewpoints in ways that feel coherent, authentic, and autonomous. To enable these youth to cope with the value integration task successfully, parents and teachers may need to be particularly understanding and supportive of their children's need to examine values and goals gradually and thoroughly. Thus, the practice of SVE might be particularly important in the case of modern Orthodox Jewish youth.

Cohen-Malayev and her colleagues (e.g., Assor, Cohen-Melayev, et al., 2005; Cohen-Malayev, 2009) conducted two quantitative studies and one qualitative study. The quantitative study was based mainly on free-response questionnaires asking participants coming from a modern Orthodox Jewish background to describe their experiences, feelings, and thoughts on religion, challenges they face in this domain, and ways of coping with these challenges. In addition, all the variables appearing in Fig. 20.3 were also assessed by questionnaires developed for this purpose (using Likert type scales). The questionnaires were validated via small space analyses (see Guttman, 1968) and correlations supporting their divergent and convergent validity relative to other measures (see Assor, Cohen-Melayev, et al., 2005; Cohen-Malayev, 2009). Results of qualitative analyses, as well as regression analyses and cluster analyses, generally supported the model presented in Fig. 20.3.

Qualitative analysis of the free response questionless indicated that contribution of SVE to the development of integrated values, perceived autonomy, and consequent positive outcomes was particularly apparent in relation to the issue of women's roles. This contribution and process is summarized in Fig. 20.4.

The issue of women's role in Jewish religion is particularly problematic for modern Orthodox Jewish women studying in nonreligious colleges because in Orthodox Judaism, women are not allowed to take leading religious roles. However, these religious norms are clearly inconsistent with the values and norms of the surrounding secular college context regarding gender roles and egalitarianism. Consistent with our general

```
Autonomy              Integration Process           Experiential and Action Outcomes
Supportive
Practices
```

Parents support the examination of religious values (SVE): Parents encourage examination of different approaches to women's role in Jewish religious practices	→	Examination of values & practices: Youth examine different religious and non religious approaches to women's role in religion and in general	→	Integrated religious values and views: Youth revise values & views concerning women's role in religion, so they fit her other values and general world view	→	Sense of autonomy: Youth feel authentic and autonomous regarding religious practices because the problem of women's role in religion is beginning to be resolved	→	Well-being, self-acceptance
							→	Enacting difficult religious practices in ways that are consistent with the revised values

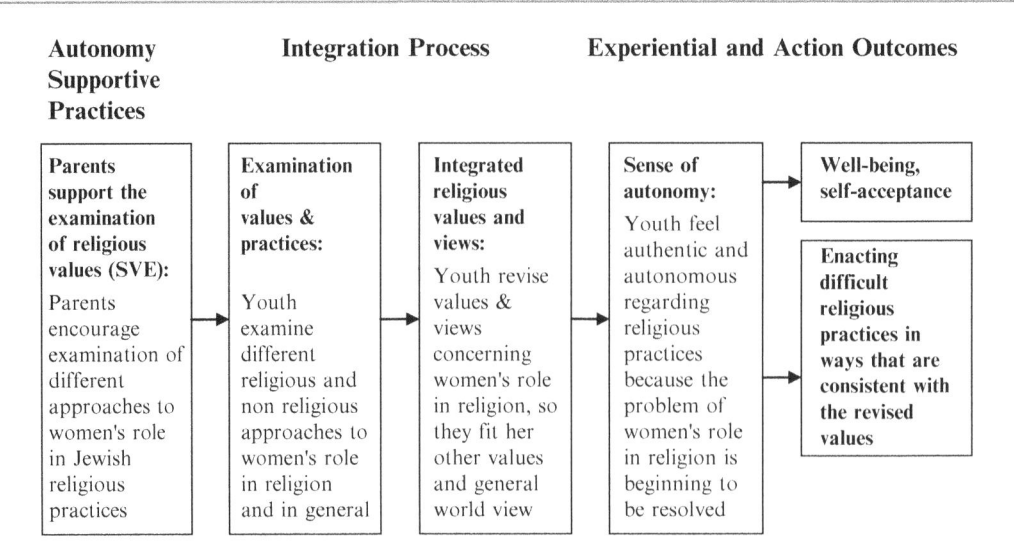

Fig. 20.4 Effects of SVE on the integration of religious values concerning women's roles and consequent outcomes in modern orthodox Jewish youth

model, we found that when parents encourage young women to examine different approaches to women's role in religion, these young women are indeed more inclined to examine this issue through talks with different people and by studying different sources (e.g., Assor, Cohen-Melayev, et al., 2005). This examination and reflection process then helps women to revise their values and views concerning women's religious role so that these values and views then fit their more liberal and egalitarian world view. For example, they now endorse a practice where women are allowed to lead prayer or sit next to men in the synagogue. As a result, these women feel more autonomous and experience better well-being and are also are more willing to enact difficult religious practices that do not pertain to women's role. Importantly, when compared to women whose parents did not support religious value examination, women whose parents did support value examination (SVE) showed a similar level of religious behavioral enactment of religious practices, but for these women (those receiving high SVE), this enactment was accompanied by a higher level of sense of autonomy and well-being.

Similar findings were obtained in relation to another difficult religious issue: women's sexual behavior and appearance. In Orthodox Judaism, women's sexual behavior is expected to be rather conservative. These religious norms are clearly inconsistent with the less conservative values and norms of the surrounding secular college context. As was the case for women's gender roles, here too parents' support for value examination promoted a value examination process that yielded values and beliefs that integrated modern secular views regarding sexual behavior with traditional Jewish Orthodox commandments. For example, women who conducted value examination in this domain allowed themselves to wear clothing items that although not seductive, are considered illegitimate in most orthodox religious circles.

While the results of our studies generally supported the proposed model, there was one unexpected, yet interesting, finding in the second quantitative study, which employed more refined measures (see Cohen-Malayev, 2009). Thus, results of separate cluster analyses yielded two types of examination: revisionist and orthodox. In revisionist value examination, there is a more comprehensive exploration of religious principles in relation to nonreligious ideas, as a result of introspection and a personal spiritual quest. For example, in revisionist examination, a woman can ask herself why is it that women are not allowed to be Rabbis. In orthodox examination, there is an examination of more practical issues, with an attempt to seek answers by consulting various religious sources. For example, a woman feels uncomfortable with various sex-related prohibitions or commandments and therefore tries to see if there is a way of doing things differently that is more in line with what she feels and yet is also acceptable to some religious authorities.

Interestingly, it was found that when SVE was associated with parents' demonstration of the intrinsic value of religious practices (IVD), it led to a more limited value examination, whereas when SVE was not accompanied by IVD, it led to the more comprehensive revisionist examination. Moreover, perhaps not surprisingly, orthodox examination was more predictive of: (a) self acceptance, (b) positive relations with other people, and (c) enactment of traditional religious practices (Cohen-Malayev, 2009).

It appears, then, that when parents provide a convincing and authentic demonstration of the practices they would like to transmit (IVD), and in addition also support value examination (SVE), youth may not feel a need to seriously challenge their parents' values and thus engage in a more limited type of value examination. This limited examination tries to modify parents' values so they fit better with offspring's everyday needs and constraints. Importantly, this limited exploration also seems to promote somewhat greater well-being in the sense of more peaceful relations with self and others. Thus, in contrast to what a romantic view of identity exploration might suggest, it is possible that for most youth, the more natural and preferred type of exploration is gradual and nonradical, that is, exploration that gradually builds on values that are already well internalized and only need minor revisions.

While the studies focusing on religious behavior did not focus on student motivation and engagement, they appear to have important implications for the domain of religious education in countries other than Israel, and in particular, religious education of youth that is exposed to the general mass media and secular ideas and lifestyles. Thus, it appears that religious schools that would support value examination in the religious domain are likely to help students to develop values and views that would enable them to feel more autonomous and more vital in relation to their religious behavior. The school's willingness to address these religious questions openly and seriously may also result in an increased willingness to attend the school and to participate in various nonreligious school activities (as was the case for the students studied by Assor and Kanat-Maymon [Assor, 2010, 2011; Kanat-Maymon & Assor, 2011]).

As we end the discussion of SVE, I would like to present one note of caution regarding this generally desirable autonomy supportive practice. Although the first studies on SVE suggest that it has fairly positive correlates, it is possible that educators support for value examination can sometimes fail to enhance perceived autonomy because the exploration is too difficult or confusing. To increase the likelihood that support for value examination would result in value and goal integration, commitment, and vitality, it appears important to support a special type of examination, which can be termed *Optimal* Support for Value Examination (OSVE). Optimal support for value examination can include:

(a) Gradual exposure of adolescents to views and experiences that might lead them to examine their goals and values
(b) Help in reflecting on the new ideas and their potentially unsettling personal implications

Future research may attempt to identify the attributes of optimal versus harmful ways of encouraging value and goal examination in youth. However, research conducted by Assor and his colleagues (Assor, 2010, 2011; Madjar, Assor, & Dotan, 2010) already identified one educational attribute that appears to increase the capacity of adolescents to engage in value examination also when this examination is difficult and confusing. This attribute is discussed in the next section.

Table 20.2 Items illustrating the three components of FIV

1. *Enhancing children's ability to withstand confusion and take their time before they make serious decisions*
   "When other kids pressure me to accept their opinion, my mom let's me feel that it is better to take the time and calm down before I decide what to do"
2. *Encouraging examination of one's authentic values and goals when faced with a difficult decision or social pressures*
   "When I have to make a tough decision, my mom encourages me to first examine what I think is the right and desirable thing to do"
3. *Encouraging consideration of alternatives and relevant information before making a decision*
   "As a child, when I had to choose what to do, my mom and me thought together on the consequences of each possible choice"

Fostering Inner-Directed Valuing Processes

FIV is another autonomy supportive practice which promotes the formation and realization of authentic direction-giving values, goals, and interests. This construct refers to a cluster of educator's behaviors which help students pay attention to their *authentic* values and needs more than to social pressures. FIV is important because it is posited to enhance youth capacity to persist in the often frustrating task of exploring one's authentic goals, values, and interests, as well as strengthen their capacity to make decisions based on their authentic values and needs. As such, FIV can be viewed as training in authentic decision making.

More specifically, FIV is assumed to include three components: (a) enhancing students' ability to withstand confusion and take their time before they make serious decisions, (b) encouraging the examination of one's values and goals when faced with a difficult decision and/or social pressures, and (c) encouraging the consideration of alternatives and relevant information before making a decision. FIV differs from general support for value examination in that it is a socializing practice that is used only when the child faces difficult decisions and social pressures, and unlike SVE, it provides a certain "training" in authentic and rational decision making under stress.

Items assessing parents, fostering of inner-directed valuing processes (FIV) are presented in Table 20.2.

Figure 20.5 shows how FIV is posited to operate together with SVE in supporting reflective value and goal examination, and consequent perceived autonomy and its positive outcomes.

Inspection of Fig. 20.5 shows that FIV and SVE are assumed to have additive influence on reflective value and goal examination. However, future research may examine the possibility that FIV may also moderate the effects of SVE on value examination. This moderating effect may occur because although SVE may foster the initial urge to engage in value examination, FIV may allow this examination to proceed when the exploration process gets difficult and confusing.

Research on the correlates and potential benefits of FIV has just begun. The first study focusing on this construct (see Assor, 2009, 2011; Madjar et al., 2010) showed that adolescents' perceptions of their parents as high on FIV were found to predict identity exploration and the formation of commitments that are experienced as autonomous. In this study, FIV was also found to predict adolescents' capacity to experience anger and anxiety without losing control or immediately suppressing these feelings, as well as their tendency to try to understand the sources of these feelings and the implications of these feelings for one's life and relationships.

So far, research did not examine the implications of FIV for engagement in studying and school activities. However, it is reasonable to assume that the increased capacity for inner valuing and for resisting social pressure would enable students to engage in studies that are less popular

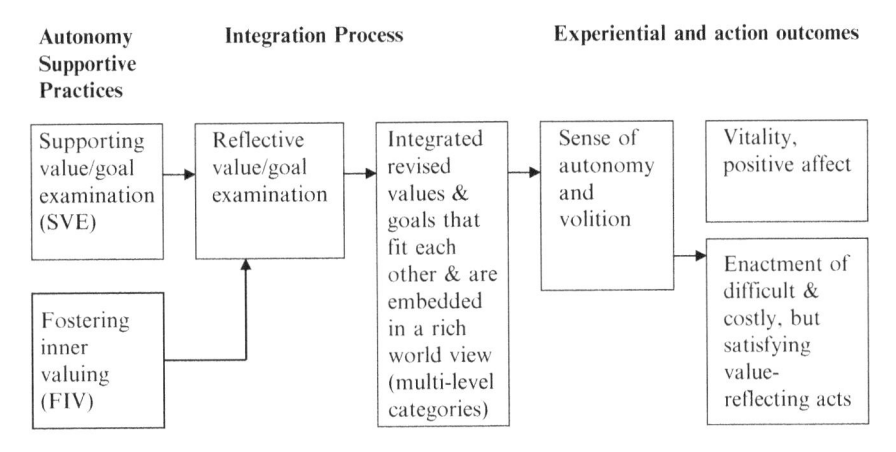

Fig. 20.5 The joint contribution of FIV and SVE to integrated values/goals and consequent positive outcomes

but are interesting for them. In addition, increased capacity to tolerate ambiguity during the exploration of one's authentic interests and values may enable students to engage in a more thorough examination of various subjects relevant to their emerging interests, goals, and values.

Conclusion

Summing up, in this chapter I focused on seven practices of autonomy support which are likely to promote two major components of the need for autonomy: (a) lack of coercion and optional choice and (b) formation and realization of an inner compass: authentic, direction-giving values, goals, and interests. A special emphasis was put on three autonomy supportive practices which are assumed to support formation and realization of authentic, direction-giving values, goals, and interests, whose impact on perceived autonomy was not sufficiently examined so far: (a) IVD – intrinsic value demonstration, (b) SVE – support for value/goal/interest examination, and (c) FIV – fostering inner-directed valuing processes. The autonomy supportive practices that foster the development of stable authentic values and goals might be especially important in western countries, in which postmodern moral relativism and the abundance of information and options make it particularly difficult for youth to form stable and authentic values and goals.

In future research, it may be interesting to examine the unique contributions to students' school engagement and well-being of the three autonomy supportive practices that were relatively underemphasized in SDT-based research: intrinsic value demonstration (IVD), support for value examination (SVE), and fostering inner valuing (FIV). In this research, it would be important to assess autonomy support practices and outcomes based on measures that are not based solely on self-reports, using longitudinal designs that can point to possible causal effects.

References

Assor, A. (1999). Value accessibility and teachers' ability to encourage independent and critical thought in students. *Social Psychology of Education, 2*, 1–24.

Assor, A. (2010). *Two under-emphasized components of autonomy support: Supporting value examination and inner valuing*. Paper presented in the 4th international conference on self determination theory, Gent, Belgium.

Assor, A. (2011). Autonomous moral motivation: Consequences, socializing antecedents and the unique role of integrated moral principles. In M. Mikulincer & P. R. Shaver (Eds.), *Social psychology of morality: Exploring the causes of good and evil*. Washington, DC: American Psychological Association.

Assor, A., Cohen-Melayev, M., Kaplan, A., & Friedman, D. (2005). Choosing to stay religious in a modern world: Socialization and exploration processes leading to an integrated internalization of religion among Israeli Jewish youth. *Advances in Motivation and Achievement, 14*, 105–150.

Assor, A., & Kaplan, H. (2001). Mapping the domain of autonomy support: Five important ways to enhance or undermine students' experience of autonomy in learning. In A. Efklides, R. Sorrentino, & J. Kuhl (Eds.), *Trends and prospects in motivation research* (pp. 99–118). Dordrecht, The Netherlands: Kluwer.

Assor, A., Kaplan, H., Kanat-Maymon, Y., & Roth, G. (2005). Directly controlling teacher behaviors as predictors of poor motivation and engagement in girls and boys: The role of anger and anxiety. *Learning and Instruction, 15*, 397–413.

Assor, A., Kaplan, H., & Roth, G. (2002). Choice is good, but relevance is excellent: Autonomy-enhancing and suppressing teaching behaviors predicting students' engagement in schoolwork. *British Journal of Educational Psychology, 27*, 261–278.

Assor, A., & Roth, G. (2005). Conditional love as a socializing approach: Costs and alternatives. *Scientific Annals of the Psychological Society of Northern Greece, 7*, 17–34.

Assor, A., Roth, G., & Deci, E. L. (2004). The emotional costs of parents' conditional regard: A self-determination theory analysis. *Journal of Personality, 72*, 47–88.

Assor, A., Roth, G., Israeli, M., & Freed, A. (2007). *The harmful costs of parental conditional regard*. Paper presented in the Society for Research in Child Development, Boston.

Assor, A., Vansteenkiste, M., & Kaplan, A. (2009). Identified versus introjected-approach and introjected-avoidance motivations in school and in sports: The limited benefits of self-worth strivings. *Journal of Educational Psychology, 2*, 482–497.

Aviram, R., & Assor, A. (2010). In defense of personal autonomy as a fundamental educational aim in liberal democracies. *Oxford Review of Education, 36*, 111–126.

Barber, B. K. (1996). Parental psychological control: Revisiting a neglected construct. *Child Development, 67*, 3296–3319.

Barber, B. K., Stolz, H., & Olsen, J. (2005). Parental support, psychological control, and behavioral control: Assessing relevance across time, culture, and method. *Monographs of the Society for Research in Child Development, 70*, 1–151.

Baumeister, R. F., & Leary, M. R. (1995). The need to belong: Desire for interpersonal attachments as a fundamental human motivation. *Psychological Bulletin, 117*, 497–529.

Berlin, I. (1969). *Four essays on liberty*. Oxford, UK: Oxford University Press.

Cohen-Malayev, M. (2009). *Religious exploration and identity – The tension between religion and religiosity: Examination of the internalization process of Jewish religious values in modern-orthodox context*. Doctoral dissertation, Ben Gurion University, Be'er-Sheva, Israel.

Cohen-Malayev, M., Assor, A., & Kaplan, A. (2009). Religious exploration in a modern world: The case of Modern-Orthodox Jews in Israel. *Identity: An International Journal of Theory and Research, 9*, 233–251.

Cordova, D. I., & Lepper, M. R. (1996). Intrinsic motivation and the process of learning: Beneficial effects of contextualization, personalization and choice. *Journal of Educational Psychology, 88*, 715–730.

Deci, E. L., Eghrari, H., Patrick, B. C., & Leone, D. R. (1994). Facilitating internalization: The self-determination theory perspective. *Journal of Personality, 62*, 119–142.

Deci, E. L., Koestner, R., & Ryan, R. M. (1999). A meta-analytic review of experiments examining the effects of extrinsic rewards on intrinsic motivation. *Psychological Bulletin, 125*, 627–668.

Deci, E. L., & Ryan, R. M. (1985). *Intrinsic motivation and self-determination in human behavior*. New York: Plenum Press.

Eisenberg, N., Fabes, R. A., & Spinrad, T. L. (2006). Prosocial development. In R. M. Lerner, N. Eisenberg, & W. Damon (Eds.), *Handbook of child psychology: Vol. 3. Social, emotional and personality development* (pp. 646–718). New York: Wiley.

Elliot, A. J., & Dweck, C. S. (2005). *Handbook of competence and motivation*. New York: Guilford Press.

Epley, A., Morewedge, C. K., & Keysar, B. (2004). Perspective taking in children and adults: Equivalent egocentrism but differential correction. *Journal of Experimental Social Psychology, 40*, 760–768.

Erikson, E. (1950). *Childhood and society*. New York: W. W. Norton.

Erikson, E. (1968). *Identity: Youth and crisis*. New York: W. W. Norton.

Fromm, E. (1941). *Escape from freedom*. New York: Rinehart.

Gottfried, A. E., Marcoulides, G. A., Gottfried, A. W., Oliver, P. H., & Guerin, D. W. (2007). Multivariate latent change modeling of developmental decline in academic intrinsic math motivation and achievement: Childhood through adolescence. *International Journal of Behavioral Development, 31*, 317–327.

Grolnick, W. S., Deci, E. L., & Ryan, R. M. (1997). Internalization within the family: The self-determination theory perspective. In J. E. Grusec & L. Kuczynski (Eds.), *Parenting and children's internalization of values* (pp. 135–161). New York: Wiley.

Guttman, L. (1968). A general nonmetric technique for finding the smallest coordinate space for a configuration of points. *Psychometrika, 33*, 469–506.

Iyengar, S. S., & Lepper, M. R. (2000). When choice is demotivating: Can one desire too much of a good thing? *Journal of Personality and Social Psychology, 79*, 995–1006.

Kasser, T., & Ryan, R. M. (1996). Further examining the American dream: Differential correlates of intrinsic and extrinsic goals. *Personality and Social Psychology Bulletin, 22*, 80–87.

Kanat-Maymon, M., & Assor, A. (2010). Perceived Maternal Control and Responsiveness to Distress as Predictors of Young Adults' Empathic Responses. *Personality and Social Psychology Bulletin, 36*, 33–46.

Kanat-Maymon, Y. & Assor, A. (2011). Supporting Value Exploration: Another Important Aspect of Autonomy Support. Ben GUrion University, Israel: Unpublished manuscript.

Katz, I., & Assor, A. (2007). When choice motivates and when it does not. *Educational Psychology Review, 19*, 429–442.

Koestner, R., Ryan, R. M., Bernieri, F., & Holt, K. (1984). Setting limits on children's behavior: The differential effects of controlling versus informational styles on children's intrinsic motivation and creativity. *Journal of Personality, 54*, 233–248.

Madjar, N., & Assor, A. (in press). Two types of perceived control over learning: Perceived efficacy and perceived autonomy. In J. A. C. Hattie & E. M. Anderman (Eds.), *International handbook of student achievement*. New York: Routledge.

Madjar, N., Assor, A., & Dotan, L. (2010). *Fostering inner valuing processes in adolescents*. Paper presented in the convention of the American Educational Research Association, Denver, CO.

Marcia, J., Waterman, A., Matteson, D., Archer, S., & Orlofsky, J. (1993). *Ego identity*. New York: Springer.

Patall, E. A., Cooper, H., & Robinson, J. C. (2008). The effects of choice on intrinsic motivation and related outcomes: A meta-analysis of research findings. Psychological Bulletin, 134, 270–300.

Reeve, J. (2006). Teachers as facilitators: What autonomy-supportive teachers do and why their students benefit. *The Elementary School Journal, 106*, 225–236.

Reeve, J., & Assor, A. (2011). Do social institutions necessarily suppress individuals' need for autonomy? The possibility of schools as autonomy promoting contexts across the globe (pp. 111–132). In V. Chirkov, A. M. Ryan, & K. Sheldon (Eds.), *Personal autonomy in cultural context: Global perspectives on the psychology of freedom and people's well-being*. New York: Springer.

Reeve, J., & Jang, H. (2006). What teachers say and do to support students' autonomy during a learning activity. *Journal of Educational Psychology, 98*, 209–218.

Reynolds, P. L., & Symons, S. (2001). Motivational variables and children's text search. *Journal of Educational Psychology, 93*, 14–22.

Roth, G., & Assor, A. (2000). *The effect of conditional parental regard and intrinsic value demonstration on academic and pro-social motivation*. Paper presented at the conference of the European Association for Learning and Instruction (EARLI), Malmoe, Sweden.

Roth, G., Assor, A., Niemiec, P. C., Ryan, R. M., & Deci, E. L. (2009). The negative consequences of parental conditional regard: A comparison of positive conditional regard, negative conditional regard, and autonomy support as parenting strategies. *Developmental Psychology, 4*, 1119–1142.

Ryan, R. M., & Deci, E. L. (2000). Self-determination theory and the facilitation of intrinsic motivation, social development, and well-being. *American Psychologist, 55*, 68–78.

Soenens, B., Elliot, A. J., Goossens, L., Vansteenkiste, M., Luyten, P., & Duriez, B. (2005). The intergenerational transmission of perfectionism: Parents' psychological control as an intervening variable. *Journal of Family Psychology, 19*, 358–366.

Soenens, B., & Vansteenkiste, M. (2010). A theoretical upgrade of the concept of parental psychological control: Proposing new insights on the basis of self-determination theory. *Developmental Review, 30*, 74–99.

White, R. W. (1959). Motivation reconsidered: The concept of competence. *Psychological Review, 66*, 297–333.

Zuckerman, M., Porac, J., Lathin, D., Smith, R., & Deci, E. L. (1978). On the importance of self-determination for intrinsically motivated behavior. *Personality and Social Psychology Bulletin, 4*, 443–446.

The Engaging Nature of Teaching for Competency Development

21

Rosemary Hipkins

Abstract

Teachers' curricular intentions and the manner they construct learning opportunities in the classroom have an impact on engagement. This chapter is set in the context of a curriculum intention to develop senior high school students' competencies/capabilities, which has implications for the manner in which teachers 'talk up' reasons for engaging with learning. Differences in perceptions of the learning affordances their teachers offer are described for the students' most and least enjoyed subjects, with enjoyment standing as a proxy for emotional engagement. The responses of the teachers of each student's two classes add to the rich contextual picture of more and less engaging classroom learning contexts and point to the importance of creating spaces for metacognitive conversations about learning, and of supporting students to more actively link current learning to their personal lives. This is practically useful knowledge because many of the dimensions of engagement discussed can arguably be influenced by teachers' actions and beliefs.

Introduction

This chapter explores students' engagement with learning in their final years of schooling. Engagement is framed as active *participation* in learning with *competency* development in mind. The link to competencies is intended to capture the sense of engagement as 'energy in action' (Russell, Ainley, & Frydenberg, 2005). Following one much-cited literature review (Fredricks, Blumenfeld, & Paris, 2004), the scope of engagement is taken to encompass behavioural, cognitive and emotional dimensions of participation in learning. Motivation, by contrast, is taken to be about '*energy* and *direction*, the reasons for behaviour, why we do what we do' (Russell et al., 2005, p.3, emphasis in the original).

The nature of engaging classrooms is explored through the complementary lenses of 'opportunities to learn' (as orchestrated by the teacher) and 'affordances' that support and enable learning (as perceived by the student). Whether tacitly assumed or explicitly identified, teachers create

R. Hipkins, Ph.D. (✉)
New Zealand Council for Educational Research,
Wellington, New Zealand
e-mail: Rose.hipkins@nzcer.org.nz

opportunities for students to engage in class through the purposes they envision for learning. These purposes in turn influence their selection of curriculum content, their choice of learning resources, the instructional processes they deploy, and how they 'talk up' and generally prepare students for any subsequent assessment events. Assuming all these choices are coherent and broadly appropriate to the learning needs of the students, the opportunities to learn that the teacher shapes are *necessary* for learning, but a sociocultural framing posits that they are not *sufficient* to ensure the engagement of all or even necessarily most of the students in the class (Haertel, Moss, Pullin, & Gee, 2008).

Opportunities to learn, as envisaged and enacted by the teacher, may or may not be recognised by the students as offering *affordances* for their personal learning. Gee (2008) described affordances as 'action possibilities posed by objects or features in the environment' (p.81). To name just a few, affordances could include students' understanding of what the learning is really about and for; their estimations of their likely success in completing the tasks in relation to their motivation to do so; their personal interest in and connections to the contexts of learning, including prior knowledge and experiences on which they might draw; and any possibilities for social and intellectual interaction as students learn together. Thus opportunities to learn are realised only when individual students see ways to transform the intended learning into action and are willing to invest the necessary effort to do so.

Within the scope just outlined, discussions of engagement include considerations of the broader purposes that frame learning at any specific stage of schooling. This chapter is set in the context of the final years of high school, when students are preparing for and being assessed to gain exit qualifications, all the while making choices that take into account their likely options for work or further study in the immediate post-school years. Traditionally, teachers have used the necessity to prepare for high-stakes examinations as a means of keeping the majority of students engaged at a stage of their learning when adolescents can become restless, ready as they see it for adult life and perhaps pushing back against the strictures of school. However, contexts for schooling are changing in ways that unsettle tidy relationships where examination prescriptions become de facto curriculum, teaching is directed towards content acquisition, and traditional exit examinations assess the extent to which the prescribed content has been acquired and understood (Bolstad & Gilbert, 2008).

Outside of education, rapidly changing social and economic conditions are creating new uncertainties. It is no longer possible to assume a 'known future, a known set of options to choose between, each requiring a known set of skills and aptitudes, and therefore a known – and well-trodden – pathway' (Bolstad & Gilbert, 2008, p.35). With global changes and uncertainties in mind, this chapter argues that new ways of thinking about keeping students engaged in the final years of schooling are now needed. It draws on data from the longitudinal study Competent Children/Competent Learners (Wylie & Hodgen, 2012) to describe student and teacher views of classroom learning conditions at age 16 and to discuss implications for changes in pedagogy. The survey items discussed in the chapter were designed with New Zealand's recent curriculum and assessment reforms in mind, specifically a focus on learning as *competency* development. New Zealand's national curriculum and school exit qualification system are briefly outlined next, to provide the context for the data and discussion that follows.

Curriculum and Assessment Reform in New Zealand

In common with many other nations, New Zealand is wrestling with questions of what it means to educate students for the rapidly changing economic, environmental and social conditions that characterise life in the twenty-first century (Bolstad & Gilbert, 2008; Gilbert, 2005). The most recent New Zealand Curriculum (NZC) is a future-focused *framework* curriculum whose purpose is to provide a sense of national direction for local decision-making. Each school has to

Table 21.1 The origins of five NZC key competencies

Name given to competency by OECD	New Zealand Curriculum version (note that these are 'best matches' not 1–1 equivalents)
Acting autonomously	Managing self
Functioning in socially heterogeneous groups	Relating to others
	Participating and contributing
Using tools interactively	Using language, symbols and texts
Thinking (as a 'cross-cutting' competency that interacts with all the others)	Thinking (not identified as cross-cutting)

work out how best to build up a detailed local curriculum based on the national framework, with the identified learning needs of its own student community demonstrably addressed. A vision statement and a set of principles guide the reading and interpretation of the whole. The vision is for students to become 'confident, connected, actively involved lifelong learners' (Ministry of Education [MoE], 2007, p.8), and the principles highlight the following as key design considerations: coherence, inclusion, cultural diversity, high expectations, a future-focus, learning-to-learn and community engagement with local curriculum design and enactment, together with a focus on the Treaty of Waitangi as the foundation for bicultural relationships with the indigenous people of New Zealand.

The vision and principles are given life when schools design learning programmes that weave more traditional content with specified values and key competencies. Eight broad sets of values, identified and shaped via a national consultation exercise, are expected to be encouraged, modelled and explored. As outlined in Table 21.1, five NZC key competencies were adapted from a set of four developed by the OECD's DeSeCo project. This project defined 'key' competencies as those learners need to develop during their schooling in order to maximise their chances of living meaningfully in, and contributing to, well-functioning societies, both during and well beyond their school years (OECD, 2005). Some people use the word 'capabilities' with similar intent (Reid, 2006). Learners draw on a wide range of competencies, but those labelled as 'key' are seen to be universal rather than situation specific (Rychen & Salganik, 2003). The implication is that these competencies are transferrable across contexts and continue to develop across the life span.

Key competencies integrate knowledge and skills with attitudes and values, and are demonstrated as complex responses to any challenges learners confront as they adapt what they already know and can do to new contexts, or to more demanding aspects of familiar contexts (Rychen & Salganik, 2003). In this way, a focus on competency development draws attention to *dispositional* aspects of learning and to ideas such as *action competence*: knowing how best to respond, having the necessary knowledge and skills to do so and being disposed to use these. These dispositional aspects of learning have been characterised as being 'ready, willing and able' to undertake the learning task and confront its challenges (Carr, 2006, 2008). Engagement here is not optional but rather a necessary condition of learning. It is '*energy in action*, the connection between person and activity' (Russell et al., 2005, p.4, emphasis in the original).

If students are to strengthen their personal competencies as demonstrable outcomes of learning, schools must weave competencies together with traditional content. The latter is specified in NZC as sets of achievement objectives for eight learning areas, each differentiated into eight curriculum levels that broadly indicate progress across all the years of school from age 5 to around age 17 or 18. (Students can leave after they turn 16, but this is discouraged because by then they would be unlikely to have any qualifications that would keep them on a learning pathway). Each learning area is framed by a one-page 'essence statement' that sets out the unique contribution that this learning area makes to the enacted curriculum. Schools are expected to discuss these 'high level' ideals as they plan how to give expression to curriculum as a complex whole (Hipkins, 2011).

This local curriculum planning will ideally result in the provision of learning experiences that support all students to develop and strengthen their current competencies and to explore and model the curriculum values, all in the context of also learning the concepts and skills specified in the achievement objectives. Planning appropriate curriculum is thus a highly complex *design* task. Even with the vision and principles to provide guidance, there could be very many different ways to assemble these pieces. There are also strong implications for pedagogy: the 'how' of teaching is as important as the 'what' and both come together in the 'why', i.e. the purposes for learning that are envisaged, or perhaps simply assumed, by both students and their teachers (Hipkins, Bull, & Reid, 2010). Framing the engagement issue thus directs the inquiry focus beyond the individual student as engaged in learning or not (although that remains important) to take account of teacher-student interactions, teachers' curriculum decision-making and the classroom learning conditions they co-construct with their students – in other words, the manner in which affordances for learning play out in action.

New Zealand does not have a programme of national testing, so effectively carrying out the processes specified in NZC for local design and review is an important professional responsibility for every school. Even the school exit qualification, awarded at three levels broadly corresponding to the final 3 years of high school, the National Certificate in Educational Achievement (NCEA), has a flexible, modular structure that continues opportunities for local curriculum design right through to the end of schooling (Bolstad & Gilbert, 2008; Hipkins & Vaughan, with Beals, Ferral, & Gardiner, 2005). Standards-based assessment is underpinned by suites of 'achievement standards' that can be mixed and matched, at least in theory. Some standards are internally assessed by each school, and these typically specify types of learning that cannot be assessed in traditional examinations. Externally assessed standards do often entail examinations, but even here, some innovation is possible; for example, portfolio assessments are often used in the arts and technology learning areas. NCEA is part of a National Qualifications Framework (NQF) that extends to post-school learning pathways. Thus, there are additional curriculum design opportunities and challenges for high schools as they create coherent pathways through and beyond the senior high years. Ideally, all assessment should be competency-focused, but in practice, revising the existing suites of achievement standards to reflect discipline-specific opportunities for competency development is proving to be demanding, with considerable implications for teacher professional learning and pedagogical change.

Changing Pedagogy for Changing Times?

An *Effective Pedagogy* section included in the NZC framework provides advice about creating a supportive learning environment, encouraging reflective thought and action, enhancing the relevance of new learning, facilitating shared learning, making connections to prior learning and experience, providing students with sufficient opportunities to learn and inquiring into one's own teaching practice to ensure student learning needs are being met (MoE, 2007, p. 34). All of these aspects of pedagogy could be seen as fundamental to improving *traditional* teaching practice. None *necessarily* implies pedagogical change or curriculum transformation for new times. However, the demands of competency development do potentially bring new pedagogical imperatives. NZC defines the key competencies drawing on 'knowledge, attitudes and values *in ways that lead to action*' (MoE, 2007, p.12, emphasis added) and the dispositional challenges of competency development have already been noted. One engagement challenge here is that action contexts that are new and challenging for one learner might not offer any learning 'stretch' to another. This implies that some degree of personalisation is needed if key competencies are to be fostered via participatory learning.

The NZC notes the development of key competencies is 'both an end in itself (a goal) and a means by which other ends are achieved' (MoE, 2007, p.12). Key competencies 'enable learning' (ibid, p.38) with the clear implication that there is a strong link between the development of key competencies and learning-to-learn.

Russell et al.'s meta-analysis of engagement and motivation begins with summary of learning outcomes for the twenty-first century. Interestingly they make essentially the same learning-to-learn connection: 'Engagement in learning is both an end in itself and a means to an end' (Russell et al., 2005, p.3). They also link engagement to more dynamic learning processes and better quality educational outcomes as foundations for continuing to learn in the years beyond school. Developing learning-to-learn dimensions challenges teachers to offer opportunities that draw students into metacognitive conversations that support them and reflect on acts of meaning-making, including *how* and *why* they are learning, not just *what* they have acquired (Hipkins, 2006). For such conversations to be rich and meaningful, the learning that is planned must be intellectually engaging for both students and the teacher, and the teacher must be clear about the nature of the 'big picture' to which the learning is making a contribution.

NZC further notes that social contexts are important enablers of progress in developing key competencies; the manner in which competencies develop over time is shaped by students' 'interactions with people, places, ideas and things' (MoE, 2007, p.12). The sociocultural idea of *affordances* is cued by these words, as is the related idea that learning is *mediated* by whether and how students understand and take up these affordances (Wertsch, 1998). Thus a sociocultural framing for learning that fosters competency development positions learning as social, contextually bound and *emergent* (Davis & Sumara, 2010). Competencies come into view during learning interactions that vary according to the demands of the specific subject, the affordances that the planned learning offers individual students, and the various new contextual links that become apparent. This description stands in contrast to a more universalist view of learning where competency might be seen as a relatively stable characteristic, separately owned by discrete individuals (Delandshere & Petrosky, 1998). A sociocultural interpretation implies that key competencies cannot be taught generically: they have to be explored from a disciplinary perspective by teachers in every subject area, and there is an element of unpredictability in their outcomes. Teachers need to be sufficiently confident to be responsive to students' ideas and reactions, and to follow new learning possibilities as these unfold.

This chapter is not intended to argue for competency development per se. Rather, it uses the idea of key competencies as a lens for re-examining curriculum assumptions and pedagogical practices, and ensuring that any initiatives intended to strengthen student engagement take the whole learning context into account, including adopting a more nuanced view of opportunities to learn and how these are impacted by the classroom environment and teacher's actions. Many teachers are unfamiliar with sociocultural theories of learning and so are likely to miss the subtle language cues in NZC. If they think about learning as being mainly the individual acquisition of knowledge and skills, they are likely to miss the part played by the affordances of learning environment they are responsible for orchestrating for their students. If they are unaware of constructivist theories of learning, the very possibility that different students will perceive different purposes for the new learning offered, and hence create different links to what they already know and can do, might pass the teacher by. The research presented in this chapter did not engage explicitly with teachers' reasoning, but rather with the manner in which their (likely tacit) curriculum and pedagogical beliefs were translated into the opportunities to learn that they offered in their classes.

Determining Engagement as a Situated and Mediated Construct

This section of the chapter introduces the engagement data drawn from the longitudinal Competent Children, Competent Learners project. This project has tracked around 500 New Zealand students from pre-school education through their school years and on into the world of work or further education. Well before the OECD key competencies were developed, the prescient decision was taken to focus on competency development as children moved through school (see Wylie & Hodgen, 2012 for a more detailed project description). At age 16, when the students were in a wide range of high schools, they were invited to respond to a set of items that described aspects of the learning they experienced during classes in the subjects they most and least enjoyed, as well as in English which they would all have been studying. This chapter focuses on data about most and least enjoyed subjects. Thus, self-reported enjoyment of learning in a class is the situated measure used in this chapter to determine comparative engagement of an individual student in two different settings, each with a different teacher.

The construct of 'most enjoyed' subjects directs attention to *emotional* components of engagement (Fredricks et al., 2004). It could be argued that focusing on enjoyment is not a good proxy for engagement because students may well enjoy subjects that make few demands on them cognitively or even behaviourally – they can have a good time and not do much work. However, the student responses outlined shortly do not bear out this sceptical view. Also, there is evidence in the Competent Learners project that enjoyment was linked to experiencing academic success (Wylie, Hipkins, & Hodgen, 2009; Wylie & Hodgen, 2012), which implies that both cognitive and behavioural dimensions of engagement are also present when students indicate positive affective responses to their learning. A second possible objection to the use of enjoyment as a proxy for engagement runs the opposite way. Students may be cognitively and behaviourally engaged in subjects they do not enjoy, especially if they are motivated by strongly held instrumental reasons for choosing these. Indeed, in other research, we have found instances of students taking physics 'under sufferance' because they need it for pre-entry courses leading to limited-entry study pathways into highly valued professions such as medicine (Hipkins, Roberts, Bolstad, & Ferral, 2006).

Many studies that include a classroom component compare different context/cohort combinations and hence conflate two sets of variables (different settings/different students). The Competent Learner study provided an illuminating lens on classroom contexts when teachers of the two classes nominated by a student were contacted and invited to complete a survey that included questions about both the class and the student. We see two different classes through the eyes of the same student, but also as perceived by the teacher of each of those classes. One part of the survey addressed opportunities to learn through the teacher's eyes. This part comprised 32 items that described the general learning conditions in the class. A 5-point Likert scale (strongly agree to strongly disagree with neutral in the middle) was provided for the teacher to indicate how well the item description accorded with the class in question. Other parts of the survey asked the teacher to respond to questions about the named student as a learner. One bank of 36 Likert-scaled items asked the teacher to estimate how often the student did what the item described (never, occasionally, sometimes, often, or always) while learning in the nominated class. Another bank of 13 items described aspects that imply motivational underpinnings for engagement (e.g. 'always strives for excellence') and asked the teacher to judge how well that item applied to the student on a 5-point Likert scale (strongly agree to strongly disagree with neutral in the middle). A full discussion of all these rich data can be accessed in the project report (Wylie et al., 2009).

The selection of teacher items for inclusion in this chapter was informed by a consideration of their potential to illuminate aspects of competency development, and by being able to match them to student items that broadly encompassed the same idea. Students completed questions about learning conditions in their most and least enjoyed classes. For each class, they responded to a bank of 58 items (X is a class where…) using a 5-point Likert scale (strongly agree to strongly disagree with neutral in the middle). Some of the items concerned the affordances they perceived in that class setting. Table 21.2 matches these to teacher items related to opportunities to learn. Other student items concerned their personal behaviour in the class. Table 21.3 matches these responses to corresponding teacher perceptions about the student as a learner in that class.

Note that the distinction teachers were asked to draw between the student as an individual and

Table 21.2 Comparing teachers' perceptions of opportunities to learn with students' perceptions of the affordances offered in these classes

Item set no	Most enjoyed class = 418 students and teacher of each student / Least enjoyed class = 417 students and teacher of each student	% agree or strongly agree — Most enjoyed	Least enjoyed	Difference
1	Student view: The teacher uses examples that are relevant to my experience	77	27	50
	Student view: My teacher knows what interests us	72	20	52
	Teacher view: *I relate the context to students' experiences*	77	66	11
2	Student view: We have a lot of hands-on practical activities	73	24	49
	Teacher view: *Students do a lot of practical activities*	72	38	34
3	Student view: The teacher gives me useful feedback on my work that helps me see what I need to do next and how to do it	86	40	46
	Teacher view: *Feedback I give students shows them their next steps*	84	75	9
4	Student view: I can try out new ideas/ways of doing things	81	35	46
	Student view: We discuss different ways of looking at things/interpretations	65	27	38
	Student view: I get to think about ideas and problems in new ways	67	30	37
	Teacher view: *Students are given time to reflect on their learning*	65	57	8
5	Student view: I get time to think and talk about how I'm learning	62	17	45
	Teacher view: *I encourage students to think and talk about how they are learning (the methods they are using)*	57	52	5
6	Student view: Students help and support each other	78	44	34
	Teacher view: *Students can work out problems together*	74	78	−4
7	Student view: I can make mistakes and learn from them without getting into trouble	84	50	34
	Teacher view: *Students can make mistakes and learn from them without getting into trouble*	92	92	–
8	Student view: We do projects about real things/issues	54	25	29
	Teacher view: *Students have the opportunity to act on issues that concern them*	50	33	17
9	Student view: We assess each other's work and give feedback	47	20	27
	Teacher view: *Students are encouraged to assess each others' work and give feedback*	39	30	9
10	Student view: We learn things outside the classroom, e.g. on fieldtrips	41	14	27
	Teacher view: *Students interact with people outside school as part of their school work*	43	23	20
11	Student view: I work with other students on group tasks	71	52	19
	Teacher view: *Students do a lot of group activities and discussions*	54	37	14
12	Student view: We can choose the topics we want to do	28	10	18
	Teacher view: *Students are encouraged to lead group projects/class activities*	37	25	12
	Teacher view: *Students are given input into the context and direction of learning activities*	64	52	12

the class as a whole does not apply to student responses – they were who they were in that setting, and hence all their items comprised one large bank. Note also that each student completed the same item set for both their most and least enjoyed subjects. Unless they had the same teacher for both these subjects (which in view of the differences about to be reported seems fairly unlikely), the corresponding teacher items for most and least enjoyed subjects will have been completed by two different teachers. A further caution concerns the likelihood that the items were not interpreted in comparable ways by the student and the teacher. Notwithstanding these cautions, the following data patterns paint a compelling picture of opportunities to strengthen competencies that can make a positive contribution to student engagement.

Table 21.3 Comparing teachers and student perceptions of the student as a learner in the class

Item set no	Most enjoyed class = 418 students and teacher of each student, Least enjoyed class = 417 students and teacher of each student	Students:% agree or strongly agree Teachers:% happens often or always		
		Most enjoyed	Least enjoyed	Difference
1	Student item: I learn things that are challenging	86	22	64
	Teacher item: Where there is a choice, chooses work that allows him/her to gain further knowledge and skills	44	27	17
2	Student item: My teacher is interested in my ideas	85	27	58
	Teacher item: Clearly explains things so you get a very good idea of what is happening and what s/he is thinking	60	37	23
3	Student item: I get totally absorbed in my work	64	13	51
	Teacher item: Has a good concentration span when working	59	40	19
4	Student item: I organise my time so I get things done	64	24	40
	Teacher item: Finishes all class work	70	45	35
	Teacher item: Is organised and well prepared for assessments	61	43	18
	Teacher item: Finishes all homework	58	38	20
5	Student item: When I finish my work, I check and make changes if needed before handing it in	68	29	39
	Teacher item: Assess his/her work and makes improvements before completing or handing it in	47	31	16
6	Student item: I expect to get lots of NCEA credits	71	32	39
	Teacher item: S/he is realistic about likely achievement in assessment tasks	68	60	8
7	Student item: We discuss different ways of looking at things/interpretations	65	27	38
	Teacher item: Aware that there are different ways of interpreting knowledge	42	30	12
8	Student item: I meet any goals I set myself	64	27	37
	Teacher item: Meets any goals s/he sets her/himself	57	39	18
9	Student item: I can make mistakes and learn from them without getting into trouble	84	50	34
	Teacher item: Learns from mistakes/experience	65	47	18
10	Student item: When I'm doing something I think about whether I understand what I'm doing	74	47	27
	Teacher item: Asks questions so s/he understands	63	41	22
11	Student item: Students can safely express different views from each other	79	53	26
	Teacher item: Respects other points of view or different ways of doing things	71	60	11
12	Student item: I work with other students on group tasks	71	52	19
	Teacher item: Takes full part in a group that is working to complete a learning task together	58	36	22
13	Student item: I can choose which assessments I want to do for NCEA	17	14	3
	Teacher item: S/he makes strategic decisions not to do assessments	5	8	3
	Teacher item: S/he makes impulsive decisions not to do assessments	8	12	4

Engaging Students in Whole-Class Settings

Table 21.2 documents 12 matched sets of items, ranked by the size of the difference between students' perceptions of the learning conditions in their most and least enjoyed classes. Each set of items shows overall frequencies for the affordances of the class as the students perceived these, matched to overall frequencies for opportunities to learn as perceived by the teacher of each student in those same classes. To illustrate, item set

1 shows that three-quarters of the students (77%) perceived that the teacher of their most enjoyed subject used examples relevant to their experiences. Congruent with this, 72% believed that this teacher knew what interested them. By contrast only 27% of these same students thought the teacher of their least enjoyed classes used relevant experiences and just 20% thought this teacher knew what interested students. Three-quarters of the teachers of the nominated most enjoyed classes (77%) thought they related contexts of learning to students' experiences, as did 66% of those who taught in students' least enjoyed classes. Thus the frequency difference between the perceptions of teachers of most and least enjoyed classes that they orchestrated opportunities to draw links between current learning and students' wider experiences was just 11%, compared to a 50% difference in students' recognition of such linking as an affordance of the learning in most and least enjoyed classes. A similar pattern holds for all the item sets in Table 21.2.

Note that some item sets in Table 21.2 are closely matched, with only a slight change of wording for teacher and student versions. However, some groupings bring together items with similar intent but different descriptions. For example, item set 4 contrasts one teacher item that asked about reflection as a general activity with three student items that each described a different possibility for reflecting on learning. Similarly, item set 12 explores students' perceptions of choice as residing in actual selection of topics and opportunities to show leadership in class. By contrast, the matched teacher item cues student 'input' which need not imply the same level of freedom, or ultimate determination of curriculum topics and directions. This difference doubtless explains the atypically large difference in item set 12 between teachers of most enjoyed classes and students' views of learning in those classes.

The pattern of responses in Table 21.2 suggests that enjoyment of learning, as a proxy for engagement in learning, is associated with a range of opportunities to be *actively participating* as a learner. In addition to a traditional focus on 'hands-on' learning, students were more likely to be active in all of the following ways in their most enjoyed classes:

- Taking part in reflective conversations about the meaning of new learning (item set 4), looking ahead to next learning steps (item set 3) and discussing acts of learning per se (item set 5), with all three item sets showing close to 50% differences in frequency of occurrence in most and least enjoyed classes
- Building connections between school and life beyond school (item set 1), learning in contexts beyond the classroom (item set 10) and engaging with real issues (item set 8)
- Interacting with peers, both during learning (item sets 6 and 11) and when assessing learning (item set 9)
- Making and correcting one's own mistakes (item set 7) and exercising some autonomy over learning directions and/or showing leadership in class (item set 12)

In the most enjoyed classes, frequencies for student recognition of the various affordances were largely matched by teacher perceptions of opportunities to learn in those classes. The pattern is very different when student responses are compared with those for teachers of least enjoyed classes. In these least enjoyed classes, the opportunities teachers perceived they offered were not recognised as affordances by many of the students. It may be that some of the teachers of the least enjoyed classes did not make certain opportunities to learn as visible to students as they thought they did. It is also possible that some teachers of these classes were out of touch with students' interests and learning needs, or perhaps simply not focused on students as individual learners, which could be the case for a teacher with a very strong content orientation, for example. Alternatively, students might be less active in seeking connections, perceiving relevance and participating actively when they are not enjoying a class. Either way, it seems less likely that opportunities to participate actively in learning will be recognised or embraced in students in their less enjoyed classes.

One caveat for the comparisons in Table 21.2 is that teachers were thinking about that class as a whole, whereas each student was focused on their personal learning. We have no way of knowing if all the students in any one class would have answered the survey in a similar way. What we can say is that not enjoying a class is often linked to having a teacher who appears less attuned to a specific student's personal learning needs, compared to the teacher of their most enjoyed class. This is borne out by a comparison of items that did apply specifically to an individual student, as discussed next.

Associations Between Expectations and Engagement

Table 21.3 follows a similar format to Table 21.2, but here the teacher is responding to items about the student as a named individual in their class. Some of the student items have already been introduced, but here, they are matched to teacher items specifically related to them personally. Where the wording matches closely, the item set draws a contrast between how the student sees themselves as a learner and how their two teachers see them. Some item sets are not as closely matched but have been paired because they inform the same opportunity or learning challenge. For example, item set 2 probes student perceptions that their teachers are interested in what they think, whereas the matched teacher item asks about how well the student can express what they think (the teacher Likert scale changes accordingly). This pairing assumes that teacher awareness of the relevant behaviours is actually linked to opportunities to demonstrate these. Item set 6 is different again. This item set contrasts students' expectations of gaining credits from their NCEA (qualifications) assessments with the teacher's view of whether or not those expectations are likely to be realistic.

Again we see, through the students' eyes, much lower frequencies of occurrence in their least enjoyed classes of the various potential affordances described. For most item sets, the teacher-reported frequencies of occurrence were also considerably lower in least enjoyed classes than in those the students most enjoyed. Keep in mind here that these are comparisons of the *same* students, as they variously engage with learning in two different settings. Classes that were seen as least enjoyable by these students were associated with:

- Lack of intellectual challenge (item set 1), or learning 'stretch' as indicated by getting totally absorbed in a task (item set 3), or getting involved in conversations about ideas (item set 2), where for all three items again we see student frequency differences of 50% or more between most and least enjoyed classes
- Lack of opportunities for learning from mistakes (item set 9), safely exploring alternative views and ways of interpreting knowledge (item sets 7 and 11), and asking questions to develop a better understanding (item set 10)
- Not valuing the work sufficiently to take care over its completion (item set 4), or checking it for potential improvements (item set 5); not working purposefully in class (item set 8), including with other students (item set 12); and the slightly greater likelihood (at least from the teacher's perspective) of skipping an NCEA assessment (item set 13)
- Not expecting to gain intrinsic rewards in the form of personal goals met (item set 8) or the extrinsic reward of assessment credits gained towards an NCEA qualification (item set 6)

Interestingly, students' intellectual involvement tended to be underestimated by teachers in most enjoyed classes, compared to students' own perceptions. For example, whereas 86% of students thought learning was challenging in their most enjoyed classes, just 44% of the teachers of those classes thought students would choose work that allowed them to gain further knowledge and skills (and hence, by implication, would be more challenging). It may be simply that some teachers felt they lacked the evidence to comment, but then that could be indicative of lacking overt opportunities to make the relevant observations during class. Alternatively, it may be that students overestimate the extent of their active meaning-making or simply do not see the challenges that the teacher sees to be inherent in learning implied by some items. What we can say is that, from the students' perspectives, there are indications that opportunities for active and challenging meaning-making are associated with greater enjoyment of learning. Both Tables 21.2 and 21.3 show such items at the top of the student rankings for frequency differences between most and least enjoyed classes. This in turn suggests that for many respondents, 'enjoyment' did not signal a preference for taking an easy route in class.

Comments made by some of the teachers of least enjoyed classes suggested they saw it as unreasonable to be expected to know personal attributes of individual students. Non-response or choice of 'neutral' in this part of the survey was correspondingly higher than for returns from teachers of favourite classes. Notice too that these teachers were consistently more pessimistic in their expectations of students' likely learning effort and success. Elsewhere in the survey, teachers were asked to predict students' likely highest level of qualification in their post-school years. The teacher of a student's most enjoyed class typically indicated a higher qualification than the teacher of the same student's least enjoyed class (Wylie et al., 2009). Students also held lower expectations of success in their least enjoyed classes, and in this instance overall frequencies for their views were much closer to those of their teachers. One student item simply stated 'I do well [in this class]'. Most students (89%) agreed this was so in their most enjoyed class, compared to 34% in their least enjoyed class.

Notice that active participation of students in making decisions about assessment for NCEA, as opposed to learning in general, was not seen by most students as something they could or would do, nor did their teachers see this as an option open to the students. Unlike almost every other item set reported in this chapter, there was no substantive difference for most and least enjoyed classes (item set 13). NCEA is built from standards-based modules, and so students have a degree of choice in shaping the composition of their certificates, at least in theory (Hipkins et al., 2005). Our 16 year olds *could* be supported to develop considerable autonomy in charting their course through NCEA, but it appears that this seldom happens. In a recent national survey, just 10% of high school teachers said they always or quite often involved their students in building NCEA assessment plans (Hipkins, 2010a).

If students perceived that NCEA did in fact offer them the affordance of making strategic assessment choices, would this enhance their enjoyment in the same way that perceptions of greater autonomy in other aspects of their learning appear to do? What would need to change for teachers to perceive that they can in fact support students to take up this opportunity, which already exists in principle? Would both they and their students experience rewards in the form of greater enjoyment of learning in the parts of the curriculum in which they choose to aspire for assessment success? These are questions that bear further investigation. Some pointers to the challenges that teachers face as practice imperatives change are implied by a small but growing body of research on teaching for competency development.

The Engaging Nature of Competency Development

A recent analysis of the challenges of integrating key competencies with learning in one very simple science topic [the water cycle] (Hipkins, 2010b) identified the following four key points of difference from traditional teaching of this topic. First, the teacher must hold a clear 'big picture' purpose in mind, so that the learning matters for something more than just acquisition of new content knowledge. Second, the learning should be set in context and linked to students' life experiences, and where possible, these links should be sufficiently open that students can personalise the connections to what matters to them. Third, acts of meaning-making within the discipline of science should be an explicit focus of learning, not just something that happens serendipitously (or not). Finally, students' ideas should be used in ways that establish and sustain their connection to the intended learning while also setting up new challenges that strengthen their learning-to-learn capabilities (Hipkins). It will be evident that all four of these areas of potential difference align with the aspects of pedagogy highlighted in Tables 21.2 and 21.3 as more likely to be happening in students' most enjoyed classes.

Notwithstanding these strong potential links between teaching for competency development and student engagement with learning, a growing body of key competencies research has revealed that they are likely to be interpreted, at least initially, as requiring only a surface level changes to pedagogy, and perhaps a strengthening of current 'good practice' (Hipkins, 2011). For example, the title 'managing self' underplays the intent of the OECD equivalent 'acting autonomously' (see Table 21.1). As cued by its NZC title, managing self has been widely interpreted to entail involving students in goal setting and managing routines of learning such as arriving at class on time and with the necessary materials, in contrast to the OECD definition that includes aspects such as 'acting within the big picture' (Rychen, 2004). Some items reported in Table 21.3 are set at this surface level of competency development, yet even this is sufficient to impact enjoyment, and hence by implication engagement with learning.

Self-managing behaviours certainly create conditions where school learning can be initiated, but they will not necessarily strengthen students' ability to apply some self-direction to their learning, or to develop self-awareness of a learning-to-learn nature. Arguably, the combination of the key competencies 'thinking' and 'using language symbols and texts' *could* refocus learning in ways that make acts of learning per se a focus of classroom conversations. On a surface level, 'thinking' might be envisaged as teaching a set of skills (Harpaz, 2007), while 'using language, symbols and texts' has been characterised by some as the 'literacy and numeracy' competency (Hipkins, 2007). While basic academic skills are foundational to other learning, a skill-based generic interpretation seriously underestimates the intellectual challenge that these competencies can add to learning. In combination, these two key competencies could invoke semiotic dimensions that require meaning-making to be explicitly addressed within different disciplinary conventions (i.e. addressing the 'nature' of the subject, not just the content). One competency identified as a specific challenge for twenty-first century learning that could be developed here is the willingness and intellectual means to explore *ideas as ideas,* not just as received wisdom (Bereiter & Scardamalia, 2006). Tables 21.2 and 21.3 include items that could be read as entailing active this type of meaning-making, although it is again likely they were not read very deeply by many respondents. Even so, the tables reveal considerable differences between the affordances that student perceive their least and most enjoyed classes offer for: exploring ideas, discussing multiple interpretations of knowledge, and thinking and talking about acts of learning.

The DeSeCo definition of competency development draws attention to the need to mobilise knowledge and skills for use in challenging new contexts (Rychen & Salganik, 2003). At the very least, the key competency 'participating and contributing' implies that students need to be able to make personally meaningful links between theory and action and between classroom learning and life beyond school (Bolstad, Roberts, Boyd, & Hipkins, 2009). 'Contribution' also implies giving something in exchange for learning, which is suggestive of an action component where appropriate. The items included in Table 21.2 tend to position teachers as the orchestrators of opportunities for learners to be active, rather than supporting students to be proactive for themselves. Nevertheless, there are clear indications in both tables that enjoyment of learning is linked to opportunities for some level of active participation in practical activities, addressing real-life issues and in conversation and interaction with other learners.

The final key competency in the NZC set of five is titled 'relating to others'. At a surface level, this competency can be seen as being about appropriate interpersonal behaviour in class and at school. With the OECD equivalent 'functioning in socially heterogeneous groups' in mind, pairing this competency with 'managing self' points towards building greater self-awareness in relation to diverse others and the need to modify personal cultural expectations and behaviours in different contexts. Taking a different tack, pairing 'relating to others' with 'participating and contributing' draws attention to other people as a learning resource, and to the need to strengthen skills for interacting and developing ideas in the spaces between learners, which is often cited as important for 'knowledge work' in the twenty-first century (Gilbert, 2005; Bereiter & Scardamalia, 2006). The items presented in Tables 21.2 and 21.3 are more clearly aligned with the latter pairing, again with the caveat that they may not have been read particularly deeply by respondents. Regardless of the level of interpretation and application in the classroom, the potential of teaching for competency development to impact engagement is again evident in clear differences between the opportunities that teachers offer and students perceive as affordances in their most and least enjoyed classes.

Items that describe practices that hint at fostering greater learner autonomy ranked lower in teachers' estimation of the opportunities they offer and students' estimation of the affordances available to them, even in most enjoyed classes. Just 39% of teachers in most enjoyed classes said that students were encouraged to assess each others' work and give feedback, and 37% said students could sometimes lead classroom learning. Just 28% of students said they could choose study topics in their most enjoyed classes, and only 17% perceived they could make choices about the NCEA assessment they would undertake. These options were hardly available at all in least enjoyed classes. If teachers are serious about fostering greater student autonomy, they need to scaffold opportunities for greater self-determination of learning pathways, greater self-awareness of purposes, habits and progress in strengthening competencies as a learner and as a citizen in a diverse and rapidly changing world. If the imperative for greater self-direction in combination with greater participation is not to be misrepresented as a relativistic 'anything goes and nothing matters' view of curriculum (Hipkins et al., 2010), many teachers of high school students will need to gain greater clarity around multiple potential purposes for learning, while also reframing their subjects as disciplinary tools that do specific sorts of work in the world, within certain agreed conventions. That is, they will need to become more 'literate' about the nature of their specialist subjects, so they can help their students do the same (Hipkins, 2010b). Given the data presented in this chapter, we could hypothesise that any shifts to affording students greater autonomy in their learning will also help strengthen student engagement. Whether the complex inter-related changes sketched in this section happen more widely in practice remains to be seen.

Advancing Teacher Conversations About Student Engagement

This chapter has explored student engagement in relation to the opportunities for learning that teachers say they offer and the affordances for learning that senior high school students perceive to be available to them in most and least enjoyed classes. Framing learning in terms of developing or strengthening key competencies adds a critical curriculum dimension to the discussion and aligns curriculum change imperatives with pedagogical change. The analysis has presented teacher and student data separately in order to contrast differences in perceptions, but, in reality, engagement is co-constructed in the classroom moment as interactions play out between teacher and students, and between the students themselves. This section of the chapter proposes a complex, dynamic framing of the relationships between teacher and student actions, motivations and engagement and identifies some implications for teacher professional learning.

As well as having separate teacher and learner components, there is an element of *simultaneity* to engagement as it emerges in the classroom moment (Davis & Sumara, 2010). Davis and Sumara noted that it is unhelpful to debate the merits of either student-centred or teacher-centred learning *as if* they are an inevitable duality. Learning is simultaneously both individual and situated. The classroom environment is anticipated and orchestrated by the teacher in the first instance but ultimately co-created by all those present. Engagement also has temporal dimensions. It emerges in the flow of time, building on past experiences and looking to possible futures. Within a complex framing such as this, the choice of feelings about individual subjects is a useful proxy for engagement because it is likely to include aspects of all three temporal dimensions (past, present, future), whether students and teachers are aware of the impact of these or not.

For the student, the identification of a subject as 'most enjoyed' is likely to relate at least in part to their *personal* interests and preferences, underpinned by the goals and aspirations that motivate them, which are grounded in past learning experiences and in all the other factors that impact on their general engagement trajectory across the years of school (Wylie & Hodgen, 2012). Although the chapter has focused on overall frequency differences between most and least enjoyed subjects, there is evidence that some students' perceptions of specific affordances did not differ for the two classes they nominated. Selecting two of the more metacognitive statements, 'I get time to think and talk about how I'm learning', and 'I like to reflect on how I've learned something', we cross-tabulated students' responses for each class. We found that the manner in which individuals responded in these two settings was significantly more likely to be similar than different. Students who agreed that they got time for reflecting on their learning in their most enjoyed class were also more likely to agree that this time was also available in their least enjoyed class. Those who selected the neutral response for one class were also more likely to select it for the other, suggesting perhaps that they were not sure what these items were about. Interestingly, the pattern did not hold at the very strong level of response: students who totally agreed they got this time in their most enjoyed class were as likely to totally disagree about their least enjoyed class as to totally agree. The relationship between individual and contextual dimensions of engagement in class is clearly complex and could well be the subject of a further level of analysis of the data set reported here.

Believing that learning that is worth the investment of effort and time doubtless acts as a continuing personal motivation, while also increasing the likelihood that opportunities offered by the teacher will be recognised as affordances for learning by the student and hence taken up. However, the clear student *and teacher* differences between most and least enjoyed subjects point to the strong influence teachers can exert on students' personal preferences in the moment. As they focus and shape the learning possibilities offered, teachers influence cognitive engagement. Interestingly, the *cognitive* quality of interactions is the pedagogical dimension where the data show the strongest differences between most and least enjoyed subjects. Students do appear to be engaged by challenging learning that stretches them (see also Wylie & Hodgen, 2012), especially when metacognitive dimensions such that learning-to-learn are also in the frame. Teachers can help students envisage *new* personal and collective learning possibilities here.

Teachers also help enlarge personal perceptions of relevance when they support students to look beyond the personal to interpersonal differences in perspectives and outwards again to the world beyond school. Again the data show strong associations with engagement. Most enjoyed classes are participatory spaces where students interact safely and enjoyably with each other, and where learning is meaningfully linked to their life experiences and to issues that concern them. With competency development in view, the purposes for learning that teachers 'talk up' need not be limited to near-horizon possibilities such as passing examinations but can extend to the sorts of young people students wish to become and the sorts of futures they could potentially help build for themselves and others (Bolstad et al., 2009). This framing illustrates why some define engagement as '*energy in action*, the connection between person and activity' (Russell et al., 2005, p.3).

The Competent Learners research shows that teachers who are more successful at engaging students appear able to make more realistic assessments of the opportunities they offer and that students take up. They know their students better and in general hold higher expectations of their achievement. One powerful implication from the findings is that teachers need not simply accept students' feelings about their class. They can take the lead in co-creating a learning environment that is more engaging and simultaneously more likely to build students' competencies in powerful and useful ways. However, in order to do so, they may need to let go of some control of the learning action, affording more space for students to create links of personal relevance to them and in which they can exercise responsible choices about learning options and pathways. In one recent case study project, we found that making these types of pedagogical changes appeared to be easier for some teachers than for others (Bolstad et al., 2005). Why is that? This question bears further investigation. There are implications for professional learning in relation to extending teachers' pedagogical repertoire, but also in relation to challenging them to rethink their views of curriculum and of purposes for learning.

This chapter has positioned key competencies as potential drivers of profound curriculum change, albeit with modest success so far in New Zealand. Doubtless other similar initiatives could achieve the same impetus by addressing the same pedagogical (and perhaps curriculum) differences between classes that students enjoy and those that they do not. This chapter is not an argument for foregrounding competency development per se but for re-examining curriculum assumptions and pedagogical practices and ensuring that any initiatives intended to strengthen student engagement take the whole learning context into account. This must include adopting a more nuanced view of opportunities to learn and how these are impacted by the classroom environment and teacher's actions.

References

Bereiter, C., & Scardamalia, M. (2006). Education for the knowledge age: Design centered models of teaching and instruction. In P. Alexander & P. Winne (Eds.), *Handbook of educational psychology* (2nd ed., pp. 695–713). Mahwah, NJ: Lawrence Erlbaum Associates.

Bolstad, R., Boyd, S., & Hipkins, R. (2005). *Students as lifelong learners: Reflections on student data from the Curriculum Innovations Projects*. Paper presented at the New Zealand Association for Research in Education annual conference, Dunedin, New Zealand, December. Retrieved November 25, 2010, from http://www.nzcer.org.nz/default.php?products_id=2714

Bolstad, R., & Gilbert, J. (2008). *Disciplining and drafting, or 21st century learning? Rethinking the New Zealand senior secondary curriculum for the future*. Wellington, New Zealand: New Zealand Council for Educational Research.

Bolstad, R., Roberts, J., Boyd, S., & Hipkins, R. (2009). *Kick starts; Key competencies: Exploring the potential of participating and contributing*. Wellington, New Zealand: NZCER Press.

Carr, M. (2006). *Dimensions of strength for key competencies*. Retrieved February 10, 2008, from http://nzcurriculum.tki.org.nz/curriculum_project_archives/references

Carr, M. (2008). Can assessment unlock and open the doors to resourcefulness and agency? In S. Swaffield (Ed.), *Unlocking assessment. Understanding for reflection and application* (pp. 36–54). London/New York: Routledge.

Davis, B., & Sumara, D. (2010). "If things were simple…": Complexity in education. *Journal of Evaluation in Clinical Practice, 16*, 856–860.

Delandshere, G., & Petrosky, A. (1998). Assessment of complex performances: Limitations of key measurement assumptions. *Educational Researcher, 27*(2), 14–24.

Fredricks, J., Blumenfeld, P., & Paris, A. (2004). School engagement: Potential of the concept, state of the evidence. *Review of Educational Research, 74*(1), 59–109.

Gee, J. (2008). A sociocultural perspective on opportunity to learn. In P. Moss, D. Pullin, J. Gee, E. Haertel, & L. Young (Eds.), *Assessment, equity and opportunity to learn* (pp. 76–108). Cambridge, UK/New York/Melbourne, Australia/Madrid, Spain/Cape Town, South Africa/Singapore/Sao Paulo, Brazil/Delhi, India: Cambridge University Press.

Gilbert, J. (2005). *Catching the knowledge wave? The knowledge society and the future of education*. Wellington, New Zealand: NZCER Press.

Haertel, E., Moss, P., Pullin, D., & Gee, J. (2008). Introduction. In P. Moss, D. Pullin, J. Gee, E. Haertel, & L. Young (Eds.), *Assessment, equity and opportunity to learn* (pp. 1–16). Cambridge, UK/New York/Melbourne, Australia/Madrid, Spain/Cape Town, South Africa/Singapore/Sao Paulo, Brazil/Delhi, India: Cambridge University Press.

Harpaz, Y. (2007). Approaches to teaching thinking: Towards a conceptual mapping of the field. *Teachers College Record, 109*(8), 1845–1874.

Hipkins, R. (2006). *The nature of the key competencies. A background paper*. Wellington, New Zealand: New Zealand Council for Educational Research. Retrieved November 25, 2010, from http://keycompetencies.tki.org.nz/Resourcebank/Introducing-key-competencies2/Key-resources

Hipkins, R. (2007). *Assessing key competencies: Why would we? How could we?* Retrieved February 10, 2009, from http://nzcurriculum.tki.org.nz/implementation_packs_for_schools/assessing_key_competencies_why_would_we_how_could_we

Hipkins, R. (2010a). *The evolving NCEA*. Wellington, New Zealand: New Zealand Council for Educational Research. Retrieved November 25, 2010, from http://www.nzcer.org.nz/default.php?products_id=2529

Hipkins, R. (2010b). *More complex than skills: Rethinking the relationship between key competencies and curriculum content*. Paper presented at the international conference on Education and Development of Civic Competencies, Seoul, South Korea, October. Retrieved November 25, 2010, from http://www.nzcer.org.nz/default.php?products_id=2713

Hipkins, R., & Boyd, S. (2011). The recursive elaboration of key competencies as agents of curriculum change. *Curriculum Matters, 7,* 70–86.

Hipkins, R., Bull, A., & Reid, A. (2010). Some reflections on the philosophical and pedagogical challenges of transforming education. *Curriculum Journal, 21*(1), 109–118.

Hipkins, R., Roberts, J., Bolstad, R., & Ferral, H. (2006). *Staying in science 2: Transition to tertiary study from the perspectives of New Zealand Year 13 science students*. Wellington, New Zealand: Report prepared for New Zealand Ministry of Research, Science and Technology (MoRST). Retrieved November 25, 2010, from http://www.nzcer.org.nz/pdfs/14605.pdf

Hipkins, R., Vaughan, K., with Beals, F., Ferral, H., & Gardiner, B. (2005). *Shaping our futures: Meeting secondary students' learning needs in a time of evolving qualifications* (Final report of the Learning Curves project). Wellington, New Zealand: New Zealand Council for Educational Research. Retrieved November 25, 2010, from http://www.nzcer.org.nz/default.php?products_id=1583

Ministry of Education. (2007). *The New Zealand curriculum*. Wellington, New Zealand: Learning Media.

OECD. (2005). *The definition and selection of key competencies: Executive summary*. Retrieved November 25, 2010, from http://www.oecd.org/dataoecd/47/61/35070367.pdf

Reid, A. (2006). Key competencies: a new way forward or more of the same? *Curriculum Matters, 2,* 43–62.

Russell, J., Ainley, M., & Frydenberg, E. (2005). *Issues digest: Motivation and engagement*. Canberra, Australia: Australian Government: Department of Education, Science and Training.

Rychen, D. (2004). *An overarching conceptual framework for assessing key competences in an international context: Lessons from an interdisciplinary and policy-oriented approach*. Retrieved November 25, 2010, from http://www.cedefop.europa.eu/etv/Upload/Projects_Networks/ResearchLab/ResearchReport/BgR1_Rychen.pdf

Rychen, D., & Salganik, L. (Eds.). (2003). *Key competencies for a successful life and a well-functioning society*. Cambridge, MA: Hogrefe and Huber.

Wertsch, J. (1998). *Mind as action*. New York: Oxford University Press.

Wylie, C., Hipkins, R., & Hodgen, E. (2009). *On the edge of adulthood: Young people's school and out-of-school experiences at 16*. Wellington, New Zealand: Ministry of Education. Retrieved November 25, 2010, from http://www.nzcer.org.nz/content/competent-learners-edge-adulthood.pdf

Wylie, C., & Hodgen, E. (2012). Trajectories and patterns of student engagement: Evidence from a longitudinal study. In S. L. Christenson, A. L. Reschly, & C. Wylie (Eds.), *Handbook of research on student engagement* (pp. 585–599). New York: Springer.

Assessment as a Context for Student Engagement

Sharon L. Nichols and Heather S. Dawson

Abstract

The purpose of this chapter is to examine the ways in which assessment-related instructional practices empirically and theoretically link to student motivation and engagement. We discuss these links in three sections. First, we briefly look at the history of standardized testing in America's schools, drawing connections between the use of testing in practice and student motivation. Next, we look at research on classroom-based assessment practices to discuss how they connect to student motivation. We organize our discussion according to summative and formative distinctions, concluding that summative testing systems tend to connect with traditional motivation processes such as goals and efficacy-related beliefs, whereas formative systems tend to connect with engagement-related processes such as self-regulated learning and self-determination. In the last section, we extrapolate from lessons learned in previous sections to hypothesize on the ways in which high-stakes testing practices may undermine student motivation and engagement.

Introduction and Chapter Overview

The cornerstone of a teacher's job is to assess and evaluate their students' academic status and progress. Using a variety of tools and activities, teachers are constantly collecting information about their students' level of understanding so that they can adjust instruction accordingly. These assessment-related tools and activities come in a variety of forms and serve many different purposes, but all feed the same goal of informing the teacher of students' academic progress so that they can construct meaningful daily lessons that target learners' academic strengths and weakness (McMillan, 2001).

The term *assessment* is used to describe any activity, tool, or interaction, planned or unplanned, that provides teachers with academic-related information about students. Assessments include formal, structured activities such as tests, strategically designed small group activities or whole-class question-and-answer sessions, as well as informal, unstructured activities such as

S.L. Nichols, Ph.D. (✉)
Department of Educational Psychology,
University of Texas, San Antonio, TX, USA
e-mail: Sharon.nichols@utsa.edu

H.S. Dawson, Ph.D.
Department of Educational Policy and Leadership,
The Ohio State University, Columbus, OH, USA
e-mail: dawson.282@osu.edu

impromptu discussions that emerge naturally and spontaneously throughout a school day (Stiggins & Conklin, 1992). Structured and unstructured assessment activities are equally critical components of effective teaching practice (Good & Brophy, 2008; Peterson & Walberg, 1979).

Assessment-related activities pervade teaching and learning, and yet there is a paucity of research examining the connection between these activities and students' motivation or engagement. One explanation rests with the fact that assessment contexts are difficult to operationalize and measure due to their inherent complexities. Brookhart (2004) put it this way,

> The reason the field [classroom assessments] is a bit scattered at present is that classroom assessment sits at intersections in both theory and practice and that the resulting array of relevant practical and theoretical material creates tensions for those who try to chart this territory (p. 429).

Another challenge is that teachers vary widely in the ways in which they construct, implement, and utilize assessment-related devices in their classrooms, making it difficult to extract generalizable data about how these activities connect with student motivation and engagement. Further, the nested nature of such data (students in classrooms, in schools) also makes it difficult to isolate cause-effect relationships among assessment and motivation variables (Miller & Murdock, 2007; Murdock & Miller, 2009).

Another challenge in studying the connection between assessment and student motivation rests with evolving definitions of what student motivation is or entails. Throughout the past century, presumptions about the core mechanisms of motivated action have evolved. McCaslin and DiMarino-Linnen (2000), for example, argued that earlier views were seemingly more complex and inclusive in that they tended to involve biologically based variables (needs, motives) as they simultaneously interacted with achievement-related dispositions (expectancy, values, goals) (Hull, 1943, 1952; McClelland, 1980, 1985). Later, Atkinson's achievement motivation theory (Atkinson, 1974, 1981a, b) prompted a significant shift in theorizing when he translated Hull's biologically based variables of habit and drive into their cognitive representations that later became Expectancy X Value Theory (Feather, 1982; McClelland, 1985; Wigfield & Eccles, 1992). Cognitive approaches dominate current theorizing about motivation.

The concept of student "engagement" emerged from the cognitive revolution in motivational theorizing. In our view, student "engagement" is a specific type of motivation that involves cognitive, affective, and self-regulatory processes (Corno & Mandinach, 2004; Elliot & Dweck, 2005). In contrast to the term "motivation" that encompasses many different theories for explaining human behavior, engagement refers to a particular view of motivated action that presumes students' active involvement in and appropriation of effort related to learning and achievement outcomes.

Chapter Goals and Structure

In spite of the challenges of isolating specific assessment-related practices (Brookhart, 2004) and the evolving conceptions of motivation, there have been some meaningful efforts aimed at understanding their connections (Black & Wiliam, 1998, 2006; Brookhart, 1997; Crooks, 1988; Natriello, 1987). Our goal is to try to bridge ideas gleaned from assessment and motivation/engagement fields and to discuss tests (especially high-stakes tests) as *contexts of learning* and to trace the ways in which these contexts empirically and theoretically connect to student motivation and engagement. We begin with a discussion of low-stakes standardized tests in American education. Their rise in popularity and use in classroom contexts prompted a wave of research investigating their effects on teacher practice. Although direct links to student motivation are lacking, we extrapolate indirect links between standardized test scores and student motivation from the teacher expectation literature.

Next we turn to classroom-based (teacher-made) assessment practices. In this chapter, "classroom-based tests" and "teacher-made tests" are used interchangeably to refer to those tests developed and administered by individual teachers. We also refer to "classroom-based" or "teacher-made" assessment *practices* as a way to discuss all of the activities subsumed within the development, administration, and evaluation of those tests. We organize this section of the chapter according to summative and formative distinctions made in the measurement literature, drawing connections to student motivation and engagement, respectively. Finally, we discuss high-stakes standardized testing. Drawing from lessons learned from studies with low-stakes standardized tests as well as with classroom-based assessments, we hypothesize on the effects of high-stakes testing and student motivation and engagement. We conclude with recommendations for future research, practice, and policy implementation.

Assessment Contexts

An essential component of a teacher's job is to *assess* (evaluate) the academic progress of their students through "structured" and "spontaneous" activities designed to inform instructional decision-making. Structured assessments include activities that are planned and purposeful such as pencil-and-paper teacher-made tests, standardized tests, and performance-based activities, homework, and teacher-student question-and-answer sessions (Crooks, 1988; Rodriguez, 2004; Stiggins & Conklin, 1992;). By contrast, "spontaneous" assessments emerge "from the naturally occurring classroom environment and lead the teacher to a judgment about an individual student's level of development" (Stiggins & Conklin, 1992, p. 33). Thus, classrooms are naturally evolving assessment contexts in which teachers use planned and unplanned activities as data to inform their teaching.

Tests are a familiar form of structured assessment activity that assume a variety of roles and purposes in the classroom (Black & Wiliam, 1998; Brookhart, 1997; Crooks, 1988). Tests are either teacher-made or standardized and can be either high or low stakes. Teacher-made tests have varied formats (multiple choice, essay, short answer, performance assessments), roles (graded, ungraded, quiz, unit test), and purposes (to diagnose student needs, clarify achievement expectations, motivate, and evaluate instructional effectiveness) and are used frequently by teachers to influence instructional decision-making (Crooks, 1988; Stiggins & Bridgeford, 1985; Stiggins & Conklin, 1992). For most students, teacher-made tests are a low-stakes situation since passing/failing a single classroom test does not lead to life-altering consequences (i.e., students have multiple opportunities throughout any given year to demonstrate proficiencies). Standardized tests by contrast, can be either high or low stakes, are developed outside of the classroom, are administered infrequently, and have historically had a minimal influence on teacher practice (Stiggins & Bridgeford, 1992).

Standardized Tests and Testing

Standardized tests emerged in the late eighteenth century at the same time psychologists were becoming increasingly interested in developing scientific methods for measuring human qualities such as intelligence (Gamson, 2007; Sacks, 1999). The widespread use of such tests, however, was not popularized until the construction of the "National Intelligence Test" spearheaded by Edward Thorndike, Lewis Terman, and Robert Yerkes in the early 1900s (Giordano, 2005). Following several prototypes, this National Test included ten tasks (such as printed directions, comparison, picture completion, vocabulary) that were organized into a booklet "that could be applied to any child in the elementary school who could read well enough to participate in a group examination" (Whipple, 1921, p. 17, as cited in Giordano, 2005, p. 21).

Growing familiarity with these standardized tests ignited debates about how best to assess students' academic success in school settings. Proponents, skeptical of subjective teacher grading systems (Starch & Elliott, 1912, as referenced in Giordano, 2005), believed that standardized tests were the perfect way to elicit meaningful and reliable data about students. Opponents worried about test bias and their limited capacity to adequately account for student differences (e.g., race, income). These familiar worries about the appropriate *use* of standardized tests have persisted since their inception (Sacks, 1999). In spite of ongoing debates regarding the fundamental purposes of schools (and therefore, use of tests, e.g., Cuban, 1988; Tyack & Cuban, 1997), proponents of standardized tests were convinced of their necessity and role. Eminent psychologist and respected psychometrician E. L. Thorndike put it this way,

> Educational science and educational practice alike need more objective, more accurate and more convenient measures...Any progress toward measuring how well a child can read with something of the objectivity, precision, commensurability, and convenience which characterize our measurement of how tall he is, how much he can lift with his back or squeeze with his hand, or how acute his vision is, would be of great help in grading, promoting, testing the value of methods of teaching and in every other case where we need to know ourselves and to inform others how well an individual or a class or a school population can read (Thorndike, 1923, p. 1–2).

Since Thorndike's time, the form and function of standardized tests have expanded swiftly and have been used for many purposes over the years (Sacks, 1999). Norm-referenced tests (e.g., IQ) gave us a way to rank students according to aptitude. Criterion-referenced tests provided measures of students' progress against externally defined standards. Other standardized tests gave us a way to make predictions about students' academic potential (e.g., SAT, GRE) (Giordano, 2005; Herman & Haertel, 2005; Moss, 2007; Sacks, 1999).

Until the 1990s, performance on any one of these types of tests had relatively low stakes for students and essentially no stakes for teachers. Although some states and districts have a history of experimenting with high-stakes testing as a way to reform and improve schools, this practice was inconsistent and relatively inconsequential for large groups of students (Allington & McGill-Franzen, 1992; Tyack, 1974). This has changed radically over the past few decades as the rhetoric of public schools in "crisis" expanded (Berliner & Biddle, 1995; Glass, 2008; National Commission for Excellence in Education [NCEE], 1983), culminating with the No Child Left Behind Act (NCLB, 2002) that mandated the use of high-stakes testing in all schools for all students. Consequential standardized testing systems pervade modern American classrooms (Herman & Haertel, 2005; Orfield & Kornhaber, 2001), creating a particular type of assessment context that we will visit in the second half of this chapter. First, we explore some data indicating how low-stakes standardized tests may connect to student motivation.

Low-Stakes Standardized Tests: Student-Teacher Connections

Research in the teacher expectation tradition provides some initial clues about how teachers' knowledge of their students' standardized test scores may impact students' motivation (e.g., Good, 1981; Good & Brophy, 1972; Kellaghan, Madaus, & Airasian, 1982). In their seminal work, *Pygmalion in the Classroom*, Rosenthal and Jacobson (1968) imposed ability-level expectations on teachers by informing them that a special test taken by their students at the beginning of the year revealed which students were about to "bloom" and which were not. At the end of the year, Rosenthal and Jacobson found that those randomly identified as "bloomers" had higher grades than those not so identified by the end of the school. From this data, they concluded that teachers' initial impressions of student abilities somehow had created a self-fulfilling prophecy effect—transforming perceived "bloomers" into actual ones by the end of the year.

Methodological inadequacies in this original study were addressed in subsequent observational studies in which teacher interactions with their students were measured after imposed (or natural) expectations were induced (or measured) (Good & Brophy, 1972, 1974; Good & Thompson, 1998). A growing literature on expectation effects revealed that teachers treated students differentially and according to their perceptions of students' ability. For example, teachers often gave their perceived high-ability students more time to think when they were asked a question, whereas perceived low-ability learners were given less time and were treated in ways in which the teacher attempted to "protect" their esteem on tasks (Good, 1981).

Importantly, we learned that students are aware of their teachers' beliefs of them. One fourth grader put it this way,

> Like half the class is pretty smart and...the other half isn't. And these people...that's not smart, she'll just let 'em go, she won't really care what they do. 'Cause she knows they don't care. And the rest of the people, she'll just push and push, and says, We gotta have some survive, you know (as quoted in Weinstein, 2002, p. 89).

Not surprisingly, then, data seem to suggest that teachers' expectations may relate to students' self-esteem and motivation (e.g., Brophy, 1998; Meichenbaum & Smart, 1971; Weinstein, 2002). However, the link of standardized test scores and student attitudes is fuzzy at best. Among all the sources of information teachers use to form impressions about their students, the role of tests in influencing teachers' treatment of students may be minimal. Kellaghan et al. (1982, p. 16) note,

> [standardized] Test information is of itself insufficient to overcome the effects of other factors such as the information teachers glean from assignments completed by students and from a knowledge of students' home backgrounds...test information is merely a part, and probably a relatively small part, of the pressure exerted on students by the educational environment. Even if expectancy processes operate in the classroom, test information is only one factor in the network that creates such expectancies, and any possible role it may have to play in affecting students has to be considered in this context.

Thus, in spite of all we know about expectation effects and students (Brophy, 1998; Weinstein, 2002), we know little about the *specific* role standardized testing data play in teachers' interactions with students and subsequently students' motivation.

Classroom-Based Tests and Testing

Classroom-based (CB) or teacher-made (TM) tests are used to evaluate students' academic understanding as it pertains to specific topics or units of instruction and can be either summative or formative in nature. Summative tests (measures *of* learning) are given at the end of units, the results of which inform teachers of students' learning. Formative assessments (measures *for* learning) are given more frequently throughout a unit or topic, the results of which inform ongoing teaching decisions and learner assessments. Both forms of classroom-based assessments are important sources of information to teachers, each with distinct purposes and with potential to influence student motivation and engagement (Black & Wiliam, 1998, 2006; Brookhart, 2004; McInerney, Brown, & Liem, 2009).

Summative Tests and Student Motivation

Summative tests are those given at the end of units or topic areas and are typically used to assign grades. They consist of test items designed to gauge how well students may (or may not) have mastered a given content area. We review data demonstrating that the use of these tests can influence student motivation in two primary ways: (a) test content influences students' effort and value formation, and (b) grading/feedback systems influence students' goal adoption.

Tests Inform Students What to Value

According to Expectancy X Value Theory, motivation is the result of students' perceptions of task outcome and value. Expectancies are typically defined as "individuals' beliefs about how well they will do on upcoming tasks, either in the immediate or longer-term future" (Eccles & Wigfield, 2002, p. 119), whereas value involves four types: attainment, intrinsic, utility, and cost (Eccles, 1983; Wigfield & Eccles, 1992, 2000, 2002). *Attainment value* refers to the importance an individual places on the task, resulting in the individual adjusting self-beliefs accordingly. *Intrinsic value* refers to the amount of enjoyment the student acquires from the task. *Utility value* refers to the perception of usefulness the task has to the student. *Cost* addresses the sacrifices the student must accept in order to engage in the task.

Studies have shown that the form and content of tests exerts a powerful influence on what is important to learn (i.e., informing students what to *value*). According to Rogers (1969, as stated in Crooks, 1988, p. 445),

Examinations tell them [students] our real aims, at least so they believe. If we stress clear understanding and aim at a growing knowledge of physics, we may completely sabotage our teaching by a final examination that asks for numbers to be put into memorized formulas. However loud our sermons, however intriguing the experiments, students will judge by that examination—and so will next year's students who hear about it.

Research also suggests that test content may influence students' study habits and effort (Natriello & Dornbusch, 1984; Snyder, 1971). For example, Snyder noticed that although classroom curricula may emphasize meaning, depth, and problem solving, if the test emphasized rote memorization, then students, wanting to perform well on tests, would often disregard classroom activities focusing on problem-oriented learning and focus on rote memorization to optimize time, effort, and academic success on tests (see also Fredericksen, 1984).

Tests are important mechanisms that convey to students not only *what* they should know but also *how* they should know it (Bloom, 1956; Krathwohl, 2002). Research suggests, for example, that students vary in their capacity to recognize the level of processing demands made by a test as well as their ability to adapt to those demands. Miller and Parlett (1974) found that some students were highly adept "cue seekers"— those who actively noticed the features of test questions and adapted their study habits accordingly to maximize their test performance. By contrast, others were "cue conscious," less active in seeking out test features but still relatively conscious about test-related cues that were handed to them (i.e., by the teacher). Others have shown that students who generally use "surface level" processing approaches (rote memorization) to tests have difficulty adjusting when deeper-level processing is necessary (Martin & Ramsden, 1987). But perhaps more worrisome are data that suggest students capable of deeper-level processing switch to surface-level approaches when faced with surface-level learning environments (i.e., in classrooms that emphasize rote memorization) (Crooks & Mahalski, 1986).

Elsewhere, Entwistle and Kozeski (1985) examined the question of how curriculum content and evaluation practices set forth through national policy prescriptions impact student study habits in two different countries: Britain and Hungary. At the time, Britain's educational culture was steeped in a summative standardized testing system that emphasized "correctness," whereas Hungarian culture had prioritized creativity and higher-order processing in their schools. Using surveys to measure students' study strategies with approximately 1,200 thirteen to seventeen-year olds in Hungary (n=579) and Britain (n=614), Entwistle and Kozeski found main effect differences in how students approached studying. Britain's students were more apt to employ surface-level strategies in learning (memorization) while Hungarian students were more likely to emphasize deeper learning strategies. Entwistle and Kozeski cautiously conclude that educational assessment environments may influence students' approach to learning.

From this data, it seems as if tests' inherent utility value as a doorway to academic advancement and personal satisfaction (e.g., doing well leads to better grades, pleases the teacher) connects to students' effort and study strategies. Students seem to adapt their study strategies according to the nature and content of the test they face and want to pass. Of course, students do not respond in a monolithic way. Some students engage in adaptive, deep-processing study strategies even if the test promotes memorization and rote learning (Crooks & Mahalski, 1986). Still, testing content conveys important message to students about what the culture values, and many adjust their efforts accordingly.

Tests Influence Student Goals and Classroom Goal Structures

Achievement goal research has dominated much of the motivation literature in recent decades. Relying heavily on self-report measures, this literature has yielded some important constructs for understanding how students' beliefs about themselves and the task at hand influence outcomes such as persistence and achievement (grades). Prior to discussing how goals intersect with tests, it seems useful to briefly review some of the main findings from this literature base.

Goals

Students' achievement goals are an integrated pattern of beliefs, attributions, and affect that produces the intentions of behavior (Weiner, 1986, see also Ames, 1992; Ames & Archer, 1988; Elliott & Dweck, 1988, 2005). Achievement goals vary according to the context, or are context specific, and vary between individuals (Ames & Archer, 1988; Kaplan, 2004). A mastery (learning) goal orientation for learning purports that the individual's purpose is to *develop* competence (Ames, 1992; Kaplan & Maehr, 2007). Students with a mastery orientation are more invested in learning for learning's sake, gaining a genuine understanding of the material, and acquiring the skills necessary to succeed at a given task (Kaplan & Maehr). Mastery-oriented students typically also have higher self-efficacy, greater persistence for a task, prefer challenges, are more self-regulated, and have a greater sense of well-being (Ames, 1992; Elliot, 1999; Kaplan & Maehr, 2007; Kaplan, Middleton, Urdan, & Midgley, 2002). Mastery goals also elicit greater effort, elaborative processing strategies, and intrinsic motivation (Elliot).

While a mastery orientation for achievement describes the individual's focus on *developing* competence, the performance orientation describes the individual's focus on *demonstrating* competence. Performance orientations toward academic achievement lend themselves to a more prominent focus on ability, the desire to achieve with little effort, and desire to avoid demonstrating lack of ability (Ames, 1992; Ames & Archer, 1988). The individual with a performance orientation is more concerned with appearing adequate. This implies that a student with this orientation will succeed or fail based upon their desire to appear competent or avoid appearing incompetent in front of their peers or mentors. Performance-oriented students attribute their success and failure to their ability rather than to the amount of effort they invested and believe ability is fixed, often referred to as an "entity" view of intelligence (Kaplan et al., 2002).

There has been research that shows that performance goals are associated with positive outcomes such as increased self-efficacy (Elliot, 1999; Urdan, 1997), and other research to show that performance goals are associated with less adaptive outcomes such as use of surface-level cognitive strategies, avoiding help seeking, and low knowledge retention (Kaplan & Maehr, 2007; Midgley, Kaplan, & Middleton, 2001). The mixed findings regarding the effects of performance goals on outcomes contributed to the development of the approach-avoid distinction for performance goals (Elliot).

Performance-approach goals are often associated with positive and negative outcomes in the literature (Elliot, 1999; Midgley et al. 2001), whereas performance-avoid goals are more clearly maladaptive in nature (Kaplan & Maehr, 2007). Performance-approach goals have been associated with positive (persistence, positive affect, and grades, Elliot, 1999; Kaplan & Maehr, 2007) and negative (anxiety, disruptive behavior, and less knowledge retention, Kaplan & Maehr, 2007; Midgley et al. 2001) outcomes. By contrast, performance-avoidant goals are consistently associated with negative outcomes including low efficacy, anxiety, avoidance of help seeking, self-handicapping, and low grades and share similarities with the work-avoidant goals, although these two goal orientations stem from different cognitive-affective frameworks (Kaplan & Maehr). Performance-avoidant goals were the only type of goal orientation to inhibit motivation (Elliot & Harackiewicz, 1996). There is evidence to support the notion that the performance-avoidant goal orientation stems from a fear of failure rather than from the desire to manage impressions that others hold about the individual (Elliot & Church, 1997).

Summative Feedback and Goals

Summative tests yield data that highlight performance comparisons among students. After all, the whole point of a summative test is to highlight what students know and/or do not know. The way in which teachers formulate their feedback on the basis of summative testing results can directly influence students' goal adoption (Black & Wiliam, 1998). In a study by Butler (1988) of 48 eleven-year-old Israeli students, participants were given different types of feedback following a series of structured paired tasks. One-third of the group was given individual comments and feedback, one-third given grades only as feedback, and one-third were given comments and grades combined. Results showed the "comments only" group did significantly better than the "grades only" or "comments plus" groups of students. Butler concludes that normative feedback can undermine motivation and that *informational* feedback enhances motivation and achievement.

Schunk's (1996) work has revealed similar patterns. In one study, he randomly assigned 44 nine to ten-year olds to one of four conditions. Half of the students were assigned to tasks where teachers emphasized performance goals and the other half into tasks where teachers emphasized learning goals. Then, within each of these conditions, students were randomly assigned to one of two subsequent conditions: half were asked to be self-reflective at the conclusion of the task, whereas the rest were only asked to fill out a questionnaire. Participants assigned to the performance goal group with no self-evaluation scored lower in skills and efficacy, while participants assigned to the mastery goal group with frequent evaluation scored higher on motivation and achievement outcomes. Feedback which "draws attention away from the task and towards self-esteem can have a negative effect on attitudes and performance" (Black & Wiliam, 1998, p. 13; see also Bangert-Drowns, Kulik, & Morgan, 1991).

Competition and Cooperation

Tests and other tasks or classroom activities can also be viewed as competitive or cooperative events. In general, classroom activities, tasks, and/or feedback systems that promote competition tend to be associated with lower student achievement than classes that promote cooperation (Johnson & Johnson, 1985, 1999). Good and Brophy (2008) argued that if students become preoccupied with "winning" or "losing" the competitive activity, they may lose sight of important instructional objectives and content. From the student's perspective, performance then takes precedence over learning. Further, inherent in the practice of competition is the necessity for someone to lose. If the same students lose over and over despite their best efforts, they may come to see the world as unfair and are likely to give up when faced with challenging academic tasks, as they have learned that failure will be the outcome no matter how hard they try to succeed. Conversely, students who routinely win at competitive tasks may lose interest in the instructional material and over time may put forth the minimal amount of effort required to outperform other students rather than maximizing effort in order to master the task or material.

Competition-oriented classrooms may promote the development of performance goals rather than mastery goals (Ames, 1984). Similarly, competition and performance goals may decrease intrinsic motivation toward academic tasks because students rely on rewards from others to motivate them to complete tasks rather than completing tasks for the reward of building competence and skills (Henderlong & Lepper, 2002; Lepper, Corpus, & Iyengar, 2005). Competition in the classroom also might distract students from learning: they become so focused on performing better than peers that they get distracted from learning or anxious about losing. In short, the quality and content of summative test feedback may promote students' performance (or learning), goal orientation, and/or competitive (or collaborative) contexts which in turn may impede (or enhance) students' motivation.

Classroom Goal Structures

In addition to individual teacher-student interaction, teachers also communicate to the whole class, establishing rules and feedback systems that impact all students. Reciprocally, these events influence students' interactions with one another, which in turn also influence teacher practice.

Classroom goal structures emerge throughout the many layers of the teaching process including the type of tasks assigned (difficulty, variety), the nature of student evaluations (norm-based or criterion-based), and the way teacher authority is communicated (e.g., Ames, 1992; Blumenfeld, 1992).

Classroom goals are often measured by aggregating individual students' perceptions of the types of goals emphasized in their classes[1] and fall into the familiar categories of mastery- or performance-based classroom goals. Tasks promote performance orientation when they prompt students to compare their abilities with other students. Similarly, evaluation systems (i.e., grades, achievement feedback) that stress social comparison in achievement are associated with performance goal classroom structures (Ames, 1984; Johnson & Johnson, 1985). And authority systems or classroom management techniques that restrict student autonomy and control are related to performance-based goal structures. Studies also suggest that classrooms with a performance goal structure are associated with higher levels of student cheating when compared to classroom with a mastery structure (Anderman, 2007).

Formative Tests and Student Engagement

Student engagement is a type of motivation that involves cognitive and affective processes that unfold over time. This dynamic view of motivation is more consistent with formative approaches to assessment because they both conceptualize learning as a process instead of a product. To explore these connections, we focus on two approaches to the concept of student engagement: self-regulated learning and self-determination.

Self-Regulation

Growing attention to the concept of self-regulation emerged in the 1970s with the advent of process-product research constructed to understand how teachers' instructional practice and use of time correlated with student outcomes (Good, 1987; Peterson & Walberg, 1979). During this period, observational research was flourishing, and researchers were beginning to understand the important connections between specific instructional activities and successful student engagement and achievement (Berliner, 1979). At the same time, researchers were focusing on teacher practice (Good & Brophy, 1972, 1974) and others were becoming more concerned with student motivation variables (e.g., Corno & Mandinach, 1983). If there were "optimal" ways teachers might distribute their time during instruction, then researchers wanted to know what were the "optimal" ways students might also be engaged in their own learning.

Corno and Mandinach (1983) described "self-regulated learning" (SRL) as one of the "most sophisticated forms of engagement that students could display in school-related (academic) activities and events" (Corno & Mandinach, 2004, p. 300). According to Corno and Mandinach (1983, 2004), SRL involved not just effective cognitive processing skills (e.g., appropriate use of knowledge and critical thinking) but also conative (willful or purposeful striving) and affective components. Since 1983, conceptions of student engagement have broadened over time, moving from a focus on the individual to a focus on social processes that support or impede engagement and self-regulated learning. Research has also grown more sophisticated to allow for the interacting influences of in- and out-of-school contexts while examining both short- and long-time impacts on academic engagement and outcomes (Boekaerts, Pintrich, & Zeidner, 2000; Corno & Mandinach, 1983, 2004; Csikszentmihalyi, Abuhamdeh, & Nakamura, 2005).

Most models of self-regulation assume that optimization involves students' active participation in and commitment to the learning activity. Boekaerts and Corno (2005) note,

---

[1] Studies of classroom goal structures have been heavily critiqued on methodological and theoretical grounds. For example, Miller and Murdock (2007) cautioned that aggregating students' perceptions undermined the validity of any classroom-based measure. Similarly, they argued that personal goals and classroom goal structures should not be viewed as orthogonal contributors to individual student effort. Using linear modeling techniques, they argued that when entered at level 2 instead of level 1, the effects of the classroom mastery goal structure are much smaller, suggesting that these are mediated by their effects on students' personal goals. Loosely translated, this suggests that a mastery goal orientation may be a product of both personality and classroom structures (Murdock & Miller, 2009).

All theorists assume that students who self-regulate their learning are engaged actively and constructively in a process of meaning generation and that they adapt their thoughts, feelings, and actions as needed to affect their learning and motivation. Similarly, models assume that biological, developmental, contextual, and individual difference constraints may all interfere with or support efforts at regulation (p. 201).

In spite of these common assumptions, different theoretical models emphasize different components. For example, Corno (2001) considers the role of volition (or will), Winne (1995) emphasizes the cognitive aspects of self-regulation, and McCaslin (2009) looks at sociocultural processes. Others are beginning to advocate a view of engagement as an inherently developmental process related to identity that unfolds and emerges over time, through academic-related interactions in the classroom (Kaplan & Flum, 2009). Common to all of these approaches to self-regulation is the notion of student will, volition, or "buy-in."

Self-Determination

Another form of student engagement comes from self-determination theory (Deci & Ryan, 1995). A distinguishing characteristic of self-determination theory (SDT) is the extent to which an individual is acting of their own volition or whether their intent is being controlled to some extent (Deci, Vallerand, Pelletier, & Ryan, 1991). The individual acting "wholly volitionally" is self-determined, meaning the person perceives the locus of causality to be internal. The individual acting without volition perceives the locus of causality to be external to them. These differences are significant and possess different components of regulation; that is, the self-determined individual possesses a regulatory process of choice, while the controlled individual possesses a regulatory process that is compliant (Deci et al., 1991).

SDT incorporates needs-based aspects of human life in its framework. There are three innate psychological needs each human possesses, according to the theory (Deci et al., 1991). They are the *need for competence*, the *need for relatedness*, and the *need for autonomy* or *self-determination*. Competence is an individual's need for attainment of various outcomes and efficacy for doing so; relatedness is an individual's need for secure and satisfying connections with others; and autonomy is the ability to regulate one's own actions and behaviors (Deci et al.). Needs are central to human behavior, and, therefore, opportunities to satisfy these needs contribute to the likelihood to be motivated.

Formative Assessment Links to Engagement Processes

Formative assessment practices are ideally suited for enhancing (or impeding) engagement-related processes. Whereas summative tests are one-time experiences that provide specific data about student performance, formative assessments are given over time and are used to inform the learning and teaching *process*. Importantly, summative tests are designed and controlled by the teacher, whereas formative assessments require active participation of students. According to Black and Wiliam (1998, p. 11),

> The core of the activity of formative assessment lies in the sequence of two actions. The first is the perception by the learner of a gap between a desired goal and his or her present state (of knowledge, and/or understanding, and/or skills). The second is the action taken by the learner to close that gap in order to attain the desired goal.

Teachers and students play equally important roles in actualizing this sequence of events. According to Black and Wiliam (1998), for the first event to occur,

> The prime responsibility for generating the information may lie with the student in self-assessment, or with another person, notably the teacher, who discerns and interprets the gap and communicates a message about it to the student. Whatever the procedures by which the assessment message is generated, in relation to action taken by the learner it would be a mistake to regard the student as the passive recipient of a call to action. There are complex links between the way the message is received, the way in which that perception motivates a selection amongst different courses of action, and the learning activity which may or may not follow.

Formative assessment practices, therefore, become a venue through which engagement-related beliefs and actions emerge and are sustained.

Studies suggest that formative assessment approaches, which inherently emphasize engagement-related processes such as self-reflection and self-determination, are more effective than summative assessment practices in promoting persistence and academic achievement. For example, Frederiksen and White (1997) compared achievement outcomes among middle school science students, half of whom were exposed to self-reflective assessment activities and half who were not. Their results demonstrate that students who participate in self-reflective assessment practices understand curriculum better than those not prompted to self-reflect. Similarly, formative assessment practices provide students with greater opportunities to demonstrate autonomy and choice through feedback processes that are more informational than controlling, thus enhancing engagement-related action and beliefs (Deci & Ryan, 1995; Grolnick & Ryan, 1987). In general, efforts made to draw students' attention to their own learning progress through activities such as self-reflection and self-evaluation enhance learning and achievement outcomes (Black & Wiliam, 1998; Thomas, 1993).

The Popularization of High-Stakes Standardized Tests

High-stakes standardized testing has increasingly assumed a more dominant role in American classrooms (Giordano, 2005; Herman & Haertel, 2005; Stiggins, 2001). Part of its rise in popularity has been due to rapid advances in technology (allowing for easier distribution and scoring) and psychometric techniques. But another influence has been political—attaching stakes to standardized test performance (i.e., high-stakes testing) has become a convenient policy position for the advocacy of evaluating, monitoring, and judging the perceived inadequacies of a public school system (Berliner & Biddle, 1995; Cuban, 1988; Good, 1996; Herman & Haertel, 2005; McDonnell, 2005; NCEE, 1983; Tyack & Cuban, 1997). The passage of NCLB in 2002 mandated use of high-stakes testing as a way to hold teachers, students, and schools accountable for learning.

Since the passage of the No Child Left Behind Act (NCLB), students are immersed in testing and test-related activities at unprecedented levels. Prior to NCLB, data suggested that standardized tests took up little time and had only minimal impact on teachers and students (Sacks, 1999). The advent of high-stakes testing accountability, however, has radically changed this educational landscape such that teachers rely more heavily on standardized test results than ever before and in ways that are largely detrimental to instructional practice (Herman & Haertel, 2005; Nichols & Berliner, 2007).

The theory of action undergirding the practice of high-stakes testing is that when faced with large incentives and threatening punishments, teachers will be more effective, students will be more motivated, and parents will become more involved (e.g., Amrein & Berliner, 2002; McDonnell, 2005; Raymond & Hanushek, 2003). In short, it is believed that the pressure of doing well on a test will spur everyone into action, thus improving American public schools significantly (Peterson & West, 2003; Phelps, 2005). Yet, 7 years after NCLB was enacted, there is no convincing evidence that student learning has increased in any significant way (e.g., Nichols, 2007). By contrast, there is a wealth of documentation that this carrot-and-stick approach to school reform has resulted in educationally deleterious side effects (e.g., Jones & Egley, 2004; Jones, Jones, & Hargrove, 2003; Orfield & Kornhaber, 2001; Pedulla et al., 2003; Valenzuela, 2005). These side effects and the pursuant collateral damage to student motivation and engagement are the focus of the next section in the chapter.

High-Stakes Tests and Student Motivation: Some Correlational Data

Students and teachers are immersed in high-stakes tests. Data reveal that in addition to taking standardized tests, teachers spend large amounts of time preparing students for tests (Nichols & Berliner, 2007). For example, survey research found that 80% of elementary teachers in North Carolina reported that they spent more than 20% of their total teaching time practicing for high-stakes tests (Jones et al., 1999). This is about the equivalent of 36 days of test preparation. Further, the survey found that 28% of those teachers reported spending more than 60% of their time practicing for the state's tests—amounting to over 100 of the typical 180 days of instruction spent in various forms of test preparation.

In spite of the overwhelming amount of time teachers and students spend engaged with high-stakes standardized tests, there is shockingly little data on the impact it has (or may have) on student motivation. One exception is a set of correlation studies from the early 1990s. Paris, Turner, and Lawton (1990, as cited in Paris, Lawton, Turner, & Roth, 1991) surveyed nearly 1,000 students in states then practicing high-stakes testing (Florida, Michigan, California, and Arizona) at the time. This cross-sectional correlational analysis of students' views of tests revealed a pattern in which younger students viewed these standardized tests as useful and valid representations of what they know. By contrast, older students demonstrated "disillusionment" in their perceptions in that they felt tests were not valuable or valid and that the growing preoccupation with tests seemed to undermine their views of their teachers.

A decade later, Paris and colleagues followed up with another set of longitudinal analyses of students' perceptions of the value of high-stakes testing (e.g., Paris, Roth, & Turner, 2000; Wong & Paris, 2000) as well as the effect of tests on teachers and schools (Paris & Urdan, 2000). Both cross-sectional and longitudinal survey data revealed that students generally view high-stakes tests negatively and that there are developmental differences between sixth and eighth graders in their views. Specifically, older students tend to hold more negative views of tests and testing, and report increasing cynicism about achievement tests and increasing worries about teachers devaluing them as a result of their test performance (Paris et al., 2000). By contrast, fifth graders held more positive views of testing (saw tests as more valuable and useful and felt more positively about them) than their eighth-grade peers.

At issue, then, is what explains these developmental trends, and there are two probable explanations. On the one hand, a rich literature already informs us that students' motivation generally declines as they move from elementary into middle and high school (e.g., Eccles & Midgley, 1989; Wigfield & Guthrie, 1997; Wigfield & Wagner, 2005). Further, there is a wealth of data to show that students' sense of self-competency also declines over time (Anderman & Maehr, 1994; Eccles et al., 1989; Wigfield, Eccles, MacIver, Reuman, & Midgley, 1991; Wigfield & Wagner, 2005). Thus, growing "disillusionment" with tests could simply be a by-product of a naturally occurring developmental trend whereby students generally grow disenchanted with school. On the other hand, it could be that there is an accumulation effect brought upon by excessive test-taking experiences. Data suggest that when it comes to test-related pressures, there emerges a "cumulative, negative impact on students that can be summarized in three general trends: growing disillusionment about tests, decreasing motivation to give genuine effort, and increasing use of inappropriate [test-taking] strategies" (Paris et al., 1991, p. 14).

High-Stakes Tests: Exaggerated Emphasis of Tests

Survey and anecdotal data suggest that as the pressure to perform well on the test rises, teachers and administrators increasingly emphasize its importance to students (Abrams, Pedulla, & Madaus, 2003). One way this has emerged is in the surge in test-day pep rallies. For example, in one NY school, the principal holds pep rallies every spring where students come together and sing "inspiring" songs such as "I've been working on my writing," and "I'm a believer" (Toy, 2006). Elsewhere in Texas, school walls are adorned with "inspirational" guidance to students to "Beat the TAKS" (Texas Assessment of Knowledge and Skills) and students meet every spring for a rally complete with a full dinner and cheerleaders leading everyone in chants such as "let's beat the TAKS" and "Use our skills!" (Foster, 2006 as reported in Nichols & Berliner, 2007). The advent of high-stakes testing has influenced schools to rally students in ways that exaggerate the importance of the test in students' lives.

High-stakes tests become overexaggerated when they change what is taught in schools. Data reveal that high-stakes testing systems are increasingly narrowing the curriculum; content that will appear on the test is emphasized while content that is not tested is eliminated from the curriculum. We know, for example, that the arts (music and art) as well as physical education are being cut at high rates (Nichols & Berliner, 2007; Vasquez Heilig, Cole, & Aguilar, 2010). One study revealed that 71% of districts surveyed had reduced instructional time in at least one other subject to make more time for reading and mathematics, the subjects tested under NCLB (Center on Education Policy [CEP], 2006). In some districts, struggling students received double periods of reading, math, or both. Data suggested that the narrowed curriculum disproportionately impacted poor and minority students. According to the CEP report, 97% of high-poverty districts (where more than 75% of students are eligible for free or reduced price lunch) compared with 55–59% of lower-poverty districts had policies that restricted curriculum offerings (CEP, 2006).

Teachers have confirmed this trend (Taylor, Shepard, Kinner, & Rosenthal, 2003). One teacher from Colorado noted, "I eliminated a lot of my social studies and science. I eliminated Colorado History. What else? Electricity. Most of that because it's more stressed that the kids know the reading and the math, so, it was pretty much said, you know, you do what you gotta do." Another teacher reiterated the point, "[I] eliminated curriculum such as novels I would teach, we didn't have time to go to the library, we didn't have time to use the computer labs because they had to cut something. [I] Cut things I thought we could live without. [I] Cut presentations, anything that takes very much time, I cut film. We have been cutting like crazy."

It is unclear how the overexaggeration of tests conveyed by test pep rallies, curriculum narrowing, and other forms of instructional manipulation in the current high-stakes testing climate impacts student motivation. But anecdotal data from students reveals something ominous. In Texas, for example, where the stakes are relatively high compared to most other states (Nichols, Glass, & Berliner, 2006), students are jaded. One high school junior notes the following (San Antonio Express-News, 2007):

> In Texas, many public school districts have found raising their standardized testing averages to be the No. 1 goal of classroom curriculum. Consequently, school is no longer a forum where students can discuss the effects of alcohol, or the best method to achieve a life filled with value and pleasure, or the simple antics of their daily life. Instead, learning institutions have become places where multiple-choice tests, quadratic equations, and the size of a cell are deemed as significant pieces of knowledge which students are required to know in order to survive.

Or, as another student stated,

> I know what it's like to be tested over and over and over and over again from the time you're in third grade until you're a junior in high school. I know what it's like having to go over multiple-choice questions for two weeks straight right before TAKS. I know how incredibly boring it is to sit in a classroom with 29 other people and wait for the rest of the school to finish the test.

Elsewhere, nefarious retention practices were revealed when administrators described practices that seemingly pushed low-achieving students out of school (Vasquez Heilig & Darling-Hammond, 2008):

> I think that the kids are being forced out of school. I had a kid who came here from [school name] and said, "Miss, I if I come here, could I ever take the [exit exam]?" and I said, "What do you mean? If you come here, you must take the [exam]." And he said, "Well, every time I think I'm going to take the test, they either say, 'You don't have to come to school tomorrow or you don't have to [take the test]'…we're told different things." (p. 99)

Students understand not only how important the test is but also how valuable they are (or are not) to the school simply on the basis of how they score on the test. These implicit and explicit messages about tests and student value have potential to seriously erode students' motivation over time (Nichols & Berliner, 2007; Perlstein, 2007).

The Dropout Crisis

There is perhaps no greater evidence of lowered motivation for school than when a student drops out of school. Tragically, data suggest that the pressures associated with high-stakes testing are related to students' decisions to leave school. Perhaps the most revealing trend on the impact of high-stakes testing and poor, minority youth emerges in dropout/graduation rate data. Data are relatively clear that when students have to pass a test to receive a diploma, poor and minority students are at greater risk of dropping out of school all together (e.g., Orfield, 2004; Orfield, Losen, Wald, & Swanson, 2004; Warren, Jenkins, & Kulick, 2006). Graduation rate data demonstrate a similar trend where poor students and those who are African-American, Latino/a, ELL, and/or who have disabilities graduate at a much lower rate than their white, more advantaged peers (Gayler, Chudowsky, Hamilton, Kober & Yeager, 2004). This connection demonstrates that for certain groups of students, testing pressures not only diminish their motivation but undermine it completely. Thus, for many students, but especially for poor minority students, the repeated failures on a test that might be their last obstacle to obtaining a high school diploma may directly undermine their motivation to stay in school and to keep trying.

There is also growing data on troubling practices emerging in high-stakes testing contexts which indirectly impact poor, minority students' motivation. For example, Vasquez Heilig and Darling-Hammond (2008) found that a disproportionate number of ninth-grade minority students were held back in order to avoid their test participation during an accountability year. One student shared her perspective, "I have a friend that was in ninth grade for 2 years, and she was 19 or 20 years old. She did not pass algebra, and the school told her that if she didn't improve her grades, they were going to drop her since she was older. So she…dropped out of school" (p. 98). Haney's research in Florida revealed that increases in students' test performance were not the result of learning gains, but the result of manipulation. He found that, "Florida started flunking more students—including disproportionately high numbers of minority students—and requiring them to repeat grade three" (Haney, 2008, p. 94). Over and over, evidence suggests that in response to high-stakes testing pressures, efforts are made to game the system (retain/flunk low-scoring students, manipulate data, lower performance standards) with these effects disproportionately impacting poor, minority students (see also Darling-Hammond, 2007; Madaus, Russell & Higgins, 2009; Nichols & Berliner, 2007; Ryan, 2004; Valenzuela, 2005).

These effects also impact high-achieving students. McNeil, Coppola, Radigan, and Vasquez Heilig (2008) found that African-American honor students noticed significant shifts in the curriculum and in the ways in which their teachers interacted with them relating to the test. One student shared,

> Instead of teaching us the real life things that we are going to need for college and stuff, they started zeroing in just on that test. So it makes everybody nervous, and it threw everybody off. So, like, our curriculum is thrown off, 'cause what they originally were teaching us in the subjects, all of the sudden they switched, and then they were just zeroing into this test (McNeil et al., 2008, p. 28).

Another African-American honors senior added this, "Some teachers are so scared and don't know what to expect on the test, that they zero in on that test and it bugs us just hearing about this test" (p. 29). Students of all achievement levels notice how their teachers respond to the test. It seems that for these students, who otherwise are extremely motivated, teachers' preoccupation with tests present missed opportunities for authentic learning experiences.

High-stakes testing pressures are also connected with lowered graduation rates (another indicator of dropout trends). Jacob (2001) for example, looked at dropout data as well as twelfth-grade achievement data in reading and math as reported on the National Educational Longitudinal Survey (NELS) in states with and without high school graduation exams. After accounting for prior achievement and other background characteristics (e.g., SES, ethnicity), Jacob found no significant differences in students' achievement between states with mandatory testing and those without. However, students, especially lower-ability students, were more likely to drop out when faced with mandatory graduation exams than students in states without such an exam. Marchant and Paulson (2005) looked at the effect of high school graduation exams on state-level graduation rates, aggregated SAT scores, and individual student SAT scores. By comparing graduation rates and SAT scores in states with a graduation exam against states without a graduation exam, they also found that states with graduation exams had lower graduation rates and lower aggregate SAT scores. These findings have been replicated in other studies (e.g., Nichols et al., 2006; Orfield et al., 2004), with the caution that the data are correlational and the measures of graduation vary (Mishel & Roy, 2006).

High-stakes standardized testing practices now pervade American classrooms. The resultant pressure on teachers and students to pass the test "or else" has yielded noticeable shifts in teacher practice that theoretically may erode student motivation and engagement. For example, the exaggerated importance of this test in students' lives draws attention not only to how students perform but also to how they perform in relation to their peers. Feedback systems that encourage performance comparisons are associated with maladaptive motivational orientations. Further, the summative nature of high-stakes testing precludes formative assessment relationships between teachers and students. The pressure to perform on a single test undermines teachers' capacities to encourage and promote engagement-related processes such as self-reflection and self-direction.

Conclusion

In this chapter, we have attempted to draw links between assessment-related practices and student motivation and engagement. The complexity of the terrain in both the assessment and motivational literature makes it exceedingly difficult to emerge with meaningful conclusions. Still, there have been some data to provide us with a glimpse of the ways in which teachers' use of tests may coincide with and/or influence students' motivation.

We organized our review by test type, focusing first on what we have learned about the role and use of standardized tests in American classrooms. Although the literature on low-stakes standardized testing systems in America is vast (Sacks, 1999), the most pertinent data for our topic comes from how standardized test scores influence teachers expectation effects (Good & Brophy, 1974). A rich literature on teacher expectations informs us that norm-referenced standardized aptitude tests may influence how teachers treat students, subsequently influencing student motivation. Importantly, these links are loosely understood at best and, therefore, cannot make any substantive references to standardized test practices and student motivation.

Next, we reviewed some of what we know about how classroom-based assessment practices (teacher-made tests, summative and formative uses) might connect with motivation and engagement. Test content and feedback systems associated with summative testing practices have strong associations with effort and student and classroom-level goal orientations/structure. Classroom goal structures and feedback systems that emphasize performance comparisons are largely detrimental to student motivation, whereas emphasis on learning goals enhances motivation and achievement.

We also reviewed formative assessment practices and discussed their links with student engagement. We view engagement in terms of self-regulation and self-determination theories, both of which presume students' active involvement in and reflection on their own learning. In contrast to summative assessment, formative assessment practices are well suited for enhancing students' engagement-related behaviors. Using tests as feedback systems from which students can learn to identify their own strengths and weaknesses, as well as their own learning-related successes and failures, is ideal for promoting student ownership, responsibility, and, ultimately, student achievement. Lastly, we reviewed some of the classroom conditions associated with high-stakes standardized testing practices. We discussed data showing how high-stakes testing is changing educational practice and the ways in which these changes impact student motivation—largely for the worse.

Implications

High-stakes testing systems have created a very specific type of learning context. One worry about their effects on student motivation has to do with the onslaught of messages regarding ability. Students who repeatedly fail or struggle are cast as problem students and treated differently. Ironically, educators worried 100 years ago about the cumulative effect of repeated test failures. In 1913, Dougherty (1913) cautioned teachers "when a child fails continually on test after test if he is conscious of his own failure, as he must sometimes be in spite of the examiner's efforts to encourage him, it is not wise to proceed until he merely fails from habit" (p. 339). Thus, educators have long worried about the cumulative effects of chronic failure on summative tests.

We believe the pervasive use of high-stakes standardized testing in American schools (Giordano, 2005) is deleterious to student motivation and engagement. When students are told over and over that learning is only as good as their test scores (Boohrer-Jennings, 2005; Jones et al., 1999, 2003; Nichols & Berliner, 2007; Perlstein, 2007), it seems likely that their beliefs about the value of learning become compromised. When students learn for extrinsic reasons, their motivation is likely to diminish (Deci, Koestner, & Ryan, 1999; Deci, Ryan, & Koestner, 2001). And the costs manifest in a multitude of ways. Struggling students might become less equipped to handle failure and frustration. Talented students might become bored and therefore fail to notice opportunities that might otherwise provide new ways of learning (Carver & Scheier, 2005). Similarly, high-achieving students, noticing teachers' preoccupations with tests, may lose motivation to persist. After all, if it is only about tests and testing (and if tests are easy for me), then why try?

Needed Research for Practice and Policy

We need more research to understand how assessment-related instructional practice relates to student motivation (Stiggins, 2001). But we especially need data on how high-stakes testing systems influence teachers and in turn, how that influence impacts students. Our review of extant data casts a looming shadow over the use of high-stakes testing and its largely deleterious influence on student motivation. However, more research is needed to more clearly identify the particular assessment-related practices that enhance or impede students' developing motivation and engagement. For example, what role does test-related pressure play in the types of motivation-related messages teachers communicate to students? How do students interpret these messages? Is there a relationship between the magnitude of the pressure and the type of feedback teachers provide to students? In what ways do teacher-student relationships change as a function of test-related pressure?

We also need to better understand the effect of the testing culture on student achievement, including literacy, deeper-level cognition and reasoning, strategy use, or complex problem solving. Research is beginning to look at these questions, but there has been little empirical work to connect these important skills to policy development and implementation. As the United States and other countries grapple with ways to reform education, and as tests increasingly grow in popularity, it seems more imperative than ever for researchers to examine the potential motivational and learning costs associated with the continuance of high-stakes testing systems.

References

Abrams, L., Pedulla, J. J., & Madaus, G. (2003). Views from the classroom: Teachers' opinions of statewide testing programs. *Theory into Practice, 42*(1), 18–28.

Allington, R., & McGill-Franzen, A. (1992). Unintended effects of educational reform in New York. *Educational Policy, 6*(4), 397–414.

Ames, C. (1984). Competitive, cooperative, and individualistic goal structures: A cognitive-motivational analysis. In R. E. Ames & C. Ames (Eds.), *Research on motivation in education: Vol. I. Student motivation*. New York: Academic.

Ames, C. (1992). Classrooms: Goals, structures, and student motivation. *Journal of Educational Psychology, 84*(3), 261–271.

Ames, C., & Archer, J. (1988). Achievement goals in the classroom: Students' learning strategies and motivation processes. *Journal of Educational Psychology, 80*(3), 260–267.

Amrein, A., & Berliner, D. (2002). High-stakes testing, uncertainty, and student learning. *Educational Policy and Analysis Archives, 10*(8). Retrieved from http://www.epaa.asu.edu/epaa/v10n18

Anderman, E. M., & Maehr, M. L. (1994). Motivation and schooling in the middle grades. *Review of Educational Research, 64*(2), 287–309.

Anderman, E. (2007). The effects of personal, classroom, and school goal structures on academic cheating (pp. 87–106). In E. M. Anderman & T. B. Murdock (Eds.), Psychology of academic cheating. NY: Elsevier.

Atkinson, J. W. (1974). Motivational determinants of intellective performance and cumulative achievement. In J. W. Atkinson & J. O. Raynor (Eds.), *Motivation and achievement*. Washington, DC: V. H. Winston.

Atkinson, J. W. (1981a). Studying personality in the context of an advanced motivational psychology. *American Psychologist, 36*(2), 117–128.

Atkinson, J. W. (1981b). Thematic apperceptive measurement of motivation in 1950 and 1980. In G. D'Ydewalle & W. Lens (Eds.), *Cognition in human motivation and learning* (pp. 159–198). Hillsdale, NH: Erlbaum.

Bangert-Drowns, R. L., Kulik, J. A., & Morgan, M. T. (1991). The instructional effect of feedback in test-like events. *Review of Educational Research, 61*, 213–238.

Berliner, D. C. (1979). Tempus educare. In P. L. Peterson & H. J. Walberg (Eds.), *Research on teaching: Concepts, findings, and implications* (pp. 120–135). Berkeley, CA: McCutchan Publishing.

Berliner, D. C., & Biddle, B. J. (1995). *The manufactured crisis: Myths, fraud, and the attack on America's public schools*. Reading, MA: Addison-Wesley.

Black, P., & Wiliam, D. (1998). Assessment and classroom learning. *Assessment in Education: Principles, Policy and Practice, 5*(1), 7–74.

Black, P., & Wiliam, D. (2006). Developing a theory of formative assessment. In J. Gardner (Ed.), *Assessment and learning* (pp. 81–100). London: Sage.

Bloom, B. S. (Ed.). (1956). *A taxonomy of educational objectives: Handbook I, the cognitive domain*. New York: Longman.

Blumenfeld, P. C. (1992). Classroom learning and motivation: Clarifying and expanding goal theory. *Journal of Educational Psychology, 84*(3), 272–281.

Boekaerts, M., & Corno, L. (2005). Self-regulation in the classroom: A perspective on assessment and intervention. *Applied Psychology: An International Review, 54*(2), 199–231.

Boekaerts, M., Pintrich, P. R., & Zeidner, M. (Eds.). (2000). *Handbook of self-regulation*. San Diego, CA: Academic.

Boohrer-Jennings, J. (2005). Below the bubble: 'Educational triage' and the Texas accountability system. *American Educational Research Journal, 42*(2), 231–268.

Brookhart, S. M. (1997). A theoretical framework for the role of classroom assessment in motivating student effort and achievement. *Applied Measurement in Education, 10*, 161–180.

Brookhart, S. M. (2004). Classroom assessment: Tensions and intersections in theory and practice. *Teachers College Record, 106*(3), 429–458.

Brophy, J. (Ed.). (1998). *Advances in research on teaching. Expectations in the classroom* (Vol. 7, pp. 273–308). Greenwich, CT: JAI.

Butler, R. (1988). Enhancing and undermining intrinsic motivation: The effects of task-involving and ego-involving evaluation on interest and performance. *British Journal of Educational Psychology, 58*, 1–14.

Carver, C. S., & Scheier, M. F. (2005). Engagement, disengagement, coping, and catastrophe. In A. J. Elliot & C. S. Dweck (Eds.), *Handbook of competence and motivation* (pp. 527–547). New York: Guilford Press.

Center on Education Policy. (2006). *From the capital to the classroom: Year four of the No Child Left Behind Act*. Washington DC: Author. http://www.cep-dc.org/nclb/Year4/CEP-NCLB-Report-4.pdf

Corno, L. (2001). Volitional aspects of self-regulated learning. In B. J. Zimmerman & D. H. Schunk (Eds.), *Self-regulated learning and academic achievement: Theoretical perspectives* (2nd ed., pp. 191–226). Mahwah, NJ: Erlbaum.

Corno, L., & Mandinach, E. B. (1983). The role of cognitive engagement in classroom learning and motivation. *Educational Psychologist, 18*(2), 88–108.

Corno, L., & Mandinach, E. B. (2004). What we have learned about student engagement in the past twenty years. In D. M. McInerney & S. V. Etten (Eds.), *Big theories revisited* (pp. 299–328). Greenwich, CT: Information Age Publishing.

Crooks, T. J. (1988). The impact of classroom evaluation practices on students. *Review of Educational Research, 58*, 438–481.

Crooks, T. J., & Mahalski, P. A. (1986). Relationships among assessment practices, study methods, and grades obtained. In J. Jones & M. Horsburgh (Eds.), *Research and development in higher education* (Vol. 8). Sydney, Australia: Higher Education Research and Development Society of Australasia.

Csikszentmihalyi, M., Abuhamdeh, S., & Nakamura, J. (2005). Flow. In A. J. Elliot & C. S. Dweck (Eds.), *Handbook of competence and motivation* (pp. 598–608). New York: Guilford Press.

Cuban, L. (1988). Constancy and change in schools (1880s to the present). In P. W. Jackson (Ed.), *Contributing to educational change: Perspectives on research and practice*. Berkeley, CA: McCutchan Publishing.

Darling-Hammond, L. (2007). Race, inequality, and educational accountability: The irony of 'No Child Left Behind'. *Race Ethnicity and Education, 10*(3), 245–260.

Deci, E. L., Koestner, R., & Ryan, R. M. (1999). A meta-analytic review of experiments examining the effects of extrinsic rewards on intrinsic motivation. *Psychological Bulletin, 125*, 627–668.

Deci, E. L., & Ryan, R. M. (1995). Human autonomy: The basis for true self-esteem. In M. Kernis (Ed.), *Efficacy, agency, and self-esteem* (pp. 31–49). New York: Plenum Publishing Co.

Deci, E. L., Ryan, R. M., & Koestner, R. (2001). The pervasive negative effects of rewards on intrinsic motivation: Response to Cameron (2001). *Review of Educational Research, 71*(1), 43–51.

Deci, E. L., Vallerand, R. J., Pelletier, L. G., & Ryan, R. M. (1991). Motivation and education: The self-determination perspective. *Educational Psychologist, 26*(3&4), 325–346.

Dougherty, M. L. (1913). Report on the Binet-Simon tests given to four hundred and eighty-three children in the public schools of Kansas City, Kansas. *Journal of Educational Psychology, 4*, 338–352.

Eccles, J. S. (1983). Expectancies, values, and academic behavior. In J. T. Spencer (Ed.), *Achievement and achievement motivation* (pp. 75–146). San Francisco: W. H. Freeman.

Eccles, J. S., & Midgley, C. (1989). Stage/environment fit: Developmentally appropriate classrooms for early adolescents. In R. E. Ames & C. Ames (Eds.), *Research on motivation in education* (Vol. 3, pp. 139–186). New York: Academic.

Eccles, J. S., & Wigfield, A. (2002). Motivational belief, values, and goals. *Annual Review of Psychology, 53*, 109–132.

Eccles, J. S., Wigfield, A., Flanagan, G., Miller, G., Reuman, D., & Yee, D. (1989). Self-concepts, domain values, and self-esteem: Relations and changes at early adolescence. *Journal of Personality, 57*, 283–310.

Elliot, A. (1999). Approach and avoidance motivation and achievement goals. *Educational Psychologist, 34*(3), 169–189.

Elliot, A. J., & Church, M. A. (1997). A hierarchical model of approach and avoidance achievement motivation. *Journal of Personality and Social Psychology, 72*, 218–232.

Elliot, A. J., & Dweck, C. S. (Eds.). (2005). *Handbook of competence and motivation*. New York: Guilford Press.

Elliot, A. J., & Harackiewicz, J. M. (1996). Approach and avoidance achievement goals and intrinsic motivation: A mediational analysis. *Journal of Personality and Social Psychology, 70*(3), 461–475.

Elliott, E. S., & Dweck, C. S. (1988). Goals: An approach to motivation and achievement. *Journal of Personality and Social Psychology, 54*, 5–12.

Entwistle, N. J., & Kozeski, B. (1985). Relationship between school motivation, approaches to studying, and attainment, among British and Hungarian adolescents. *British Journal of Educational Psychology, 55*, 124–137.

Feather, N. T. (Ed.). (1982). *Expectations and actions: Expectancy-value models in psychology*. Hillsdale, NJ: Erlbaum.

Foster, S. (2006). *How Latino students negotiate the demands of high-stakes testing: A case study of one school in Texas*. Unpublished doctoral dissertation, Arizona State University, Tempe, AZ.

Fredericksen, N. (1984). The real test bias: Influences of testing on teaching and learning. *American Psychologist, 39*, 193–202.

Frederiksen, J. R., & White, B. J. (1997). *Reflective assessment of students' research within an inquiry-based middle school science curriculum*. Paper presented at the annual meeting of the American Educational Research Association, Chicago.

Gamson, D. (2007). Historical perspectives on democratic decision making in education: Paradigms, paradoxes, and promises. In P. Moss (Ed.), *Evidence and decision making: 106th yearbook of the National Society for the Study of Education, Part I* (pp. 15–45). Malden, MA: Blackwell Publishing.

Gayler, K., Chudowsky, N., Hamilton, M., Kober, N., & Yeager, M. (2004). *State high school exit exams: A maturing reform*. Washington, DC: Center on Education Policy. Retrieved June 5, 2007, from http://www.cep-dc.org/highschoolexit/ExitExamAug2004/ExitExam2004.pdf

Giordano, G. (2005). *How testing came to dominate American schools: The history of educational assessment*. New York: Peter Lang.

Glass, G. V. (2008). *Fertilizers, pills, and magnetic strips: The fate of public education in America*. Charlotte, NC: Information Age Publishing.

Good, T. L. (1981). Teacher expectations and student perceptions: A decade of research. *Educational Leadership, 38*, 415–423.

Good, T. L. (1987). Two decades of research on teacher expectations: Findings and future directions. *Journal of Teacher Education, 38*(4), 32–47.

Good, T. L. (1996). Educational researchers comment on the educational summit and other policy proclamations from 1983–1997. *Educational Researcher, 25*(8), 4–6.

Good, T. L., & Brophy, J. E. (1972). Behavioral expression of teacher attitudes. *Journal of Educational Psychology, 63*, 617–624.

Good, T. L., & Brophy, J. E. (1974). Changing teacher and student behavior: An empirical investigation. *Journal of Educational Psychology, 66*, 390–405.

Good, T. L., & Brophy, J. E. (2008). *Looking in classrooms* (10th ed.). Boston: Pearson.

Good, T. L., & Thompson, E. K. (1998). Research on the communication of performance expectations: A review of recent perspectives. In J. Brophy (Ed.), *Advances in research on teaching: Expectations in the classroom* (Vol. 7, pp. 273–308). Greenwich, CT: JAI Press.

Grolnick, W. S., & Ryan, R. M. (1987). Autonomy in children's learning: An experimental and individual different investigation. *Journal of Personality and Social Psychology, 52*, 890–898.

Haney, W. (2008). Evidence on education under NCLB (and How Florida boosted NAEP scores and reduced the race gap). In G. L. Sunderman (Ed.), *Holding NCLB accountable: Achieving accountability, equity, and school reform* (pp. 91–102). Thousand Oaks, CA: Corwin Press.

Henderlong, J., & Lepper, M. R. (2002). The effects of praise on children's intrinsic motivation: A review and synthesis. *Psychological Bulletin, 128*(5), 774–795.

Herman, J. L., & Haertel, E. H. (Eds.). (2005). *Uses and misuses of data for educational accountability and improvement: The 104th yearbook of the National Society for the Study of Education, part II*. Malden, MA: Blackwell.

Hull, C. (1943). *Principles of behavior*. New York: Appleton.

Hull, C. (1952). *A behavior system*. New Haven: Yale University Press.

Jacob, B. (2001). Getting tough? The impact of high school graduation exams. *Educational Evaluation and Policy Analysis, 23*(2), 99–121.

Johnson, D. W., & Johnson, R. T. (1985). Motivational processes in cooperative, competitive, and individualistic learning situation. In C. Ames & R. Ames (Eds.), *Research on motivation in education: Vol. 2. The classroom milieu*. New York: Academic.

Johnson, D. W., & Johnson, R. T. (1999). *Learning together and alone: Cooperative, competitive, and individualistic learning* (5th ed.). Boston: Allyn & Bacon.

Jones, B. D., & Egley, R. J. (2004, August 9). Voices from the frontlines: Teachers' perceptions of high-stakes testing. *Education Policy Analysis Archives, 12*(39). Retrieved December 2, 2004, from http://epaa.asu.edu/epaa/v12n39/

Jones, M. G., Jones, B. D., Hardin, B., Chapman, L., Yarbrough, T., & Davis, M. (1999). The impact of high-stakes testing on teachers and students in North Carolina. *The Phi Delta Kappan, 81*(3), 199–203.

Jones, M. G., Jones, B. D., & Hargrove, T. (2003). *The unintended consequences of high-stakes testing*. Lanham, MD: Rowman & Littlefield.

Kaplan, A. (2004). Achievement goals and intergroup relations. In P. R. Pintrich & M. L. Maehr (Eds.), *Advances in research on motivation and achievement: Vol. 13: Motivating students, improving schools: The legacy of Carol Midgley* (pp. 97–136). Oxford, UK: Elsevier.

Kaplan, A., & Flum, H. (Guest Eds.). (2009). Motivation and identity [Special issue]. *Educational Psychologist, 44*(2).

Kaplan, A., & Maehr, M. L. (2007). The contributions and prospects of goal orientation theory. *Educational Psychology Review, 19*, 141–184.

Kaplan, A., Middleton, M. J., Urdan, T., & Midgley, C. (2002). Achievement goals and goal structures. In C. Midgley (Ed.), *Goals, goal structures, and patterns of adaptive learning* (pp. 21–53). Mahwah, NJ: Lawrence Erlbaum Associates.

Kellaghan, T., Madaus, G. F., & Airasian, P. W. (1982). *The effects of standardized testing*. Boston: Kluwer-Nijhoff.

Krathwohl, D. R. (2002). A revision of Bloom's Taxonomy: An overview. *Theory into Practice, 41*(4), 212–218.

Lepper, M. R., Corpus, J. H., & Iyengar, S. S. (2005). Intrinsic and extrinsic motivational orientations in the classroom: Age differences and academic correlates. *Journal of Educational Psychology, 97*(2), 184–196.

Madaus, G., Russell, M., & Higgins, J. (2009). *The paradoxes of high-stakes testing: How they affect students, their parents, teachers, principals, schools, and society*. Charlotte, NC: Information Age Publishing.

Marchant, G. J., & Paulson, S. E. (2005, January 21). The relationship of high school graduation exams to graduation rates and SAT scores. *Education Policy Analysis Archives, 13*(6). Retrieved June 30, 2006, from http://epaa.asu.edu/epaa/v13n6/

Martin, E., & Ramsden, P. (1987). Learning skills and skill in learning. In J. T. E. Richardson, M. W. Eysenck, & D. W. Piper (Eds.), *Student learning: Research in education and cognitive psychology*. Milton Keynes, England: Open University Press & Society for Research into Higher Education.

McCaslin, M. (2009). Co-regulation of student motivation and emergent identity. *Educational Psychologist, 44*(2), 137–146.

McCaslin, M., & DiMarino-Linnen, E. (2000). Motivation and learning in school: Societal contexts, psychological constructs, and educational practices. In T. Good (Ed.), *Schooling in America: Yesterday, today, and tomorrow. 100th yearbook of the National Society for the Study of Education* (pp. 84–151). Chicago: University of Chicago Press.

McClelland, D. C. (1980). Motive disposition: The merits of operant and respondent measures. In L. Wheeler (Ed.), *Review of personality and social psychology* (Vol. 1). Beverly Hills, CA: Sage.

McClelland, D. C. (1985). How motives, skills, and values determine what people do. *American Psychologist, 40*(7), 812–825.

McDonnell, L. (2005). Assessment and accountability from the policymaker's perspective. In J. L. Herman & E. H. Haertel (Eds.), *Uses and misuses of data for educational accountability and improvement: The 104th yearbook of the National Society for the Study of Education, Part II*. Malden, MA: Blackwell.

McInerney, D. M., Brown, G. T. L., & Liem, G. A. D. (Eds.). (2009). *Student perspectives on assessment: What students can tell us about assessment for learning*. Charlotte, NC: Information Age Publishing.

McMillan, J. H. (2001). *Classroom assessment: Principles and practice for effective instruction* (2nd ed.). Boston: Allyn & Bacon.

McNeil, L. M., Coppola, E., Radigan, J., & Vasquez Heilig, J. (2008). Avoidable losses: High-stakes accountability and the dropout crisis. *Education Policy Analysis Archives, 16*(3). Retrieved March 16, 2009, from http://epaa.asu.edu/epaa/v16n3/

Meichenbaum, D. H., & Smart, T. (1971). Use of direct expectancy to modify academic performance and attitudes of college students. *Journal of Counseling Psychology, 18*, 531–535.

Midgley, C., Kaplan, A., & Middleton, M. J. (2001). Performance-approach goals: Good for what, for whom, under what circumstances, and at what cost? *Journal of Educational Psychology, 93*, 77–86.

Miller, A. D., & Murdock, T. B. (2007). Modeling latent true scores to determine the utility of aggregate student perceptions as classroom indicators in HLM: The case of classroom goal structures. *Contemporary Educational Psychology, 32*, 83–104.

Miller, C. M. L., & Parlett, M. (1974). *Up to the mark: A study of the examination game*. London: Society for Research into Higher Education.

Mishel, L., & Roy, J. (2006). *Rethinking high school graduation rates and trends*. Washington, DC: Economic Policy Institute.

Moss, P. (Ed.). (2007). *Evidence and decision making. The 106th yearbook of the National Society for the Study of Education, Part 1*. Malden, MA: Blackwell Publishing.

Murdock, T. B., & Miller, A. D. (2009). Specification issues in the use of multilevel modeling to examine the effects of classroom context. In M. Wosnitza, S. A. Karabenick, A. Efklides, & P. Nenniger (Eds.), *Contemporary motivation research: From global to local perspectives* (pp. 249–264). Cambridge, MA: Hogrefe.

National Commission for Excellence in Education. (1983). *A nation at risk: The imperatives for educational reform*. Washington, DC: Author.

Natriello, G. (1987). The impact of evaluation processes on students. *Educational Psychologist, 22*(2), 155–175.

Natriello, G., & Dornbusch, S. M. (1984). *Teacher evaluative standards and student effort*. New York: Longman.

Nichols, S. L. (2007). High-stakes testing: Does it increase achievement? *Journal of Applied School Psychology, 23*(2), 47–64.

Nichols, S., & Berliner, D. C. (2007). *Collateral damage: How high-stakes testing corrupts America's schools*. Cambridge, MA: Harvard Education Press.

Nichols, S. L., Glass, G. V., & Berliner, D. C. (2006). High-stakes testing and student achievement: Does accountability pressure increase student learning? *Education Policy Analysis Archives, 14*(1). Retrieved July 20, 2009, from http://epaa.asu.edu/epaa/v14n1/

No Child Left Behind (NCLB) Act of 2001, 20 U.S.C.A. § 6301 *et seq.* (2002).

Orfield, G. (Ed.). (2004). *Dropouts in America: Confronting the graduation rate crisis*. Cambridge, MA: Harvard Education Press.

Orfield, G., & Kornhaber, M. L. (Eds.). (2001). *Raising standards or raising barriers? Inequality and high stakes testing in public education*. New York: The Century Foundation Press.

Orfield, G., Losen, D., Wald, D., & Swanson, C. (2004). *Losing our future: How minority youth are being left behind by the graduation rate crisis*. Cambridge, MA: The Civil Rights Project at Harvard University.

Paris, S. G., Lawton, T. A., Turner, J. C., & Roth, J. L. (1991). A developmental perspective on standardized achievement testing. *Educational Researcher, 20*, 12–20.

Paris, S. G., Roth, J. L., & Turner, J. C. (2000). Developing disillusionment: Students' perceptions of academic achievement tests. *Issues in Education, 6*(1/2), 17–46.

Paris, S. G., Turner, J. C., & Lawton, T. A. (1990, April). *Students' views of standardized achievement tests*. Paper presented at Educational Research Association, Boston.

Paris, S. G., & Urdan, T. (2000). Policies and practices of high-stakes testing that influence teachers and schools. *Issues in Education, 6*(1/2), 83–108.

Pedulla, J. J., Abrams, L. M., Madaus, G. F., Russell, M. K., Ramos, M. A., & Miao, J. (2003, March). *Perceived effects of state-mandated testing programs on teaching and learning: Findings from a national survey of teachers*. Boston: Boston College, National Board on Educational Testing and Public Policy. Retrieved January 7, 2004, from http://www.bc.edu/research/nbetpp/statements/nbr2.pdf

Perlstein, L. (2007). *Tested: One American school struggles to make the grade*. New York: Henry Holt & Co.

Peterson, P. L., & Walberg, H. J. (Eds.). (1979). *Research on teaching: Concepts, findings, and implications*. Berkeley, CA: McCutchan Publishing.

Peterson, P. E., & West, M. R. (Eds.). (2003). *No Child Left Behind? The politics and practice of school accountability*. Washington, DC: Brookings Institute.

Phelps, R. P. (Ed.). (2005). *Defending standardized testing*. Mahwah, NJ: Erlbaum.

Raymond, M. E., & Hanushek, E. A. (2003, Summer). High-stakes research. *Education Next, 3*(3), 48–55. Retrieved from http://www.educationnext.org/

Rodriguez, M. C. (2004). The role of classroom assessment in student performance on TIMSS. *Applied Measurement in Education, 17*(1), 1–24.

Rogers, E. M. (1969). Examinations: Powerful agents for good or ill in teaching. *American Journal of Physics, 37*, 954–962.

Rosenthal, R., & Jacobson, L. (1968). *Pygmalion in the classroom*. New York: Holt, Rinehart & Winston.

Ryan, J. (2004). The perverse incentives of the No Child Left Behind Act. *New York University Law Review, 79*, 932–989.

Sacks, P. (1999). *Standardized minds: The high price of America's testing culture and what we can do to change it*. Cambridge, MA: Perseus Publishing.

San Antonio Express-News (2007, March 9). Teen talk: Tackling TAKS. *San Antonio Express-News*, p. 1F.

Schunk, D. H. (1996). Goal and self-evaluative influences during children's cognitive skill learning. *American Educational Research Journal, 33*, 359–382.

Snyder, B. R. (1971). *The hidden curriculum*. Cambridge, MA: M.I.T. Press.

Starch, D., & Elliott, E. C. (1912). Reliability of the grading of high-school work in English. *School Review, 20*, 442–457.

Stiggins, R. J. (2001). The unfulfilled promise of classroom assessment. *Educational Measurement: Issues and Practice, 20*(3), 5–15.

Stiggins, R. J., & Bridgeford, N. J. (1985). The ecology of classroom assessment. *Journal of Educational Measurement, 22*(4), 271–286.

Stiggins, R. J., & Conklin, N. F. (1992). *In teachers' hands: Investigating the practices of classroom assessment*. Albany, NY: State University of New York Press.

Taylor, G., Shepard, L., Kinner, F., & Rosenthal, J. (2003). *A survey of teachers' perspectives on high-stakes testing in Colorado: What gets taught, what gets lost* (CSE Technical Report 588). Los Angeles: University of California.

Thomas, J. W. (1993). Promoting independent learning in the middle grades: The role of instructional support practices. *The Elementary School Journal, 93*, 575–591.

Thorndike, E. L. (1923). *Education: A first book*. New York: Macmillan.

Toy, V. (2006, January 1). Elmont's school success is a lesson to others. *New York Times*, p. 14L.

Tyack, D. (1974). *The one best system: A history of American urban education*. Cambridge, UK: Harvard University Press.

Tyack, D., & Cuban, L. (1997). *Tinkering toward utopia: A century of public school reform*. Cambridge, MA: Harvard University Press.

Urdan, T. (1997). Achievement goal theory: Past results, future directions. In M. L. Maehr & P. R. Pintrich (Eds.), *Advances in motivation and achievement* (Vol. 10, pp. 99–141). Greenwich, CT: JAI.

Valenzuela, A. (Ed.). (2005). *Leaving children behind: How "Texas-style" accountability fails Latino youth*. Albany, NY: State University of New York Press.

Vasquez Heilig, J., Cole, H., & Aguilar, A. (2010). From Dewey to No Child Left Behind: The evolution and devolution of public arts education. *Arts Education Policy Review, 111*, 136–145.

Vasquez Heilig, J., & Darling-Hammond, L. (2008). Accountability Texas-style: The progress and learning of urban minority students in a high-stakes testing context. *Educational Evaluation and Policy Analysis, 30*(2), 75–110.

Warren, J. R., Jenkins, K. N., & Kulick, R. B. (2006). High school exit examinations and state-level completion and GED Rates, 1975 through 2002. *Educational Evaluation and Policy Analysis, 28*(20), 131–152.

Weiner, B. (1986). *An attributional theory of motivation and emotion*. New York: Springer.

Weinstein, R. S. (2002). *Reaching higher: The power of expectations in schooling*. Cambridge, MA: Harvard University Press.

Whipple, G. M. (1921). The national intelligence tests. *The Journal of Educational Research, 4*, 16–31.

Wigfield, A., & Eccles, J. (1992). The development of achievement task values: A theoretical analysis. *Developmental Review, 12*, 265–310.

Wigfield, A., & Eccles, J. (2000). Expectancy x value theory of achievement motivation. *Contemporary Educational Psychology, 25*, 68–81.

Wigfield, A., Eccles, J., MacIver, D., Reuman, D., & Midgley, C. (1991). Transitions at early adolescence: Changes in children's domain-specific self-perceptions and general self-esteem across the transition to junior high school. *Developmental Psychology, 27*, 552–565.

Wigfield, A., & Eccles, J. S. (2002). The development of competence beliefs, expectancies for success, and achievement values from childhood through adolescence. In A. Wigfield & J. S. Eccles (Eds.), *Development of achievement motivation* (pp. 91–120). San Diego, CA: Academic.

Wigfield, A., & Guthrie, J. T. (1997). Relations of children's motivation for reading to the amount and breadth of their reading. *Journal of Educational Psychology, 89*, 420–432.

Wigfield, A., & Wagner, A. L. (2005). Competence and motivation during adolescence. In A. J. Elliott & C. S. Dweck (Eds.), *Handbook of competence and motivation* (pp. 222–239). New York: Guilford Press.

Winne, P. H. (1995). Inherent details in self-regulated learning. *Educational Psychologist, 30*, 173–187.

Wong, C. A., & Paris, S. G. (2000). Students' beliefs about classroom tests and standardized tests. *Issues in Education, 6*(1/2), 47–6677.

Part III Commentary: Socio-Cultural Contexts, Social Competence, and Engagement at School

Kathryn Wentzel

Abstract

A highly regarded motivation researcher, Kathryn Wentzel, shared her perspectives in a commentary on the chapters in Part III. Wentzel explored questions relating to student competence including its definition, relation to engagement, and the role of support from important contexts (home, school, peers, and community) in fostering competence and engagement. The chapter concludes with directions for future research.

The social contexts and interactions that define children's lives can have a profound effect on their ability and willingness to engage in the academic life of schools. As illustrated clearly and convincingly in the chapters in this section of the *Handbook on Engagement*, interpersonal relationships, family and peer group dynamics, instruction-based social interactions, and indicators of competence all determine to some extent how and why students strive to achieve academic success. Beyond this recognition that learning is embedded in social contexts, however, how might a social-ecological approach help scholars and educators better understand children's engagement at school? One strategy is to bring to the forefront the notion that educational and intellectual endeavors are inherently social in nature and in doing so, consider more explicitly how and why advances in learning and cognitive development might reflect aspects of social competence.

In support of this approach are traditional developmental perspectives that recognize the interdependent relations of cognitive and social functioning in descriptions of intellectual development (e.g., Piaget, 1983; Vygotsky, 1978). More recently, scholars also have argued convincingly that the ability to excel at tasks designed to assess cognitive abilities is highly dependent on broad-level social influences that reflect cultural belief systems and practices (e.g., Greenfield, 1997), as well as intra-individual differences in social and emotional skills and self-regulation (e.g., Durlak, Weissberg, Dymnicki, Taylor, & Schellinger, 2011). If scholars adopt this ecological perspective, however, questions arise as to what it means to be a socially competent student, how social competence supports various forms of intellectual engagement, and how competence development can be supported across multiple contexts of home, school, peer group, and community.

K. Wentzel (✉)
Department of Human Development and Quantitative Methodology, University of Maryland, College Park, MD, USA
e-mail: wentzel@umd.edu

In this commentary, I focus on three central issues that reflect these questions. The first concerns the notion that social competencies contribute to successful academic and learning-related outcomes. Implicit in this notion are fundamental questions concerning how to define social competence and understand it within the context of schooling. Second, issues surrounding the socially-valued goals and objectives that are relevant for understanding school adjustment are considered. Indeed, if social competence is an integral part of school success, how do we identify and examine the socially-valued goals that we would like students to achieve? Finally, processes of influence and theoretical issues related to social contexts and schooling are discussed. If sociocultural contexts are important for students' school-based competencies, how and why might this be so? I close with some general conclusions and provocations for future research in this area.

Defining Social Competence at School

In the social developmental literature, social competence has been described from a variety of perspectives ranging from the development of individual skills to more general adaptation within a particular setting. In these discussions, social competence frequently is associated with person-level outcomes such as effective behavioral repertoires, social problem-solving skills, positive beliefs about the self, achievement of social goals, and positive interpersonal relationships (see Rose-Krasnor, 1997). In addition, however, central to many definitions of social competence is the notion that social contexts play an integral role in providing opportunities for the development of these outcomes as well as in defining the appropriate parameters of children's social accomplishments (e.g., Bronfenbrenner, 1989). In this view, social competence reflects a more systemic phenomenon in which a balance is achieved between the accomplishment of positive outcomes for the individual and context-specific effectiveness.

Support for defining social competence as person-environment fit can be found in the work of several theorists (e.g., Bronfenbrenner, 1989; Eccles & Midgley, 1989; Ford, 1992). Bronfenbrenner (1989) argued that competence is a product of personal attributes such as goals, values, self-regulatory skills, and cognitive abilities, and of ways in which these attributes contribute to meeting situational requirements and demands. Bronfenbrenner further suggested that competence is facilitated by contextual supports that provide opportunities for the growth and development of these personal attributes, including communications concerning what is expected by the social group. Ford expanded on this notion by specifying dimensions of social competence that are framed within a model in which personal and context-specific goals are coordinated to address the needs of the individual as well as those of the social group.

The application of these ecologically-based models of social competence to the realm of schooling results in a multi-faceted description of children who are engaged in the social and academic life of their school. First, competent students are engaged in achieving goals that are personally valued as well as those that are valued by others. Second, the goals they pursue result in social integration as well as in positive developmental outcomes for the student. Socially-integrative outcomes are those which promote the smooth functioning of social groups at school (e.g., cooperative behavior) and are reflected most proximally in social acceptance and socially interdependent actions; student-related outcomes reflect healthy development of the self (e.g., perceived social competence, feelings of self-determination) and feelings of emotional well-being (Bronfenbrenner, 1989; Ford, 1992).

The systemic nature of this approach highlights the fact that a student's school-based competencies are a product of social reciprocity between themselves, their teachers and their classmates. Just as students must behave in ways that meet the expectations of others, so must teachers and peers provide support for the achievement of a student's multiple goals. In this regard, the authors in this section reflect on the potential threats to children's social, emotional, and intellectual engagement when a balance between the goals and needs of the student and those valued by others is not achieved. This can occur at the level of a students' broader cultural background and community (Bempechat & Shernoff, 2012), within the peer group (Juvonen, Espinoza, & Knifsend, 2012), or when teachers and students do not achieve common purpose (Assor, 2012; Hipkins, 2012).

From this work, it is clear that a central tenet of an ecological approach to understanding student engagement is that achieving a balanced "fit" between the needs of the individual and those of the broader educational environment requires a focused consideration of the goals that children expect and are expected to achieve when they are at school. Assuming that socially competent students and responsive social systems contribute in meaningful ways to academic learning and achievement, an essential task is to identify the goals for education that we hold for students and consider their contribution to effective and sustainable engagement. This issue is discussed in the following section.

Social Goals and Objectives for Education

Surprisingly, research on educational goals is sparse. On the one hand, public schools were initially developed with an explicit function of educating children to become healthy, moral, and economically productive citizens; social outcomes in the form of moral character, conformity to social rules and norms, cooperation, and positive styles of social interaction have been promoted consistently by policy makers as goals for students to achieve (see Wentzel, 1991, for a review). On the other hand, researchers rarely have asked parents and teachers about their specific goals for students, although teachers often describe their "ideal" students with regard to outcomes in social (e.g., sharing, helping, and following rules), motivational (e.g., persistence, being intrinsically interested), and performance (e.g., earning high grades) domains (Wentzel, 2003). Similarly, the social and academic classroom goals that students themselves wish to achieve and would like their classmates to achieve are not well-documented (cf., Dowson & McInerney, 2003).

Given this lack of empirical work on educational goals, several issues are especially relevant for future research on engagement. With respect to adults, perhaps the most important task for understanding the socio-cultural contexts of learning is to come to terms with the fundamental questions central to the education of children: As parents and educators, what are our educational goals for our children? As Nichols and Dawson (2012) suggest, do we want to teach simply to the test or nurture our children in ways that will help them become productive and healthy adults and citizens? By the same token, what are the goals that children bring with them to school and how can we accommodate these goals in educational settings? Do they strive to excel academically, to satisfy their curiosities, to establish relationships with others, or simply to feel safe? Finally, how can we support children's willingness to engage in academic pursuits and create learning environments in which all of these outcomes can be achieved?

In addressing the latter question, Raftery, Grolnick, and Flamm (2012) suggest that parental practices reflecting involvement, autonomy support, and structure can be instrumental in building a strong foundation for meeting students' goals that support engagement. Hipkins (2012) also highlights the importance of identifying curricular goals that afford students the opportunity to relate learning to their personal lives and interests. Assor (2012) discusses similar classroom practices that support the internalization of personal goals while also providing opportunities for students to achieve more fundamental needs for relatedness, competence, and autonomy. Practices that promote effective goal pursuit, that are common across socialization contexts as well as unique to particular settings, clearly deserve systematic exploration and further clarification.

In addition, the role of peers in helping students define social competence for themselves and each other should not be ignored when trying to address these questions. As Juvonen et al. (2012)

illustrate, a consideration of self-enhancing as well as socially-integrative outcomes as dual components of social competence is especially important because the achievement of personal goals and social acceptance are not always compatible. Indeed, the process of achieving optimal levels of engagement will always include negotiations, compromise, and coordination of the multiple and often conflicting goals of teachers, peers, students themselves, and their parents. It is imperative that we identify ways to help students coordinate these often antagonistic goals to achieve a healthy balance of multiple objectives.

Finally, just as we need to specify further the socially valued goals we would like students to achieve, it is important that definitions of engagement also reflect these socially-derived outcomes more explicitly. For example, behavioral engagement is routinely defined as behavior specific to learning tasks such as effort and persistence (Fredricks, Blumenfeld, & Paris, 2004; Skinner, Kindermann, Connell, & Wellborn, 2009). In contrast, Pianta, Hamre, and Allen (2012) offer a more systemic approach, defining behavioral engagement as a process, embedded in relationships and social interactions (see also Hipkins, 2012). This more inclusive approach to behavioral engagement is especially valuable given that being successful at school requires children to perform a range of social as well as academic competencies.

In fact, displays of prosocial (e.g., helping and sharing) and socially responsible (e.g., following rules) behavior are essential for developing positive relationships with teachers and peers, and have been associated positively and consistently to a range of academically-related outcomes, including motivation and academic performance (see Wentzel, 1999, 2005, 2009 for reviews). Similarly, establishing and maintaining healthy relationships with teachers and peers has been related positively to a range of academic outcomes, including motivation and engagement (Wentzel, 1999, 2005, 2009). Therefore, if efforts to develop and maintain interpersonal relationships and to display positive forms of social behavior are important for understanding school success, defining desirable forms of engagement to include more behavioral and process-oriented activities can only enhance our understanding of school-based competence.

Processes of Influence

In addition to issues concerning the nature of social competence and what it is that we would like students to engage in at school, the authors in this section remind us that it also is necessary to understand how and why social and contextual supports can facilitate active engagement. In this regard, many authors reflect on the ongoing social interactions that children have with parents, teachers, and peers, with a specific focus on the opportunities and resources that these relationships provide to support or hinder academic engagement (see chapters by Raftery et al.; Juvonen et al.; & Pianta et al.). These discussions, however, also highlight the need for more precise understanding of the nature of interpersonal relationships and the mechanisms whereby the supports they provide have influence on students' engagement at school. More specifically, they call into question what it is that we mean when we refer to a relationship, and what it is about a relationship that promotes positive engagement in children.

Defining Interpersonal Relationships

Relationships are typically defined as enduring connections between two individuals, uniquely characterized by degrees of continuity, shared history, and interdependent interactions across settings and activities (Collins & Repinski, 1994; Hinde, 1997). Definitions also are frequently extended to include the qualities of a relationship, as evidenced by levels of trust, intimacy, and sharing; the presence of positive affect, closeness, and affective tone; and the content and quality of communication (Collins & Repinski, 1994; Laible & Thompson, 2007). Along each of these dimensions, relationships can evoke positive as well as negative experiences (see also, Juvonen et al., 2012).

In addition, relationships are often thought of in terms of their influence and what they provide the individual. From a developmental perspective, relationships are believed to be experienced through the lens of mental representations developed over time and with respect to specific experiences (Bowlby, 1969; Laible & Thompson, 2007). Early representations of relationships with caregivers are believed to provide the foundation for developing relationships outside the family context, with the quality of parent-child relationships (i.e., levels of warmth and security) often predicting the quality of peer and teacher relationships in early and middle childhood (see Wentzel & Looney, 2007). Mental representations that associate relationships with a personal sense of power and agency, predictability and safety, useful resources, and reciprocity are believed to be optimal for the internalization of social influence (see Kuczynski & Parkin, 2007; Raftery et al., 2012). Researchers also have focused on the additional benefits of relationships, such as emotional well-being, a sense of cohesion and connectedness, instrumental help, knowledge of what is expected, and a sense of identity for promoting positive developmental outcomes (Bukowski & Hoza, 1989).

Of relevance for the current discussion is that research on students' relationships with others rarely captures the conceptually rich nature of these definitions or the developmental implications of their influence. Expanding models and assessment strategies to include these multiple aspects of interpersonal relationships would undoubtedly enhance our understanding of how they support engagement at school. A description and discussion of illustrative models follows in the next section.

Elaborating on Models of Influence

Similar to socialization perspectives, the models used to guide research on the influence of interpersonal relationships on engagement described in this section propose causal pathways by which the affective quality of relationships (e.g., those that are emotionally close and secure), have influence primarily by promoting a positive sense of self and emotional well-being, and motivation to engage with the environment (see chapters by Bempechat & Shernoff; Juvonen et al.; Lam, Wong, Yang, & Liu, 2012).

An additional strategy has been to consider relationships as serving a broader range of functions that contribute to students' competence at school (see chapters by Pianta et al.; Raftery et al.; see also, Wentzel, 2004, 2005; Wentzel, Russell, Garza, & Merchant, 2011). Although the affective tone of interpersonal interactions is a central focus of these models, additional dimensions of relationships that reflect levels of predictability and structure, instrumental resources, and concern with a student's emotional and physical well-being also are considered. In line with ecological perspectives on competence development, Wentzel's model (2004) described how teacher-student and peer interactions along these dimensions can promote student motivation and academic performance. The utility of this model for guiding work on engagement lies in a differentiated definition of social support and a more complete picture of how perceived supports might influence academic engagement and learning in the classroom.

As depicted in Fig. 23.1, Wentzel's model predicts that multiple social supports promote positive engagement in the social and academic life of the classroom in part, by influencing the psychological and emotional functioning of students. Specifically, Wentzel suggested that students will come to value and subsequently pursue academic and social goals valued by teachers and peers when they perceive their interactions and relationships with them as providing clear direction concerning goals that should be achieved; as facilitating the achievement of their goals by providing help, advice, and instruction; as being safe and responsive to their goal strivings; and as being emotionally supportive and nurturing. These dimensions reflect essential components of social support discussed in this volume, in that: (1) information is provided concerning what is expected and valued in the classroom (Bempechat & Shernoff; Nichols & Dawson; Raftery et al.); (2) attempts to achieve these valued outcomes are

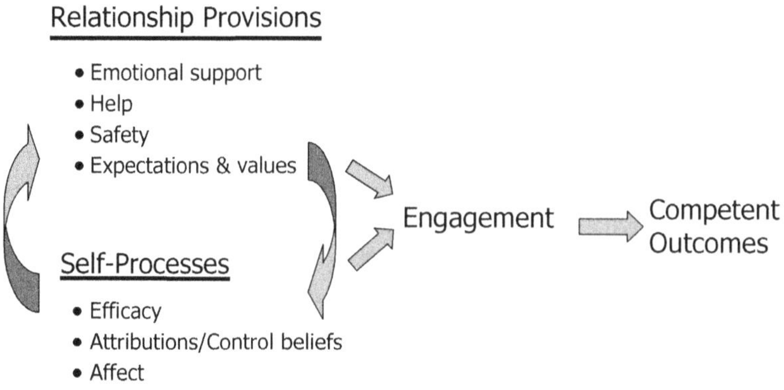

Relationship Provisions
- Emotional support
- Help
- Safety
- Expectations & values

Self-Processes
- Efficacy
- Attributions/Control beliefs
- Affect

→ Engagement → Competent Outcomes

Fig. 23.1 A Model of Social Supports and Classroom Competence

met with help and instruction (Assor; Bempechat & Shernoff; Pianta et al.; Raftery et al.); (3) attempts to achieve outcomes can be made in a safe, non-threatening environment (Juvonen et al.); and (4) individuals are made to feel like a valued member of the group (Bempechat & Shernoff; Juvonen et al.; Pianta et al.).

As a set of interacting processes, these dimensions create a climate within which specific instructional practices and academic content are delivered. Moreover, the degree to which these practices and content result in tangible learning outcomes depends on the quality of the relationship climate (see Darling & Steinberg, 1993). In other words, the affective quality of these educational climates will determine the effectiveness of other contextual supports such as communication of expectations and instrumental help in promoting engagement. With regard to classrooms, therefore, engagement in socially-valued activities, including academic pursuits, will be more likely to occur if students believe that others care about them and want them to engage (e.g., Wentzel, Baker, & Russell, 2012; Wentzel, Russell, Garza, & Merchant, 2012).

The model shown in Fig. 23.1 suggests that these various aspects of social support can promote classroom engagement indirectly by having an impact on students' beliefs about themselves. Several belief systems are likely to be critical in this regard, including self-perceptions of academic efficacy (Bandura, 1986), perceived control and autonomy (e.g., Ryan & Deci, 2000), and affect associated with academic pursuits (e.g., negative arousal or anxiety or a positive sense of well-being) (Meece, Wigfield, & Eccles, 1990; Pekrun, 2009). Each of these self-perceptions are central to theories of motivation and engagement and are consistent predictors of student goals, values, interests, and positive forms of classroom behavior (see, Wentzel & Wigfield, 2009).

Finally, this model predicts that social supports and self-perceptions are related to academic outcomes by way of classroom engagement in social and academic outcomes that are central to the learning process. These outcomes can take many forms, including the active pursuit of socially valued goals such as to behave appropriately and to learn, effort and persistence at academic tasks, displays of appropriate classroom behavior, and focused attention on learning and understanding subject matter (e.g., Wentzel, 1994, 1997, 1998, 2002). Students' pursuit of academic and social goals that are personally as well as socially valued should then serve as a mediator between opportunities afforded by positive interactions with teachers and peers, and their academic and social accomplishments.

Wentzel's model provides an example of a more complex set of processes that link process model of interpersonal relationships to engagement that can move the field forward. In addition, however, greater focus on broader-level context supports also is needed. For example, within the context of schools, structural features such as school and class size, teacher:student ratios, and funding can influence the amount and quality of social and instructional resources and opportunities available to students. Similarly, additional research on classroom reward structures (Nichols & Dawson, 2012; Slavin, 2012), organizational culture and climate (Roeser, Urdan, & Stephens, 2009), and person-environment fit (Bempechat & Shernoff, 2012; Eccles & Midgley, 1989) also might inform our understanding of how the social institutions and contexts within which learning takes place can motivate children to engage in learning activities and positive forms of social interaction.

Finally, work that clearly delineates the processes and mechanisms whereby contexts and relationships can be improved warrants careful attention. To illustrate, work in the area of peer relationships has provided evidence that teachers' beliefs and behaviors, classroom organization, and school-wide structure, composition, and climate affects students' choice of friends, their general propensity to make friends, and levels of peer acceptance and friendship networks in classrooms (Juvonen et al., 2012; Pianta et al., 2012; see also, Wentzel, Baker, & Russell, 2009). Similar work on teacher-student relationships has been less frequent although professional development efforts to improve teachers' classroom management strategies (Evertson & Weinstein, 2006), disciplinary strategies (Developmental Studies Center), and interpersonal interactions and relationships with students (Pianta, 2006; Pianta et al., 2012) have shown promise. Finally, in this volume, chapters by Bempechat and Shernoff (2012), Raftery et al. 2012, highlight ways in which families and schools can build stronger and more interdependent connections. These are excellent examples of work that is challenging but necessary to move the field forward.

Final Provocations for the Field

The nested quality of socio-cultural contexts described by the authors in this section provides interesting and provocative challenges for future research. Many of these challenges have already been noted, However, several remaining issues deserve comment. First, as noted by many of the authors in this volume, models of school-based engagement and competence also need to account for a diversity of student backgrounds and experiences (e.g., chapters by Bempechat & Shernoff; Raftery et al.). Indeed, much of what we know about these processes comes from studies of White, middle-class children. In addition to the research described herein, other researchers have found that supportive relationships with teachers might benefit minority students and girls in achieving positive behavioral and academic outcomes to a greater extent than Caucasian students and boys (e.g., Crosnoe & Needham, 2004). Studies of adolescent peer groups have documented that some African-American youth might face disproportionate levels of conflict between parental and peer values, with the potential to have a negative impact on academic achievement (Steinberg, Brown, & Dornbusch, 1996). Hispanic adolescents are more likely than their non-Hispanic peers to be highly connected to parents and family members, with levels of family interdependence and closeness being related positively to healthy academic and social functioning (e.g., Phinney, Kim-Jo, Osorio, & Vilhjalmsdottir, 2005).

Along these lines, the moderating effects of broader contextual factors requires further study. For instance, in response to findings reported by the NICHD Child Care Study, researchers have argued that when childcare variables are assessed in more diverse samples that include a broader range of SES and ethnicity, different results are obtained (e.g., Sagi, Koren-Karie, Gini, Ziv, & Joels, 2002). Researchers of older children also have found that race moderates relations between dropping out of school and features of their schools and families, such that the SES of families and schools predicts dropping out for White and Hispanic adolescents but not for African-American students (Rumberger, 1995). Some studies also have demonstrated differential teacher treatment of students as a function of student gender, race (Irvine, 1986), and behavioral styles (Chang, 2003), with these differences sometimes attributed in part, to teachers' own race and gender (Saft & Pianta, 2001). Expanding research to incorporate the experiences of all students would provide valuable information about the generalizability of extant theories and empirical findings, and provide practitioners with needed guidance for working with diverse populations of students.

In addition to studying ways in which families, communities, and cultures can support student engagement, additional research on ways in which schools can have effects on children by way of their positive impact on the economic and political life of communities also is warranted (e.g., Sederberg, 1987; Reynolds, 1995). School-to-work and service learning programs provide excellent examples of school-based resources that have the potential to provide positive benefits to communities and families by engaging adults and children in activities outside of the classroom. The notion that community and family effects might mediate the impact of schools on children is intriguing, but rarely studied in systematic fashion. Therefore, a necessary next step is the development of conceptual models that consider ways in which children and the various social systems in which they develop, including home, peer groups, communities, and schools, interact to support the development of school-related competence. How the coordination of these systems changes as children develop and ways in which they jointly contribute to children's developing school-related goals should be a primary target of researchers' efforts.

Finally, identifying ways in which social contexts promote the development of social and academic competencies at school requires systematic experimental research over time. However, experimental studies designed to examine processes that support social competence development in schools are rare. Moreover, most school reform efforts focus on improving achievement test scores and other academic outcomes (e.g., No Child Left Behind Act of 2001), without consideration of the social and psychological consequences of these efforts. Given the strong inter-relations among school success, qualities of relationships with teachers and peers, classroom climate, and school cultures, it seems essential that reform initiatives involving experimentation in schools and evaluation of student progress incorporate assessments of processes and outcomes informed by a broader socio-cultural perspective.

In closing, the authors of chapters in this section are to be applauded for their extremely rich and insightful work on socio-cultural contexts and student engagement. The goal of this commentary has been to provide some additional thoughts and insights into the nature of school-related competence and how it might be supported by students' experiences within broader socio-cultural contexts, including relationships with their parents, teachers and peers, social aspects of learning structures, and the value and belief systems that define school cultures and the communities they live in. In conjunction with the other chapters in this volume, my hope is to provide a strong foundation to explore further the role of social experiences and contexts in supporting the social and intellectual accomplishments of all children.

References

Assor, A. (2012). Allowing choice and nurturing an inner compass: Educational practices supporting students' need for autonomy. In S. L. Christenson, A. L. Reschly, & C. Wylie (Eds.), *Handbook of research on student engagement* (pp. 421–439). New York: Springer.

Bandura, A. (1986). *Social foundations of thought and action: A social cognitive theory*. Englewood Cliffs, NJ: Prentice-Hall.

Bempechat, J., & Shernoff, D. J. (2012). Parental influences on achievement motivation and student engagement. In S. L. Christenson, A. L. Reschly, & C. Wylie (Eds.), *Handbook of research on student engagement* (pp. 315–342). New York: Springer.

Bowlby, J. (1969). *Attachment and loss. Attachment* (Vol. 1). New York: Basic Books.

Bronfenbrenner, U. (1989). Ecological systems theory. In R. Vasta (Ed.), *Annals of child development* (Vol. 6, pp. 187–250). Greenwich, CT: JAI.

Bukowski, W. M., & Hoza, B. (1989). Popularity and friendship: Issues in theory, measurement, and outcome. In T. J. Berndt & G. W. Ladd (Eds.), *Peer relationships in child development* (pp. 15–45). New York: Wiley.

Chang, L. (2003). Variable effects of children's aggression, social withdrawal, and prosocial leadership as functions of teacher beliefs and behaviors. *Child Development, 74*, 535–548.

Collins, W. A., & Repinski, D. J. (1994). Relationships during adolescence: Continuity and change in interpersonal perspective. In R. Montemayor, G. Adams, & T. Gullotta (Eds.), *Personal relationships during adolescence* (pp. 7–36). Thousand Oaks, CA: Sage.

Crosnoe, R., & Needham, B. (2004). Holism, contextual variability, and the study of friendships in adolescent development. *Child Development, 75,* 264–279.

Darling, N., & Steinberg, L. (1993). Parenting style as context – An integrative model. *Psychological Bulletin, 113,* 487–496.

Developmental Studies Center (n.d.). Retrieved August 2, 2007, from www.devstu.org/

Dowson, M., & McInerney, D. M. (2003). What do students say about their motivational goals?: Towards a more complex and dynamic perspective on student motivation. *Contemporary Educational Psychology, 28,* 91–113.

Durlak, J. A., Weissberg, R. P., Dymnicki, A. B., Taylor, R. D., & Schellinger, K. B. (2012). The impact of enhancing students' social and emotional learning: A meta-analysis of school-based universal interventions. *Child Development, 82,* 405–432.

Eccles, J. S., & Midgley, C. (1989). Stage-environment fit: Developmentally appropriate classrooms for young adolescents. In C. Ames & R. Ames (Eds.), *Research on motivation in education* (Vol. 3, pp. 139–186). New York: Academic Press.

Evertson, C., & Weinstein, C. (2006). *Handbook of Classroom Management – Research, Practice, and Contemporary Issues.* Mahwah, NJ: Erlbaum.

Ford, M. E. (1992). *Motivating humans: Goals, emotions, and personal agency beliefs.* Newbury Park, CA: Sage.

Fredricks, J. A., Blumenfeld, P. C., & Paris, A. H. (2004). School engagement: Potential of the concept, state of the evidence. *Review of Educational Research, 74,* 59–109.

Greenfield, P. M. (1997). You can't take it with you – Why ability assessments don't cross cultures. *American Psychologist, 52,* 1115–1124.

Hinde, R. A. (1997). *Towards understanding relationships.* London: Academic Press.

Hipkins, R. (2012). The engaging nature of teaching for competency development. In S. L. Christenson, A. L. Reschly, & C. Wylie (Eds.), *Handbook of research on student engagement* (pp. 441–456). New York: Springer.

Irvine, J. J. (1986). Teacher-student interactions: Effects of student race, sex, and grade level. *Journal of Educational Psychology, 78,* 14–21.

Juvonen, J., Espoinoza, G., & Knifsend, C. (2012). The role of peer relationships in student academic and extracurricular engagement. In S. L. Christenson, A. L. Reschly, & C. Wylie (Eds.), *Handbook of research on student engagement* (pp. 387–401). New York: Springer.

Kuczynski, L., & Parkin, M. (2007). Agency and bidirectionality in socialization: Interactions, transactions and relational dialectics. In J. Grusec & P. Hastings (Eds.), *Handbook of social development* (pp. 259–283). New York: Guilford.

Laible, D., & Thompson, R. A. (2007). Early socialization: A relationship perspective. In J. Grusec & P. Hastings (Eds.), *Handbook of social development* (pp. 181–207). New York: Guilford.

Lam, S., Wong, B. P. H., Yang, H., & Liu, Y. (2012). Understanding student engagement with a contextual model. In S. L. Christenson, A. L. Reschly, & C. Wylie (Eds.), *Handbook of research on student engagement* (pp. 403–419). New York: Springer.

Meece, J. L., Wigfield, A., & Eccles, J. S. (1990). Predictors of math anxiety and its influence on young adolescents' course enrollment intentions and performance in mathematics. *Journal of Educational Psychology, 82,* 60–70.

Nichols, S., & Dawson, H. (2012). Assessment as a context for student engagement. In S. L. Christenson, A. L. Reschly, & C. Wylie (Eds.), *Handbook of research on student engagement* (pp. 457–477). New York: Springer.

Pekrun, R. (2009). Emotions at school. In K. R. Wentzel & A. Wigfield (Eds.), *Handbook of motivation at school* (pp. 575–604). New York: Taylor & Francis.

Phinney, J. S., Kim-Jo, T., Osorio, S., & Vilhjalmsdottir, P. (2005). Autonomy and relatedness in adolescent-parent disagreements: Ethnic and developmental factors. *Journal of Adolescent Research, 20,* 8–39.

Piaget, J. (1983). Piaget's theory. In P. H. Mussen (Ed.), *Handbook of child psychology* (Vol. 1, pp. 103–128). New York: Wiley.

Pianta, R. (2006). Classroom management and relationships between children and teachers: Implications for research and practice. In C. Evertson & C. Weinstein (Eds.), *Handbook of classroom management – Research, practice, and contemporary issues* (pp. 685–710), Mahwah, NJ: Erlbaum

Pianta, R. C., Hamre, B., & Allen, J. P. (2012). Teacher-student relationships and engagement: Conceptualizing, measuring, and improving the capacity of classroom interactions. In S. L. Christenson, A. L. Reschly, & C. Wylie (Eds.), *Handbook of research on student engagement* (pp. 365–386). New York: Springer.

Raftery, J. N., Grolnick, W. S., & Flamm, E. S. (2012). Families as facilitators of student engagement: Toward a Home-School Partnership Model. In S. L. Christenson, A. L. Reschly, & C. Wylie (Eds.), *Handbook of research on student engagement* (pp. 343–364). New York: Springer.

Reynolds, D. R. (1995). Rural education: Decentering the consolidation debate. In E. N. Castle (Ed.), *The changing American countryside: Rural people and places* (pp. 451–480). Lawrence, KS: University Press of Kansas.

Roeser, R., Urdan, T., & Stephens, J. (2009). School as a context of student motivation and achievement. In K. R. Wentzel & A. Wigfield (Eds.), *Handbook of motivation at school* (pp. 381–410). New York: Taylor & Francis.

Rose-Krasnor, L. (1997). The nature of social competence: A theoretical review. *Social Development, 6,* 111–135.

Rumberger, R. W. (1995). Dropping out of middle school: A multilevel analysis of students and schools. *American Educational Research Journal, 32,* 583–625.

Ryan, R. M., & Deci, E. L. (2000). Self-determination theory and the facilitation of intrinsic motivation, social development, and well-being. *American Psychologist, 55,* 68–78.

Saft, E. W., & Pianta, R. C. (2001). Teachers' perceptions of their relationships with students: Effects of child age, gender, and ethnicity of teachers and children. *School Psychology Quarterly, 16*, 125–141.

Sagi, A., Koren-Karie, N., Gini, M., Ziv, Y., & Joels, T. (2002). Shedding further light on the effects of various types and quality of early child care on infant-mother attachment relationship: The Haifa study of early child care. *Child Development, 73*, 1166–1186.

Sederberg, C. H. (1987). Economic role of school districts in rural communities. *Research in Rural Education, 4*, 125–130.

Skinner, E. A., Kindermann, T. A., Connell, J. P., & Wellborn, J. P. (2009). Engagement and disaffection as organizational constructs in the dynamics of motivational development. In K. R. Wentzel & A. Wigfield (Eds.), *Handbook of motivation at school* (pp. 223–246). New York: Taylor & Francis.

Slavin, R. (2011). Instruction based on cooperative learning. In R. Mayer & P. Alexander (Eds.), *Handbook of research on learning and instruction* (pp. 344–360). New York: Routledge.

Steinberg, L., Brown, B. B., & Dornbusch, S. M. (1996). *Beyond the classroom: why school reform has failed and what parents need to do*. New York: Simon & Schuster.

Vygotsky, L. S. (1978). *Mind in society: The development of higher psychological processes*. Cambridge, MA: Harvard University Press.

Wentzel, K. R. (1991). Social competence at school: Relations between social responsibility and academic achievement. *Review of Educational Research, 61*, 1–24.

Wentzel, K. R. (1994). Relations of social goal pursuit to social acceptance, classroom behavior, and perceived social support. *Journal of Educational Psychology, 86*, 173–182.

Wentzel, K. R. (1997). Student motivation in middle school: The role of perceived pedagogical caring. *Journal of Educational Psychology, 89*, 411–419.

Wentzel, K. R. (1998). Social support and adjustment in middle school: The role of parents, teachers, and peers. *Journal of Educational Psychology, 90*, 202–209.

Wentzel, K. R. (1999). Social-motivational processes and interpersonal relationships: Implications for understanding students' academic success. *Journal of Educational Psychology, 91*, 76–97.

Wentzel, K. R. (2002). Are effective teachers like good parents? Interpersonal predictors of school adjustment in early adolescence. *Child Development, 73*, 287–301.

Wentzel, K. R. (2003). School adjustment. In W. Reynolds & G. Miller (Eds.), *Handbook of psychology, Vol. 7: Educational Psychology* (pp. 235–258). New York: Wiley.

Wentzel, K. R. (2004). Understanding classroom competence: The role of social-motivational and self-processes. In R. Kail (Ed.), *Advances in child development and behavior* (Vol. 32, pp. 213–241). New York: Elsevier.

Wentzel, K. R. (2005). Peer relationships, motivation, and academic performance at school. In A. Elliot & C. Dweck (Eds.), *Handbook of competence and motivation* (pp. 279–296). New York: Guilford.

Wentzel, K. R. (2009). Students' relationships with teachers as motivational contexts. In K. Wentzel & A. Wigfield (Eds.), *Handbook of motivation at school* (pp. 301–322). Mahwah, NJ: LEA.

Wentzel, K. R., & Wigfield, A. (2009). *Handbook of motivation at school*. New York, NY: Taylor Francis.

Wentzel, K. R., Baker, S. A., & Russell, S. (2009). Peer relationships and positive adjustment at school. In R. Gillman, S. Huebner, & M. Furlong (Eds.), *Promoting wellness in children and youth: A handbook of positive psychology in the schools* (pp. 229–244). Mahwah, NJ: Erlbaum.

Wentzel, K. R., & Looney, L. (2007). Socialization in school settings. In J. Grusec & P. Hastings (Eds.), *Handbook of social development* (pp. 382–403). New York: Guilford.

Wentzel, K., Russell, S., & Baker, S. (2011). Multiple goals of teachers, parents, and peers as predictors of young adolescents' goals and affective functioning. Unpublished manuscript, University of Maryland, College Park.

Wentzel, K. R., Russell, S., Garza, E., & Merchant, B. (2011). Understanding the role of social supports in Latina/o adolescents' school engagement and achievement. In N. Cabrera, F. Villarruel, & H. Fitzgerald (Eds.), *Volume of Latina/o adolescent psychology and mental health: Vol. 2: Adolescent development*. (pp.195–216). Santa Barbara, CA: ABC-CLIO.

Wentzel, K. R., Baker, S. A., & Russell, S. L. (2012). Young adolescent's perceptions of teachers' and peers' goals as predictors of social and academic goal pursuit. *Applied Psychology*.

Part IV

Student Engagement: Determinants and Student Outcomes

The Relationship Between Engagement and High School Dropout

Russell W. Rumberger and Susan Rotermund

Abstract

This chapter first reviews some prominent models of dropping out and the role that individual factors, including engagement, and contextual factors play in the process. It then reviews empirical research related to those factors, with a focus on engagement-related factors. Scholars have proposed a number of models to explain the process of dropping out of school. While there is a fair amount of overlap in the models, they differ with respect to the specific factors that are thought to exert the most influence on dropping out and the specific process that leads to that outcome. The review of conceptual models of the empirical research literature leads to several conclusions about why students drop out. First, no single factor can completely account for a student's decision to continue in school until graduation. Just as students themselves report a variety of reasons for quitting school, the research literature also identifies a number of salient factors that appear to influence the decision. Second, the decision to drop out is not simply a result of what happens in school. Clearly, students' behavior and performance in school influence their decision to stay or leave. But students' activities and behaviors outside of school—particularly engaging in deviant and criminal behavior—also influence their likelihood of remaining in school. Third, dropping out is more of a process than an event.

---

*Much of the material for this chapter comes from a book by the first author, *Dropping Out: Why Students Quit School and What Can Be Done About It* (Cambridge, MA: Harvard University Press, 2011). We would like to thank the editors, Sandra Christenson and Cathy Wylie, for their helpful feedback on an earlier version of this paper.

R.W. Rumberger (✉)
Graduate School of Education, University of California, Santa Barbara, CA, USA
e-mail: russ@education.ucsb.edu

S. Rotermund
MPR Associates, Berkeley, CA, USA
e-mail: srotermund@mprinc.com

The problem of high school dropouts in the United States has been characterized as a national crisis and a "silent epidemic" (Bridgeland, DiIulio, & Morison, 2006). According to *Education Week*, the nation's leading education periodical, 1.3 million students from the high school class of 2010 will fail to earn a high school diploma (Education Week, 2010). This means that the nation's schools are losing almost 7,200 students each school day. Moreover, the problem is getting worse. Nobel laureate economist James Heckman examined the various sources of data used to calculate dropout and gradation rates and, after correcting for errors in previous calculations, concluded that the high school graduation rate in the USA is currently 77%, lower than it was 40 years ago (Heckman & LaFontaine, 2010).

Dropping out of school has consequences for both dropouts and the larger society. Dropouts face bleak economic futures. They are the least educated workers in the labor market and thus have the poorest job prospects compared to more educated workers. This means they are less likely to find jobs and when they do find jobs, the jobs generally pay the lowest wages. For example, in 2008, the median annual earnings of high school dropouts were 28% less than the earnings of high school graduates (Snyder & Dillow, 2010, Table 385). Over their working lives, the US Census Bureau estimates that dropouts will earn about $200,000 less than high school graduates (Day & Newburger, 2002, Figure 3). Dropouts are more likely to engage in crime and, consequently, are more likely to be arrested and incarcerated (Pettit & Western, 2004). They also have poorer health and, as a result, have shorter life spans than persons with more education (Currie, 2009).

The negative impacts from dropping out not only affect dropouts themselves. They also impact the larger society. The fact that dropouts have lower employment and earnings means they make smaller contributions to their local and state economies as well as the national economy. It also means they pay fewer taxes. At the same time, they are more likely to require public assistance in the form of unemployment benefits, welfare, and public health care. Dropouts generate further social costs because of their increased criminal activity. These costs are not simply related to the additional costs from law enforcement and incarceration, but also the costs borne by the victims of crime in the form of property damage, hospitalization, and loss of life. One recent study estimated that each new high school graduate would generate more than $200,000 in government savings, and that cutting in half the dropout rate from a single cohort of dropouts would generate more than $45 billion in savings for the economy (Belfield & Levin, 2007).

Understanding why students drop out of school is the key to designing effective interventions to help solve this critical and costly problem. Yet identifying the causes of dropping out is extremely difficult. Like other forms of educational achievement, such as test scores and grades, dropping out of school is likely influenced by an array of factors, some immediately preceding departure from high school and others occurring years earlier in middle and even elementary school. These factors may be related to the characteristics and experiences of the students themselves as well as the characteristics and features of their environment—their families, their schools, and the communities where they live.

To understand why students drop out, it is most useful to consider dropping out as a process that culminates in students quitting or finishing high school (Rumberger, 2011). Researchers have developed a number of models to explain the process of dropping out and the underlying factors that contribute to it. In fact, some scholars have also characterized dropping out as "symptom" in recognition of the role and importance of these underlying factors:

> Dropping out of high school is overrated as a *problem* in its own right—it is far more appropriately viewed as the end result or *symptom* of other problems which have their origin much earlier in life (Bachman, Green, & Wirtanen, 1971, P. 169).

Researchers have also developed models to explain some of the factors that figure prominently into the process of dropping out. One of the most prominent factors found in many of these models is student engagement. Finally, researchers have examined the role of context or settings in shaping various aspects of adolescent development, including engagement and dropping out.

This chapter first reviews some prominent models of dropping out and the role that individual factors, including engagement, and contextual factors play in the process. It then reviews empirical research related to those factors, with a focus on engagement-related factors.

Conceptual Models of Dropout and Engagement

Models of Dropping Out

Scholars have proposed a number of models to explain the process of dropping out of school. Some models focus specifically on dropping out while others attempt to explain student outcomes in general, with dropping out representing simply one. Most of the models focus on an individual perspective and identify a number of general types of factors: prior school experiences, particularly academic performance (grades, test scores, etc.); behaviors, including academic (e.g., doing homework), cognitive (exerting effort toward academic ends), social (getting along with teachers and classmates); and psychological conditions, such as self-esteem and identification with school. While there is a fair amount of overlap in the models, they differ with respect to the specific factors (italicized in the discussion below) that are thought to exert the most influence on dropping out and the specific process that leads to that outcome. In some cases, the models are developed from a review of the literature, but not tested empirically; in other cases, the models are derived from a specific empirical study.

Finn's Models

In a widely cited review of the literature, Finn proposed two alternative, developmental models to explain dropping out (Finn, 1989). The first, which he labeled the "frustration-self-esteem" model, posits that the initial antecedent to school withdrawal is early *school failure*, which, in turn, leads to low *self-esteem* and then *problem behaviors* (skipping class, truancy, disruptive behavior, and juvenile delinquency). Over time, problem behaviors further erode school performance, which leads to further declines in self-esteem and increases in problem behaviors. Eventually, students either voluntarily quit school or are removed from school because of their problematic behavior.

The second model Finn labels the "participation-identification" model. In this model, the initial antecedent to withdrawal is the lack of *participation* in school activities (classroom participation, homework, and participation in the social, extracurricular, athletic, and governance aspects of the school), which, in turn, leads to *poor school performance* and then to less *identification* (a sense of "belonging" and "valuing") with school. Over time, the lack of identification with school leads to less participation, poorer school performance, less identification with school, and eventually dropping out of school.

Both of Finn's models include three types of factors: school performance, behaviors, and psychological conditions. The models differ in the specific behavioral and psychological factors they highlight: the "frustration-self-esteem" model focuses on problem behaviors (skipping class, truancy, disruptive behavior, and juvenile delinquency, as well as dropping out) and self-esteem; while the "participation-identification" model focuses on participation and identification with school.

Life Course Models

A number of long-term longitudinal studies have been conducted in the USA that have tracked the educational experiences and outcomes of small, local samples of children. These studies have developed and tested empirical models of the dropout process to determine the direct and indirect effects of various early and late factors on whether students dropped out or completed high school. Because of their long-term perspective, some scholars refer to these as life course models.

In their study of 1,242 children who were enrolled as first graders in pubic and parochial schools in the poor, black community of Woodlawn in Chicago in the 1966–1967 school year, Ensminger and Slusarcick found that variables in five domains—family background, family educational expectations and values, parent-child interaction concerning school, the social integration of the family in terms of school, and the child's cognitive and behavioral performance in school—predicted whether children dropped out or graduated from high school (Ensminger & Slusarcick, 1992).

In their study of 205 Euro-American families with varied living arrangements (two-parent families, single mothers, cohabitating couples, and commune and group living arrangements) from California that started in 1974–1975, Garnier, Stein, and Jacobs found that nonconventional family lifestyles and values, cumulative family stresses, and family socioeconomic status (SES) affected school performance and motivation, adolescent stress and substance use, and, ultimately, school dropout (Garnier, Stein, & Jacobs, 1997).

In their study based on data from the Beginning Baltimore Study (BBS), a panel study of 661 children who entered first grade in 20 Baltimore city schools in the fall of 1982—Alexander and Entwisle present and test a model of dropping out from a life course perspective that views dropping out as a long-term "process of progressive academic disengagement" (Alexander, Entwisle, & Kabbini, 2001). Their model identified three types of factors—students' school experiences (school performance, grade retention, and track-like placements), students' personal resources (what they labeled "engagement behaviors" and "engagement attitudes"), and parental attitudes, behaviors, and support—in several developmental periods of students' school careers—first grade, elementary years (grades 5–8), middle school (grades 6–8), and early high school (grade 9)—that predicted whether students dropped out or stayed in school.

In two studies based on data from the Chicago Longitudinal Study—an ongoing investigation of 1,569 low-income, minority children born in 1979 or 1980 who grew up in high-poverty neighborhoods of Chicago—Reynolds, Ou, and Topitzes developed a conceptual model of the various pathways that preschool participation affects such long-term outcomes as educational attainment and juvenile delinquency (Reynolds, Ou, & Topitzes, 2004). They found that preschool participation directly affected school performance (cognitive ability, retention), social adjustment, and family support which, in turn, affected school quality, persistence, and motivation in middle grades which, in turn, affected educational attainment and delinquency in later adolescence.

Tinto Model

Another theoretical perspective that is useful in explaining dropout behavior is a widely acknowledged theory of institutional departure at the postsecondary level developed by sociologist Vincent Tinto (Tinto, 1987, 1994). Tinto focused on the role of the institutional environment in influencing students' adjustment and ultimately their departure decision. The process of departure is first influenced by a series of personal attributes, which predispose students to respond to different situations or conditions in particular ways. These personal attributes include *family background*, *skills and abilities*, and *prior school experiences*, including *goals* (intentions) and *motivation* (commitments) to continue their schooling. Once students enroll in a particular school, two separate dimensions of that institution influence whether a student remains there: a social dimension that deals with the *social integration* of students with the institution and the value of schooling; and an academic dimension that deals with the *academic integration* or engagement of students in meaningful learning. Both dimensions are influenced by the informal as well as the formal structure of the institution. For example, academic integration may occur in the formal system of classes and in the informal system of interactions with faculty in other settings.

These two dimensions can have separate and independent influences on whether students leave an institution, depending on the needs and attributes of the student, as well as external factors. To remain in an institution, students must become integrated to some degree in either the social system or the academic system. For example, some students may be highly integrated into the academic system of the institution, but not the social system. Yet as long as their social needs are met elsewhere and their goals and commitment remain the same, such students will remain in the same institution. Likewise, some students may be highly integrated into the social system of the institution, but not the academic system. But again, as long as they maintain minimum academic performance and their goals and commitment remain the same, such students will remain in the same institution.

Tinto's model offers several insights into the process of institutional departure, which can involve either transferring to another school or quitting school altogether. First, it distinguishes between the commitment to the goal of finishing college and the commitment to a particular institution, and how these commitments can be influenced by students' experiences in school over time. Some students who are not sufficiently integrated into their current college may simply transfer to another educational setting rather than drop out, if they can maintain their goals and commitment to schooling more generally. Other students, however, may simply drop out rather than transfer to another school if their current school experiences severely diminish their goals and commitment to schooling. Second, it suggests that schools can have multiple communities or subcultures to accommodate and support the different needs of students. Third, it acknowledges the importance of external factors that can influence student departure. For example, external communities, including families and friends, can help students better meet the academic and social demands of school by providing necessary support. External events can also change a student's evaluation of the relative costs and benefits of staying in a particular school if other alternatives change (e.g., job prospects).

Wehlage and Colleagues' Model

Drawing on their research on at-risk students and programs as well as Tinto's model, Gary Wehlage and his colleagues developed a model to explain dropping out and other high school outcomes that focuses on the contribution of school factors (Wehlage, Rutter, Smith, Lesko, & Fernandez, 1989). In this model, student outcomes are jointly influenced by two broad factors: *school membership* (or social bonding) and *educational engagement*.

Social bonding, which is critical to connecting students to the school, has four aspects: "A student is socially bonded to the extent that he or she is attached to adults and peers, committed to the norms of the school, involved in school activities and has belief in the legitimacy and efficacy of the institution" (p. 117). Drawing on Tinto's work, they then identified four common impediments to school membership: *adjustment* to a new and often larger and more impersonal school setting; *difficulty* in doing more rigorous academic work; *incongruence* between students' values, experiences, and projected future and the goals and rewards of the school; and *isolation* from teachers and peers in both academic and social experiences, something very similar to Tinto's concept of academic and social integration.

Educational engagement for Wehlage et al referred to the "psychological investment required to comprehend and master knowledge and skills explicitly taught in school" (p. 177). They identified three impediments to educational engagement: (1) schoolwork is not extrinsically motivating for many students because achievement is not tied to any explicit and valued goal; (2) the dominant learning process pursued in schools is too abstract, verbal, sedentary, individualistic, competitive, and controlled by others (and therefore not intrinsically motivating) as opposed to concrete, problem-oriented, active, kinesthetic, cooperative, and autonomous; and (3) classroom learning is often stultifying because educators are obsessed with the "coverage" of the subject matter, which makes school knowledge superficial and also intrinsically unsatisfying, preventing students from gaining a sense of competence (p. 179).

Models of Deviance

While most of the models reviewed thus far have focused on student attitudes and behaviors within school, social scientists in such fields as psychology, sociology, economics, and criminology have focused on a range of deviant behaviors of adolescents outside of school—including juvenile delinquency, drug and alcohol abuse, teenage parenting and childbearing—and their relationship to school dropout (Lerner & Galambos, 1998).

Sara Battin-Pearson and her colleagues identified five alternative theories of dropout that conceptualize the process and the salient influences of dropping out differently (Battin-Pearson et al., 2000). The first model, *academic mediation theory*, posits that all predictors of dropping out, including deviant behavior, low social bonding, and family background, are mediated by poor academic achievement. In the remaining four models, poor academic achievement only mediates some of the effects of the other predictors, so that at least some predictors also exert a direct influence on dropping out. In the second model, *general deviance theory*, several types of deviant behavior—juvenile delinquency, drug and alcohol use, smoking, and teenage pregnancy—exert a direct influence on dropping out. In the third model, *deviant affiliation theory*, bonding with antisocial or delinquent friends exerts a direct influence on dropping out. In the fourth model, *family socialization theory*, poor family socialization, as related to parental expectations, family stress, and parental control, exerts a direct influence on dropping out. And in the fifth model, *structural strains theory*, demographic factors such as race, ethnicity, and family socioeconomic status, exert a direct influence on dropping out. In addition to general models of deviance, criminologists have developed a number of alternative theories to explain why involvement with the juvenile justice system may be detrimental or beneficial to subsequent delinquent behavior and school dropout (Sweeten, 2006).

The models reviewed in this section identify a number of factors and processes to explain why students drop out. They suggest the process of dropping out is complex, influenced by a number of factors in and out of school and over time. Some factors, such as school performance, are common to virtually all the models, while other factors, such as misbehavior or attitudes toward school, are found in only some models. The models are not necessarily competitive, but rather may be useful in identifying different patterns or types of dropouts.

The Role of Engagement

Student engagement figures prominently in the process of dropping out. In fact, in an early review of the research literature published in 1987, Rumberger suggested, "dropping out itself might be better viewed as a process of disengagement from school, perhaps for either academic or social reasons, that culminates in the final act of leaving" (Rumberger, 1987, p. 111). Similarly, in her study of students in two California continuation high schools, Kelly preferred to use the term *disengagement* to either the term *dropout*, which she argued put inordinate blame on the student's agency, or *pushout*, which put inordinate blame on schools (Kelly, 1993). Student engagement is also an important precursor to other aspects of school performance, particularly academic performance in the classroom. Because of its importance, scholars have proposed a number of models to explain student engagement.

In a follow-up to his work on at-risk students and programs, Gary Welhage and his colleagues, Fred Newman and Susie Lamborn, developed a model of student engagement in academic work, which they define as "the student's *psychological investment* in and *effort* directed toward learning, understanding, or mastering the knowledge, skills, or crafts that academic work is intended to promote" (Newmann, 1992, p. 12). As they point out, because engagement is an inner quality of concentration and effort, it is not readily observed, so it must be inferred from indirect indicators such as the amount of *participation in academic work* (attendance, amount of time spent on academic work), and *interest* and *enthusiasm* exhibited by students. They further suggest that engagement is related to but differs from motivation, a subject of longstanding concern to educational psychologists:

> Academic motivation usually refers to a general desire or disposition to succeed in academic work and in the more specific tasks of school. Conceivably a student can be motivated to perform well in a general sense without being engaged in the specific tasks of school. Engagement in specific tasks may either precede or presume general motivation to succeed. By focusing on the extent to which students demonstrate active interest, effort, and concentrations in the specific work that teachers design, engagement calls special attention to the contexts that help activate underlying motivation, and also to the conditions that may generate new motivation (p. 13).

They posit that engagement in academic work is largely influenced by three major factors: "students' underlying *need for competence*, the extent to which students experience *membership* in the school, and the *authenticity* of the work they are asked to complete" (p. 17). They identify a number of factors that influence school membership and authentic work similar to those identified by Wehlage and his colleagues in their model of student dropout.

In 2004, the National Research Council issued a report, *Engaging Schools: Fostering High School Students' Motivation to Learn*, which similarly made the distinction between motivation and engagement in schoolwork (National Research Council, Committee on Increasing High School Students' Engagement and Motivation to Learn [NRC, CIHSSEML], 2004). The committee that issued the report stated that engagement involved both observable behaviors (active participation in class, completing work, taking challenging classes) and unobservable behaviors (effort, attention, problem solving, and the use of metacognitive strategies) as well as emotions (such as interest, enthusiasm, and pride in success), similar to how Newmann, Wehlage, and Lamborn characterized it. But unlike Newmann and his colleagues, the committee developed a model that suggested the impact of the educational context (such as instruction, school climate, school organization, school composition, and school size) is mediated by three psychological variables: students' beliefs about their *competence* and *control* (*I can*), their *values* and *goals* (*I want to*), and their sense of *social connectiveness* or *belonging* (*I belong*). This model incorporates more explicit aspects of student motivation from the research literature. Connell, for example, postulated that the more students perceive the school setting as meeting their psychological needs for *autonomy*, *competence*, and *relatedness*, the more engaged they will be in school activities (Connell, 1990).

Both the Wehlage and NRC models focus on engagement in academic work. But as Tinto and Finn suggested in their models, participation and integration in school can take place in other arenas besides the classroom. So while academic engagement may be sufficient to improve academic achievement, engagement in other areas of the school, such as extracurricular activities, may be equally valuable in getting students to stay in school (although not necessarily sufficient to have them improve their academic performance or to graduate).

In their extensive review of research literature, Fredricks, Blumenfeld, and Paris (2004) identified three dimensions of this broader concept of engagement: (1) *behavioral engagement*, which represents behaviors that demonstrate students' attachment and involvement in both the academic and social aspects of school, such as doing homework and participating in extracurricular activities like athletics or student government; *emotional engagement*, which refers to students' affective reactions to their experiences in school and in their classes, such as whether they are happy or bored; and *cognitive engagement*, which represents mental behaviors that contribute to learning, such as trying hard and expending effort on academic tasks. Their review went on to examine both the outcomes and the antecedents to engagement. The antecedents include school-level factors, such as school size, communal structures, and disciplinary practices; and classroom-level factors, such as teacher support, peers, classroom structure, and task characteristics. In a more recent review, Appleton, Christenson, and Furlong (2008) identified a myriad of definitions and measures of engagement that help illuminate the various dimensions of the concept, but also make it difficult to collect and use consistent information on engagement to design interventions.

The Role of Context

The models presented thus far focus largely on dropping out as a process influenced by a broad array of individual factors, including attitudes, behaviors, and school performance. Yet these factors and students' experiences more generally are shaped by three settings or contexts where youths spend their time: families, schools, and communities. Increasingly, social scientists have come to realize the importance of these settings in shaping child and adolescent development. In psychology, for example, Bronfenbrenner's influential book, *The Ecology of Human Development* (1979), helped to focus attention of psychologists on how the various contexts of the family, schools, peer groups, and communities shape all aspects of adolescent development—physical, psychological, cognitive and social—as well as how the relationship between context and development change over time (Bronfenbrenner, 1979; Lerner & Galambos, 1998; Steinberg & Morris, 2001). The importance of context was further emphasized by the National Research Council Panel on High-Risk Youth in their 1993 report, *Losing Generations: Adolescents in High-risk Settings*, which argued that too much emphasis had been placed on high-risk youth and their families, and not enough on the high-risk settings in which they live and go to school:

> The work of this panel began as an attempt to better understand why some adolescents are drawn to risky life-styles while others, similarly situated, engage in only normal adolescent experimentation. As our work progressed, however, we became convinced that a focus on individual characteristics of adolescents would contribute to the overemphasis of the last two decades on the personal attributes of adolescents and their families at the expense of attention to the effects or settings or context. We concluded that it was important to right the balance by focusing on the profound influence that settings have on the behavior and development of adolescents (p. 1).

Social scientists have long recognized the critical role that context plays in understanding such phenomena as poverty, racial inequality, gang behavior, and unwed motherhood (Edin & Kefalas, 2005; Evans, 2004; Sullivan, 1989; Wilson, 1987).

Although a wide variety of contextual factors have been shown to influence adolescent development and school performance, they can be categorized into four major areas: (1) *composition*, such as the characteristics of the persons within the setting or context; (2) *structure*, such as size and location; (3) *resources*, such as physical, fiscal and human resources; and (4) *practices*, such as parenting practices within families and instructional practices within schools.

A Conceptual Model of Student Performance in High School

These models can be used to construct a comprehensive conceptual framework for understanding the process of dropping out and graduation, as well as the salient factors underlying that process. The framework, illustrated in Fig. 24.1, considers dropping out and graduation as specific aspects of student performance in high school and identifies two types of factors that influence that performance: individual factors associated with students, and institutional factors associated with the three major contexts that influence students—families, schools, and communities.

Individual factors can be grouped into four areas or domains: educational performance, behaviors, attitudes, and background. Although the framework suggests a causal ordering of these factors, from background to attitudes to behaviors to performance, the various models of dropout and engagement discussed earlier indicate a less linear relationship. In particular, the relationship between attitudes and behaviors is generally considered to be more reciprocal; for example, initial attitudes may influence behaviors, which, in turn, may influence subsequent attitudes (as suggested by Tinto's model). But the purpose of this framework is not to suggest a particular model of the dropout process, but simply a framework for organizing a review of the literature. The factors listed within each group represent conceptual categories that may be measured by one or more specific indicators or variables

The first domain is educational performance. The framework posits three inter-related dimensions of educational performance: (1) academic achievement, as reflected in grades and test scores, (2) educational persistence, which reflects whether students remain in the same school or transfer (school mobility) or remain enrolled in school at all (dropout), and (3) educational attainment, which is reflected by progressing in school (e.g., earning credits and being promoted from one grade to another) and completing formal education by earning of degrees or diplomas. The framework suggests that high school graduation is dependent on both persistence and achievement. That is, students who either interrupt their schooling by dropping out or changing schools, or who have poor academic achievement in school, are less likely to progress in school and to graduate.

The second domain consists of a range of behaviors that are associated with educational

Conceptual Model of High School Performance

	BACKGROUND	ATTITUDES	BEHAVIORS	PERFORMANCE
Individual Factors	Demographics Health Prior performance Past experiences	Goals Values Self-perceptions	Engagement Coursework Deviance Peers Employment	Achievement Persistence Attainment

	FAMILIES	SCHOOLS	COMMUNITIES
Institutional Factors	Structure Resources Practices	Composition Structure Resources Practices	Composition Resources

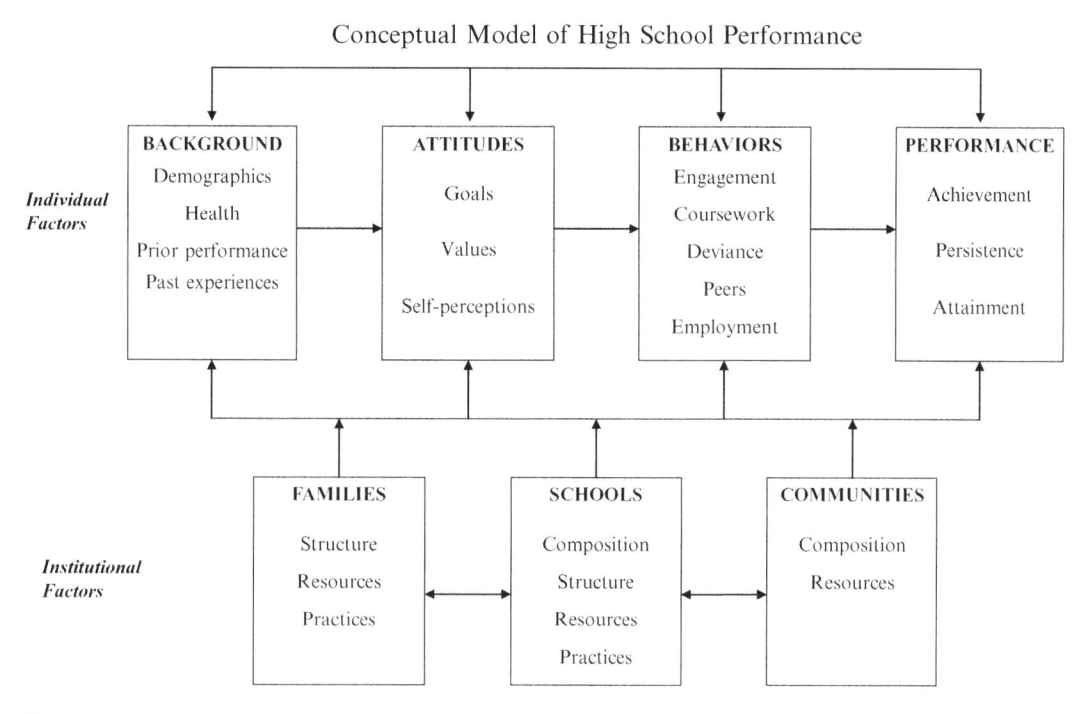

Fig. 24.1 Conceptual model of high school performance

performance. The first factor is student engagement, which we list in the behavioral group even though some conceptions of engagement, as discussed earlier, can have attitudinal (emotional) as well as behavioral components. Other behaviors that have been identified in the research literature include coursetaking, deviance (misbehavior, drug and alcohol use, and childbearing), peer associations, and employment.

The third domain consists of attitudes, which we use as a general label to represent a wide range of psychological factors including expectations, goals, values, and self-perceptions (e.g., perceived competence, perceived autonomy, and perceived sense of belonging).

The last domain consists of student background characteristics, which include demographic characteristics, health, prior performance in school, and past experiences, such as participation in preschool, after-school activities, and summer school.

The framework further posits that these individual-level characteristics are influenced by three institutional contexts—families, schools, and communities—and several key features within them: composition, structure, resources, and practices. This conceptual framework can be used to review the empirical research on high school dropouts.

Empirical Research

Scholars have conducted literally hundreds of studies to understand how and why students drop out or graduate from high school. They have also employed a wide range of research methodologies, from in-depth case studies of students and schools designed to understand the process of dropping out and the salient factors that contribute to that process (Fine, 1991; Flores-Gonzalez, 2002; Kelly, 1993; Romo & Falbo, 1996; Valenzuela, 1999) to large-scale statistical studies designed to identify the unique contribution of specific factors on whether students drop out or graduate from high school (Bryk & Thum, 1989;

Lee & Burkam, 2003; Rumberger, 1995; Rumberger & Thomas, 2000).

It should be pointed out that scholars, for the most part, are unable to establish definitively that any specific factor "causes" students to drop out. Even complex, statistical models with large numbers of variables are often unable to control for other, unobservable factors that may contribute to the dropout process and that may mediate the effects of other variables. However, in recent years, new research designs and statistical models do allow stronger, more causal inferences to be made (Schneider, Carnoy, Kilpatrick, Schmidt, & Shavelson, 2007). Yet because most existing studies do not employ these techniques, it is more accurate to refer to these various factors as "predictors" or "influences" rather than "causes" of dropping out.

Because the empirical research is extensive, in this section we only provide a short review of the literature on high school dropouts. The review focuses on engagement-related predictors of dropping out at the individual level and then a short summary of the predictors at the family and school levels. The discussion below draws heavily on a 2008 review of the research literature by Rumberger and Lim that examined 389 separate analyses found in 203 statistical dropout studies published in academic journals between 1983 and 2007 (Rumberger & Lim, 2008). The review identified specific factors that the studies found had a direct effect on dropping out or graduation, controlling for other factors. As a result, the review did not examine indirect effects or total effects. The review also only examined whether the factors were statistically significant, not the size of the effects.

Individual Factors

A range of individual factors encompasses various aspects of engagement. We first review behavioral factors, then attitudes, and finally composite measures of risk, which often include engagement measures.

Behaviors

In the earlier discussion about the process of dropping out, engagement emerged as an important part of the educational process and a powerful precursor to dropping out. Students who are engaged in school, whether in the academic arena or the social arena, are more likely to attend, to learn, and eventually to finish high school; students who are disengaged are not. Research studies have measured engagement in several ways, but no matter how it is measured, it predicts dropping out.

One of the most direct and visible indicators of engagement is attendance. To graduate, students must not only enroll in school, they must attend school. Yet some students have poor attendance and such students are more likely to drop out of school. In our review of the literature, 13 of the 19 analyses of attendance found that high absenteeism predicted dropping out (Rumberger & Lim, 2008, p. 41).

Another indicator of engagement is participation in extracurricular activities. Most, but not all, middle and high school students participate in extracurricular activities. In 2002, more than 50% of second-year high school students reported participating in athletics, 11% in cheerleading and drill teams, 22% in music, and 10% in hobby clubs (Cahalan, Ingles, Burns, Planty, & Daniel, 2006, Tables 23 and 24). In 2007, 59% of eighth graders reported participating in sports, 40% in drama or music, and 32% in clubs (Walston, Rathbun, & Huasken, 2008, Table 4). In our review of the literature, 14 of the 26 analyses found that participation in extracurricular activities reduced the odds of dropping out (with most of the other studies showing non-significant effects). At the middle school level, only two out of seven analyses found that involvement in extracurricular activities reduced the odds of dropping out of high school. Participation in sports, especially among males, shows more consistent effects than participation in other extracurricular activities or participation in extracurricular activities more generally (McNeal, 1995; Pittman, 1991; Yin & Moore, 2004).

Other research studies created multiple indicators of student engagement often based on information from student and teacher questionnaires. For example, one recent study of high school sophomores (second-year high school students) created an index of academic engagement based on four questions from the student questionnaire:

- How many times during the first semester or term were you late to school?
- How many times during the first semester or term did you cut or skip class?
- How many times during the first semester or term were you absent from school?
- How much do you agree or disagree that the subjects you're taking are interesting and challenging? (Dalton, Glennie, & Ingels, 2009, p. A-22)

The least engaged students (those who ranked in the bottom third of this index) were five times more likely to drop out (12.1% v. 2.5%) as the most engaged students (those who ranked in the top third) (Dalton et al., 2009, Table 7).

Of the 35 analyses that examined various composite measures of student engagement in high school in Rumberger and Lim's review of the literature, 24 found that higher levels of engagement reduced the likelihood of dropping out or increased the likelihood of graduating from high school. Of the 31 analyses that examined student engagement in middle school, 10 analyses found engagement reduced dropout and increased graduation from high school. At the elementary level, only one of three analyses found that engagement reduced the odds of dropping out of high school (Alexander et al., 2001). The fact that high school measures of engagement are more reliable predictors of dropping out than middle and elementary predictors is consistent with the growing literature on early warning systems that shows proximal (high school) indicators are more powerful predictors than middle and elementary school predictors (Allensworth & Easton, 2005; Meyer, Carl, & Cheng, 2010).

Another indicator of engagement is school misbehavior. In Rumberger and Lim's review, 49 analyses examined the relationship between misbehavior and dropping out, with most of the analyses focusing on the high school level. Among the 31 analyses at the high school level, 14 found that misbehavior was significantly associated with higher dropout and lower graduation rates (Rumberger & Lim, 2008, Table 2). Of the 17 analyses at the middle school level, 14 found that misbehavior in middle school was significantly associated with higher dropout and lower graduation rates in high school. The one analysis that focused on the elementary school level found that misbehavior in elementary school increased the odds of dropping out of high school (Ou, Mersky, Reynolds, & Kohler, 2007). It is interesting to note that misbehavior in middle school was a more consistent predictor of dropping out than high school misbehaviour, while academic performance in high school is a more consistent predictor than academic performance in middle school.

Misbehavior may contribute to dropping out in at least three ways. Students who misbehave may be suspended or even expelled, as Sullivan documents in his study of youth crime and work in three neighborhoods of Brooklyn (Sullivan, 1989, p. 56). They also may be transferred to alternative school settings. Two-thirds of the boys in Kelly's study of two continuation high schools were sent to the schools because of discipline problems (Kelly, 1993, Table 3). Finally, misbehavior in elementary or middle school could lead to misbehavior in high school.

A final behavior indicator of engagement is student mobility. The research literature shows that student mobility, at least during middle and high school, affects school dropout and graduation. At the high school level, ten of 14 analyses in Rumberger and Lim's review of the literature found that student mobility increased the odds of dropping out or decreased the odds of graduating. At the middle school level, nine of 13 analyses found a positive impact of student mobility. At the elementary level, eight of 14 analyses found a significant relationship. One possible reason for the impact at the middle and high school levels is that secondary students are more sensitive to the disruptions to their friendship networks (Ream, 2005; Ream & Rumberger, 2008). Of course, the significant association between mobility and dropout may not be causal; instead, it could be due to preexisting, common factors, such as academic achievement or misbehavior, which influence both mobility and dropout. Nonetheless, even studies that control for a host of preexisting factors, such as student achievement, conclude that some causal association between mobility and educational performance is likely (Pribesh & Downey, 1999). The impact also depends on the reasons students change schools. Students who change schools in a purposeful way—to find a more suitable school environment—may have more positive impacts than students who change schools in a reactive way, such as getting into trouble and being asked or even forced to find a new school (Ream, 2005; Rumberger, Larson, Ream, & Palardy, 1999).

Attitudes

Students' beliefs, values, and attitudes are related to both their behaviors and to their performance in school. These psychological factors include motivation, values, goals, and a range of students' self-perceptions about themselves and their abilities. These factors change over time through students' developmental periods and biological transformations, with the period of early adolescence and the emergence of sexuality being one of the most important and often the most difficult period for many students:

> For some children, the early-adolescent years mark the beginning of a downward spiral leading to academic failure and school dropout. Some early adolescents see their school grades decline markedly when they enter junior high school, along with their interest in school, intrinsic motivation, and confidence in their intellectual abilities. Negative responses to school increase as well, as youngsters become more prone to test anxiety, learned helplessness, and self-consciousness that impedes concentration on learning tasks (Eccles, 1999, p. 37).

Although there is a substantial body of research that has explored a wide range of student beliefs, values, and attitudes, far less research has linked them to student dropout (Eccles & Wigfield, 2002).

One exception is a detailed longitudinal study of a cohort of first-grade students from the Baltimore Beginning School Study (BSS) that began in the fall of 1982 (Alexander et al., 2001). That study collected a wide range of attitudinal and behavioral information on students in grades 1–9 from student self-reports, teachers' reports, and school report cards. The attitudinal information included self-expectations for upcoming grades, educational attainment, self-ability and competence, and measures of psychological engagement ("likes school") and school commitment (pp. 810–812). The attitudinal items (as well as the behavioral items) were all combined into a single construct for grade 1, grades 2–5, grades 6–8, and grade 9. This allowed the researchers to examine not only the relative effects of student attitudes and behaviors overall relative to other predictors, but also their relative effects over different grade levels or stages of schooling. The authors found that while the effects of behavioral engagement on school dropout appear in grade 1, even after controlling for the effects of school performance and family background in grade 1, student attitudes do not demonstrate a separate effect on school dropout until grade 9, with behavioral engagement still showing the stronger effect (Alexander et al. 2001, Table 9). Interestingly, the authors also find that the correlation between attitudes and behaviors increases from grade 1 to grade 9 (p. 796).

Goals

To succeed in school, students must value school. That is, they have to believe that it will be instrumental in meeting their short-term or long-term goals (Eccles & Wigfield, 2002). Most students, as well as their parents, believe that education is the key to a better job and a better life. Yet some youths, such as those profiled in Sullivan's study of youth crime and work in Brooklyn, were more ambivalent about whether finishing high school would lead them into better jobs in their neighborhoods where such jobs were scarce and their fathers and older brothers were employed in jobs that did not require educational credentials (Sullivan, 1989, p. 54).

Most students and their parents also expect to not only complete high school, but to finish college. In 2002, more than 80% of high school sophomores (and their parents) expected that they would earn a bachelor's degree or more advanced college degree (Dalton et al., 2009, Table 5).

Students who expect to graduate from college are much less likely to drop out of high school than students who only expect to finish high school. Among 2002 high school sophomores who expected to earn a bachelor's degree, only 4% dropped out of high school, compared to 21% for students who only expected to complete high school (Ibid.). These findings are confirmed in other research studies. In our review of the research literature, we identified 82 analyses that examined the relationship between educational expectations and school dropout. At the high school level, 33 of the 41 analyses found that higher levels of educational expectations were associated with lower dropout rates, even after controlling for academic performance. At the middle school level, 23 of the 38 analyses found the same relationship. Three analyses examined educational expectations in elementary school and none found a significant effect on high school dropout or graduation.

Self-perceptions

To be successful in school, students not only must value school, they must believe they are capable of achieving success. Students' perceptions of themselves and their abilities are a key component of achievement motivation and an important precursor of student engagement (NRC, CIHSSEML, 2004).

Research studies have examined a number of self-perceptions and their relationship to high school dropout and graduation. All of these perceptions are constructed as composite measures based on student responses to a number of questions about themselves. One such construct is self-concept. Self-concept is basically a person's conception of himself or herself (Bong & Skaalvik, 2003). Although self-concept can be viewed and measured as a general construct, scholars have come to realize that it is multidimensional and that it should be measured with respect to a particular domain, such as academic self-concept or self-concept with respect to reading. A related construct is self-esteem, which measures self-assessments of qualities that are viewed as important (Ibid.). Another construct is locus of control, which measures whether students feel they have control over their destiny (internal control) or not (external control). Poor self-perceptions can undermine motivation, thereby increasing the risk of dropping out.

Although such perceptions are a central component of motivation for remaining in school, relatively few studies have found a direct relationship between any of these self-perceptions and dropping out, suggesting that the effects are most likely mediated by academic performance. The most studied has been locus of control. Of the 22 analyses of locus of control in Rumberger and Lim's review, only three analyses in three studies found a direct, significant relationship with dropout, with students who had an external locus of control—the feeling of little control over one's destiny—even as early as first grade, showing a higher propensity to drop out (Alexander et al., 2001; Ekstrom, Goertz, Pollack, & Rock, 1986; Rumberger, 1983).

Combining Factors

While it is useful to identify individual predictors of dropping out, it is also useful to understand how various factors jointly contribute to the process of dropping out. Researchers have used three approaches for combining factors: creating a composite index of risk; creating taxonomies to identify different types of dropouts; and testing structural models that link factors together.

Risk Factors

Instead of examining the effects of individual student predictors on dropping out, a number of studies combined a series of factors into a composite index of risk. Some studies only included student factors (Connell, Halpern-Felsher, Cliffor, Crichlow, & Usinger, 1995; Lee & Burkam, 1992), while other studies included both student and family factors (Benz, Lindstrom, & Yovanoff, 2000; Cabrera & La Nasa, 2001; Croninger & Lee, 2001). For example, one study based on a national longitudinal study of eighth grade students, created a "social risk" index based on five demographic factors (poverty, language minority status, ethnic minority, single-parent household, and having a dropout parent) and an "academic risk" index based on five school performance factors (grades below C, retained between grades 2 and 8, educational expectations no greater than high school, sent to the office at least once in the first semester, and parents notified at least once of a problem with their child during the first semester) (Croninger & Lee, 2001). The study found that about one third of the students had at least one academic risk factor and those students were twice as likely to drop out as students with no academic risk factors, whereas having at least one social risk factor increased the odds of dropping out by 50% both for academically at-risk student and students who were not academically at risk. Another study based on institutional data from the Philadelphia Public Schools created an index based on four factors measured in the sixth grade that indicated whether the student: (1) attended school 80% or less of the time; (2) failed math; (3) failed English; and (4) received an out-of-school suspension (Balfanz, Herzog, & Mac Iver, 2007). This study found that odds of graduating declined precipitously with each additional risk factor—one risk factor reduced the percentage graduating by one-third, two risk factors reduced the percentage by one-half, and three risk factors reduced the percentage by three-fourths. All five studies in our review of the statistical research found that academic (and in some cases academic and family) risk was a significant predictor or whether students graduated or dropped out of high school (Rumberger & Lim, 2008, Table 2).

Typologies

Another approach is to use various factors to create a typology that distinguishes different types or profiles of dropouts. One study of high school students in Montreal, Canada identified four types of dropouts: (1) *quiet* dropouts (40% of dropouts) who demonstrated moderate to high levels of commitment and no evidence of school misbehavior; (2) *maladjusted* dropouts (40%) who demonstrated low commitment and poor school performance; (3) *disengaged* dropouts (10%) who demonstrated low commitment, average performance, and average to low level of school misbehavior; and (4) *low-achiever* dropouts (10%) who demonstrated low commitment, very poor performance, average to low level of school misbehavior, and very poor school performance (Janosz, LeBlanc, Boulerice, & Tremblay, 2000).

Structural Models

Another approach for examining how various factors jointly influence the dropout process is to construct and test a structural model using a statistical technique know as structural equation modeling (Kline, 2010). This technique allows researchers to examine the strength of the direct and indirect relationships among predictors and to estimate how well the resulting model "fits" the data. One recent study estimated a model based on the NRC report, *Engaging Schools*, which suggested dropping out is influenced by student engagement and a set of psychological antecedents (Rotermund, 2010). The study, based on a national longitudinal study of tenth grade students who were tracked for 2 years, found that that only two tenth grade factors directly influenced dropping out in high school: student achievement and behavioral engagement (not absent, late, skipping classes, or getting into trouble). Both behavioral engagement and cognitive engagement (works hard, puts forth effort) also influenced dropping out through their effects on grades, while affective engagement (likes school, finds classes interesting and challenging) affected both cognitive and behavioral engagement. Finally, three psychological antecedents—perceived competence, valuing school and a sense of belonging—influenced the three dimensions of engagement. A number of other studies have estimated models of dropping out using this technique, including studies that incorporate predictors from early childhood (Archambault, Janosz, Fallu, & Pagani, 2009; Battin-Pearson et al., 2000; Ensminger & Slusacick, 1992; Garnier et al., 1997; Reynolds et al., 2004). Together, these studies support the notion that dropping out is indeed a long-term process influenced by a wide variety of factors, including engagement factors.

Institutional Factors

While a large array of individual attitudes, behaviors, and aspects of educational performance influence dropping out and graduating, these individual factors are shaped by the institutional settings or contexts where children live—families, schools, and communities. Research has identified a number of factors within students' families, schools, and communities that influence whether students dropout or graduate from high school. As in the case of individual factors, it is difficult to verify a causal connection between institutional factors and dropping out, but research has demonstrated that a number of factors affect the odds that students will drop out or graduate from high school, as well as the antecedents to dropout and graduation, including engagement factors. Due to space limitations, the review will only highlight some of the research findings.

Families

Family background has long been recognized as the single most important contributor to success in school (Coleman et al., 1966; Jencks et al., 1972). What is less clear is what aspects of family background matter and how they influence school achievement (Hoover-Dempsey & Sandler, 1997; Pomerantz, Moorman, & Litwack, 2007). Although the research literature has identified a wide array of family factors that contribute to dropping out, three aspects appear to be most important: (1) structure, (2) resources, and (3) practices.

Structure

Family structure generally refers to the number and types of individuals in a child's household. In 2005, 67% of families in the United States with children under 18 were married-couple families, 25% were female-headed families, and 8% were male-headed families (KewalRamani, Gilbertson, & Fox, 2007, Table 3). The research finds that students living with both parents had lower dropout rates and higher graduation rates compared to students living in other family living arrangements, even controlling for the effects of family income (Perreira, Harris, & Lee, 2006; Rumberger, 1995; Rumberger & Lim, 2008, Table 3). There is less consistent evidence that family size matters.

Resources

Family resources are critical for supporting the emotional, social, and cognitive development of children. The most widely used indicator of family resources is *socioeconomic status* (SES), which is typically constructed as a composite index based on several measures of financial and human resources, such as both parents' years of education, both parents' occupational status, and family income. A national study of high school sophomores found that students from the lowest quartile of SES were five times more likely to drop out of school (12.4% v. 1.8%) as students from the highest quartile of SES (Dalton et al., 2009, Table 1). The majority of studies in Rumberger and Lim's review found that students from high SES families were less likely to drop out than students from low SES families (Rumberger & Lim, 2008, Table 3).

Practices

Fiscal and human resources simply represent the means or the capacity to improve the engagement and educational outcomes of children. This capacity is realized through the actual practices and behaviors of parents. These practices, manifested in the relationships parents have with their children, their schools, and the communities, are what sociologist James Coleman labeled *social capital* (Coleman, 1988). Other researchers have labeled such practices *parental involvement* or *parenting style* (Fan & Chen, 2001; Jeynes, 2007; Pomerantz et al., 2007; Spera, 2005). Parenting practices related to student engagement include educational expectations (how much schooling they want or expect their children to get), within-home practices (general supervision, helping with or monitoring homework), and home-school practices (participation in school activities, communication with the school).

Rumberger and Lim's review did not reveal a consistent, direct relationship between specific parenting practices and school dropout. Yet several studies found that multiple indicators of parenting practices at the secondary level reduced the risk of dropping out. One early study of 1980 high school sophomores found that four parenting practices (as reported by the students) during high school had significant effects on whether students dropped out or graduated: (1) whether their mother wanted them to graduate from college, (2) whether their mother monitored their school progress, (3) whether their father monitored their school progress, and (4) whether their parents supervised their school work (Astone & McLanahan, 1991). Another study of eighth graders from 1988 found four parenting practices that predicted whether students dropped out by grade 12: (1) parental educational aspirations for their child in grade 8, (2) parental participation in school activities in grade 8, (3) parental communication with the school in grade 12, and (4) a measure of intergenerational closure—how many parents of their children's friends they know—which is a key component of social capital that provides a source of information, norms, expectations, and standards of behavior (Carbonaro, 1998).

Schools

It is widely acknowledged that schools exert powerful influences on student achievement, including dropout rates. Using statistical techniques to disentangle institutional factors from individual factors, some studies have found that about 20–25% of the variability in student outcomes can be attributed to the characteristics of the schools that students attend (Li, 2007; Rumberger & Palardy, 2004). Nonetheless, as in the case of individual factors, it is hard to verify a causal relationship between school factors and dropout rates without using sophisticated statistical techniques (Pohl, Steiner, Eisermann, Soellner, & Cook, 2009; Schneider et al., 2007). Four school factors have been shown to influence dropout and graduation rates: (1) student composition (2) structure, (3) resources, and (4) practices.

Student Composition
Student characteristics not only influence student achievement at an individual level, but also at an aggregate or social level (Gamoran, 1992). Social composition may affect student achievement in two ways: first, by serving as a proxy for other characteristics of schools—for example, high-poverty and high-minority schools generally have more inexperienced teachers and suffer from high teacher turnover (Clotfelter, Ladd, Vigdor, & Wheeler, 2007; Hanushek, Kain, & Rivkin, 2004; Reed, 2005); second, by influencing motivation, engagement, and achievement directly through interactions with peers (Jencks & Mayer, 1990; Kahlenberg, 2001; Ryan, 2000). A number of studies have found that several dimensions of student composition—the average socioeconomic status of the students attending the school, the proportion of at-risk students (students who get poor grades, cut classes, have discipline problems, or were retained) (Rumberger, 1995; Rumberger & Thomas, 2000), the proportion of racial or linguistic minorities (Rumberger, 1995; Sander, 2001), the proportion of students who had changed schools or residences (Sander, 2001), the proportion of students from non-traditional (not both parents) families—affect dropout rates above and beyond other school characteristics (Bryk &Thum, 1989; McNeal, 1997; Rumberger, 1995; Rumberger & Palardy, 2005; Rumberger &Thomas, 2000; Sander, 2001).

Structure
Several structural characteristics of schools contribute to student performance—school location (whether the school is located in an urban, suburban, or rural location), school size, and type of school (public comprehensive, public charter, and private).

Research evidence is inconsistent on the relationship between high school size and dropout or graduation rates. Some studies found that students were more inclined to drop out of large (greater than 1,200 and less than 1,500 students) high schools (Lee & Burkam, 2003; Marsh, 1991; Rumberger &Palardy, 2005) other analyses found that students were less likely to drop out of large schools (Pirog & Magee, 1997; Rumberger & Thomas, 2000); and still others found that school size had no significant effects (Bryk &Thum, 1989; Grogger, 1997; McNeal, 1997; Pittman & Haughwout, 1987; Rumberger, 1995; Sander, 2001; Van Dorn, Bowen, & Blau, 2006).

One reason for the mixed effects is that the relationship between school size and student outcomes may be non-linear, with middle-size schools (500–1,200 students) more effective than either small or large schools (Lee & Burkam, 2003). Another reason is that there may be offsetting features of schools associated with size, with large schools offering more curriculum and program options, but also having a poorer social climate (Pittman & Haughwout, 1987). School size may have different and conflicting effects on different school outcomes; one recent study found larger schools had greater improvement in student learning, perhaps because of curricular benefits, but they also had higher dropout rates, perhaps because of poorer climate (Rumberger & Palardy, 2005).

There is also mixed evidence on the effects of school type. Research has not found that private schools as a whole have consistently higher graduation rates than public schools (Rumberger & Lim, 2008), but the evidence is stronger that dropout rates are lower and graduation rates higher in Catholic schools, even after controlling for student background characteristics and other school inputs (Evans & Schwab, 1995; Rumberger & Larson, 1998; Rumberger & Palardy, 2005; Rumberger & Thomas, 2000; Sander, 1997; Sander & Krautmann, 1995; Teachman, Paasch, & Carver, 1997). Some of those studies also find that the Catholic school effect is mediated by school practices, which further supports the claim that Catholic schools provide a more rigorous academic and supportive school environment compared to public and other private schools (Coleman & Hoffer, 1987; Lee & Burkam, 2003; Rumberger & Palardy, 2005; Rumberger & Thomas, 2000). Yet empirical studies have also found that students from private and Catholic schools typically transfer to public schools instead of or before dropping out, meaning that student turnover rates in private schools are not statistically different than turnover rates in public schools (Lee & Burkam, 2003; Rumberger & Thomas, 2000).

The research is also mixed on the effectiveness of charter schools—publicly funded schools run by for-profit and non-profit organizations largely free from public school regulations. A 2008 review of 14 studies as well as several recent large-scale studies have found that some charter schools outperform public schools and some do not (Betts & Tang, 2008; Center for Research on Education Outcomes (CREDO), 2009; Gleason, Clark, Tuttle, & Dwoyer, 2010; Zimmer et al., 2009), although one of the studies found that in Florida and Chicago "attending a charter high school is associated with statistically significant and substantial increases in the probability of graduating and attending college" (Zimmer et al., 2009, pp. xii–xv).

Resources

Another area of considerable debate concerns the extent to which school resources contribute to school effectiveness (Greenwald, Hedges, & Laine, 1996; Hanushek, 1989, 1994, 1997; Hanushek & Jorgenson, 1996; Hedges, Laine, & Greenwald, 1994). A number of studies have examined the relationship between various types of school resources—average expenditures per pupil, teacher salaries, the number of students per teacher, and measures of teacher quality, such as the percentage of teachers with advanced degrees—and dropout or graduation rates. Overall, relatively few studies in Rumberger and Lim's review found significant effects (Rumberger & Lim, 2008, Table 3). Several additional studies that used district- and state-level data, along with more sophisticated statistical techniques to better control for unobserved factors, found that higher per-pupil expenditures or higher teacher salaries were associated with lower dropout rates (Li, 2007; Loeb & Page, 2000; Warren, Jenkins, & Kulick, 2006). For example, one study that used a more sophisticated model of teacher salaries, which took into account the non-monetary job characteristics and alternative employment opportunities in the local job market (what economists refer to as "opportunity costs"), found that raising teacher wages by 10% reduced high school dropout rates by 3–4% (Loeb & Page, 2000).

Practices

School policies and practices affect student persistence in two ways. One way is through policies and practices that lead to students' disengaging from school and eventual *voluntary* withdrawal—either dropping out or transferring—from school.

The other way is through policies and conscious decisions that cause students to *involuntarily* withdraw from school through suspensions, expulsions, or forced transfers (Bowditch, 1993; Fine, 1986, 1991). Some scholars argue that the social relationships or ties among students, parents, teachers, and administrators—which have been characterized as *social resources* or *social capital*—are a key component of effective and improving schools (Ancess, 2003; Bryk & Schneider, 2002; Elmore, 2004; Hoy, Tarter, & Hoy, 2006).

A number of indicators of school practices have been shown to influence dropout and graduation rates. One study, which created a single composite indicator of school climate from student responses to questions about various aspects of the school, such as school loyalty and student behavior (i.e., fighting, cutting class), found that a positive school climate reduced the likelihood of dropping out, net of other factors (Worrell & Hale, 2001). Another study found that schools with higher attendance rates, a school-level measure of student engagement—had lower dropout rates (Rumberger & Thomas, 2000). Several studies found that students were less likely to drop out if they attended schools with a stronger academic climate, as measured by more students in the academic track (versus general or vocational) or taking academic courses, and students reporting more hours of homework—another school-level measure of engagement (Bryk & Thum, 1989; Lee & Burkam, 2003; Rumberger & Palardy, 2005). Some studies have found that students were more likely to drop out in schools with a poor disciplinary climate, as measured by student reports of student disruptions in class or discipline problems in the school (Pittman, 1991; Rumberger, 1995; Rumberger & Palardy, 2005), or in schools where students reported feeling unsafe (Bryk & Thum, 1989; Pittman, 1991; Rumberger, 1995; Rumberger & Palardy, 2005). Several studies have found that positive relationships between students and teachers—an aspect of school social capital—reduced the risk of dropping out, especially among high-risk students (Croninger & Lee, 2001; Rumberger & Palardy, 2005).

Summary and Conclusion

Understanding why students drop out of high school is critical for informing efforts to address this critical educational problem. Our review of conceptual models of dropping out and of the empirical research literature leads to several conclusions about why students drop out.

First, no single factor can completely account for a student's decision to continue in school until graduation. Just as students themselves report a variety of reasons for quitting school, the research literature also identifies a number of salient factors that appear to influence the decision.

Second, the decision to drop out is not simply a result of what happens in school. Clearly, students' behavior and performance in school influence their decision to stay or leave. But students' activities and behaviors outside of school—particularly engaging in deviant and criminal behavior—also influence their likelihood of remaining in school.

Third, dropping out is more of a process than an event. For many students, the process begins in early elementary school. A number of long-term studies that tracked groups of students from preschool or early elementary school through the end of high school were able to identify early indicators that could significantly predict whether students were likely to drop out or finish high school. The two most consistent indicators were early academic performance and students' academic and social engagement (behaviors) in school.

Fourth, contexts matter. The research literature has identified a number of factors within families, schools, and communities that affect whether students are likely to drop out or graduate from high school. These include access to not only fiscal and material resources, but also social resources in the form of supportive relationships in families, schools, and communities.

Finally, there is no single model that fully explains the dropout process for all dropouts. Rather, because students drop out of school for different reasons, some factors are more salient for some students than for others. For example, boys are more likely to drop out because of behavior problems, while girls are more likely to "silently" disengage from school by skipping class or being absent.

One implication of this review is that there are numerous leverage points for addressing the problem of high dropout rates. Clearly, early intervention in preschool and early elementary school is warranted. Rigorous experimental evaluations have proven that high quality preschool programs and small classes in early elementary school improve high school graduation rates (Barnett & Belfield, 2006; Finn, Gerber, & Boyd-Zaharias, 2005). Such programs are also cost-effective—they generate two to four dollars in economic benefits for every dollar invested (Belfield & Levin, 2007). But there are other leverage points as well. Even high school is not too late—both small programs serving a limited number of high-risk students and comprehensive school reform models have been proven to improve graduation rates (Ibid.).

References

Alexander, K. L., Entwisle, D. R., & Kabbini, N. S. (2001). The dropout process in life course perspective: Early risk factors at home and school. *Teachers College Record, 103*, 760–882.

Allensworth, E., & Easton, J. Q. (2005). *The on-track indicator as a predictor of high school graduation*. Chicago: Consortium on Chicago School Research, University of Chicago. Retrieved December 20, 2010, from http://ccsr.uchicago.edu/content/publications.php?pub_id=10

Ancess, J. (2003). *Beating the odds: High schools as communities of commitment*. New York: Teachers College Press.

Appleton, J. J., Christenson, S. L., & Furlong, M. J. (2008). Student engagement with school: Critical conceptual and methodological issues of the construct. *Psychology in the Schools, 45*, 369–386.

Archambault, I., Janosz, M., Fallu, J.-S., & Pagani, L. S. (2009). Student engagement and its relationship with early high school dropout. *Journal of Adolescence, 32*, 651–670.

Astone, N. M., & McLanahan, S. S. (1991). Family structure, parental practices and high school completion. *American Sociological Review, 56*, 309–320.

Bachman, J. G., Green, S., & Wirtanen, I. D. (1971). *Youth in transition, Vol. III: Dropping out: Problem or symptom?* Ann Arbor, MI: Institute for Social Research, The University of Michigan.

Balfanz, R., Herzog, L., & Mac Iver, D. J. (2007). Preventing student disengagement and keeping students on the graduation path in urban middle-grades schools: Early identification and effective interventions. *Educational Psychologist, 42*, 223–235.

Barnett, W. S., & Belfield, C. R. (2006). Early childhood development and social mobility. *The Future of Children, 16*, 73–98.

Battin-Pearson, S., Newcomb, M. D., Abbott, R. D., Hill, K. G., Catalano, R. F., & Hawkins, J. D. (2000). Predictors of early high school dropout: A test of five theories. *Journal of Educational Psychology, 92*, 568–582.

Belfield, C., & Levin, H. M. (Eds.). (2007). *The price we pay: Economic and social consequences of inadequate education*. Washington, DC: Brookings Institution Press.

Benz, M. R., Lindstrom, L., & Yovanoff, P. (2000). Improving graduation and employment outcomes of students with disabilities: Predictive factors and student perspectives. *Exceptional Children, 66*, 509–529.

Betts, J. R., & Tang, Y. E. (2008). *Value-added and experimental studies of the effect of charter schools on student achievement*. Seattle, WA: University of Washington Bothell, Center on Reinventing Public Education, National Charter School Research Project. Retrieved August 19, 2010, from http://www.crpe.org/cs/crpe/view/csr_pubs/253

Bong, M., & Skaalvik, E. M. (2003). Academic self-concept and self-efficacy: How different are they really? *Educational Psychology Review, 15*, 1–40.

Bowditch, C. (1993). Getting rid of troublemakers: High school disciplinary procedures and the production of dropouts. *Social Problems, 40*, 493–509.

Bridgeland, J. M., DiIulio, J. J., Jr., & Morison, K. B. (2006). *The silent epidemic: Perspectives on high school dropouts*. Washington, DC: Civil Enterprises.

Bronfenbrenner, U. (1979). *The ecology of human development*. Cambridge, MA: Harvard University Press.

Bryk, A. S., & Schneider, B. (2002). *Trust in schools: A core resource for improvement*. New York: Russell Sage.

Bryk, A. S., & Thum, Y. M. (1989). The effects of high school organization on dropping out: An exploratory investigation. *American Educational Research Journal, 26*, 353–383.

Cabrera, A. F., & La Nasa, S. M. (2001). On the path to college: Three critical tasks facing America's disadvantaged. *Research in Higher Education, 42*, 119–149.

Cahalan, M. W., Ingles, S. J., Burns, L. J., Planty, M., & Daniel, B. (2006). *United States high school sophomores: A twenty-two year comparison, 1980-2002*. (NCES 2006-327). Washington, DC: National Center for Education Statistics.

Carbonaro, W. J. (1998). A little help from my friend's parents: Intergenerational closure and educational outcomes. *Sociology of Education, 71*, 295–313.

Center for Research on Education Outcomes (CREDO). (2009). *Multiple choice: Charter school performance in 16 states*. Stanford, CA: CREDO, Stanford University. Retrieved December 20, 2010, from http://credo.stanford.edu/

Clotfelter, C. T., Ladd, H. F., Vigdor, J. L., & Wheeler, J. (2007). High poverty schools and the distribution of teachers and principals. *North Carolina Law Review, 85*, 1345–1379.

Coleman, J. S. (1988). Social capital in the creation of human capital. *American Journal of Sociology, 94*, S95–S120.

Coleman, J. S., Campbell, E. Q., Hobson, C. J., McPartland, J., Mood, A. M., Weinfeld, F. D., & York, R. L. (1966). *Equality of educational opportunity*. Washington, DC: U.S. Government Printing Office.

Coleman, J. S., & Hoffer, T. (1987). *Public and private high schools: The impact of communities*. New York: Basic Books.

Connell, J. P. (1990). Context, self and action: A motivational analysis of self-system processes across the life span. In D. Cicchetti & M. Beeghly (Eds.), *The self in transition: Infancy to childhood* (pp. 61–97). Chicago: University of Chicago Press.

Connell, J. P., Halpern-Felsher, B. L., Cliffor, E., Crichlow, W., & Usinger, P. (1995). Hanging in there: Behavioral, psychological, and contextual factors affecting whether African-American adolescents stay in high school. *Journal of Adolescent Research, 10*, 41–63.

Croninger, R. G., & Lee, V. E. (2001). Social capital and dropping out of high school: Benefits to at-risk students of teachers' support and guidance. *Teachers College Record, 103*, 548–581.

Currie, J. (2009). Healthy, wealthy, and wise: Socioeconomic status, poor health in childhood, and human capital development. *Journal of Economic Literature, 47*, 87–122.

Dalton, B., Glennie, E., & Ingels, S. J. (2009). *Late high school dropouts: Characteristics, experiences, and changes across cohorts*. (NCES 2009-307). Washington, DC: U.S. Department of Education. Retrieved December 20, 2010, from http://nces.ed.gov/pubsearch/pubsinfo.asp?pubid=2009307

Day, J. C., & Newburger, E. C. (2002). *The big payoff: Educational attainment and synthetic estimates of work-life earnings*. Washington, DC: U.S. Census Bureau.

Eccles, J. S. (1999). The development of children ages 6 to 14. *The Future of Children, 9*, 30–44.

Eccles, J. S., & Wigfield, A. (2002). Motivational beliefs, values, and goals. *Annual Review of Psychology, 53*, 109–132.

Edin, K., & Kefalas, M. (2005). *Promises I can keep: Why poor women put motherhood before marriage*. Berkeley, CA: University of California Press.

Education Week. (2010, June 10). *Diplomas Count 2010: Graduation by the numbers: Putting Data to work for student success*. Washington, DC: Education Week. Retrieved August 28, 2010, from http://www.edweek.org/ew/toc/2010/06/10/index.html

Ekstrom, R. B., Goertz, M. E., Pollack, J. M., & Rock, D. A. (1986). Who drops out of high school and why? Findings from a national study. *Teachers College Record, 87*, 356–373.

Elmore, R. F. (2004). *School reform from the inside out*. Cambridge, MA: Harvard Education Press.

Ensminger, M. E., & Slusacick, A. L. (1992). Paths to high school graduation or dropout: A longitudinal study of a first-grade cohort. *Sociology of Education, 65*, 95–113.

Evans, G. W. (2004). The environment of childhood poverty. *American Psychologist, 59*, 77–92.

Evans, W. N., & Schwab, R. M. (1995). Finishing high school and starting college: Do Catholic schools make a difference? *The Quarterly Journal of Economics, 110*, 941–974.

Fan, X., & Chen, M. (2001). Parental involvement and students' academic achievement: A meta-analysis. *Educational Psychology Review, 13*, 1–22.

Fine, M. (1986). Why urban adolescents drop into and out of public high school. *Teachers College Record, 87*, 393–409.

Fine, M. (1991). *Framing dropouts: Notes on the politics of an urban public high school*. Albany, NY: State University of New York Press.

Finn, J. D. (1989). Withdrawing from school. *Review of Educational Research, 59*, 117–142.

Finn, J. D., Gerber, S. B., & Boyd-Zaharias, J. (2005). Small classes in the early grades, academic achievement, and graduating from high school. *Journal of Educational Psychology, 97*, 214–223.

Flores-Gonzalez, N. (2002). *School kids/street kids: Identity development in Latino students*. New York: Teachers College Press.

Fredricks, J. A., Blumenfeld, P. C., & Paris, A. H. (2004). School engagement: Potential of the concept, state of the evidence. *Review of Educational Research, 74*, 59–109.

Gamoran, A. (1992). Social factors in education. In M. C. Alkin (Ed.), *Encyclopedia of Educational Research* (pp. 1222–1229). New York: Macmillan.

Garnier, H. E., Stein, J. A., & Jacobs, J. K. (1997). The process of dropping out of high school: A 19-year perspective. *American Educational Research Journal, 34*, 395–419.

Gleason, P., Clark, M., Tuttle, C. C., & Dwoyer, E. (2010). *The evaluation of charter school impacts: Final report*. (NCEE 2010-4029). Washington, DC: National Center for Education Evaluation and Regional Assistance, Institute of Education Sciences, U.S. Department of Education. Retrieved August 20, 2010, from http://ies.ed.gov/ncee/pubs/20104029/index.asp

Greenwald, R., Hedges, L. V., & Laine, R. D. (1996). The effect of school resources on student achievement. *Review of Educational Research, 66*, 361–396.

Grogger, J. (1997). Local violence and educational attainment. *The Journal of Human Resources, 32*, 659–682.

Hanushek, E. A. (1989). The impact of differential expenditures on school performance. *Educational Researcher, 18*, 45–62.

Hanushek, E. A. (1994). Money might matter somewhere: A response to Hedges, Laine, and Greenwald. *Educational Researcher, 23*(4), 5–8.

Hanushek, E. A. (1997). Assessing the effects of school resources on student performance: An update. *Educational Evaluation and Policy Analysis, 19*, 141–164.

Hanushek, E. A., & Jorgenson, D. W. (Eds.). (1996). *Improving America's schools: The role of incentives.* Washington, DC: National Academy Press.

Hanushek, E. A., Kain, J. F., & Rivkin, S. G. (2004). Why public schools lose teachers. *Journal of Human Resources, 39*, 326–354.

Heckman, J. J., & LaFontaine, P. A. (2010). The American high school graduation rate: Trends and levels. *The Review of Economics and Statistics, 92*, 244–262.

Hedges, L. V., Laine, R. D., & Greenwald, R. (1994). Does money matter? A meta-analysis of studies of the effects of differential school inputs on student outcomes. *Educational Researcher, 23*(3), 5–14.

Hoover-Dempsey, K. V., & Sandler, H. M. (1997). Why do parents become involved in their children's education? *Review of Educational Research, 67*, 3–42.

Hoy, W. K., Tarter, C. J., & Hoy, A. W. (2006). Academic optimism of schools: A force for student achievement. *American Educational Research Journal, 43*, 425–446.

Janosz, M., LeBlanc, M., Boulerice, B., & Tremblay, R. E. (2000). Predicting different types of school dropouts: A typological approach with two longitudinal cohorts. *Journal of Educational Psychology, 92*, 171–190.

Jencks, C., & Mayer, S. E. (1990). The social consequences of growing up in a poor neighborhood. In L. Lynn Jr. & M. G. H. McGeary (Eds.), *Inner-City Poverty in the United States* (pp. 111–186). Washington, DC: National Academy Press.

Jencks, C., Smith, M., Acland, H., Bane, M. J., Cohen, D., Gintis, H., Heyns, B., & Michelson, S. M. (1972). *Inequality: A reassessment of the effects of family and schooling in America.* New York: Basic Books.

Jeynes, W. H. (2007). The relationship between parental involvement and urban secondary school student academic achievement—A meta-analysis. *Urban Education, 42*, 82–110.

Kahlenberg, R. D. (2001). *All together now: Creating middle-class schools through public school choice.* Washington, DC: Brookings Institution.

Kelly, D. M. (1993). *Last chance high: How girls and boys drop in and out of alternative schools.* New Haven: Yale University Press.

KewalRamani, A., Gilbertson, L., & Fox, M. A. (2007). *Status and trends in the education of racial and ethnic minorities.* (NCES 2007-039). Washington, DC: National Center for Education Statistics. Retrieved December 20, 2010, from: http://nces.ed.gov/pubsearch/pubsinfo.asp?pubid=2007039

Kline, R. B. (2010). *Principles and practice of structural equation modeling* (3rd ed.). New York: Guilford Publications.

Lee, V. E., & Burkam, D. T. (1992). Transferring high schools: An alternative to dropping out? *American Journal of Education, 100*, 420–453.

Lee, V. E., & Burkam, D. T. (2003). Dropping out of high school: The role of school organization and structure. *American Educational Research Journal, 40*, 353–393.

Lerner, R. M., & Galambos, N. L. (1998). Adolescent development: Challenges and opportunities for research, programs, and policies. *Annual Review of Psychology, 49*, 413–46.

Li, M. (2007). Bayesian proportional hazard analysis of the timing of high school dropout decisions. *Econometric Reviews, 26*, 529–556.

Loeb, S., & Page, M. E. (2000). Examining the link between teacher wages and student outcomes: The importance of alternative labor market opportunities and non-pecuniary variation. *The Review of Economics and Statistics, 82*, 393–408.

Marsh, H. W. (1991). Employment during high school: Character building or a subversion of academic goals. *Sociology of Education, 64*, 172–189.

McNeal, R. B. (1995). Extracurricular activities and high school dropouts. *Sociology of Education, 68*, 62–80.

McNeal, R. B. (1997). High school dropouts: A closer examination of school effects. *Social Science Quarterly, 78*, 209–222.

Meyer, R., Carl, B., & Cheng, H. E. (2010). *Accountability and performance in secondary education in Milwaukee public schools.* Washington, DC: Council of Great City Schools.

National Research Council, Panel on High-Risk Youth. (1993). *Losing generations: Adolescents in high-risk settings.* Washington, DC: National Academies Press.

National Research Council, Committee on Increasing High School Students' Engagement and Motivation to Learn. (2004). *Engaging schools: Fostering high school students' motivation to learn.* Washington, DC: The National Academies Press.

Newmann, F. M. (Ed.). (1992). *Student engagement and achievement in American secondary schools.* New York: Teachers College Press.

Ou, S.-R., Mersky, J. P., Reynolds, A. J., & Kohler, K. M. (2007). Alterable predictors of educational attainment, income, and crime: Findings from an inner-city cohort. *Social Service Review, 81*, 85–128.

Perreira, K. M., Harris, K. M., & Lee, D. (2006). Making it in America: High school completion by immigrant and native youth. *Demography, 43*, 511–536.

Pettit, B., & Western, B. (2004). Mass imprisonment and the life course: Race and class inequality in US incarceration. *American Sociological Review, 69*, 151–169.

Pirog, M. A., & Magee, C. (1997). High school completion: The influence of schools, families, and adolescent parenting. *Social Science Quarterly, 78*, 710–724.

Pittman, R. B. (1991). Social factors, enrollment in vocational/technical courses, and high school dropout rates. *Journal of Educational Research, 84*, 288–295.

Pittman, R. B., & Haughwout, P. (1987). Influence of high school size on dropout rate. *Educational Evaluation and Policy Analysis, 9*, 337–343.

Pohl, S., Steiner, P. M., Eisermann, J., Soellner, R., & Cook, T. D. (2009). Unbiased causal inference from an observational study: Results of a within-study comparison. *Educational Evaluation and Policy Analysis, 31*, 463–479.

Pomerantz, E. M., Moorman, E. A., & Litwack, S. D. (2007). The how, whom, and why of parents' involvement in children's academic lives: More is not always better. *Review of Educational Research, 77*, 373–410.

Pribesh, S., & Downey, D. B. (1999). Why are residential and school moves associated with poor school performance? *Demography, 36*, 521–534.

Ream, R. K. (2005). *Uprooting children: Mobility, social capital, and Mexican American underachievement*. New York: LFB Scholarly Publishing.

Ream, R. K., & Rumberger, R. W. (2008). Student engagement, peer social capital, and school dropout among Mexican American and non-Latino white students. *Sociology of Education, 81*, 109–139.

Reed, D. (2005). *Educational resources and outcomes in California, by race and ethnicity*. San Francisco: Public Policy Institute of California.

Reynolds, A. J., Ou, S.-R., & Topitzes, J. W. (2004). Paths of effects of early childhood intervention on educational attainment and delinquency: A confirmatory analysis of the Chicago Child-Parent Centers. *Child Development, 75*, 1299–1328.

Romo, H. D., & Falbo, T. (1996). *Latino high school graduation: Defying the odds*. Austin, TX: University of Texas Press.

Rotermund, S. L. (2010). *The role of psychological antecedents and student engagement in a process model of high school dropout*. Doctoral dissertation. Santa Barbara, CA: Gevirtz Graduate School of Education, University of California, Santa Barbara.

Rumberger, R. W. (1983). Dropping out of high school: The influence of race, sex, and family background. *American Educational Research Journal, 20*, 199–220.

Rumberger, R. W. (1987). High school dropouts: A review of issues and evidence. *Review of Educational Research, 57*, 101–121.

Rumberger, R. W. (1995). Dropping out of middle school: A multilevel analysis of students and schools. *American Educational Research Journal, 32*, 583–625.

Rumberger, R. W. (2011). *Dropping out: Why students quit school and what can be done about it*. Cambridge, MA: Harvard University Press.

Rumberger, R. W., & Larson, K. A. (1998). Student mobility and the increased risk of high school drop out. *American Journal of Education, 107*, 1–35.

Rumberger, R. W., Larson, K. A., Ream, R. K., & Palardy, G. A. (1999). *The educational consequences of mobility for California Students and Schools*. Berkeley, CA: Policy Analysis for California Education.

Rumberger, R. W., & Lim, S. A. (2008). *Why students drop out of school: A review of 25 years of research*. Santa Barbara, CA: California Dropout Research Project. Retrieved December 20, 2010, from http://cdrp.ucsb.edu/dropouts/pubs_reports.htm#15

Rumberger, R. W., & Palardy, G. J. (2004). Multilevel models for school effectiveness research. In D. Kaplan (Ed.), *Handbook of quantitative methodology for the social sciences* (pp. 235–258). Thousand Oaks, CA: Sage Publications.

Rumberger, R. W., & Palardy, G. J. (2005). Test scores, dropout rates, and transfer rates as alternative indicators of high school performance. *American Educational Research Journal, 41*, 3–42.

Rumberger, R. W., & Thomas, S. L. (2000). The distribution of dropout and turnover rates among urban and suburban high schools. *Sociology of Education, 73*, 39–67.

Ryan, A. M. (2000). Peer groups as a context for the socialization of adolescents' motivation, engagement, and achievement in school. *Educational Psychologist, 35*, 101–111.

Sander, W. (1997). Catholic high schools and rural academic achievement. *American Journal of Agricultural Economics, 79*, 1–12.

Sander, W. (2001). Chicago public schools and student achievement. *Urban Education, 36*(1), 27–38.

Sander, W., & Krautmann, A. C. (1995). Catholic schools, dropout rates and educational attainment. *Economic Inquiry, 33*, 217–233.

Schneider, B., Carnoy, M., Kilpatrick, J., Schmidt, W. H., & Shavelson, R. J. (2007). *Estimating causal effects using experimental and observations designs*. Report from the Governing Board of the American Educational Research Association Grants Program. Washington, DC: American Educational Research Association.

Snyder, T. D., & Dillow, S. A. (2010). *Digest of Education Statistics 2009*. (NCES 2010-013). U.S. Department of Education, National Center for Education Statistics. Washington, DC: U.S. Government Printing Office. Retrieved December 20, 2010 from http://nces.ed.gov/pubsearch/pubsinfo.asp?pubid=2010013

Spera, C. (2005). A review of the relationship among parenting practices, parenting styles, and adolescent school achievement. *Educational Psychological Review, 17*, 120–146.

Steinberg, L., & Morris, A. S. (2001). Adolescent development. *Annual Review of Psychology, 52*, 83–110.

Sullivan, M. L. (1989). *"Getting paid": Youth crime and work in the inner city*. Ithaca, NY: Cornell University Press.

Sweeten, G. (2006). Who will graduate? Disruption of high school education by arrest and court involvement. *Justice Quarterly, 23*, 462–480.

Teachman, J. D., Paasch, K., & Carver, K. (1997). Social capital and the generation of human capital. *Social Forces, 75*, 1343–1359.

Tinto, V. (1987). *Leaving college: Rethinking the causes and cures for student attrition*. Chicago: University of Chicago Press.

Tinto, V. (1994). *Leaving college: Rethinking the causes and cures for student attrition* (2nd ed.). Chicago: University of Chicago Press.

Valenzuela, A. (1999). *Subtractive schooling: U.S.-Mexican youth and the politics of caring*. Albany, NY: State University of New York Press.

Van Dorn, R. A., Bowen, G. L., & Blau, J. R. (2006). The impact of community diversity and consolidated inequality on dropping out of high school. *Family Relations, 55*, 105–118.

Walston, J., Rathbun, A., & Huasken, E. G. (2008). *Eighth grade: First findings from the final round of the Early Childhood Longitudinal Study, Kindergarten Class of 1998-99 (ECLS-K)*. Washington, DC: U.S. Department of Education. Retrieved December 20, 2010, from http://nces.ed.gov/pubsearch/pubsinfo.asp?pubid=2008088

Warren, J. R., Jenkins, K. N., & Kulick, R. B. (2006). High school exit examinations and state-level completion and GED rates, 1975-2002. *Educational Evaluation and Policy Analysis, 28*, 131–152.

Wehlage, G. G., Rutter, R. A., Smith, G. A., Lesko, N., & Fernandez, R. R. (1989). *Reducing the risk: Schools as communities of support*. New York: Falmer Press.

Wilson, W. J. (1987). *The truly disadvantaged: The inner city, the underclass, and public policy*. Chicago: The University of Chicago Press.

Worrell, F. C., & Hale, R. L. (2001). The relationship of hope in the future and perceived school climate to school completion. *School Psychology Quarterly, 16*, 370–388.

Yin, Z. N., & Moore, J. B. (2004). Re-examining the role of interscholastic sport participation in education. *Psychological Reports, 94*, 1447–1454.

Zimmer, R., Gill, B., Booker, K., Lavertu, S., Sass, T. R., & Witte, J. (2009). *Charter schools in eight states: Effects on achievement, attainment, integration, and competition*. Santa Monica, CA: Rand.

High School Reform and Student Engagement

Marcia H. Davis and James M. McPartland

Abstract

This chapter describes how internal high school reforms can be aimed at six different dimensions of student motivation and engagement. Students will respond to more accessible immediate rewards such as good grades and teacher praise when high schools improve with focused extra help for needy students and other interventions to narrow skill gaps or recognize individual progress. Students will benefit from embedded intrinsic interest in their school program when innovations are introduced to challenge their minds and creativity. Students will find more functional relevance in their studies when high schools integrate academic and career education. Students will enjoy a more positive interpersonal climate for learning when high schools use smaller learning communities with teacher teams and advisors. Students will find opportunities to exercise their own personal nonacademic talents when schools provide more diverse electives and extracurricular activities. Students will feel more connected to shared communal norms when high schools practice fair disciplinary procedures and provide for some shared decision-making. Different combinations and sequences of high school reforms are discussed in terms of implementation strategies and the interactions of the six dimensions of student motivation and engagement. High school reform can be aimed at either the external constraints and incentives for school improvement or the internal conditions for student engagement and learning. This chapter puts reforms of the internal conditions in the context of alternative strategies for improving American high schools and examines six different aspects of student engagement in high school and how specific internal reform efforts can activate and maximize each component.

M.H. Davis (✉) • J.M. McPartland
Center for Social Organization of Schools,
Johns Hopkins University, Baltimore, MD, USA
e-mail: marcy@jhu.edu; jmcpartland@jhu.edu

External and Internal Conditions of High School Reform

Most high school reform proposals focus on the external conditions that set the boundaries and incentives for improved student achievement (Clark, 2009), when changes within the school and classroom walls can be more closely linked to student engagement with their school program and their motivation to learn (American Youth Policy Forum, 2000; National Association of Secondary School Principals, 1996, 2002; National Research Council and the Institute of Medicine, 2004).

External conditions for reforms include parental choice of public or charter schools, high standards of curriculum coverage and associated achievement testing, direct accountability of school principals and teachers for student success, and the reallocation of financial resources to schools with different student populations and needs. While these issues of school governance, parental choice, district teacher and union prerogatives, assessments and their consequences, and curriculum coverage can set the terms and incentives for how different adult interests and stakeholders may address high school reform, evidence is still weak connecting them to actual improvements in student outcomes. In contrast to such external policy levers, students themselves are more likely to be responsive to how the relationships and daily learning activities within their schools and classrooms are presented. Indeed, high school reforms will touch student motivation and engagement only when their proximate learning environment is improved.

Motivation and Engagement

We make a distinction between student motivation and engagement according to the timing relative to a particular event or activity. Student motivation occurs before participation as a precursor to the actual experience. It involves students' anticipations in terms of potential enjoyment, challenge, or usefulness. A student will be positively motivated if he or she looks forward to the experience and expects to do well and benefit from the participation. On the other hand, a student may have no prior attitudes going into an experience or may approach it in negative ways such as fear of failure or unpleasant outcomes. There are numerous ways that student motivation may develop the expectations about a new opportunity or challenge, including from past experiences in similar situations, through formal or informal preparatory activities, or by way of social influences from friends or those in authority.

Student engagement occurs during the actual experience of an activity or event. Engagement is positive when the individual finds the experience to be enjoyable, is successful in meeting the demands and fulfilling the roles, or appreciates the value to be derived for personal goals and fulfillment. Student engagement can sometimes be a mixed bag of both positive and negative dimensions with a particular experience, where the net balance can determine whether the individual persists in the activity with strong energy or gradually withdraws emotionally or physically.

Student motivation and engagement can interact in different ways. An individual who approaches a task or activity with strong positive motivation will be more alert to seek out and appreciate those positive aspects of actual participation that can result in powerful engagement for high energy and sustained commitment. On the other hand, a well-motivated student's expectations may be either disappointed or frustrated when the actual experience occurs, so engagement is weak and future motivation is threatened.

At the same time, strong positive student engagement need not assume a parallel positive motivation going into the activity. A student without any vivid preconceptions can take the experience on its own terms and decide to become positively engaged or not depending upon how well the actual activities offer satisfactions, can be handled successfully, or excite other worthwhile payoffs. Even a student who approaches an activity with negative motivation by expecting difficulties or punishments may be pleasantly surprised that the participation itself proves to be the opposite and becomes engaged with the enjoyment, fulfillment or follow-up benefits actually experienced.

Framework of Reforms and Engagement

We will use a framework of six dimensions of student motivation and engagement that can be activated by certain high school reforms that either prepare students for or offer them actual opportunities to experience different sources of satisfaction, stimulation, or benefits.

We will consider how high school reforms can address six dimensions of student motivation and engagement:

1. Immediate rewards for school work are made more accessible for all students, such as good grades, respect and recognition from teachers, and timely grade promotions and graduation.
2. Intrinsic interest is embedded in more learning tasks, so students get a sense of accomplishment and self-improvement from their classroom activities.
3. Functional relevance of the curriculum and program of studies is strengthened, so students appreciate how working hard at their studies can pay off for personal interests and career goals.
4. A positive climate for learning with good adult-student relationships is established, so students look forward to coming to school each day in a safe, serious, and sensitive environment.
5. Personal nonacademic strengths are explored and reinforced at school, so that the full range of human talents can also flourish in high school along with the strictly academic subjects and pursuits.
6. A positive climate of trust in school governance and fairness of disciplinary rules exists, so students feel part of a shared community with appropriate responsibilities and decision-making opportunities.

Table 25.1 outlines the kinds of high school reforms we will discuss that are associated with each dimension of student motivation or engagement.

Table 25.1 Dimensions of student engagement and associated high school reforms

Dimension of student motivation or engagement	Associated high school reforms
1. Accessible Immediate Awards	– Different course sequences without tracking – Levels of focused extra help – Multiple criteria for grades and recognition
2. Embedded Intrinsic Interest	– Thinking skills for problem solving and influence – Content literacy and disciplinary thinking – Project-based learning
3. Direct Functional Relevance	– Career Academies or majors – Integration of academic and career education
4. Positive Interpersonal Climate	– Small learning communities – Interdisciplinary teacher teams – Adult mentors and advisors
5. Alternative Talent Development	– Career and nonacademic skill explorations – Elective courses – Extracurricular activities
6. Shared Communal Engagement	– Firm and fair rules – Student participation in decision-making – Trust and self-regulating norms

We will use examples from the Talent Development High School model, a comprehensive reform approach developed at Johns Hopkins University, to show how different organizational, instructional, and governance improvements relate to dimensions of student motivation and engagement.

Immediate Rewards for School Success Become Accessible to All Students

The biggest barrier to students' engagement with their high school program is likely to be their failure to obtain good or even passing grades in their courses and the other immediate rewards attached to success at school work. Missing out on the positive incentives of good course grades can become accompanied by absence of teacher's esteem for the student, unwelcome pressure from home, and lower status from some peers. Repeated failures in their courses can leave students in a state of learned helplessness, where they believe that they will not be able to improve no matter how hard they try (Mark, 1983). When course failures build up, the negative consequences of being left back to repeat a grade in high school often leads to dropping out, the ultimate case of student disengagement. Research on Philadelphia data indicated that students who failed English in the sixth grade were 42% less likely to graduate than students who did not fail English. Students who failed math in sixth grade were 54% less likely to graduate (Balfanz, Herzog, & Mac Iver, 2007).

But even when students manage to get by with mostly low grades, the daily struggle to keep up with the school learning standards can be a significant source of discouragement and alienation. Each time these struggling students put some effort to manage the material in their class they are often presented with poor grades for their efforts. Within a behavioral learning theory view, following the Operant Conditioning framework of B.F. Skinner, the poor grades serve as a punishment for not turning in work at the level of the other students in the class (Skinner, 1953). Punishments work to decrease the behavior preceding the punishments. Therefore, poor grades will decrease the behavior of the students, which, in this case is trying to honestly complete an assignment. After their efforts are paired with the consequence of bad grades often enough, they will eventually change their behavior to avoid feeling bad about receiving poor grades. This can show up as weak daily attendance, as struggling students choose to avoid the negative experiences of being a weak student. Instead of always receiving poor grades as a consequence of trying, teachers should be setting up types of positive reinforcement for even small attempts at understanding their course material. By giving these students time to understand the material and by giving opportunities to show their understanding of the material in multiple ways, their attempts at understanding will be reinforced rather than punished. As positive reinforcements increase, students will place more value on these immediate incentives and their pursuit.

Three high school reforms are approaches to make immediate school success and the associated good grades and positive esteem as a learner more accessible to every student. Students' chances of doing well at school work to earn positive immediate rewards can be improved both by more transitional courses as preparation for high-standards requirements and also by focused extra help when needed to pass high-standards courses. In addition, grading practices themselves may be modified to reward elements of student success that now go unrecognized.

Transitional Preparation Courses Without Tracking

Many students enter high school poorly prepared for a high-standards curriculum. They are not ready for Algebra in mathematics and classic novels and plays in English, as well as demanding content in history and science. In the past, high schools used program tracking to deal with student diversity of prior preparations. Under tracking, only selected students would enter an Academic or College Preparatory program with all high-standards course offerings. Those students who did not qualify for the top track would enter a Vocational or Business program where many occupational courses took up the schedule, or a General program where less demanding academic courses were taken, such as Consumer Math instead of Algebra and Remedial English emphasizing basic grammar skills rather than literature appreciation. But such comprehensive program tracking is no longer part of educational policy, since limited exposure to a challenging curriculum has been shown to be a major factor in poor student achievement test scores and is seen as an unfair lack of equal educational opportunities (Lucas, 1999; Oakes, Gamoran, & Page, 1992). Further, tracking has been shown to exacerbate racial and ethnic achievement gaps (Burris, Wiley, Welner, & Murphy, 2008; Chambers, Hugins, & Scheurich, 2009; Gamoran, Nystrand, Berends, & LePore, 1995).

Yet, the problems of major student differences in academic preparation for high school remain, with the prospects for extensive student course failures when a high-standards curriculum is required for all (Balfanz, McPartland, & Shaw, 2002). A reform is to revise the curriculum scheduling so needy students can get more class time to succeed at the required high-standards courses, often with transition courses to address prerequisite skill gaps taken before the required courses are attempted (Balfanz et al., 2002).

This approach is often called the "double dose" of math or English courses, where twice as much time is scheduled in these core academic subjects. The extra time can include a "transition" course that precedes and prepares students for success in the required courses, or added time can "stretch" the required course time itself so a teacher can interrupt with background learning when necessary or adjust to the actual learning pace of the class. Research has found small positive benefits on student learning gains and course pass rates from adding transition courses or from increasing the time to cover a core course (Gamoran, Porter, Smithson, & White, 1997). Another study to compare transition courses with stretch courses in algebra is underway with early indications that both approaches have similar beneficial effects on success in algebra grades and achievement tests, while students receiving transition-course experiences had the highest gain in general math skills and knowledge (Neild, Byrnes, & Sweet, 2010).

One example of using transition courses is the Talent Development High School reform model. This model was initially developed in 1992 in Baltimore and Philadelphia high schools and is currently used in more than 120 sites across America to provide double doses of time in math and English for most students in ninth, tenth, and eleventh grades. Using an extended period block schedule of 90 daily class minutes in each subject throughout the school year, a transition course is offered in the first 18-week term to prepare for the high standards required course in the second term. In mathematics, pre-algebra and pre-geometry courses have been developed as first-term transitional offerings that establish a firm foundation of both the conceptual understandings and procedural fluencies that are the prerequisites for success in the high-standards requirements. In English, the transition course takes into account students' current reading levels by using high-interest low-frustration novels, short stories, and nonfiction to practice comprehension strategies before, during, and after reading. A study of ten matched pairs of high schools in Philadelphia found statistically significant positive benefits from transition courses on ninth grade students' mathematics achievement gains with a 10% decrease in students scoring below basic on their eleventh grade scores on the Pennsylvania System of School Assessment compared to a 4% decrease in control schools (Kemple, Herlihy, & Smith, 2005). An evaluation of the ninth grade transition courses in English with 64 high schools across the nation showed a statistically significant moderate positive relationship between implementation quality of the program and reading comprehension gains over a school year (Davis & McPartland, 2009).

Since not all students or all schools may need a transition course in high school math or English, there are concerns that this approach is just another form of unfair tracking when students are separated into groups with different need levels. But no student is being withheld from the opportunity to learn the same high-standards math or English curriculum, which is the usual definition of program tracking. The grouping of students for transition courses is aimed to give all a better chance to succeed at high standards after preparation gaps are first addressed. Moreover, when an entire school is scheduled with double-dose offerings in English and math, because all students can profit from the transition courses, there should be no stigma as in other tracking. Still, the issues of heterogeneous or homogeneous student groupings can still remain, when some classrooms enroll more far-behind students to better focus the transition preparations. Some studies indicate lower achievement expectations of both teachers and students are inevitable in classrooms where poorly prepared students predominate (Hallinan, 1990; Oakes et al., 1992; Slavin, 1990), but other research shows nevertheless that skill gaps can be significantly narrowed or closed when needy students are gathered together for additional focused "catch up" classes (Balfanz, Legters, & Jordan, 2004; Gamoran, 1992, 1993).

Levels of Focused Extra Help

The double-dose transition-course approach is one instance of a more general reform strategy using different levels of student intervention based upon earlier indicators of specific student needs. Often discussed as an example of "response to intervention" (RTI) that was developed in special education programs (Duffy, 2007), high schools are being reformed to offer different levels and intensities of help to students with various academic and behavioral needs. It is a strategy to help all students achieve the immediate rewards of good school work by dealing directly with the individual needs that may stand in the way of success at school (U.S. General Accounting Office, 1993).

This approach can be aimed at preventing high school dropouts, the ultimate stage of student disengagement, where learning difficulties in academic courses are only one potential problem source that needs to be addressed. Dropout risks also include students with poor attendance habits, disciplinary problems, and personal issues of immaturity, weak sense of personal responsibility, low self-confidence as a learner, or interferences with school work from outside issues of substance abuse or serious family problems (Roderick & Camburn, 1999).

A high school reform model that uses early warning signs from elementary and middle grades to prescribe the levels of extra help needed by different students is the Diplomas Now approach currently being evaluated in multiple sets of schools across the country. Diplomas now defines three different levels of support for needy students and draws extra resources from volunteer and community agencies to address particular student issues and to provide more intensive support.

The first level of support is school-wide interventions for large segments of the student enrollment that come poorly prepared for high school success. Diplomas Now combines the school-wide high school reform program developed under the Talent Development model, with extra services from two existing national school support entities, City Year and Communities in Schools. With financial support from a large federal Investing in Innovation (i3) grant, Diplomas Now will be implemented in 65 high schools with middle school feeders across America in 2010 through 2015. Diplomas Now draws upon the Talent Development model to provide a double-dose curriculum and interdisciplinary teams of teachers sharing the same student group for improving attendance and discipline.

The second level of intervention is for smaller subsets of students who receive small group interventions to address academic or other personal difficulties. For example, at this level, a "triple dose" of academic interventions is used, such as a pull-out course for remedial math or English having a small class enrollment and using different instructional interventions like computers or project-based learning. Likewise, a small group intervention can be used to improve students' coping skills where they have had serious disciplinary encounters, or to shape behavior where substance abuse is a serious problem.

The third level of intervention is at the individual level, where help needs to be very focused and intense because of the seriousness of academic or personal needs. For example, tutoring in word attack skills may address an unusual high school student need that stands in the way of good reading. Or personal counseling to find direction and enhance personal responsibility and positive choices may be unavoidable for certain troubled youth.

Enhancing Criteria for Grades and Recognition

High school students' positive behaviors may go unmeasured and unrewarded, especially when the conventional basis for course grades and public recognition leaves many without sources of pride for future engagement.

The conventional way of assigning course grades in US schools is to record how well a student ranks in class or performs relative to an absolute standard in the subject, which leaves many students who are consistently below average with little chance for high marks and the associated positive recognitions. Many students' positive motivation and engagement must surely suffer under a grading system that leaves little room for top rewards except to those who can beat all the rest in class rank or national norms. But these same low-ranking students are frequently learning well in terms of progressing in knowledge and skills across the term, without any indication at report card time of these accomplishments. Even their teachers may not appreciate these students' efforts and results when at grading time all attention is to standing in class or meeting very high standards. So while a conventional grade tells a student where he or she stands according to an acknowledged standard (which is useful information), it will not serve as a source of motivation for those who have little chance even with heroic efforts to significantly move up in class. For sure, just avoiding a course failure is an incentive for some students, but school reforms to give every student a realistic chance of a top grade should offer a stronger incentive to all students' efforts.

Some high schools are attempting more responsive grading, by adding a progress score or an effort score to the usual skills grade. The progress score is to reward growth in course skills from the individual student's own starting point so gains in knowledge and skills from the beginning of the term will be recognized. Even if a student does not move up in class rank or has yet to meet a high achievement standard, a good progress score should motivate a student with the recognition that he or she has improved themselves over the time of the course. Likewise, a good effort score for a student who attends every day, completes the assignments, and tries hard to learn can be earned by anyone regardless of the achievement standing in class, and may have a positive effect on motivation.

Meta-analytic research on extrinsic motivation has indicated that responsive rewards, such as progress scores, can increase intrinsic motivation for uninteresting tasks (Cameron, Banko, & Pierce, 2001; Deci, Koestner, & Ryan, 1999) and for interesting activities when "participants are verbally praised for their work, when tangible rewards are presented in an informational manner, when rewards signify competence at an activity, and when the rewards are offered and given for achieving performance standards or goal" (Cameron et al., 2005, p. 642). The reason rewards presented in this manner could potentially increase motivation is because they help children form or maintain their self-efficacy for a task. If recognition and praise is given for meeting small tasks, self-efficacy may increase and the student may try a more difficult task in the future.

Teachers can use different behavioral and subjective indicators for progress or effort grades, including parallel tests at the start and end of a marking period, records on good attendance and completed assignments, as well as judgments from students' performance in class or in conferences with the teacher. But the progress or effort scores should be separately added grades so they can highlight and reward individual student accomplishments, rather than combined together in a single grade including class achievement standing which muddles the message and dilutes the potential rewards. Research remains limited on the practical approaches for more responsive grading and the effects on student engagement. But since immediate rewards for classwork can be so motivating for students, developing more responsive grading practices where all students can earn positive recognition seems to be a promising new direction (Trumbull & Farr, 2000).

Increase Intrinsic Interest of School Work

Students will be more engaged in learning tasks that are inherently satisfying rather than the more mundane drill and practice exercise to master individual skills. For example, a student who enjoys reading mystery novels in her spare time is motivated primarily from the enjoyment of reading these books and not from an outside influence, such as for a school grade or to impress her teacher. This enjoyment will still be present even when reading a mystery novel is a school task. This enjoyment and motivation that comes from within a person is called intrinsic motivation (Cordova & Lepper, 1996; Eccles & Wigfield, 2002; Ryan & Deci, 2000). Activities will be more intrinsically motivating when a student is using skills that bring pleasure in themselves, such as using the mind to solve a challenging problem or to create a novel product, or when a student is responsible for a project from beginning to end that has an outcome to be proud of. In these cases, a student will be working not so much to earn a good grade as to learn or improve oneself for his or her own sake. High intrinsic motivation for academic tasks leads to increases in learning and academic achievement (Fredricks, Blumenfeld, & Paris, 2004).

Students who are intrinsically motivated in a task are more likely to set mastery goals as opposed to performance goals. Mastery goals are made by students who want to learn and improve their abilities and who are not as concerned about what others think of their performance as they are learning (Pintrich & Schunk, 2002). They see the end result of an academic task as increased knowledge or skills. Performance goals, however, are made by those who want to look good for others and get good grades. Although a student may have a mix of both of these goals, mastery goals are more related to help seeking, deep strategy use, and confidence (Midgley, 2001). To support mastery goals, teachers need to de-emphasize the importance of grades and have a classroom climate that supports, rather than punishes, student mistakes and errors as they attempt to learn difficult material in their classrooms.

Three examples illustrate instructional reforms that should bring more intrinsic interest to school work: teaching for conceptual understanding; distinguishing disciplinary thinking in each subject, and project-based learning.

Teaching for Conceptual Understanding

In recent years, curriculum specialists in both English and mathematics have been arguing about the proper instructional emphasis between procedural knowledge and conceptual understanding in each subject. Sometimes called the "reading wars" or the "math wars," strong opinions have been held on each side of the issue. In early reading, proponents of phonics-based instruction where mastery of word attack skills are emphasized have conflicted with whole language advocates who recommend immersing young readers in real books to learn as they enjoy the experiences. In mathematics, one side urges an instructional concentration on basic arithmetic and other operational skills including memorizing multiplication tables and fraction-percent equivalencies, while others recommend an emphasis on understanding core concepts through discovery activities, so that students understand the ratio basis for thinking when working with fractions rather than the counting framework for whole number arithmetic, for example. The outcome of these disagreements is important for student engagement as well as for learning, since the mental challenges of conceptual understanding should be more intrinsically motivating.

A balance of both instructional elements is now emerging among high school reformers in both English and mathematics. A middle ground to the reading wars, balanced literacy instruction, is becoming more accepted where basic word attack skills as well as comprehension strategies are being taught (National Reading Panel, 2000; Pressley, 1998, 2000). A similar phenomenon has occurred in high school math to encourage the math educator not to overly focus on basic math skills without an emphasis on thinking and problem solving (National Council of Teachers of Mathematics, 2009).

In high school reading instruction, reading fluency to process text with ease and automaticity is being developed by giving students regular opportunities for extensive reading, often of books of their own choice. This should appeal to students' intrinsic motivation by offering enjoyable learning experiences where each individual can take some initiative. Reading comprehension instruction teaches students to actively think along with the author and to regularly check for understanding with corrective strategies. This has potential for intrinsic satisfaction by challenging students to use their minds while reading, including making proper inferences to fully appreciate an author's intentions and to be an active participant in understanding the material.

In high school mathematics instruction, students are still expected to remember basic facts and formulas but primarily as tools for mathematical reasoning and problem solving. Even when they do not immediately recognize the algorithm to apply with a math problem, students learn how to get started toward a solution with various thinking strategies. Students will learn how to use handheld calculators and other technologies, but also to have the mental estimation skills to determine whether they have arrived at a reasonable answer. Students will build their confidence that they can reason as a mathematician to frame a formulation that uses the symbolic language and tools to model a complex process or to solve an interesting problem. Intrinsic motivation should be strong for these learning experiences that challenge the mind and encourage analytic thinking (National Research Council, 2000).

Disciplinary Thinking

High school reformers are also recommending that instruction in each of the core academic subjects plays close attention to the unique disciplinary thinking of each case, so the intrinsic interest becomes clear (Newman, 1992; Nystrand & Gamoran, 1992; Resnick, 2010). Students in history should not only learn the events and sequences of important periods, but also how historians use primary sources to make judgments about causations and long-term consequences in writing historic narratives (Brown, 2009; Lattimer, 2008). Likewise, science students need to learn major processes and laws of nature, but at the same time understand how scientists combine empirical evidence with alternative theories to advance knowledge at different points of time (Zimmerman, 2007). Literature and writing classes should help students grow in their appreciation of the writer's craft within the various genres of fiction and forms of nonfiction, so that their own writing can improve for different goals and audiences. Mathematics students should learn how the symbolic language and reasoning tools can be applied in problem formulation and solutions (Kilpatrick, 2001; Yore, Pimm, & Tuan, 2007). Intrinsic motivation should be strengthened when students assume the role of specialists in each discipline and appreciate the unique discourse and thinking patterns of each subject.

The centrality of disciplinary thinking has also recently emerged in "content literacy," with instruction on how to read for understanding in each of the major subjects (Heller & Greenleaf, 2007; Lee & Spratley, 2010; Shanahan & Shanahan, 2008). Besides teaching students useful strategies to use in all subjects before, during, and after reading, it is important for them to learn how the text structures and presentation of information reflect the unique discourse patterns and disciplinary aspects of each separate subject. Upgrading instruction in each subject to include disciplinary thinking should enhance the intrinsic motivation for learning. When students are expected to use their minds as an expert would in each subject and to participate in relevant thinking activities, the learning challenges should be more exciting and satisfying as they are mastered.

Project-Based Learning

Project-based learning is also a growing feature under high school reforms, where students learn by conducting an extended interdisciplinary project. These projects are meant to be authentic, complex problem-solving tasks (Bell, 2010; Blumenfeld et al., 1991). The need for authentic tasks dates back to Dewey's philosophy on learning through practical experiences.

Project-based learning can take many forms. Sometimes students work in teams to complete a project, but individual project assignments are also used (Johnson & Johnson, 1985). The length from beginning to end of a project can also vary from 1 or 2 days to a couple of weeks or more. The product of a project may be a written outcome, a performance or presentation, a business enterprise or simulation, or a construction using artistic or practical materials. The content of a project may be an application or example from a single subject such as science, history, literature, or mathematics or a combination of disciplinary contributions to the final product. Students can be part of the selection of the driving question or problem as well as determining the nature of the final product. Studies on project-based learning show a benefit of this approach for standardized and state assessments (Geier et al., 2008).

The instructional benefits of applying disciplinary skills and tools for a practical outcome also contribute to the intrinsic motivation appeals. Student should draw satisfaction from a task that demonstrates the actual usefulness of one or more of their academic courses.

The project task itself and outcome also has intrinsic motivation components (Blumenfeld et al., 1991). An individual who works through a complex sequence of connected activities should derive satisfaction from the mature planning and coordination required. Also, producing an end product can deliver a sense of accomplishment and pride that is often a defining characteristic of intrinsic motivation. Many projects involve collaboration which is motivating for some students. Finally, since project-based instruction should be student-based, students have the opportunity to make choices and have more control over their learning which is more motivating than teacher-directed activities (Deci & Ryan, 1987). Students' intrinsic motivation for a project, however, will depend to an extent on their teacher's intrinsic motivation during project-based learning (Lam, Cheng, & Ma, 2009). Teachers need to constantly monitor and support motivation throughout a lengthy project.

Functional Relevance of Learning

School work will also be more engaging for high school students when it is clearly connected to an individual's personal long-range goals or when it feeds into current personal concerns and coping skills (Schneider & Stevenson, 1999). The relevance of school work for a student's long-run or short-run needs should be explicit or easily understood to have most value for increased student engagement. Motivational psychologists say that a task has "utility value" when a person understands how a task will help him or her reach their goals (Eccles & Wigfield, 2002; Eccles, Wigfield, & Schiefele, 1998). If the "utility value" of the task is strong, the person will value the outcome of the task greatly and will put in more effort.

Compare a student who is always asking his or her teachers "Why are you making us learn this stuff?" to one who has chosen a program of studies because it makes sense for personal career goals and interests. In the first case, engagement with learning will be weak because no useful connection is readily seen between school work and the student's personal needs or goals. In the latter case, we expect this student to come to school each day anticipating a useful learning experience that is directly relevant for personal career expectations, and to be regularly engaged with a program of choice.

The integration of academic and career education is an element of high school reform to enhance the functional relevance of learning for student engagement. Two ways this can be accomplished are through a Career Academy structure with appropriate elective courses and experiences or by merging career applications into core academic courses.

Career Academies

Career Academies may be an organizational component of comprehensive reform models such as Talent Development and Diplomas Now, or a stand-alone innovation to integrate academic and occupational education in high schools (Maxwell & Rubin, 2000; Stern, Dayton, & Raby, 2010; Stern, Raby, & Dayton, 1992). Career Academies are usually self-contained units within a high school with an instructional program centered around a broad occupational cluster—such as science or health, arts and expression, business and data management, construction or engineering—which a student has selected to attend based on a careful exploration of individual career interests, strengths, and goals. Each different Career Academy may cover three or more high school grades, such as 10–12, and enroll enough students to require its own teaching faculty for all academic and career courses (usually 350 or more students for three grades). The instructional program includes the core college preparatory academic subject courses as well as a sequence of elective career education courses that can lead to a special credential at graduation. The program also offers some experiential learning opportunities, where students pursue activities off-site at an actual business or agency or where on-site career simulations or enterprises are established for students to practice career roles.

When separate Career Academies are formed within a high school, precautions should be taken to offset informal forces to make undesirable distinctions about selectivity and academic standards (Lee & Ready, 2007). Career Academies should be available for every student, so a residual program does not exist as the college preparatory track. Likewise, each Career Academy should be open to all students and have a complete set of college preparatory academic courses including a share of advanced placement electives, so informal distinctions of different standards and outcomes can be avoided. Sometimes, career education is introduced for all students in a high school without separate Academies in their own space, when students choose a career major and add elective courses to their program from career cluster offerings (Grubb, 1995). But career majors without a complete Academy structure will not provide the full integration of academic and career education in all courses that would otherwise be possible.

Student engagement is strengthened by career academies in multiple ways. The program of studies has functional relevance for the student by including elective courses and additional learning experiences focused on the career themes of strong personal interest to the individual. The opportunity to choose among alternative Career Academies personifies the practical usefulness of the curriculum and represents a personal commitment to the program of studies. Attending classes with like-minded students who selected the same Career Academy also can bring some shared pride in the program and reinforces its functional relevance. The chance to earn an additional credential at graduation for completion of the Career Academy program is another symbol of its functional value.

Several studies have demonstrated the value of curriculum programs like Career Academies that integrate academic and career education in a relevant learning experience. In a field experiment across 30 high schools in five districts where students were randomly assigned to programs using career academies or not, the evaluation firm of MDRC has published several reports on short-term and long-term effects (Kemple & Snipes, 2000; Kemple & Willner, 2008). The most impressive outcomes found were the benefits after high school graduation for career academy students, who were more likely to succeed in college and in holding well-paying jobs in their selected occupational area. In separate research using national high school survey and records data, Plank (2001) found positive short-term benefits during the high school years for students who enrolled in a combined academic and career program of studies. The results on the relationship between percentage of career courses taken and the risk of dropping out suggested a U-shaped pattern in that students with a mix of both career and academic courses had a lower risk for dropping out than students who took primarily either career or academic courses.

Blending Career Applications

Even without a complete program of studies to focus on the career relevance of school work, each individual academic course can demonstrate its useful relevance by including interesting career and practical applications.

Perhaps mathematics instruction provides the most opportunities to include various practical applications for most of the course units and topics. For example, a unit on exponential functions can cover applications to several fields, including compound interest in business, epidemic growth or drug decay in health, or population dynamics in history and social studies. Although most high school math textbooks include some brief, practical examples and exercises, some packages of more extensive career applications that encourage discovery and extended student discussions are available for high school reformers.

Language arts courses also have room for various practical applications, such as writing assignments for various career goals and audiences, or coordinated reading experiences that overlap characters or situations from selected industries or occupations. Likewise, science knowledge and procedure can be used to address current affairs issues and debates through applications in selected science courses. The mode of presentations using tables, graphs, and trend lines found in mathematics and social studies courses can also be employed for parallel practical applications in understanding daily newspaper and popular media accounts.

Positive Teacher-Student Relations

Students are likely to be more engaged with their high school when they have a personal and respectful relationship with the teachers and administrators they encounter during the school day (Baker, Terry, Bridges, & Winsor, 1997; Furrer & Skinner, 2003; Hallinan, 2005; Wentzel, 1997, 2009). If instead a student is largely anonymous to the adults of the school, because the school size is large and teachers have too many different students to get to know each one well, few human connections outside of one's own student peer group will exist to socially connect to the school. As students move up in grades and have more teachers during the day, their sense of school belonging decreases (Anderman, 1999).

Research on teacher involvement and caring notes that the effective teachers show affection and appreciation for their students, know a lot about their students, dedicate time and energy to their students, and are dependable (Skinner & Belmont, 1993). Some have argued that good teaching practice is similar to good parenting styles, with consistent enforcement of rules, high and reasonable expectations, democratic communication, nurturance, and an emphasis on self-reliance (Baumrind, 1971; Wentzel, 2002).

Positive social connections with the adult educators are valuable for student engagement with the school for several reasons. Students will be more eager to earn respect and praise for good work and accept the goals set for them from teachers and administrators who know them well and demonstrate real care for their success (Grusec & Goodnow, 1994). Teachers and staff who can communicate on a personal basis with all the students they interact with in the halls and classrooms will be better able to establish and enforce a proper disciplinary climate that is safe and serious.

High school reforms that can foster good teacher-student relations and a positive climate conducive to learning include schools organized into smaller learning communities, teachers working in interdisciplinary teams that share the same group of students, and adults who serve over multiple years as the mentor and advisor to a limited number of individual students.

Small Learning Communities

Very large high schools pose special problems for establishing positive teacher-student relations (Lee, 2000; Louis & Marks, 1998). The sheer number of students and staff make it likely that traffic in the halls, stairways, and cafeteria will involve many anonymous encounters. Likewise, teachers who have many different students each day in their courses will find it difficult to get to know each one well along with his or her individual motivational and learning needs. Large student enrollments can also make the enforcement overwhelming of school regulations about absenteeism, tardiness, class cutting, or deportment, when the number of detentions and other punishments each day are hard to monitor and follow up if frequently ignored by students. As a consequence, the climate in large schools can often be chaotic in the halls and public spaces, absent of the safe feeling of adults-in-charge, and haphazard in the chances of close, respectful individual adult-student relationships.

A strong reform movement for smaller high school learning communities has been pursued for several years around the turn of the twentieth century, with major backing from the Bill and

Melinda Gates Foundation and other funders. Sometimes this involved starting new small high schools of 400 students or less, or breaking up a large facility into several separate self-contained high schools (called "multiplex" high schools at times). Another common arrangement is a "schools-within-the-school" organization where a large high school would create several smaller learning communities or "houses" defined by grade level or by curriculum focus. The Talent Development High School model created a separate Ninth Grade Success Academy and several Career Academies, each covering grades 10–12 with about 300 students or less. In this case, each Academy has its own contiguous building space, preferably with its own entrance door, as well as its own Academy Principal and administrative staff and its own teaching faculty for all required and elective courses. Research studies of this model have shown the Academy's structure can turn around a weak school climate or enhance a strong one, as well as foster widespread positive student-teacher relations (Legters, Balfanz, Jordan, & McPartland, 2002). An evaluation of 123 small schools of choice (SSC) in New York City where students were randomly enrolled to these sites in comparison to other students who were not admitted in the random lottery process showed positive benefits between 2002 and 2010 on timely progression across the grades and graduation rates. A difference of 10 percentage points in favor of SSC students was found in being on track toward graduation over 3 years as well as an overall 6.8% advantage in actual graduation rates, which is equivalent to one-third of the city-wide gap between white students and students of color (Bloom, Thompson, & Unterman, 2010).

Interdisciplinary Teacher Teams

Another threat to student engagement is when initial problems with attendance, course grades, or discipline go unattended and grow into major barriers to grade promotion and graduation. In many high schools, there are no early warning systems with corrective actions, so troubled students can "fall between the cracks" with eventual major negative consequences. Ninth grade students during their transition year into high school are especially prone to having early missteps escalate to severe problems before anyone notices and effectively intervenes.

Interdisciplinary teams of teachers that share the same group of students and have regular common planning time is a high school reform to personalize the learning experience, take notice of individual students in difficulty and address their problems. In the Ninth Grade Success Academy of the Talent Development High School model, two or more teams of four or five teachers, including an English, math, science, and history/social studies teacher, serve the same group of 120–150 students for all of their major instruction. Each team has a common planning period every day when all their students are in an elective course, to monitor individual student problems and to pursue corrective action plans. Thus, not only do the numbers involved make detailed personal knowledge possible in all teacher-student relationships, time is available for adults to be proactive in short circuiting student difficulties. When working well, the teacher team takes responsibility for individual student success without shifting authority to school-wide principals and disciplinary officials except in the most extreme cases.

Evaluation research has demonstrated how the use of such teacher teams has significant positive impacts on improved student attendance, course passing, and grade promotions, and reduced disciplinary incidents and removals, as well as on measures of positive school climate and caring and respectful adult-student relationships (McPartland, Balfanz, Jordan, & Legters, 1998).

Adult Mentors and Advisors

Student engagement with their high school program can also be better ensured when every individual has their own adult mentor or advisor in the school who can advocate in various ways for their success. To work well, the individual student "case load" for each participating adult should not be too large, and the time to get to know one another well should be sufficient.

Some high schools establish an expanded pool of adults to serve the mentor-advisor role, including nonteaching department heads, counselors, coaches, and specialist staff as well as the total teaching faculty. Sometimes, schools strive to maintain each adult as mentor for several years of the same students, including all 4 years of high school. Schools will schedule time for advising and mentoring in different ways, such as a short advisory period each week or at the start of each day, as well as selected periods for private discussions at report card time or other junctures for "taking stock" on how things are going with school life and outcomes.

A study of 94 ninth grade high school students, half of whom were randomly assigned to receive adult mentoring services, showed positive differences on not dropping out of school (9% compared with 30%) and on earning significantly more course credits toward high school graduation (Sinclair, Christenson, Evelo, & Hurley, 1998). In general, research shows that positive relationships with adults in the school, including teachers, relates to more interest in school ($\beta=.33, p<.001$) (Wentzel, 1998), classroom engagement ($\beta=.46, p<.01$) (Furrer & Skinner, 2003), and academic effort ($\beta=.31, p<.001$) (Wentzel, 1997).

Opportunities for Personal Expression and Nonacademic Interests

Another source for strong student engagement with their high school derives from the range of nonacademic talents that individual students come with and the degree to which schools can respond to these diverse strengths. Nonacademic talents include not only the athletic skills and music or art abilities that can flourish in extracurricular teams and clubs but also the other dimensions of human talents that vocational and learning psychologists have identified that could find expression in some high school courses and classroom activities.

Vocational psychologists have defined six categories of human talents or personalities that match different occupational requirements, where individual satisfaction and success are maximized when there is a good match between the two (Rottinghaus, Hees, & Conrath, 2009). Under the categorization developed by Holland (1997), some students may be particularly adept at building or fixing mechanical things, while others are especially good in working with others in team or helping roles. In addition, individual student nonacademic strengths may be in areas of creative imagination and expression. Figuring out how things work and thinking like a scientist can characterize other students. Fascination with business or financial affairs and organizing data for decision-making can be other sets of strengths.

The idea of multiple intelligences (Gardner, 1983, 1999) is another conceptualization of the different skills and talents that individuals can bring to learning tasks. Gardner posited eight different intelligences including logical-mathematical, linguistic, musical, spatial, bodily-kinesthetic, interpersonal, intrapersonal, and naturalist. Later he introduced the idea that there may even be spiritual and existential intelligences. In the USA, most school systems place the highest value on both linguistic (verbal) and logical-mathematical intelligences. However, others such as bodily-kinesthetic and musical intelligences are not as valued, although they could be used in the classroom to strengthen learning. For example, students with high musical intelligence may be able to compose a song to summarize information in science or a student high in bodily-kinesthetic ability could be asked to act out a scene as a soldier in World War 1.

Some high school reforms, such as the Talent Development High School model, are based in part on the concept that there are many talents, in addition to the academic competencies which are the focus of most achievement tests and grades, that should also be identified and developed during the secondary grades because of their importance in adult life. Indeed, while academic grades and test scores may be important for advancing to higher levels of education, research has found them to be a weak predictor of adult occupational success. After controlling for the level of educational attainment, the relationship of grades and test scores obtained earlier in life do not explain much of the variation in adult job status or income (Jencks, 1975). Moreover, studies of renowned high accomplishment in various fields of business, law, creative design or performance, governmental and community leadership, and humanitarian service frequently identify outstanding examples who had ordinary academic records but possessed other personal traits that were the foundation of their exemplary careers (Coyle, 2009; Scott, 2007). Economists have also successfully used the diversity of human cognitive and noncognitive skills to estimate models of adult accomplishment (Cunha & Heckman, 2008). Apparently, there are a wide range of other nonacademic talents that society needs and rewards, but go largely unnoticed and unrewarded in American high schools' preoccupation with traditional academic achievement goals. Moreover, it is likely that every individual in high school has personal nonacademic strengths and interests which could be further developed as a source of engagement in high school and as an investment for successful adult occupational careers or satisfying personal pursuits.

High school reforms that may increase student engagement by appealing to nonacademic skills and talents include personal exploration opportunities, elective courses, and extracurricular activities.

Personal Exploration

An initial high school reform to engage students through nonacademic talents is to acknowledge the range of human talents and to help each individual student to explore their own personal strengths and interests. This would help students understand that each of them has strong personal strengths in which to take pride, even if they are not a top student in academic course grades and tests. When exploring the range of human traits, more students would see school as a means to exercise and enjoy their own special talents and as a route to preparing for later success and satisfaction.

Several instruments and experiences are available for high schools to help their students collect and organize data about their personal nonacademic strengths and interests. Among the vocational interest inventories that high school students can take, the Self-Directed Search (SDS) is based upon Holland's six types of careers and associated personality profiles. The SDS is a booklet where students report and score their own experiences, preferences, strengths, and interests along each broad dimension. This information is then organized into a resulting two- or three-letter code which summarizes each student's nonacademic personal priorities. Students understand that the SDS is not a test but a method for organizing their own personal information for further awareness of personal nonacademic strengths and interests.

The personal exploration continues with various possible implications and planning options that derive from the individual's nonacademic or career codes. Students learn that there are many educational levels for different occupations within the same code. They see that different orderings of their own codes reveal a variety of alternative careers that would respond to their own strengths and interests. They find supplementary materials about specific careers of potential interest to them and the kinds of people who have been leaders or have found success in these careers. The SDS with follow-up activities is used to motivate Career Academy choices in Talent Development high schools. There are also other useful tools available for student explorations (Gottfredson, 1986).

Course Planning and Selection

Individual explorations of nonacademic strengths and interests can also be included in a student's high school planning process. In a Career Academy high school, as described above, information about the alternative choices can be connected to a student's own codes for nonacademic and career interests. An informed choice will have the appeal of new opportunities for using personal strengths, as well as reinforcing student engagement for personal long-term goals.

Even in high schools without a Career Academy structure, students can leverage their awareness of personal nonacademic strengths with elective course opportunities. When a student finds electives that overlap with their personal strengths, the school experience should be more engaging as a way to further develop one's individuality. At its best, well-informed students may find course offerings and sequences where their own passions for learning are welcomed and stimulated.

Extracurricular Activities

High school reforms should also not overlook the out-of-class opportunities to allow a wide variety of students' nonacademic strengths to flourish and further develop. Some students may draw their strongest points of school engagement from the teams or clubs where they can exercise their personal strengths and contribute to group or individual accomplishments. Numerous research studies have identified extracurricular activities as a positive setting for personal growth and for strengthening students' engagement at school (Eccles & Barber, 1999; Fredricks & Eccles, 2005; Gilman, Meyers, & Perez, 2004).

The Talent Development High School model is using the benefits for personal growth by extending extracurricular activities beyond the traditional teams and clubs as after-school entities. Several Talent Development sites have added a daily period at the end of each day for personal exploration and activities that use artists, musicians, dancers, circus performers, political debaters, and other creative individuals from the community to lead the classroom activities. A goal is to expand the school curriculum so that every student gets a wide variety of nonacademic experiences that may expand interests for some and reinforce personal strengths in others. In addition, Career Academies in many of the Talent Development high schools are providing learning experiences for students in community enterprises and agencies to appreciate how skills from academic courses combine with more specialized abilities for success in adult occupations (Epstein, 2001; Pearson, 2002).

School Governance, Disciplinary Practices, and Communal Engagement

Communal engagement is another way students can become attached to their high schools, which will be affected by how the school as a whole is governed (Lee, Bryk, & Smith, 1993; Shouse, 1997). Communal engagement is connected by the concepts of relational trust and social capital that sociologists have developed to describe the quality of social exchanges in key role relationships (Bryk & Schneider, 2002) and the power of relational ties within a social system (Coleman, 1988). A school with high levels of relational trust and social capital has individuals who strongly value their membership in this community, are willing to work together with others for the common good, and to look out for one another's legitimate interests. The school members share common norms about how individuals should behave ("do what is right") in their organizational community, expect mutual caring, and respect and personally identify with and take pride in "my school" (Bryk & Schneider, 2002). Students who have had the experiences to develop relational trust and to rely upon the social capital of their school we define to have communal engagement with the school.

Communal engagement is valuable in its own right as students enjoy the experiences of a close-knit supportive community, and it can also benefit students' academic learning processes and be a source of their general citizenship socialization. We discussed above how positive teacher-student relationships can enhance the incentives for students to exert effort at school work to earn recognition from a valued adult, and these roles can lead to further learning benefits when embedded in a school with strong social ties where all adults are sensitive to each student's needs. In this case, teachers will share information with one another to monitor and improve individual student behaviors, just as neighbors in a small community with strong social capital will watch out for each other's children and help them grow up well (Coleman, 1988). Moreover, students who participate in a well-governed school where authority is clearly exercised for the common good and each individual has community responsibilities, can be expected to develop general appreciation for good citizenship and shared values in broader society.

Students will be more likely to feel positively attached to a school that is largely governed by shared norms of civility and trust, where the necessary rules are legitimized by participatory decision-making, and infractions are adjudicated and discussed as learning experiences (Osterman, 2000; Webb, Covington, & Guthrie, 1993). In contrast, students can feel estranged and alienated from their schools if rules seem excessive and arbitrary, and discipline appears inconsistent and without recourse even for harsh penalties such as suspensions or expulsions.

To be sure, some high schools are more difficult to manage because of large size, awkward traffic patterns in stairways and corridors, student bodies that are more prone to mischief or group tensions, or reputations for chaotic behavior. Indeed, getting a high school under control that has unsafe or disorderly climates is usually the first priority of a reform program (McPartland et al., 1998). Two aspects of effective school governance closely tied to student engagement are the school rules and disciplinary practices themselves as well as opportunities for student participation in school governance and disciplinary enforcement.

Rules and Disciplinary Practices

A national survey to analyze school-wide disciplinary practices from a stratified random sample of 848 public and private schools, sponsored by the US Department of Justice, was completed in 2000 (Gottfredson et al., 2000, 2004). When the quality of disciplinary practices was scored, most schools had good communications and documentation practices, but much fewer were adequate in the consistency and predictability of their disciplinary enforcements or in the range of responses to misconduct and to desirable conduct.

Almost all schools have established a set of school rules and policies with the consequences for different misbehaviors that are made known to the student population, especially for dangerous misconduct such as possession of a weapon at school. Most schools are also good at keeping records of the disciplinary actions taken during a school year. These rules usually distinguish between crimes and other very serious infractions, such as having weapons in school, possession of drugs or alcohol, and criminal attacks, versus other misbehaviors, such as use of profane or abusive language, tobacco possession, and truancy and some physical fighting. But most schools fall down on how well the rules are applied and on the range of responses made to both desired and inappropriate conduct.

Although potential consequences of breaking school rules might extend from detention, reprimands, notifying parents, brief exclusion from class, loss of privileges, and school or community service, to removal from school for short or long suspensions or even permanent expulsion, the survey found that about three quarters of the schools used the same one or two responses to all offenses. Indeed, the more extreme punishment of disciplinary removals was often found to be the prominent and initial responses in many high schools to both dangerous and less consequential student offenses. Likewise, a wide range of positive responses, if any at all, for positive student behaviors was found missing in most secondary schools. The praise or recognition, material or privilege rewards, or other potential reinforcements of good student behavior were used in combination by only 20% of the surveyed schools.

Students are more likely to appreciate "firm but fair" enforcement of school rules, but the survey showed that the quality of disciplinary practice is often poor. Less than half of secondary schools were found to practice consistent discipline, where punishments do not depend upon what teacher makes the referral or what kind of student is involved. Less than one-third were predictable in their disciplinary decision-making, where both teachers and students are clear about the specific disciplinary consequences that follow each kind of infraction.

Thus, student engagement with their school is frequently threatened when they perceive school rules as too harsh or capricious and school use of punishments to far outweigh rewards for good conduct as the usual official responses to their behavior. Students who feel that the discipline system of their school is ineffective or unfair are less likely to participate in class and attend school (Finn & Voelkl, 1993; Osher, Bear, Sprague, & Doyle, 2010) and more likely to drop out of school (Fine, Valenzuela, & Bowditch, 1993; Wehlange & Rutter, 1986).

Student Involvement in Decision-Making

Student engagement is also likely to be a function of their own opportunities to influence how rules are established and enforced and other decisions about school life are made.

Student opportunities to help shape disciplinary rules can occur at both the classroom level and school wide. At the beginning of the term, a teacher can invite the students to help shape the rules that will guide classroom behavior, including how discussions and interactions with peers and adults are to proceed, and how school discipline policies will be applied. Similarly, student representatives from the elected grade or school councils or from appointed committees can help set disciplinary policies and priorities to govern student behavior throughout the building and grounds (Rosenberg & Jackman, 2003).

Some high schools have also used student participation in the enforcement of school rules, through student courts where students are given a hearing before punishment for an offense, or by way of peer mediation services where conflicts between individuals are worked out through face-to-face discussions facilitated by other student helpers. Student monitors in halls and cafeterias can also be a way to involve others in the maintenance of an orderly and respectful environment.

But how students are treated for disciplinary purposes in their relationship to school adults and authorities can also determine how often strong informal norms of good behavior develop and make frequent official reactions less necessary. As discussed earlier, a self-regulating school can develop when individual teachers seek to address most student behavioral issues without sending a student to the office for an official disciplinary officer to take action. Teachers working in teams can organize a sequence of responses that bring in other adults who share responsibility for a student to discuss a disciplinary issue with the individual and seek solutions. Even when a student referral is made to a school authority for disciplinary reasons, the manner in which discussions proceed for learning experiences can shape how the student views rules as legitimate and worthy of adherence. The concept of "mutual trust" has been cited as a feature of a good problem-solving and self-regulating school that leads to strong student engagement (Bryk & Schneider, 2002).

Interaction of Dimensions of High School Student Motivation and Engagement

The six dimensions of student motivation and engagement discussed in this chapter can interact with one another and the associated high school reforms. Different dimensions call for certain preparatory actions to establish a motivational foundation for later student engagement with each reform. Some dimensions may be more dependent on others, with implications for planning the order and sequence of different reforms. Different combinations of school improvements can enhance one another for a total impact on student engagement, which highlights the needs for comprehensive high school reform.

Preparing for Student Motivation and Engagement

Using the distinction between student motivation that is established before participating in activities and student engagement that is activated during experiences, sets of the six dimensions and associated high school reforms seem to require particular anticipatory preparations for motivation to lead to engagement.

Helping students gain insight into their own personal strengths and career interests can be valuable preliminary activities to set up strong student motivation under the two dimensions of the functional relevance and the opportunities for talent development of their school program. When early on in their high school years students have the opportunities to explore what they bring in terms of personal strengths to be further developed and what they hope to accomplish in terms of building new skills and a record of accomplishment for goals after graduation, a motivational foundation can be established for actually experiencing their school program with high interest and energy. For example, a student who is helped to appreciate that she or he is especially interested in working with others as a career goal is ready to choose a Career Academy program and to seek out extracurricular activities that can foster this emphasis. Likewise, a student who understands that she or he has major strengths in building or fixing things and especially enjoys figuring out how things work can get strongly involved with curriculum choices and out-of-class learning opportunities that build on these personal talents. In these and other parallel cases, preparatory activities and choices can establish the motivational fulcrums to leverage student engagement with reforms that bring functional relevance and opportunities for talent development to the school program and activities.

Preparatory activities can also strengthen student motivation for responding to the reforms' dimensions of shared communal engagement and positive interpersonal climate. When students are initially invited to help establish the school rules for school discipline with opportunities to participate in their enforcement, important first steps can be made toward a school governance climate of trust and self-regulation. Likewise, when students are assigned to teacher teams that spend up front time building group spirit and ways for students to seek adult guidance and assistance, a motivational platform can occur that supports student engagement with reforms for an ongoing learning environment of positive interpersonal relations.

The motivational stage can also be set to foster student engagement with the two reform dimensions regarding either immediate rewards or embedded intrinsic interest of their learning activities. Students can receive valuable orientations toward high school learning that balance the performance goals of earning good grades and the mastery goals of improving one's own skills and understandings. When students begin with the belief that their teachers want them to pass and earn good grades and will provide extra help when needed for these accomplishments, they will be more likely to value these immediate rewards and work hard for them. At the same time, when the initial motivational orientation for learning can set the overriding goal of self-improvement and the growth of the mind, students will also be ready for engagement in the thinking challenges of their course and the intrinsic satisfactions of project-based learning.

Setting Reform Priorities and Sequences

Three dimensions of student engagement we have described in this chapter are aspects of students' daily classroom learning activities: accessible immediate awards, embedded intrinsic interest, and direct functional relevance. The other three dimensions are more concerned with the school-level factors that cover the general climate for learning and personal development at the school: positive interpersonal climate, opportunities for alternative talent development, and governance for communal engagement.

Often, high schools begin reforms with the school-level factors because good student attendance and a positive learning climate that derive from these factors must be established first before any other reforms can take hold.

Good student attendance is a necessary condition for improved learning. If a student does not come to school every day, there is no way he and she can take full advantage of improved classroom instruction and learn better. Moreover, a student usually needs good attendance to earn passing grades regardless of individual achievement levels because most teachers will require adequate attendance as a major criterion for report card credits. As discussed earlier, reforms aimed at good attendance can make a significant difference when teacher teams reach out to absentees (positive interpersonal climate), when students are drawn to a school program that addresses their own goals and interests (alternative talent development), and when the school is perceived to be safe and considerate (shared communal engagement).

Likewise, the learning environment of the school cannot be a distraction from serious educational purposes nor a situation where students feel estranged or uncared for, before any other improvements can occur. If discipline in the school building is weak, with chaotic behavior in the halls and stairways, and lack of mutual respect between teachers and students in the classrooms, adult energies will be drawn to enforcing school rules and managing classroom deportment and away from inspiring educational ambitions and motivating good learning. If teachers and students do not get to know each other well and develop respectful and caring relationships, both will be deprived of the foundations for learning activities that can be both challenging and joyful. Thus, troubled high schools will often begin with reforms for positive learning environments that encourage positive interpersonal relationships, provide student choices of activities in and outside of class that coincide with personal interests, and govern the school for common norms of good behavior and mutual trust. So, if a high school is afflicted with a dangerous or unruly disciplinary environment or a pattern of high student absenteeism, reform priorities will be the school organization dimensions that are aimed at the student engagement factors related to a safe and serious school climate, programmatic opportunities for personal fulfillment, and a communal environment of shared beliefs and goals.

Once an environment conducive to good attendance and serious learning has been established at the school level, the reforms for motivation and engagement in classroom instructional activities can proceed. Instructional arrangements can be made to provide extra help focused on particular student needs, so every learner has a good chance to earn good grades and positive feedback for skill improvements. At the same time, teachers can work to improve the motivational challenges to students of their daily learning tasks, by emphasizing intrinsically interesting aspects of using thinking skills in each major subject and applying new knowledge to useful projects. Moreover, time can be devoted to integrating career and academic learning in course offerings and classroom applications to reinforce students' engagement through the functional relevance of their program of studies.

Giving priorities to student attendance and school learning environment highlights the value of assessing a high school's starting point before reforms to target student engagement. If a school is fortunate enough to begin with high levels of student attendance and can assume a climate that is safe, serious, and sensitive to individual students, major school-level reforms may not be needed to organize smaller units with teacher teams, to expand nonacademic options, or to revise school rules and decision-making. Such a school would not have to delay instructional improvements until the school-level factors are gotten under control and could begin with a campaign to engage students more in learning activities, while perhaps also making the school dimensions even more attractive. However, a different very troubled school with serious discipline and attendance problems would establish its reform credibility by the early victories of an improved school climate and better student attendance that can be achieved from school organization changes. Once these improvements are achieved, the prospects for successful reforms of the instructional program to engage students will have a firm foundation.

Comprehensive Reforms

While each dimension of student engagement plays a separate role in how an individual approaches the daily learning activities and life in school, improvements in one dimension can strengthen others. For example, if a student believes major long-run payoffs will follow completion of their school studies because of the functional relevance of their courses, she or he may be able to endure possible less motivating aspects of their instruction when they cannot earn high grades or find many of their classes tedious or boring. On the other hand, a student may be turned on by courses that are intellectually challenging and intrinsically interesting, even if the links to practical applications are weak or the chances for high grades are difficult. But, when a learning opportunity combines all sources of satisfaction, with activities of intrinsic interest, very accessible recognition for good work and clear connections to personal goals, the total impact on student engagement is likely to be more than just the sum of the parts. This argues for comprehensive high school instructional reforms that address multiple dimensions, and teacher professional development that prepares them for all aspects. Not only should extra help be timely and focused to help all students earn passing grades, the learning tasks also should have high appeal themselves as worthy of a strong and inquisitive mind and with clear relevance for practical use and long-term goals.

Individual school-level reforms aimed at practical dimensions of student engagement can also have synergistic value to one another in a comprehensive program of change. School governance of student participation for firm and fair discipline is important in its own right, but can also improve the chances that positive student-teacher relations can emerge from smaller learning communities with stronger aspects of mutual respect and caring. Likewise, school-wide opportunities for individual students to explore and engage their own nonacademic strengths and interests can flourish best in a setting with a stable and supportive learning environment. Thus, comprehensive school-level reforms can create positive feedbacks where different dimensions of student engagement are collectively enhanced.

Comprehensive high school reforms can also address both the more basic dimensions of student engagement, where individuals strive in a safe environment to meet the formal success requirement of passing grades and a good disciplinary record, with the deeper dimensions of student engagement, where individuals pursue their own learning passions, can work in a caring and supportive environment, and experience fulfillment of personal growth and strong preparation for a desired future. Thus, a program of high school reform can begin with changes to make the school safe and extra instructional help available to those in need, so no one needs to drop out before earning a high school diploma. By continuing with a reform program to develop and engage individual students' personal strengths and interests and to establish a supportive human environment for individual exploration and investments in diverse learning opportunities, a comprehensive package of school and classroom reforms can address a wide set of dimensions for student engagement.

Some important needs of further research and development on high school reform for student engagement are indicated by next steps being taken with the Talent Development model. Because the dropout problem is so severe in many high schools, reforms must be intensified to reach all the students, even those with very debilitating individual circumstances. We will be evaluating how adding strong community resources and intensive tutoring services to the school-wide Talent Development organizational and instructional reforms may be successful in eliminating the dropout problem. Studies of student engagement across the full-grade spectrum are needed, so early warning signs at elementary or middle grades can also be used for more timely responses to individual student needs before ultimate risks of school dropouts can develop. Besides this focus on the most needy students, we are also studying how stronger instructional reforms can more successfully challenge all students' critical thinking skills in each high school subject with the additional benefits of strengthening their intrinsic motivations for learning. And while priority is given to internal high school reforms for increasing student motivation and engagement, some future attention should return to external factors such as the kinds of curriculum requirements, assessment tests, and teacher accountability mechanisms that either confine or enable the best internal improvements.

References

American Youth Policy Forum. (2000). *High schools of the millennium*. Washington, DC: American Youth Policy Forum.

Anderman, L. H. (1999). Classroom goal orientation, school belonging and social goals as predictors of students' positive and negative affect following the transition to middle school. *Journal of Research and Development in Education, 32*, 131–147.

Baker, J., Terry, T., Bridger, R., & Winsor, A. (1997). Schools as caring communities: A relational approach to school reform. *School Psychology Review, 26*, 586–602.

Balfanz, R., Herzog, L., & Mac Iver, D. J. (2007). Preventing student disengagement and keeping students on the graduation path in urban middle-grades schools: Early identification and effective interventions. *Educational Psychologist, 42*(4), 223–235.

Balfanz, R., Legters, N., & Jordon, W. (2004). Catching up: Effects of the Talent Development ninth-grade instructional interventions in reading and mathematics in high-poverty high schools. *NASSP Bulletin, 88*, 3–30.

Balfanz, R., McPartland, J., & Shaw, A. (2002). Re-conceptualizing extra help for high school students in a high standards era. *Journal of Vocational Special Needs Education, 25*, 24–41.

Baumrind, D. (1971). Current patterns of parental authority. *Developmental Psychology Monograph, 4*(1, Pt. 2), 1–103.

Bell, S. (2010). Project-based learning for the 21st century: Skills for the future. *Clearing House: A Journal of Educational Strategies, Issues and Ideas, 83*(2), 39–43.

Bloom, H. S., Thompson, S. L., & Unterman, R. (2010). *Transforming the high school experience: How New York City's new small schools are boosting student achievement and graduation rates.* New York: MDRC.

Blumenfeld, P. C., Soloway, E., Marx, R. W., Krajcik, J. S., Guzdial, M., & Palincsar, A. (1991). Motivating project-based learning: Sustaining the doing, supporting the learning. *Educational Psychologist, 26*(3–4), 369–398.

Brown, S. D. (2009). History circles: The doing of teaching history. *The History Teacher, 42*(2), 191–203.

Bryk, A. S., & Schneider, B. (2002). *Trust in schools.* New York: Russell Sage.

Burris, C. C., Wiley, E., Welner, K. G., & Murphy, J. (2008). Accountability, rigor, and detracking: Achievement effects of embracing a challenging curriculum as a universal good for all students. *Teachers College Record, 110*(3), 571–607.

Cameron, J., Banko, K. M., & Pierce, W. D. (2001). Pervasive negative effects of rewards on intrinsic motivation: The myth continues. *Behavior Analyst, 24*(1), 1–44.

Cameron, J., Pierce, W. D., Banko, K. M., & Gear, A. (2005). Achievements-based rewards and intrinsic motivation: A test of cognitive mediators. *Journal of Educational Psychology, 97*(4), 641–655.

Chambers, T. T. V., Hugins, K. S., & Scheurich, J. J. (2009). To track or not to track: Curricular differentiation and African American students at Highview High School. *Journal of Cases in Educational Leadership, 12*(1), 38–50.

Clark, D. (Ed.). (2009). *Improving No Child Left Behind: Linking world-class education standards to America's economic recovery.* The Aspen Institute Congressional Program: Washington, DC.

Coleman, J. S. (1988). Social capital and the creation of human capital. *The American Journal of Sociology, 94*, 95–120.

Cordova, D., & Lepper, M. (1996). Intrinsic motivation and the process of learning: Beneficial effects of contextualization, personalization, and choice. *Journal of Educational Psychology, 88*, 715–730.

Coyle, D. (2009). *The talent code: Greatness isn't born. It's grown. Here's how.* New York: Bantam.

Cunha, F., & Heckman, J. J. (2008). Formulating, identifying and estimating the technology of cognitive and non-cognitive skill formation. *Journal of Human Resources, 43*, 738–782.

Davis, M. H., & McPartland, J. (2009). *Supporting high school teachers to close adolescent literacy gaps.* Paper presented at the American Educational Research Association, San Diego, CA.

Deci, E. L., Koestner, R., & Ryan, R. M. (1999). A meta-analytic review of experiments examining the effects of extrinsic rewards on intrinsic motivation. *Psychological Bulletin, 125*, 627–668.

Deci, E. L., & Ryan, R. M. (1987). The support of autonomy and the control of behavior. *Journal of Personality and Social Psychology, 53*, 1024–1037.

Duffy, H. (2007). *Meeting the needs of significantly struggling learners in high school: A look at approaches to tiered intervention.* Washington, DC: National High School Center.

Eccles, J. S., & Barber, B. L. (1999). Student council, volunteering, basketball, or marching band: What kind of extracurricular involvement matters? *Journal of Adolescent Research, 14*(1), 10–43.

Eccles, J. S., & Wigfield, A. (2002). Motivational beliefs, values, and goals. *Annual Review of Psychology, 53*, 109–132.

Eccles, J., Wigfield, A., & Schiefele, U. (1998). Motivation to succeed. In W. Damon (Series Ed.) & N. Eisenberg (Vol. Ed.), *Handbook of child psychology: Vol. 3. Social, emotional, and personality development* (5th ed., pp. 1017–1095). New York: Wiley.

Epstein, J. L. (2001). *School, family, and community partnerships: Preparing educators and improving schools.* Boulder, CO: Westview Press.

Fine, M., Valenzuela, A., & Bowditch, C. (1993). Getting rid of troublemakers: High school disciplinary procedures and the production of dropouts. *Social Problems, 40*, 493–509.

Finn, J. D., & Voelkl, K. E. (1993). School characteristics related to student engagement. *The Journal of Negro Education, 62*(3), 249–268.

Fredricks, J. A., Blumenfeld, P. C., & Paris, A. H. (2004). School engagement: Potential of the concept, state of the evidence. *Review of Educational Research, 74*(1), 59–109.

Fredricks, J. A., & Eccles, J. S. (2005). Developmental benefits of extracurricular involvement. Do peer characteristics mediate the link between activities and youth outcomes? *Journal of Youth and Adolescence, 34*, 507–520.

Furrer, C., & Skinner, E. (2003). Sense of relatedness as a factor in children's academic engagement and performance. *Journal of Educational Psychology, 95*, 148–162.

Gamoran, A. (1992). The variable effects of high school tracking. *American Sociological Review, 57*, 812–828.

Gamoran, A. (1993). Alternative uses of ability grouping in secondary schools: Can we bring high-quality instruction to low-ability classes? *American Journal of Education, 102*, 1–22.

Gamoran, A., Nystrand, M., Berends, M., & LePore, P. C. (1995). An organizational analysis of the effects of ability grouping. *American Educational Research Journal, 32*, 687–715.

Gamoran, A., Porter, A. C., Smithson, J., & White, P. A. (1997). Upgrading high school mathematics instructions: Improving learning opportunities for low-achieving, low-income youth. *Educational Evaluation and Policy Analysis, 19*, 325–338.

Gardner, H. (1983). *Frames of mind: The theory of multiple intelligences*. New York: Basic Books.

Gardner, H. (1999). Are there additional intelligences? In J. Kane (Ed.), *Education, information, and transformation: Essays on learning and thinking* (pp. 111–131). Upper Saddle River, NJ: Prentice-Hall.

Geier, R., Blumenfeld, P. C., Marx, R. W., Krajcik, J. S., Fishman, B., Soloway, E., et al. (2008). Standardized test outcomes for students engaged in inquiry-based science curricula in the context of urban reform. *Journal of Research in Science Teaching, 45*(8), 922–939.

Gilman, R., Meyers, J., & Perez, L. (2004). Structured extracurricular activities among adolescents: Findings and implications for school psychologists. *Psychology in the Schools, 41*, 31–41.

Gottfredson, G. D., Gottfredson, D. C., Czeh, E. R., Cantor, D., Crosse, S. B., & Hantman, I. (2000). *National study of delinquency prevention in schools*. Ellicott City, MD: Gottfredson Associates.

Gottfredson, G. D., Gottfredson, D. C., Czeh, E. R., Cantor, D., Crosse, S. B., & Hantman, I. (2004). *Toward safe and orderly schools – The national study of delinquency prevention in schools*. Washington, DC: National Institute of Justice, U.S. Department of Justice.

Gottfredson, L. S. (1986). Occupational Aptitude Patterns Map: Development and implications for a theory of job aptitude requirements. *Journal of Vocational Behavior, 29*, 254–291.

Grubb, W. N. (1995). Coherence for all students: High schools with career clusters and majors. In W. N. Grubb (Ed.), *Education through occupations in American high schools: Approaches to integrating academic and vocational education: Vol. 1* (pp. 97–113). New York: Teachers College Press.

Grusec, J. E., & Goodnow, J. J. (1994). Impact of parental discipline methods on the child's internalization of values: A reconceptualization of current points of view. *Developmental Psychology, 30*, 4–19.

Hallinan, M. (2005). The normative culture of a school and student socialization. In L. V. Hedges & B. Schneider (Eds.), *The social organization of schooling* (pp. 129–146). New York: Russell Sage.

Hallinan, M. T. (1990). The effects of ability grouping in secondary schools: A response to Slavin's best-evidence synthesis. *Review of Educational Research, 60*, 501–504.

Heller, R., & Greenleaf, C. L. (2007). *Literacy instruction in the content areas*. Washington, DC: Alliance for Excellent Education.

Holland, J. L. (1997). *Making vocational choices: A theory of vocational personalities and work environments* (3rd ed.). Odessa, FL: Psychological Assessment Resources.

Jencks, C. S. (1975). Effects of high schools on their students. *Harvard Educational Review, 45*(3), 273–324.

Johnson, D., & Johnson, R. (1985). Motivational process in cooperative, competitive, and individualistic learning situations. In C. Ames & R. Ames (Eds.), *Research motivation in education: Vol. II. The classroom milieu* (pp. 249–286). Orlando, FL: Academic.

Kemple, J., & Snipes, J. (2000). *Career academies: Impacts on student engagement and performance in high school*. New York: MDRC.

Kemple, J. J., Herlihy, C. M., & Smith, T. J. (2005). *Making progress toward graduation: Evidence from the Talent Development High School model*. New York: MDRC.

Kemple, J. J., & Willner, C. J. (2008). *Career academies: Long-term impacts on labor market outcomes, educational attainment, and transitions to adulthood*. New York: MDRC.

Kilpatrick, J. (2001). Where's the evidence? *Journal for Research in Mathematics Education, 32*(4), 421–427.

Lam, S., Cheng, R. W.-Y., & Ma, W. Y. K. (2009). Teacher and student intrinsic motivation in project-based learning. *Instructional Science, 37*(6), 565–578.

Lattimer, H. (2008). Challenging history: Essential questions in the social studies classroom. *Social Education, 72*(6), 326–329.

Lee, C. D., & Spratley, A. (2010). *Reading in the disciplines: The challenges of adolescent literacy*. New York: Carnegie Corporation of New York.

Lee, V., Bryk, A., & Smith, J. (1993). The organization of effective secondary schools. *Review of Research in Education, 19*, 171–268.

Lee, V. E. (2000). School size and the organization of secondary schools. In M. T. Hallan (Ed.), *Handbook of sociology of education* (pp. 327–344). New York: Kluwer Academic/Plenum.

Lee, V. E., & Ready, D. D. (2007). *Schools within schools*. New York: Teachers College Press.

Legters, N. E., Balfanz, R., Jordan, W. J., & McPartland, J. M. (2002). *Comprehensive reform for urban high school: A Talent Development approach*. New York: Teachers College Press.

Louis, K., & Marks, H. (1998). Does professional community affect the classroom? Teachers' work and student experiences in restructuring schools. *American Journal of Education, 106*, 532–575.

Lucas, S. R. (1999). *Tracking inequality: Stratification and mobility in American high schools*. New York: Teachers College Press.

Maxwell, N., & Rubin, V. (2000). *High school career academies: A pathway to educational reform in urban school districts*. Kalamazoo, MI: W.E. Upjohn Institute.

Mark, S. F. (1983). To succeed or not to succeed: A critical review of issues in learned helplessness. *Contemporary Educational Psychology, 8*(1), 1–19.

McPartland, J., Balfanz, R., Jordan, W., & Legters, N. (1998). Improving school climate and achievement in a troubled urban high school through the Talent Development Model. *Journal of Education for Students Placed at Risk, 3*(4), 337–361.

Midgley, C. (2001). A goal theory perspective on the current status of middle level schools. In T. Urdan & F. Pajares (Eds.), *Adolescence and education: Vol. I* (pp. 33–59). Greenwich, CT: Information Age Publishing.

National Association of Secondary School Principals. (1996). *Breaking ranks: Changing an American institution*. Reston, VA: NASSP.

National Association of Secondary School Principals. (2002). *What the research shows: Breaking ranks in education*. Reston, VA: NASSP.

National Council of Teachers of Mathematics. (2009). *Focus in high school mathematics: Reasoning and sense making*. Reston, VA: NCTM.

National Reading Panel. (2000). *Report of the National Reading Panel: Teaching people to read*. Washington, DC: National Institute of Child Health and Human Development.

National Research Council. (2000). *How people learn: Brain, mind, experience, and school, Expanded edition*. In J. D. Bransford, A. L. Brown, & R. R. Cocking (Eds.), Committee on Developments in the Science of Learning, Committee on Learning Research and Educational Practice, Commission on Behavioral and Social Sciences and Education. Washington, DC: National Academy Press.

National Research Council and the Institute of Medicine. (2004). *Engaging Schools: Fostering high school students' motivation to learn*. Committee on Increasing High School Students' Engagement and Motivation to Learn. Board on Children, Youth and Families, Division of Behavioral and Social Sciences and Education. Washington, DC: The National Academies Press.

Neild, R., Byrnes, V., & Sweet, T. (2010, March). *Early results from a randomized trial of two sequences for helping underprepared students to master algebra*. Paper presented at the Annual Conference of the Society for Research on Educational Effectiveness, Washington, DC.

Newman, F. (1992). *Student engagement and achievement in American secondary schools*. New York: Teachers College Press.

Nystrand, M., & Gamoran, A. (1992). Instructional discourse and student engagement. In D. H. Schunk & J. Meece (Eds.), *Student perceptions in the classroom* (pp. 149–179). Hillsdale, NJ: Lawrence Erlbaum.

Oakes, J., Gamoran, A., & Page, R. (1992). Curriculum differentiation: Opportunities, outcomes, and meanings. In P. Jackson (Ed.), *Handbook of research on curriculum* (pp. 570–608). New York: Macmillan.

Osher, D., Bear, G. G., Sprague, J. R., & Doyle, W. (2010). How can we improve school discipline? *Educational Researcher, 39*, 48–58.

Osterman, K. F. (2000). Students' need for belonging in the school community. *Review of Educational Research, 3*, 323–367.

Pearson, S. S. (2002). *Finding common ground: Service learning and education reform*. Washington, DC: American Youth Policy Forum.

Pintrich, P. R., & Schunk, D. H. (2002). *Motivation in education: Theory, research, and applications* (2nd ed.). Upper Saddle River, NJ: Merrill/Prentice-Hall.

Plank, S. (2001). *Career and technical education in the balance: An analysis of high school persistence, academic achievement, and post secondary destinations*. Minneapolis, MN: National Research Center for Career and Technical Education.

Pressley, M. (1998). *Reading instruction that works: The case for balanced teaching*. New York: Guilford Press.

Pressley, M. (2000). What should comprehension instruction be the instruction of? In M. L. Kamil, P. B. Mosenthal, P. D. Pearson, & R. Barr (Eds.), *Handbook of reading research: Vol. III* (pp. 545–561). Mahwah, NJ: Lawrence Erlbaum.

Resnick, L. B. (2010). Nested learning systems for the thinking curriculum. *Educational Researcher, 39*, 183–197.

Roderick, M., & Camburn, E. (1999). Risk and recovery from course failure in the early years of high school. *American Educational Research Journal, 36*(2), 303–343.

Rosenberg, M. S., & Jackman, L. A. (2003). Development, implementation, and sustainability of comprehensive school-wide behavior management systems. *Intervention in School and Clinic, 39*(1), 10–21.

Rottinghaus, P. J., Hees, C. K., & Conrath, J. A. (2009). Enhancing job satisfaction perspectives: Combining Holland themes and basic interests. *Journal of Vocational Behavior, 75*, 139–151.

Ryan, R. M., & Deci, E. L. (2000). Intrinsic and extrinsic motivations: Classic definitions and new directions. *Contemporary Educational Psychology, 25*, 54–67.

Schneider, B., & Stevenson, D. (1999). *The ambitious generation: America's teenagers, motivated but directionless*. New Haven, CT: Yale University Press.

Scott, S. (2007). Do grades really matter? *Maclean's, 120*(35/36), 70–74.

Shanahan, T., & Shanahan, C. (2008). Teaching disciplinary literacy to adolescents: Rethinking content-area literacy. *Harvard Educational Review, 78*(1), 40–59.

Shouse, R. D. (1997). Academic press, sense of community, and student achievement. In J. S. Coleman, B. Schneider, S. Plank, K. S. Schiller, R. Shouse, & H. Wang (Eds.), *Redesigning American education* (pp. 60–86). Boulder, CO: Westview Press.

Sinclair, M. F., Christenson, S. L., Evelo, D. L., & Hurley, C. M. (1998). Dropout prevention for youth with disabilities: Efficacy of a sustained school engagement procedure. *Exceptional Children, 65*(1), 7–21.

Skinner, B. F. (1953). *Science and human behavior*. New York: Macmillan.

Skinner, E. A., & Belmont, M. J. (1993). Motivation in the classroom: Reciprocal effects of teacher behavior and student engagement across the school year. *Journal of Educational Psychology, 85,* 571–581.

Slavin, R. E. (1990). Achievement effects of ability grouping in secondary schools: A best-evidence synthesis. *Review of Educational Research, 60,* 471–499.

Stern, D., Dayton, C., & Raby, M. (2010). *Career academies: A proven strategy to prepare high school students for college and careers.* Berkeley, CA: Career Academy Support Network.

Stern, D., Raby, M., & Dayton, C. (1992). *Career academies: Partnerships for reconstructing American high schools.* San Francisco: Jossey-Bass.

Trumbull, E., & Farr, B. (Eds.). (2000). *Grading and reporting student progress in an age of standards.* Portland, OR: Christopher-Gordon.

U.S. General Accounting Office. (1993). *School linked human services: A comprehensive strategy for aiding students at risk of school failure* (Report to the Chairman, Committee on Labor and Human Resources). Washington, DC: Department of Health and Human Services.

Webb, F. R., Covington, M. V., & Guthrie, J. W. (1993). Carrots and sticks: Can school policy influence student motivation? In T. M. Tomlinson (Ed.), *Motivating students to learn* (pp. 99–124). Berkeley, CA: McCutchan.

Wehlange, G. G., & Rutter, R. A. (1986). Dropping out: How much do schools contribute to the problem? *Teachers College Record, 87*(3), 374–392.

Wentzel, K. R. (1997). Student motivation in middle school: The role of perceived pedagogical caring. *Journal of Educational Psychology, 89,* 411–419.

Wentzel, K. R. (1998). Social relationships and motivation in middle school: The role of parents, teachers, and peers. *Journal of Educational Psychology, 90*(2), 202–209.

Wentzel, K. R. (2002). Are effective teachers like good parents? Teaching styles and student adjustment in early adolescence. *Child Development, 73,* 287–301.

Wentzel, K. R. (2009). Students' relationships with teachers as motivational contexts. In K. R. Wentzel & A. Wigfield (Eds.), *Handbook on motivation at school* (pp. 301–322). New York: Routledge.

Yore, L. D., Pimm, D., & Tuan, H. (2007). The literacy component of mathematical and scientific literacy. *International Journal of Science and Mathematics Education, 5*(4), 559–589.

Zimmerman, C. (2007). The development of scientific thinking skills in elementary and middle school. *Developmental Review, 27*(2), 172–223.

The Power of Mindsets: Nurturing Engagement, Motivation, and Resilience in Students

26

Robert Brooks, Suzanne Brooks, and Sam Goldstein

Abstract

In this chapter, three interrelated concepts—student engagement, motivation, and resilience—are examined through the lens of "mindsets." Mindsets are assumptions that we possess about ourselves and others that guide our behavior. The mindset that educators hold about the factors that contribute to student engagement, motivation, and resilience determines their expectations, teaching practices, and relationships with students. We identify the key components of these three concepts, highlighting those that overlap. We distinguish between extrinsic and intrinsic motivation and the ways in which the latter is more closely attuned with student engagement and resilience than the former. We encourage the ongoing discussion of mindsets at staff meetings so that teachers become increasingly aware of the mindset of engaged, motivated learners and consider how to nurture this mindset in the classroom. We offer many strategies to facilitate the enrichment of this mindset in all students.

In this chapter, we will describe the close link among three interrelated concepts: motivation, student engagement, and resilience. We will examine these concepts through the lens of "mindsets." Mindsets may be understood as assumptions that we possess about ourselves and others that guide our behavior. The mindsets that educators hold about the basic components of motivation and engagement will determine their expectations, teaching practices, and relationships with students (Brooks, 2001, 2004; Brooks & Goldstein, 2001, 2004, 2007, 2008; Goldstein & Brooks, 2007).

The concept of mindsets has become an increasingly prominent area of study, especially with the emergence of the field of "positive psychology." As examples, Carol Dweck authored a book titled *Mindset* (2006) in which she distinguished between a "fixed" and "growth" outlook; the research of Martin Seligman and his

R. Brooks (✉)
Department of Psychiatry, Harvard Medical School,
Boston, MA, USA
e-mail: contact@drrobertbrooks.com

S. Brooks
Weston Public Schools, Weston, MA, USA
e-mail: Suzbrooks@comcast.net; Brooks@mail.weston.org

S. Goldstein
University of Utah School of Medicine,
Salt Lake City, UT, USA
e-mail: info@samgoldstein.com; sam@samgoldstein.com

colleagues about "learned helplessness" and "learned optimism" as well as resilience (Reivich & Shatte, 2002; Seligman, 1990) have underpinnings in attribution theory, which is basically about mindsets, examining how we understand the reasons for our successes and setbacks (Weiner, 1974).

Educators bring assumptions about student behavior into all of their interactions with those in their classrooms and schools. The more aware they are of these assumptions, the more they can change those beliefs that may work against the creation of a positive classroom environment. Even those assumptions about which we may not be cognizant have a way of being expressed to students. For example, a teacher may be annoyed or frustrated with a child without realizing that the anger is rooted in the teacher's assumption that the child's constant asking of questions is an intentional ploy to distract the class. In addition, the teacher may not be aware that his annoyance is not as disguised as he believes and is being communicated through facial expressions and tone of voice.

In contrast, another teacher with the same student may assume that the child's ongoing questions represent an attempt to understand the material being presented. This teacher is more likely to express positive verbal and nonverbal messages and to offer assistance, perceiving the child as being vulnerable and motivated rather than being oppositional.

The impact that the mindset of educators has in determining their approach to students and the extent to which they nurture motivation, student engagement, and resilience is apparent in the following example:

> Parents of a high school student, John, contacted the first author several years ago. They asked Bob to serve as a consultant to John's school program. An earlier evaluation revealed that John was struggling with learning disabilities and academic demands. When Bob met with John's teachers and requested that they share their perceptions of him, one immediately responded with obvious anger, "John is one of the most defiant, oppositional, lazy, unmotivated, irresponsible students we have at this school!"
>
> Another teacher seemed surprised by the harshness of this assessment. In a manner that maintained respect of her colleague's opinion, she said, "I have a different view. I think John is really struggling with learning and he feels very vulnerable every day when he enters the school. I think that as a staff we should figure out a different way of teaching him because what we are doing now is a prescription for failure."

In listening to these two descriptions of the same student, one could not help but conclude that the teachers were offering opinions of two distinctly different youngsters. It would not be surprising to discover that these vividly contrasting opinions or mindsets and the teacher behaviors they triggered would likely contribute to John having markedly different mindsets and responses to each of these two teachers. In fact, this was the case.

After the meeting, Bob interviewed John and asked him to describe his teachers, not revealing what they had said about him. In describing the teacher who had portrayed him very negatively, John said with noticeable force, "She hates me, but that's okay because I hate her. And I won't do any work in her class."

John continued, "And don't tell me that I'm only hurting myself by not doing work (he must have heard that advice on numerous occasions). What you don't understand, Dr. Brooks, is that in her eyes I am a failure. Whatever I do in her class is never going to be good enough. She doesnt' expect me to pass, so why even try?" He said that from the first day of class he felt "angry vibes" from her.

She just didn't like me and soon I didn't like her. I could tell she didn't want me in her class just by the way she spoke to me. Right away she seemed so angry at me. I really don't know why she felt that way. So after a while I knew there was no way I could succeed in her class so I just decided that I wouldn't even try. It would just be a waste of time. She told me I was lazy, but if she was honest she would have to admit that she doesn't think I could ever get a good grade in her class.

John's face lit up as he described the teacher who thought that the primary issues that should be addressed were his struggles with learning and his sense of vulnerability. He said, "I love her. She went out of her way the first week of school to tell me something. She said that she knew I was having trouble with learning, but she thought I was smart and she had to figure out the best way to teach me. She said that one of the reasons she became a teacher was to help all students learn. She's always there to help."

In hearing John's perception or mindset of these two teachers, it is not difficult to appreciate why he was a discipline problem with the first teacher but not the second. His behavior with each of them reflected what he believed were their mindsets and expectations for him. We recognize that it typically takes "two to tango," and most likely at some point, John bore some responsibility for adding fuel to the "angry vibes," thereby confirming the first teacher's negative perceptions of him. However, it is essential for educators to identify and modify those features of their mindset that work against student motivation and student engagement and serve as barriers to students becoming more optimistic and resilient.

Guiding Questions for Consideration

Given the power of mindsets in determining the social-emotional and learning climate created in classrooms, several key questions can be raised:
- What are the characteristics of the mindset of students who are motivated and engaged?
- What are the characteristics of the mindset of resilient students? How do resilient students see themselves differently from their peers who are not resilient? In what ways does a "resilient mindset" overlap with the mindset of motivated, engaged students?
- What are the characteristics of the mindset of educators who are most effective in nurturing motivation, engagement, and resilience in students?
- What specific strategies or interventions can teachers with positive mindsets develop and implement to nurture motivation, engagement, and resilience in their classrooms?

To answer these questions, one must also examine the following related question:

What are the main components housed in the concepts of motivation, student engagement, and resilience?

Characteristics of Students

The Mindset of Engaged, Motivated Students

Goldstein and Brooks (2007) have identified five major characteristics of the mindset of motivated students. They include:
1. To perceive the teacher as a supportive adult. We place this first to capture the essential relationship that teachers form with students in promoting motivation. As has often been expressed, "Students don't care what you know until they first know you care." Motivated students feel that teachers genuinely care about them as individuals and want them to learn and to succeed (Klem & Connell, 2004; McCombs & Pope, 1994; Middleton & Pettit, 2010; Wagner, Kegan, Lahey, & Lemons, 2005). When struggling with an academic task or with nonacademic issues, the successful student feels comfortable in taking the initiative and asking the teacher for assistance. They do not perceive requesting help as a weakness, but rather as an integral feature of the classroom environment.
2. To believe that whether they learn as students is based in great part on their own motivation, perseverance, and effort (Adelman & Taylor, 1983; Brooks, 1991; Deci, Hodges, Pierson, & Tomassone, 1992; DiCintio & Gee, 1999; Seligman, 1995; Weiner, 1974). This does not minimize the role that teachers play, but if students do not view themselves as active participants in the learning process, but rather as passive recipients of what is being taught, their interest, enthusiasm, and involvement for learning will be greatly diminished.
3. To recognize that making mistakes and not immediately comprehending certain concepts or material are expected features of the learning process. Students who persist when confronted with challenging learning tasks are those who believe that mistakes serve as the basis for future learning and that mistakes invite new learning strategies (Andrews & Debus, 1978; Canino, 1981; Dweck, 1986, 2006). This outlook is in sharp contrast to students who interpret their mistakes as an indication that they are not very intelligent and thus, they are incapable of correcting the situation. If they believe that any efforts they make to learn will not eventuate in success, they will not persevere in that activity, demonstrating what Seligman (1990) labeled as "learned helplessness."
4. To have a clear understanding of their learning strengths and learning vulnerabilities. It is essential that learning strengths and vulnerabilities be identified for students (Levine, 2003).

As students gain insight into their learning profile, the more they can develop and apply effective strategies to learn successfully (Schunk & Rice, 1993). When students do not understand why they are struggling with learning or when they believe they are dumb or stupid or lazy, they are more vulnerable to engage in self-defeating ways of coping represented by noncompliant behaviors.
5. To treat classmates with respect and avoid teasing or bullying, recognizing that such behaviors work against a positive school climate and adversely affect the learning of all students (Davis, 2003; Olweus, 1994). Students must realize that maintaining a caring, respectful classroom and school is the responsibility of each member of that classroom and school.

The Mindset of Resilient Children and Adolescents

Brooks and Goldstein (2001) have defined resilience as the capacity to cope effectively and positively with past or present adversity. They have identified the outlook and skills associated with a "resilient mindset." They include:

1. To be able to set realistic goals and expectations for themselves.
2. To believe that they have the ability to solve problems and make thoughtful decisions and thus are more likely to view mistakes, setbacks, and obstacles as challenges to confront rather than as stressors to avoid.
3. To rely on effective coping strategies that promote growth and are not self-defeating.
4. To be aware of and not deny their weaknesses and vulnerabilities. They do not view these vulnerabilities as flaws but rather as areas for improvement. They also realistically accept when certain tasks may be beyond their abilities at the present time but open to change in the future.
5. To recognize, enjoy, and engage in their strong points and talents.
6. To possess a self-concept that is filled with images of strength and competence or what we have referred to as "islands of competence" (Brooks, 2004; Brooks & Goldstein, 2001).
7. To feel comfortable relating with others and to rely on effective interpersonal skills with peers and adults alike. This enables them to seek out assistance and nurturance in a comfortable, appropriate manner from adults who can provide the support they need.
8. To believe that there is a purpose to their existence and that they are making a positive difference in the lives of others.
9. To define the aspects of their lives over which they have control and to focus their energy and attention on those rather than on factors over which they have little, or any, influence.

Numerous researchers and clinicians have studied and articulated different features of this mindset (Masten, 2001; Masten & Coatsworth, 1998; Rutter, 1987; Seligman, 1995; Sheridan, Eagle, & Dowd, 2005; Shure, 1996, 2003; Werner & Smith, 1992, 2001; Wright & Masten, 2005). As will be apparent, many of these features overlap with those associated within the mindset of motivated learners.

It is our belief that educators can nurture mindsets associated with increased motivation, engagement, and resilience as a natural part of their classroom teaching practices. It is important to note that reinforcing social-emotional skills should not be perceived as an "extra curriculum" that ciphers already limited time from teaching academic subject matter. In fact, our position is that the more secure and engaged students are, the more motivated they will be to meet academic requirements.

Let us turn now to examining the concepts and components of motivation and student engagement before identifying the mindset and practices of teachers who are skilled in nurturing these qualities in students.

Motivation, Student Engagement, and Resilience

Motivation: Intrinsic or Extrinsic— Autonomous or Controlled

There is no simple answer to the question, "What is the relationship between student engagement and motivation?" As we shall see, not only is the concept of student engagement multidimensional (Appleton, Christenson, & Furlong, 2008; Appleton, Christenson, Kim, & Reschly, 2006; Christenson & Anderson, 2002) but so too is motivation, which without wishing to simplify things has primarily been cast as residing in two broad camps, namely, motivation that is intrinsically or extrinsically driven.

To capture the key dimensions of intrinsic and extrinsic motivation, psychologists Edward Deci and Richard Ryan at the University of Rochester in New York have advanced "self-determination theory" (SDT) (Deci & Flaste, 1995; Deci, Koestner, & Ryan, 2001; Deci & Ryan, 2000). Instead of the words intrinsic and extrinsic, they prefer to use the concepts autonomous and controlled.

They distinguish autonomous from controlled in the following way (Deci & Flaste, 1995):

> To be autonomous means to act in accord with one's self—it means feeling free and volitional in one's actions. When autonomous, people are fully willing to do what they are doing, and they embrace the activity with a sense of interest and commitment. Their actions emanate from their true sense of self so they are being authentic. In contrast, to be controlled means to act because one is being pressured. When controlled, people act without a sense of personal endorsement. Their behavior is not an expression of the self, for the self has been subjugated to the controls. In this condition, people can reasonably be described as alienated (p. 2).

As we attempt to understand the relationship between motivation and student engagement and consider the two main types of motivation spotlighted by Deci and Ryan, we might be better served to ask the questions, "Does intrinsic (autonomous) or extrinsic (controlled) motivation contribute more to the enrichment of student engagement? Or, is there any difference at all? Or can aspects of intrinsic motivation be applied even when extrinsic motivation is used?"

We would argue that the variables associated with intrinsic motivation are much more closely aligned with both student engagement and resilience than those embedded within extrinsic motivation. To take this argument a step further, it is our belief that practices predicated upon extrinsic motivation may, at times, actually work against students becoming more engaged with learning tasks or becoming more resilient unless features of intrinsic motivation are incorporated within the practices of extrinsic motivation.

Lepper, Greene, and Nisbett (1973) conducted a study in the early 1970s that generated much dialogue about those factors involved in motivating children to engage in particular activities. Their research is often cited in the literature about motivation, not simply as a result of the topic it examined, but because their findings were counterintuitive to what many anticipated.

Lepper, Greene, and Nisbett observed a preschool class and identified those children who chose to draw during their "free time" play. Then, they designed an experiment to discover what happens when you reward an activity that the children already enjoyed doing. The researchers divided the children into three groups. The first was called the "expected-award" group. They showed each of the children in this group a "Good Player" certificate featuring a blue ribbon and the child's name; they told these children that they would receive an award for drawing. The second group was designated the "unexpected award" group. These children were asked if they wanted to draw, and if they did, they were given one of the "Good Player" certificates when the session concluded. They did not know in advance that they would receive an award. The third group was the "no award" group. These preschoolers were asked if they wanted to draw, but they were neither promised a certificate prior to drawing nor given one at the end.

Two weeks later, the teachers of the preschoolers put out paper and markers during the "free play" period while the researchers secretly observed the students. A central question being studied was whether being involved in one of the three groups 2 weeks earlier would have any impact on the child's behavior now. If so, what would it be? One prediction was that an award given 2 weeks earlier would not impact appreciably or at all on the child's behavior today. Another possibility, strongly rooted in what Pink (2009) called "The Motivation 2.0 Operating System," would be that the children who received awards for engaging in drawing would display even greater interest in and motivation to draw since they were rewarded for that behavior. Motivation 2.0 is based on the premise that the way you motivate people to do what you want is to reward them for the behavior you seek and punish them for behavior you do not want to appear. It is predicated on extrinsic motivation.

The tenets of Motivation 2.0 would lead one to assume that those children told in advance they would receive a reward for drawing would be most motivated 2 weeks later to engage in this activity since it had been rewarded previously. This seemed to be a logical conclusion, based on the notion that providing external rewards for accomplishing particular tasks would increase involvement in these tasks. It was basically the model articulated by famed psychologist B. F. Skinner in which the occurrence of certain behaviors was either increased or decreased by the use of rewards and punishment.

However, what those subscribing to an extrinsic motivation model may have hypothesized was not in keeping with what Lepper, Greene, and Nisbett discovered. Children in the "unexpected-award" and "no award" groups drew just as much and with the same enthusiasm as they had before the experiment. But children in the first group—the ones who had expected and then been given an award—displayed much less interest and spent much less time drawing. Even 2 weeks later, the prizes—so common in many classrooms—had seemingly transformed play into work. It is important to point out that it was not necessarily the rewards themselves that reduced the children's interest since when children did not expect a reward, receiving one had little impact on their intrinsic motivation. Only *contingent* rewards—if you do this, then you will get that—had the negative effect.

The results of this study invite the question of why did not the so-called "extrinsic motivators" heighten interest in drawing? Also, do the results represent an anomaly not to be replicated in other studies? Pink (2009), in reviewing the literature, cited many other examples of the negative impact of rewarding particular behaviors.

An explanation for these unexpected findings may be found in the position advanced by Deci and Ryan (2000) who contended that there are three basic, innate, psychological needs that we all possess: the need to belong or feel connected, the need to feel competent, and the need for autonomy or self-determination. Deci and Ryan asserted that when these needs are satisfied, motivation and productivity are increased, but when they are not met, motivation and satisfaction are diminished.

Ryan observed, "This is a really big thing in management. When people aren't producing, companies typically resort to rewards or punishment. What they haven't done is the hard work of diagnosing what the problem is. You're trying to run over the problem with a carrot or a stick" (Pink, 2009, p. 72). Deci added that self-determination theory does not unequivocally oppose the use of rewards. "Of course, they're necessary in workplaces and other settings, but the less salient they are made, the better" (Pink, 2009, p. 72).

Pink (2009) summarized the limited conditions under which extrinsic motivation may be beneficial. "For routine tasks, which aren't very interesting and don't demand much creative thinking, rewards can provide a small motivational booster shot without harmful side effects. In some ways, that's just common sense" (p. 62). Pink recommended that even routine tasks can be made more enticing by lessening control and introducing autonomy. "Allow people to complete the task their own way. Think autonomy not control. State the outcome you need. But instead of specifying precisely the way to reach it, give them freedom over how they do the job" (2009, p. 64).

Appleton and colleagues (2008) captured the complexity of both SDT and the concepts of extrinsic and intrinsic motivation. They highlighted at least two features of SDT that are especially relevant for educators. First, similar to Pink's contention that even seemingly external demands can be offered in a way that provide a modicum of internal control, SDT posited that in those situations in which the catalyst for behavior is external to oneself, aspects of internal control can be established (Ryan & Deci, 2000). In support of this position, Appleton et al. wrote, "The theory (SDT) specifies qualitative differences in the level of self-determination associated with external motivation; situates these levels along a continuum; and contends that external expectations can be internalized, integrated, and result in highly autonomous functioning" (p. 378).

The second aspect of SDT Appleton et al. (2008) identified that is highly relevant for teaching practices is related to the first feature. It highlighted the importance of contextual factors and suggested that teachers have greater power than they may recognize to accentuate and reinforce autonomous behaviors in the school environment even when external demands appear to dominate the school arena. In the face of educational requirements and curricula that seem fixed or perhaps rigid, teachers are empowered to ask, "How can I implement teaching strategies that integrate intrinsic motivation principles within a more controlled environment?" This question encourages educators to reflect upon and appreciate the impact they have on enhancing student motivation and engagement even within a more restrictive educational milieu.

Appleton et al. (2008) provided some guidance for moving toward greater autonomy regardless of the environmental restraints. "Educators can facilitate student self-determination with extrinsically motivated tasks by using relationships, setting up students for success in course tasks (via scaffolding of lessons and attention to developmental level), and orchestrating student opportunities for decision making and other authentically autonomous experiences" (pp. 378–379). Support for this position is found in a number of research studies (Grolnick, Ryan, & Deci, 1991; Maehr & Meyer, 1997; Miserandino, 1996; Vansteenkiste, Simons, Lens, Sheldon, & Deci, 2004).

In considering SDT, Pink (2009) reframed to some extent Deci and Ryan's three basic needs of autonomy, belonging, and competence, casting autonomy as the essential component, but describing "mastery" and "purpose" as two other dimensions of intrinsic motivation. Mastery is viewed as the pleasure that accrues from being engaged in a task that is exciting and challenging. Csikszentmihalyi (1975, 1998) introduced the concept of *flow*, a state in which people are absorbed and challenged by what they are doing. A key quality producing *flow* is the level of the challenge of the task. A task that is either too easy or too difficult given the skills of the individual will not permit the experience of *flow* to emerge.

The concept of *flow* as proposed by Csikszentmihalyi is linked to both motivation and engagement and houses major implications for the teaching style and curriculum presented by teachers. If students are to experience flow, they must be challenged to move beyond their current levels of competence in activities that are interesting and relevant to them and that encourage their input and feedback.

In addition to autonomy and mastery, the third nutriment of motivation emphasized by Pink is purpose, which relates to commitment, meaning, and the belief that one's activities are of benefit to others. This sense of purpose and commitment has been identified as a notable feature of resilience (Rutter, 1980; Werner, 1993) and of a resilient mindset (see point #8 above and Brooks & Goldstein, 2001). As we shall see later in this chapter, purpose and commitment also serve as a foundation for becoming stress hardy (Kobasa, Maddi, & Kahn, 1982). Pink (2009) wrote, "Autonomous people working toward mastery perform at very high levels. But those who do so in the service of some greater objective can achieve even more. The most deeply motivated people—not to mention those who are most productive and satisfied—hitch their desires to a cause larger than themselves" (p. 133).

Earlier, we expressed our position that in comparison with extrinsic or controlled motivation, the components of intrinsic or autonomous motivation were most in accord with nurturing resilient, engaged students. Let us turn our attention to the concept of "student engagement" to understand the basis for this position.

Student Engagement: A Multidimensional Concept

Christenson and her colleagues articulated the various dimensions of engagement in schools and developed the Student Engagement Instrument (SEI) (Anderson, Christenson, Sinclair, & Lehr, 2004; Appleton et al., 2006,

2008; Christenson et al., 2008). They noted that the distinction between motivation and engagement remains an ongoing issue. As a point of illustration, they identified one conceptual framework in which motivation is cast in terms of the direction and intensity of one's energy (Maehr & Meyer, 1997). In this framework, motivation is linked to underlying psychological processes such as autonomy, belonging or connectedness, and competence and is perceived to answer the question of "why" for a given behavior.

In contrast, engagement has been described as "energy in action," the connection between person and activity (Russell, Ainley, & Frydenberg, 2005, p. 1), and reflects a person's active involvement in a task or activity. Appleton et al. (2006) wrote, "Although motivation is central to understanding engagement, the latter is a construct worthy of study in its own right" (p. 428).

Engagement, achievement, and school behavior were found to be associated with each other. Low student engagement heightened the likelihood of students dropping out of school. Check & Connect is one illustration of a targeted intervention program designed to promote student engagement (Appleton et al., 2006; Christenson & Thurlow, 2004; Sinclair, Christenson, & Thurlow, 2005). Key components of Check & Connect are closely related to the features of a resilient mindset, perhaps the most important of which is a mentor who works with students and their families for a minimum of 2 years. Mentors promote problem-solving skills, persistence, and learning within a supportive relationship. Mentors also focus on nurturing their mentee's sense of autonomy, belonging, and competence, which parallel the main ingredients of SDT proposed by Deci and Ryan (2000).

Finn (1989) advanced the view that engagement can be conceptualized as being comprised of two main components: behavioral (e.g., participation in school activities) and affective (e.g., identifying oneself with the school, having a sense of belonging and connectedness). More recent reviews of the literature have posited that engagement is made up of three variables: behavioral (e.g., appropriate demeanor, effort, active participation), cognitive (e.g., self-regulation, developing and adhering to learning goals), and emotional or affective (e.g., showing an interest in and positive attitude toward learning, having a sense of belonging and connectedness) (Fredricks, Blumenfeld, & Paris, 2004; Jimerson, Campos, & Greif, 2003).

Christenson and her colleagues (Betts, Appleton, Reschly, Christenson, & Huebner, 2010; Christenson & Anderson, 2002; Reschly & Christenson, 2006) proposed a taxonomy for defining student levels of engagement as well as for identifying the goodness of fit between the student, the learning environment, and factors that impact upon the fit. They viewed engagement as comprised of four subtypes: academic, behavioral, cognitive, and psychological. Appleton et al. (2006) elaborated on this taxonomy:

> There are multiple indicators for each subtype. For example, academic engagement consists of variables such as time on task, credits earned toward graduation, and homework completion, while attendance, suspensions, voluntary classroom participation, and extra-curricular participation are indicators of behavioral engagement. Cognitive and psychological engagement includes less observable, more internal indicators, such as self-regulation, relevance of schoolwork to future endeavors, value of learning, and personal goals and autonomy (for cognitive engagement), and feelings of identification or belonging, and relationships with teachers and peers (for psychological engagement) (p. 419).

Appleton et al. (2006) also emphasized the importance of the context in which these subtypes occur such as relationships with adults at school, encouragement from family members, and support from peers. In addition, they wrote that while the majority of research has been directed toward the academic and behavioral components of student engagement since they tend to lend themselves to more precise observation, "measuring cognitive and psychological engagement is relevant because there is an overemphasis in school practice on indicators of academic and behavioral engagement. Such overemphasis ignores the budding literature that suggests that cognitive and psychological engagement indicators are associated with positive learning outcomes, related to motivation, and increase in response to specific teaching strategies" (p. 431). The SEI was developed to

Table 26.1 Common components or beliefs (mindset) associated with student engagement, motivation, and resilience

- I believe that adults are encouraging and supportive rather than judgmental and accusatory
- I am connected to and welcome in the school environment
- My opinion is respected, that I have, within reason, some say or input into my own education
- I am accountable for my actions
- My interests and strengths ("islands of competence") are identified and reinforced
- Academic demands are challenging, but in keeping with my abilities; my teachers and I are aware of my learning strengths and vulnerabilities
- Mistakes are perceived as *expected* and *accepted*. I never feel criticized because of these mistakes, but rather I use mistakes as the basis for future learning
- I am provided with opportunities to contribute to the well-being of both the school community and beyond
- All members of the school community are respectful toward each other

measure both cognitive and psychological engagement, which has subsequently been labeled affective engagement (Appleton et al., 2008).

The International Center for Leadership in Education (ICLE), which researched and developed a model of teaching based on the concepts of rigor and relevance, advanced the view that student engagement is an essential underpinning of these dimensions of the learning process (Jones, Marrazo, & Love, 2007). Jones (2009) asserted that while student engagement is not an exact science, it can be planned, measured, and enriched. He described student engagement as the:

> Positive behaviors that indicate full participation by the student in the learning process. When students are engaged, we can hear, see, or feel their motivation in completing a task, taking pride in their work, or going beyond the minimum work required. Engaged students demonstrate a feeling of belonging by the way they act, the positive things they say about school, and through their passionate involvement in class activities (p. 1).

Based on a review of the literature and research conducted by ICLE, Jones identified those factors that contribute to a school milieu in which student engagement is nurtured. Many of these factors are similar to those described above for the mindset of motivated, resilient learners. They include:

1. Interactions between and among students, teachers, administrators, parents, etc., are respectful, collegial, and warm.
2. There is an atmosphere of mutual accountability; people feel a sense of responsibility to one another and to the larger school community.
3. Signs of positive community identity and a sense of belonging permeate the school.
4. Students take leadership roles in representing and "owning" the school, exhibiting energy and enthusiasm about their institution.
5. The physical space is clean and safe.
6. Regular forums, structures, and interactions acknowledge and celebrate school and individual success.
7. The school actively involves and engages family and community members in the life of the school.
8. The school promotes and supports student activism by helping students engage in community change (pp. 37–38).

Commonalities Among Motivation, Engagement, and Resilience

If educators are to nurture motivation, engagement, and resilience in students, they should attend to and reinforce the common components associated with the mindset of each of these concepts. There are many commonalities, especially if the underpinnings of intrinsic motivation as opposed to extrinsic motivation are used in the comparison. A summary of the common beliefs (mindset) are included in Table 26.1.

It is important to emphasize that each of the beliefs listed in Table 26.1 are part of the foundations of student engagement, motivation, and resilience. They are also part of a student's mindset and therefore open to reinforcement. Teachers who are most effective in reinforcing these beliefs in students and thereby creating a school climate in which motivation, engagement, and resilience are nurtured are guided by their own specific beliefs and mindsets, a topic to which we now turn.

Educators' Beliefs and Practices

The Mindset of Effective Educators

A consideration of the mindset of students who are motivated, engaged, and resilient invites several other questions, including two listed earlier: What are the characteristics of the mindset of educators who are most effective in nurturing motivation, engagement, and resilience in students? What specific strategies or interventions can teachers with positive mindsets develop and implement to nurture motivation, engagement, and resilience in their classrooms?

It is essential for educators to appreciate that the assumptions they hold for themselves and their students, often unstated, have profound influence in determining effective teaching practices, the quality of relationships with students, and the positive or negative climate that is created in the classroom and school building. It is also essential that teachers discuss and examine the mindsets of effective, motivated learners and consider how to nurture this mindset in the classroom.

The following are assumptions and beliefs held by educators about students that appear most likely to eventuate in practices that nurture student motivation, engagement, and resilience (Goldstein & Brooks, 2007):

1. To appreciate that they have a lifelong impact on students, including on their sense of hope and resilience.
2. To believe that the level of motivation and learning that occurs in the classroom and the behavior exhibited by students has as much, if not more, to do with the influence of teachers than what students might bring into the situation.
3. To believe that all students yearn to be successful, and if a student is not learning, educators must ask how they can adapt their teaching style and instructional material to meet student needs.
4. To believe that attending to the social-emotional needs of students is not an "extra curriculum" that draws time away from teaching academic subjects, but rather a significant feature of effective teaching that enriches learning.
5. To recognize that if educators are to relate effectively to students, they must be empathic, always attempting to perceive the world through the eyes of the student and considering the ways in which students view them.
6. To appreciate that the foundation for successful learning and a safe and secure classroom climate is the relationship that teachers forge with students.
7. To recognize that students will be more motivated to learn and more engaged in the classroom when they feel a sense of ownership or autonomy for their own education.
8. To understand that one of the main functions of an educator is to be a disciplinarian in the true sense of the word, namely, to perceive discipline as a teaching process rather than as a process of intimidation and humiliation. Disciplinary practices should reinforce self-discipline, which is a critical behavior associated with resilience.
9. To realize that one of the greatest obstacles to learning is the fear of making mistakes and feeling embarrassed or humiliated and to take active steps to minimize this fear.
10. To subscribe to a strength-based model, which includes identifying and reinforcing each student's "islands of competence."
11. To develop and maintain positive, respectful relationships with colleagues and parents.

Themes and Exercises to Nurture a Positive Mindset in Educators

Information can be imparted to teachers, and exercises can be introduced to articulate and reinforce these beliefs associated with nurturing student motivation, engagement, and resilience. The goal is for all faculty and staff in a school to share within reason a common perspective or mindset.

The following are suggested themes for discussion and exercises to facilitate this task:

The focus on a student's social/emotional development and well-being is not an extra curriculum that takes time away from teaching academic skills and content. As we noted earlier in this chapter, it is unfortunate that a dichotomy has arisen in many educational quarters prompting some educators to perceive that attending to a student's emotional and social health is mutually exclusive from the goal of teaching academic material. This dichotomy has been fueled, in part, by the emergence of high stakes testing and an emphasis on accountability. The following refrain is heard in many schools: "We barely have time to get through the assigned curriculum. We really don't have the time to focus on anything else."

We are not opposed to assessment or accountability. We welcome research conducted to define effective teaching practices. However, what we question is relegating a student's emotional life to the background and not appreciating its important role in the process of learning. This attitude was captured at one of our workshops. A high school science teacher challenged our viewpoint by contending: "I am a science teacher. I know my science and I know how to convey science facts to my students. Why should I have to spend time thinking about a student's emotional or social life? I don't have time to do so and it will distract me from teaching science."

While many teachers and school administrators would take issue with the views expressed by this science teacher, others might not. We believe that strengthening a student's feeling of well-being, self-esteem, and dignity is not an extra curriculum. If anything, a student's sense of belonging, security, and self-confidence in the classroom provides the scaffolding that supports the foundation for enhanced learning, engagement, motivation, self-discipline, responsibility, and the ability to deal more effectively with obstacles and mistakes (Brooks, 1991, 2004; Cohen, 2006; Cohen & Sandy, 2003; Elias, Zins, Graczyk, & Weissberg, 2003).

To highlight this point, educators can be asked to reflect on their own teachers and think about those from whom they learned most effectively. It has been our experience that the teachers they select are those who not only taught academic content but, in addition, supported the emotional well-being of students and were interested in the "whole child." Very importantly, as educators reflect upon their teachers as well as their own teaching practices, they can be asked to consider the following question: "Do you believe that developing a positive relationship with your students enhances or detracts from teaching academic material? Please offer examples."

Examples should be encouraged whether the answer is yes, no, or maybe. It is important for educators to give serious consideration to this question. In our experience, most educators are able to offer examples of "small gestures" on their part (or on the part of their teachers) that took little, if any, time, but communicated to students a message of respect and caring (Brooks, 1991). If teachers contend they would like to develop more meaningful relationships with students, but are unable to allot the time to do so, other educators who have been able to accomplish this task can offer specific suggestions.

Educators have a lifelong impact on students and their resilience. Closely associated with this previous point is the belief of teachers that what they say and do each day in their classroom can have a lifelong influence on their students (Brooks, 1991; Brooks & Goldstein, 2001). While most teachers appreciate that they are and will continue to be influential in the lives of their students for years to come, many are not aware of the extent of their impact.

It is important that teachers are acquainted with research findings from the resilience literature to highlight this impact. Such knowledge will add meaning and purpose to their role as teachers and lessen disillusionment and burnout. In the past 25 years, there has been an increased effort to define those factors that help children and adolescents to deal more effectively with stress, to overcome adversity, and to become resilient (Brooks, 1994; Brooks & Goldstein, 2001; Goldstein & Brooks, 2005; Katz, 1997; Werner & Smith, 1992). We highlight that schools have been spotlighted as environments in which self-esteem, hope, and resilience can be fortified, frequently quoting the late psychologist Julius Segal (1988) who wrote:

> From studies conducted around the world, researchers have distilled a number of factors that enable such children of misfortune to beat the heavy odds against them. One factor turns out to be the presence in their lives of a charismatic adult—a person with whom they can identify and from whom they gather strength. And in a surprising number of cases, that person turns out to be a teacher (p. 3).

It is important for teachers to recognize that they are in a unique position to be a "charismatic adult" in a student's life and that even seemingly small gestures can have a lifelong impact. A smile, a warm greeting, a note of encouragement, a few minutes taken to meet alone with a student, and an appreciation of and respect for different learning styles are but several of the activities that define a "charismatic teacher" (Brooks, 1991).

Teachers are often unaware that they are or have been "charismatic adults" in the life of a student. To emphasize this issue, faculty can be asked if they have ever received unexpectedly, a note from a former student thanking them for the positive impact they had on the student's life. While many have been fortunate to be the recipient of such a note, others have not although they are equally deserving of such feedback.

We frequently ask participants at our workshops if there are teachers who had a significant influence on their lives whom they have failed to acknowledge via a note or letter. It is not unusual for many teachers to voice regret they have not thanked several such "charismatic adults." Some have written notes to the latter following the workshop.

We use these exercises to suggest that while we may not receive formal confirmation that we have worn the garb of "charismatic adults," if we approach each day with the belief that today may be the day we say or do something that directs a student's life in a more positive path, we will be more optimistic about our role, and our students will be the beneficiaries of more realistic, hopeful expectations. The belief that we can serve as "charismatic adults" serves as one of the major motivating forces described by Pink (2009) in his elaboration of SDT, namely, the existence of "purpose" in our lives.

All students wish to learn and to succeed, and if they seem unmotivated or disengaged, they may believe they lack the ability to achieve in school. We often hear teachers refer to students as lazy or unmotivated. As we have noted, once these accusatory labels are used and a negative mindset dominates, educators are more likely to respond to these students with annoyance. The mindset of an effective educator constantly echoes, "I believe that all students come to school desiring to learn. If they are disinterested and feel defeated, we must figure out how best to reach and teach them."

Subscribing to this view has a profound impact on the ways in which we respond to students, especially those who are struggling. When students lose faith in their ability to learn and when feelings of hopelessness pervade their psyche, they are vulnerable to engaging in counterproductive or self-defeating ways of coping. They may quit at tasks, clown around, pick on other students, or expend little time and effort in academic requirements. When a student feels that failure is a foregone conclusion, it is difficult to muster the energy to consider alternative ways of mastering learning demands.

Teachers who observe such counterproductive behaviors may easily reach the conclusion that the student is unmotivated or lazy, or not caring about school. As negative assumptions and mindsets dominate, teachers are less likely to consider more productive strategies for reaching the student. Instead, thoughts turn to punitive actions; for example, what punishments would finally get through to the student. However, if educators subscribe to the belief that each student wishes to succeed, negative assumptions are less likely to prevail.

A shift in perspective was obvious in a consultation Bob did about Sarah, a problematic high school student. One of her teachers began by asking, "Don't you think it's okay for a 16 1/2-year-old to drop out of school?" The agenda was clear. These teachers, who typically displayed a caring and encouraging attitude, were very frustrated and angry with Sarah to the extent of wishing her to drop out of school. The teachers elaborated that Sarah was a student who "sabotaged" all of their efforts. "Even if Sarah agrees to do something, she doesn't follow through. It's obvious that she dislikes school and she's disruptive and disrespectful. She couldn't care less about how she does in school."

As we shall see, Sarah cared a great deal about wanting to achieve in school, but entertained little hope for doing so. It was only when her teachers truly accepted that each student desperately wants to succeed that a positive mindset emerged, which permitted them to consider new solutions. A turning point occurred when Bob empathized with the teachers about their frustration but then asked, "Can anyone tell me how you think Sarah feels each day when she enters the school building?"

After several moments of silence, one teacher responded, "How Sarah feels. I never really thought about that before." Another teacher followed, "I never really thought about that before either, but as I'm doing so now, only one word comes to mind, defeated. I think everyday when Sarah comes in to the school building she feels defeated."

As this teacher shared her observation, the shift in mindset that permeated the room was palpable, highlighted by one teacher asking Bob, "You've written a lot about helping kids be more confident and resilient in the school setting. So what can we do to help a student who feels defeated begin to feel less defeated?" A lively, creative discussion ensued, filled with ideas that had not been considered previously, including having Sarah, who relished being helpful, assist in the office. The teachers also shifted their focus from what punitive action to take to a desire to "get to know" Sarah, not via a tense, confrontational meeting but rather by having lunch with her.

This new approach prompted Sarah to be more responsible, and a positive cycle was set in motion. The catalyst for this new cycle was when her teachers shifted their mindset, no longer viewing Sarah's behaviors as oppositional, but rather as a reflection of the despair and defeatism she experienced. They adopted the assumption that students wish to succeed, but at times, obstacles appear on the road to success—obstacles that teachers working in concert with students could remove.

If our strategies are not effective, we must ask, "What is it that I can do differently?" rather than continuing to wait for the student to change first. A basic underpinning of motivation and resilience is the belief of "personal control," namely, that we are the "authors of our own lives," and it makes little sense to continue to do the same thing repeatedly if our actions are not leading to positive results (Brooks & Goldstein, 2004). While many educators and others say they subscribe to this assumption, their actions frequently belie their assertion. For example, it is not unusual to hear the following statements offered by educators at consultations we have conducted: "This student is unmotivated to change. She just won't take responsibility for her behavior."

Or, "We've been using this strategy with this student for five months. He's still not responding. He's resistant and oppositional." We believe in perseverance, but if a staff has been employing the same approach for 5 months without any positive outcome, one can ask, "Who are the resistant ones here?"

As one perceptive teacher emphasized, "Asking what is it that we can do differently should not be seen as blaming ourselves but rather as a source of empowerment." She continued, "Isn't it better to focus on what we can do differently rather than continue to wait for someone else to change first? We may have to wait forever and continue to be frustrated and unhappy." This same teacher summarized her belief with the statement, "If the horse is dead, get off." We have found that there are many dead horses strewn on the grounds of a school.

The assumption of personal control should be addressed directly at staff meetings. Teachers should recognize that a change in strategy on their part is not the equivalent of "giving in" (this is a belief that often crops up), but rather as a sign that we are seeking a more productive intervention. If change on a teacher's part is interpreted as acquiescing to the student, any new strategy will be tainted by feelings of resentment.

A helpful exercise to illustrate the power of personal control and the need to change "negative scripts" that exist in our lives is to ask educators to think about one or two instances when they changed their usual script and to consider what resulted as a consequence of their new script. Many educators, such as those involved with Sarah, are able to describe very positive results. Unfortunately, others report less satisfactory results, often believing that they had gone out of their way for students, but the students did not reciprocate. When the outcome of a change in script is not positive, a problem-solving attitude should be introduced by asking, "With hindsight, is there anything you would do differently today to lessen the probability of an unfavorable result?"

The possibility that a modification of a script may not eventuate in a positive outcome should be addressed. When a new script is implemented, educators should have one or two backup scripts in mind should the first prove ineffective. Having a backup script conveys the positive message that if a strategy that sounds promising does not yield the results we wish, rather than feel exasperated or defeated, we should learn from the experience and be prepared with alternative actions. We must keep in mind that a new script may create the conditions that encourage students to change their behaviors.

Empathy is an essential skill for effective teaching and relationships with students as well as parents and colleagues. Empathic educators are able to place themselves inside the shoes of their students and others and perceive the world through their eyes, just as Sarah's teachers attempted to do, eventually understanding that she felt defeated. Goleman (1994) highlighted empathy as a major component of emotional intelligence.

Being empathic invites educators to ask, "Would I want anyone to say or do to me what I have just said or done to this student (or parent or colleague)?" or "Whenever I say or do things with students (parents or colleagues), what is my goal and am I saying or doing these things in a way that my students will be most likely to hear and respond constructively to my message?"

As an example, a teacher may attempt to motivate a student who is not performing adequately by exhorting the student to "try harder." While the teacher may be well-intentioned, the comment is based on the assumption that the student is not willing to expend the time and energy necessary to succeed. Thus, such a remark is frequently experienced as accusatory and judgmental. When students feel accused, they are less prone to be cooperative. Consequently, the teacher's comment is not likely to lead to the desired results, which, in turn, may reinforce the teacher's belief that the student is unmotivated and not interested in "trying." In contrast, an empathic teacher might wonder, "If I were struggling in my role as a teacher, would I want another teacher or my principal to say to me, 'If you just tried a little harder you wouldn't have this problem'?" When we have offered this question at workshops, many teachers laugh and say they would be very annoyed if they were accused of not trying. The question prompts them to reflect upon how their statements are interpreted by their students.

There are several exercises that can be introduced at staff meetings to reinforce empathy. A favorite is to have teachers think of a teacher they liked and one that they did not like when they were students and then to describe each in several words. Next, they can be reminded, "Just as you have words to describe your teachers, your students have words to describe you." They can then consider these questions: What words would you hope your students used to describe you? What have you done in the past month so they are likely to use these words? What words would they actually use to describe you? How close would the words you hope they use parallel the words they would actually use? (One teacher jokingly said, "I would love my students to use the word 'calm,' but I don't think they would since I feel I have been raising my voice a great deal the past month or two and not showing much patience").

Another exercise that educators have found useful in reinforcing empathy revolves around our own memories of school. Teachers can be requested

at workshops to share with their colleagues their response to the following questions:
- Of all of the memories you have as a student, what is one of your favorite ones, something that a teacher or school administrator said or did that boosted your motivation and self-dignity?
- Of all of the memories you have as a student, what is one of your worst ones, something that a teacher or school administrator said or did that lessened your motivation and self-dignity?
- As you reflect upon both your positive and negative memories of school, what did you learn from both, and do you use these memories to guide what you are doing with your students today?

Recounting one's own positive and negative memories of school with one's colleagues often proves very emotional and leads teachers to ask: What memories are my students taking from their interactions with me? Are they the memories I would like them to take? If not, what must I change so that the memories they will take will be in accord with the memories I hope they take? These exercises to nurture empathy often prompt teachers to consider how best to obtain feedback from students to gain a realistic picture of how they are perceived. We will address this question in the next point.

Ongoing feedback and input from students enhances empathy and promotes a sense of engagement, responsibility, and ownership in students. Effective teachers not only welcome the input of students, but they appreciate that such input must be incorporated on a regular basis. When students feel their voice is being heard, they are more likely to be engaged in academic requirements, work more cooperatively with teachers, and demonstrate greater motivation to meet academic challenges. Eliciting student opinion reinforces a feeling of personal control and responsibility—essential ingredients of a positive school climate; encouraging student input is also a basic feature of motivation, engagement, and resilience (Adelman & Taylor, 1983; Cohen, 2006; Deci et al., 1992; DiCintio & Gee, 1999; Henderson & Milstein, 1996; Jacobson, 1999; Thomsen, 2002).

There are various ways for teachers to obtain student feedback and input. For instance, teachers can request anonymous feedback from students. One high school teacher asked students to draw him, describe him, list what they liked about his teaching style and the class, and what they would recommend he change. While one of his colleagues scoffed at this practice, contending that such feedback was not important and took valuable time from teaching, the outcome of the exercise proved the colleague wrong. The exercise actually increased achievement scores and cooperation; this was not surprising since the students felt respected. Another teacher requested that students complete a one-page report card about him whenever he filled out report cards on them. The students actually developed the report card, which evaluated the teacher on such dimensions as discipline style, response to student questions, teaching style, and fairness toward all students. Recommendations for change were elicited.

Ownership in students can also be reinforced by engaging students in a discussion about the benefits or drawbacks of educational practices that are typically seen as "givens," including such activities as tests, reports, and homework. In addition, educators can strengthen a feeling of student ownership by incorporating a variety of choices in the classroom, none of which diminishes a teacher's authority but rather empowers students to feel a sense of control over their own education.

Choice and ownership can also be applied to disciplinary practices by asking students to consider such questions as:
- What rules do you think we need in this classroom for all students to feel comfortable and learn best? (It is not unusual for teachers to report that the rules recommended by students often parallel those of the teacher).
- Even as your teacher, I may forget a rule. If I do, this is how I would like you to remind me. (Teachers can then list one or two ways they would like to be reminded). Now that I have mentioned how I would like to be reminded, how would you like me to remind you? (When students inform teachers how they would like to be reminded should they forget a rule, they

are less likely to experience the reminder as a form of nagging and more likely to hear what the teacher has to say. It is easier for students to consider ways of being reminded if teachers first serve as models by offering how they would like to be reminded).

- What should the consequences be if we forget a rule? (We have heard teachers report, especially when asking these questions to angry students, that the consequences suggested by the students are more severe than any teacher would use).

These questions pertaining to disciplinary practices encourage a sense of ownership for rules and consequences, thereby promoting responsibility and self-discipline in students.

The second author regularly reinforces a sense of control in her therapy sessions with children who have problems in school. For instance, Anna, an 8-year-old, was burdened by social anxiety. Although she was willing to talk with Suzanne about her interests, she became frozen whenever the discussion turned to friends and school. Her teacher told Suzanne that Anna frequently struggles to enter groups of two or more children, particularly on the school playground. Suzanne applied a very effective, well-known therapeutic technique involving the use of "displacement." She told Anna that she knew a little boy who was having a problem talking with friends and did not know how to help him. Anna immediately replied, "Does he have a hard time on the playground?" Suzanne responded, "Yes, the playground is where he has the most trouble."

Anna continued, "Is he scared to talk with other children?" Eventually, the discussion led her to assert, "I think he might be worried they will make fun of him."

Once this worry was verbalized, Suzanne engaged Anna in considering strategies for helping the boy deal with his problems, which, of course, were the same strategies that Anna could implement to deal with her own problems. In essence, Anna was placed in a position of control, which encouraged her to discuss her own struggles more directly, leading to a lessening of her anxiety.

Each student has different "islands of competence" and learning styles that must be identified, respected, and reinforced. This belief is at the core of a strength-based approach to education and overlaps with many of the other points reviewed in this chapter. Effective teachers appreciate that one must move beyond a philosophy that fixates on a student's problems and vulnerabilities and affords equal, if not greater space, to strengths and competencies.

Researchers and clinicians have emphasized the significance of recruiting selected areas of strength or "islands of competence" in building self-confidence, motivation, and resilience (Deci & Flaste, 1995; Katz, 1994; Rutter, 1985). Rutter, in describing resilient individuals, observed, "Experiences of success in one arena of life led to enhanced self-esteem and a feeling of self-efficacy, enabling them to cope more successfully with the subsequent life challenges and adaptations" (p. 604). Katz noted, "Being able to showcase our talents, and to have them valued by important people in our lives, helps us to define our identities around that which we do best" (p. 10).

Understanding How You Learn Best

One of the most obvious guideposts for assisting students to feel competent is to teach them in ways in which they can learn best. Educators must appreciate that each student has different learning strengths and vulnerabilities (Gardner, 1983; Levine, 2002). This requires that teachers familiarize themselves with such topics as multiple intelligences and learning styles.

At the beginning of the school year, teachers can meet with each student for a few minutes and ask, "What are you interested in? What do you like to do? What do you think you do well?" While some students will respond eagerly, others may simply say, "I don't know." In that case, teachers can respond, "That's okay, it often takes time to figure out what you're good at. I'll try to be of help."

When the second author evaluates students referred for learning difficulties, she always asks them how they prefer to learn. Some students are not able to answer immediately, and many are surprised by the question, perhaps expecting that testing will only highlight their weaknesses. To encourage students to reflect upon their learning style, Suzanne often raises more specific questions. For example, she asked Noah, a 15-year-old high school freshman who was described by his parents as "highly intelligent and curious but completely unmotivated in school and often distracted in class," if he had ever gone on a trip that he really enjoyed and still thinks about.

Noah's expression, which had previously been rather flat and tired looking, lit up as he began to describe his trip to China with his family last summer. He talked about the landscape, the culture, and the people with much excitement. Suzanne used his response to discuss the different ways we learn and to note that he appeared to be an "experiential learner." Noah, with obvious excitement in his voice, said, "That's it. Is that why I'm so bored in class all the time?" Suzanne explained that although most of our learning occurs in the classroom, we could consider ways to supplement his learning with hands-on experiences once he reaches high school to make school feel less boring. Noah loved this idea, and as it turned out, the high school he will attend has a practicum option for students, which connects what they are learning in the classroom with real-life experiences. By asking Noah how he learned best, Suzanne was not only able to understand his struggles more clearly but in addition was able to develop a plan that would in essence adapt more traditional teaching methods to fit with his learning style. By encouraging his input, she also reinforced his sense of ownership in the school environment.

A high school teacher noted that given all of the students attending his classes, he did not have the time to meet with each individually at the beginning of the year. Instead, he devised a questionnaire that he sent out to each student a week before school began. He told them that it was not mandatory that they complete the questionnaire, but if they did, it would help him to be a more effective teacher. The questionnaire focused on a number of areas, several of which asked students to list what they perceived to be their strengths and weaknesses and how they learned best. In the 7 years in which he has sent out the questionnaire, not one student has failed to return it. This teacher found the information he obtained to be an invaluable resource in connecting with students.

Providing Opportunities to Help Others

Another strategy to enhance a sense of competence is to provide students with an opportunity to help others. Students experience a more positive attachment to school and are more motivated to learn if they are encouraged to contribute to the school milieu (Brooks, 1991; Rutter, 1980; Werner, 1993). Examples include older students with learning problems reading to younger children; a hyperactive child being asked to assume the position of "attendance monitor," which involved walking around the halls to take attendance of teachers while the latter were taking attendance of students; and the use of cooperative learning in which students of varying abilities work together as a team bringing their own unique strengths to different projects.

Lessening the Fear of Failure

One of the most powerful approaches for reinforcing a feeling of competence in students is to lessen their fear of failure. Many students equate making mistakes with feeling humiliated and, consequently, will avoid learning tasks that appear very challenging. There are students who would rather be bullies or quit at tasks or assert the work is dumb rather than engage in a learning activity that they feel may result in failure and embarrassment. In a desperate attempt to avoid failure, they journey down a path that takes them farther away from possible success.

The fear of making mistakes and failing permeates every classroom, and if it is not actively addressed, it remains an active force, compromising the joy and enthusiasm that should be part of the learning process. Effective educators can begin to overcome the fear of failure by identifying and openly addressing it with students. One technique for doing so is for teachers to ask their class at the beginning of the school year, "Who feels they are going to make a mistake and not understand something in class this year?" Before any of the students can respond, teachers can raise their hand as a way of initiating a discussion of how the fear of making mistakes affects learning.

It is often helpful for teachers to share some of their own anxieties and experiences about making mistakes when they were students. They can recall when they were called upon in class, when they made mistakes, or when they failed a test. This openness often invites students to share some of their thoughts and feelings about making mistakes. Teachers can involve the class in problem solving by encouraging them to suggest what they can do as teachers and what the students can do as a class to minimize the fear of failure and appearing foolish. Issues of being called on and not knowing the answer can be discussed.

One middle school English teacher frequently uses a method he refers to as "playing dumb" when he is seeking their responses to a book that was read. He starts by saying, "I completely forgot what happens in the end, does anyone remember?" He has found that this question is typically followed by an enthusiastic show of hands with students explaining the ending to their teacher. Although his questioning may seem contrived, this technique empowers students to take risks through the acknowledgement that even teachers can forget information and make mistakes. Effective teachers recognize that when the fear of failure and humiliation are actively addressed in the classroom, students will be more motivated to take realistic risks and to learn.

To realize that one must strive to become stress hardy rather than stressed out. At the conclusion of one of our workshops, a teacher said, "I love your ideas, but I'm too stressed out to use them." While the remark had a humorous tone, it also captured an important consideration.

At first glance, the remark seems paradoxical since numerous educators have informed us that the strategies we advocate do not take time away from teaching, but rather help to create a classroom environment that is more conducive to learning and less stressful. Yet, we can appreciate their frustration that change requires additional time, a commodity that is not readily available.

Some are hesitant to leave their "comfort zone" even when this zone is filled with stress and pressure. They would rather continue with a known situation that is less than satisfying than engage in the task of entering a new, unexplored territory that holds promise but also uncertainty.

If educators are to be effective in applying many of the ideas described in this chapter for nurturing motivation, engagement, and resilience in students, they must venture from their "comfort zone" by utilizing techniques for dealing with the stress and pressure that are inherent in their work. Each teacher can discover his or her own ways for managing stress. For instance, some can rely on exercise, others on relaxation or meditation techniques, all of which can be very beneficial. In addition to these approaches, there has been research conducted by Kobasa and her colleagues (Kobasa et al., 1982; Kobasa & Puccetti, 1983) under the label of "stress hardiness" that examines the characteristics or mindset of individuals who experience less stress than their colleagues while working in the same environment. Kobasa's work has been applied to the teaching profession (Holt, Fine, & Tollefson, 1987; Martinez, 1989).

This mindset involves three interrelated components: commitment, challenge, and control ("3Cs"). When we describe them at our workshops, we encourage educators to reflect upon how they might apply this information to lessen stress and burnout.

The first C represents "commitment." Stress-hardy individuals do not lose sight of why they are doing what they are doing. They maintain a genuine passion or purpose for their work, which as we have seen is a critical dimension of intrinsic motivation. While we may all have "down" days, it is sad to observe educators who basically say to themselves each morning in a resigned way, "I've got to go to school. I've got to see those kids." Once a feeling of "I've got to" or "being forced to" pervades one's mindset, a sense of commitment and purpose is sacrificed, replaced by feelings of stress and burnout. As an antidote to burnout, a staff meeting might be dedicated to sharing why one became a teacher, a school administrator, a counselor, a nurse, or a psychologist. Such an exercise helps staff to recall and invigorate their dreams and goals.

The second C is for "challenge." Educators who deal more effectively with stress have developed a mindset that views difficult situations as opportunities for learning and growth rather than as stress to avoid. For example, a principal of a school faced a challenging situation. Her school was located in a neighborhood that had changed in a few short years from a middle class population with much parent involvement to a neighborhood with a lower socioeconomic makeup and less parent involvement. There were several key factors that contributed to the decrease in parent involvement, including less flexibility for many parents to leave work in order to attend a school meeting or conference as well as many parents feeling unwelcome and anxious in school based upon their own histories as children in the school environment.

Instead of bemoaning this state of affairs and becoming increasingly upset and stressed, this particular principal and her staff realized that the education of their students would be greatly enhanced if parents became active participants in the educational process; consequently, they viewed the lack of involvement as a challenge to meet rather than as a stress to avoid. Among other strategies, they scheduled several staff meetings in the late afternoon and moved the site of the meetings from the school building to a popular community house a few blocks away. These changes encouraged a number of the parents to attend the meetings since the new time was more accommodating to their schedules and the new location helped them to feel more comfortable since it was held on their "turf." The relationship between parents and teachers was greatly enhanced, and the children were the beneficiaries.

The third C is "control" or what we earlier referred to as "personal control" since some individuals may mistakenly view the word control as a form of controlling others. Control, as used in stress hardiness theory, implies that individuals who successfully manage stress and pressure focus their time and energy on factors over which they have influence rather than attempting to change things that are beyond their sphere of control. Although many individuals believe they engage in activities over which they have influence or control, in fact, many do not. We worked with a group of teachers who were feeling burned out. We reviewed the basic tenets of stress hardiness theory and asked if they focused their energies on factors within their domain of control. They replied in the affirmative.

We then asked them to list what would help their jobs to be less stressful. Their answers included, "If the students came from less dysfunctional families, if they came to school better prepared to learn, if they had more discipline at home." After a few moments, one of the teachers smiled and said, "We first said that we focus on what we have control over, but everything that we are mentioning to help us feel less stressed are things over which we have little control." After the teacher said this, the group engaged in a lively discussion focusing on what educators might do to create classroom climates that nurtured learning and engagement even if the students came from home environments that were less than supportive of education. One teacher astutely noted, "We are expecting our students to come to school excited about learning and when they do not we get frustrated and annoyed. Instead, what I'm hearing is that we must ask, 'What can we do differently to help motivate students who are not motivated and what can we do to help students who feel hopeless about learning to feel more hopeful? As the discussion continued, the teachers recognized that by focusing on what they could do differently to improve the learning environment was empowering and lessened stressful feelings. The mood of pessimism and burnout that had pervaded the room began to change.

Concluding Thoughts

The concept of mindsets can help us to understand the underpinnings of three interrelated concepts: motivation, student engagement, and resilience. Future research can evaluate the outcome of implementing within the school culture different components of the mindset that cut across these three concepts. For instance, educators can examine the impact of introducing a mentoring system and the specific activities of the mentors (such as offered by the Check & Connect program; Sinclair et al., 2005), increasing student input and ownership by having students regularly attend parent-teacher conferences, or engaging students to contribute to the welfare of others.

When these interventions are introduced, researchers can study changes in a number of variables including: learning and achievement, student attendance, dropout rates, acts of bullying, occurrence of behavioral problems, and teacher retention. Well-researched and field-tested assessment instruments such as the Comprehensive School Climate Inventory (CSCI) developed by the National School Climate Center (formerly the Center for Social and Emotional Education [CSEE]) can be used to obtain input from students, parents, and school personnel to measure changes in school climate when mindsets for motivation, student engagement, and resilience are reinforced in a systematic way (Cohen, 2006).

The more aware educators are of the mindset of motivated, engaged, resilient students and the more aware they are of their own mindset, the more capable they will be in implementing strategies to develop this mindset in all students. The result will be classroom environments filled with excitement, safety, eagerness to learn, engagement, self-discipline, respect, and resilience. Both faculty and students will thrive in such an environment.

References

Adelman, H. S., & Taylor, L. (1983). Enhancing motivation for overcoming learning and behavior problems. *Journal of Learning Disabilities, 16*, 384–392.

Anderson, A. R., Christenson, S. L., Sinclair, M. F., & Lehr, C. A. (2004). Check & Connect: The importance of relationships for promoting engagement with school. *Journal of School Psychology, 42*, 95–113.

Andrews, G. R., & Debus, R. L. (1978). Persistence and the causal perceptions of failure: Modifying cognitive attributions. *Journal of Educational Psychology, 70*, 154–166.

Appleton, A. R., Christenson, S. L., & Furlong, M. J. (2008). Student engagement with school: Critical conceptual and methodological issues of the construct. *Psychology in the Schools, 45*, 369–386.

Appleton, J. J., Christenson, S. L., Kim, D., & Reschly, A. L. (2006). Measuring cognitive and psychological engagement: Validation of the Student Engagement Instrument. *Journal of School Psychology, 44*, 427–445.

Betts, J. E., Appleton, J. J., Reschly, A. L., Christenson, S. L., & Huebner, E. S. (2010). A study of the factorial invariance of the Student Engagement Instrument (SEI): Results from middle and high school students. *School Psychology Quarterly, 25*, 84–93.

Brooks, R. (1991). *The self-esteem teacher*. Loveland, OH: Treehaus Communications.

Brooks, R. (1994). Children at risk: Fostering resilience and hope. *The American Journal of Orthopsychiatry, 64*, 545–553.

Brooks, R. (2001). To touch a student's heart and mind: The mindset of the effective educator. In *Proceedings of the 1999 Plain Talk conference sponsored by the Center for Development and Learning*, New Orleans (pp. 167–177). Cambridge, MA: Educators Publishing Service.

Brooks, R. (2004). To touch the hearts and minds of students with learning disabilities: The power of mindsets and expectations. *Learning Disabilities: A Contemporary Journal, 2*, 9–18.

Brooks, R., & Goldstein, S. (2001). *Raising resilient children*. New York: McGraw-Hill.

Brooks, R., & Goldstein, S. (2004). *The power of resilience*. New York: McGraw-Hill.

Brooks, R., & Goldstein, S. (2007). *Raising a self-disciplined child*. New York: McGraw-Hill.

Brooks, R., & Goldstein, S. (2008). The mindset of teachers capable of fostering resilience in students. *Canadian Journal of School Psychology, 23*, 114–126.

Canino, F. (1981). Learned helplessness theory: Implication for research in learning disabilities. *Journal of Special Education, 15*, 471–484.

Christenson, S. L., & Anderson, A. R. (2002). Commentary: The centrality of the learning context for students' academic enabler skills. *School Psychology Review, 31*, 378–393.

Christenson, S. L., Reschly, A. L., Appleton, J. J., Berman, S., Spanjers, D., & Varro, P. (2008). Best practices in fostering student engagement. In A. Thomas & J. Grimes (Eds.), *Best practices in school psychology* (5th ed., pp. 1099–1119). Bethesda, MD: National Association of School Psychologists.

Christenson, S. L., & Thurlow, M. L. (2004). School dropouts: Prevention considerations, interventions, and challenges. *Current Directions in Psychological Science, 13*(1), 36–39.

Cohen, J. (2006). Social, emotional, ethical, and academic education: Creating a climate for learning, participation in democracy, and well-being. *Harvard Educational Review, 76*, 201–237.

Cohen, J., & Sandy, S. (2003). Perspectives in social-emotional education: Theoretical foundations and new evidence-based developments in current practice. *Perspectives in Education, 21*, 41–54.

Csikszentmihalyi, M. (1975). *Beyond boredom and anxiety: Experiencing flow in work and play*. San Francisco: Jossey-Bass.

Csikszentmihalyi, M. (1998). *Finding flow: The psychology of engagement with everyday life.* New York: Basic Books.

Davis, S. (2003). *Schools where everyone belongs.* Wayne, ME: Stop Bullying Now.

Deci, E. L., & Flaste, R. (1995). *Why we do what we do: Understanding self-motivation.* New York: Penguin.

Deci, E. L., Hodges, R., Pierson, L., & Tomassone, J. (1992). Autonomy and competence as motivational factors in students with learning disabilities and emotional handicaps. *Journal of Learning Disabilities, 25,* 457–471.

Deci, E. L., Koestner, R., & Ryan, R. M. (2001). Extrinsic rewards and extrinsic motivation in education: Reconsidered once again. *Review of Educational Research, 71,* 1–27.

Deci, E. L., & Ryan, R. M. (2000). The "what" and "why" of goal pursuits. Human needs and the self-determination of behavior. *Psychological Inquiry, 11,* 227–268.

DiCintio, M. J., & Gee, S. (1999). Control is the key: Unlocking the motivation of at-risk students. *Psychology in the Schools, 36,* 231–237.

Dweck, C. S. (1986). Motivational processes affecting learning. *American Psychologist, 41,* 1040–1048.

Dweck, C. S. (2006). *Mindset: The new psychology of success.* New York: Random House.

Elias, M. J., Zins, J. E., Graczyk, P. A., & Weissberg, R. P. (2003). Implementation, sustainability, and scaling up of social-emotional and academic innovations in public schools. *School Psychology Review, 32,* 303–319.

Finn, J. D. (1989). Withdrawing from school. *Review of Educational Research, 59,* 117–142.

Fredricks, J. A., Blumenfeld, P. C., & Paris, A. H. (2004). School engagement: Potential of the concept, state of the evidence. *Review of Educational Psychology, 74,* 59–109.

Gardner, H. (1983). *Frames of mind.* New York: Basic Books.

Goldstein, S., & Brooks, R. (Eds.). (2005). *Handbook of resilience in children.* New York: Springer.

Goldstein, S., & Brooks, R. (2007). *Understanding and managing classroom behavior: Creating resilient, sustainable classrooms.* New York: Wiley.

Goleman, D. (1994). *Emotional intelligence.* New York: Bantam.

Grolnick, W. S., Ryan, R. M., & Deci, E. L. (1991). Inner resources for school achievement: Motivational mediators of children's perceptions of their parents. *Journal of Educational Psychology, 83,* 508–517.

Henderson, N., & Milstein, M. (1996). *Resiliency in schools: Making it happen for students and educators.* Thousand Oaks, CA: Corwin.

Holt, P., Fine, M., & Tollefson, N. (1987). Mediating stress: Survival of the hardy. *Psychology in the Schools, 24,* 51–58.

Jacobson, L. (1999). Three's company: Kids prove they have a place at the parent-teacher conference. *Teacher Magazine, 11,* 23.

Jimerson, S. R., Campos, E., & Greif, J. L. (2003). Toward an understanding of definitions and measures of school engagement and related items. *California School Psychologist, 8,* 7–27.

Jones, R. D. (2009). *Student engagement: Teacher handbook.* Rexford, NY: International Center for Leadership in Education.

Jones, R. D., Marrazo, M. J., & Love, C. J. (2007). *Student engagement: Creating a culture of academic achievement.* Rexford, NY: International Center for Leadership in Education.

Katz, M. (1994, May). From challenged childhood to achieving adulthood: Studies in resilience. *Chadder,* 8–11.

Katz, M. (1997). *On playing a poor hand well.* New York: Norton.

Klem, A., & Connell, R. (2004). Relationships matter: Linking teacher support to student engagement and achievement. *Journal of School Health, 74,* 262–273.

Kobasa, S., Maddi, S., & Kahn, S. (1982). Hardiness and health: A perspective inquiry. *Journal of Personality and Social Psychology, 42,* 168–177.

Kobasa, S., & Puccetti, M. (1983). Personality and social resources in stress resistance. *Journal of Personality and Social Psychology, 42,* 839–850.

Lepper, M. R., Greene, D., & Nisbett, R. E. (1973). Undermining children's intrinsic interest with extrinsic rewards: A test of the "overjustification" hypothesis. *Journal of Personality and Social Psychology, 28,* 129–137.

Levine, M. D. (2002). *A mind at a time.* New York: Simon & Schuster.

Levine, M. D. (2003). *The myth of laziness.* New York: Simon & Schuster.

Maehr, M. L., & Meyer, H. A. (1997). Understanding motivation and schooling: Where we've been, where we are, and where we need to go. *Educational Psychology Review, 9,* 371–408.

Martinez, J. (1989). Cooling off before burning out. *Academic Therapy, 24,* 271–284.

Masten, A. S. (2001). Ordinary magic: Resilience processes in development. *American Psychologist, 56,* 227–238.

Masten, A. S., & Coatsworth, J. D. (1998). The development of competence in favorable and unfavorable environments: Lessons from successful children. *American Psychologist, 53,* 205–220.

McCombs, B. L., & Pope, J. E. (1994). *Motivating hard to reach students.* Washington, DC: American Psychological Association.

Middleton, K., & Pettit, E. A. (2010). *Simply the best: 29 things students say the best teachers do around relationships.* Bloomington, IN: Author House.

Miserandino, M. (1996). Children who do well in school: Individual differences in perceived competence and autonomy in above-average children. *Journal of Educational Psychology, 88,* 203–214.

Olweus, D. (1994). *Bullying at school: What we know and what we can do.* Malden, MA: Blackwell Publishers.

Pink, D. H. (2009). *Drive: The surprising truth about what motivates us.* New York: Riverhead Books.

Reivich, K., & Shatte, A. W. (2002). *The resilience factor: 7 keys to finding your inner strength and overcoming life's hurdles.* New York: Random House.

Reschly, A. L., & Christenson, S. L. (2006). Prediction of dropout among students with mild disabilities: A Case for the inclusion of student engagement variables. *Remedial and Special Education, 27,* 276–292.

Russell, V. J., Ainley, M., & Frydenberg, E. (2005). School issues digest: Student motivation and engagement. From: http://dest.gov.au/setors/school_education/publication_resources/schooling_issues_digest_motivation_engagement.htm

Rutter, M. (1980). School influences on children's behavior and development. *Pediatrics, 65,* 522–533.

Rutter, M. (1985). Resilience in the face of adversity: Protective factors and resistance to psychiatric disorder. *The British Journal of Psychiatry, 147,* 598–611.

Rutter, M. (1987). Psychosocial resilience and protective factors. *The American Journal of Orthopsychiatry, 57,* 316–331.

Ryan, R. M., & Deci, E. L. (2000). Self-determination theory and the facilitation of intrinsic motivation, social development, and well-being. *American Psychologist, 55,* 68–78.

Schunk, D. H., & Rice, J. M. (1993). Strategy fading and progress feedback: Effects on self-efficacy and comprehension among students receiving remedial reading services. *The Journal of Special Education, 27,* 257–276.

Segal, J. (1988). Teachers have enormous power in affecting a child's self-esteem. *Brown University Child Behavior and Development Newsletter, 10,* 1–3.

Seligman, M. E. P. (1990). *Learned optimism: How to change your minds and life.* New York: Pocket Books.

Seligman, M. E. P. (1995). *The optimistic child.* New York: Houghton Mifflin.

Sheridan, S. M., Eagle, J. W., & Dowd, S. E. (2005). Families for contexts for children's adaptation. In S. Goldstein & R. Brooks (Eds.), *Handbook of resilience in children* (pp. 165–180). New York: Kluwer Academic/Plenum Publishers.

Shure, M. B. (1996). *Raising a thinking child: Help your young child resolve everyday conflicts and get along with others.* New York: Pocket Books.

Shure, M. B. (2003). A problem-solving approach to preventing early high-risk behaviors in children and preteens. In D. Romer (Ed.), *Preventing adolescent risk* (pp. 85–92). Thousand Oaks, CA: Sage.

Sinclair, M. F., Christenson, S. L., & Thurlow, M. L. (2005). Promoting school completion of urban secondary youth with emotional or behavioral disabilities. *Exceptional Children, 71*(4), 465–482.

Thomsen, K. (2002). *Building resilient students: Integrating resiliency into what you already know and do.* Thousand Oaks, CA: Corwin.

Vansteenkiste, M., Simons, J., Lens, W., Sheldon, K. M., & Deci, E. L. (2004). Motivating learning, performance, and persistence: The synergistic effects of intrinsic goal contents and autonomy-supportive contexts. *Journal of Personality and Social Psychology, 87,* 246–260.

Wagner, T., Kegan, R., Lahey, L. L., & Lemons, R. L. (2005). *Change leadership: A practical guide to transforming our schools.* San Francisco: Jossey-Bass.

Weiner, B. (1974). *Achievement motivation and attribution theory.* Morristown, NJ: General Learning Press.

Werner, E. E. (1993). Risk, resilience, and recovery: Perspectives from the Kauai Longitudinal Study. *Development and Psychopathology, 5,* 503–515.

Werner, E. E., & Smith, R. (1992). *Overcoming the odds: High risk children from birth to adulthood.* Ithaca, NY: Cornell University Press.

Werner, E. E., & Smith, R. (2001). *Journeys of childhood to midlife: Risk, resilience, and recovery.* Ithaca, NY: Cornell University Press.

Wright, M. O., & Masten, A. S. (2005). Resilience processes in development. In S. Goldstein & R. Brooks (Eds.), *Handbook of resilience in children* (pp. 17–37). New York: Kluwer Academic/Plenum Publishers.

The Relations of Adolescent Student Engagement with Troubling and High-Risk Behaviors

Amy-Jane Griffiths, Elena Lilles, Michael J. Furlong, and Jennifer Sidhwa

Abstract

Nearly one third of secondary school students report decreased engagement in school during their teen years. When considering the emotional or psychological aspects of engagement, which are routinely associated with high-risk behaviors, a student must somehow conclude that, at a minimum, at least one specific person at their school truly cares about him or her not only as a student, but as a person. This caring individual, be it a teacher, coach, administrator, or counselor, does not simply express respect, concern, and trust in the student as part of their job, but also the student comes to believe that this person sees intrinsic value in him or her as a human being. In this chapter we underscore the association between student engagement and high-risk behaviors in adolescence. Although all aspects of student engagement are important to the full development of youth, the salience of student engagement when considering troubling and high-risk behaviors in schools warrants educators' attention. We summarize research in this area and provide an overview of system-level

---

A.-J. Griffiths, Ph.D. (✉)
The Help Group, Sherman Oaks, CA, USA
e-mail: agriffiths@thehelpgroup.org

E. Lilles, M.Ed.
University of Oregon, Santa Barbara, CA, USA
e-mail: elilles@education.ucsb.edu

M.J. Furlong, Ph.D.
Department of Counseling, Clinical,
and School Psychology, University of California
Santa Barbara, Santa Barbara, CA, USA
e-mail: mfurlong@education.ucsb.edu

J. Sidhwa, B.A.
Educational Leadership and Organizations Program,
Gevirtz Graduate School of Education, University
of California Santa Barbara, Santa Barbara, CA, USA
e-mail: jsidhwa@education.ucsb.edu

interventions and strategies to build bonding and connectedness, particularly for those students who engage in high-risk behaviors. We conclude that clear definitions and unified research in the area of student engagement can allow for continued advancements in understanding how to best engage students, specifically high-risk students, and yield positive academic and life outcomes for youth.

Introduction

We approach the topic of adolescent student engagement, particularly considering high-risk behaviors, from the perspective that engagement research is incomplete if it only considers students' individual academic behaviors or personal scholastic incentives. In our view, the student and his or her personal beliefs and perceptions about school and the schooling process are central to engagement considerations. When considering the emotional or psychological aspects of engagement, which are routinely associated with high-risk behaviors, a student must somehow conclude that, at a minimum, at least one specific person at their school truly cares about him or her not only as a student but as a person (Murray & Malmgren, 2005). This caring individual, be it a teacher, coach, administrator, or counselor, does not simply express respect, concern, and trust in the student as part of their job (Johnson, 2009), but also the student comes to believe that this person sees intrinsic value in him or her as a human being. As was stated by one of the teachers in Gregory and Ripski's (2008) study of student trust, "The one thing that seems to mean the most to her (the student) is my affection and my caring about her as a person" (p. 343).

Literature reviewed in this chapter underscores the association between student engagement and high-risk behaviors in adolescence. To examine this topic, we first define the engagement terms presented in the chapter and provide brief comments to address the three common topics in each chapter of this volume by (a) providing our definition of engagement and motivation, (b) describing the framework and theory we use to study and explain engagement and motivation, and (c) defining the role of context in explaining student engagement. We then summarize research about the identified relations between student engagement and troubling and high-risk behaviors. Finally, we provide an overview of system level interventions and strategies to build bonding and connectedness, particularly for those students who engage in high-risk behaviors. We hope reader will recognize the importance of this research, noting that the topic of this chapter applies to many students because nearly one third of secondary school students report decreased engagement during their teen years (Archambault, Janosz, Morizot, & Pagani, 2009). In addition, even for the majority of students who are generally involved in their schooling experience, affective engagement is lower than behavioral and cognitive engagement (Archambault et al., 2009).

Definitions of Engagement

Various aspects of student engagement have been studied under a variety of terms including school connectedness, teacher support, school bonding, school climate, school engagement, and more recently student engagement (Blum & Libbey, 2004; O'Farrell & Morrison, 2003). Researchers have suggested that the term represents a multifaceted construct that involves student thoughts, beliefs, emotions, and behaviors as it relates to school. Researchers have recently organized the conceptualization of engagement into three subtypes: behavioral, cognitive, and emotional or affective (Fredricks, Blumenfeld, & Paris, 2004; Jimerson et al., 2003). However, Appleton, Christenson, and Furlong (2008) made a convincing argument for four components of student engagement: academic, behavioral, cognitive, and psychological. These four components are based on a comprehensive review of literature related to student engagement and particularly the work of Finn (1989), Connell (Connell, Halpern-Felsher, Clifford, Crichlow, & Usinger, 1995; Connell & Wellborn, 1991), and McPartland (1994).

Academic engagement includes variables such as points earned, homework completion, and time on task. *Behavioral engagement* may include variables such as attendance, the absence of disruptive behaviors, adhering to school rules, extracurricular activities participation, and student participation in learning and academic assignments (Fredricks et al., 2004). *Emotional engagement* is the student's emotional reactions at school that includes interest, boredom, happiness, sadness, and anxiety (Fredricks et al., 2004). Otherwise labeled as psychological engagement, this may include relationships with teachers and peers, as well as feelings of belonging. *Cognitive engagement* may include indicators such as personal goal development, self-regulation relevance of schoolwork to future goals, and the value of learning. Fredricks et al., 2004 suggested cognitive engagement can be described as the students' investment in learning, self-regulation, and the use of strategies to gain knowledge and skills.

Engagement and Motivation

How does one know if a student is motivated? When others "see" motivation, they describe what a student does, the products he or she produces (quality and quantity), and perhaps mention comments that the student makes, from which attitudes, goals, and dreams are inferred. That is, the student's behaviors signal that he or she values schoolwork and is striving to do it well, perhaps to fulfill higher life aspirations. These are inferences made by others rather than motivation. By its nature, motivation is an internal, personal experience. In our view, motivation is the psychological driving force that increases the probability that a student engages in behaviors that lead toward desired scholastic goals. In this regard, engagement is the more visible manifestation of such motivational tendencies. Students who are motivated to learn and do well in school can be observed doing the "work" of a student (Schaufeli, Martinez, Pinto, Salanova, & Bakker, 2002). This describes what has been labeled the "behavioral" and "academic" aspects of engagement (Appleton et al., 2008; Fredricks et al., 2004). Among the markers that have been used to assess behavioral engagement—the student is at school nearly every day, completes tasks in a timely manner, is attentive to and responsive to teacher questions, and asks teachers how they did on assignments—all suggest personal commitment to the schooling process. From our view, confusion arises between the terms motivation and engagement because (a) motivation is an internal experience that can only be inferred indirectly by others and (b) the evolution of the term engagement has expanded to include both behavioral components and internal psychological ones (affective and cognitive). The term engagement implies some level of involvement and activity: Are you doing the work of a student? Do you value the work being done? Are you in it for the long haul? When we speak of motivation, we see it as being the combination of these three key questions. As has been conceptualized by others (Appleton et al., 2008), the behavioral and cognitive components also clearly address these key questions. What then distinguished the historical conceptualization of engagement from motivation is the affective component that can be understood as the link between the student as an individually motivated learner and the student as a member of a social network that encompasses both one-on-one relationships (e.g., student-teacher and friend-friend) and being the part of larger social networks (e.g., classroom, social groups, school-wide climate). In this chapter, we will focus on the affective elements of engagement, utilizing various terms seen in the literature, such as school engagement, student engagement, school connectedness, and school bonding. The term school bonding is the oldest term and connotes the personal and relational links associated with reduced participation in risky behaviors.

The Engagement Process

Social development researchers (e.g., Hawkins, Guo, Hill, Battin-Pearson, & Abbott, 2001) have suggested that student engagement develops in the individual as they are provided the opportunity for behavioral involvement, social skills training, and rewards for using these social skills in interpersonal situations. Extending this model to include the various terms that have been used in the student engagement literature, Furlong et al. (2003) offered the PACM model. *Participation* (behavioral involvement) contributes to the formation of interpersonal *Attachments* (social bonding), which in turn results in a student developing a sense of personal *Commitment* (valuing of education), and ultimately to incorporating school *Membership* (identification as a school community citizen) as part of his or her self-identity (P → A → C → M). Such a model is relevant to all students, particularly those considered to be "high risk." This model, if used as the basis for educational practice, has the potential to structure overall school improvement efforts.

O'Farrell, Morrison, and Furlong (2006) reviewed five levels of engagement supported within the school environment. First, schools can conduct school-wide activities (e.g., clubs, sports) that *reaffirm* relationships with the majority of students who are not at risk. Second, schools can reach out to and *reconnect* with students who are marginally involved with school and may not respond to universal strategies. Third, schools may need to *reconstruct* relationships with students who show serious emotional and behavioral difficulties through intensive interventions such as family therapy or behavioral assessments and interventions. Fourth, for a small group of students, schools will need to *repair* the relationships of students who may have been marginalized, and/or victims of serious or chronic violence at school and require interventions to *renew* a sense of school safety and membership. For marginalized students, opportunities to repair bonds across various social contexts may be of particular importance. If a student is significantly disengaged from school and possibly other environments (home and community), it may be necessary to use multiple agencies to intervene and create opportunities for attachment and the development of self-efficacy. We will focus on reconstruction and repair of relationships for youth engaging in high-risk behavior.

The Engaged and Disengaged Student

In this section, we offer the distinction between active and positive engagement in school and active and negative disengagement; that is, disengagement is not merely the absence of engagement. Guthrie (2001), for example, described an engaged reader in this way,

> Devoted students are intent on reading to understand. They focus on meaning and avoid distractions. Strategies such as self-monitoring and inferencing are used with little effort. These readers exchange ideas and interpretations with fellow students. We refer to these students who are intrinsically motivated to read for knowledge and enjoyment as 'engaged' readers (p. 2).

In this regard, cognitive engagement focuses on how deeply the student participates in the tasks of being a student and on using academic tasks for broader personal skill development and enhancing self-efficacy. However, researchers (Abbott et al., 1998; Hirschi, 1969) have long recognized that some students do not participate in such personally facilitative ways in the academic context. Drawing from resilience research (Catalano, Hawkins, & Smith, 2001; Herrenkohl, Hawkins, Chung, Hill, & Battin-Pearson, 2000), models show that youth with the accumulation of multiple challenges (e.g., poverty, inconsistent parenting experiences) are at an increased risk of negative developmental outcomes. These life experiences may make it more difficult for a youth to be able to focus on and be behaviorally engaged at school. These youth are seen as being, in fact, more likely to be "disengaged," "disconnected," or at best inconsistently committed to the educational values and mission of the school.

Such students are likely to be less motivated by task mastery or performance goals (Eccles & Wigfield, 2002; Finn, 1989, 1993). They are more likely to be suspended from school for behaviors such as defiance, disobedience, or disrespect directed toward the teacher (Morrison & Skiba, 2001), which can strain the formation of a caring supportive relationship and undermines the legitimacy of a teacher's authority for the student (Gregory & Ripski, 2008). In fact, disengaged students may not just ignore or disregard teachers and other school authority figures, but if they conclude that school is not a place that is accepting and inclusive, they can actively resist teacher directives (Solorzarno & Delgado Bernal, 2001). It is not just that disengaged students may believe that their teachers and others at school do not have positive regard for them, but they conclude that the school context actively rejects them and does not promote or have a supportive caring climate (Noddings, 1995).

A number of organizations and measures focus on student and community assets. The Search Institute is one of these organizations, which uses their framework of 40 developmental assets and the relationship of these assets to negative outcomes, to inform asset building in communities. The Search Institute has partnered with cities and schools to utilize these data to assist in the development of programs that target student engagement. The Search Institute has led a multiyear study of developmental assessment among school-aged youth and linked asset profiles to the students' individual school records. The results of this research show that low assets are associated with increased participation in high-risk behaviors such as substance use and aggressive behavior (Roehlkepartain, Benson, & Sesma, 2003).

In addition, California Healthy Kids Survey (CHKS) data provide information about the relations between student engagement and risky behaviors. The CHKS includes sections about violence, perceptions of safety, harassment, bullying, and the use of alcohol and other drugs. The CHKS also has a *Resilience Youth Development Module* to measure external resources (protective factors). RYDM external assets items measure students' perceptions of caring relationships, high expectations, and opportunities for meaningful participation in school. Hanson and Kim (2007) conducted several factor analyses and found that the six items from the Caring Relationship and High Expectation subscales combined to form one factor that they called "school support" with the three meaningful participation items holding together in a separate factor.

We examined the CHKS sample of 92,600 students collected during the 2006–2007 and 2007–2008 school years who were in grades 9 (52%) and 11 (48%). These students were from 50 of the 58 California counties. Students were placed into one of three groups, as shown in Table 27.1. The first

Table 27.1 Percentage of California students in grades 9 and 11 reporting troubling and high-risk behaviors by perceptions of school support (caring adult relations and high expectations) and opportunities for meaningful participation in school activities (N=92,600)

Troubling and high-risk behaviors	High[a] level of meaningful participation and school supports (%)	All other students (%)	Low[b] level of meaningful participation and school supports (%)
Any past 30-day cigarette use	6	9	16
Any past 30-day marijuana use	8	12	20
In past 30-days had at least 1 alcoholic drink	12	19	37
Any past 30-day binge drinking	12	16	23
Any past 12-month fighting at school	13	16	25
Any past 30-day carried gun at school	2	3	8
Any past 12-month skipped school or cut class	31	38	49
Self-report gang member	6	7	12

Note: **School supports** is the total of the following six items: *At my school, there is a teacher or some other adult… (1 = Not at All True, 2 = A Little True, 3 = Pretty Much True, 4 = Very Much True)* who really cares about me, who tells me when I do a good job, who notices when I am not there, who always wants me to do my best, who listens to me when I have something to say, and who believes that I will be a success. **Meaningful participation** is the total of the following three items: *At school… (1 = Not at All True, 2 = A Little True, 3 = Pretty Much True, 4 = Very Much True)*, I do interesting activities; I help decide things like class activities or rules; I do things that make a difference (see Furlong et al., 2009; Hanson & Kim, 2008 for more information on the CHKS survey and these scales). Missing responses for each item ranged from 0.5% to 1.0%
[a] z-Scores > 1.0
[b] z-Scores < 1.0

group included youth whose z-scores on the School Supports and Meaningful Participation scales were both more than one standard deviation above the means for the entire sample. These students perceived their relationships with teachers to be very positive and caring, and they believed they had ample opportunities to participate in meaningful activities at school. In brief, these students reported being highly connected and engaged with school (note that this was only about 6% of 9th graders and 8% of 11th graders). At the other end of the connectedness continuum, a second group included youth whose z-scores on the School Supports and Meaningful Participation scales were both more than one standard deviation below the means for the entire sample. These students were generally disengaged (note that this was about 21% of 9th graders and 18% of 11th graders in this sample). The remaining students were somewhere in between these two extreme exemplar groups. As shown in Table 27.1, about one in five students who reported low levels of connectedness and engagement also consistently reported higher rates of involvement in substance use and aggression-related behaviors. The students who reported being disengaged from school typically reported engaging in risky behaviors about twice as often as highly engaged students. It is inaccurate to conclude that these behaviors are typical for most students, but they do illustrate that when students are able to form positive relationships with adults at school, they are less likely to report engaging in troubling and risky behaviors.

The Impact of Student Engagement

Student Engagement and Troubling and High-Risk Behaviors

When youth consider engaging in risky and troubling behaviors (i.e., if they are not acting on impulse), various factors can influence their choices—the behavior's danger, excitement, legality, morality, and, of relevance to this chapter's topic, the opinions of peers and adults (Abbott-Chapman, Denholm, & Wyld, 2008). Of these considerations, which aspects of engagement are most salient when considering students who might otherwise be unmotivated or disengaged from school? Most of the research on adolescents and their involvement in troubling and high-risk behaviors has identified the affective component of engagement as being particularly important. This research has multidisciplinary origins (public health, education, development, psychopathology), but has coalesced to encompass the core notion that adolescents' perceptions of the commitment and caring of adults at school are associated with reduced involvement in troubling and high-risk behaviors.

Research has established positive relations between student engagement and student developmental outcomes including academic achievement (Fredricks et al., 2004; Lee & Smith, 1995), substance use, physical and mental health problems (Carter, McGee, Taylor, & Williams, 2007), school dropout (National Research Council and Institute of Medicine, 2004; Perry, 2008), as well as conduct problems and violence (Henrich, Brookmeyer, & Shahar, 2005; Loukas, Suzuki, & Horton, 2006). This section reviews both short-term and long-term benefits of student engagement as well as the negative correlates of student disengagement.

Academic Achievement

According to the National Research Council and Institute of Medicine (2004), one of the most consistently documented correlates of student engagement is student academic achievement. Research has found a strong positive relation between the level of student engagement and student academic achievement as measured by scores on standardized assessments (e.g., Finn & Voelkl, 1993; Lee & Smith, 1995; Roeser, Midgley, & Urdan, 1996). This relation has been found to be consistent across demographic variables including gender, race/ethnicity, and socioeconomic status, and was found to be a positive correlate for academic achievement among high-risk students (Finn, 1993; Finn & Rock, 1997).

Student engagement has been identified to function as a key mediator of academic achievement through academic performance, grade promotion, and grade retention (Perry, 2008; Perry, Liu, & Pabian, 2010). Among a sample of 1,803 high-risk students, Finn and Rock (1997) identified engagement to be a significant component of "academic resilience" even after controlling for background and psychological characteristics. Results indicated a significant effect size of .78 ($p = .001$) when examining the teacher report of student engagement of students who dropped out of school compared to students who completed school. Students who are better engaged with various aspects of their schooling show higher academic achievement compared to disengaged students (Fredricks et al., 2004). Anderman and Anderman (1999) found that student sense of school belonging was associated with motivation and focus toward academic tasks, which subsequently yielded academic achievement. Similarly, disengaged students attend school irregularly, do not complete coursework, and subsequently learn less than their academically engaged peers. This disengaged pattern of behavior results in lower levels of overall academic achievement (National Research Council and Institute of Medicine, 2004) and likely leads to reduced opportunities for positively engaging adults at school and subsequently developing positive relationships.

The relation between a student's level of school engagement and academic achievement is evident even in primary grades (Alexander, Entwisle, & Dauber, 1993); however, the consequences of disengagement may not be observed until later years (i.e., middle school and high school; Roscigno & Ainsworth-Darnell, 1999). Early achievement researchers have found that engagement in early primary grades predicts long-term scholastic growth (Ladd & Dinella, 2009). Alexander and colleagues (1993) and Alexander, Entwisle, and Dauber (1996) found that teachers' ratings of student school engagement based on student interest and participation in the classroom in the first grade of school were related to later achievement, as observed through academic test scores (direct effect coefficients of .33 in reading and .28 in math, $p = .01$), and grades over the first 4 years of school (direct effect coefficients of .37 in year 1 to .20 in year 4, $p = .01$).

Early problems with school engagement, or school disengagement, have long-term effects and put students at risk for academic achievement difficulties. Research findings suggest that student engagement continues to parallel achievement patterns through high school (Roscigno & Ainsworth-Darnell, 1999).

Finn (1989) described the long-term effects of student engagement on academic achievement through a participation-identification model. This model suggests that early disengagement from school (e.g., lack of behavioral participation) leads to unsuccessful academic outcomes. These poor school outcomes lead to student withdrawal and lack of identification with the school. This lack of identification results in nonparticipation in school-related activities, which, in turn, results in negative academic outcomes. The participation-identification model is a cyclical process, meaning that school participation and school identification reciprocally influence each other over time. Overall, literature suggests that engagement with the school community and academic schoolwork is a proximate determinant of both current and future student academic achievement.

Substance Use and Physical and Mental Health Correlates

Student engagement has also been identified as having an impact on substance use and physical and mental health outcomes among adolescents. Student disengagement during the teenage years may lead to the failure to acquire basic proficiencies needed to survive in society. A lack of such skill sets put individuals at risk for poor overall health outcomes (National Research Council and Institute of Medicine, 2004). Unhealthy behaviors that begin during adolescence are more often found among students with low levels of engagement compared to students with high levels of engagement. These behaviors can have lifelong negative consequences. A key study by Resnick and colleagues (1997) generated unique, substantial interest in the potential protective role of what they called "school connectedness" with adults at school. Resnick et al. (1997) conducted a study to identify various risk and protective factors both inside and outside of the school setting. The researchers performed cross-sectional analysis on interview data of 12,118 (of 90,118) high school and middle school students who participated in the National Longitudinal Study of Adolescent Health (ADD Health). When analyzing the data separately for the adolescents in grades 7–8 and 9–12, respectively, they found that high levels of school connectedness and use of cigarettes were negatively correlated at a magnitude of −.19 ($p<.001$) for students in grades 7–8 and −.25 ($p<.001$) for students in grades 9–12. The use of alcohol was negatively correlated at a magnitude of −.23 ($p<.001$) for students in grades 7–8 and −.21 ($p<.001$) for students in grades 9–12. In other words, students with high levels of school engagement were significantly less likely to use cigarettes and alcohol. Similarly, high levels of school connectedness for the two groups were associated with less frequent marijuana use. School engagement and marijuana use were correlated at a magnitude of −.22 ($p<.001$) for students in grades 7–8 and −.24 ($p<.001$) for students in grades 9–12. As might be expected, they found that parent/family connectedness was associated with the frequency of substance use, but that positive school social connections explained unique variance in risk-related behavior patterns.

Additionally, student engagement is associated with student mental health and well-being. Students with high levels of engagement were found to have reduced risk of depression and suicidal ideation compared to students with low engagement (Carter et al., 2007). Highly engaged students were found to report better overall mental health and well-being outcomes compared to disengaged youth (Holdsworth & Blanchard, 2006). A high level of student engagement was found to be related to healthy behaviors, for example, high engagement related to higher levels of physical activity, better eating habits and nutrition, safer sex, and cycle helmet use (Carter et al., 2007). Strong student engagement was also found to be associated with a decreased likelihood of pregnancy among teenage girls (Manlove, 1998).

School Dropout

School dropout is one of the most visible outcomes of pervasive student disengagement (Alliance for Excellent Education, 2009; National Research Council and Institute of Medicine, 2004). In a review of research on outcomes associated with student engagement, Fredricks and colleagues (2004) found that student disengagement from school including low academic participation, poor attendance, minimal work involvement, and displays of negative conduct is a precursor of school dropout (Barrington & Hendricks, 1989; Fredricks et al., 2004). It is clear that students who are not engaged in school are at a greater risk for low academic achievement and school failure and subsequently exhibit higher dropout rates compared to high achieving students (Bridgeland, DiJulio, & Morison, 2006; Janosz, Archambault, Morizot, & Pagani, 2008; National Research Council and Institute of Medicine, 2004; Perry, 2008). Janosz and colleagues (2008) found that out of a sample of 13,300 students between the ages of 12 and 16, those students who were identified as demonstrating negative or inconsistent school engagement patterns were between 10 and 80 times more at risk for dropping out of school than peers who exhibited typical school engagement patterns.

Consequences of being disengaged from school are serious for high-risk youth who may not have other resources available to help counterbalance the effects of school failure. Disengaged students from challenging backgrounds (e.g., poverty) in urban school settings are more likely to drop out than disengaged students who are not from disadvantaged backgrounds (Perry, 2008). However, just as student disengagement can lead to student dropout, student engagement can act as a protective factor against academic failure (Fredricks et al., 2004). Students with high levels of engagement are more likely to exhibit high academic achievement and are less likely to drop out of school (Crosnoe, Mistry, & Elder, 2002). A student's perception of his or her connection to the school, teachers, and peers can act as a protective factor that keeps high-risk children in school (Fine, 1991; Finn & Rock, 1997; Fredricks et al., 2004; Mehan et al., 1996).

Conduct Problems/Violence

Many forms of community and school violence have been perpetrated by students who had a history of social alienation and detachment at school (Sandhu, Arora, & Sandhu, 2001). Students with high levels of engagement were identified as exhibiting lower levels of problem behaviors (Finn & Rock, 1997; Gutman & Midgley, 2000). Students with low levels of engagement were more likely than engaged peers to display negative behaviors or conduct problems such as fighting which leads to additional negative consequences including school suspension and further disengagement from school (Carter et al., 2007; Fredricks et al., 2004). Along this same vein, high levels of student engagement are correlated to a lower likelihood of being involved in violent behaviors for ethnically and socioeconomically diverse male and female adolescents in grades 7–12 (Henrich et al., 2005; Loukas et al., 2006). Furthermore, student engagement has been identified as a protective factor against weapon carrying for ethnically diverse males and African-American females (Kodjo, Auinger, & Ryan, 2003). Last, students who feel more engaged in school, empowered by their teachers, and supported by their teachers and peers are less likely to bully others or be victimized by peers (Brookmeyer, Fanti, & Henrich, 2006). These findings hold true for both urban and suburban, ethnically diverse adolescents.

Summary of Recent Studies: Hybrid Risk and Protective Factors

Student disengagement from school is associated with considerable negative academic, behavioral, and physical outcomes. Similarly, strong student engagement has been identified as a protective and promotive factor contributing to both academic and overall success. Recent research on student engagement and compatible terms (e.g., school connectedness, school bonding) continue to highlight the positive outcomes associated with a positive relationship between students and school community, and the negative effects associated with student disengagement. Table 27.2 summarizes the findings of key studies published within the past decade that evaluate student engagement and the associated outcomes. This table serves as a reference guide to review both positive and negative outcomes associated with student engagement and disengagement from school.

Prevention and Intervention: What Can Be Done?

Although all aspects of student engagement are important to the full development of youth, the salience of student connectedness when considering troubling and high-risk behaviors in schools is recognized in a vast body of research. Research evidence supporting the recommendation to promote positive and caring relationships among students parents and staff is substantial and is strongly backed by randomized control trials (Langberg et al., 2006, 2008; Molina et al., 2008; Murray & Malgren, 2005; Sinclair, Christenson, Evelo, & Hurley, 1998; Sinclair, Christenson, & Thurlow, 2005), quasi-experimental studies (Gottfredson, Gerstenblith, Soule, Womer, & Lu, 2004) and single case studies (Hawken & Horner, 2003; Moore, Cateledge, & Heckaman, 1995), and single case studies (Hawken & Horner, 2003; Moore, Cateledge, & Heckaman, 1995). Most of these studies were specifically designed to improve the school relationships of students who were at risk or had already exhibited behavior problems.

Although contexts outside the school setting contribute to student engagement, schools still need to consider ways to engage students, avoid disengaging students, as well as reconstruct and repair relationships with students who have disengaged. Fortunately, research indicates that alterable school-based assets influence student engagement for youth at all levels of family risk, even when individual traits are considered (Sharkey, You, & Schnoebelen, 2008). Furlong and colleagues (2003) suggested that student engagement can be conceptualized as a set of behaviors along a continuum from high to low levels of school involvement. Therefore, intervention strategies to encourage student engagement

Table 27.2 Key studies of relations between school connectedness/student engagement/school bonding and its effect on alcohol use, cigarette use, marijuana use, dropping out, and conduct disorder/violence among adolescents

Authors/year	Term and measure used	Alcohol	Cigarettes	Marijuana	Dropout	Conduct problems	Findings
Substance use							
Resnick et al. (1997)	School connectedness ADD Health Scale[a]	X	X	X			High levels of school connectedness related to less frequent alcohol, cigarette, and marijuana use
Simons-Morton (2004)	School engagement Three items about school in general[b]	X					Students engaged in school were less likely to start drinking alcohol
Rasmussen, Damsgaard, Holstein, and Poulsen (2005)	School connectedness (Danish) Health Behavior in School-Aged Children National Study[c]		X				Students connected to school were less likely to smoke cigarettes
Henry (2008)	School attachment Five items about teacher, safety, and enjoyment[d]	X	X	X			Low levels of school attachment were positively correlated to involvement with friends who use drugs, which was related to use or intention to use alcohol and drugs

Students who are more engaged in school are less likely to start using alcohol than less engaged students. In addition, those who are more engaged use alcohol, marijuana, and cigarettes at a lower rate than their less engaged peers. These effects are found for both males and females from grades 6 through 12 in both rural and urban communities. Findings suggest that student engagement may be a protective factor against substance use in other first world countries as well. Moreover, low student engagement is related to involvement with friends who use drugs, which is subsequently related to using drugs (alcohol, cigarettes, marijuana).

Authors/year	Term and measure used	Alcohol	Cigarettes	Marijuana	Dropout	Conduct problems	Findings
Dropout							
Croninger and Lee (2001)	Teacher-based social capital National Educational Longitudinal Study[e]				X		Students who receive less "teacher-based" social capital had a higher likelihood of dropping out of high school
Janosz et al. (2008)	Student engagement Three-dimensional factor structure[f]				X		Students with normative levels of student engagement were less likely to drop out than those with varying levels of engagement. Also, students with an overall reduction in levels of student engagement were more likely to drop out
Archambault et al. (2009)	Student engagement Behavior, affective, and cognitive engagement[g]				X		Adolescents with high global or behavioral student engagement were less likely to drop out of school compared to adolescents with lower levels of student engagement

Students who feel more supported by their teachers are less likely to drop out of school compared to those who do not. Behavioral, affective, and cognitive engagement (compliance to rules, enjoyment of school, and willingness to learn) together are related to lower rates of school dropout. However, when examining the parts separately, only behavioral engagement by itself is a protective factor against dropping out of school. Lastly, students with consistent levels of student engagement are less likely to drop out than those who had varying levels, including decreasing, increasing, or both. Also, those with lower baseline levels and those who experience an overall reduction are at a higher risk for dropping out of school. These findings are nationally representative of the USA and some French provinces in Canada.

Conduct problems/violence

Study	Measure		
Kodjo et al. (2003)	School connectedness ADD Health Scale[a]	X	High levels of school connectedness significantly reduced weapon carrying for all adolescent males and for African-American females
Henrich et al. (2005)	School connectedness ADD Health Scale[a]	X	Adolescents who were more connected to school were less likely to commit a violent crime than those less connected to school
Brookmeyer et al. (2006)	School engagement ADD Health Scale[a]	X	Adolescents who reported high levels of student engagement participated in less violent behavior over time than those who reported lower levels of school connectedness
Loukas et al. (2006)	School connectedness ADD Health Scale[a]	X	Adolescents more connected to school were involved in less conduct problems than those who were not as connected to school
Frey et al. (2008)	School attachment Attachment to School Scale[b]	X	Boys who showed consistently elevated levels of school attachment during the transition from grade 8 to 9 exhibited lower levels of violent behavior
Nation, Vieno, Perkins, and Santinello (2008)	Empowerment with teachers and classmates Teacher and Classmate Support Scale[i]	X	Disempowered relationships with teachers predicted both bullying and victimization among youth
Flaspohler, Elfstrom, Vanderzee, Sink, and Birchmeier (2009)	Teacher and social support Child and Adolescent Social Support Scale[j]	X	Students who were not involved in bullying (perpetrator or victim) felt more supported by their teachers and peers than those who bullied others or were victimized

Student engagement is a protective factor against weapon carrying for ethnically diverse males and African-American females. In addition, high levels of student engagement are correlated to a lower likelihood of being involved in violent behaviors for diverse (ethnic and socioeconomic) male and female adolescents in grades 7–12. One study found a similar relationship that also included lying and cheating as conduct behaviors. Lastly, students who feel more engaged in school, empowered by their teachers, and supported by their teachers and peers are less likely to bully others or be victimized. These findings hold true for both urban and suburban, ethnically diverse adolescents.

(continued)

Table 27.2 (continued)

Authors/year	Term and measure used	Alcohol	Cigarettes	Marijuana	Dropout	Conduct problems	Findings
Hybrid risks							
Dornbusch, Erikson, Laird, and Wong (2001)	School connectedness ADD Health Scale[a]	X	X	X		X	High levels of school connectedness predicted less delinquent behaviors on a whole. Specifically, school connectedness predicted a decline in cigarette use and less violent behavior
McNeely and Falci (2004)	School connectedness ADD Health Scale[a]	X	X	X		X	Strong school connectedness was correlated to less initiation and low escalation of drinking alcohol, smoking marijuana, and smoking cigarettes. Likewise, strong school connectedness was related to less participation in delinquent and violent behaviors
Bond et al. (2007)	School connectedness The Communities That Care Youth Survey Scale[k]	X	X	X	X		High levels of school connectedness were related to low levels of substance use and a better chance of completing school
Simons-Morton, Crump, Haynie, and Saylor (1999)	School-bonding and perception of school climate School bonding index[l] and instrument to measure school climate[m]	X	X	X		X	High levels of school bonding and perceived school climate were negatively associated with several problem behaviors

High levels of student engagement are correlated with less substance use, dropping out, and problem behaviors such as fighting, bullying, stealing, weapon carrying, and vandalizing. This was found for both male and female students of diverse ethnicities and socioeconomic statuses. The association between school engagement and hybrid risks became more refined when separating school engagement into two parts: teacher support and social belonging. Teacher support and social belonging are protective against cigarette smoking initiation and escalation from occasional to regular smoking. Teacher support decreases drinking initiation and escalation from being an occasional drinker to a regular drinker, while social belonging does not. Teacher support also acts as a buffer for marijuana initiation, but not escalation to regular use. In addition, adolescents who feel supported by their teachers are less likely to engage in violent behaviors and more likely to cease violent participation if they have been violent in the past.

Note: Measurement scales for student engagement used in studies

[a]Resnick et al. (1997), [b]Simons-Morton (2004), [c]Currie et al. (2000), [d]Henry (2008), [e]Ingels et al. (1994), [f]Fredricks et al. (2004), [g]Archambault et al. (2009), [h]Weissberg et al. (1991), [i]Simons-Morton and Chen (2009), [j]Malecki et al. (2000), [k]Arthur et al. (2002), [l]Torsheim, Wold, and Samdal (2000), [m]Pyper et al. (1987)

can occur in multiple systems. Sharkey et al. (2008) argued that school administrators may need to be encouraged to focus on relationship building, school safety, and school climate in order to promote positive outcomes. Providing youth with opportunities for meaningful school involvement and reinforcing this involvement can lead to the development of facilitative school bonds (Catalano, Kosterman, Hawkins, Newcomb, & Abbott, 1996).

Intervention and Engaging Protective Mechanisms

Based on research indicating that high-risk behavior is related to numerous contextual influences ranging from individual factors to social/community factors, it will be important to take all of these into account when understanding how to intervene, engage protective mechanisms in their school environment, and provide these children with an ability to attain positive outcomes. Rutter (1987) described four protective mechanisms. The first mechanism is the reduction of risk impact, meaning the negative impact may be reduced by preparing the child for the situation, exposing the child when he or she can handle the situation, decreasing exposure to the risk factor, providing the child with practice in coping, and reducing the demands of the risk factor. The second mechanism is the reduction of negative chain reactions (the snowball effect), by implementing interventions that prevent a chain of reactions that perpetuate the risk effects in the future. The third mechanism is described as the development of self-esteem and self-efficacy so that the child feels that he or she has the ability to deal with life's challenges, is satisfied with his or her social relationships, and feels success in the completion of some tasks. Finally, the fourth mechanism described is the opening of opportunities. These four mechanisms are child-focused but may be implemented throughout the various systems.

An effective intervention strategy may be to organize and activate positive institutions or systems that will promote healthy development and potentially alter a child's negative trajectory. Some of these systems may include fostering positive attachment relationships (i.e., with teachers), increasing youth's self-regulation skills (i.e., teaching appropriate behaviors and self-monitoring), or providing opportunities for the child to experience success in order to increase self-efficacy and motivation to succeed in life (i.e., acknowledging students and pointing out successes through reinforcement). Other strategies may be employed to increase the resources required for children to build competence. Providing additional tutoring, free extracurricular activities, and providing job programs for parents may lead to an increase in the resources available to at-risk youth (Benson, Galbraith, & Espeland, 1995; Benson, Scales, Leffert, & Roehlkepartain, 1999).

Utilizing System Level Interventions

Given the importance of activating protective mechanisms across multiple systems, schools may begin to intervene with high-risk and troubling behaviors from a systems perspective. Those students who have been involved in the juvenile justice system or who have exhibited antisocial behavior represent a unique population who are at a greater risk of school and lifelong problems. The use of system-wide proactive approaches to prevent further problems will be especially important to decrease problem behavior and increase student achievement, although information to support the effectiveness of these strategies with high-risk populations is limited.

Schools should be able to use specific behavioral strategies, practices, and processes beyond the individual student and apply them to the whole school with integrity. Specific to implementing a behavioral program, Mayer (1995) provided three factors in schools that are related to antisocial behavior. These factors include (a) unclear rules and policies, (b) inconsistent staff (i.e., lack of staff agreement on policies, inconsistent with rules, staff do not support one another), and (c) lack of allowances for individual differences (i.e., academic and social skills of students vary, the selection of reinforcers, and punishers is not individualized). Overall, academic programs that successfully manage behavior adjust their programs to the student's level of functioning and build skills in areas of struggle. This adjustment allows the student to be successful and work in a positive environment. Implementing these strategies has been associated with a decrease in dropout rates and suspensions (Griffiths, Parson, Burns, & VanDerHeyden, 2007).

School-Wide and Targeted Interventions

School-wide intervention programs may be an effective strategy to increase student engagement (Maddox & Prinz, 2003), particularly for those youth engaging in high-risk behaviors. These programs may help students bond with their schools and experience fewer negative outcomes. Despite the research available on school-wide interventions, there is limited research supporting the use of these interventions for the high-risk population discussed in this chapter. Scott et al. (2002) provide a description of how Positive Behavior Interventions and Supports (PBIS) may be used in alternative education settings as a means of prevention of problem behavior for youth who are at a greater risk. Increasingly, alternative education programs have been identified as schools for disruptive youth (Foley & Pang, 2006). Already socially marginalized, these students have failed to meet the expectations of traditional schools and most likely experienced difficulty developing positive connections with peers and adults at these schools. These schools are often located outside of mainstream school campuses so as to not "distract others" from learning; however, they continue to perpetuate the social marginalization of these students (Munoz, 2004).

One of the fundamental aims of PBIS is to prevent violence and substance abuse among young people. Within most school systems, acts of violence are most often punished by suspensions or expulsions, which remove the student from the learning environment and at times place them into an alternative setting. PBIS programs are intended to reduce the number of both in-school and out-of-school suspensions by preventing disruptive behaviors from occurring, although little is known about the impact of these types of programs on youth with extreme behavior disorders or those already placed in more restrictive educational programs. According to the PBIS Brief Guide (n.d.), the school district staff noted that PBIS implementation has had an overall positive effect on school climate by improving the positive interactions among staff, which provides a positive model for students to follow, although there is little empirical evidence to support this statement.

Recently, Griffiths (2010) investigated the application of school-wide positive behavior support (PBIS) in an alternative school setting. The main purpose of this 1-year evaluation case study was to evaluate the impact of a high school PBIS model on school-wide discipline outcomes (incident reports, teacher reports of student behavior). A secondary aim was to gain an increased understanding of the psychological well-being, engagement, and adjustment of students in the alternative education setting, specifically as it relates to individual student's participation in or response to this particular intervention (PBIS). The impact of intervention implementation was measured using quantitative and qualitative methods. The overall level of implementation of PBIS during the first year of implementation reached 69%, as measured by the School-Wide Evaluation Tool.

The results indicated that the overall number of incident reports did not significantly differ between the baseline year and the implementation year. However, there were some significant reductions in defiance-related behaviors ($z = 2.46$, $p < .05$). Based on student participation in the program, students were divided into two groups: "responders" and "nonresponders." Between these groups, students' responses to a number of measures (obtained prior to intervention) assessing student perception of individual, school, social/community, and home systems were compared. Results indicated that the individual system model and the school system model were able to distinguish between responders and nonresponders. Specifically, a one-way between-groups multivariate analysis of variance

(MANOVA) was performed to explore the difference between groups (responders and nonresponders) on hostility, destructive expression of anger, hope, life satisfaction, depression, and sense of inadequacy. There was a statistically significant difference between responders and nonresponders on the combined variables (F (1, 38) = 3.28, p = .012; Wilks' lambda = .63; partial eta squared = .374). When the results for the variables were considered separately, the univariate differences to reach statistical significance were hostility, destructive expression of anger, and depression. An inspection of the mean scores indicated increased scores on all of these variables for nonresponders.

Within the school system model, there was a statistically significant difference between responders and nonresponders on the combined variables (F (1, 38) = 3.20, p = .035; Wilks' lambda = .794; partial eta squared = .206). When the results for the univariate analyses were considered, the differences to reach statistical significance were academic self-concept, attitude to teachers, and attitude to school. An inspection of the mean scores indicated increased scores (indicating a problem) on the attitude to teachers and attitude to school subtests for nonresponders. Responders had higher mean scores on academic self-concept.

A logistic regression revealed that hostility, destructive expression of anger, depression, academic self-concept, attitude to school, and attitude to teachers, as a group, were able to distinguish responders from nonresponders (χ^2 (6, N = 40) = 12.58, p = .05). These findings seem to indicate that PBIS had some impact on improving outcomes for specific behavior types (defiance) for some students in alternative school settings. However, it must be considered that given the path these students have been on to get to an alternative school, they have likely developed an ingrained distrust and negative attitude toward school and teachers that may require more intensive intervention. In addition, these students, particularly those classified as "nonresponders," tend to experience numerous mental health concerns and contextual risk factors, and will require more intensive supports in conjunction with universal interventions.

An example of a small group intensive intervention program is Check & Connect (C&C), a targeted intervention used to facilitate student engagement and school completion for a small group of students already identified to be at risk. The C&C model includes the core elements of relationship building, routine monitoring of alterable risk factors, individualized intervention, continuous monitoring of targeted students, teaching problem-solving skills, building affiliation with school, and a persistent reinforcement of academic behaviors. Within this program, data are systematically used to guide intervention plans and improve the program at each school site (Sinclair, Christenson, Lehr, & Anderson, 2003). In an evaluation of C&C, 80 elementary and middle school students involved in the program served as participants. Results indicated that after accounting for student risks and prior attendance, intervention staff and student perceptions of the quality and closeness of their relationship were positively correlated with the behavioral engagement indicator of school attendance. The implementers' perception of their relationship with students was related to teacher-rated academic engagement, which includes being prepared for class, work completion, and persistence (Anderson, Christenson, Sinclair, & Lehr, 2004).

Classroom-Based Interventions and Student-Teacher Relationships

In addition to considering school-wide variables and targeted interventions, a variety of classroom variables may be manipulated to increase a student's sense of belonging to a positive learning community and may lead to an increase in student engagement (Furlong et al., 2003). These factors include the use of cooperative learning instructional strategies, positive student-teacher relationships, and promotion of mutual respect within the classroom.

Some classroom interventions may include reducing or eliminating visible academic competition among peers, as it may improve engagement of students of varying academic achievement levels but for various reasons. For example, Wehlage and Rutter (1986) found that students who were average achieving and found their secondary schools to be interpersonally unsupportive and academically frustrating were more likely to drop out of school. By minimizing competition and privileges for honor roll students and high achievers, perceptions of frustration and defeat may be altered (Wehlage & Rutter, 1986). Recently, Morgan (2006) reviewed studies that examined preference and choice making as classroom interventions for increasing behavioral task engagement. These 15 reviewed studies supported the hypothesis that preference assessment and choice making improve the behavior and academic performance of students. Morgan concluded that teachers who use preference assessment, in addition to choice making, are more likely to improve the students' engagement than those using choice-making procedures alone.

Teaching techniques are crucial to increasing engagement. Reeve, Jang, Carrell, Jeon, and Barch (2004) examined the use of autonomy support in a teacher motivation style as a way to promote engagement during instruction. Two aspects of engagement were measured: task involvement (attention, effort, verbal participation, persistence, and positive emotion) and influence attempts (teacher and student verbal and nonverbal attempts to influence the behavior or decision of the other party in a constructive manner). Teachers trained in these techniques displayed more autonomy-supportive behaviors than teachers who were not trained. The more teachers used autonomy support, the more the students were engaged.

With regard to student-teacher relationships, Gregory and Ripski (2008) found that student trust mediated the relation between teacher relational (personal) discipline approaches and both student and teacher reported defiant behavior. In this study, the teachers purposefully sought to make a personal emotional connection with students, and their students reciprocated. In other words, even at the classroom level, the development of a positive trusting student-teacher relationship is associated with decreases of troubling behaviors (Gregory & Ripski, 2008). In a related study, Suldo et al., (2009) found that middle school students' perceptions of teacher emotional support were related to their global subjective well-being. On the other hand, behaviors such as noncompliance may damage student-teacher relationships and result in missed opportunities for learning (Walker & Walker, 1991). Students who exhibit defiant behavior may frequently engage in a negative pattern of interactions with teachers, with noncompliance being a frustrating experience for teachers. Based on observations, children considered to be noncompliant and aggressive or disruptive spend less time on task than comparison students and experience a disruption in academic skills development (Shinn, Ramsey, Walker, O'Neill, & Steiber, 1987).

Although the link between adolescent students' perceptions of the quality of their relationships with teachers and classroom behavior is proximal (e.g., classroom behavior), other researchers report that it is associated with more distal high-risk behaviors that are of concern to educators and parents such as substance use (Rostosky, Owens, Zimmerman, & Riggle, 2003), aggressive/conduct disorder behavior (Frey, Ruchkin, Martin, & Schawb-Stone, 2008), and school dropout (Christenson & Thurlow, 2004). These relations are particularly important for those students who already engage in high-risk behaviors. Many students who engage in high-risk behaviors have had multiple experiences of failure in the school setting, as well as a series of negative interactions with adults at school, at home, and in the community.

When further examining relationships between students and their teachers, Hughes and Kwok (2007) investigated the influence of student-teacher and parent-teacher relationships on engagement and achievement. Their model suggests that the quality of teacher's relationships with students and their parents explained the relation between students' background and student engagement. Engagement, in turn, mediated the relations between student-teacher and parent-teacher relatedness and student achievement the following year. Results indicated that African-American children and their parents had less supportive relationships with teachers when compared with Latino and Caucasian children and their parents. Schools should not only work on parental involvement in school but also develop the relationship between parents and teachers, particularly with the families of low-income and minority students. Teachers may need training in how to build successful relationships with parents and how to create a supportive classroom environment.

Interventions Beyond the School Context

Given the multiple risk factors present in the lives of "high-risk youth," it is likely that intervention should extend beyond the immediate school setting. However, interventions that are useful and impact more than one environment for the child may be identified by school professionals. Multisystemic therapy has shown some promise in making changes for these youth (Timmons-Mitchell, Bender, Kishna, & Mitchell, 2006). This speaks to the importance of understanding each child within the context of the systems within which he or she is embedded. Understanding these students' needs on both a broad and in-depth level will allow school professionals to measure the student's current status, set goals for the student, coordinate services, and evaluate whether or not the interventions were effective. Rather than pouring multiple resources into an individual without a precontemplated outcome or plan, coordination of services may prove to be effective, economical, and efficient.

Summary of Strategies to Build Bonding and Connectedness

When it comes to high-risk behaviors, it is well established that positive family relatedness and other factors can be both promotive and protective factors against involvement in high-risk behaviors such as substance use, aggression, and other externalizing behavior problems (Witherspoon, Schotland, Way, & Hughes, 2009). In addition, it is known that students who report that they have formed a generalized belief that adults at their school care about them are at substantially lower risk of involvement in troubling externalizing behaviors. Positive connectedness to adults at school may serve as a barrier to high-risk or troubling behaviors. It is almost as if when faced with choices related to high-risk behaviors, a student would consider the question of "Who at this school would I disappoint if I engaged in this behavior?" This highlights the importance of schools focusing on system-wide programs and intensive interventions that provide the opportunity to reconstruct and repair bonds with marginalized students across various contexts.

In addition, one must consider that most youth do not engage in serious troubling or risky behaviors whether or not they are bonded or connected to school. There are other protective forces in youth lives such as extended family members, community organizations, mentors, music teachers, and many others. As Masten (2009) suggested, youth seem to need, and benefit from having, life conditions that include the caring attention of adults. For many youth, a natural, meaningful context for this to occur is in the school with teachers and other adults who are engaged with them on a daily basis, often over several years.

A final point that merits some attention is that of which aspects of affective engagement are the focus of research. Since the Resnick et al., (1997) article appeared in the *Journal of the American Medical Association* and refocused attention on what was called "school connectedness," it has been cited more than a 1,000 times by other publications indexed in the PsyInfo database. This study led to a special journal issue in the *Journal of School Health*, September 2004, with articles focusing on school connectedness (Blum & Libbey, 2004). In addition, the Centers for Disease Control and Prevention (CDC, 2009) released a document that specifically summarizes research-supported strategies to build school connectedness. As defined in the CDC document, connectedness is a "…belief by students that adults in the school care about their learning as well as about them as individuals" (CDC, 2009, p. 3). However, as used in practice, the same scale used in the Resnick et al. (1997) study and called school connectedness has been used in other studies (e.g., Anderman, 2002) and called "school bonding." This imprecision in the labeling of the latent traits of interest is not trivial. If researchers interested in the forces that have a protective influence on youth aim to examine student-teacher relationships, then the term that makes the most sense is "caring adult relationships." This contrasts with researchers who are interested in whether a student broadly perceives his or her school environment to be one that is accepting and to which they feel included in as a member of the school community (Shochet, Smith, Furlong, & Homel, 2011). This latter notion of student engagement has been called school bonding or, when the student personally identified as being a "citizen" of the school community, "school membership" (Finn, 1989; Goodenow, 1993; Wehlage, 1989). This is what Wehlage defined as "more than simple technical enrollment in the school. It means that students have established a social bond between themselves, the adults in the school, and the norms governing the institution" (Wehlage, 1989, p. 10).

Future research examining the salvative effects of the affective component of student engagement, in our view, will be enhanced by more precision in the latent traits being examined and assuring that the measures being used actually measure those traits (see You, Ritchey, Furlong, Shochet, & Boman, 2011; and Furlong, O'Brennan, & You, 2011 for more discussion of this topic). Unified research in the area of student engagement can allow for continued advancements in understanding how to best engage students, specifically high-risk students, and yield positive academic and life outcomes for youth.

References

Abbott, R. D., O'Donnell, J., Hawkins, J. D., Hill, K. G., Kosterman, R., & Catalano, R. F. (1998). Changing teaching practices to promote achievement and bonding to school. *The American Journal of Orthopsychiatry*, 68, 542–552. doi:10.1037/h0080363.

Abbott-Chapman, J., Denholm, C., & Wyld, C. (2008). Social support as a factor inhibiting teenage risk-taking: Views of students, parents and professionals. *Journal of Youth Studies*, 11, 611–627. doi:10.1080/13676260802191938.

Alexander, K. L., Entwisle, D. R., & Dauber, S. L. (1993). First grade classroom behavior: Its short- and long-term consequences for school performance. *Child Development*, 64, 801–814. doi:10.2307/1131219.

Alexander, K. L., Entwisle, D. R., & Dauber, S. L. (1996). Children in motion: School transfers and elementary school performance. *The Journal of Educational Research*, 90, 3–12.

Alliance for Excellent Education. (2009). *The high cost of high school dropouts: What the nation pays for inadequate high schools*. Available at http://www.all4ed.org/.

Anderman, E. M. (2002). School effects on psychological outcomes during adolescence. *Journal of Educational Psychology*, 94, 795–809. doi:10.1037//0022-0663.94.4.795.

Anderman, L. H., & Anderman, E. M. (1999). Social predictors of changes in students' achievement goal orientations. *Contemporary Educational Psychology*, 24, 21–37. doi:10.1006/ceps.1998.0978.

Anderson, A. R., Christenson, S. L., Sinclair, M. F., & Lehr, C. A. (2004). Check & Connect: The importance of relationships for promoting engagement with school. *Journal of School Psychology*, 42, 95–113. doi:10.1016/j.jsp.2004.01.002.

Appleton, J. J., Christenson, S. L., & Furlong, M. J. (2008). Student engagement with school: Critical conceptual and methodological issues of the construct. *Psychology in the Schools*, 45, 369–386. doi:10.1002/pits.20303.

Archambault, I., Janosz, M., Morizot, J., & Pagani, L. (2009). Adolescent behavioral, affective, and cognitive engagement in school: Relationship to dropout. *The Journal of School Health*, 79, 408–415. doi:10.1111/j.1746-1561.2009.00428.x.

Arthur, M. W., J.D. Hawkins, J. D., Pollard, J. A., Catalano, R. F., & Baglioni, A. J. (2002). Measuring risk and protective factors for substance use, delinquency, and other adolescent problem behaviors: The Communities That Care Youth Survey. *Evaluation Review*, 26, 575–603. doi:10.1177/019384102237850.

Barrington, B. L., & Hendricks, B. (1989). Differentiating characteristics of high school graduates, dropouts, and nongraduates. *The Journal of Educational Research*, 82, 309–319.

Benson, P. L., Galbraith, J., & Espeland, P. (1995). *What kids need to succeed*. Minneapolis, MN: Free Spirit.

Benson, P. L., Scales, P. C., Leffert, N., & Roehlkepartain, E. C. (1999). *A fragile foundation: The state of developmental assets among American youth*. Minneapolis, MN: Search Institute.

Blum, R. W., & Libbey, H. P. (2004). School connectedness: Strengthening health and educational outcomes for teenagers. Executive summary. *The Journal of School Health*, 74, 231–232.

Bond, L., Butler, H., Deip, E., Dip, G., Lydnal, T., Carlin, J., et al. (2007). Social and school connectedness in early secondary school as predictors of late teenage substance use, mental health, and academic outcomes. *Journal of Adolescent Health*, 40, e9–e18. doi:10.1016/j.jadohealth.2006.10.013.

Bridgeland, J. M., DiIulio, J., & Morison, K. B. (2006, March). *The silent epidemic: Perspectives of high school dropouts*. Washington, DC: Civic Enterprises, LLC.

Brookmeyer, K., Fanti, K., & Henrich, C. (2006). Schools, parents, and youth violence: A multilevel ecological analysis. *Journal of Clinical Child and Adolescent Psychology, 35*, 504–514. doi:10.1207/s15374424jccp3504_2.

Carter, M., McGee, R., Taylor, B., & Williams, S. (2007). Health outcomes in adolescence: Associations with family, friends and school engagement. *Journal of Adolescence, 30*, 51–62.

Catalano, R. F., Hawkins, J. D., & Smith, B. H. (2001). Delinquent behavior. *Pediatrics in Review, 23*, 387–392.

Catalano, R. F., Kosterman, R., Hawkins, J. D., Newcomb, M. D., & Abbott, R. D. (1996). Modeling the etiology of adolescent substance use: A test of the social development model. *Journal of Drug Issues, 26*, 429–455.

Centers for Disease Control and Prevention. (2009). *School connectedness: Strategies for increasing protective factors among youth*. Atlanta, GA: U.S. Department of Health and Human Services.

Christenson, S. L., & Thurlow, M. L. (2004). School dropouts: Prevention considerations, interventions, and challenges. *Current Directions in Psychological Science, 13*, 36–39. doi:10.1111/j.0963-7214.2004.01301010.x.

Connell, J. P., Halpern-Felsher, B. L., Clifford, E., Crichlow, W., & Usinger, P. (1995). Hanging in there: Behavioral, psychological, and contextual factors affecting whether African American adolescents stay in high school. *Journal of Adolescent Research, 10*, 41–63.

Connell, J. P., & Wellborn, J. G. (1991). Competence, autonomy, and relatedness: A motivational analysis of self-system processes. In M. R. Gunnar & L. A. Sroufe (Eds.), *Self processes and development* (Vol. 23). Hillsdale, NJ: Lawrence Erlbaum.

Croninger, R. G., & Lee, V. E. (2001). Social capital and dropping out of high school: Benefits to at-risk students of teacher's support and guidance. *Teachers College Record, 103*, 548–581. doi:10.1111/0161-4681.00127.

Crosnoe, R., Mistry, R. S., & Elder, G. H., Jr. (2002). Economic disadvantage, family dynamics, and adolescent enrollment in higher education. *Journal of Marriage and the Family, 64*, 690–702. doi:10.1111/j.1741-3737.2002.00690.x.

Currie, C., et al. (Eds.). *Health and health behaviour among young people. health behaviour in school-aged children: a WHO Cross-National Study (HBSC), International Report*. Copenhagen: WHO, 2000. Available, from http://www.hbsc.org/downloads/Int_Report_00.pdf.

Dornbusch, S., Erikson, K., Laird, J., & Wong, C. (2001). The relation of family and school attachment to adolescent deviance in diverse groups and communities. *Journal of Adolescent Research, 16*, 396–422. doi:10.1177/0743558401164006.

Eccles, J. S., & Wigfield, A. (2002). Motivational beliefs, values, and goals. *Annual Review of Psychology, 53*, 109–132. doi:10.1146/annurev.psych.53.100901.135153.

Fine, M. (1991). *Framing dropouts: Notes on the politics of an urban public high school*. Albany, NY: State University of New York Press.

Finn, J. D. (1989). Withdrawing from school. *Review of Educational Research, 29*, 141–162. doi:10.3102/00346543059002117.

Finn, J. D. (1993). *School engagement and students at risk*. Washington, DC: National Center for Education Statistics.

Finn, J. D., & Rock, D. A. (1997). Academic success among students at risk. *Journal of Applied Psychology, 82*, 221–234. doi:10.1037/0021-9010.82.2.221.

Finn, J. D., & Voelkl, K. E. (1993). School characteristics related to student engagement. *The Journal of Negro Education, 62*, 249–268. doi:10.2307/2295464.

Flaspohler, P., Elfstrom, J., Vanderzee, K., Sink, H., & Birchmeier, Z. (2009). Stand by me: The effects of peer and teacher support in mitigating the impact of bullying on quality of life. *Psychology in the Schools, 46*, 636–649. doi:10.1002/pits.20404.

Foley, R. M., & Pang, L. S. (2006). Alternative education programs: Program and student characteristics. *The High School Journal, 89*, 10–21.

Fredricks, J. A., Blumenfeld, P. C., & Paris, A. H. (2004). School engagement: Potential of the concept, state of the evidence. *Review of Educational Research, 74*, 59–109. doi:10.3102/00346543074001059.

Frey, A., Ruchkin, V., Martin, A., & Schawb-Stone, M. (2008). Adolescents in transition: School and family characteristics in the development of violent behaviors entering high school. *Child Psychiatry and Human Development, 40*, 1–13. doi:10.1007/s10578-008-0105.

Furlong, M. J., O'Brennan, L., & You, S. (2011). Psychometric properties of the Add Health School Connectedness Scale for 18 sociocultural groups. *Psychology in the Schools, 48*, 986–997.

Furlong, M. J., Ritchey, K., & O'Brennan, L. (2009). Developing norms for the California Resilience Youth Development Module: Internal assets and school resources subscales. *The California School Psychologist, 14*, 35–46.

Furlong, M. J., Whipple, A. D., St. Jean, G., Simental, J., Soliz, A., & Punthuna, S. (2003). Multiple contexts of school engagement: Moving toward a unifying framework for educational research and practice. *The California School Psychologist, 8*, 99–114.

Goodenow, C. (1993). The psychological sense of school membership among adolescents: Scale development and educational correlates. *Psychology in the Schools, 30*, 79–90. doi:10.1002/1520-6807(199301)30:1<79::AID-PITS2310300113>3.0.CO;2-X.

Gottfredson, D. C., Gerstenblith, S. A., Soule, D. A., Womer, S. C., & Lu, S. (2004). Do after school programs reduce delinquency? *Prevention Science: The Official Journal of the Society for Prevention Research, 5*, 253–266. doi:10.1023/B:PREV.0000045359.41696.02.

Gregory, A., & Ripski, M. B. (2008). Adolescent trust in teachers: Implications for behavior in the high school classroom. *School Psychology Review, 37*, 337–353.

Griffiths, A. J. (2010). *Positive behavior support in the alternative education setting: A case study*. Unpublished doctoral dissertation, University of California, Santa Barbara, Santa Barbara, CA.

Griffiths, A. J., Parson, L. B., Burns, M. K., & VanDerHeyden, A. M. (2007). *Response to intervention: Research for practice*. Alexandria, VA: National Association of State Directors of Special Education.

Guthrie, J. T. (2001, March). Contexts for engagement and motivation in reading. *Reading Online, 4*(8). Available, from http://www.readingonline.org/articles/art_index.asp?HREF=/articles/handbook/guthrie/index.html.

Gutman, L. M., & Midgley, C. (2000). The role of protective factors in supporting the academic achievement of poor African American adolescents during the middle school transition. *Journal of Youth and Adolescence, 29*, 223–248. doi:10.1023/A:1005108700243.

Hanson, T. L., & Kim, J. O. (2007). *Measuring resilience and youth development: The psychometric properties of the Healthy Kids Survey* (Issues & Answers Report, REL 2007–No. 034). Washington, DC: U.S. Department of Education, Institute of Education Sciences, National Center for Education Evaluation and Regional Assistance, Regional Educational Laboratory West.

Hawken, L. S., & Horner, R. H. (2003). Implementing a targeted intervention within a school-wide system of behavior support. *Journal of Behavioral Education, 12*, 225–240. doi:10.1023/A:1025512411930.

Hawkins, J. D., Guo, J., Hill, K. G., Battin-Pearson, S., & Abbott, R. D. (2001). Long-term effects of the Seattle Social Development intervention on school bonding trajectories. In J. Maggs & J. Schulenberg (Eds.), *Applied developmental science: Special issue: Prevention as altering the course of development, 5*, 225–236. doi:10.1207/S1532480XADS0504_04.

Henrich, C., Brookmeyer, K., & Shahar, G. (2005). Weapon violence in adolescence: Parent and school connectedness as protective factors. *Journal of Adolescent Health, 37*, 306–312. doi:10.1016/j.jadohealth.2005.03.022.

Henry, K. L. (2008). Low prosocial attachment, involvement with drug-using peers, and adolescent drug use: A longitudinal examination of meditational mechanisms. *Psychology of Addictive Behaviors, 22*, 302–308. doi:10.1037/0893-164X.22.2.302.

Herrenkohl, T. I., Hawkins, J. D., Chung, I.-J., Hill, K. G., & Battin-Pearson, S. (2000). School and community risk factors and interventions. In R. Loeber & D. P. Farrington (Eds.), *Child delinquents: Development, intervention, and service needs* (pp. 211–246). Thousand Oaks, CA: Sage.

Hirschi, T. (1969). *Causes of delinquency*. Berkeley, CA/Los Angeles: University of California Press.

Holdsworth, R., & Blanchard, M. (2006). Unheard voices: Themes emerging from studies of the views about school engagement of young people with high support needs in the area of mental health. *Australian Journal of Guidance and Counselling, 16*, 14–28. doi:10.1375/ajgc.16.1.14.

Hughes, J., & Kwok, O. (2007). Influence of student-teacher and parent-teacher relationships on lower achieving readers' engagement and achievement in the primary grades. *Journal of Educational Psychology, 99*, 39–51. doi:10.1037/0022-0663.99.1.39.

Ingels, S. J., Dowd, K. L., Stipe, J. L., Baldridge, J. D., Bartot, V. H., & Frankel, M. R. (1994, October). Second follow-up: Dropout component data file user's manual. Washington, DC: U.S. Department of Education, Office of Educational Research and Improvement. Available, from http://nces.ed.gov/pubsearch/pubsinfo.asp?pubid=94375.

Janosz, M., Archambault, I., Morizot, J., & Pagani, L. (2008). School engagement trajectories and their differential predictive relations to dropout. *Journal of Social Issues, 64*, 21–40. doi:10.1111/j.1540-4560.2008.00546.x.

Jimerson, S. R., Campos, E., & Greif, J. L. (2003). Toward an understanding of definitions and measures of school engagement and related terms. *California School Psychologist, 8*, 7–27. Retrieved from www.csa.com.

Johnson, L. S. (2009). School contexts and student belonging: A mixed methods study of an innovative high school. *The School Community Journal, 19*, 99–118.

Kodjo, C., Auinger, P., & Ryan, S. (2003). Demographic, intrinsic, and extrinsic factors associated with weapon carrying at school. *Archives of Pediatric Adolescent Medicine, 157*, 96–103.

Ladd, G. W., & Dinella, L. M. (2009). Continuity and change in early school engagement: Predictive of children's achievement trajectories from first to eighth grade. *Journal of Educational Psychology, 101*, 190–206. doi:10.1037/a0013153.

Langberg, J. M., Epstein, J. N., Urbanowicz, C. M., Simon, J. O., & Graham, A. J. (2008). Efficacy of an organization skills intervention to improve the academic functioning of students with attention-deficit/hyperactivity disorder. *School Psychology Quarterly, 23*, 407–417. doi:10.1037/1045-3830.23.3.407.

Langberg, J. M., Smith, B. H., Bogle, K. E., Schmidt, J. D., Cole, W. R., & Pender, C. A. S. (2006). A pilot evaluation of small group challenging horizons program (CHP): A randomized trial. *Journal of Applied School Psychology, 23*, 31–58. doi:10.1300/J370v23n01_02.

Lee, V. E., & Smith, J. B. (1995). Effects of high school restructuring and size on early gains in achievement and engagement. *Sociology of Education, 68*, 241–270. doi:10.2307/2112741.

Loukas, A., Suzuki, R., & Horton, K. (2006). Examining school connectedness as a mediator of school climate effects. *Journal of Research on Adolescence, 16*, 491–502. doi:10.1111/j.1532-7795.2006.00504.x.

Maddox, S. J., & Prinz, R. J. (2003). School bonding in children and adolescents: Conceptualization, assessment, and associated variables. *Clinical Child and Family Psychology Review, 6*, 31–49. doi:10.1023/A:1022214022478.

Malecki, C. K., Demaray, M. K., & Elliott, S. E. (2000). The Child and Adolescent Social Support Scale. DeKalb: Northern Illinois University.

Manlove, J. (1998). The influence of high school dropout and school disengagement on the risk of school-age pregnancy. *Journal of Research on Adolescence, 8*, 187–220. doi:10.1207/s15327795jra0802_2.

Masten, A. S. (2009). Ordinary magic: Lessons from research on resilience in human development. *Education Canada, 49*, 28–32.

Mayer, G. R. (1995). Preventing antisocial behavior in the schools. *Journal of Applied Behavior Analysis, 28*, 467–478.

McNeely, C., & Falci, C. (2004). School connectedness and the transition into and out of health-risk behavior among adolescents: A comparison of social belonging and teacher support. *The Journal of School Health, 74*, 284–292. doi:10.1111/j.1746-1561.2004.tb08285.x.

McPartland, J. M. (1994). Dropout prevention in theory and practice. In R. J. Rossi (Ed.), *Schools and students at risk: Context and framework for positive change* (pp. 255–276). New York: Teachers College.

Mehan, H., Villanueva, I., Hubbard, L., Linz, A., Okamato, D., & Adams, J. (1996). *Constructing school success: The consequences of untracking low achieving students*. Cambridge, UK: Cambridge University Press.

Molina, B. S. G., Flory, K., Bukstein, O. G., Greiner, A. R., Baker, J. L., Krug, V., et al. (2008). Feasibility and preliminary efficacy of an after school program for middle schoolers with ADHD: A randomized trial in a large public middle school. *Journal of Attention Disorders, 12*, 207–217. doi:10.1177/1087054707311666.

Moore, R. J., Cartledge, G., & Heckaman, K. (1995). The effects of social skill instruction and self-monitoring on game-related behaviors of adolescents with emotional or behavioral disorders. *Behavioral Disorders, 20*, 253–266.

Morgan, P. L. (2006). Increasing task engagement using preference or choice making: Some behavioral and methodological factors affecting their efficacy as classroom interventions. *Remedial and Special Education, 27*, 176–187. doi:10.1177/07419325060270030601.

Morrison, G., & Skiba, R. (2001). Predicting violence from school misbehavior: Promises and perils. *Psychology in the Schools, 38*, 173–184. doi:10.1002/pits.1008.

Munoz, J. S. (2004). The social construction of alternative education: Re-examining the margins of public education for at-risk Chicano/a students. *The High School Journal, 88*, 3–22.

Murray, C., & Malmgren, K. (2005). Implementing a teacher-student relationship program in a high poverty urban school: Effects on social, emotional, and academic adjustment and lessons learned. *Journal of School Psychology, 43*, 137–152. doi:10.1016/j.jsp. 2005.01.003.

Nation, M., Vieno, A., Perkins, D., & Santinello, M. (2008). Bullying in school and adolescent sense of empowerment: An analysis of relationships with parents, friends, and teachers. *Journal of Community & Applied Social Psychology, 18*, 211–232. doi:10.1002/casp. 921.

National Research Council and Institute of Medicine. (2004). *Engaging schools: Fostering high school students' motivation to learn*. Committee on increasing high school students' engagement and motivation to learn. Washington, DC: The National Academies Press.

Noddings, N. (1995). Teaching themes of care. *Phi Delta Kappa, 76*, 675–679.

O'Farrell, S., Morrison, G. M., & Furlong, M. J. (2006). School engagement. In G. Bear & K. Minke (Eds.), *Children's needs III* (pp. 45–58). Bethesda, MD: National Association of School Psychologists.

O'Farrell, S. L., & Morrison, G. M. (2003). A factor analysis exploring school bonding and related constructs among upper elementary students. *The California School Psychologist, 8*, 53–72.

PBIS Brief Guide. (n.d.). Retrieved May 2, 2008, from www.pbis.org.

Perry, J. C. (2008). School engagement among urban youth of color. *Journal of Career Development, 34*, 397–422. doi:0.1177/0894845308316293.

Perry, J. C., Liu, X., & Pabian, Y. (2010). School engagement as a mediator of academic performance among urban youth: The role of career preparation, parental career support, and teacher support. *The Counseling Psychologist, 38*, 269–295. doi:10.1177/0011000009349272.

Pyper, R., Freiberg, H. J., Ginsburg, M., & Spuck, D. W. (1987). Instruments to measure teacher, parent, and student perceptions of school climate. In L. W. Barber (Ed.), *School climate* (pp. 87–96). Bloomington, IN: Center on Evaluation, Phi Delta Kappa.

Rasmussen, M., Damsgaard, M., Holstein, B., & Poulsen, L. P. (2005). School connectedness and daily smoking among boys and girls: The influence of parental smoking norms. *European Journal of Public Health, 2005*(15), 607–612. doi:10.1093/eurpub/cki039.

Reeve, J., Jang, H., Carrell, D., Jeon, S., & Barch, J. (2004). Enhancing students' engagement by increasing teachers' autonomy support. *Motivation and Emotion, 28*, 147–169. doi:10.1023/B:MOEM.0000032312.95499.6f.

Resnick, M. D., Bearman, P. S., Blum, R. W., Bauman, K. E., Harris, K. M., Jones, J., et al. (1997). Protecting adolescents from harm: Findings from the National Longitudinal Study on Adolescent Health. *Journal of the American Medical Association, 278*, 823–832. doi:10.1001/jama.278.10.823.

Roehlkepartain, E. C., Benson, P. L., & Sesma, A. (2003). *Signs of progress in putting children first: Developmental assets among youth in St. Louis Park, 1997–2001*. Prepared by Search Institute for St. Louis Park's Children First Initiative, Minneapolis, MN.

Roeser, R., Midgley, C., & Urdan, T. C. (1996). Perception of the school environment and early adolescents' psychological and behavioral functioning in school: The mediating role of goals and belonging. *Journal of Educational Psychology, 88*, 408–422. doi:10.1037/0022-0663.88.3.408.

Roscigno, V. J., & Ainsworth-Darnell, J. W. (1999). Race and cultural/educational resources: Inequality, micropolitical processes, and achievement returns. *Sociology of Education, 72*, 158–178. doi:10.2307/2673227.

Rostosky, S. S., Owens, G. P., Zimmerman, R. S., & Riggle, E. D. B. (2003). Associations among sexual attraction status, school belonging, and alcohol and marijuana use in rural high school students. *Journal of Adolescence, 26*, 741–751. doi:10.1016/j.adolescence.2003.09.002.

Rutter, M. (1987). Psychosocial resilience and protective mechanisms. *The American Journal of Orthopsychiatry, 57*, 316–331.

Sandhu, D. S., Arora, M., & Sandhu, V. S. (2001). School violence: Risk factors, psychological correlates, prevention and intervention strategies. In D. Sandhu (Ed.), *Faces of violence: Psychological correlates, concepts and intervention strategies* (pp. 45–71). Huntington, NY: Nova Science.

Schaufeli, W. B., Martinez, I., Pinto, A. M., Salanova, M., & Bakker, A. (2002). Burnout and engagement in university students: A cross-national study. *Journal of Cross-Cultural Psychology, 33*, 464–481. doi:10.1177/0022022102033005003.

Scott, T. M., Nelson, C. M., Liaupsin, C. J., Jolivette, K., Christle, C. A., & Riney, M. (2002). Addressing the needs of at-risk and adjudicated youth through positive behavior support: Effective prevention practices. *Education and Treatment of Children, 25*, 532–551.

Sharkey, J. D., You, S., & Schnoebelen, K. J. (2008). The relationship of school assets, individual resilience, and student engagement for youth grouped by level of family functioning. *Psychology in the Schools, 45*, 402–418. doi:10.1002/pits.20305.

Shinn, M. R., Ramsey, E., Walker, H. M., O'Neill, R., & Steiber, S. (1987). Antisocial behavior in school settings: Initial differences in an at-risk and normal population. *Journal of Special Education, 2*, 69–84.

Shochet, I. M., Smith, C. L., Furlong, M. J., & Homel, R. (2011). A prospective study investigating the impact of school belonging factors on negative affect in adolescents. *Journal of Clinical Child & Adolescent Psychology, 40*, 586–595. http://dx.doi.org/10.1080/15374416.2011.581616.

Simons-Morton, B. (2004). Prospective association of peer influence, school engagement, drinking expectancies, and parent expectations with drinking initiation among sixth graders. *Addictive Behaviors, 29*, 299–309. doi:10.1016/j.addbeh.2003.08.005.

Simons-Morton, B., & Chen, R. (2009). Peer and parent influences on school engagement among early adolescents. *Youth and Society, 41*, 3–25. doi:10.1177/0044118X09334861.

Simons-Morton, B., Crump, A., Haynie, D., & Saylor, K. (1999). Student-school bonding and adolescent problem behaviors. *Health Education Research, 14*, 99–107. doi:10.1093/her/14.1.99.

Sinclair, M. F., Christenson, S. L., Evelo, D. L., & Hurley, C. M. (1998). Dropout prevention for youth with disabilities: Efficacy of a sustained school engagement procedure. *Exceptional Children, 65*, 7–21.

Sinclair, M. F., Christenson, S. L., Lehr, C. A., & Anderson, A. R. (2003). Facilitating student engagement: Lessons learned from Check & Connect longitudinal studies. *The California School Psychologist, 8*, 29–42.

Sinclair, M. F., Christenson, S. L., & Thurlow, M. L. (2005). Promoting school completion of urban secondary youth with emotional or behavioral disabilities. *Exceptional Children, 71*, 465–482.

Solorzano, D. G., & Delgado Bernal, D. (2001). Examining transformational resistance through a critical race and LatCrit theory framework: Chicana and Chicano students in an urban context. *Urban Education, 36*, 308–342. doi:10.1177/0042085901363002.

Suldo, S. M., Friedrich, A. A., White, T., Farmer, J., Minch, D., & Michalowski, J. (2009). Teacher support and adolescents' subjective well-being: A mixed-methods investigation. *School Psychology Review, 38*, 67–85.

Timmons-Mitchell, J., Bender, M. B., Kishna, M. A., & Mitchell, C. C. (2006). An independent effectiveness trial of multisystemic therapy with juvenile justice youth. *Journal of Clinical Child and Adolescent Psychology, 35*, 227–236. doi:10.1207/s15374424jccp3502_6.

Torsheim, T., Wold, B., & Samdal, O. (2000). The teacher and classmate support scale: Factor structure, test–retest reliability and validity in samples of 13- and 15-year-old adolescents. School Psychology International, *21*, 195–212. doi:10.1177/0143034300212006.

Walker, H. M., & Walker, J. T. (1991). *Coping with noncompliance in the classroom: A positive approach for teachers*. Austin, TX: Pro-Ed.

Wehlage, G. (1989). Dropping out: Can schools be expected to prevent it? In L. Weise, E. Farrar, & H. Petrie (Eds.), *Dropouts from school*. Albany, NY: State University of New York Press.

Wehlage, G. G., & Rutter, R. A. (1986). Dropping out: How much do schools contribute to the problem? *Teachers College Record, 87*, 374–392. doi:10.2307/1164483.

Weissberg, R. P., Caplan, M., & Harwood, R. L. (1991). Promoting competent young people in competence-enhancing environments: A systems-based perspective on primary prevention. Journal of Consulting and Clinical Psychology, 59, 830–841. doi:10.1037/0022-006X.59.6.830.

Witherspoon, D., Schotland, M., Way, N., & Hughes, S. (2009). Connecting the dots: How connectedness to multiple contexts influences the psychological and academic adjustment of urban youth. *Applied Developmental Science, 13*, 199–216. doi:10.1080/10888690903288755.

You, S., Ritchey, K., Furlong, M. J., Shochet, I., & Boman, P. (2011). Examination of the latent structure of the Psychological Sense of School Membership Scale. *Journal of Psychoeducational Assessment, 29*(3), 225–237. doi:10.1177/0734282910379968.

Trajectories and Patterns of Student Engagement: Evidence from a Longitudinal Study

28

Cathy Wylie and Edith Hodgen

Abstract

Longitudinal study of student engagement patterns is relatively rare but sheds useful light on the factors that contribute to different levels of student engagement in school and its role in student achievement. This chapter uses data from a New Zealand study to focus on changes in student engagement patterns between the ages of 10 and 16, to show (a) the range of individual trajectories of student engagement that lie behind overall declines, and (b) how these different trajectories are related to differences in competency levels and to activities and relationships outside school in ways that compound the patterns of engagement in learning in the school environment and vice versa. Looking at student engagement longitudinally raises the question of whether decline in student engagement levels overall is related to transitions between schools or occurs more as part of general human development that may be better supported by different learning opportunities than schools currently provide. The chapter ends with the case for more longitudinal research into the nature and role of student engagement across different schooling contexts.

Introduction

Student engagement in school is important to student outcomes because of the co-productive nature of learning. School success is receiving ever-increasing emphasis as an essential component of moving into productive adulthood, as opportunities for employment without school qualifications grow tighter. The link between disengagement in school and eventually dropping out of school, or leaving without a qualification that will allow meaningful employment and further education opportunities, is now well established (Finn, 1989; Rumberger & Rotermund, 2012). The bar has also been raised on expectations of schools that they succeed with a majority, or all, of their students, as evident in policies such as No Child Left Behind in the United States. Systematic focus on patterns of student engagement in school provides a lens for schools to gauge how well they are activating student energy, interest and self-regulation.

C. Wylie, Ph.D. (✉) • E. Hodgen
New Zealand Council for Educational Research,
Wellington 6040, New Zealand
e-mail: cathy.wylie@nzcer.org.nz;
Edith.hodgen@nzcer.org.nz

Much of the research focus on student engagement in school as a whole (rather than engagement in particular learning tasks, at a more micro-level) has focused on those at the disengaged end of the spectrum. Janosz, Archambault, Morizot, and Pagani (2008) questioned whether there is in fact a uniform trajectory of disengagement culminating in dropping out—and therefore, whether there was also a uniform trajectory of engagement—using two analyzes of longitudinal data which show a range of patterns. Categorization of the close to a third of a sample of 1,582 Montreal high school students who had not completed high school by age 22 showed that 40% had had high levels of school motivation—the '*quiet* dropouts' (Janosz, LeBlanc, Boulerice, & Tremblay, 2000). Analysis of student engagement trajectories between ages 12 and 16 of 13,280 students from 69 middle and high schools serving low-socioeconomic areas in Quebec showed seven different pathways. Three of these pathways were relatively stable, accounting for 91% of the students. Fourteen percent had high engagement levels throughout the period. Just over half (53%) had somewhat high levels of engagement, with a slight decline over the period. Twenty-four percent had a 'stable moderate' trajectory of engagement, at lower levels than the first two groups. The other four groups comprised those whose student engagement decreased over the period (2%); those whose engagement increased (1%); those whose engagement was low at age 12, increased at 14, then became low again at age 16 (3%); and those whose engagement was moderate at age 12, decreased to low levels at age 14, then returned to moderate levels at age 16 (3%). This last group was most likely to drop out—42% did so. By contrast, only 1% of the first three groups dropped out of school. However, because most students were in the first three groups, 21% of the dropouts in fact came from the group with the stable student engagement trajectories.

Janosz et al. (2008) found that those whose engagement trajectories were unstable over this adolescent period were more likely to have lower self-reported grades or be in special classes; they had also began the period with lower levels of engagement. The authors suggested that the differences found between the stable and unstable patterns of engagement were likely to reflect levels of stability in individuals, their families and school environments, and in the match between these.

This chapter aims to build on this important contribution to the deepening understanding of the development and role of student engagement by exploring another longitudinal data-set from a different country. This data-set, from the *Competent Learners* study, allows us to start a little earlier, before adolescence (age 10), to track engagement levels in relation to competency levels over time and to situate student engagement in school in relation to student engagement in activities outside school, including risk behaviour, friendships and relations with family, as well as learning opportunities in the final years of high school.

We start with a brief description of the *Competent Learners* study to provide a context for the way student engagement and motivation are operationalized in this chapter. Next, the overall pattern of student engagement from ages 10 to 16 is charted, before the trajectories found for this New Zealand sample are described. Then we outline the links between different trajectories of student engagement and competency levels, high school qualifications and post-school learning experiences up to age 20. A closer look at two different dimensions of student engagement in school at ages 14 and 16 follows, to explore their relative weight in relation to student competency levels and high school qualifications and out-of-school experiences and relationships. The conclusion discusses implications of the findings, with some suggestions for further longitudinal research.

The Competent Learners Study

The *Competent Learners* study originated in the early 1990s to analyze the impact of early childhood education and, if Ministry of Education funding continued for more than 3 years, to provide a second cohort for a linked study on the impact of policy changes which increased family choice of school and school competition. The linked study did not continue, but the *Competent Learners* study did, as an exploratory study of the roles of education and home in the development of competencies. Data collection

Table 28.1 Competent Learners study: data collection

Age of participants	Number in study	Number of early childhood education (ECE) services or schools	Data collected
Near 5	307 (Full study)	87 ECE services	Assessment tasks, observations of children's activities in ECE centre, parent interview, teacher rating of child's attitudinal competencies, ECE director interview, ECE service quality rating
Near 5	767 (Light interview)	56 ECE services	Education participation, family resources, home activities (from parent and teacher survey)
6	298 (Full study)	121 schools	Assessment tasks, child interview, parent interview, teacher rating of child's attitudinal competencies, and contextual information
8	523 (Full study + 242 from light interview)	168 schools	Assessment tasks, child interview, parent interview, teacher rating of child's attitudinal competencies, and contextual information
10	507	185 schools	Assessment tasks, child interview, parent interview, teacher rating of child's attitudinal competencies, and contextual information
12	496	129 schools	Assessment tasks, child interview, parent interview, teacher rating of child's attitudinal competencies, and contextual information
14	476	76 schools	Assessment tasks, student interview, student self-report, parent interview, teacher rating of student's attitudinal competencies (3), dean survey
16	447, 420 at school (school is compulsory until age 16)	74 schools	Assessment tasks, student interview, student self-report, parent interview, teacher rating of student's attitudinal competencies (3), dean survey
20	401	None	Young person interview, on-line self-report

began when the participants were aged near 5 and in their final months of early childhood education (children start school in New Zealand on their individual fifth birthdays). Table 28.1 sets out the data collection phases of the study.

When the study began, there were few longitudinal studies of 'everyday' early childhood education (as compared with early childhood education as an intervention, such as the Perry Preschool). Most studies of the 'impact' of early childhood education had little information about its wider context, such as learning experiences in homes. Existing studies also tended to either focus on academic or on socio-emotional outcomes. This study aimed to cover both kinds of outcomes, calling them 'competencies', and to include the wider context of children's lives as well as their formal educational context. The theoretical framework that informed the initial conceptualization of the study came from Bronfenbrenner's ecological framing of human development (Bronfenbrenner, 1979) and Vygotsky's work on the role of previous experiences in the scaffolding of learning (Vygotsky, 1978); it was also informed by Sartre's concepts of praxis and project in the constitution of the self (Craib, 1976; Sartre, 1965).

This study did not set out, then, with an explicit focus on student engagement as such. When we sought to gain information on student experiences and reactions to school, we did not have a distinct measure for engagement. In our items asked of students about their school experiences, we did touch on what have since been described (Fredricks, Blumenfeld, & Paris, 2004) as distinct, if interwoven, aspects of engagement: behavioral (e.g. 'I skip classes'), emotional (e.g. 'I like my teachers'), and cognitive (e.g. 'I get tired of trying'), as well as aspects of support, fair treatment and a sense of belonging at school. We also touched on some aspects of cognitive engagement in a set of items asking what information students used to think about the progress they were making (e.g. 'I learn something interesting'). At high school level, where students have different teachers for different subjects, we asked them items about three different classes; the items included aspects of their own engagement (behavioral, cognitive, emotional), as well as the opportunities for learning. Findings on the relationship between student engagement and opportunities for learning provided in classes are described in Hipkins (2012). In this chapter, we focus on student engagement as effort and enjoyment of learning, including both behavioral and cognitive aspects, and experience of supportive relationships with teachers.

Motivation in this longitudinal study of overall development is treated in terms of whether education—school—is seen to serve a purpose that lies beyond the day-to-day effort and attendance, and the future beyond school. This is akin to the Maehr and Meyer (1997) conceptualization, summarized by Appleton, Christenson and Furlong (2008, p. 379), as 'answering the question of "why am I doing this?"'.

To operationalise this concept of motivation, we used a cluster analysis undertaken in the age-14 phase of the Competent Learners study (Wylie & Hipkins, 2006). This analysis included student answers across a range of different questions at the age-14 phase, including how long they thought they would stay at school (whether past the age of 16, when school attendance is no longer compulsory), whether they thought they were gaining useful knowledge for their future in each of the three compulsory subjects (English, mathematics, science), what they wanted to do when they left school, and the kind of work they thought they might do (related to the kinds of qualifications they might need). Thus, our operational definition of motivation is reasonably instrumental and long term.

Overall Patterns of Student Engagement in School from Ages 10 to 16

To compare patterns of student engagement from the end of elementary school through middle school (48% of New Zealand Year 7 and 8 students attend a 2-year middle school, called 'intermediate', commonly between the ages of 11 and 13) and high school, we have used items from a wider set of items that were asked at ages 10, 12, 14 and 16. These items had the stem 'School is a place where…', and students were asked to rate how often the experience (e.g. 'I enjoy learning') occurred for them, on a 4-point scale at age 10 (*always, often, sometimes* and *never*), a 3-point scale at age 12 (*usually, occasionally, rarely/never*) and a 4-point scale at ages 14 and 16 (*almost always/always, usually, occasionally, rarely/never*). To enable comparison across the ages, the age-12 engagement measure was calculated as if the responses were on a scale with values 1, 2.5 and 4 rather than 1, 2, 3.

Initially, we tried a set of only six items, defining student engagement only in terms of effort and reaction, indicating behavioral and cognitive aspects of student engagement. While this set of six items showed a reasonable level of coherence (reliability) at ages 14 and 16 (Cronbach's alpha of 0.71 and 0.72, respectively), it did not at ages 10 and 12 (Cronbach's alpha of 0.54 and 0.56, respectively). This difference in coherence may relate to slight changes in wording over the period, but it may also indicate that the items and the rating levels mean different things to students in high school and those at the end of elementary school or in middle school. It would be interesting to research this further, with even younger students. Preliminary analysis of the draft *Me and My School* student engagement survey for New Zealand students in Years 4–6 in relation to the *Me and My School* survey for Years 7–10 suggested that there may be some differences in meaning (Darr, 2012).

To get a measure of student engagement that had more coherence, we needed to add another dimension. Our data allowed us to add one aspect of the dimension of emotional engagement, with material on student views of their relationships with teachers. The final measure of student engagement used in this chapter has ten items, as listed below:
I enjoy myself/I enjoy learning.
I could do better work if I tried.
I get bored.
I get tired of trying.

Table 28.2 Student engagement: mean scores on the student engagement items from ages 10 to 16 ($n = 401$)

Age	Mean item score for the 10-item measure (1 = highest level, 4 = lowest)	SD	Median item score for the 10-item measure
10	1.465	0.408	1.400
12	1.787	0.439	1.750
14	2.120	0.438	2.100
16	2.187	0.448	2.167

I feel restless.
I keep out of trouble.
I like my teacher(s).
Teacher(s) listens to what I have to say/is interested in my ideas.
Teacher(s) treats me fairly in class.
I get all the help I need.

This multidimensional measure of student engagement had reasonable coherence (reliability), and again, more coherence at the high school level than at the elementary or middle school levels (Cronbach's alphas of 0.68, 0.70, 0.81 and 0.81 for ages 10, 12, 14 and 16, respectively). Overall student engagement levels for the sample as a whole, as indicated by the mean score for the ten items comprising the measure, did decrease over time (Table 28.2).

However, while a comparison of age 10 with age 16 engagement scores would show decline happens between ages 10 and 14—there is little difference in the mean engagement level of students aged 14 and 16, between the early and middle years of high school. Yazzie-Mintz (2009) also found little difference in student engagement levels within high school, across grades 9–12 in the USA (ages 14–18). However, Archambault, Janosz, Morizot, and Pagani (2009) showed some decline for most of the engagement trajectory groups between ages 14 and 16 in a sample of students from Quebec.

Darr (2012), with a larger New Zealand sample covering the ages 12–14 (school Years 7, 8, 9 and 10), and a more comprehensive scale of student engagement, *Me and My School,* found a drop in engagement levels between Years 8 (when many students are aged 12) and 9, the first year of high school (when many students are aged 13), but little difference between Years 7 and 8, and Years 9 and 10. The change from one level of schooling to another, from the largely single-teacher format of elementary and intermediate schools to the multiteacher format of high schools, seems a self-evident reason for the drop. But without comparable data from further back in schooling careers, as we report here, locating change in engagement in change in schooling level may be misleading. Further analysis of the *Competent Learners* patterns showed no significant differences in the mean scores on the student engagement scale we use here between students who attended intermediate school and those who did not, at ages 12, 14 and 16, suggesting that transitions into another school or another schooling level do not per se alter engagement levels.

Longitudinal analysis of changes in engagement levels raises the question of whether there may be different reasons for changes in overall levels of student engagement at different schooling levels. For example, preliminary analysis of the *Me and My School* trial survey for younger New Zealand students, in Years 4–6, with two separate samples, indicated a drop in average scores between Years 4 and 5, when most students remain in the same school (C. Darr, personal communication, 2010; R. Dingle, personal communication, 2010). One reason for this may be the 'fourth grade slump', as some students struggle with moving from 'learning to read' to 'reading to learn' (Chall, 1996).

The overall patterns we found in the *Competent Learners* study raise questions about changes in the experience of education, as well as education's place in what children experience in different contexts. Does the rate of change in engagement levels evident in this sample reflect changing understanding or reference points as children grow into adolescence? Do mid-adolescents understand the items relating to engagement as effort differently from those who are younger? Does the context of high school give a different meaning to these items? Do students expect different things of education as they grow older, or do their views reflect changes in the nature of their schooling experiences? Is there a growing mismatch between their developmental needs and how school is framed (Eccles, 1999)?

Looking at changes in individual items over time suggests a mixture of these possible reasons, as well as differences for individuals. Enjoyment of learning declined somewhat (from 84% of the age-10 students to 70% of the age-14 and age-16 students), but experiences of boredom increased between ages 12 and 14, from 12% to 34%. Feeling they could do better work if they tried was reported as usually or more often the experience for much the same proportion of 10- and 12-year olds, around 30%, increasing to 46% of the 14-year olds, and again to 57% of the 16-year olds, as the students encountered more assessment at high school, including the national qualifications. *Usually* or *almost always* feeling restless doubled from 4% of the 10-year olds, to 8% of the 12-year olds, to 16% of the 14-year olds, and then increased less markedly to 25% of the 16-year olds.

The New Zealand data on student engagement, whether using the small set of indicators we have used in this analysis, or the more comprehensive *Me and My School* measure (Darr, 2012), show more changes between early adolescence (age 12) and mid-adolescence (age 14) than between ages 14 and 16. This is consistent with the pattern of less continuity between the ages of 12 and 14 than between the ages of 14 and 16 in individuals' activities outside school, values and friendships that we have found in the *Competent Learners* study, suggesting that the years of early adolescence may be the more volatile, and the ones where support to encourage engagement in learning and productive time use outside school may be particularly critical (Wylie, Hipkins, & Hodgen, 2008; Wylie & Hodgen, 2011).

Trajectories of Student Engagement

Yet this overall pattern of student engagement over time masks variation within—and between—individuals. Correlations between individuals' scores at different ages on this measure of student engagement were not strong, though they did increase over time: $r=0.36$ between ages 10 and 12, $r=0.49$ between ages 12 and 14, and $r=0.54$ between ages 14 and 16. To some extent, this lack of marked individual consistency on the measure we used may simply reflect immediate experiences colouring overall views. It would be very interesting to ask students to rate their engagement in school a number of times over the course of a school year, or to ask students to describe why they chose the rating they did after they had completed it, to see just what role immediate experiences play or whether they carry more weight for some students than others.

We found nine different trajectories for individual students by dividing scores on the engagement measure for each year into quartile groups and categorising the resulting patterns. We regrouped these to provide meaningful larger groups that we could use in cross tabulation with other data, so that we could explore differences in experiences, relationships and competency levels that might be associated with differences in student engagement trajectories.

Seventeen percent of the sample showed a stable high level of student engagement (comparable with the 13% reported in the Quebec analysis, using a different measure of student engagement, Janosz et al., 2008). Thirteen percent showed a stable low level of student engagement. In between came those who showed a stable moderately high level and those who showed some variability around a moderate level (21%); those whose engagement was at a moderately low level throughout or decreased (24%) and those whose engagement was variable or increased (26%). Figure 28.1 shows these five trajectories.

Social Characteristics of Different Student Engagement Trajectories

Student engagement trajectories do reflect some differences in the family resources available, both at an early age and when they attended high school, gender and ethnicity, with the differences most evident between those at either end of the student engagement spectrum. So, students whose trajectory was low between ages 10 and 16 were more than twice as likely as those whose trajectory was high to have come from homes that were low income as they approached school starting age (38% and 14%, respectively) and six

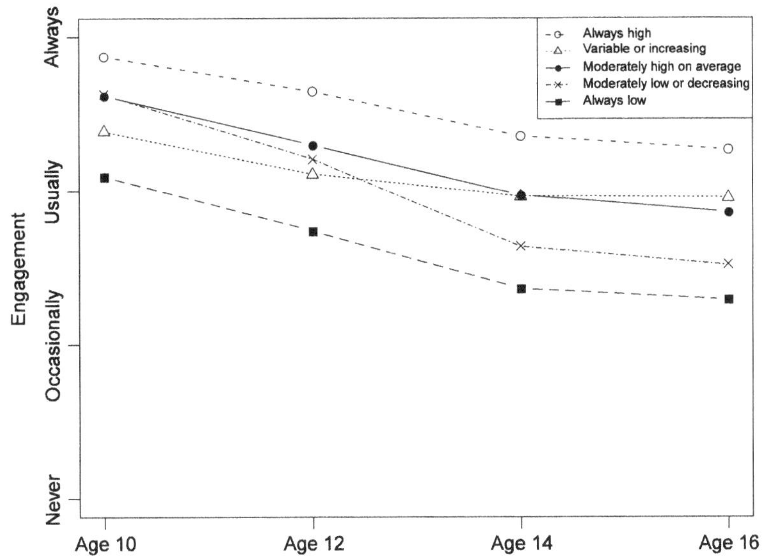

Fig. 28.1 Student engagement trajectories

times as likely to come from homes in difficult financial situations when they were age 14 (30% compared to 6% of the high trajectory group). Only 6% of the low trajectory group had mothers with a university qualification compared with 36% of those in the high trajectory group. Males were more likely to be in the low or variable/increasing trajectory groups (56% of these groups compared to 33% of the high trajectory group). Māori (New Zealand's indigenous people) or Pasifika students were least likely to be in the high trajectory group (5%, where they comprised 13% of the sample).

Links with Early Enjoyment of School

When the sample was aged 6, 8 and 10, we asked their parents an open-ended question about how their child liked school. At age 6, almost all the parents thought their children were enthusiastic. At age 8, most parents thought their child showed enthusiasm about going to school (73%), but some differences related to these later student engagement trajectories were evident (84% of the later high trajectory group showed enthusiasm at age 8, compared to 67% of those in the variable/increasing group, and 66% of the low trajectory group). Mixed feelings about school at age 8 were most likely among those who later had low engagement levels, or who were in the variable/increasing group, or the moderately low/decreasing group. These patterns were also evident in parent responses when the sample was aged 10. What is interesting also about parent perspectives—at least as indicated at this broad level—is that many of those with children whose age-10 self-report suggests a low student engagement level described them as enjoying school.

Links with Competency Levels, School Qualifications and Post-school Learning

Competency Levels

The different trajectories of student engagement show some marked differences in student competency levels, both prior to age 10 and during the age 10–16 period. The competencies measured in the *Competent Learners* study are twofold. The first set we describe as 'cognitive' comprises reading, writing, mathematics and the Raven's Standard Progressive Matrices (New Zealand Council for Educational Research, 1984; Raven, 2000), all assessed through age-appropriate standardised assessments. The second set we describe

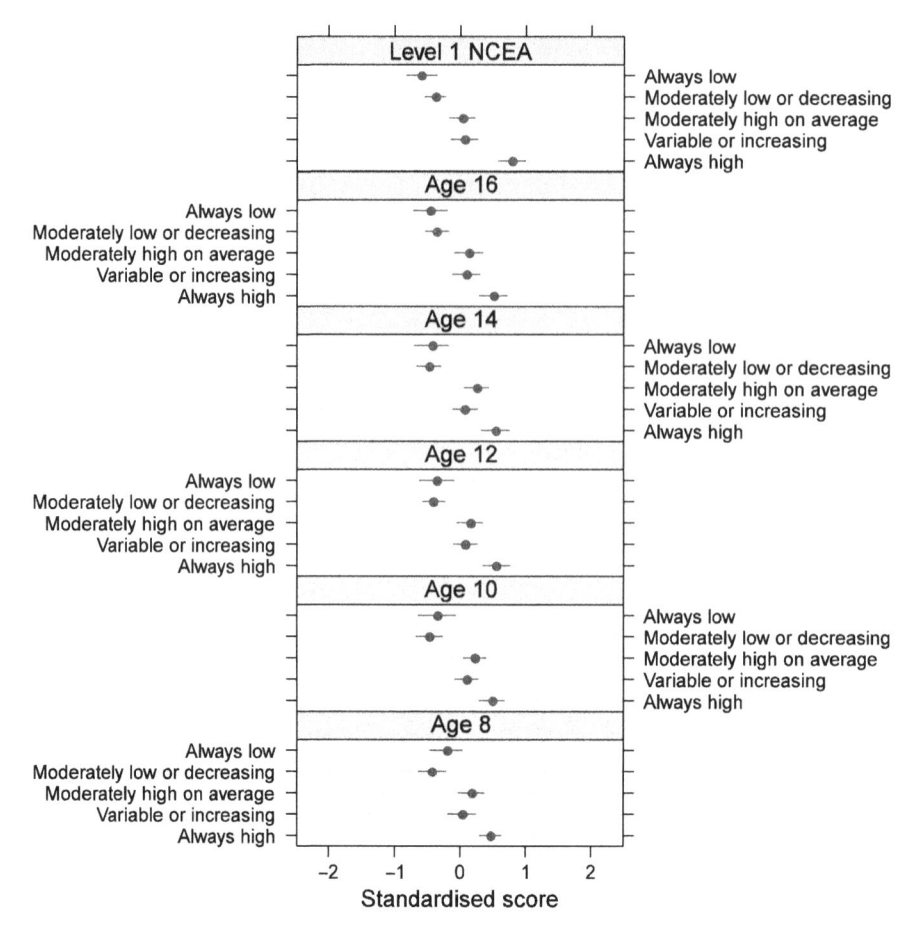

Fig. 28.2 Student engagement trajectories and levels on cognitive competencies over time

as 'attitudinal' was originally derived from thinking about the purpose of early childhood education and thinking of its role as the entrance to formal learning, a platform for developing skills and understandings that would enable ongoing learning in other contexts. The 'attitudinal' competencies comprise communication (expressive and receptive oral language), curiosity, perseverance, social skills (with adults and with peers) and self-management. These areas were among those later identified by the Organisation for Economic Development and Co-operation (OECD)'s DeSeCo project identifying key competencies that allow the use of learning in ways that positively contribute to personal well-being and support social participation (Hipkins, 2011; Rychen, 2004).

Figures 28.2 and 28.3 show the average scores for the five student engagement trajectory groups on standardised scores of the composite measures of each of these two sets of competencies from ages 8 to 16 and in relation to their achievement level on the first tier of the New Zealand three-level secondary qualification, the National Certificate of Educational Achievement (NCEA). New Zealand has a criterion-referenced high school qualification, the NCEA, with three levels. Level 1 is usually the goal of Year 11 students (aged 14–15); Level 2 usually the goal of Year 12 students (aged 15–16); and Level 3, the goal of Year 13 students (aged 17–18).

The five engagement trajectory groups show three different trends. The high engagement trajectory group had above average mean scores on the cognitive competency composite measure. However, this group was not clearly distinct from the stable moderate trajectory group or the variable/increasing trajectory group. The latter two

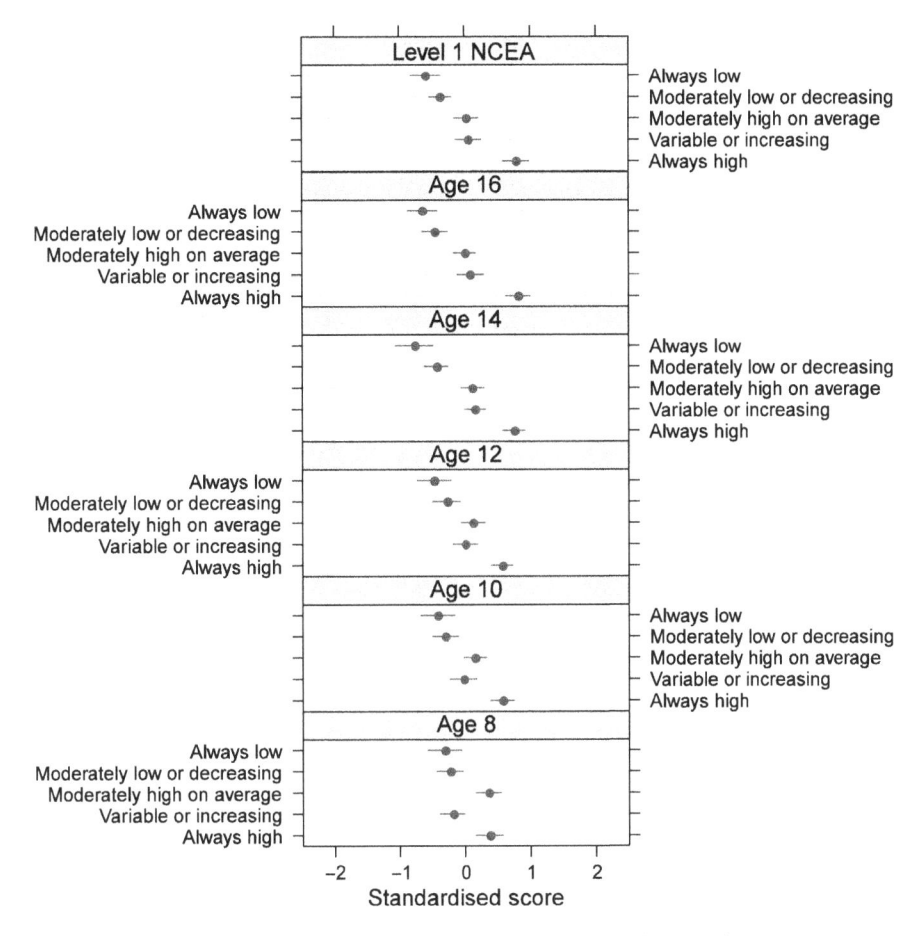

Fig. 28.3 Student engagement trajectories and levels on attitudinal competencies over time

groups sat in the middle of the average cognitive competency score spectrum, and at age 10, started to be distinct from the two groups at the other end of the spectrum, those in the always low trajectory or moderately low/decreasing trajectory groups. These tripartite trends are not quite so distinct for the attitudinal composite measure until age 14.

This tendency for differences to show first on the cognitive composite and then on the attitudinal composite is evident in other analyzes we have done (Wylie, with Ferral, 2005), suggesting that early school success, or conversely a sense of failure, has a bearing on attitudes and skills; this is consistent with the research on the development of competence beliefs (Eccles, Wigfield, & Schiefele, 1998). Structural equation modelling of the relationship between the attitudinal and cognitive competencies between the ages of 8 and 16 also showed that cognitive competency levels at one age made a separate contribution to attitudinal competency levels at the next age but not vice versa, as shown in Fig. 28.4. Gaining understanding from the reading given in school when one is aged 10, for example, feeds into helpful levels of perseverance, curiosity and communication at age 12, which are then of use in tackling more complex reading and analysis.

School Leaving Age and Highest School Qualification

The trends are slightly different when looking at school leaving age and school qualification, with sometimes more success among those whose engagement level had been at the low end of moderate and then decreased than among those whose engagement level had remained low between ages 10 and 16. Schooling is compulsory

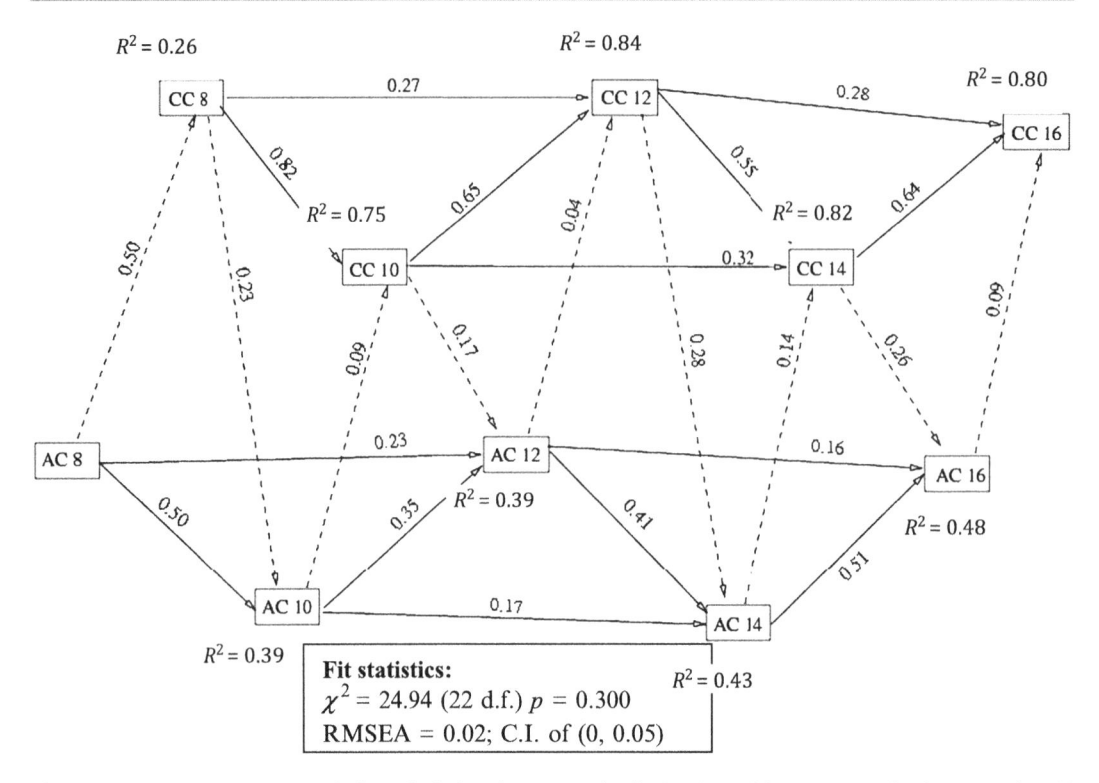

Fig. 28.4 Structural equation modelling of relations between attitudinal and cognitive competencies from ages 8 to 16 (*CC* cognitive composite, *AC* attitudinal composite)

in New Zealand until a student turns 16, though it has been possible to be granted an 'early exemption' if a student had evidence of full-time employment or tertiary study. As one might expect, those in the consistently low engagement trajectory group were most likely to be among those who left as soon as they legally could (29% of this group). Early school leaving rates were more than twice as high for the moderately low and decreasing engagement trajectory group and the variable or increasing group than for the moderately highly engaged group or the high engagement trajectory group (19%, 15%, 7% and 6%, respectively).

Level 2 NCEA is now spoken of as the minimal qualification that New Zealand students need for a secure adult future. Almost half of those (45%) in the low engagement trajectory group left school without this qualification, as did 28% of those in the moderate-decreasing trajectory group, 19% of those in the variable-increasing group, 14% of those in the moderately high on average group, and 1% of those in the high trajectory group.

These links between student engagement trajectories—as the effort put in and the perception of supportive teacher-student relationships over a 6-year period—and academic school outcomes are quite marked. This is consistent with our finding that it was higher scores on the attitudinal composite measure that distinguished students who gained a Level 2 NCEA from those who gained only Level 1 NCEA, or no qualification, not higher scores on the cognitive composite measure (Wylie & Hodgen, 2011).

Motivation Levels

Motivation levels—here defined as seeing a long-term purpose in schooling at the age of 14—were clearly linked with different engagement trajectories. Fifty-one percent of the high trajectory group also had high motivation levels compared to 11% of the low trajectory group and 20% of the moderately low-decreasing trajectory group, with the other two groups in between the latter and the high trajectory group. A similar pattern was evident in relation to a factor focused on whether students gauged their progress in learning through interest in mastery and through self-regulation.

Post-school Study

Different levels of student engagement at school do not always lead on predictably or uniformly to patterns of post-school learning. For example, at the age of 20, 22% of the high student engagement trajectory group had *not* gone on to undertake further study, and 26% of the low student engagement trajectory group were enrolled for a bachelor's degree. However, just under half (47%) of the low and moderate-decreasing groups did no further formal study once school was behind them. A quarter of those in the low trajectory group had left a post-school course without completing it, as had 17% of those in the moderately low-decreasing trajectory group. Student engagement levels in school also seemed to have a bearing on post-school learning approaches, with lower scores for the low and the moderately low-decreasing trajectory groups on our measure of 'disciplined approaches to learning', and the least need for support to learn among the high trajectory group. Thus, relying on 'second chance' education to make up for missed learning and qualifications at the school level may not be realistic for young adults who have not brought with them habits of engaging in learning.

Student Engagement in School and Experiences of Engagement Out of School

How do patterns of student engagement in school fit with experiences of engagement out of school? Can activities at home and in the wider community counter a lack of student engagement in school—or does it become harder to engage in other activities if school does not provide productive avenues to sharpen knowledge, attitudes and skills that support confidence and a sense of efficacy? Our data show considerable overlaps between school and out-of-school engagement patterns. Enjoyment of reading between the ages of 8 and 14 shows the most consistency for those in the high student engagement trajectory group: 75% enjoyed reading all through this period. Reading enjoyment consistency matches pretty well with the other trajectory groups, too, from 53% of those in the middling/variable trajectory group to 15% of those in the low trajectory group. We found a similar pattern, with smaller gaps between the trajectory groups, for time spent watching television over the 8–14 age period. At age 14, the low trajectory group were most likely to include those who either had no particular leisure interests or who spent time on electronic games, and the high and middling/variable trajectory groups were most likely to include those who had creative leisure interests. The low trajectory group was least likely to include those whose values (when thinking of what was important to them in the future) we summarized as 'anchored and achieving' (an emphasis on having an interesting job, a good education, being with family, being helpful or kind, and enjoying the things they did) and most likely to include those who wanted to 'stand out' (have lots of money to spend, lots of friends, wear the right clothes or look cool, and have an important job). Thus, low levels of student engagement in school may also be further weighed down by lack of engagement in activities outside school which could also provide goals for effort and experiences of absorption and achievement related to effort.

Relations with others are also related to engagement trajectories. Over the period between age 10 and 14, the low trajectory group was much more likely than the high trajectory group to report some experience of bullying (as victim, bully or both), 83% compared to 55%, with the other three trajectory groups in between these two. Similar patterns are evident in relation to having friends with risky behaviour and undertaking risky behaviour (using alcohol, having sex) oneself at the age of 14, and, not unrelated, having less experience of good family communication and inclusion, and reporting more pressure from family—and, by parent account, more friction in parent–child relationships.

This relative consistency of experience in and out of school in approaches to activity—the depth and manner of engagement—and then the kinds of relationships which are likely to accompany or be triggered by different approaches to activity, points to dialectical rather than unidirectional or passive relationships between individuals and the contexts in which they form themselves. Shiner and Caspi (2003, p. 14) wrote of the ways in which individuals build continuity of personality 'not merely through the constancy of behaviour across time and diverse circumstances, but also through the consistency over time in the ways that persons characteristically modify their changing contexts as a function of their behaviour'. We take this to mean in thinking about engagement that young people's behaviour can elicit responses from family, peers and teachers that may compound their habits: the ways they spend time, the ways they engage in learning, and the avenues open to them as a result.

Engagement in Learning and Belonging in School

Relationships are often mentioned in relation to student engagement in learning. Teacher-student interactions, particularly responsiveness to individual students, active guidance and encouragement in activities, joining in children's play and asking open-ended questions, were enduring aspects of early childhood education experience that multivariate analysis showed still making a contribution to cognitive and social skills competency levels at age 16 in the *Competent Learners* study, after taking into account family income and maternal qualification levels (Wylie & Hodgen, 2007). Of interest in thinking about how student engagement in learning can be developed and improved are two other strands in our analysis of high school experiences.

The first strand is the dimension of belonging at school, feeling safe and treated as an individual. In both the age-14 and age-16 phases exploratory factor analysis of our large set of items, items relating to this dimension were identified within a separate factor from a factor that brought together items related to engagement in schoolwork. The correlation between these two factors, school belonging and engagement in schoolwork, was a moderate 0.58. Thus, while it was likely that a 16-year-old student who was comfortable in the school environment would also put energy into the work of learning, it did not always follow, and vice versa. School belonging and engagement in schoolwork were both associated with student reports of being absorbed in their learning, with positive classroom learning activities and with positive relations with teachers. But each factor also had some different associations with family, peers and events. Having a supportive family, friendships which contained some challenge as well as support, and experiences of being praised for achievement were more likely to be associated with belonging in school than with engagement in schoolwork. Risky behaviour, friends with risky behaviour, family pressure and experience of adverse events in the past year were more likely to be negatively associated with engagement in schoolwork than with feelings of belonging in school; school can be a place for social reinforcement as well as learning. Belonging in school had a much lower correlation with performance levels on the first level of NCEA than did student engagement in schoolwork (0.36 compared to 0.57). But the proportion of variance in each of these factors accounted for by age-14 motivation levels was slightly higher for belonging in school than for student engagement (11.2% compared to 7%). Thus, both school belonging and engagement in schoolwork were playing a role in student attachment to school.

However, if one is interested in improving student achievement through improving student engagement levels, then the interaction between learning opportunities and what individuals bring with them warrants attention. A second strand of this study shows that student perceptions that they were offered the kinds of learning opportunities that develop self-regulation and thinking (see Hipkins, 2012) were closely correlated with positive views of teachers. Both aspects of student engagement analyzed here (engagement with schoolwork and feelings of belonging) had higher correlation levels ($r=0.43$ and 0.51, respectively) with these reports of learning opportunities to develop self-regulation than did experience of adverse events or relations with family and friends (with the exception of similar correlation levels [negative] with student engagement as effort and friends with risky behaviour).

Conclusion

Longitudinal patterns of student engagement, when they can be related to academic performance and to both school and out-of-school contexts, do confirm that student self-reports of their engagement, here operationalized as effort and support, are worth attending to. Student self-reports of engagement do provide reasonable indicators of competency levels and, probably through that link, to likely later academic performance and post-school learning. There was an almost linear relationship between the five engagement trajectory patterns (at low, middle and high levels) and school achievement. The patterns described here also point to the importance of student engagement in school—in the work of school—for the use of attention and effort in the activities, interests and relationships outside school that also form identity. If nothing else, then, the importance of formal education for the whole of life is evident. The relationships between formal education experiences and experiences outside school are not unidirectional—but reinforcing and shaping the attention and effort likely to be made in either sphere.

Yet while longitudinal patterns of student engagement show consistencies, they also show some fluidity—only three of the original nine trajectories we found remained stable over the 6-year period from when students were aged 10 to when they were aged 16. The most consistent patterns found in this study were for those who by the age of 10 had experienced school success at a reasonably high level and, conversely, for those who at that age were struggling with school work. Those with high engagement levels by age 10 appear most likely to maintain those levels; but others with moderate or low levels are more open to change (both down and upward). Students play a role in shaping their learning through the effort they put in and the responses of others as a result, but their effort is also susceptible to changing learning opportunities (some classes offer more in the way of experiences that build engagement) and events (such as accidents, loss of family or friends).

Decline of student engagement over ages 10–16 raises some questions which are important in thinking about how to improve student engagement. Is the pattern we found with a New Zealand sample universal? Are there universal developmental differences, as Eccles (1999) suggests in her discussion of the importance of the fit between individual psychological needs and the opportunities students had in school and with their families, particularly through middle-childhood years? Eccles identified the 'key psychological challenges' for middle-childhood as self-awareness, social comparison and self-esteem. The key psychological challenges she identified for early adolescence were more to do with 'a drive for autonomy paired with a continuing need for close, trusting relationships with adults' (Eccles, 1999, p. 41).

Longitudinal studies of student engagement in context are still rare, but as the field grows, we need more studies that follow students over time to find out more about the role of different contexts and different learning opportunities in different levels and trajectories of engagement and to find out more about how different aspects of engagement are related. Ideally, a longitudinal study of student engagement and its links with student achievement would use a single scale with strong psychometric properties that could be used across different ages and one that contained sub-scales of behavioral, emotional and cognitive dimensions of engagement, so that the way these are related and whether these relationships change over time could also be investigated in relation to theories of human development. Archambault et al. (2009) provided a very interesting analysis of changes in student engagement over ages 12–16, separately for behavioral, cognitive and affective engagement and for different trajectories of engagement over that period. They suggested that it would be valuable to include in such analysis more information on cognitive engagement, for example, the use of self-regulation strategies. We would agree and go further. A comprehensive investigation of changes in student engagement over time would need to include measures of learning opportunities in student classrooms, based on the research about the kinds that are linked with student engagement, learning enjoyment and the development of self-regulation and metacognitive skills. Such an investigation would need a more complex measure of motivation than the somewhat utilitarian one we used in this study. It would also need to include measures of student achievement and competencies, so that we could gain a full picture of the dynamic relations between engagement dimensions, achievement (including and extending what we covered here in the attitudinal competencies) and learning opportunities. Material would be collected on activities and values beyond school, and relations with family and friends, to deepen our understanding of the circumstances in which learning identities become consistent in positive, or negative ways, within and beyond school, and of the ways in which these constituents of individual identity and source of action can be combined differently to markedly and durably alter declining or low student engagement in learning. Longitudinal analysis shows that while earlier patterns of student engagement contribute to later patterns, student engagement levels are not immutable and do respond to different opportunities.

References

Appleton, J. J., Christenson, S. L., & Furlong, M. J. (2008). Student engagement with school: Critical conceptual and methodological issues of the construct. *Psychology in the Schools, 45*, 369–386.

Archambault, I., Janosz, M., Morizot, J., & Pagani, L. (2009). Adolescent behavioral, affective, and cognitive engagement in school: Relationship to dropout. *Journal of School Health, 79*, 408–415.

Bronfenbrenner, U. (1979). *The ecology of human development: Experiments by nature and design.* Cambridge, MA: Harvard University Press.

Chall, J. S. (1996). *Stages of reading development* (2nd ed.). Fort Worth, TX: Harcourt Brace.

Craib, I. (1976). *Existentialism and sociology: A study of Jean-Paul Sartre.* Cambridge, UK: Cambridge University Press.

Darr, C. (2011). Measuring student engagement: The development of a scale for formative use. In S. L. Christenson, A. L. Reschly, & C. Wylie (Eds.), *Handbook of research on student engagement.* New York: Springer.

Eccles, J. S. (1999). The development of children ages 6 to 14. *The Future of Children. When School is Out, 9*, 30–44.

Eccles, J. S., Wigfield, A., & Schiefele, U. (1998). Motivation to succeed. In W. Damon (Series Ed.) & N. Eisenberg (Vol. Ed.), *Handbook of child psychology* (5th ed., pp. 1017–1095). New York: Wiley.

Finn, J. (1989). Withdrawing from school. *Review of Educational Research, 59*, 117–142.

Fredricks, J. A., Blumenfeld, P. C., & Paris, A. (2004). School engagement: Potential of the concept, state of the evidence. *Review of Educational Research, 74*, 59–109.

Hipkins, R. (2012). The engaging nature of teaching for competency development. In S. L. Christenson, A. L. Reschly, & C. Wylie (Eds.), *Handbook of research on student engagement* (pp. 441–456). New York: Springer.

Janosz, M., Archambault, I., Morizot, J., & Pagani, L. S. (2008). School engagement trajectories and their differential predictive relations to dropout. *Journal of Social Issues, 64*(1), 21–40.

Janosz, M., LeBlanc, M., Boulerice, B., & Tremblay, R. E. (2000). Predicting types of school dropouts: A typological approach with two longitudinal samples. *Journal of Youth and Adolescence, 26*, 733–759.

Maehr, M., & Meyer, H. (1997). Understanding motivation and schooling: Where we've been, where we are, and where we need to go. *Educational Psychology Review 9*, 371–409.

New Zealand Council for Educational Research. (1984). *Standard progressive matrices: New Zealand norms supplement.* Wellington, New Zealand: NZCER.

Raven, J. (2000). The Raven's progressive matrices: Change and stability over culture and time. *Cognitive Psychology, 41*, 1–48.

Rumberger, R. A., & Rotermund, S. (2011). The relationship between engagement and high school dropout. In S. L. Christenson, A. L. Reschly, & C. Wylie (Eds.), *Handbook of research on student engagement.* New York: Springer.

Rychen, D. S. Tiana, A., & Ferrer, A. T. (Eds.), (2004). Key competencies for all: An overarching conceptual frame of reference. In *Developing key competencies in education: Some lessons for international and national experience* (pp. 5–34). Paris: UNESCO International Bureau of Education.

Sartre, J. P. (1965). *The philosophy of Jean-Paul Sartre.* Edited and introduced by R. Denoon Cumming. New York: Random House.

Shiner, R., & Caspi, A. (2003). Personality differences in childhood and adolescence: Measurement, development, and consequences. *Journal of Child Psychology and Psychiatry, 44*, 2–32.

Vygotsky, L. S. (1978). *Mind in society.* Cambridge, MA: Harvard University Press.

Wylie, C., with Ferral, H. (2005). Patterns of cognitive and personality development: Evidence from the longitudinal Competent Children/Learners study. In J. Low & P. Jose (Eds.), *Lifespan development – New Zealand perspectives* (pp. 90–100). Auckland: Pearson Education.

Wylie, C., & Hipkins, R. (2006). *Growing independence: Competent learners @ 14.* Wellington, New Zealand: Ministry of Education.

Wylie, C., Hipkins, R., & Hodgen, E. (2008). *On the edge of adulthood: Young people's school and out-of-school experiences at 16.* Wellington, New Zealand: Ministry of Education.

Wylie, C., & Hodgen, E. (2007). *The continuing contribution of early childhood education to young people's competency levels.* Wellington, New Zealand: Ministry of Education.

Wylie, C., & Hodgen, E. (2011). *Forming adulthood. Past, present and future in the experiences and views of the competent learners @ 20.* Wellington, New Zealand: Ministry of Education.

Yazzie-Mintz, E. (2009). *Engaging the voice of students: A report on the 2007 & 2008 high school survey of student engagement.* http://www.indiana.edu/~ceep/hssse/images/HSSSE_2009_Report.pdf.

Instructional Contexts for Engagement and Achievement in Reading

John T. Guthrie, Allan Wigfield, and Wei You

Abstract

In this chapter, we review research on students' engagement in reading activities and how classroom instructional practices influence engagement in reading and other academic activities. We define engaged readers as motivated to read, strategic in their approaches to reading, knowledgeable in their construction of meaning from text, and socially interactive while reading. We present a conceptual model of reading engagement linking classroom practices directly and indirectly to students' motivation to read, behavioral engagement in reading, and reading achievement. A major premise of this model is that behavioral engagement in reading mediates the effects of classroom practices on reading outcomes. We present evidence from a variety of experimental and correlational studies documenting the direct and indirect links among classroom practices, motivation, behavioral engagement, and achievement outcomes. One reading comprehension instructional program on which we focus is Concept-Oriented Reading Instruction. This program integrates strategy instruction and instructional practices to foster students' reading motivation, and teaches reading, in particular, in content domains such as science and social studies.

*The project described was supported by Grant Number R01HD052590 from the National Institute of Child and Human Development. The content is solely the responsibility of the authors and does not necessarily represent the official views of the National Institute of Child Health and Human Development or the National Institutes of Health.

J.T. Guthrie (✉) • A. Wigfield
Department of Human Development
and Quantitative Methodology, University of Maryland,
College Park, MD, USA
e-mail: jguthrie@umd.edu; awigfiel@umd.edu

W. You
Department of Curriculum & Instruction,
University of Maryland, College Park, MD, USA
e-mail: weiyou@umd.edu

Defining Engagement

The construct of engagement is increasingly prominent in the educational and developmental psychology literatures and is defined generally as involvement, participation, and commitment to some set of activities. Skinner, Kindermann, Connell, and Wellborn (2009a) described engagement as a reflection or manifestation of motivated action and noted that action incorporates emotions, attention, goals, and other psychological processes along with persistent and effortful behavior. Fredricks, Blumenfeld, and Paris

(2004) defined behavioral, emotional, and cognitive aspects of school engagement. Behavioral engagement is direct involvement in a set of activities and includes positive conduct, effort and persistence, and participation in extracurricular activities. Emotional engagement covers both positive and negative affective reactions (e.g., interest, boredom, anxiety, frustration) to activities, as well as to the individuals with whom one does the activities (teachers, peers). It also comprises identification with school. Cognitive engagement means willingness to exert the mental effort needed to comprehend challenging concepts and accomplish difficult tasks in different domains, as well as the use of self-regulatory and other strategies to guide one's cognitive efforts.

We have focused on students' engagement in reading activities and defined reading engagement as interacting with text in ways that are both strategic and motivated (Guthrie & Wigfield, 2000). More broadly, we and our colleagues have described engaged readers as motivated to read, strategic in their approaches to comprehending what they read, knowledgeable in their construction of meaning from text, and socially interactive while reading (Guthrie, McGough, Bennett, & Rice, 1996; Guthrie & Wigfield, 2000; Guthrie, Wigfield, & Perencevich, 2004; see also Baker, Dreher, & Guthrie, 2000). In this review, we introduce the construct of behavioral engagement to this set of engagement processes. Specific indicators of behavioral engagement of reading include students' report of effort and persistence (Skinner, Kindermann, & Furrer, 2009b), students' report of time spent reading (Guthrie, Wigfield, Metsala, & Cox, 1999), and teachers' observations of students' reading behaviors (Wigfield et al., 2008).

Students' engagement in reading is enhanced when the contexts in which reading occurs foster it. There are a variety of instructional practices that foster students' reading engagement, and we discuss them below. We believe that engagement in reading is crucial to the development of reading comprehension skills and reading achievement; we present evidence documenting this point throughout the chapter. By focusing on reading, we address an urgent problem in education which is that high proportions of students are disaffected with reading. They overwhelmingly shun books in science, history, and math that carry the substance of their education. In other words, in elementary and secondary education, disengagement from reading is a national dilemma (Grigg, Ryan, Jin, & Campbell, 2003; Perie, Grigg, & Donahue, 2005).

Engagement and motivation are related terms that sometimes are used interchangeably in the literature (e.g., National Research Council, 2004), but we believe the constructs should be distinguished from one another (see also Fredricks et al., 2004; Skinner et al., 2009a, 2009b for distinctions between these constructs). As just noted, engagement is a multidimensional construct that includes behavioral, cognitive, and affective attributes associated with being deeply involved in an activity such as reading; indeed, Fredricks et al. (2004) called engagement a meta-construct. By contrast, motivation is a more specific construct that relates to engagement but can be distinguished from it. Motivation is what energizes and directs behavior and often is defined with respect to the beliefs, values, and goals individuals have for different activities (Eccles & Wigfield, 2002; Wigfield, Eccles, Schiefele, Roeser, & Davis-Kean, 2006).

Motivation often is domain specific; in the reading domain, we defined reading motivation as follows: "Reading motivation is the individual's personal goals, values, and beliefs with regard to the topics, processes, and outcomes of reading" (Guthrie & Wigfield, 2000, p. 405). Motivation also is important for the maintenance of behavior, particularly when activities are cognitively demanding (Wolters, 2003). Reading is one such activity, as many different cognitive skills are involved. These range from processing individual words to generating meaning from complex texts. Furthermore, although reading is required for many school tasks and activities, it is also something students can choose to do or not; "Am I going to read or do something else?" Given these characteristics, motivation is especially crucial to reading engagement. Like Skinner et al. (2009a, 2009b), then, we believe that engagement reflects motivated action. When students are positively motivated to read, they will be more engaged in reading. We discuss how specific aspects of motivation relate to engagement later in this chapter.

Engagement Perspective on Reading

We (Guthrie & Wigfield, 2000) developed an engagement perspective on reading that connects classroom instructional practices to students' motivations, strategy use, conceptual knowledge, and social interactions, and ultimately to their reading outcomes. Students' motivation includes multifaceted aspects such as goals, intrinsic and extrinsic motivation, values, self-efficacy, and social motivation. These motivational aspects of the reader propel students to choose to read and to use cognitive strategies to comprehend. The *strategies* in the model refer to students' multiple cognitive processes of comprehending, self-monitoring, and constructing their understanding and beliefs during reading. *Conceptual knowledge* refers to the notion that reading is knowledge-driven. *Social interactions* include collaborative practices in a community and the social goals of helping other students or cooperating with a teacher. These in turn influence students' reading achievement, knowledge gained from reading, and the kinds of practices in which they engage.

We chose the instructional practices in the model for two primary reasons. First, each practice has been shown to relate to students' motivation and achievement in a variety of correlational and classroom-based studies (see Guthrie & Humenick, 2004, for a meta-analytic review of the work on a number of these practices). Second, several of the practices are included in Concept-Oriented Reading Instruction (CORI), a reading comprehension instruction program that combines reading strategy instruction, support for student motivation, and connections to content areas (Guthrie, Wigfield, & Perencevich, 2004; Guthrie et al., 1996). As the instructional practices have been described fully elsewhere (e.g., Guthrie, McRae, & Klauda, 2007), we briefly mention them here and present an example lesson later in this chapter.

Learning and knowledge goals refer to core learning goals for particular topic areas that provide students with compelling cognitive reasons for learning the material.

Real-world interactions are connections between the academic curriculum and the personal experiences of the learners and, more specifically, are stimulating activities that connect students to the content they are learning. These real-world interactions also provide motivation for students to read more about what they are learning.

Instructional Practices

- *Autonomy support* is based on premises from self-determination theory (Ryan & Deci, 2009) that giving students some control over their own learning is motivating.
- *Interesting texts* refers to the practice of providing an abundance of high interest texts in the classroom.
- *Strategy instruction* concerns the kinds of reading strategies teachers teach; in CORI, a set of strategies shown to have strong empirical support (National Reading Panel, 2000) are the strategies used in the program.
- *Collaboration* is the social discourse among students in a learning community that enables them to see perspectives and to socially construct knowledge from text (Johnson & Johnson, 2009).
- *Praise and rewards* involve the ways in which teachers provide feedback to students (Brophy, 1981). Rewards are often used in reading instruction and other instructional programs as a way to build students' motivation (Gambrell & Marniak, 1997).
- Students are *evaluated* in classrooms in a myriad of ways. Some methods of evaluation can provide meaningful information about student

learning and actually can support student motivation (Afflerbach, 1998).

- Finally, *teacher involvement* represents the teacher's knowledge of individual learners, caring about their progress and pedagogical understanding of how to foster their active participation (Skinner & Belmont, 1993).

Guthrie and Wigfield (2000) reviewed evidence for the connections of each of these practices to reading outcomes.

A crucial assumption in this model is that the effects of instructional practices on the student outcomes of achievement, knowledge, and reading practices are mediated by the engagement processes (see also Skinner & Belmont, 1993). That is, classroom contexts only affect student outcomes to the extent that they produce high levels of student engagement. Behavioral engagement is one of these processes and is increased by CORI.

Conceptual Framework for Engagement Processes in Reading

Purposes of the Framework

Figure 29.1 presents our current framework on engagement that depicts both the direct and indirect (or mediated) effects of classroom practices and conditions on student reading outcomes, particularly their reading competence. Our aim in building this framework is to describe how instruction, motivation, behavioral engagement, and achievement are related. The classroom practices and conditions in the box at the left of the figure include many of those incorporated in Guthrie and Wigfield's (2000) engagement model of reading development, and others that are particularly relevant to middle school reading, the focus of our current research project on enhancing adolescents' engagement in reading (Guthrie, Klauda, & Morrison, 2012; Guthrie, Mason-Singh, & Coddington, 2012). Our framework is consistent with the perspective of Appleton, Christenson, and Furlong (2008) in that we seek the characteristics of classrooms that are sufficiently powerful to impact variables for which educators are held accountable, such as achievement on major tests as well as experimental measures. Furthermore, we attempt to identify and document the engagement processes that serve as links between the practices of teachers and students' outcomes.

Depicted in this graphic are the engagement processes in reading consisting of motivations to read, behavioral engagement in reading, and reading competence, along with classroom contexts. Many of the studies we review in this chapter show that behavioral engagement in reading impacts reading competence, and motivations to read impact behavioral engagement in reading. Our rationale for considering these all to be engagement processes is that they represent motivational, behavioral, and cognitive dimensions of

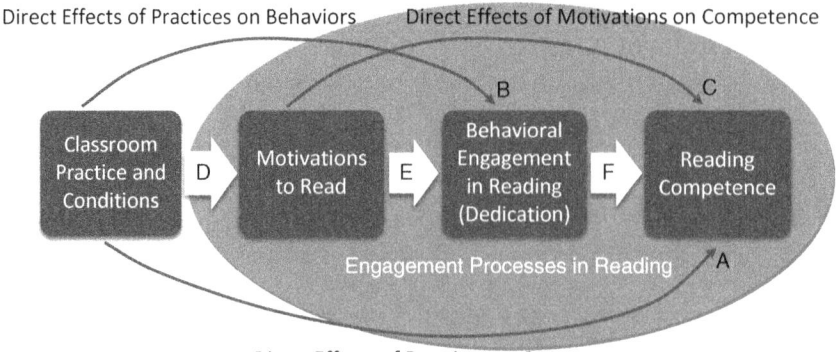

Fig. 29.1 Model of reading engagement processes within classroom contexts

interacting with text. On the far left of the graphic, classroom practices and conditions are shown to represent their role in impacting motivations, behavioral engagement, and reading competence. We will review empirical evidence documenting that classroom practices have both direct effects on competence and indirect effects mediated by motivations and behavioral engagement. In this graphic, the capital letters represent pathways from classroom practices through engagement processes to reading competence. Although empirical research is likely to reveal reciprocal pathways throughout this model, we do not include them here because they have not been widely studied in reading and the current evidence for them is limited. We do not address emotional engagement or affective processes because they have not been studied frequently in reading, and space constraints prevent us from examining them here. We do address cognitive engagement, such as the use of strategies for reading, because it is important to control for them statistically when investigating the associations of behavioral engagement and reading achievement. This review of context effects is organized by reviewing evidence for each pathway, beginning with the effects of behavioral engagement on reading competence, and then discussing each pathway in the model. In several instances, a particular study provides evidence for more than one pathway in the model. We discuss these studies in each pathway where it supplies documentation.

Behavioral Engagement Impacts Reading Competence

Our rationale for linking behavioral engagement in reading and reading competence (Path F) is grounded in cognitive science (van den Broek, Rapp, & Kendeou, 2005; Walczyk et al., 2007). Experimental studies show that acquiring declarative knowledge from text demands the complex system of rapid, automatic processes at the word and sentence level integrated with effortful, deliberate processes of inferencing and reasoning (Kendeou, van den Broek, White, & Lynch, 2007). As facilitators of reading competence, these processes may be termed "cognitive engagement." These processes demand effort and attention sustained over substantial amounts of time during which this cognitive system is acquired to a level of expertise (Ericsson, Krampe, & Tesch-Romer, 1993).

While students are expending effort in the behavior of reading, motivational processes are occurring simultaneously. If the book is interesting, the reading act may be intrinsically motivating. If the book is perceived as important, the reading behavior may contribute to a student's sense of identification with reading in school. It is during this passage of time that motivations impact students' cognitive proficiencies. When motivations are positive (intrinsic motivation), cognitions increase; when motivations are negative (avoidance or disaffection), behaviors become aversive, leading to a gradual decline in cognitive proficiency. It is evident that cognitive expertise cannot be attained without sustained behaviors, and the absence of reading behaviors is a precursor to cognitive decline.

Evidence for the Effects of Behavioral Engagement on Competence in Reading

In this section, we document that time, effort, and persistence in reading behaviors impacts a variety of indicators of reading competence. The studies for this section are presented in Table 29.1. However, this documentation cannot be simple. A student who spends a high amount of time reading and also has high competence, according to standardized test scores, is likely to have a variety of correlated characteristics. Most basically, this student is likely to have high amounts of background knowledge about the topic or genre of the reading behavior. The relationship of behavioral engagement and achievement is confounded by many variables. For example, a behaviorally engaged student with high reading competence is likely to have high levels of motivation, such as self-efficacy and intrinsic motivation for reading, and so these variables must be taken into account in analyses. Guthrie et al. (1999)

Table 29.1 Effects of behavioral engagement on competence in reading

Citation[a]	Number of participants	Grade levels	Dependent variables	Independent variables[b]	Strength of association[c]
Duckworth et al. (2007a)	1,545 Adults aged 25 and older	NA	1. Grit	(a) Age (b) Educational attainment	$\eta^2 = 0.05^{***}$ for educational attainment
Duckworth et al. (2007b)	690 Adults aged 25 and older	NA	1. Grit	(a) Age (b) Educational attainment	$\eta^2 = 0.05^{***}$ for educational attainment
Duckworth et al. (2007c)	139 Undergraduate students	NA	1. GPA	(a) Grit (b) SAT	$r_{1a} = 0.34^{***}$ after SAT scores were held constant
Duckworth et al. (2007d)	1,218 Freshman in the US Military Academy, West Point	NA	1. Summer retention 2. First-year academic GPA 3. Military performance score (MPS)	(a) Grit (b) Self-control (c) Whole Candidate Score	$\beta_{1a} = 0.44^{**d}$ after self-control and Whole Candidate Score were held constant, partial $r_{2a} = -0.01$, ns; partial $r_{3a} = 0.09^{**}$
Duckworth et al. (2007e)	1,308 Freshman in the US Military Academy, West Point	NA	1. Summer retention	(a) Grit (b) Conscientiousness (c) Whole Candidate Score	$\beta_{1a} = 0.39^{*e}$
Duckworth et al. (2007f)	175 National Spelling Bee finalists from 7 to 15 years old	NA	1. Final round 2. Prior competition 3. Study time	(a) Grit (b) Self-control (c) Verbal IQ Score (d) Study time (e) Prior competition	$\beta_{1a} = 0.62^{*f}$ $\beta_{3a} = 0.28^{***g}$ $\beta_{1d} = 0.30^{***h}$ Study time was a mediator between grit and performance $\beta_{2a} = 0.48^{*i}$ $\beta_{1c} = 1.21^{***j}$ Prior final competition was a mediator between grit and performance
Duckworth and Seligman (2005a)	140	8	1. Final GPA	(a) Self-discipline (b) First-making-period GPA	$r_{1a} = 0.55^{***}$ $R^2 = 0.85^{***k}$ $\beta_{1a} = 0.10^{*}$
Duckworth and Seligman (2005b)	164	8	1. Final GPA	(a) Self-discipline (b) First-making-period GPA (c) IQ (d) April achievement test scores	$r_{1a} = 0.67^{***}$ $R^2 = 0.90^{***l}$ $\beta_{1a} = 0.08^{*}$
Fredricks et al. (2004)	Review				
Guthrie, Klauda, et al. (2012)	1,200	7	1. Reading achievement 2. Avoidance of reading information books for school	(a) Amount of school reading (b) Amount of out-of-school reading (c) FARMS status (d) Amount of information book reading (e) Devaluing (f) Perceived difficulty	$r_{1a} = 0.20^{**}$ with FARMS status partialed out $r_{1b} = 0.19^{**}$ with FARMS status partialed out $r_{1d} = 0.04$ (ns) with FARMS status partialed out $\beta_{2e} = 0.75^{***}$ $\beta_{2f} = 0.14^{***}$

Study	N	Age/Grade	Outcomes	Predictors	Statistics
Guthrie et al. (1999a)	271	3, 5	1. Passage comprehension 2. Conceptual learning from multiple texts	(a) Past achievement (b) Prior knowledge (c) Motivation (d) Self-efficacy (e) Reading amount	$\Delta R^2 = 0.015^m$ for reading amount $\beta_{1e} = 0.126^*$ $\Delta R^2 = 0.022^m$ for reading amount $\beta_{2e} = 0.150^*$
Guthrie et al. (1999b)	17,424	10	1. Text comprehension	(a) Reading amount (b) Past reading comprehension achievement (c) Reading efficacy (d) Reading motivation (e) SES	$\beta_{1a} = 0.12^{***}$ $r_{1a} = 0.29^{***}$ $\Delta R^2 = 0.014^m$ for reading amount
Jang (2008)	136 College students	NA	1. Conceptual learning 2. Identified Regulation 3. Engagement 4. Interest regulation	(a) Rationale	Model 1: $\beta_{13} = 0.45^{*n}$ $R^2 = 0.20$ Model 2: $\beta_{13} = 0.44^*$ $R^2 = 0.20$ Model 3: $\beta_{13} = 0.44^*$ $R^2 = 0.20$
Ladd and Dinella (2009)	383 Children	Ages 5.5–13.5	1. Initial levels of achievement (achievement intercepts) 2. Growth in scholastic achievement from first through eighth grade (achievement slopes)	(a) Changes in school liking-avoidance from first through third grade (b) Changes in cooperative-resistant classroom participation from first through third grade (c) Average school liking-avoidance from first through third grade (d) Average cooperative-resistant classroom participation from first through third grade	$\beta_{2b} = 0.31^{**o}$ $\beta_{2d} = 0.37^{**}$
Orvis et al. (2009)	274	College students	1. Learning	(a) Off-task attention (b) Training satisfaction (c) Training motivation (d) Goal orientation (e) Learner control	$\beta_{1a} = -0.15^{*p}$
Reeve et al. (2002a)	141	College students	1. Identification experience (perceived importance and perceived self-determination as the indicator variables) 2. Effort	(a) Reason to try	$\beta_{1a} = 0.26^{**}$ $\beta_{21} = 0.59^{**}$
Reeve et al. (2002b)	70	College students	1. Identification experience 2. Pre-lesson identified regulation 3. Effort	(a) Reason to try	$\beta_{1a} = 0.34^{**}$ $\beta_{21} = 0.54^{**}$ $\beta_{13} = 0.45^{**}$

(continued)

Table 29.1 (continued)

Citation[a]	Number of participants	Grade levels	Dependent variables	Independent variables[b]	Strength of association[c]
Salamonson et al. (2009)	126 Second-year nursing students	NA	1. Academic performance in pathophysiology	(a) Overall homework completion (b) Overall lecture attendance (c) Hours spent in part-time employment	$R^2 = 0.381$[q] $\beta_{1a} = 0.44$*** $\beta_{1b} = 0.21$* $\beta_{1c} = -0.26$***
Schwinger et al. (2009)	231	11, 12	1. GPA	(a) Motivational regulation strategies (b) Effort management (c) Intelligence	$\beta_{1b} = 0.29$**[r] $R^2 = 0.11$

*$p<0.05$, **$p<0.01$, ***$p<0.001$

Notes

[a] We only included the studies documenting path F in Fig. 29.1
[b] We did not include those variables which the authors reported as covariates or as control variables in their analyses
[c] We only reported the effect sizes of behavioral engagement on outcomes of our interest
[d] The effect size reported in this study is the standardized beta coefficient in the final model in which three predictors (grit, self-control, and Whole Candidate Score) were simultaneously entered to predict summer retention
[e] The effect size reported in this study is the standardized beta coefficient in the final model in which three predictors (grit, conscientiousness, and Whole Candidate Score) were simultaneously entered to predict summer retention
[f] The effect size reported here is the beta coefficient in the model in which three predictors (grit, self-control, and age) were simultaneously entered to predict final round
[g] The effect size reported here is the beta coefficient in the model in which two predictors (grit and age) were simultaneously entered to predict study time
[h] The effect size reported here is the beta coefficient in the model in which three predictors (grit, study time, and age) were simultaneously entered to predict final round
[i] The effect size reported here is the beta coefficient in the model in which two predictors (grit and age) were simultaneously entered to predict prior competition
[j] The effect size reported here is the beta coefficient in the model in which three predictors (grit, number of prior competition, and age) were simultaneously entered to predict 2005 final round
[k] The effect size reported here is R^2 for the overall regression with two predictors (self-discipline and first-making-period GPA)
[l] The effect size reported here is R^2 for the overall regression with four predictors (self-discipline, IQ, April achievement test scores, and first-making-period GPA)
[m] The effect size reported here ΔR^2 was the unique contribution of reading amount to the outcome above and beyond the other predictors in the model
[n] The effect sizes reported in this study are standardized coefficients in structural equation modeling
[o] The effect sizes reported in this study are path coefficients in path analysis
[p] The effect sizes reported in this study are standardized path coefficients in structural equation modeling
[q] The effect sizes reported in this study is R^2 for the overall regression with seven predictors (overall homework completion, overall lecture attendance, hours spend in part-time employment, study time on pathophysiology, age, sex, and non-English speaking at home)
[r] The effect sizes reported in this study is R^2 of GPA predicted by effort management

found that third- and fifth-grade students' self-report of amount of time spent reading in school and out of school was associated with competency tests of students' reading comprehension, even when controlling for background knowledge, previous grades, intrinsic motivation, and self-efficacy. This finding appeared not only for single passages but for acquisition of knowledge from text in a 2-day learning activity. They also found in a nationally representative sample of tenth-grade students that behavioral engagement in reading (assessed by time spent) was correlated with reading comprehension test scores, when the potentially confounding variables of past achievement, SES, and self-efficacy were controlled statistically. Thus, behavioral engagement impacted reading competence for samples of elementary and secondary students, when potentially confounding cognitive and motivational variables were statistically controlled.

As indicated previously, students' aversion to reading information texts in secondary school is a widespread crisis. In middle school, the highest achievers overwhelmingly rate information text to be uninteresting (Guthrie, Klauda, et al., 2012). In this light, it is valuable to understand the variables that influence students' competence in reading uninteresting text (Reeve, Jang, Hardre, & Omura, 2002). In one experimental study, Jang (2008) gave one group of college students the task of reading some text about statistical correlations, which was not interesting to them, with the rationale that the text was important to their professions. The behavioral engagement of this group increased compared to a group not told that this material was beneficial to them. After reading the texts, the group given the "importance rationale" was superior in conceptual understanding of the text. Thus, experimentally increasing behavioral engagement enhanced students' conceptual learning. Note that this study also provides evidence for other pathways in our model; we discuss this evidence later. In a longitudinal study with children ages 5–13, Ladd and Dinella (2009) examined the effect of behavioral engagement on a wide variety of reading achievement tests. Some students showed high behavioral engagement of interest, attention, and participation in classwork. Other students showed behavioral disengagement consisting of resistance by not performing tasks, not completing homework, and acting defiantly toward academic activities. Statistically controlling for reading achievement in grade 1, the gain in reading from grades 1 to 8 was higher for students whose behavioral engagement increased in grades 1–3 than for students whose resistance and behavioral disengagement increased in grades 1–3. In other words, increasing behavioral engagement produced the positive slope for achievement, whereas decreasing behavioral engagement produced a less positive slope in measured reading competence.

A variety of studies document the generalizability of this effect of behavioral engagement in reading on reading competence, using different indicators of engagement. Schwinger, Steinmayr, and Spinath (2009) measured 11th- and 12th-grade German high school students' effort management as an indicator of behavioral engagement. Investigators used items such as "I study hard whether I am interested or not." Such behavioral engagement predicted students' GPAs, although intelligence also predicted GPA and the behavioral engagement effect was not statistically controlled. Salamonson, Andrew, and Everett (2009) used homework completion in a nursing program, which consisted of textbook reading, as an indicator of behavioral engagement; this variable likely reflected time spent reading. Controlling for age and ethnicity, this indicator was a positive predictor of academic performance in a course on pathophysiology. In an electronic learning environment, off-task attention was an indicator of behavioral disengagement from learning, which predicted subsequent posttest scores (Orvis, Fisher, & Wasserman, 2009). Although statistical controls were often absent, these studies suggest that behavioral engagement is a robust variable impacting competence for a variety of reading tasks at a variety of ages.

In related research, students' reports of effort and perseverance have been referred to as self-discipline (Duckworth, Peterson, Matthews, & Kelly, 2007). In characterizing self-discipline, they used items such as "I am a hard worker," "I finish whatever I begin," and "I have achieved a goal that took years of work." Using this measure in a series of six studies, the investigators found that this measure of self-discipline correlated significantly with GPAs, even when SAT scores were held constant for college students. Duckworth and Seligman (2005) used a similar measure of self-discipline in a study of eighth-grade students and found that it predicted GPA more strongly than did IQ. Furthermore, this indicator of behavioral engagement predicted GPA when controlling for previous IQ scores. The authors concluded that the duration and direction of effort predict the development of expertise more fully than indicators of talent or aptitude. One limitation of this research was that the motivational sources of behavioral engagement were not explicitly investigated. However, such sources have been examined in the engagement literature.

Motivations Impact Behavioral Engagement in Reading

We turn next to a consideration of Path E, links of motivation with behavioral engagement. The studies for this section are presented in Table 29.2. Our argument in this section is that motivations such as self-efficacy, intrinsic motivation, and valuing that are related to reading increase an individual's reading behaviors, that is, the effort, attention, time spent, concentration, and long-term persistence in reading activities. As discussed earlier, we distinguish motivations from behavioral engagement because they are referring to goals, values, beliefs, and dispositions rather than physical behaviors (Wigfield & Guthrie, 2010). In the literature that relates motivation to reading, motivational constructs have been drawn from four theoretical perspectives including expectancy value theory (Wigfield & Eccles, 2002), social cognitive theory (Bandura & Schunk, 1981), goal theory (Maehr & Zusho, 2009), and self-determination theory (Ryan & Deci, 2000). Relations of key constructs from these theories to reading are portrayed in Guthrie and Coddington (2009).

In attempting to characterize a relationship between motivations and behavioral engagement in reading, it is beneficial to consider controlling potentially confounding variables. For example, both motivation and behavioral engagement are likely to be correlated with achievement, as indicated by test scores or grades, and declarative knowledge of the world, which facilitates comprehension and is associated with motivation for reading. As discussed earlier, Guthrie et al. (1999) reported that intrinsic motivation predicted behavioral engagement measured by students' self-reported frequency and breadth of reading activities, even when students' prior knowledge, past achievement, and self-efficacy in reading were controlled. Thus, while controlling for self-efficacy and the cognitive variables of background knowledge and school achievement, intrinsic motivation was associated with behavioral engagement in reading for both elementary and secondary level students. These results extended previous findings by Wigfield and Guthrie (1997) that intrinsic motivation constructs such as challenge, curiosity, and involvement correlated with students' amount and breadth of reading behaviors.

Students' behavioral engagement in reading, according to their self-reported frequency and breadth of reading activities, has further been associated with multiple motivations. Lau (2009) found that 11–18-year olds' intrinsic motivation and social motivation each made unique contributions to their amount of reading, although self-efficacy and extrinsic motivation for reading, which were also included in the model, did not make significant contributions. While this finding appeared for younger secondary students, only intrinsic motivation uniquely contributed to amount of reading when the other motivational constructs were controlled in the model for older secondary students. Thus, intrinsic motivation, which was measured as enjoying reading, appeared to predominate as a predictor of behavioral engagement in reading for both age groups when several other motivational constructs were statistically controlled.

As discussed earlier, Jang (2008) found that when college students were required to perform the aversive task of reading uninteresting material, the extent to which they valued the content of the text determined the extent of their behavioral

Table 29.2 Effects of motivations on behavioral engagement and on reading competence[a]

Citation[a]	Number of participants	Grade levels	Dependent variables	Independent variables[b]	Strength of association[c]
Anmarkrud and Bråten (2009)	104	9	1. Reading comprehension	(a) Topic knowledge (b) Deeper strategies (c) Surface strategies (d) Reading efficacy (e) Reading task value (f) Previous semester social studies grades	$r_{1e} = 0.46***$ $\beta_{1e} = 0.24*$ $\Delta R^2 = 0.06**$ for reading efficacy and reading task value on reading comprehension[d]
Baker and Wigfield (1999)	371	5, 6	1. Students' reports of their reading activity 2. Gates-MacGinitie Reading Comprehension Test Scores 3. CTBS reading 4. Performance assessment	(a) Challenge (b) Self-efficacy (c) Curiosity (d) Involvement (e) Social (f) Importance (g) Recognition (h) Grades (i) Competition (j) Work avoidance (k) Compliance	$r_{1a} = 0.51***$ $r_{1b} = 0.43***$ $r_{1c} = 0.43***$ $r_{1d} = 0.51***$ $r_{1e} = 0.46***$ $r_{2j} = -0.26***$ $r_{3j} = -0.24***$ $r_{4j} = -0.13*$ $r_{4k} = 0.21***$ $r_{4h} = 0.14*$ $r_{4g} = 0.14*$
Chan (1994)	338	5, 7, 9	1. Reading comprehension 2. Use of reading strategies 3. Knowledge of reading strategies	(a) Perceived cognitive competence (b) Belief in personal control (c) Learned helplessness	For grade 5, $\beta_{1c} = -0.32$ For grade 7, $\beta_{1b} = 0.24$ For grade 9, $\beta_{2a} = 0.22$ $\beta_{2a} = 0.44^e$ $\beta_{2a} = 0.20$ $\beta_{2b} = 0.29$
Durik et al. (2006)	606	4, 10	1. Time per week spent reading for pleasure in 10th grade 2. Number of language arts courses per year of high school 3. Reading relatedness of 12th-grade career aspirations	(a) Tenth-grade self-concept of ability (b) Tenth-grade importance (c) Tenth-grade intrinsic value (d) Fourth-grade self-concept of ability (e) Fourth-grade importance (f) Fourth-grade intrinsic value (g) Third-grade reading grade (h) Eighth-grade English grade	$\beta_{1a} = 0.22^f$ $\beta_{2a} = 0.18$ $\beta_{2d} = 0.13$ $\beta_{2b} = 0.19$ $\beta_{2e} = 0.23$ $\beta_{1c} = 0.16$ $\beta_{2c} = 0.18$ $\beta_{1f} = 0.18$
Greene et al. (2004)	220	High school students	1. Percentage of course points in the English class, which is a combination of exams, projects, and homework assignments	(a) Self-efficacy (b) Perceived instrumentality (c) Autonomy support (d) Motivating tasks	$r_{1a} = 0.47**$ $r_{1b} = 0.245**$ $r_{1c} = 0.24**$ $r_{1d} = 0.20**$
Guthrie, Klauda, et al. (2012)	1,200	7	1. Information text comprehension	(a) Perceived difficulty (b) Self-efficacy	$r_{1a} = -0.22**$ $r_{1b} = 0.18**$

(continued)

Table 29.2 (continued)

Citation[a]	Number of participants	Grade levels	Dependent variables	Independent variables[b]	Strength of association[c]
Guthrie et al. (1999a)	271	3, 5	1. Passage comprehension 2. Conceptual learning from multiple texts 3. Reading amount	(a) Past achievement (b) Prior knowledge (c) Reading motivation (d) Self-efficacy (e) Reading amount (f) Intrinsic motivation (g) Extrinsic motivation	$\beta_{3c}=0.383***$ $\Delta R^2=0.138$[g] $\beta_{3f}=0.333***$ $\Delta R^2=0.107$ $\beta_{3g}=0.364***$ $\Delta R^2=0.124$
Guthrie et al. (1999b)	17,424	10	1. Text comprehension 2. Reading amount	(a) Reading amount (b) Past reading comprehension achievement (c) Reading efficacy (d) Reading motivation (e) SES	$r_{2a}=0.29****$ $r_{1d}=0.59****$ $\beta_{1d}=0.419***$ $\Delta R^2=0.229$[g] $\beta_{2d}=0.266***$ $\Delta R^2=0.083$
Guthrie, Wigfield, Barbosa, et al. (2004a)	361	3	1. Multiple text comprehension 2. Passage comprehension	(a) Motivation composite, including self-efficacy, challenge, involvement, and curiosity	$r_{1a}=0.76*$ $r_{2a}=0.82**$
Guthrie, Wigfield, Barbosa, et al. (2004b)	524	3	1. Gates-MacGinitie Reading Comprehension Test 2. Passage comprehension	(a) Intrinsic motivation (b) Self-efficacy (c) Extrinsic motivation	$r_{1a}=0.88**$ $r_{1b}=0.81**$ $r_{2a}=0.75**$ $r_{2b}=0.75**$
Guthrie, Hoa, et al. (2007)	31	4	1. Gates-MacGinitie Reading Comprehension Test 2. Multiple text comprehension	(a) Interest (b) Choice (c) Involvement (d) Efficacy (e) Social motivation	$\Delta R^2=0.12$ for interest[b] $\Delta R^2=0.22$ for choice $\Delta R^2=0.12$ for involvement $\Delta R^2=0.03$ for efficacy $\Delta R^2=0.06$ for social motivation
Jang (2008)	136 College students	NA	1. Conceptual learning 2. Identified regulation 3. Engagement 4. Interest regulation	(a) Rationale	Model 1: $\beta_{32}=0.33*; R^2=0.19$ Model 2: $\beta_{32}=0.25*$ $\beta_{3a}=0.22*$ $R^2=0.16$ Model 3: $\beta_{32}=0.32*; R^2=0.19$
Lau (2009)	1,146	11–18 years of age	1. Reading amount 2. Self-efficacy 3. Intrinsic motivation 4. Extrinsic motivation 5. Social motivation	(a) Perception of reading instruction	$\beta_{3a}=0.49$ $\beta_{3a}=0.55$ $\beta_{2a}=0.44$ $\beta_{4a}=0.46$ $\beta_{15}=0.28$ $\beta_{15}=0.26$
Legault et al. (2006a)	351	12–18 years of age	1. Academic amotivation	(a) Value of task[j] (b) Ability beliefs[j] (c) Task characteristics[j] (d) Effort beliefs[j]	$r_{ab}=0.36***$ $r_{ac}=0.66***$ $r_{ad}=0.51***$ $r_{bc}=0.30***$ $r_{bd}=0.55***$ $r_{cd}=0.64***$

Study	N	Grade	Outcome measures	Predictor variables	Effect sizes
Legault et al. (2006b)	349	12–18 years of age	1. Academic performance 2. Time spent studying 3. Intention to drop out	(a) Value of task[j] (b) Ability beliefs[j] (c) Task characteristics[j] (d) Effort beliefs[j]	$r_{1a} = -0.12*$ $r_{2a} = -0.33***$ $r_{3a} = 0.46***$ $r_{1b} = -0.42**$ $r_{2b} = -0.18**$ $r_{3b} = 0.36***$ $r_{1d} = -0.15**$ $r_{2d} = -0.23***$
Legault et al. (2006c)	741	12–19 years of age	1. Academic performance 2. Problem behaviors 3. Academic self-esteem 4. Intention to drop out	(a) Value of task[j] (b) Ability beliefs[j] (c) Task characteristics[j] (d) Effort beliefs[j]	$\beta_{1b} = -0.39*^k$ $\beta_{1d} = -0.34*$ $\beta_{2a} = 0.21*$ $\beta_{2d} = 0.38*$ $\beta_{3b} = -0.65*$ $\beta_{4a} = 0.49***$ $\beta_{4b} = 0.28*$
Morgan and Fuchs (2007)	Review				
Nolen (1988)	50	8	1. Use of deep processing strategies	(a) General task orientation (b) Task-specific task involvement (c) Perceived value of deep processing strategy (d) Perceived ability (e) Science grade	$\beta_{1a} = 0.31**^l$ $\beta_{1b} = 0.39***$ $\beta_{1c} = 0.18$ $\beta_{ac} = 0.40***$ $\beta_{ab} = 0.28*$
Pintrich and de Groot (1990)	173	7	1. Cognitive strategy use 2. Self-regulation 3. Student performance on seatwork 4. Student performance on exams/quizzes 5. Student performance on essays/reports 6. Student performance on average grade for the course	(a) Self-efficacy (b) Intrinsic value (c) Test anxiety	$r_{1b} = 0.63***$ $r_{2b} = 0.73***$ $r_{1a} = 0.33***$ $r_{2a} = 0.44***$ Partial $r_{23} = 0.18*$ Partial $r_{24} = 0.26***$ Partial $r_{25} = 0.22***$ Partial $r_{6a} = 0.18*$ Partial $r_{6c} = 0.22**$
Rapp and van den Broek (2005)	Review				
Schiefele (1999)	Review				
Schunk and Zimmerman (2007)	Review				
Strambler and Weinstein (2010)	111	1–5	1. 2004–2005 Language arts score. 2. 2004–2005 Math score	(a) Academic valuing (b) Academic devaluing (c) Alternative ID	$\beta_{1b} = -0.41*^m$ $\beta_{2b} = -0.45*$

(continued)

Table 29.2 (continued)

Citation[a]	Number of participants	Grade levels	Dependent variables	Independent variables[b]	Strength of association[c]
Wang and Guthrie (2004)	187 US students and 197 Chinese students	4	1. Text comprehension 2. Enjoyment reading amount 3. School reading amount	(a) Intrinsic motivation (curiosity, involvement, and preference for challenge) (b) Extrinsic motivation (recognition, grades, social, competition, and compliance)	$\beta_{1a} = 0.64$[n] $\beta_{1b} = -0.57$ $\beta_{2a} = 0.85$ $\beta_{2b} = -0.44$ $\beta_{3a} = 0.26$ $\beta_{3b} = 0.04$
Wigfield and Guthrie (1997)	105	4, 5	1. Reading amount 2. Reading breadth	(a) Reading efficacy (b) Curiosity (c) Involvement (d) Recognition (e) Grades (f) Social (g) Challenge (h) Intrinsic composite (i) Extrinsic composite	$r_{1a} = 0.36**$ $r_{2a} = 0.30**$ $r_{1b} = 0.24*$ $r_{2b} = 0.22*$ $r_{1c} = 0.24*$ $r_{2c} = 0.35**$ $r_{1d} = 0.24*$ $r_{2d} = 0.25*$ $\Delta R^2 = 0.07$ for extrinsic composite on children's reading amount[o] $\Delta R^2 = 0.15$ for intrinsic composite on children's breadth of reading[p]

$*p < 0.05$, $**p < 0.01$, $***p < 0.001$, $****p < 0.0001$

Notes

[a] We only included the studies documenting paths E and C in Fig. 29.1
[b] We did not include those variables which the authors reported as covariates or as control variables in their analyses
[c] We only reported the effect sizes of motivations on behavioral engagement (path E) and motivations on reading competence (path C)
[d] This ΔR^2 was the unique contribution of reading efficacy and reading task value to reading comprehension above and beyond gender, prior achievement, topic knowledge, deeper strategies, and surface strategies
[e] All the effect sizes reported in this study are path coefficients in path analysis
[f] All the beta coefficients reported in this study are standardized path coefficients in structural equation modeling
[g] All the ΔR^2 reported in this study are the unique contributions of the variable of interest to the outcome, after controlling for the other variables in the model
[h] All the ΔR^2 reported in this study are the unique contributions of the variables of interest to Gates-MacGinitie Reading Comprehension Test in December, after controlling for prior reading achievement in September
[i] All the beta coefficients reported in this study are standardized path coefficients in structural equation modeling
[j] These variables are negatively coded in these studies, with high scores representing high levels in the four dimensions of academic amotivation and low scores representing low levels in the four dimensions of academic amotivation
[k] All the beta coefficients reported in this study are standardized path coefficients in structural equation modeling
[l] All the effect sizes reported in this study are causal correlations obtained in path analysis
[m] All the beta coefficients reported in this study are standardized path coefficients in structural equation modeling
[n] All the effect sizes reported in this study are the direct effects of the variables of interest on the outcomes, which were obtained from the decomposition of effects for structural paths. Due to the space limit, we only reported the effects sizes for the US students
[o] This ΔR^2 was the unique contribution of spring extrinsic composite to 1993 reading amount above and beyond 1992 reading amount, fall intrinsic composite, fall extrinsic composite, and spring intrinsic composite
[p] This ΔR^2 was the unique contribution of spring intrinsic composite to children's spring reading breadth above and beyond their fall reading breadth, fall intrinsic composite, fall extrinsic composite, and spring extrinsic composite

engagement in the reading activity. Behavioral engagement was optimized for students who showed identified regulation, which referred to believing that the text content was beneficial to their professional work. Students high on identified regulation believed that the task was important and worthwhile to them. In this context, identified regulation (perceived value) contributed to behavioral engagement, but interest in the text did not significantly contribute to behavioral engagement in reading the texts. Consequently, although intrinsic motivation is consistently associated with behavioral engagement in academic reading tasks, when those reading tasks are inherently uninteresting, valuing the content for personal reasons other than intrinsic motivation is likely to be associated with behavioral engagement in reading.

To this point, we have documented that intrinsic motivation and valuing contribute to the behavioral engagement in reading in terms of its quantity, such as amount of time spent, frequency of behavioral activities, and breadth of reading. In addition, motivations are associated with the quality of behavioral engagement. To oversimplify a range of cognitive science phenomena (Rapp & van den Broek, 2005), reading can be deep or superficial. Deep processing strategies consist of making inferences, forming summaries, integrating diverse elements, and monitoring one's comprehension during reading. Superficial strategies are typified by underlining, memorizing, and seeking to complete tasks rather than comprehending fully. Nolen (1988) investigated motivations that were associated with deep processing strategies of eighth graders who were asked to read expository passages. Intrinsic motivation for learning (or the goal of understanding and learning for its own sake) was positively associated with the use of deep processing strategies for text comprehension. In contrast, ego orientation (the goal of demonstrating high ability in comparison to others) was positively related to use of surface-level strategies only. This finding confirmed reports of Pintrich and de Groot (1990) that intrinsic motivation for classwork in reading/language arts was associated with deep processing strategies for text comprehension. Thus, it is evident that motivational constructs not only increase the amount of behavioral engagement but also influence the quality of behavioral engagement by activating cognitive strategies that are productive for full comprehension of complex text.

Behavioral engagement in reading can be expanded to choices that students make during school and leisure time. In a longitudinal study of students from grades 3 to 12, Durik, Vida, and Eccles (2006) tracked the extent to which motivational constructs influenced behavioral engagement in the form of selection of courses and the pursuit of leisure reading. Behavioral engagement was characterized by the number of language arts classes students took per year, including composition, American literature, speech, and humanities. In a longitudinal path model, students' valuing (ratings of importance for reading and language arts) in grade 4 predicted the behavioral engagement in terms of the number of courses selected in grade 10. Self-efficacy in grade 4 predicted number of courses taken in grade 10, but intrinsic value for reading in grade 4 did not predict number of courses directly but was mediated by intrinsic valuing for reading in grade 10. In comparison, the behavioral engagement of leisure reading out of school was predicted by intrinsic motivation in grade 4, although leisure reading was not predicted by valuing or self-efficacy in grade 4.

In summary, it is evident that motivations (such as valuing) activated in a brief laboratory activity increased behavioral engagement in an assigned reading task (Jang, 2008), and more sustained, wide-ranging intrinsic motivation for reading in elementary grades predicted amount of participation in reading intensive courses in high school (Durik et al., 2006). The linkage between motivation and behavioral engagement in reading appears to be viable within highly situated classroom contexts and across a broad sweep of time and place of reading in the schooling process.

Motivations Impact Reading Competence

Figure 29.1 includes a direct pathway from motivations to read to reading competence. In the schematic, it is labeled Path C: Direct Effects of Motivations on Competence. This refers to studies that document the association between a variety of motivations and reading competence; the studies relevant to this path are summarized in Table 29.2. Similar to other constructs in the model, motivations and reading competence are both likely to be correlated with other variables (Chan, 1994). These variables need to be controlled to examine clearly the relations of motivation to reading competence, as Guthrie et al. (1999) did in their study showing that intrinsic reading motivation predicted text comprehension more highly than SES, past achievement, reading amount, or self-efficacy, although the controlling variables were all statistically significant.

The potential mediation of the effect of motivation on reading competence by behavioral engagement was investigated by Jang (2008). In his classroom study with college students, he reported that valuing the content of the text increased test scores reflecting reading comprehension. This effect was mediated by the amount and quality of students' behavioral engagement in the reading activity; thus, valuing impacted reading competence through the activation of competence-relevant reading behaviors. Anmarkrud and Bråten (2009) examined how reading task value predicted ninth-grade students' social studies reading comprehension. Reading competence was measured by a test of reading comprehension containing inferential and literal items. Reading task value, which consisted of perceived importance and utility of reading, predicted text comprehension while controlling for the variables of gender, grades, topic knowledge, deep strategy use, surface strategy use, and self-efficacy in reading. This shows that valuing was associated with reading competence, even when multiple cognitive and motivational variables that may have been present in the Jang study were statistically controlled.

Interest in reading is a motivational construct that has frequently been associated with reading competence. In a review of the empirical literature, Schiefele (1999) observed that interest is akin to intrinsic motivation, but interest is more tightly tied to a particular text. Students rarely have an interest in all texts and all genres. However, ratings of interestingness for a particular text are highly associated with the outcome of rich conceptual understanding from reading. Although such deep understanding is highly correlated with amount of background knowledge, Schiefele's studies showed that interest has a unique contribution to reading competence after background has been controlled either statistically or experimentally. Although Schiefele's studies were based on measures of self-reported interest in text, other investigators have determined interest through questionnaires and interviews. In one interview study, students' interests were based on their positive affect toward texts, topics in texts, authors, or series of books. Reliable rubrics were used to gauge levels of interest based on two 30-min interviews. With this measure, fourth graders' interest in reading in September of the academic year predicted their growth in reading comprehension from September to December. Interest in reading explained 12% of the variance in reading comprehension in December after September levels of reading comprehension were controlled. In addition, a person-centered profile analysis showed that students who increased in motivation from September to December showed higher reading comprehension growth than students who did not increase in motivation during that time period. In other words, not only does high interest in reading forecast comprehension growth, but an increase in the motivations of self-efficacy and involvement in reading forecast reading growth as well (Guthrie, Hoa, et al., 2007).

Self-efficacy is argued to contribute to reading competence through its effect on students' self-regulation (Schunk & Zimmerman, 2007). These authors said that "Self-efficacy refers to learners' perceived capabilities for learning or performing actions at designated levels, while self-regulation refers to self-generated thoughts, feelings, and actions that are systematically designed to affect one's learning of knowledge and skills" (p. 7). In other words, self-efficacy is expected to influence the quality of students' behavioral engagement with reading tasks, which will consequently have a positive influence on reading competence. Consistent with this formulation, self-efficacy is correlated with reading comprehension in many studies (Baker & Wigfield, 1999; Greene, Miller, Crowson, Duke, & Akey, 2004; Guthrie et al., 1999; Guthrie, Wigfield, Barbosa, et al. 2004). In addition, the highly related measure of perceived difficulty in reading has been observed to correlate with reading competency measures in middle school students. For example, for the total sample, perceived difficulty correlated −.22 with information text comprehension, whereas self-efficacy correlated .18 with the same variable when other motivations and gender were statistically controlled (Guthrie, Klauda, et al., 2012).

Another motivational variable associated with reading competence is devaluing. Legault, Green-Demers, and Pelletier (2006) defined devaluing as the rejection of importance or utility of academic work and disidentification with schooling. Strambler and Weinstein (2010) studied devaluing of language arts among African American and Hispanic students. Devaluing was characterized by questionnaire items such as the following: "I don't care about learning." "I don't care about getting a bad grade." In a path analysis, devaluing negatively predicted language arts test scores significantly at −.45 when positive valuing and alternative identification (seeking to be popular, fashionable, cool) were statistically controlled (Strambler & Weinstein, 2010).

The relationship between motivations and competence is almost certainly reciprocal. As Morgan and Fuchs (2007) documented, when end of year achievement in reading is controlled for beginning of year levels, motivations are associated with end of year performance. Simultaneously, when end of year motivations are controlled for beginning of year levels of motivation, reading comprehension is associated with end of year motivation levels. In other words, achievement predicts motivation growth and motivation predicts achievement growth simultaneously. These findings appear for motivational constructs of task orientation (interest in reading), self-efficacy, and perceived difficulty. By contrast, Guthrie, Hoa, et al. (2007) reported that while reading motivation levels (interest in reading books for enjoyment) predicted reading comprehension growth, reading comprehension levels did not predict motivation growth for students in the later elementary grades. However, this issue has not been fully examined for later elementary and secondary students or for special groups of lower or higher achievers.

Classroom Practices Impact Students' Motivations

We turn next to the direct path from classroom practices to students' motivation (Path D). The studies for this section are presented in Table 29.3. In this chapter, we characterize the classroom context in terms of teachers' explicit teaching activities and practices. A widely promoted and documented classroom practice that impacts students' motivation is autonomy support (Green et al., 2004; Reeve, Jang, Carrell, Jeon, & Barch, 2004; Zhou, Ma, & Deci, 2009). This construct, based in self-determination theory (Ryan & Deci, 2009), refers to the instructor taking the students' perspectives, acknowledging students' feelings, and providing them with opportunities for choice or self-direction. Such teaching minimizes the use of controlling pressures and demands. Across a range of subjects including English, students who were afforded autonomy support by the teacher were more likely than other students to report placing a high value on reading (identified regulation) or intrinsically motivated reading (integrated regulation). The identified student believes that school activities and materials such as books are important and useful, whereas the integrated student is intrinsically motivated to read, which involves "doing an activity out of interest because it is rewarding in its own right" (Zhou et al., 2009, p. 492). Thus, autonomy support fosters valuing and intrinsic motivation. In elementary school, autonomy support may assume the form of providing challenging and interesting texts for reading (Miller & Meece, 1999).

In our current study with middle school readers, we increasingly are focused on the teaching practice of relevance along with autonomy support (Guthrie, Mason-Singh, et al., in press). Relevance means instructional activities that are related to students' lives. Perceived relevance is associated with self-efficacy and social motivation

Table 29.3 Effects of classroom practices on motivations, behavioral engagement, and competence

Citation[a]	Number of participants	Grade levels	Dependent variables	Independent variables[b]	Strength of association[c]
Assor et al. (2002)	862	3–8	1. Behavioral and cognitive engagement	(a) Intruding (b) Suppressing criticism (c) Fostering relevance (d) Allowing criticism (e) Providing choice (f) Fostering understanding and interest (g) Forcing meaningless activities	$\beta_{1c} = 0.25^{***[d]}$ for grades 3–5 $R^2 = 0.15$ $\beta_{1c} = 0.24^*$ for grades 6–8 $R^2 = 0.19$ $r_{be} = -0.44^{**}$ $r_{eg} = -0.25^{**}$ $r_{fg} = -0.18^{**}$ $r_{ac} = -0.31^{**}$ $r_{af} = -0.49^{**}$
Decker et al. (2007)	44	K–6	1. Student-report social skills 2. Student-report engagement 3. Teacher-report social skills 4. Teacher-report engagement 5. Academic engaged time 6. Behavioral referrals 7. Suspensions	(a) Teachers' perspective of the student-teacher relationship (b) Student perspective—psychological proximity seeking (c) Student perspective—emotional quality	$\Delta R^2_{1a} = 0.14^e$ $\Delta R^2_{2a} = 0.18$ $\Delta R^2_{3a} = 0.22$ $\Delta R^2_{4a} = 0.14$ $\beta_{5a} = -0.37^*$ $\beta_{5c} = 0.49^{**}$ $\beta_{6b} = 0.36^*$ $\beta_{6c} = -0.41^{**}$ $\beta_{7a} = -0.38^{**}$ $\beta_{7c} = -0.31^*$
Dill and Boykin (2000)	72	5	1. Text-recall performance 2. Evaluative item: liked the learning period 3. Evaluative item: would do the project again 4. Evaluative item: cared about peer	(a) Learning context: communal (b) Learning context: peer (c) Learning context: individual (d) Gender	$\eta^2 = 0.112$ Between learning context and recall $M_{1a} > M_{1b}{}^* M_{1a} > M_{1c}{}^{*f}$ $r_{3a} = 0.478^{**}$ $r_{4a} = 0.596^{**}$ $r_{2b} = 0.406^{**}$ $r_{4b} = 0.467^{**}$
Filaka and Sheldon (2008)	220 College students	NA	1. Course approval 2. Instructor approval 3. Grade prediction 4. Need satisfaction 5. Student self-determined motivation	(a) Teacher autonomy support	$\beta_{5a} = 0.35^{**g}$ $\beta_{4a} = 0.76^{**}$ $\beta_{45} = 0.26^{**}$ $\beta_{14} = 0.74^{**}$ $\beta_{24} = 0.72^{**}$ $\beta_{34} = 0.28^{**}$
Furrer and Skinner (2003)	641	3–6	1. Teacher-report student behavioral engagement 2. Child-report student behavioral engagement 3. Changes in child-report engagement from the beginning to the end of the school year	(a) Relatedness to teacher (b) Relatedness to peer (c) Overall relatedness in the fall	$\beta_{1a} = 0.14^{**h}$ $\Delta R^2 = 0.01$ $\beta_{1b} = 0.11^*$ $\Delta R^2 = 0.01$ $\beta_{2a} = 0.26^{**}$ $\Delta R^2 = 0.05$ $\beta_{2b} = 0.16^{**}$ $\Delta R^2 = 0.02$ $\beta_{3c} = 0.12^{**}$ $R^2 = 0.59$

Study	N	Grade	Measure	Construct	Result
Greene et al. (2004)	220	High school students	1. Percentage of course points in the English class, which is a combination of exams, projects, and homework assignments 2. Self-efficacy 3. Mastery goals 4. Performance-approach goals	(a) Autonomy support (b) Self-efficacy (c) Strategy use	$\beta_{2a} = 0.22*$ $\beta_{1b} = 0.38*$ $\beta_{1c} = 0.15*$ $\beta_{4b} = 0.24*$ $\beta_{4b} = 0.22*$
Guthrie, Klauda, et al. (2012)	1,200	7	1. Dedication in reading 2. Self-efficacy	(a) Relevance (b) Choices (c) Collaboration (d) Success (in text) (e) Thematic unit	$r_{1a} = 0.36**$ $r_{1b} = 0.19**$ $r_{1d} = 0.23**$ $r_{2d} = 0.61**$
Guthrie, Mason-Singh, et al. (in press)	1,200	7	1. Social motivation 2. Self-efficacy 3. Intrinsic motivation 4. Value	(a) Collaboration (b) Thematic unit (c) Reading awareness	$\beta_{1a} = 0.30*$ For African American students $\beta_{2b} = 0.46**$ For African American students $\beta_{2b} = 0.24**$ For European American students $\beta_{4c} = 0.29*$ For African American students $\beta_{4c} = 0.38*$ For European American students $\beta_{3c} = 0.32*$ For European American students
Guthrie, McRae, et al. (2007)	Review				
Guthrie, Wigfield, Barbosa, et al. (2004a)	361	3	1. Multiple text comprehension 2. Passage comprehension	(a) Motivation composite, including self-efficacy, challenge, involvement, and curiosity	$r_{1a} = 0.76*$ $r_{2a} = 0.82**$
Guthrie, Wigfield, Barbosa, et al. (2004b)	524	3	1. Gates-MacGinitie Reading Comprehension Test 2. Passage comprehension	(a) Intrinsic motivation (b) Self-efficacy (c) Extrinsic motivation	$r_{1a} = 0.88**$, $r_{1b} = 0.81**$ $r_{2a} = 0.75**$, $r_{2b} = 0.75**$
Hamre and Pianta (2005)	908	5–6 Years of age	1. Achievement (Woodcock-Johnson)	(a) Instructional support (b) Emotional support (c) Maternal education (d) High functional risk (e) Maternal education × instructional support (f) High functional risk × emotional support	$\eta^2 = 0.02**$ For maternal education × instructional support $\eta^2 = 0.01*$ For high functional risk × emotional support

(continued)

Table 29.3 (continued)

Citation[a]	Number of participants	Grade levels	Dependent variables	Independent variables[b]	Strength of association[c]
Jang (2008)	136 College students	NA	1. Conceptual learning 2. Identified regulation 3. Engagement 4. Interest regulation	(a) Rationale (b) Identified regulation (c) Engagement (d) Interest regulation	Model 1:[j] $\beta_{2a}=0.42*$ $\beta_{32}=0.33*$ $\beta_{13}=0.45*$ Model 2: $\beta_{4a}=0.41*$ $\beta_{34}=0.25*$ $\beta_{13}=0.44*$ Model 3: $\beta_{2a}=0.41*$ $\beta_{32}=0.32*$ $\beta_{13}=0.44*$ $\beta_{2b}=0.41*$
Lau (2009)	1,146	11–18 years of age	1. Reading amount 2. Self-efficacy 3. Intrinsic motivation 4. Extrinsic motivation 5. Social motivation	(a) Perception of reading instruction	$\beta_{3a}=0.49^k$ $\beta_{3a}=0.55$ $\beta_{2a}=0.44$ $\beta_{4a}=0.46$ $\beta_{13}=0.28$ $\beta_{15}=0.26$
Miller and Meece (1999)	24	3	1. Students' value ratings of academic task	(a) Academic task (high/low challenge) (b) Type of value question: liking and interest in an academic task (c) Exposure (maximum/minimum) (d) Achievement (high/average/low)	Main effect $F(1, 36)=5.04*$, indicating students expressing a greater liking and interest in the high-challenge academic tasks
Perry et al. (2007)	257	1	1. Math achievement 2. Interpersonal behavior 3. Intrapersonal behavior 4. Self-perceived competence	(a) Child-centered practices	$\gamma_{1a}=3.17**{[l]}$ $\gamma_{2a}=-12.39*$ $\gamma_{3a}=-15.94*$ $\gamma_{4a}=0.09**$
Ponitz et al. (2009)	171	K	1. Spring reading 2. Behavioral engagement	(a) Classroom quality (b) Fall reading (c) Sociodemographic risk	$\beta_{2a}=0.16*{[m]}$ $\beta_{12}=0.18*$
Reeve et al. (2004)	20 High school teachers	NA	1. Teacher's autonomy-supportive behaviors 2. Students' engagement: task involvement (third observation) 3. Students' engagement: influence attempts (third observation)	(a) Teacher exposure to information on how to support students' autonomy (b) Teacher's autonomy support (third observation)	Unique $R^2_{2b}=0.37^n$ $\beta_{2b}=0.61**$ Unique $R^2_{3b}=0.29$ $\beta_{3b}=0.54**$
Ryan and Deci (2009)	Review				
Schunk and Zimmerman (2007)	Review				

Study	N	Grade	Variables	Predictors	Statistics
Shih (2008)	343	8	1. Behavioral engagement: involvement 2. Behavioral engagement: persistence 3. Behavioral engagement: participation 4. Behavioral engagement: avoiding 5. Behavioral engagement: ignoring	(a) Perceived autonomy support (b) Mastery-approach goal (c) Mastery-avoidance goal (d) Performance-approach goal (e) Performance-avoidance goal (f) Controlled motivation (g) Autonomous motivation	$\beta_{1a}=0.24^{***o}$ $\beta_{1b}=0.30^{***}$ $\beta_{1f}=-0.20^{***}$ $\beta_{1g}=0.35^{***}$ $\beta_{2b}=0.39^{***}$ $\beta_{2e}=0.31^{***}$ $\beta_{3a}=0.17^{***}$ $\beta_{3h}=0.23^{**}$ $\beta_{3g}=0.26^{***}$ $\beta_{3h}=-0.34^{***}$ $\beta_{4e}=0.24^{***}$ $\beta_{4f}=0.19^{**}$ $\beta_{4g}=-0.23^{**}$ $\beta_{5a}=-0.17^{**}$ $\beta_{5h}=-0.29^{**}$ $\beta_{5f}=0.17^{**}$
Skinner and Belmont (1993)	144	3, 4, 5	1. Student perception of structure 2. Student perception of autonomy support 3. Student perception of involvement 4. Student behavioral engagement 5. Student emotional engagement	(a) Teacher involvement (b) Teacher autonomy support (c) Teacher structure (d) Teacher perception of student behavioral engagement (e) Teacher perception of student emotional engagement	$\beta_{1a}=0.28^{**p}$ $\beta_{2a}=0.25^{***}$ $\beta_{3a}=0.25^{**}$ $\beta_{4i}=0.33^{***}$ $\beta_{53}=0.20^{**}$ $\beta_{cd}=0.28^{**}$ $\beta_{bd}=0.72^{***}$ $\beta_{ad}=0.61^{***}$
Skinner et al. (2008)	805	4–7	1. Changes in engaged behavior from fall to spring 2. Changes in disaffected behavior from fall to spring	(a) Student report of teacher support (b) Teacher report of teacher support	$\beta_{1a}=0.23^{***}$ $R^2=0.37$ $\beta_{2a}=-0.12^{***}$ $R^2=0.46$ $\beta_{1b}=0.07^{*}$
Skinner et al. (2009b)	1,018	3–6	1. Student reports of engagement in spring of year 3 2. Teacher reports of engagement in spring of year 3	(a) Teacher warmth (b) Teacher structure (c) Teacher autonomy support	$r_{1a}=0.55^{**}$ $r_{1b}=0.55^{**}$ $r_{1c}=0.47^{**}$ $r_{2a}=0.26^{**}$ $r_{2b}=0.28^{**}$ $r_{2c}=0.20^{**}$
Souvignier and Mokhlesgerami (2006)	593	5	1. Reading comprehension 2. Understanding the use of reading strategies 3. Application of reading strategies 4. Self-efficacy 5. Motivational orientation	(a) Instructional group: MSR+strat+CSR (b) Instructional group: strat+CSR (c) Instructional group: strat (d) Instructional group: control	$T_{a-b}=2.25^{*q}$ For reading comprehension in retention $d_{a-d}=0.82$ For understanding the use of reading strategies in retention $T_{a-b}=2.20^{*}$ For application of reading strategies in retention $d_{a-d}=1.12$ For application of reading strategies in retention $T_{a-b}=2.20^{*}$ For motivational orientation in retention

(continued)

Table 29.3 (continued)

Citation[a]	Number of participants	Grade levels	Dependent variables	Independent variables[b]	Strength of association[c]
Strambler and Weinstein (2010)	111	1–5	1. 2004–2005 Language arts score 2. 2004–2005 Math scores	(a) Academic valuing (b) Academic devaluing (c) Alternative ID	$\beta_{1b} = -0.41^{*r}$ $\beta_{2b} = -0.45^{*}$
Vansteenkiste et al. (2004a)	200 College students	NA	1. Autonomous motivation 2. Superficial processing 3. Deep processing 4. Test performance 5. Persistence	(a) Intrinsic goal framing vs. extrinsic goal (b) Autonomy-supportive context vs. controlling contexts	$\eta^2_{1a} = 0.59^{***s}$ $\eta^2_{3a} = 0.42^{***}$ $\eta^2_{4a} = 0.21^{***}$ $\eta^2_{5a} = 0.12^{***}$
Vansteenkiste et al. (2004b)	377 College students	NA	1. Autonomous motivation 2. Superficial processing 3. Deep processing 4. Underlining 5. Test performance 6. Persistence	(a) Intrinsic goal framing vs. extrinsic goal (b) Autonomy-supportive context vs. controlling contexts	$\eta^2_{1a} = 0.59^{***s}$ $\eta^2_{3a} = 0.35^{***}$ $\eta^2_{4a} = 0.17^{***}$ $\eta^2_{6a} = 0.12^{***}$
Vansteenkiste et al. (2004c)	224	10, 11	1. Autonomous motivation 2. Test performance 3. Persistence	(a) Intrinsic goal framing vs. extrinsic goal (b) Autonomy-supportive context vs. controlling contexts	$\eta^2_{1a} = 0.50^{***s}$ $\eta^2_{2a} = 0.16^{***}$ $\eta^2_{3a} = 0.09^{***}$
Vansteenkiste et al. (2005a)	130	5, 6	1. Perceived autonomy 2. Conceptual learning T1 3. Rote learning T1 4. Conceptual learning T2 5. Rote learning T2	(a) Goal orientation (intrinsic, extrinsic) (b) Communication style (autonomy support, internal control, external control)	Main effect: $\eta^2 = 0.13^{***t}$ for goal orientation $\eta^2 = 0.30^{***}$ for communication style $\eta^2_{4a} = 0.05^{*}$
Vansteenkiste et al. (2005b)	113	11- to 12- year-olds	1. Perceived autonomy 2. Conceptual learning T1 3. Conceptual learning T2	(a) Goal orientation (intrinsic, extrinsic) (b) Communication style (autonomy support, internal control)	Main effect: $\eta^2 = 0.25^{***}$ for goal orientation $\eta^2 = 0.52^{***}$ for communication $\eta^2_{3a} = 0.30^{***u}$
Vansteenkiste et al. (2005c)	80	11- to 12- year-olds	1. Conceptual learning 2. Task involvement 3. Relative autonomy	(a) Goal orientation (intrinsic, extrinsic) (b) Communication style (autonomy support, internal control)	Main effect: $\eta^2 = 0.31^{***t}$ for goal orientation $\eta^2_2 = 0.87^{***}$ for communication $\eta^2_{1a} = 0.07$ $\eta^2_{2a} = 0.15^{***}$
Wentzel (2009)	Review				

Study	N	Grade	Measures	Variables of interest	Effect sizes
Wigfield et al. (2008)	315	4	1. Gates-MacGinitie Reading Comprehension 2. Multiple text comprehension 3. Strategy composite	(a) Instructional groups (CORI, SI, TI) (b) Engagement	Main effect of instructional group: $F_{(8, 18)} = 4.10^{**}$ b(CORI) > b(SI)** b(CORI) > b(TI)* With engagement as covariate, main effect of instructional group: $F_{(3, 6)} < 1$ ns
Zhou et al. (2009a)	195	4–6	1. Interest 2. Perceived competence 3. Perceived choice	(a) Autonomous motivation (b) Controlled motivation (c) Interaction term	$\beta_{1a} = 0.60^{**}$ $R^2 = 0.36^{****w}$ $\beta_{2a} = 0.58^{***}$ $R^2 = 0.39^{***}$ $\beta_{3a} = 0.38^{***}$ $R^2 = 0.20^{***}$
Zhou et al. (2009b)	48	4, 5	1. Autonomous motivation at time 2 2. Controlled motivation at time 2 3. Perceived competence at time 2 4. Perceived choice at time 2 5. Interest at time 2	(a) Autonomous motivation at time 1 (b) Controlled motivation at time 1 (c) Perceived competence at time 1 (d) Perceived choice at time 1 (e) Interest at time 1 (f) Change in perceived teacher autonomy support from time 1 to time 2	$\beta_{1f} = 0.31^{*x}$ $\beta_{5f} = 0.50^{***}$

$*p < 0.05$, $**p < 0.01$, $***p < 0.001$, $****p < 0.0001$

Notes

[a] We only included the studies documenting paths A, B, and D in Fig. 29.1

[b] We did not include those variables which the authors reported as covariates or as control variables in their analyses

[c] We only reported the effect sizes of classroom practices on motivations (path D), behavioral engagement (path B), and reading competence (path A)

[d] The effect sizes reported in this study are the standardized beta coefficients obtained in simultaneous multiple regressions. The R^2 refers to the contributions of the five predictors (intruding, suppressing criticism, fostering relevance, allowing criticism, providing choice) to the outcome

[e] The effect sizes reported in this study are the standardized beta weights in multiple regressions. ΔR^2 are the unique contributions of each predictor to the outcomes

[f] The post hoc analysis indicated that students assigned to communal learning ($M = 6.67$) context outperformed students assigned to both the peer ($M = 4.29$) and individual ($M = 4.21$)

[g] All the effect sizes reported in this study are path coefficients in path analysis

[h] All the effect sizes reported in this study are beta coefficients in multiple regressions. The ΔR^2 were the unique contributions of the variable of interest to the outcomes

[i] The effect sizes reported here are standardized beta coefficients in stepwise multiple regression

[j] All the effect sizes reported in this study are standardized coefficients in structural equation modeling

[k] Due to the space limit, we only reported the effects sizes for junior secondary students. All the effects sizes reported in this study are significant path coefficients in path analysis

(continued)

Table 29.3 (continued)

[l]The effect sizes reported in this study are the gamma coefficients in hierarchical linear modeling

[m]The effect sizes reported in this study are standardized coefficients in structural equation modeling

[n]Due to space limit, we only reported the effect sizes for the third observation. The ΔR^2 is the unique contribution of teacher autonomy support (during the third observation) to student engagement outcomes, after controlling for students' engagement and teachers' autonomy support at the second observation

[o]The effect sizes reported in this study are the standardized beta coefficients in multiple regressions

[p]The effect sizes reported in this study are standardized regression coefficients in path analysis

[q]The original study reported the effect sizes in both posttest and retention. Due to the space limit, we only reported the effect sizes in retention

[r]All the effect sizes reported in this study are standardized coefficients in structural equation modeling

[s]Due to the space limit, we only reported the effect sizes for goal content

[t]Due to the space limit, we only reported the effect sizes for goal content. η^2_{3a} was the effect of intrinsic goal on long-term conceptual learning after controlling for short-term conceptual learning

was the effect of intrinsic goal on long-term conceptual learning after controlling for short-term conceptual learning

[u]Due to the space limit, we only reported the effect sizes for goal content

[v]Due to the space limit, we only reported the effect sizes for goal content

[w]The effect sizes reported in this study are beta coefficients in multiple regressions. The R^2 are the contributions of the three predictors (autonomous motivation, controlled motivation, interaction term) to each outcome

[x]These effect sizes reported in this study are the beta coefficients in hierarchical regressions. Time 2 motivation and self-perception variables were regressed onto the corresponding variables in time 1 and then onto the residual scores of perceived teacher autonomy support at time 2 in the math and English classes, while controlling for time 1 autonomy support from their previous math or English classroom teachers

(Assor, Kaplan, & Roth, 2002; Lau, 2009). Providing students with an awareness of the benefits of reading increases their valuing of reading work in the classroom. For example, Jang (2008) told prospective teachers that reading about complications of statistical analyses would benefit their professions, which increased their perceived value for reading texts about statistics. Likewise, providing middle school students with an awareness that reading about science is important to their ability to explain their world and succeed in school increased students' valuing of information books such as science texts (Guthrie, Mason-Singh, et al., 2012).

Another important classroom characteristic is the quality of teacher-student relationships. When teachers emphasize collaboration and positive interpersonal relationships (between themselves and students and among students in the classroom), students' motivation increases for school in general and for reading. When students believe their teachers think they are important, they are likely to participate more socially in the classroom (Furrer & Skinner, 2003). As both teacher and student reports of the quality of teacher-student relationships increase, there are also enhancements in positive social interactions and engagement outcomes (Decker, Dona, & Christenson, 2007). For African American students in particular, collaborative learning environments enhance students' recall of stories and desire to participate in similar activities in the future (Dill & Boykin, 2000). Across a range of contexts, explicit arrangements for student collaborations in reading and writing increased students' satisfaction with the classroom (Guthrie, Mason-Singh, et al., in press).

Support for students' self-efficacy in reading and other subjects is crucial because self-efficacy is exceptionally low for struggling students. As portrayed by Schunk and Zimmerman (2007), several explicit teaching practices increase students' self-efficacy. The self-efficacy-fostering framework consists of providing students with process goals, which consists of steps for performing academic tasks successfully. Teachers provide feedback for success in the process goals rather than the students' products or outcomes. That is, teachers give specific direction to students about the effectiveness of their strategy for performing work and help students set realistic goals in their learning domain. Experimental studies summarized by these researchers confirm that these practices increase students' belief in their capacity, perceived competence, and eventually, their achievement in reading tasks. Also beneficial to students' self-efficacy in reading is their perception of coherence in the texts and tasks of instruction. When students can identify the links across specific domains of knowledge in their reading and perceive themes in the substance of their reading materials, they gain a belief that they can succeed in reading and writing about text (Guthrie, Mason-Singh, et al., in press).

Effects of teachers' practices on students' motivations are sufficiently powerful that they can have deleterious effects. Some teachers behave in ways that are devaluing for students. For example, negative feedback from teachers may be devaluing for students. When teachers consistently scold or make students feel bad for having the wrong answers, they respond by devaluing academic work, as indicated by their expressions that they do not care about learning or grades (Strambler & Weinstein, 2010). In addition, middle school students who experience no choices or limited choices in reading in Language Arts or Science classes show losses of intrinsic motivation for reading, according to self-report questionnaires. Likewise, when books are extremely difficult to read, students report declines in self-efficacy for reading. When books are irrelevant, as indicated by students' failure to report being able to connect the content to their prior knowledge or their life experiences, they report low levels of interest or dedication to reading (Guthrie, Klauda, et al., 2012). What this shows is that classroom practices are a sword that cuts in two directions. Affirming practices may foster positive affect and motivational growth, while at the same time undermining practices, such as negative feedback, controlling instruction, and irrelevance, may generate decreases in motivation. These findings are consistent with the correlational findings reported by Assor et al.

(2002) and reciprocal relationships between classroom instruction and student motivations found by Skinner and Belmont (1993).

Direct Effects of Classroom Practices on Behavioral Engagement

This assertion is represented in the schematic as Path B, which forms a connection between explicit practices and observed behavioral engagement. The studies for this section are presented in Table 29.3. In three studies with high school and college students, Vansteenkiste, Simons, Lens, Sheldon, and Deci (2004) examined the effects of intrinsic goal framing as an instructional practice. The definition of intrinsic goal framing is that the purpose for reading relates to the students' personal interests and goals. For prospective teachers, intrinsic goal framing consisted of stating that reading the text will "help you teach toddlers well" or "help you make the world a better place." For adolescents with obesity issues, intrinsic goal framing consisted of showing that reading would enable students to improve their health and lose weight. In contrast, extrinsic goal framing consisted of stating that students should read to learn how to save money or improve one's physical image. In several experiments, students were given texts to read with one of the two goal frames. They were then given measures of reading comprehension that reflected either deep processing or surface memorizing. Finally, students were given a measure of behavioral engagement, which was an opportunity to persist in reading more about this topic following the experimental reading task and the assessment. Results showed that intrinsic goal framing increased deep processing of text (conceptual learning) and persistence, as indicated by time spent reading related materials. The effect of intrinsic goal framing on the behavioral indicator of engagement, which was persistence, was mediated by students' autonomous motivation, which was a composite of their valuing and interest in the texts. In sum, this set of studies confirms experimentally that intrinsic goal framing increased behavioral engagement, and its effect was mediated by autonomous motivation which combined interest and valuing for the content of the reading materials (Vansteenkiste, Simons, Lens, Soenens, & Matos, 2005).

Lau (2009) found middle and high school students' perception of instruction as relevant because it was related to their lives, useful for their goals, and interesting, showing higher volumes of reading activity (more reading engagement) than students who perceived the instruction as less relevant to them. The effect of relevance as a teaching practice was on behavioral engagement, as measured by amount of reading, and was fully mediated by intrinsic motivation and social motivation for younger secondary students. The effect of relevance of instruction was mediated for older secondary students by intrinsic motivation only. The behavioral engagement impacted by this instruction was educationally significant because highly engaged students were reading eight times more than disengaged students on a scale that measured frequency, time spent, and breadth of materials. These findings are similar to Vansteenkiste and colleagues' (2005) findings on intrinsic framing and were obtained in actual classroom contexts. In both cases, Path B in the model was affirmed, showing that the quality of classroom practices impacted behavioral engagement in reading mediated by intrinsic motivation and, in the latter case, also social motivation.

Another characteristic of the classroom context that is related to behavioral engagement is teacher support. This global indicator emphasizes students' perceptions of teacher involvement (warmth, knowledge, and dependability) and classroom structure (clarity of goals and expectations) (Skinner et al., 2009b). In this line of research, teacher support represents student-centeredness of instruction and contrasts with a domineering or controlling approach by the teacher. Furrer and Skinner (2003) found that teacher support is associated with increases in student engagement from fall to spring for students in grades 3–6. Students' behavioral engagement referred to their self-reported effort, attention, and persistence while participating in classroom learning activities. Consistent with this finding, Skinner, Furrer, Marchand, and Kindermann (2008) reported that in grades 4–7, students' behavioral disaffection decreased from fall to spring as a consequence of teacher support. This decrease consisted of a reduction in students' lack of effort or withdrawal from learning activities. Although teacher support is not a specific practice, but rather a broad attribute that may be associated with a number of specific practices such as assuring success, providing relevance, offering choices, arranging collaborations, and providing themes for learning, it was strongly associated with students' increases in behavioral engagement (standardized regression coefficient of .23 ($p<.001$)) and decreases in behavioral disaffection (standardized regression coefficient of $-.12$ ($p<.001$)). The researchers did not examine the possible mediation by motivations of the relationship between teacher support and engagement.

Akin to these findings, Shih (2008) reported that Taiwanese eighth graders who reported perceptions of autonomy support from their teachers were likely to show relatively high levels of behavioral engagement in the form of listening carefully in class, persisting with hard problems, and participating in class discussions, while not ignoring classroom activities or avoiding hard challenges. In this case, perceived autonomy referred to the instructors' openness and acceptance of students.

Classroom Practices Impact Student Competence

In the graphic representation of the model of reading engagement processes with classroom contexts, we present classroom practices and conditions on the far left. The purpose of this location is to indicate that these contextual variables may influence students' motivations, behavioral engagement, and reading competence. At the most general level, a number of studies have shown that contextual variables of the classroom such as instructional practices, teacher support, and other conditions may directly impact students' reading competence; we denote this with Path A in the model. Although we believe that the effects of classroom practices on achievement are fully mediated by motivations and engagement, in the initial portion of this section, we briefly review research that has addressed the direct effect of motivational practices in the classroom on reading competence. In the second portion of the section, we identify a more limited set of contextual variables that have been shown to affect competence mediated either by students' motivations or their behavioral engagements in reading or both.

A number of studies based in self-determination theory (Ryan & Deci, 2009) document the effects of two forms of autonomy support on students' conceptual learning. It is reasonable to include those studies in this chapter on reading because the conceptual learning outcome has referred to knowledge gained from students' interaction with text. We discussed above Vansteenkiste and colleagues' (2005) experimental work on intrinsic framing, which refers to reasons for reading and studying texts that are personally significant to students, and also Jang's (2008) study on how giving students a rationale for reading uninteresting texts about statistics that will benefit students' careers and professional effectiveness increased students' conceptual learning from text. In some cases, the control condition of extrinsic framing increased factual memory and surface processing of text. Consequently, the effects of these practices on reading competence are firmly established experimentally. One limitation of these investigations is that they are short term, with brief interventions and limited measures of conceptual learning that may not be generalizable to academically significant success. A second limitation is that they have been performed mainly with college students.

Studies of classroom practices that increase students' motivation have also been performed with elementary and middle school students in Reading and Language Arts classrooms over periods from 6 to 36 weeks. We and our colleagues have examined how Concept-Oriented Reading Instruction (CORI) influences third-, fourth-, fifth-, and seventh-grade students' reading comprehension and engagement in reading (Guthrie,

Wigfield, Barbosa, et al. 2004; see Guthrie, McRae, et al., 2007, for review of the findings). CORI includes the classroom practices of providing relevance, choices, collaboration, leveled texts, and thematic units. This cluster of practices is designed to increase intrinsic motivation, self-efficacy, social motivation, and valuing for reading (Guthrie, Wigfield, & Perencevich, 2004).

To exemplify CORI, a synopsis of a lesson is presented next. The CORI goal is to teach reading comprehension with motivation support. This lesson is from a 6-week CORI unit that teaches the reading strategies of inferencing, summarizing, and concept mapping to foster seventh graders' comprehension of information text. Using the conceptual theme "Diversity of Life," this is lesson 9 which occurs in week 2.

The teacher posts the question for the day: "What are some special features of wetland plants that enable them to survive in their environment?" To begin, students view a 5-minute video about aquatic plants, showing their locations, stems, root systems, and leaf varieties. (This video supports intrinsic motivation by providing relevance for the texts that follow). Individuals record their observations of the video in a journal and share them with a partner. Partners then select one of two texts on aquatic plants. Together they locate a 2–4-page section that addresses the day's question (partnerships support social motivation; choice of texts supports students' autonomy).

Teachers guide students to select 2–5 key words that represent the main idea of the text, which they enter into their journals. Then teachers guide students to identify 3–4 supporting facts for each key word (scaffolding of the summarizing process enables students to learn a widely applicable strategy for summarizing information text—the essence of comprehension instruction; this scaffolding also assures success in grappling with complex information text, giving students support for increasing self-efficacy in reading these texts).

Next, the teacher gives students the choice of showing their understanding about "special features of wetland plants" by either writing a summary or drawing and labeling a diagram (choice of knowledge expression is autonomy supportive). Pairs of students select an option for self-expression and complete the task, entering it in their portfolio.

Teacher closes the lesson by asking, "What choices did you have today and how did they help you?" (In this 5-minute reflection, the students' awareness of autonomy support enhances their perception that the instruction affirms their motivational development as well as their acquisition of cognitive expertise in reading.)

Guthrie, Hoa, et al. (2007) performed a meta-analysis of CORI's effects across 11 experiments with 75 effect sizes. CORI was found to surpass comparison treatments in increasing students' competence according to standardized tests of reading comprehension ($ES = .90$), 2-day reading and writing tasks ($ES = .93$), passage comprehension ($ES = .73$), and reading fluency ($ES = .59$), as well as word recognition ($ES = .75$). CORI also fostered students' self-reported reading motivation ($ES = 1.2$) and teacher-reported students' engagement in reading ($ES = 1.0$), as well as amount of reading ($ES = .49$). This confirms that an integrated cluster of motivational practices over extended time can increase students' performance on educationally significant measures of reading comprehension. The bulk of the evidence shows that CORI impacted reading comprehension outcomes, although the one study that examined the issue also showed that this instructional effect was mediated by behavioral engagement (Wigfield et al., 2008; see further discussion below). Furthermore, these effects were confirmed by investigators who showed that an intervention that added motivational supports to instruction in self-regulation increased students' self-regulated reading more effectively than instruction that did not include motivational practices (Souvignier & Mokhlesgerami, 2006).

A burgeoning literature exists documenting the effect of perceived emotional support from teachers on students' academic performance (Wentzel, 2009). The outcomes of these studies are often grades rather than test scores, which may reflect students' motivational and social attributes in addition to their reading competence. In these studies, teacher support refers to students' relationships with teachers that enable them to perceive the goals of teaching clearly, belief that their teachers will help them attain the goals efficiently, and that the students are in a safe and trusting environment. The findings range from grade 1 (Hamre & Pianta, 2005; Perry, Donohue, & Weinstein, 2007) to college classrooms (Filaka & Sheldon, 2008). For example, teacher support was found to increase competence in reading words and passages in the middle of first grade for students placed at risk due to low maternal education. The instructional effect of motivation practices was stronger than the effect of excellent pedagogy in word recognition for at-risk students (consisting of direct instruction in phonological knowledge and letter sound correspondences) (Hamre & Pianta, 2005).

One dominant construct in the teacher support literature is teacher caring, which correlates positively with academic achievement in reading and English courses (Wentzel, 2009). However, the specific ways in which teachers express caring for students have been little studied. It also is unclear how teacher caring relates to some of the other practices discussed earlier, such as helping students to see the relevance of instruction, make meaningful choices during learning, interact with classmates for academic purposes, enjoy the acquisition of expertise, and learn in meaningful, coherent themes; this remains an important topic for future research.

Indirect Effects of Classroom Practices on Students' Reading Competence

A few of the studies documenting the effects of classroom motivation practices on reading competence have attempted to quantify the mediation of these effects by students' motivations or behavioral engagements. As previously stated, we are proposing that under a majority of conditions, classroom practices and conditions that support student motivation in the classroom context are most likely to impact students' reading competence by virtue of their effects on students' motivations, which are then expected to increase behavioral engagement in reading, which is the proximal variable that influences cognitive competence in reading. The Jang (2008) study that we have discussed in this chapter documents this double mediation. All three pathways (D, E, and F) were tested in the study, illustrating that classroom practices impacted motivations, which increased behavioral engagements, which influenced reading competence. Jang found that college students who were given a rationale emphasizing the value of reading an uninteresting statistics text passage perceived the text as more important than did students not given the rationale; Jang stated that the students who received the value rationale increased in their identified regulation. Students whose perceived importance/identified regulation increased also showed enhanced behavioral engagement. According to the reports of external raters who observed students during their reading and learning, behaviorally engaged students were attentive, on task, effortful, and persistent in the face of challenges. Behaviorally disengaged students tended to be off task, passive, and give up quickly on the reading activity. In addition, highly behaviorally engaged students gained deeper conceptual understanding than less behaviorally engaged students, although behavioral engagement did not influence students' learning of minor facts. This confirms the proposition that the classroom practice of affording students a value rationale for learning increased students' perceived importance/identified regulation, which in turn increased their behavioral engagement during the reading activity, which enhanced their performance on the conceptual learning aspect of a reading test on this text. It should be noted that intrinsic motivation was not a mediator in this study. Although the effect of the value rationale on reading comprehension was mediated by students' values (identified regulation), it was not significantly mediated by students' intrinsic motivation (interest regulation). Thus, for the ecologically valid task of reading an uninteresting text, the mediating motivation was perceived importance, but not intrinsic motivation (reading interesting material), which is frequently shown to be a contributor to reading achievement.

Other investigators have shown that the impact of motivational practices on students' reading competencies is mediated by students' behavioral engagement in actual classroom contexts. Wigfield et al. (2008) reported that the effects of CORI on fourth-grade students' reading comprehension were mediated by students' behavioral engagement in reading. In this investigation, students receiving CORI showed higher reading comprehension outcomes than students in control classrooms, but the effect of instructional conditions was fully mediated by the extensiveness of their behavioral engagement in reading activities.

The effects of intrinsic goal framing on conceptual learning described previously have occasionally been examined for their mediational processes. In Vansteenkiste et al.'s (2005) study, the effect of the autonomy-supportive communication style given by the experimenters during the study was mediated by students' autonomous motivation, which referred to their value and interest in the task. In this study, young adolescents who were obese were given a text on food nutrition and health. In one case, the material was presented sympathetically from the students' perspective and explained how students who understood it could improve their health and comfort. The control experimental condition presented the material didactically as a task they should attempt to master. Students who received the autonomy-supportive communications valued the reading activity more highly and gained conceptual knowledge (although not rote information) from it more fully. The motivational practice impacted students' understanding of major concepts, but not minor material in the texts, which shows that not all learning, but primarily high-level conceptual learning, was facilitated by motivational practices.

Examples of single mediation are also provided in practical classroom learning environments. For example, in Hamre and Pianta's (2005) study of reading instruction in kindergarten, global classroom quality was assessed in terms of teachers' provision of effective instruction while building warm emotional connections with students, which includes support for students' self-regulation, a balance of activities for children's diverse skill levels, and sensitivity to students' interests. Classrooms with high global quality induced high levels of behavioral engagement, which consisted of attending to tasks, completing reading activities, following rules, persisting in the face of difficulty, and exercising control. Students with high behavioral engagement showed more gain in reading competencies than students with lower behavioral engagement and lower global quality of instruction (Ponitz, Rimm-Kaufman, Grimm, & Curby, 2009). At the other end of the educational continuum, in a college journalism course, students reported varying levels of perceived autonomy support from their laboratory instructor. They also reported intrinsic motivation for learning in the course. In this situation, the effect of autonomy-supportive instruction on students' grades was mediated by their intrinsic motivation for learning in the course (Filaka & Sheldon, 2008). These examples illustrate that the mediating processes of behavioral engagement and motivation are sufficiently prominent to be measured in research and to be functional in influencing students' grades and tested achievement in classrooms.

Limitations and Next Steps

The work reviewed in this chapter clearly documents how classroom practices and conditions impact student motivation, engagement, and competence. Equally, if not more important, there now is clear evidence that students' motivation and engagement mediate the effects of classroom practices on student achievement outcomes. That is, the impact of classroom practices on student outcomes depends upon the level of student engagement in classroom activities.

Although we have learned much about the linkages between classroom practices, motivation, engagement, and outcome as presented in Fig. 29.1, there are several limitations in this literature which should be noted. First, the large majority of studies of mediation entail structural equation modeling. In the absence of experimental designs, the inferences to causality are extremely limited. Although mediated effects are often assumed to have a causal direction, the direction of causality cannot be inferred confidently any more easily than it can be with a zero order correlation. Specifically, mediation is a procedure to characterize overlapping variances, but it does not yield strong inferences about causal relationships. Experiments of the kind conducted by Vansteenkiste et al. (2004) should be extended. Instructional supports such as relevance, choice, student-centeredness, and teachers' emotional support have very rarely been investigated with experimental designs, and thus, their causal characteristics remain unknown. Second, minority students are rarely disaggregated within these studies or serve as the target populations for investigations. Consequently, our knowledge base about African American and Hispanic students is not established, and it cannot be assumed to be identical to the knowledge base for European Americans. The exception is that Asian students, including Taiwanese, Hong Kong, Chinese, and Korean populations have been investigated from the viewpoint of effects of classroom practices on motivational outcomes (Jang, Reeve, Ryan, & Kim, 2009; Lau, 2009; Shih, 2008; Zhou et al., 2009).

Third, students who are low achieving in reading have not been the focus of a sufficient number of investigations. For example, it is unknown whether the effects of behavioral engagement on reading competence are higher, lower, or the same for low-achieving readers in comparison to average- or high-achieving readers. As noted by Quirk and Schwanenflugel (2004), most reading programs for low achievers are strongly cognitive and tend to neglect motivational practices, although researchers would agree that explicitly supporting self-efficacy would be valuable for this population.

Fourth, motivation for reading electronic text should be studied. Although students are intrinsically motivated by interacting with electronic media, relatively few studies have been conducted that examine how students' motivation and competence are impacted by reading digital text (see Mills, 2010, for review of this work). As Jang (2008) found, interest was not associated with learning from uninteresting text, and it is possible that interest regulation is not associated with learning from highly interesting electronic media due to its relatively high interest level. Because electronic text is nearly universal in schools, homes, and students' backpacks, it seems warranted examining whether motivation, behavioral engagement, and competence in the domain of electronic text interaction is subject to the same principles as traditional interaction with printed text. It is conceivable that electronic text is highly motivating due to the autonomy, efficacy, and apparent value it affords the student. If so, academic learning may be accelerated through instructional use of this medium, and properties of the medium may have motivational impacts on motivation, learning, and achievement.

References

Afflerbach, P. (1998). Reading assessment and learning to read. In J. Osborn & F. Lehr (Eds.), *Literacy for all: Issues in teaching and learning* (pp. 239–263). New York: Guilford Press.

Anmarkrud, O., & Bråten, I. (2009). Motivation for reading comprehension. *Learning and Individual Differences, 19*, 252–256.

Appleton, J. J., Christenson, S. L., & Furlong, M. J. (2008). Student engagement with school: Critical conceptual and methodological issues of the construct. *Psychology in the Schools, 45*, 369–386.

Assor, A., Kaplan, H., & Roth, G. (2002). Choice is good, but relevance is excellent: Autonomy-enhancing and suppressing teacher behaviours predicting students' engagement in schoolwork. *British Journal of Educational Psychology, 72*, 261–278.

Baker, L., Dreher, M. J., & Guthrie, J. T. (Eds.). (2000). *Engaging young readers*. New York: Guilford Press.

Baker, L., & Wigfield, A. (1999). Dimensions of children's motivation for reading and their relations to reading activity and reading achievement. *Reading Research Quarterly, 34*, 452–477.

Bandura, A., & Schunk, D. H. (1981). Cultivating competence, self-efficacy, and intrinsic interest through proximal self-motivation. *Journal of Personality and Social Psychology, 41*, 586–598.

Brophy, J. (1981). Teacher praise: A functional analysis. *Review of Educational Research, 51*, 5–32.

Chan, L. K. S. (1994). Relationship of motivation, strategic learning, and reading achievement in grades 5, 7, and 9. *The Journal of Experimental Education, 62*, 319–339.

Decker, D. M., Dona, D. P., & Christenson, S. L. (2007). Behaviorally at-risk African American students: The importance of student-teacher relationships for student outcomes. *Journal of School Psychology, 45*, 83–109.

Dill, E. M., & Boykin, A. W. (2000). The comparative influence of individual, peer tutoring, and communal learning contexts on the text recall of African American children. *Journal of Black Psychology, Special issue: African American culture and identity: Research directions for the new millennium, 26*, 65–78.

Duckworth, A. L., Peterson, C., Matthews, M., & Kelly, D. (2007). Grit: Perseverance and passion for long-term goals. *Journal of Personality and Social Psychology, 92*, 1087–1101.

Duckworth, A. L., & Seligman, M. E. P. (2005). Self-discipline outdoes IQ in predicting academic performance of adolescents. *Psychological Science, 16*, 939–944.

Durik, A. M., Vida, M., & Eccles, J. S. (2006). Task values and ability beliefs as predictors of high school literacy choices: A developmental analysis. *Journal of Educational Psychology, 98*, 382–393.

Eccles, J. S., & Wigfield, A. (2002). Motivational beliefs, values, and goals. *Annual Review of Psychology, 53*, 109–132.

Ericsson, K. A., Krampe, R. T., & Tesch-Romer, C. (1993). The role of deliberate practice in the acquisition of expert performance. *Psychological Review, 100*, 363–406.

Filaka, V. F., & Sheldon, K. M. (2008). Teacher support, student motivation, student need satisfaction, and college teacher course evaluations: Testing a sequential path model. *Educational Psychology, 28*, 711–724.

Fredricks, J. A., Blumenfeld, P. C., & Paris, A. H. (2004). School engagement: Potential of the concept, state of the evidence. *Review of Educational Research, 74*, 59–109.

Furrer, C., & Skinner, E. (2003). Sense of relatedness as a factor in children's academic engagement and performance. *Journal of Educational Psychology, 95*, 148–162.

Gambrell, L., & Marniak, B. (1997). Incentives and intrinsic motivation to read. In J. T. Guthrie & A. Wigfield (Eds.), *Reading engagement: Motivating readers through integrated instruction* (pp. 205–217). Newark, DE: International Reading Association.

Greene, B. A., Miller, R. B., Crowson, H. M., Duke, B. L., & Akey, K. L. (2004). Predicting high school students' cognitive engagement and achievement: Contributions of classroom perceptions and motivation. *Contemporary Educational Psychology, 29*, 462–482.

Grigg, W. S., Ryan, R. M., Jin, Y., & Campbell, J. R. (2003). *The nation's report card: Reading 2002* (Publication No. NCES 2003-521). Washington, DC: U. S. Government Printing Office.

Guthrie, J. T., & Coddington, C. S. (2009). Reading motivation. In K. Wentzel & A. Wigfield (Eds.), *Handbook of motivation at school* (pp. 503–525). New York: Routledge.

Guthrie, J. T., Hoa, L. W., Wigfield, A., Tonks, S. M., Humenick, N. M., & Littles, E. (2007). Reading motivation and reading comprehension growth in the later elementary years. *Contemporary Educational Psychology, 32*, 282–313.

Guthrie, J. T., & Humenick, N. M. (2004). Motivating students to read: Evidence for classroom practices that increase reading motivation and achievement. In P. McCardle & V. Chhabra (Eds.), *The voice of evidence in reading research* (pp. 329–354). Baltimore: Brookes Publishing.

Guthrie, J. T., Klauda, S. L., & Morrison, D. A. (2012). Motivation, achievement and classroom contexts for information book reading. In J. T. Guthrie, A. Wigfield, & S. L. Klauda (Eds.), http//www.corilearning.com/research-publications/ *Adolescents' engagement in academic literacy*. Sharjah, UAE: Bentham Science Publishers.

Guthrie, J. T., Mason-Singh, A., & Coddington, C. S. (in press). Instructional effects of Concept-Oriented Reading Instruction on motivation for reading information text in middle school. In J. T. Guthrie, A. Wigfield, & S. L. Klauda (Eds.), *Adolescents' engagement in academic literacy*. Sharjah, UAE: Bentham Science Publishers.

Guthrie, J. T., McGough, K., Bennett, L., & Rice, M. E. (1996). Concept-Oriented Reading Instruction: An integrated curriculum to develop motivations and strategies for reading. In L. Baker, P. Afflerbach, & D. Reinking (Eds.), *Developing engaged readers in school and home communities* (pp. 165–190). Hillsdale, NJ: Erlbaum.

Guthrie, J. T., McRae, A. C., & Klauda, S. L. (2007). Contributions of Concept-Oriented Reading Instruction to knowledge about interventions for motivations in reading. *Educational Psychologist, 42*, 237–250.

Guthrie, J. T., & Wigfield, A. (2000). Engagement and motivation in reading. In M. L. Kamil & P. B. Mosenthal (Eds.), *Handbook of reading research* (Vol. III, pp. 403–422). Mahwah, NJ: Erlbaum.

Guthrie, J. T., Wigfield, A., Barbosa, P., Perencevich, K. C., Taboada, A., Davis, M. H., et al. (2004). Increasing reading comprehension and engagement through Concept-Oriented Reading Instruction. *Journal of Educational Psychology, 96*, 403–423.

Guthrie, J. T., Wigfield, A., Metsala, J. L., & Cox, K. E. (1999). Motivational and cognitive predictors of text comprehension and reading amount. *Scientific Studies of Reading, 3*, 231–256.

Guthrie, J. T., Wigfield, A., & Perencevich, K. C. (Eds.). (2004). *Motivating reading comprehension: Concept-Oriented Reading Instruction*. Mahwah, NJ: Erlbaum.

Hamre, B. K., & Pianta, R. C. (2005). Can instructional and emotional support in the first-grade classroom make a difference for children at risk of school failure? *Child Development, 76*, 949–967.

Jang, H. (2008). Supporting students' motivation, engagement, and learning during an uninteresting activity. *Journal of Educational Psychology, 100*, 798–811.

Jang, H., Reeve, J., Ryan, R. M., & Kim, A. (2009). Can self-determination theory explain what underlies the productive, satisfying learning experiences of collectivistically oriented Korean students? *Journal of Educational Psychology, 101*, 644–661.

Johnson, D. W., & Johnson, R. T. (2009). An educational psychology success story: Social interdependence theory and cooperative learning. *Educational Researcher, 38,* 365–379.

Kendeou, P., van den Broek, P., White, M. J., & Lynch, J. (2007). Comprehension in preschool and early elementary children: Skill development and strategy interventions. In D. S. McNamara (Ed.), *Reading comprehension strategies* (pp. 27–43). New York: Erlbaum/Taylor & Francis Group.

Ladd, G. W., & Dinella, L. M. (2009). Continuity and change in early school engagement: Predictive of children's achievement trajectories from first to eighth grade? *Journal of Educational Psychology, 101,* 190–206.

Lau, K. (2009). Reading motivation, perceptions of reading instruction and reading amount: A comparison of junior and secondary students in Hong Kong. *Journal of Research in Reading, 32,* 366–382.

Legault, L., Green-Demers, I., & Pelletier, L. (2006). Why do high school students lack motivation in the classroom? Toward an understanding of academic amotivation and the role of social support. *Journal of Educational Psychology, 98,* 567–582.

Maehr, M. L., & Zusho, A. (2009). Achievement goal theory: The past, present, and future. In K. R. Wentzel & A. Wigfield (Eds.), *Handbook of motivation at school* (pp. 77–104). New York: Routledge/Taylor & Francis Group.

Miller, S. D., & Meece, J. L. (1999). Third graders' motivational preferences for reading and writing tasks. *The Elementary School Journal, 100,* 19–35.

Mills, K. A. (2010). A review of the "digital turn" in the New Literacy studies. *Review of Educational Research, 80,* 246–271.

Morgan, P. L., & Fuchs, D. (2007). Is there a bidirectional relationship between children's reading skills and reading motivation? *Exceptional Children, 73,* 165–183.

National Reading Panel. (2000). Fluency. In *Teaching children to read: An evidence-based assessment of the scientific research literature on reading and its implications for instruction.* Bethesda, MD: National Institutes of Health, National Institute of Child Health and Human Development.

National Research Council. (2004). *Engaging schools: Fostering high school students' motivation to learn.* Washington, DC: National Academies Press.

Nolen, S. B. (1988). Reasons for studying: Motivational orientations and study strategies. *Cognition and Instruction, 5,* 269–287.

Orvis, K. A., Fisher, S. L., & Wasserman, M. E. (2009). Power to the people: Using learner control to improve trainee reactions and learning in web-based instructional environments. *Journal of Applied Psychology, 94,* 960–971.

Perie, M., Grigg, W., & Donahue, P. (2005). *The nation's report card: Reading 2005* (U.S. Department of Education, National Center for Educational Statistics, NCES 2006–451). Washington, DC: U.S. Government Printing Office.

Perry, K. E., Donohue, K. M., & Weinstein, R. S. (2007). Teaching practices and the promotion of achievement and adjustment in first grade. *Journal of School Psychology, 45,* 269–292.

Pintrich, P. R., & de Groot, E. V. (1990). Motivational and self-regulated learning components of classroom academic performance. *Journal of Educational Psychology, 82,* 33–40.

Ponitz, C. C., Rimm-Kaufman, S. E., Grimm, K. J., & Curby, T. W. (2009). Kindergarten classroom quality, behavioral engagement, and reading achievement. *School Psychology Review, 38,* 102–120.

Quirk, M. P., & Schwanenflugel, P. J. (2004). Do supplemental remedial reading programs address the motivational issues of struggling readers? An analysis of five popular programs. *Reading Research and Instruction, 43,* 1–19.

Rapp, D., & van den Broek, P. (2005). Dynamic text comprehension: An integrative view of reading. *Current Directions in Psychological Science, 14,* 276–279.

Reeve, J., Jang, H., Carrell, D., Jeon, S., & Barch, J. (2004). Enhancing students' engagement by increasing teachers' autonomy support. *Motivation and Emotion, 28,* 147–169.

Reeve, J., Jang, H., Hardre, P., & Omura, M. (2002). Providing a rationale in an autonomy-supportive way as a strategy to motivate others during an uninteresting activity. *Motivation and Emotion, 26,* 183–207.

Ryan, R. M., & Deci, E. L. (2000). Self-determination theory and the facilitation of intrinsic motivation, social development, and well-being. *American Psychologist, 55,* 68–78.

Ryan, R. M., & Deci, E. L. (2009). Promoting self-determined school engagement: Motivation, learning, and well-being. In K. Wenzel & A. Wigfield (Eds.), *Handbook of motivation at school* (pp. 171–195). New York: Routledge/Taylor & Francis Group.

Salamonson, Y., Andrew, S., & Everett, B. (2009). Academic engagement and disengagement as predictors of performance in pathophysiology among nursing students. *Contemporary Nurse, 32,* 123–132.

Schiefele, U. (1999). Interest and learning from text. *Scientific Studies of Reading, 3,* 257–279.

Schunk, D. H., & Zimmerman, B. J. (2007). Influencing children's self-efficacy and self-regulation of reading and writing through modeling. *Reading & Writing Quarterly, 23,* 7–25.

Schwinger, M., Steinmayr, R., & Spinath, B. (2009). How do motivational regulation strategies affect achievement: Mediated by effort management and moderated by intelligence. *Learning and Individual Differences, 19,* 621–627.

Shih, S. (2008). The relation of self-determination and achievement goals to Taiwanese eighth graders' behavioral and emotional engagement in schoolwork. *The Elementary School Journal, 108,* 313–334.

Skinner, E. A., & Belmont, M. J. (1993). Motivation in the classroom: Reciprocal effects of teacher behavior and student engagement across the school year. *Journal of Educational Psychology, 85,* 571–581.

Skinner, E. A., Furrer, C., Marchand, G., & Kindermann, T. A. (2008). Engagement and disaffection in the classroom: Part of a larger motivational dynamic? *Journal of Educational Psychology, 100*, 765–781.

Skinner, E. A., Kindermann, T. A., Connell, J. P., & Wellborn, J. G. (2009a). Engagement and disaffection as organizational constructs in the dynamics of motivational development. In K. R. Wentzel & A. Wigfield (Eds.), *Handbook of motivation at school* (pp. 223–245). New York: Routledge/Taylor & Francis Group.

Skinner, E. A., Kindermann, T. A., & Furrer, C. J. (2009b). A motivational perspective on engagement and disaffection: Conceptualization and assessment of children's behavioral and emotional participation in academic activities in the classroom. *Educational and Psychological Measurement, 69*, 493–525.

Souvignier, E., & Mokhlesgerami, J. (2006). Using self-regulation as a framework for implementing strategy instruction to foster reading comprehension. *Learning and Instruction, 16*, 57–71.

Strambler, M. J., & Weinstein, R. S. (2010). Psychological disengagement in elementary school among ethnic minority students. *Journal of Applied Developmental Psychology, 31*, 155–165.

van den Broek, P., Rapp, D. N., & Kendeou, P. (2005). Integrating memory-based and constructionist processes in accounts of reading comprehension. *Discourse Processes, 39*, 299–316.

Vansteenkiste, M., Simons, J., Lens, W., Sheldon, K. M., & Deci, E. L. (2004). Motivating learning, performance, and persistence: The synergistic effects of intrinsic goal contents and autonomy-supportive contexts. *Journal of Personality and Social Psychology, 87*, 246–260.

Vansteenkiste, M., Simons, J., Lens, W., Soenens, B., & Matos, L. (2005). Examining the motivational impact of intrinsic versus extrinsic goal framing and autonomy-supportive versus internally controlling communication style on early adolescents' academic achievement. *Child Development, 76*, 483–501.

Walczyk, J. J., Wei, M., Griffith-Ross, D. A., Cooper, A. L., Zha, P., & Goubert, S. E. (2007). Development of the interplay between automatic processes and cognitive resources in reading. *Journal of Educational Psychology, 99*, 867–887.

Wang, J. H.-Y., & Guthrie, J. T. (2004). Modeling the effects of intrinsic motivation, extrinsic motivation, amount of reading, and past reading achievement on text comprehension between U.S. and Chinese students. *Reading Research Quarterly, 39*, 162–186.

Wentzel, K. R. (2009). Students' relationships with teachers as motivational contexts. In K. R. Wentzel & A. Wigfield (Eds.), *Handbook of motivation at school* (pp. 301–322). New York: Routledge/Taylor & Francis Group.

Wigfield, A., & Eccles, J. S. (2002). The development of competence beliefs, expectancies for success, and achievement values from childhood through adolescence. In A. Wigfield & J. S. Eccles (Eds.), *Development of achievement motivation* (pp. 91–120). San Diego, CA: Academic.

Wigfield, A., Eccles, J. S., Schiefele, U., Roeser, R. W., & Davis-Kean, P. (2006). Development of achievement motivation. In N. Eisenberg, W. Damon, & R. M. Lerner (Eds.), *Handbook of child psychology: Vol. 3, Social, emotional, and personality development* (6th ed., pp. 933–1002). Hoboken, NJ: Wiley.

Wigfield, A., & Guthrie, J. T. (1997). Relations of children's motivation for reading to the amount and breadth or their reading. *Journal of Educational Psychology, 89*, 420–432.

Wigfield, A., & Guthrie, J. T. (2010). The impact of Concept-Oriented Reading instruction on students' reading motivation, reading engagement, and reading comprehension. In J. Meece & J. S. Eccles (Eds.), *Handbook on schools, schooling, and human development* (pp. 463–477). Mahwah, NJ: Erlbaum.

Wigfield, A., Guthrie, J. T., Perencevich, K. C., Taboada, A., Klauda, S. L., McRae, A., et al. (2008). The role of reading engagement in mediating effects of reading comprehension instruction on reading outcomes. *Psychology in the Schools, 45*, 432–445.

Wolters, C. A. (2003). Regulation of motivation: Evaluating an underemphasized aspect of self-regulated learning. *Educational Psychologist, 38*, 189–205.

Zhou, M., Ma, W. J., & Deci, E. L. (2009). The importance of autonomy for rural Chinese children's motivation for learning. *Learning and Individual Differences, 19*, 492–498.

A Self-regulated Learning Perspective on Student Engagement

30

Christopher A. Wolters and Daniel J. Taylor

Abstract

Models of both self-regulated learning and student engagement have been used to help understand why some students are successful in school while others are not. The goal of this chapter is to provide greater insight into the relations between these two theoretical frameworks. The first section presents a basic model of self-regulated learning, outlining the primary phases and areas involved in that process. The next section discusses key similarities and differences between aspects of self-regulated learning and features of student engagement, drawing on both theoretical suggestions and empirical research. The final section offers ideas and avenues for additional research that would serve to better link self-regulated learning and student engagement.

Self-regulated learning and student engagement both represent research and theoretical frameworks used to understand students' functioning and performance with regard to academic contexts. Models of self-regulation, broadly speaking, have been developed with regard to a variety of domains to understand how individuals take an active, purposeful, and reflective role in their own functioning (Baumeister & Vohs, 2004; Boekaerts, Pintrich, & Zeidner, 2000). For instance, models exist to understand individuals' self-management of chronic illness, smoking, exercise, eating, shopping, and other noneducational processes (Baumeister & Vohs, 2004; Boekaerts et al., 2000). The subset of these models developed to understand and explain individuals' active management of their own motivational, behavioral, and cognitive functioning within academic settings use the term self-regulated learning. Even within this more narrowly defined domain, models of self-regulated learning have emerged from a diverse set of theoretical roots that incorporate research investigating cognitive and social development, metacognition, volition, and motivation (Zimmerman & Schunk, 2001). Across most models, self-regulated learning can be viewed as an active, constructive process through which learners set goals for their learning and then work to monitor, regulate, and control their cognition, motivation, and behavior in order to accomplish those goals (Pintrich, 2004; Wolters, Pintrich, & Karabenick, 2005).

C.A. Wolters, Ph.D. (✉) • D.J. Taylor, M.A.
Department of Educational Psychology,
University of Houston, Houston, TX, USA
e-mail: cwolters@uh.edu; djtaylor@uh.edu

The history of research on student engagement is populated mostly by school psychologists initially focused on understanding behavioral indicators of students' participation in academic settings (Jimerson, Campos, & Greif, 2003). Broadly defined, student engagement was viewed as a person's active participation in school-related endeavors and as "energy in action" (Russell, Ainley, & Frydenberg, 2005, p. 1). Over the past few decades, the concept of engagement has been expanded to incorporate the involvement produced by emotional and cognitive processes as well (Fredricks, Blumenfeld, & Paris, 2004). Hence, student engagement is now viewed by most researchers as a multidimensional construct that reflects both observable, external factors as well as less observable, internal factors (Appleton, Christenson, & Furlong, 2008; Fredricks et al., 2004; Reschly, Huebner, Appleton, & Antaramian, 2008; Skinner, Kinderman, & Furrer, 2009). The particular way in which these factors are divided varies across particular models. For instance, some models break down these facets further into academic and/or behavioral (observable, external) subtypes and cognitive and/or affective/psychological (less observable, internal) subtypes (Appleton, Christenson, Kim, & Reschly, 2006; Fredricks et al., 2004; Jimerson et al., 2003). In the present discussion, we follow the structure presented by Fredricks et al. and differentiate between behavioral, emotional, and cognitive engagement.

An initial consideration reveals a number of similarities between these two broad conceptual frameworks (i.e., self-regulated learning, student engagement). One, the research on both self-regulated learning and student engagement includes a variety of models that share key assumptions but also show variability. For instance, there are prominent models of self-regulated learning that have been spearheaded by Pintrich (2004; Pintrich & Zusho, 2002; Wolters et al., 2005), Winne (Winne & Hadwin, 1998, 2008), and Zimmerman (2000). Similarly, related but distinct models of student engagement have been proposed by Finn (1989), Skinner (Skinner & Belmont, 1993), Christenson (Christenson et al., 2008), and others (Fredricks et al., 2004). Two, self-regulated learning and student engagement are both conceptualized as multidimensional because they bring together distinct facets or subprocesses of students' academic functioning into a more global model. For example, prominent models of self-regulated learning and student engagement both attempt to account for behavioral, cognitive, and emotional processes. Third, both self-regulated learning and student engagement have been viewed as mediating processes that provide a bridge between contextual and personal factors on one side and students' academic performance or achievement on the other (Appleton et al., 2006; Christenson et al., 2008; Fredricks et al., 2004; Pintrich, 2004). Hence, student engagement and self-regulated learning both have been used to differentiate between more and less effective learners or to explain why some students are more successful in school.

Perhaps even more telling than these general similarities, definitions of self-regulated learning and student engagement often invoke terminology or concepts that are central to the other. For instance, self-regulated learners are commonly described as students who are actively engaged in their own learning (Wolters, 2003a; Zimmerman, 2002). At the same time, recent theoretical descriptions identify self-regulation as one component or facet of student engagement (Fredricks et al., 2004). That is, self-regulation or the active use of self-regulation strategies is portrayed as a key feature of what it means for students to exhibit engagement in school contexts. In sum, these many similarities suggest that self-regulated learning and student engagement should be theoretically and practically linked.

The purpose of this chapter is to advance a deeper understanding of the relations between these two theoretical frameworks or areas of research by evaluating their conceptual similarities and differences. To accomplish this goal, the remainder of the chapter is divided into three major sections. In the initial section, we briefly present a basic model of self-regulated learning. Next, we discuss similarities and differences between this view of self-regulated learning and key features of how student engagement is conceptualized. Finally, in the last section, we provide some concluding remarks and map out a few

Self-regulated Learning

We review the main components or facets of self-regulated learning using a model emerging primarily from the work of Pintrich and his colleagues (Pintrich, 2004; Pintrich & De Groot, 1990; Pintrich, Wolters, & Baxter, 2000; Pintrich & Zusho, 2002; Wolters, 2003a; Wolters et al., 2005). According to this model, self-regulated learning is characterized as involving four interdependent phases (see Table 30.1). In other models, similar dimensions have been labeled as stages, operations, subprocesses, classes, or components of self-regulated learning (Greene & Azevedo, 2007; Winne & Hadwin, 2008; Zimmerman, 2000).

Phases of Self-regulated Learning

One phase, often labeled forethought or planning (Pintrich, 2004; Zimmerman, 2000), reflects students' planning, prior knowledge activation, and other processes that frequently occur before formally initiating participation in a task. Setting goals, a core feature of all models of self-regulated learning, is one central process within this phase. As well, this phase is key to motivation because it includes the activation of students' initial attitudes and beliefs regarding the perceived importance or usefulness of the material to be learned and the interestingness of the activity. Similarly, Zimmerman (1989) stressed that this initial phase includes students' activation of their perceived self-efficacy or confidence in their ability to successfully reach a goal or complete a learning task at some given level of proficiency. Consistent with Winne and Hadwin (1998), Pintrich (2004) proposed that students initially define the task by producing perceptions about what the task entails and what limitations and resources are currently available. Once students generate these ideas, they set goals and create a plan to carry out the task. Cognitively, this phase would reflect students' efforts to consider what they already know about the topic or subject area, what they know about how to learn the type of material, and what particular learning strategies should be used to complete the task.

A second phase, called monitoring by Pintrich (2004; Pintrich et al., 2000), describes students' efforts to keep track or be aware of their ongoing progress and performance at a task or learning activity. Zimmerman (2000) included self-observation or students' tracking of their performance, the conditions of the task, and the products of their efforts. Winne and Hadwin (1998) described metacognitive monitoring that occurs during enactment of the task. As stressed by Butler and Winne (1995) an important by-product of this process is different forms of feedback including rate of progress toward the goal, effectiveness of particular strategies, and personal abilities or skills. The generation of these various forms of feedback provides the information or products needed by other processes within self-regulated learning. Monitoring also allows students to generate evaluations such as the task is too difficult or that they may not have the ability to accomplish their goals.

In addition to monitoring, a third phase or subprocess that often occurs while students participate in tasks is labeled control, management, or just regulation (Greene & Azevedo, 2007; Winne & Hadwin, 2008; Zimmerman, 2000). This process reflects what Zimmerman and others have identified as simply performance, enactment, or completion of the task. Most centrally, this phase involves students' actual use and management of the various learning strategies and tactics intended to reach the goals that have been established (Pintrich et al., 2000; Winne & Hadwin, 1998; Zimmerman, 2000). It reflects learners' efforts to actively manage, modify, or change what they are doing in order to maintain their effectiveness or progress toward their goals. Zimmerman explained how students demonstrate self-control by utilizing the specific methods or strategies they chose during the initial phase. Similarly, Corno (2001) emphasized the role that volition plays in completing a task. Once students have

Table 30.1 Phases and areas for self-regulated learning

Phases of self-regulation	Areas for self-regulation			
	Cognition	Motivation	Behavior	Context
Forethought/ planning	Setting goals for learning and understanding Activation of cognitive and metacognitive knowledge Planning/selecting cognitive strategies	Achievement goal adoption Activation of motivational beliefs and attitudes Planning/selecting motivational strategies	Setting behavioral and time management goals Recall of prior behavior and experiences Planning/selecting cognitive strategies	Considering and selecting contexts for learning Perceptions of context, situation, task Planning/selecting context-relevant strategies
Monitoring	Monitoring of cognitive processes	Monitoring of motivation and affect	Monitoring of effort, time use, behavior	Monitoring of task and context conditions Monitoring need for help
Control/ management	Enacting and regulating cognitive, metacognitive, critical thinking strategies	Enacting and regulating motivational and affective strategies	Enacting and regulating behavioral strategies	Enacting and regulating context, help-seeking strategies
Reaction/ reflection	Learning and cognitive judgments, generation of cognition-related knowledge	Affective reactions, generation of motivational and affect-related beliefs	Choice behavior, generation of behavior-related knowledge	Generation of new context-related knowledge

Note: Adapted from Pintrich (2004)

decided to undertake a learning activity, volitional processes are used to protect those intentions from distractions or possible temptations that would thwart efforts to complete the task.

The fourth phase proposed in this model, termed reaction or reflection, includes students' efforts to review and respond to the information produced through monitoring and feedback and to their experiences with a task more generally. One core aspect of this phase is the generation of new metalevel knowledge about the tasks, strategies, or self. For instance, Winne and Hadwin (1998) argued that it is through this process that students obtain object-level information used to adapt their approach to task engagement in order to reduce discrepancies between actual performance and ideal standards found during monitoring. In line with this idea, Zimmerman (2000) stated that students self-evaluate their current performance with some preset standard or goal and produce self-judgments about that performance during this phase of self-regulated learning.

As a general rule, theorists do not view these different phases as a strict time-ordered sequence or as causally connected in a linear fashion (Pintrich, 2004; Winne & Hadwin, 2008; Zimmerman, 2000). Rather, the phases simply provide a structure and emphasize that self-regulated learning is dependent on students' active engagement before, during, and after the completion of academic tasks. Self-regulated learners are expected to engage or re-engage in the processes endemic to particular phases at any time in a cyclic, flexible, and adaptive fashion so that they can efficiently and successfully complete their academic work. For example, a student might first set goals for a paper that is due in a few weeks. As the student begins to research and write, he monitors his progress and begins to realize that his initial plans for completing the paper need to be altered, so he sets new goals. Also, he wonders if outlining the paper as he continues would be beneficial, so he uses that strategy. He again monitors his progress and acknowledges that this method is useful for accomplishing his goals. After completing the paper, this student recognizes the advantages of tactics he used and resolves to utilize them again in the future.

Areas of Self-regulated Learning

As illustrated in Table 30.1, these subprocesses represented in these phases are used by students to manage their own academic functioning with regard to at least four areas of learning (Pintrich, 2004; Wolters et al., 2005). Put differently, these four areas represent different dimensions of academic learning that can be the target of regulation by the learner. One dimension, cognition, concerns the various mental processes individuals use to encode, process, or learn while participating in academic tasks (Pintrich, 2004). Most typically, this area has included students' use of cognitive and metacognitive learning strategies. For example, students monitor and control their use of rehearsal, organization, elaboration, or other information-processing strategies needed to learn new material or skills. Researchers from an information-processing perspective have stressed the significance of this cognitive dimension (Winne & Hadwin, 1998). For instance, information in long-term memory may be retrieved for use in working memory, different knowledge, ideas, or beliefs may be restructured in a manner that is beneficial for the task, or information represented in one form (e.g., an image) may be converted into another form (e.g., words). Although less often studied, this area would also include students' engagement in critical thinking, problem solving, or other forms of higher-order reasoning. Students can, that is, set goals and monitor, regulate, and reflect on their use of problem-solving strategies and efforts at critical thinking.

Motivation refers both to the process through which goal-directed behavior is instigated and sustained (Schunk, Pintrich, & Meece, 2008) as well as an individual's willingness to engage in and persist at academic tasks (Wolters, 2003a). As such, motivation represents a second dimension of learning that individuals can self-regulate (Boekaerts, 1996; Pintrich, 2004; Wolters, 2003a). In other words, their own level of motivation or motivational processing represents an important target for students who are working to manage their own learning. Motivational processes or beliefs tend to promote intentions to complete a task or to learn new information

(Corno, 2001). Students can establish goals or form expectations about the level of motivation they anticipate in a task, they can maintain an awareness of how motivated (or unmotivated) they are feeling, and they can work to control their level of motivation for completing a task. Prior work has identified several kinds of strategies that students use to sustain or improve their own motivation. These strategies include self-provided rewards, self-talk about the importance or usefulness of material, and making learning activities into a game so they are more enjoyable (Sansone & Thoman, 2006; Wolters, 2003a). Although some models of self-regulation have stressed emotional processing more exclusively (e.g., Carver & Scheier, 2000), affective processes often have been grouped together with motivation within this one area (e.g., Pintrich). In either case, models of self-regulated learning commonly assume that students can manage their emotional processes as another important dimension of their academic functioning (Corno, 1993; Schutz & Davis, 2000).

According to this model, a third area that students can self-regulate is their overt behaviors, actual participation, conduct, or other physical actions necessary for the completion of learning tasks. Time management strategies that students use to organize and control where and when they study fit into this area. Pintrich (2004) also indicated that part of time management includes students' decisions about how they will apportion their efforts to complete the task. The observation of one's own behavior is also consistent with Zimmerman's (2000) model of self-regulated learning.

A fourth dimension of learning that is a potential target of students' regulation is the context or environment (Pintrich, 2004). This area includes facets of the immediate task, classroom, or even cultural environment that students can monitor and manage. Students, for instance, might set goals and monitor and control the lighting, temperature, and noise level in their study environment. In line with this view, Corno (2001) explained that environmental control includes both changes made to task circumstances and changes made toward the actions of other people who could be involved with the task. As an example, help-seeking strategies in which students manage their learning by effectively utilizing teachers, parents, peers, or others within the social environment fit within this dimension (Newman, 1998). After a study session, students can reflect on whether a particular environment is conducive to learning or form expectations about the advantages and disadvantages of trying to do work within a particular context or in collaboration with specific people.

Although it is possible to distinguish among them conceptually, these four dimensions overlap and intertwine with one another in practice (Pintrich, 2004). Self-regulating the functioning associated with one area (e.g., motivation) may also involve changes in the functioning within the other areas (e.g., cognition, behavior). As an example, students may set a particular goal (e.g., go to the library to study for 2 h in the afternoon with classmates) based on the implications it has for their cognition (e.g., additional resources at hand if needed), motivation (e.g., studying with friends is more enjoyable), behavior (e.g., studying in the afternoon frees up time in the evening), and context (e.g., can get help from friends). Hence, students' overall efforts to plan and control where, when, and how they complete academic tasks likely involve consideration of all four of these different areas.

Comparing Self-regulated Learning and Student Engagement

In this section, we evaluate relations between self-regulated learning and student engagement. This discussion is based most directly on the model of self-regulation described above and a view of student engagement consistent with Fredricks et al. (2004). However, additional perspectives from both frameworks are also included when relevant. Initially, several conceptual similarities between the two areas of research with regard to cognitive, emotional, and behavioral functioning are discussed. These similarities indicate that, as a whole, models of self-regulated learning and student engagement appear consistent with one another with regard to the characteristics and forms of academic functioning attributed to highly effective students. Next, points on which the two frameworks differ or appear more incongruous with one another are considered.

Similarities

The extent of conceptual overlap between these two frameworks is perhaps most apparent when considering the area of cognition or cognitive engagement. One might easily argue that there is little practical difference between what researchers studying student engagement describe as high levels of cognitive engagement and what others identify as the cognitive aspects of self-regulated learning. In line with the model of self-regulated learning, one core element of student's cognitive engagement is the increased use of cognitive strategies that promote the encoding and retention of the material to be learned (Appleton et al., 2006; Fredricks et al., 2004; Reschly et al., 2008). These strategies typically include efforts at rehearsal, elaboration, summarization, organization, as well as more domain-specific learning strategies (e.g., math algorithms, writing strategies). For instance, Blumenfeld, Kempler, and Krajcik (2006) defined cognitive engagement as including students' willingness to expend effort to learn through utilizing cognitive, metacognitive, and volitional strategies that enhance understanding. They further discussed that learning strategies can be classified as either superficial or deep. Strategies involving mnemonics and rehearsal reflect more superficial cognitive engagement, whereas those for elaboration and organization reflect deeper-level thinking and engagement. In some cases, there is little empirical difference between how these processes are operationalized. For instance, as part of their measurement of cognitive engagement in high school students, Greene, Miller, Crowson, Duke, and Akey (2004) included a self-report subscale of study strategy use that is substantially parallel to items used to measure cognitive aspects of self-regulated learning (Wolters, 2004).

Also in line with the model of self-regulated learning, researchers have further characterized cognitive engagement as involving increased metacognitive awareness and use of metacognitive control strategies (Appleton et al., 2006; Fredricks et al., 2004; Furlong & Christenson, 2008). Strategies that reflect planning, goal setting, and monitoring, for instance, are staples of how theorists describe the metacognitive activities displayed by both self-regulated learners and students who are cognitively engaged (Blumenfeld et al., 2006; Fredricks et al., 2004; Pintrich, et al., 2000; Yazzie-Mintz, 2007). Even when they are not clearly labeled as metacognitive, empirical measures of students' cognitive engagement often include planning, monitoring, and other types of control strategies that do reflect this type of processing (Appleton et al., 2006; Greene et al., 2004; National Center for School Engagement, 2006).

The conceptual consistency between these two frameworks is even more obvious when researchers examining cognitive engagement explicitly define it as including students' self-regulation or use of self-regulation strategies (Appleton et al., 2008; Furlong & Christenson, 2008; Kortering & Christenson, 2009). As an example, Furlong and Christenson incorporated the idea that students self-regulate their performance as part of displaying cognitive engagement. Other researchers have even more plainly stated that being a self-regulated learner typifies cognitive engagement (Fredricks et al., 2004; Sinclair, Christenson, Lehr, & Anderson, 2003). Overall, both theoretical frameworks converge on the belief that more efficient, more effective, and higher quality engagement follows when students utilize an array of cognitive strategies and have the metacognitive knowledge and skills necessary to deploy and manage these strategies successfully.

A comparable level of conceptual agreement emerges when considering emotional and affective processes within academic contexts. Students viewed as self-regulated learners, generally, are thought to have more positive and fewer negative emotional experiences within academic settings (Linnenbrink & Pintrich, 2000; Schutz & Davis, 2000). In particular, they tend to report a constellation of emotional experiences with regard academics that includes increased enjoyment, pride, feelings of autonomy, and other positive emotions, and decreased instances of anxiety, shame, frustration, anger, or other negative emotions (Pekrun, Goetz, Titz, & Perry, 2002).

Consistent with this work, but to an even greater extent, researchers studying student engagement also portray students' emotional and affective processing as an important dimension of their academic functioning. In particular, many prominent models identify emotional or affective processing as one major form of student engagement (Finn, 1989; Fredricks et al., 2004; Skinner et al., 2009; Yazzie-Mintz, 2007). Within these models and most similar to the research on self-regulated learning, students' emotional engagement has been evidenced by their affective experiences in response to their schoolwork (Fredricks et al., 2004). For instance, positive emotions such as interest, happiness, and excitement have been studied as indicators of students' emotional engagement (Connell & Wellborn, 1991; Skinner & Belmont, 1993). In addition, emotional engagement has also been understood as a function of students' relationship with their teacher, their sense of belonging, and their general identification with school (Finn, 1989; Fredricks et al., 2004; Goodenow, 1993; Stipek, 2002). For instance, Finn described the emotional dimension of engagement as relating to identification with the school and includes the concepts of belonging and valuing. The degree to which students are attached and committed to the school indicates their emotional involvement in the school. The more the students identify with the school, the stronger emotional engagement they exhibit. Yazzie-Mintz echoed this conceptualization of emotional engagement in what he called "engagement of the heart" (p. 8). He described emotional engagement as students' feelings of where they fit in their school, how well the school functions, and their interactions with people in their school.

In addition to work examining more positive emotions, researchers examining self-regulated learning have also studied more negative emotional experiences within academic contexts. Most notably, there is extensive work examining the importance of test anxiety as one maladaptive influence on students' academic performance (Kondo, 1997; Schutz & Davis, 2000; Schutz, Davis, & Schwanenflugel, 2002). In a similar way, research on student engagement has also explicitly examined the role of negative emotions including boredom, sadness, and anxiety. For instance, Yazzie-Mintz (2007) indicated that about two out of every three students in the high schools he studied felt bored every day in school and that the vast majority also reported that they did not like the school or the teachers. Within the Skinner et al. (2009) model of student engagement, disengagement is important to conceptualize as well. This model of engagement includes the concept of disaffection which encompasses lethargic emotions (e.g., boredom, tired), alienated emotions (e.g., frustration, anger), and coerced participation. Within both frameworks, these negative forms of emotions are viewed as precursors to a host of maladaptive academic outcomes such as disaffection, withdrawal of effort, and lack of investment in school tasks.

Models of self-regulated learning and student engagement also share the view that overt behaviors represent an important facet of students' academic functioning that need to be understood and explained. Evidence that students are self-regulating their behavior is typically indicated by examining their level of effort, persistence, or time on task (Corno, 1993; Pintrich, 2004; Schunk & Zimmerman, 2003; Vrugt & Oort, 2008). Individuals' use of time management strategies to plan when and where they complete academic tasks also reflects this facet of self-regulation (Housand & Reis, 2008; Kitsantas, Winsler, & Huie, 2008; Stoeger & Ziegler, 2008).

In line with this perspective but elaborated to a greater degree, the behavioral aspect of student engagement includes three main ideas (Finn, 1989, 1993; Finn & Voelkl, 1993; Fredricks et al., 2004). In some models, forms of behavioral involvement are termed academic rather than behavioral engagement (Appleton et al., 2006; Furlong & Christenson, 2008). Whereas behavioral engagement reflects students' attendance, classroom participation, overt behavioral effort, and involvement in extracurricular activities, academic engagement refers more to time spent on learning tasks, amount of assignments completed, and credits earned in school. One dimension of behavioral engagement is evidenced when students simply attend class each day, follow school rules, abide by classroom norms, and do not participate in troublesome behaviors. This facet reflects aspects of behavior that have been described as universal in that they are expected of all students (Furlong, Whipple, St. Jean, Simental, & Punthuna, 2003).

Most similar to the research in self-regulated learning, another aspect of behavioral engagement consists of students being more involved in learning and academic tasks and displaying overt behaviors that reflect effort, persistence, and adaptive help-seeking. This aspect of behavioral engagement involves behaviors that reflect students showing initiative in their learning, displaying more enthusiasm, actively participating in classroom activities, and spending more time on their work (Finn & Rock, 1997). Finally, behavioral engagement also includes students' participation in behaviors that reflect optional forms of involvement such as band, athletics, school governance, and other extracurricular interests (Furlong et al., 2003). This final dimension suggests behavioral engagement that goes beyond what is expected of the typical student. Unlike this work on student engagement, few studies examining self-regulated learning have focused on explaining the broader educational behaviors such as enrollments, graduation, attendance, or extracurricular activities. Research examining whether self-regulated learners evidenced increased participation in extracurricular activities or whether this participation can be seen as an outgrowth of their self-regulatory functioning is particularly scarce. The important role that involvement in these activities can play with regard to adolescents' resilience to an array of risky behaviors suggests that this is a serious oversight (Feldman & Matjasko, 2005; Linver, Roth, & Brooks-Gunn, 2009).

Indicators of students' academic involvement within both frameworks also include more maladaptive forms of behavior. Research on self-regulated learning, for instance, has sought to understand procrastination, defensive pessimism, and other forms of self-handicapping as indicators of lapses in students' self-regulation (Stoeger & Ziegler, 2008; Wolters, 2003b). In line with this work, some research on student engagement has investigated students' withdrawal of efforts in learning activities, such as merely pretending to work during class (Skinner et al., 2009). In general, however, research concentrating on maladaptive behaviors leading to disengagement has investigated more global behaviors such as lack of school attendance and conduct problems, (Appleton et al., 2008; Finn & Rock, 1997; Skinner et al., 2009).

Differences

Despite these many consistencies, there also are points on which these two areas of research diverge and that counter the notion that models of self-regulated learning and student engagement can fit together seamlessly. In the following discussion, we review three particular incongruities involving conceptualization and organization across the frameworks, the centrality of personal agency, and the reach of metalevel knowledge. Within this discussion, moreover, we highlight issues involving motivation.

Most basically, it is apparent when examining the components of each framework that there are incongruities with regard to the categorizations used to differentiate among certain concepts that are very similar. As well, there are some clear differences in the particular constructs that have emerged and been examined most closely within each framework. As noted previously, for instance, there is differential treatment of constructs such as sense of belonging, identity, and help-seeking across these two areas of research. As well, there are clear differences in the attention given to behavioral forms of engagement such as course taking, graduation, and involvement in extracurricular activities. Space limitations prohibit any exhaustive review of all these differences. Instead, we focus our discussion on the differences that appear with regard to the understanding and categorization of motivation across the two frameworks.

Unlike the history of research on student engagement, motivation has been included as an important part of what it means to be a self-regulated learner from its inception. In an oft-quoted description, for instance, Zimmerman (1986) characterized self-regulated learners as metacognitively, *motivationally*, and behaviorally active participants in their own learning (emphasis added). Other early descriptions also incorporated the importance of students' motivation to the process of self-regulated learning (McCombs & Marzano, 1990; Paris & Oka, 1986; Pintrich & De Groot, 1990; Schunk, 1990). Motivation has only more recently been included in explanations of the main components of student engagement (Appleton et al., 2006; Fredricks et al, 2004; Jimerson et al., 2003).

Through its history, furthermore, the research on self-regulated learning has incorporated a wide variety of different motivational constructs. Perhaps most prominently, students' beliefs concerning their ability to successfully complete academic tasks have been highlighted as a central motivational construct within models of self-regulated learning (Pintrich, 1999; Schunk, 1990; Zimmerman, 1989). The importance of self-efficacy was presented by Bandura (1986, 1997) as vital to cognitive and behavioral functioning and to self-regulation. Focusing more specifically on self-regulated learning, self-efficacy has continued to be stressed by some of the most influential researchers in this area (Schunk & Ertmer, 2000; Zimmerman, 2000). Achievement goal theory has also been incorporated repeatedly into models of self-regulated learning (Fryer & Elliot, 2008; Pintrich, 1999; Wolters, Yu, & Pintrich, 1996). As well, others have detailed the role of motivational constructs such as value, interest, and autonomy in the process of self-regulated learning (Hidi & Ainley, 2008; Reeve, Ryan, Deci, & Jang, 2008; Wigfield, Hoa, & Klauda, 2008).

Within most of this research, motivation is conceptualized and considered distinct from other areas of functioning, especially cognition and metacognition but also behavior, context, and in some cases even emotion. At times, this differentiation of motivation from cognitive and metacognitive processing has extended to a point that motivation has been described more as a cause of self-regulation and not actually part of the process itself (Pintrich & De Groot, 1990). Motivation was seen as providing the drive, energy, or force that instigated and sustained the processes necessary for self-regulation but was not necessarily inherent to the system itself. As well, some descriptions of self-regulated learning have focused more exclusively on highlighting the cognitive, metacognitive, or information-processing aspects of the model (Winne, 2001). More recently, however, motivation has consistently been viewed as so deeply integrated and vital that it is considered part of the process of self-regulated learning and not separate from it (Pintrich, 2004; Winne & Hadwin, 2008; Wolters, 2003a). From this latter point of view, being motivated and being a self-regulated learner are irreducibly linked in a larger system that explains students' academic functioning. That is, motivational processes play a vital and ongoing role throughout the self-regulation of learning. Motivation is not simply a catalyst that ignites a process that then continues unabated and untended until a task is completed.

This distinction and relation between cognition and motivation is less well established within the research on student engagement. In this work, motivation is not often considered a separate form of involvement but is incorporated into what it means to be cognitively and emotionally engaged. For instance, according to Fredricks et al. (2004), cognitive engagement is reflected in those who value learning and exert efforts to understand or master certain knowledge or skills. Cognitively engaged students include those who espouse learning goals as opposed to performance goals, strive to understand material, master a task, and persist in challenging activities. Others have also described cognitive engagement as including concepts such as value of school in terms of future plans, goal setting, and sense of autonomy, (Appleton et al., 2006; Reschly et al., 2008). At the same time, emotional engagement is also explained in a way that incorporates motivational concepts. Skinner et al. (2009) described engaged emotions as those that indicate energized emotional states, like enthusiasm, enjoyment, and interest. Although this model includes interest as an engaged emotion, only the state of being "caught and held" (p. 495) is used in the conceptualization of emotional engagement, as opposed to including factors that catch and hold students' interest. In sum, motivation is more intricately weaved into conceptualizations of what is viewed as cognitive and emotional engagement. Consistent with most contemporary models of achievement motivation (Schunk et al., 2008), views of self-regulated learning would more typically view these as forms of motivation and therefore conceptually distinct from cognition.

Less apparent, but perhaps more acute, another distinction between the research on self-regulated learning and student engagement is the centrality that is attributed to the agency of students. Characterizing it as a core aspect of his social cognitive theory, Bandura (2006) described agency as the ability of individuals to influence their own cognitive and behavioral functioning. This view of individuals as potentially influential in their own functioning stands in contrast to more deterministic views of behavioral and academic outcomes. At their core, models of self-regulated learning adopt this assumption about human agency and focus on understanding students' academic engagement as a function of their own purposeful, planful, or goal-directed efforts (Greene & Azevedo, 2007; Winne & Hadwin, 2008; Zimmerman, 2000). From this standpoint, students ultimately qualify as self-regulated learners only to the extent that their active engagement in academic contexts is a function of agentic processes. Students coerced to finish worksheets using specific tactics rigidly dictated by a teacher may appear cognitively and behaviorally engaged but likely would not be considered self-regulated. Models of student engagement generally do recognize and incorporate this planfulness within the metacognitive aspects of cognitive engagement. However, models of self-regulated learning expand the ability to be purposeful beyond the cognitive domain into other areas, including motivation, context, and behavior. That is, models of self-regulated learning assume that students can be consciously aware and purposefully intervene to improve and reflect on their actions with regard to a wider set of processes.

The ability to set goals, monitor, reflect upon, and manage one's own motivation serves as a prime example of this distinction. Wolters (1998, 2003a, 2011), for instance, described the strategies that students use to actively and purposefully manage their motivational processing. In one study, college students were presented with 12 different situations by crossing four types of academic situations and three motivational problems. Students were asked to consider each situation and identify what they might do to overcome the motivational problem, provide effort, and complete the task. Analysis of their written responses revealed more than ten distinct types of strategies that students identified as ways of sustaining or improving their level of motivation within the situations. These strategies included efforts to give themselves rewards, use self-talk, reduce distractions, and make the task into a game (Wolters, 1998). Using a forced-choice survey based on the strategies found in this early study, additional work showing that some early adolescents have and use a variety of these motivational strategies provides further support for the importance of this type of engagement (Wolters, 1999; Wolters & Rosenthal, 2000).

Others have studied similar issues with regard to students' emotional processes during academic tasks, especially during tests (Corno, 1993; Kondo, 1997; Schutz et al., 2002). In this work, it is presumed that students can set goals about the emotions they want or expect to experience and can monitor whether they experience those emotions. As well, they can take steps to manipulate their affect and reflect on their affective experience when a task is complete. For instance, students in a testing situation might monitor their emotional state and take steps to reduce feelings of anxiety, frustration, or anger (Schutz & Davis, 2000). Finally, theoretical models of self-regulated learning propose that students also plan, monitor, control, and reflect on different aspects of their behavior. As an example, students may employ organizational and other time management strategies as a way to control their overt behaviors related to studying (Housand & Reis, 2008; Kitsantas et al., 2008; Stoeger & Ziegler, 2008).

In sum, models of self-regulated learning have highlighted the ability of students to assume a purposeful and agentic role across many different facets of their academic functioning. In contrast, beyond the importance of metacognition, models of student engagement do not stress this type of agency when considering students' academic functioning. Rather, these models focus on defining engagement as a state or event based on what students are doing, feeling, or thinking and less on the underlying explanations for why they are doing it (Furlong & Christenson, 2008). Put differently, models of student engagement are not restricted by the assumption of agency or purposefulness in students' academic functioning. Instead, these models allow that students' engagement can result from a more diverse set of influences that include contextual, social, family, and instructional factors. Models of self-regulated learning acknowledge these influences but tend to focus on how they play a role in fostering or hampering students' efforts to manage their own learning.

A third closely related, but theoretically discrete, disparity in these two frameworks is the significance and reach attributed to various types of metalevel knowledge. Researchers from both traditions agree that students' metalevel knowledge regarding their cognitive functioning is critical. Metacognitive knowledge about the self, tasks, and strategies is one basis for students' cognitive engagement and serves as a basis for effective self-regulation of cognitive functioning (Blumenfeld et al., 2006; Winne & Hadwin, 1998). Within both models, students who have greater awareness, understanding, and knowledge relevant to academic task are more likely to be engaged and efficient learners. Descriptions of self-regulated learning, however, move beyond this assumption by incorporating metalevel knowledge associated with other areas of academic functioning (Boekaerts, 1996; Pintrich, 2004; Winne & Hadwin, 2008; Wolters, 2003a). That is, self-regulated learners also are presumed to have metalevel knowledge that provides the foundation necessary for planning, monitoring, and regulating their emotional, behavioral, and motivational processing.

This more far-reaching emphasis on metalevel knowledge is well illustrated when considering motivation. For instance, Boekaerts (1996, 1997) has described how students' knowledge or domain-specific beliefs provide a foundation necessary for the regulation of motivation. In particular, she emphasized the term metamotivational to describe individuals' knowledge or understanding of their own motivation and motivational processing more generally. Metamotivational knowledge provides the awareness necessary for students' to plan, monitor, and manage their level of motivation within academic tasks. In line with this work, Wolters (2003a, 2011) also argued for the importance of this type of knowledge with regard to students' regulation of their motivation. In his view, students need declarative, procedural, and conditional knowledge about motivational strategies in order to use them effectively to sustain or improve motivation. Empirical evidence for the importance of this knowledge about motivation strategies comes from Cooper and Corpus (2009). Using interviews based on short fictional scenarios, these researchers found that adults demonstrated more knowledge of the effectiveness of motivational strategies than older elementary students who, in turn, evidenced greater understanding than younger students. In contrast to this research based on models of self-regulated learning, researchers examining student engagement have not explicitly identified these additional forms of metalevel knowledge as important or incorporated them into their models. Rather, students' conscious awareness, understanding, or metalevel knowledge regarding their functioning typically is restricted to considering metacognitive knowledge.

Concluding Remarks and Directions for Research

Overall, there is substantial overlap among researchers studying self-regulated learning and student engagement with regard to many of the characteristics that are viewed as central to students being effective, efficient, and high-performing learners. These similarities suggest that students who are characterized as self-regulated learners will exhibit the types of cognitive activities, emotional experiences, and overt behaviors that reflect increased student engagement. One obvious conclusion, therefore, is that the research on self-regulated learning and student engagement can, and should, be integrated to a greater extent. A more active integration of these two areas of research should benefit each of them separately, as well as the broader goal of understanding and improving students' functioning within academic contexts.

At the same time, there are some points on which these two theoretical frameworks show greater divergence. In many cases, however, these issues do not appear intractable but rather signify a need for greater conceptual integration and opportunities for research. Disparities in how particular constructs are labeled or the emphasis they are given within each framework reflect this type of difference. It is worth noting, furthermore, that conformity in all areas is absent even with regard to models within each framework. For instance, some models of student engagement make distinctions among three types of engagement, whereas others expand this to four types. As well, even the most prominent models show variation in the processes, skills, or abilities that are viewed as most central to self-regulated learning. In the end, it is likely that most conceptual discrepancies would not provide an insurmountable obstacle to the development of a more integrated model of self-regulated learning and student engagement.

One point that emerges when considering both the commonalities and differences across these two frameworks is the need for additional research that advances their integration. Here, we identify several recommendations that would both serve to integrate these two frameworks and advance the broader understanding of what makes students more effective, more efficient learners within academic contexts. Based on our own background, we frame these ideas for research as ways to improve the work on self-regulated learning.

One recommendation is for additional research that documents students' efforts to plan, monitor, and manage their participation in broader, larger grain, or longer term academic behaviors. Prior research demonstrates the importance of academic behaviors such as attending class and involvement in extracurricular activities (Finn & Rock, 1997; National Center for School Engagement, 2006). Yet, there is little research examining how students might actively manage their engagement in these broader types of academic behaviors. For instance, to what extent do students purposefully plan their involvement in extracurricular activities in service of learning goals? This type of research is needed to complement the ongoing efforts to examine students' self-regulated learning using relatively short-term, computerized tasks or self-reported study behaviors. These latter efforts provide valuable insights into the cognitive and metacognitive processes important to self-regulated learning with regard to small grain size behaviors. Self-regulation and engagement that plays out over more extended periods and involves all aspects of students' functioning (e.g., cognitive, motivational, emotional, behavioral) is also needed.

A second and related recommendation for additional research emerging from this evaluation is the need to expand the work on self-regulated learning to better account for the additional types of engagement shown to be important. One specific need is for work that integrates emotional forms of engagement such as sense of belonging and identity more thoroughly. Interestingly, the research on development of the self or identity has received relatively little attention by researchers examining self-regulated learners. To be sure, some researchers have stressed the importance of better understanding these aspects of being a self-regulated learner (McCombs, 1989; Paris, Byrnes, & Paris, 2001; Roeser & Peck, 2009). As well, it is clear that self-related beliefs (e.g., self-concept, self-efficacy) are central to all models of self-regulated learning. Nonetheless, few empirical studies have examined specifically how individuals' development of identity or self is connected to their ability to engage in self-regulated learning. Also, students' sense of belonging or identification with school is not well understood as either influences or outcomes of the self-regulated learning process. Yet, researchers have found that junior high school students who perceived greater interpersonal support and had a stronger sense of belonging reported higher motivation and were more likely to show increased effort in school and to obtain higher grades (Goodenow, 1993; Goodenow & Grady, 1993). Self-regulated learning processes such as planning, monitoring, and control could be instrumental as explanations for these relations.

Expanding the research examining how students' metalevel knowledge influences their engagement and self-regulated learning would also be fruitful. Past work has tended to focus on metacognitive knowledge about learning strategies. Less well understood is students' understanding, beliefs, or knowledge regarding other aspects of their learning. Questions remain about students' metalevel knowledge about motivation, emotion, behavior, and contexts (Wolters, 2003a, 2011). Assuming it is connected to students' engagement and self-regulated learning, it would also be good to better understand how it is fostered or supported by instructional practices.

Another recommendation arises from the different emphasis within these two frameworks on the purposefulness or planfulness of students' engagement. Models of self-regulated learning, more so than those concerning student engagement, have emphasized the importance of students being goal-directed or purposeful in their actions. At the same time, there is reason to question the extent to which students alone are really consciously responsible for controlling their own learning processes (Fitzsimons & Bargh, 2004; McCaslin & Hickey, 2001). These questions suggest that more research is needed to document better how often and under what conditions students' engagement in different learning processes can actually be considered as self-regulated.

As is always the case, the success of future research will depend on the availability of instruments, designs, and procedures that allow for the reliable and valid assessment of all the relevant constructs. The research on self-regulated learning, however, has often struggled with how best to assess this complex, multifaceted process (Winne & Perry, 2000). Moving forward, there is a continuing need for measures that better differentiate between the more event-like and more trait-like aspects of self-regulated learning.

A final recommendation is for a more complete treatment of context as an area that can be self-regulated. Pintrich (2000, 2004) has argued convincingly that students can and do work to manage different facets of their context in order to reach learning goals. Individuals' efforts to structure or control their environment are a distinct part of volitional accounts of self-regulation (Corno, 1993, 2001), and processes can also be found in other prominent models (Zimmerman, 2000). Whether or how this type of self-regulation of the environment fits with models of student engagement is uncertain. Ultimately, work targeting each of these issues will advance both theoretical frameworks and allow for a more robust and integrated understanding of students' self-regulated learning and engagement.

References

Appleton, J., Christenson, S., & Furlong, M. (2008). Student engagement with school: Critical conceptual and methodological issues of the construct. *Psychology in the Schools, 45*, 369–386.

Appleton, J., Christenson, S., Kim, D., & Reschly, A. (2006). Measuring cognitive and psychological engagement: Validation of the Student Engagement Instrument. *Journal of School Psychology, 44*, 427–445.

Bandura, A. (1986). Self-regulatory mechanisms. In A. Bandura (Ed.), *Social foundations of thought and action: A social–cognitive theory* (pp. 335–389). Englewood Cliffs, NJ: Prentice Hall.

Bandura, A. (1997). *Self-efficacy: The exercise of control*. New York: W. H. Freeman.

Bandura, A. (2006). Toward a psychology of human agency. *Perspectives on Psychological Science, 1*, 164–180.

Baumeister, R., & Vohs, K. (Eds.). (2004). *Handbook of self-regulation: Research, theory, and applications*. New York: Guilford Press.

Blumenfeld, P. C., Kempler, T. M., & Krajcik, J. S. (2006). Motivation and cognitive engagement in learning environments. In R. K. Sawyer (Ed.), *The Cambridge handbook of the learning sciences* (pp. 475–488). New York: Cambridge University Press.

Boekaerts, M. (1996). Self-regulated learning at the junction of cognition and motivation. *European Psychologist, 1*, 100–112.

Boekaerts, M. (1997). Self-regulated learning: A new concept embraced by researchers, policy makers, educators, teachers, and students. *Learning and Instruction, 7*, 161–186.

Boekaerts, M., Pintrich, P. R., & Zeidner, M. (Eds.). (2000). *Handbook of self-regulation: Theory, research, and applications*. San Diego, CA: Academic.

Butler, D., & Winne, P. H. (1995). Feedback and self-regulated learning: A theoretical synthesis. *Review of Educational Research, 65*, 245–281.

Carver, C. S., & Scheier, M. F. (2000). On the structure of behavioral self-regulation. In M. Boekaerts, P. Pintrich, & M. Zeidner (Eds.), *Handbook of self-regulation* (pp. 41–84). San Diego, CA: Academic.

Christenson, S. L., Reschly, A. L., Appleton, J. J., Berman, S., Spanjers, D., & Varro, P. (2008). Best practices in fostering student engagement. In A. Thomas & J. Grimes (Eds.), *Best practices in school psychology* (5th ed., pp. 1099–1120). Bethesda, MD: National Association of School Psychologists.

Connell, J. P., & Wellborn, J. G. (1991). Competence, autonomy, and relatedness: A motivational analysis of self-system processes. In M. R. Gunnar & L. A. Sroufe (Eds.), *Self processes and development* (Vol. 23, pp. 43–77). Hillsdale, NJ: Lawrence Erlbaum.

Cooper, C., & Corpus, J. (2009). Learners' developing knowledge of strategies for regulating motivation. *Journal of Applied Developmental Psychology, 30*, 525–536.

Corno, L. (1993). The best–laid plans: Modern conceptions of volition and educational research. *Educational Researcher, 22*(2), 14–22.

Corno, L. (2001). Volitional aspects of self–regulated learning. In B. Zimmerman & D. Schunk (Eds.), *Self-regulated learning and academic achievement: Theoretical perspectives* (2nd ed., pp. 191–225). Mahwah, NJ: Erlbaum Associates.

Feldman, A., & Matjasko, J. (2005). The role of school-based extracurricular activities in adolescent development: A comprehensive review and future directions. *Review of Educational Research, 75*, 159–210.

Finn, J. (1989). Withdrawing from school. *Review of Educational Research, 59*, 117–142.

Finn, J. (1993). *School engagement and students at risk*. Washington, DC: National Center for Educational Statistics.

Finn, J., & Rock, D. (1997). Academic success among students at risk for school failure. *Journal of Applied Psychology, 82*, 221–235.

Finn, J., & Voelkl, K. (1993). School characteristics related to school engagement. *The Journal of Negro Education, 62*, 249–268.

Fitzsimons, G., & Bargh, J. (2004). Automatic self-regulation. In R. Baumeister & K. Vohs (Eds.), *Handbook of self-regulation: Research, theory, and applications* (pp. 151–170). New York: Guilford Press.

Fredricks, J. A., Blumenfeld, P. C., & Paris, A. H. (2004). School engagement: Potential of the concept, state of the evidence. *Review of Educational Research, 74*, 59–109.

Fryer, J., & Elliot, A. (2008). Self-regulation and achievement goal pursuit. In D. Schunk & B. Zimmerman (Eds.), *Motivation and self-regulated learning: Theory, research, and applications* (pp. 53–75). Mahwah, NJ: Erlbaum Associates.

Furlong, M., & Christenson, S. (2008). Engaging students at school and with learning: A relevant construct for all students. *Psychology in the Schools, 45*, 365–368.

Furlong, M., Whipple, A., St. Jean, G., Simental, J., & Punthuna, S. (2003). Multiple contexts of school engagement: Moving toward a unifying framework for educational research and practice. *The California School Psychologist, 8*, 99–113.

Goodenow, C. (1993). Classroom belonging among early adolescent students: Relationships to motivation and achievement. *The Journal of Early Adolescence, 13*, 21–43.

Goodenow, C., & Grady, K. (1993). The relationship of school belonging and friends' values to academic motivation among urban adolescent students. *The Journal of Experimental Education, 62*, 60–71.

Greene, B., Miller, R., Crowson, H., Duke, B., & Akey, L. (2004). Predicting high school students' cognitive engagement and achievement: Contributions of classroom perceptions and motivation. *Contemporary Educational Psychology, 29*, 462–482.

Greene, J., & Azevedo, R. (2007). A theoretical review of Winne and Hadwin's model of self-regulated learning: New perspectives and directions. *Review of Educational Research, 77*, 334–372.

Hidi, S., & Ainley, M. (2008). Interest and self-regulation: Relationships between two variables that influence learning. In D. Schunk & B. Zimmerman (Eds.), *Motivation and self-regulated learning: Theory, research, and applications* (pp. 77–109). Mahwah, NJ: Erlbaum Associates.

Housand, A., & Reis, S. (2008). Self-regulated learning in reading: Gifted pedagogy and instructional settings. *Journal of Advanced Academics, 20*, 108–136.

Jimerson, S., Campos, E., & Greif, J. (2003). Toward an understanding of definitions and measures of school engagement and related terms. *The California School Psychologist, 8*, 7–27.

Kitsantas, A., Winsler, A., & Huie, F. (2008). Self-regulation and ability predictors of academic success during college: A predictive validity study. *Journal of Advanced Academics, 20*, 42–68.

Kondo, D. S. (1997). Strategies for coping with test anxiety. *Anxiety, Stress, and Coping, 10*, 203–215.

Kortering, L., & Christenson, S. (2009). Engaging students in school and learning: The real deal for school completion. *Exceptionality, 17*, 5–15.

Linnenbrink, E., & Pintrich, P. (2000). Multiple pathways to learning and achievement: The role of goal orientation in fostering adaptive motivation, affect, and cognition. In C. Sansone & J. Harackiewicz (Eds.), *Intrinsic and extrinsic motivation: The search for optimal motivation and performance* (pp. 195–254). San Diego, CA: Academic.

Linver, M., Roth, J., & Brooks-Gunn, J. (2009). Patterns of adolescents' participation in organized activities: Are sports best when combined with other activities? *Developmental Psychology, 45*, 354–367.

McCaslin, M., & Hickey, D. (2001). Self-regulated learning and academic achievement: A Vygotskian view.

In B. Zimmerman & D. Schunk (Eds.), *Self-regulated learning and academic achievement: Theoretical perspectives* (2nd ed., pp. 227–252). Mahwah, NJ: Erlbaum Associates.

McCombs, B. (1989). Self-regulated learning and academic achievement: A phenomenological view. In B. Zimmerman & D. Schunk (Eds.), *Self-regulated learning and academic achievement: Theory, research, and practice* (pp. 51–82). New York: Springer.

McCombs, B., & Marzano, R. (1990). Putting the self in self-regulated learning: The self as agent in integrating will and skill. *Educational Psychologist, 25*, 51–69.

National Center for School Engagement. (2006). *Quantifying school engagement: Research report.* Available at http://www.schoolengagement.org/. Accessed March 11, 2010.

Newman, R. (1998). Adaptive help-seeking: A role of social interaction in self–regulated learning. In S. Karabenick (Ed.), *Strategic help-seeking: Implications for learning and teaching* (pp. 13–37). Hillsdale, NJ: Erlbaum Associates.

Paris, S., Byrnes, J., & Paris, A. (2001). Constructing theories, identities, and actions of self-regulated learners. In B. Zimmerman & D. Schunk (Eds.), *Self-regulated learning and academic achievement: Theoretical perspectives* (2nd ed., pp. 253–287). Mahwah, NJ: Erlbaum Associates.

Paris, S., & Oka, E. (1986). Children's reading strategies, metacognition, and motivation. *Developmental Review, 6*, 25–56.

Pekrun, R., Goetz, T., Titz, W., & Perry, R. (2002). Academic emotions in students' self-regulated learning and achievement: A program of qualitative and quantitative research. *Educational Psychologist, 37*, 91–105.

Pintrich, P. (1999). The role of motivation in promoting and sustaining self-regulated learning. *International Journal of Educational Research, 31*, 459–470.

Pintrich, P. (2000). The role of goal orientation in self–regulated learning. In M. Boekaerts, P. Pintrich, & M. Zeidner (Eds.), *Handbook of self-regulation* (pp. 451–502). San Diego, CA: Academic.

Pintrich, P. (2004). A conceptual framework for assessing motivation and self–regulated learning in college students. *Educational Psychology Review, 16*, 385–407.

Pintrich, P., & De Groot, E. (1990). Motivational and self–regulated learning components of classroom academic performance. *Journal of Educational Psychology, 82*, 33–40.

Pintrich, P., Wolters, C., & Baxter, G. (2000). Assessing metacognition and self–regulated learning. In G. Schraw (Ed.), *Metacognitive assessment.* Lincoln, NE: University of Nebraska Press.

Pintrich, P., & Zusho, A. (2002). The development of academic self-regulation: The role of cognitive and motivational factors. In A. Wigfield & J. Eccles (Eds.), *Development of achievement motivation* (pp. 249–284). San Diego, CA: Academic.

Reeve, J., Ryan, R., Deci, E., & Jang, H. (2008). Understanding and promoting autonomous self-regulation: A self-determined theory perspective. In D. Schunk & B. Zimmerman (Eds.), *Motivation and self-regulated learning: Theory, research, and applications* (pp. 223–244). Mahwah, NJ: Erlbaum Associates.

Reschly, A., Huebner, E., Appleton, J., & Antaramian, S. (2008). Engagement as flourishing: The contribution of positive emotions and coping to adolescents' engagement at school and with learning. *Psychology in the Schools, 45*, 419–431.

Roeser, R., & Peck, S. (2009). An education in awareness: Self, motivation, and self-regulated learning in contemplative perspective. *Educational Psychologist, 44*, 119–136.

Russell, V. J., Ainley, M., & Frydenberg, E. (2005). *Schooling issues digest: Student motivation and engagement.* Canberra, Australia: Department of Education, Science and Training, Australian Government.

Sansone, C., & Thoman, D. (2006). Maintaining activity engagement: Individual differences in the process of self-regulating motivation. *Journal of Personality, 74*, 1697–1720.

Schunk, D. (1990). Goal setting and self-efficacy during self-regulated learning. *Educational Psychologist, 25*, 71–86.

Schunk, D., & Ertmer, P. (2000). Self-regulation and academic learning: Self–efficacy enhancing interventions. In M. Boekaerts, P. Pintrich, & M. Zeidner (Eds.), *Handbook of self-regulation* (pp. 631–649). San Diego, CA: Academic.

Schunk, D., & Zimmerman, B. (2003). Self-regulation and learning. In W. Reynolds & G. Miller (Eds.), *Handbook of psychology: Vol. 7. Educational psychology* (pp. 59–78). New York: Wiley.

Schunk, D. H., Pintrich, P. R., & Meece, J. L. (2008). *Motivation in education: Theory, research, applications* (3rd ed.). Upper Saddle River, NJ: Pearson Education.

Schutz, P., & Davis, H. (2000). Emotions and self-regulation during test taking. *Educational Psychologist, 35*, 243–256.

Schutz, P., Davis, H., & Schwanenflugel, P. (2002). Organization of concepts relevant to emotions and their regulation during test taking. *The Journal of Experimental Education, 70*, 316–342.

Sinclair, M. F., Christenson, S. L., Lehr, C. A., & Anderson, A. R. (2003). Facilitating student engagement: Lessons learned from Check & Connect longitudinal studies. *The California School Psychologist, 8*, 29–42.

Skinner, E., Kinderman, T., & Furrer, C. (2009). A motivational perspective on engagement and disaffection: Conceptualization and assessment of children's behavioral and emotional participation in academic activities in the classroom. *Educational and Psychological Measurement, 69*, 493–525.

Skinner, E. A., & Belmont, M. J. (1993). Motivation in the classroom: Reciprocal effects of teacher behavior and student engagement across the school year. *Journal of Educational Psychology, 85,* 571–581.

Stipek, D. (2002). Good instruction is motivating. In A. Wigfield & J. Eccles (Eds.), *Development of achievement motivation* (pp. 309–332). San Diego, CA: Academic.

Stoeger, H., & Ziegler, A. (2008). Evaluation of a classroom based training to improve self-regulation in time management tasks during homework activities with fourth graders. *Metacognition and Learning, 3,* 207–230.

Vrugt, A., & Oort, F. (2008). Metacognition, achievement goals, study strategies, and academic achievement: Pathways to achievement. *Metacognition and Learning, 3,* 123–146.

Wigfield, A., Hoa, L., & Klauda, S. (2008). The role of achievement values in the regulation of achievement behaviors. In D. Schunk & B. Zimmerman (Eds.), *Motivation and self-regulated learning: Theory, research, and applications* (pp. 169–195). Mahwah, NJ: Erlbaum Associates.

Winne, P. (2001). Self-regulated learning viewed from models of information processing. In B. Zimmerman & D. Schunk (Eds.), *Self-regulated learning and academic achievement: Theoretical perspectives* (2nd ed., pp. 153–189). Mahwah, NJ: Erlbaum Associates.

Winne, P., & Hadwin, A. (1998). Studying as self-regulated learning. In D. Hacker, J. Dunlosky, & A. Graesser (Eds.), *Metacognition in educational theory and practice* (pp. 277–304). Mahwah, NJ: Erlbaum.

Winne, P., & Hadwin, A. (2008). The weave of motivation and self-regulated learning. In D. Schunk & B. Zimmerman (Eds.), *Motivation and self-regulated learning: Theory, research, and applications* (pp. 297–314). Mahwah, NJ: Erlbaum Associates.

Winne, P., & Perry, N. (2000). Measuring self-regulated learning. In M. Boekaerts, P. Pintrich, & M. Zeidner (Eds.), *Handbook of self-regulation* (pp. 531–566). San Diego, CA: Academic.

Wolters, C. (1998). Self-regulated learning and college students' regulation of motivation. *Journal of Educational Psychology, 90,* 224–235.

Wolters, C. (1999). The relation between high school students' motivational regulation and their use of learning strategies, effort, and classroom performance. *Learning and Individual Differences, 11,* 281–299.

Wolters, C. (2003a). Regulation of motivation: Evaluating an underemphasized aspect of self–regulated learning. *Educational Psychologist, 38,* 189–205.

Wolters, C. (2003b). Understanding procrastination from a self-regulated learning perspective. *Journal of Educational Psychology, 95,* 179–187.

Wolters, C. (2004). Advancing achievement goal theory: Using goal structures and goal orientations to predict students' motivation, cognition, and achievement. *Journal of Educational Psychology, 96,* 236–250.

Wolters, C. (2011). Regulation of motivation: Contextual and social aspects. *Teacher's College Record, 113,* 265–283.

Wolters, C., Pintrich, P., & Karabenick, S. (2005). Assessing academic self-regulated learning. In K. Moore & L. Lippman (Eds.), *What do children need to flourish?: Conceptualizing and measuring indicators of positive development* (pp. 251–270). New York: Springer.

Wolters, C., & Rosenthal, H. (2000). The relation between students' motivational beliefs and attitudes and their use of motivational regulation strategies. *International Journal of Educational Research, 33,* 801–820.

Wolters, C., Yu, S., & Pintrich, P. (1996). The relation between goal orientation and students' motivational beliefs and self-regulated learning. *Learning and Individual Differences, 8,* 211–238.

Yazzie-Mintz, E. (2007). *Voices of students on engagement: A report on the 2006 High School Survey of Student Engagement*. Bloomington, IN: Center for Evaluation & Education Policy, Indiana University.

Zimmerman, B. (1986). Becoming a self–regulated learner: Which are the key processes? *Contemporary Educational Psychology, 11,* 307–313.

Zimmerman, B. (1989). A social cognitive view of self-regulated learning and academic learning. *Journal of Educational Psychology, 81,* 329–339.

Zimmerman, B. (2000). Attaining self-regulation: A social cognitive perspective. In M. Boekaerts, P. R. Pintrich, & M. Zeidner (Eds.), *Handbook of self-regulation: Theory, research, and applications* (pp. 13–29). San Diego, CA: Academic.

Zimmerman, B. (2002). Becoming a self-regulated learner: An overview. *Theory Into Practice, 41,* 64–70.

Zimmerman, B., & Schunk, D. (Eds.). (2001). *Self-regulated learning and academic achievement: Theoretical perspectives* (2nd ed.). Mahwah, NJ: Erlbaum.

Classroom Strategies to Enhance Academic Engaged Time

31

Maribeth Gettinger and Martha J. Walter

Abstract

A strong predictor of student achievement is the amount of time students are actively engaged in learning, or academic engaged time (AET). Sustained engagement, in turn, is influenced by the extent to which students are motivated to invest time in learning. Despite the importance of AET, studies reveal that engagement (determined by motivation) may be as low as 45–50% in some classrooms. Beginning with a model developed by Carroll in 1963, several theoretical conceptualizations of school learning have emphasized the critical role of engaged time in determining student achievement. Subsequently, empirical studies focusing on the relationship between time and learning have documented the role of the instructional context in explaining both student motivation (willingness to invest time in learning) and student engagement (actual involvement or participation in learning). In addition to discussing theory and research that implicate time in the teaching-learning process, this chapter describes three groupings of evidence-based practices that contribute to student engagement and motivation, including classroom management, instructional design, and student-mediated strategies.

Introduction and Overview

Student engagement in learning contributes to overall achievement and, in itself, is an important outcome of schooling. Various conceptualizations of student engagement have appeared in the literature, ranging from broad perspectives that view engagement as a psychological process underlying students' social and cognitive development to more narrow conceptualizations that view engagement as a behavioral index of attention to learning tasks (Marks, 2000). Notwithstanding the significant contributions to academic success made by students' cognitive, affective, and social engagement in the schooling process, the specific focus in this chapter is on time-based indices of student engagement in learning. For purposes of this chapter, student engagement is conceptualized as direct, measurable involvement or participation in learning activities.

M. Gettinger (✉) • M.J. Walter
Department of Educational Psychology,
University of Wisconsin-Madison, Madison, WI, USA
e-mail: mgetting@wisc.edu; mjwalter@wisc.edu

A strong predictor of academic achievement is the amount of time students are actively engaged in learning. The link between academic engaged time (AET) and learning is one of the most enduring and consistent findings in educational research (Gettinger & Ball, 2007). Simply put, learning requires engagement or investment of time on the part of the learner. The greater the amount of time students are engaged in learning, the higher their achievement. Student motivation is distinct from, yet highly related to, student engagement. Specifically, engagement is determined, in large part, by the extent to which students are motivated to participate in learning. In this chapter, student motivation is viewed as leading to student engagement, with engagement being the point of entry for instruction. In other words, sustained and continuous engagement in learning over time (determined by motivation) is the mechanism through which classroom instruction directly influences student outcomes.

Reliable approaches to assessing levels of engaged learning often rely on observable criteria. Thus, the amount of observed time students are actively involved in learning serves as the index of student engagement in both descriptive and empirical research on time and learning (Adelman, Haslam, & Pringle, 1996). To the extent that engagement is determined by motivation, the amount of time students choose to engage themselves in learning (i.e., under conditions of student choice or self-determined study time) has also been used as a time-based metric for students' motivation (Guthrie & Wigfield, 2000).

Despite the importance of AET, descriptive studies reveal that (a) as little as half of each school day is typically devoted to academic instruction, (b) students are engaged in learning activities only 28–56% of the total time they spend in school during a given year, and (c) the level of students' on-task behavior may be as low as 45% in some classrooms (Black, 2002; Fisher, 2009; Hollywood, Salisbury, Rainforth, & Palombaro, 1995; Rangel, 2007; Smith, 2000). In response to growing national concerns about declining levels of achievement and engagement among students, the National Education Commission on Time and Learning (NECTL) was established in 1991 to conduct a comprehensive examination of time use in American schools. In 1994, the NECTL released its report, entitled *Prisoners of Time*, which concluded, "it would be unreasonable to believe that…the quality…of American schools could be improved without substantial changes in the amount and use of time allowed for teachers and students to do their work" (p. 15). According to this report, despite longer school days, students in American schools spend less time engaged in academic instruction and learning than do students in other nations. In 2005, the NECTL updated and reissued its report to reiterate the critical need for better use of instructional time in schools and to underscore the importance of academic engaged time for enhancing achievement among all learners.

The purpose of this chapter is to address classroom strategies designed to enhance academic engaged time (AET). The chapter is predicated on the contention that AET is a useful variable for measuring instructional processes and that it plays a key role in contributing to student achievement. To examine the concept of AET, the chapter begins with a historical review of theoretical models and research paradigms that place time as a central variable in school learning, in terms of both student engagement and motivation. Next, academic engaged time is defined. The components of AET are explained, and factors that determine each AET component are delineated. Finally, research-supported practices for maximizing students' AET are reviewed, with a focus classroom management practices, instructional approaches, and student-mediated strategies.

Historical Perspectives

Both theory and research on the association between time and learning affirm that time spent in learning, a construct closely related to AET, is a crucial factor in influencing achievement. In one of the earliest reviews on the relationship between time and learning, Fredrick and Walberg (1980) found that the correlation between time spent in learning and achievement ranged from .13 to .71, depending on how time was operationalized and measured. Subsequent research on learning time during the 1980s and 1990s focused, first, on the extent to which differences in achievement among learners can be explained by time spent in learning (e.g., Gettinger, 1985, 1989) and, second, on identifying instructional factors that maximize time spent in learning and, in turn, achievement (Wang, Haertel, & Walberg, 1993; Wyne & Stuck, 1982). A review of prominent theories and research on school learning that stress the role of time in learning is provided below.

Theoretical Foundations for Academic Engaged Time

Interest in engaged learning time can be traced to several theories that implicated time in the learning process, beginning with John Carroll's original model of school learning (1963). Collectively, multiple theoretical perspectives, described briefly in the following paragraphs, provided the foundation for later empirical and applied research focusing on the construct of AET and its importance for school success.

Carroll's Model of School Learning

One of the earliest and most influential models for school learning was proposed in 1963 by John Carroll (1963, 1984, 1989). Carroll theorized about the functional relationship between time variables and measures of learning. The major premise of Carroll's model was that school learning is a function of two time variables, the amount of time students spend in learning relative to the amount of time they actually need for learning. According to Carroll, students master instructional objectives to the extent that they are allowed and are willing to invest the time required to learn the content. Carroll's model can be expressed as a simple mathematical equation: degree of learning $= f$ [time spent/time needed] (Carroll, 1963). Based on this equation, the degree to which a learner succeeds in learning a task is dependent on the amount of time she/he spends in relation to the amount of time she/he needs. The closer individuals come to achieving equilibrium between the amount of time they require for learning and the amount of time they actually engage in learning, the higher their level of mastery. As such, the primary metric for both student motivation and student engagement in Carroll's model was time.

Carroll identified five factors that influence either "time spent" or "time needed" in his model. Three factors determine time needed for learning: (a) student aptitude, (b) ability to understand instruction, and (c) quality of instruction. Specifically, the higher a learner's aptitude for learning content and ability to comprehend instruction, the less time needed for learning. Conversely, poor quality of instruction increases the amount of time needed for learning beyond what would be necessary under optimal conditions. Two factors affect time spent in learning: (a) time allocated for learning, or opportunity to learn, and (b) perseverance, or the amount of time the learner is willing to spend in learning, a variable most closely related to student motivation. According to Carroll, the relationship between these latter two factors and student learning tends to be linear. Specifically, degree of learning is higher or lower to the extent that adequate learning time is provided. Moreover, learning will be incomplete if students are not motivated to spend the necessary amount of time for learning. Thus, in Carroll's model, motivation leads to engagement. The measure Carroll proposed for opportunity to learn was the amount of time a teacher makes available for learning; the proposed measure for perseverance was engagement rate or percentage of allocated time during which students are actually on task. In the equation, allocated time is multiplied by engagement rate to produce the "time spent" numerator, or number of minutes that students are engaged in learning. In Carroll's original model, there was significant overlap between the constructs of student engagement and student motivation. Subsequent theoretical conceptualizations of time and learning (described below) drew sharper distinctions between these two time-based determinants of learning.

By placing time as a pivotal variable in school learning, Carroll's model initiated a major shift in educational thought and research on the teaching-learning process (Anderson, 1985; Ben-Peretz &

Bromme, 1990; Gettinger, 1984). Influenced by Carroll's work, researchers directed greater attention to the variable of time in student learning, acknowledging that individual differences in various time metrics (time needed, time engaged, time allocated) accounted for significant variability in educational performance (Anderson, 1984; Haertel, Walberg, & Weinstein, 1983). Carroll's work was the major impetus for subsequent models of school learning and contributed to a number of research projects designed to explicate further the relationship between time and learning.

The primary appeal of Carroll's model was his specification of measurable, time-related variables that affect individual learning. Carroll's model was viewed as an individual-differences framework in that most of the time-related variables in his model (perseverance, time needed to learn, etc.) were conceptualized as individual learner characteristics (Berliner, 1990a). Classroom learning, however, is affected by variables outside the learner, such as opportunity to learn and quality of instruction. Moreover, schooling is often organized to provide group instruction, with fixed time periods allocated to curricular content. Thus, subsequent models were developed to refine Carroll's theory and adapt it for classroom settings. These models (described below) placed greater emphasis on time factors external to the learner (including strategies to motivate learners) and incorporated features of the instructional process at the classroom level.

Bloom's Theory of School Learning

Most notable of the models that were based on Carroll's constructs and attempted to incorporate time factors within an instructional theory of classroom learning was that of Benjamin Bloom (1974). The development of the mastery learning model by Bloom and his students generated extensive research on time and school learning during the 1980s. Although developed as an instructional approach, mastery learning provided an appropriate experimental paradigm within which variation in both time needed and time spent in learning was systematically evaluated (Gettinger, 1984).

According to Bloom, the notions of fixed time and variable achievement as unavoidable conditions of school learning often pervaded educational thought. Moreover, the influence of these assumptions on educational practices was frequently counterproductive. In Bloom's mastery learning model, achievement level was held constant, and the amount of time needed to attain a targeted level of achievement was variable. As such, the goal was to fix the degree of learning at an acceptable criterion level and vary time and instructional methods, according to learner needs, so that nearly all students attained it. The mastery learning model rested on the belief that with adequate time to learn, sufficient motivation to engage in learning, and high-quality instruction, all students could learn what only a percentage of students were able to learn under traditional fixed-time instruction. In fact, mastery learning theorists proposed that 80% of students could achieve a criterion level usually attained by only about 20%, if they were given sufficient time and appropriate help to maximize their engagement in learning (Block, 1971; Block & Anderson, 1975). The success of mastery learning models rested not only on allocating time for learning but also on motivating students to be engaged in learning. According to mastery learning theorists, understanding and accommodating individual learners' need for choice, autonomy, encouragement, modeling, and feedback enable teachers to motivate students and keep them engaged with academic tasks.

There is a contrast between Carroll's conceptual notion that time needed for learning is a relatively stable student characteristic (as a function of aptitude and ability to understand instruction) and Bloom's instructional notion that time needed for learning can be reduced with appropriate teaching-learning experiences. Researchers demonstrated that variation in students' time needed for learning does, in fact, decrease across learning tasks within a mastery learning paradigm (Block, 1983; Guskey, 2001). Guskey theorized that individualized learning time and high-quality instruction within a mastery learning approach develop students' skills, resulting in increased confidence and competence. Greater confidence, in turn, motivates students to engage in learning and successfully complete academic tasks. According to Berliner (1990a), Bloom's reconceptualization of learner variables, such as time needed for learning, as malleable characteristics represented an important contribution to thinking about students and schools.

Wiley and Harnischfeger's Model of Instructional Exposure

Wiley and Harnischfeger offered another model of the teaching-learning process based on Carroll's theoretical work. Similar to Carroll's model, the Wiley-Harnischfeger model rested on the conviction that quantity of education (total amount of actual learning time) determines the degree of student learning (Wiley & Harnischfeger, 1974). Wiley and Harnischfeger, however, placed significant emphasis on the total amount of time allocated to students and for specific learning topics, which typically varied across districts, schools, and classrooms. In elaborating their model, Wiley and Harnischfeger discussed this concept of quantity of education, which they labeled "instructional exposure" (Harnischfeger & Wiley, 1976). For Wiley and Harnischfeger, Carroll's factor of opportunity to learn or time allowed, in combination with the amount and manner in which allocated time is used for instruction, comprised a major determinant of achievement. According to their model, the maximum time available for instruction is established by the length of the school year and school day, as well as individual teacher allocations and scheduling. Maximum time, however, is typically reduced by several intervening factors, such as attendance, instructional design, and time spent by teachers for disciplining or making transitions. According to Wiley and Harnischfeger, only a percentage of the allocated time becomes actual exposure time, and, in turn, only a portion of exposure time translates into usable time (i.e., time without interruptions). Thus, Carroll's factor of opportunity or time allowed was refined to the point of representing only a fraction of the total time allocated. Within the Wiley-Harnischfeger model, achievement is a function of the ratio of maximum allocated exposure time (reduced, first, to active learning time within the maximum limits, and further to usable learning time) relative to the total time needed. Because maximum allocated exposure time is amenable to manipulation and educational policy modifications, it was viewed by Wiley and Harnishfeger as the most important time variable in school learning (Karweit, 1989).

Within the Wiley-Harnischfeger's comprehensive model, achievement is determined by four time variables, including maximum exposure time, percent usable exposure time, percent active learning time, and total time needed for learning. Their conceptualization of achievement was expressed as the following equation: achievement $= f$ [(allocated time) (percent usable time) (percent active time)/time needed]. In this model, the percentage of time students are actively engaged in learning plays a prominent role in explaining achievement (Harnischfeger & Wiley, 1985). Students, in turn, are motivated to be actively engaged in learning when they have an understanding of the purpose or goal for doing so. Thus, according to Wiley and Harnischfeger, one mechanism for schools to accomplish instructional goals is to focus on the tasks in which students are engaged, ensure that students understand the purpose of those tasks, and, in turn, maximize the duration of their engagement.

Cooley and Leinhardt's Classroom-Process Model

Like Wiley and Harnischfeger, Cooley and Leinhardt proposed a refinement of Carroll's model that also underscored the importance of the use of instructional time over scheduled time per se in influencing achievement. The model of classroom processes proposed by Cooley and Leinhardt (1976) focused on the relationship between school practices (including instructional time use) and school performance. The Cooley-Leinhardt model was a revision of Carroll's model in that it provided a more precise specification of instructional processes that account for learning. Their model imposed several qualifications on the quantity of instruction, to which they referred as the "opportunity construct." Consistent with Carroll's model, opportunity was defined as the amount of time students can potentially work on specific content. Motivators, another factor in their model, are the behaviors or attitudes (e.g., self-efficacy beliefs, understanding the purpose for learning) that promote learning; these motivators include both internal factors (student interest) and external factors (e.g., teacher praise) that serve to maximize the amount of time students engage themselves in learning. Cooley and Leinhardt (1980) found that amount of time scheduled for a specific subject may bear little relation to achievement. Within their model, the efficient and effective use of allocated time is more important than allocation per se; however, as Wiley and Harnischfeger emphasized, allocation is always the upper bound of time use. In addition to opportunity, Cooley and Leinhardt identified three other constructs that explain variation in student performance under constant instructional time conditions, specifically student motivation, instructional events, and structure. All three constructs, when taken together, represent Carroll's quality of instruction variable, thereby reflecting the relative emphasis placed on this factor in determining overall degree of learning. Thus, within the Cooley-Leinhardt model, opportunity to learn, combined with motivators to encourage learning and appropriate instruction, is facilitative in promoting achievement (Leinhardt, 1978). The Cooley-Leinhardt model was the first to articulate the explicit role of student motivation in determining student engagement in learning.

Huitt Model of the Teaching-Learning Process

Huitt (1995) focused on student behavior within the classroom as well as the influence of teacher behaviors on students' engagement in learning. Specifically, in the Huitt model, academic learning time replaced the "time spent" variable in Carroll's model. According to Huitt, student behavior encompasses all actions of students in classrooms and, importantly, includes academic learning time (ALT). Within this model, ALT was specifically defined as the amount of time students are successfully covering content that will be tested. Thus, ALT was a combination of three variables: (a) content overlap, which is the percentage of the content included on a test that is actually covered by students in the classrooms and sometimes referred to as "time on target"; (b) involvement, which is the amount of time students are actively involved in the learning process and is most often equated with "time on task"; and (c) success, or the extent to which students accurately complete the assignments they have been given (Squires, Huitt, & Segars, 1983).

Summary of Theoretical Foundations

In sum, prominent theoretical conceptualizations of school learning evolved since Carroll's (1963) model that incorporated a focus on instructional time and emphasized the critical role of engaged time in determining student achievement. Whereas Carroll's original model focused primarily on the quantity of time (e.g., amount of time allocated, amount of time engaged), more recent models stress the importance of quality of time as well. Beginning with Bloom's mastery learning model, research on time and learning has devoted greater attention to the role of the instructional context, such as quality of instruction, performance feedback, or student interest in content, in explaining both student motivation (willingness to invest time in learning) and student engagement (actual involvement or participation in learning).

Process-Product Paradigm

The conceptualization of AET is integrally linked to the emergence of research during the 1970s which defined teaching effectiveness in terms of specific classroom behaviors. The primary goal of teaching-effectiveness research was to determine the relationship between classroom processes and student performance, with the intent of identifying teaching practices and behaviors associated with school learning and, in particular, student engagement (Gettinger & Stoiber, 2009). The search for relations between classroom processes (e.g., teaching behaviors) and outcomes (e.g., student achievement) came to be known as process-outcome (or process-product) research. Process-outcome research has been the most common paradigm for establishing the importance of AET for student learning and for identifying classroom variables that contribute to AET.

Within a process-outcome approach, researchers are concerned with identifying relationships between teaching behaviors and student outcomes, both of which can be defined, observed, and measured (Berliner, 1990b). Process-outcome studies use AET as an indicator or outcome of teaching effectiveness as well as a predictor of student learning. Process-outcome research can be characterized on the basis of several methodological features. In a typical study, teachers and students are observed in classrooms. Teaching processes are described in a series of low-inference behavioral categories, often mutually exclusive, such that any classroom event (e.g., giving directions for completing a task) is coded in only one way. Relationships between patterns of teaching behaviors and student outcomes (specifically, student engagement or achievement) are described as statistical correlations (Gettinger & Kohler, 2006).

One of the most significant contributions to the advent of process-outcome research has been the emphasis on measurement of classroom processes and student engagement through systematic, direct observation. With advances in observation technology, researchers are able to focus directly on the process of instruction and its effects on learning and behavior. Moreover, direct observations can be used to measure and quantify students' level of engagement in learning tasks. Although definitions vary, most observation protocols incorporate fairly broad indices to assess student engagement. The *Code for Instructional Structure and Student Academic Response* (CISSAR; Stanley & Greenwood, 1981), for example, defines engagement in terms of observable behaviors such as attending (e.g., looking at the teacher), working (e.g., reading silently), or managing learning resources (e.g., looking for a library book). Regardless of the definition of engagement, most observational procedures use some form of a time-sampling system. In these methods, observers note whether engaged behaviors are occurring or not occurring during brief observation intervals to derive an estimate of AET.

In general, process-outcome research has concluded that teachers' use of effective management and teaching strategies (classroom processes) is associated with increased student engagement and higher achievement (learner outcomes). Within process-outcome research, the concept of AET provides a way of understanding and interpreting these results. For example, process-outcome research provides correlational evidence that when teachers provide structure in their lessons (e.g., communicate expectations, monitor student work, provide feedback, etc.), their students have high achievement. The concept of AET enables researchers to offer multiple explanations for this relation. First, lesson structure helps students understand their responsibility for learning, thereby increasing their perseverance or motivation and, in turn, academic engaged time. Alternately, providing explicit structure and expectations may guard against students being engaged on the wrong task and is likely to increase their engagement and success on appropriate tasks. In other words, effective teaching (process) is linked to achievement (outcome) through its direct effect on maximizing students' AET.

The earliest and most extensive process-outcome research program to document the relationship between time and learning and to provide empirical support for the importance of AET was the Beginning Teacher Evaluation Study (BTES) conducted during the 1980s (Denham & Lieberman, 1980). Although the original purpose of the BTES was to evaluate beginning teacher competencies, the focus of the study shifted toward identifying teaching activities and classroom conditions that promote student learning. Thus, the BTES became a major study on teaching effectiveness that generated educational implications dealing with time, instructional processes, and classroom environment. Based on observations in classrooms over a 6-year period, BTES researchers developed an operational definition and measurable index of what they termed academic learning time. Specifically, they defined academic learning time (ALT) as the amount of time a student spends engaged in academic tasks of appropriate difficulty, on which they achieve 80% success or accuracy (Denham & Lieberman). The use of success rate in the BTES for determining ALT was of particular significance because it represented an attempt to provide a time metric for two variables in Carroll's original model, quality of instruction and ability to understand instruction. That is, if a students' success rate was high, then quality of instruction and/or ability to understand instruction must be high. Conversely, if success rate was low, then either or both of these variables must be low (Fisher & Berliner, 1985).

Within the process-outcome tradition, the BTES used ALT as an index of student learning. In attempting to identify the key components of effective teaching, BTES researchers also discovered that a high level of ALT can be taken as evidence of effective teaching. One of the most significant findings from the BTES project is that ALT results from specific measurable, teaching behaviors and has a strong influence on students' academic achievement. Beyond engagement in academic tasks, BTES researchers investigated how students' success rates during engagement affect later achievement. They found that the proportion of time during which academic tasks are performed with high success was positively associated with level of learning. Likewise, when students experienced low success rates in learning activities, they had lower achievement. In evaluating the interactions between teachers and students during instruction, the BTES data suggested that more frequent, substantive interactions (such as teachers presenting explicit content to be learned, closely monitoring students' work, and providing performance feedback) between the student and the teacher were associated with high levels of ALT. Higher levels of ALT, in turn, contributed to achievement. In sum, the BTES findings provided evidence that teaching behaviors and classroom processes which increase motivation and enable students to accrue high levels of ALT have a strong influence on academic learning and student achievement.

Research on the relationship between time and learning since the BTES spans at least four decades. The majority of studies have examined one of three time variables – allocated time, time on task, or academic engaged time. The inconsistent use of time indices makes it difficult to draw comparisons across studies. It also explains why there appear to be mixed findings about the degree to which time influences student learning (Karweit & Slavin, 1981). Despite this variability in measurement choices, however, the literature reveals a fairly consistent pattern. Compared to scheduled or allocated time, engaged time demonstrates the stronger relationship with achievement. As Karweit and Slavin noted, increasing the amount of scheduled time per se is an inefficient means to increase engaged time. It is more effective to strengthen instructional strategies to focus students' attention and cognitive engagement on learning tasks.

Learning time research by Gettinger (1985, 1989) also emphasized the importance of student motivation – what Carroll called perseverance – or the amount of time students are motivated to spend engaged in learning. As predicted by Carroll's model, Gettinger found that spending less time than needed in learning had a direct negative impact on both initial degree of learning and later retention. When elementary school children were permitted to self-determine their amount of study time, they spent, on average, only 68% of the time they actually needed (determined on the basis of a baseline condition in which they were required to learn material to a criterion level of accuracy). As such, Gettinger's research demonstrated the link between motivation and engagement and between engagement and learning, suggesting that student engagement can be differentiated from motivation to the extent that it mediates the relationship between motivation and learning. Although motivating students to engage in learning is important, it is ultimately student engagement (an outcome of student motivation) that contributes to achievement. Similar research conducted with adult learners evaluated the extent to which quantity of instruction influences time spent devoted to self-study (a proxy for AET) and achievement (Gijselaers & Schmidt, 1995; van den Hurk, Wolfhagen, Dolmans, & van der Vleuten, 1998). The results of these studies suggested that the association between allocated time and engaged self-study time may be described as a trade-off mechanism. Allocated instructional time proved instrumental in influencing time spent on self-study and achievement; however, increasing instructional time was only effective to the extent that students were willing to spend an increased amount of time engaged in self-study.

In other words, a higher level of student engagement (afforded by allocating more learning time) resulted only when students were motivated to actually engage in learning for longer periods of available time.

In sum, beginning with the BTES, research on time and classroom learning has consistently shown that the more time students are engaged in learning activities, the more they learn. There is a strong positive relationship between AET and student achievement. Whereas schools and teachers may schedule and allocate the appropriate amount of time for learning, descriptive studies reveal that teachers may not always ensure that students are actively engaged in learning during the allocated time (Mulholland & Cepello, 2006). In some classrooms, students spend less than 50% of the allocated time actually engaged in learning (Black, 2002). Three major factors that contribute to such low engagement are (a) instructional design, (b) classroom management, and (c) student self-study. A later section of this chapter provides a review of strategies for increasing academic engaged and active responding time.

Academic Engaged Time: Definition and Differentiation Among Key Concepts

A theoretical focus on the relationship between time and learning, combined with a research paradigm that implicates time as an index of effective teaching, has contributed to the current conceptualization and definition of AET. An explanation and distinction among several concepts is important for applying the construct of AET to classroom practices.

Research on the relationship between time and learning has been complicated by the variety of ways in which researchers have conceptualized and measured time. Learning time, from which the concept of AET is derived, is best understood as a superordinate concept which encompasses subordinate and more refined concepts of time. As such, time concepts can be ordered on a vertical continuum (see Fig. 31.1). At the top of the continuum is the most broadly described, easily measured, and directly controlled time index, i.e., the number of hours in a school day and number of days in a year. At the bottom is the time variable which is most narrowly focused, challenging to measure, and difficult to modify, i.e., the number of minutes when learning is actually taking place, or AET.

Theoretical conceptualizations of AET identify multiple constituent components along the continuum illustrated in Fig. 31.1. The first component of AET is available time, which represents the total number of hours or days that potentially can be devoted to instruction. Available time is typically established by school district policies and state requirements. The second component, scheduled or allocated time, is the amount of time determined by classroom teachers for instruction within each content domain. Scheduled time represents the upper limit of in-class opportunities for students to be engaged in learning. The process by which scheduled time is converted into productive learning time depends on classroom instruction and management practices, as well as student characteristics. Despite variation across classrooms in the amount of time scheduled for instruction, Marks (2000) found that most variability in AET is attributable to differences in individual student characteristics, not classrooms. This finding may be due to several reasons. First, as implicated in Carroll's model and demonstrated through Bloom's research, some students simply require more time for learning than do others. In fact, individual differences in the amount of time needed for learning, within a constant level of scheduled time, contribute to variable achievement more so than do differences in scheduled time (Gettinger, 1984). A second reason is that students in the same classroom often self-allocate variable time for independent or self-study. Thus, the amount of self-determined or self-scheduled learning time (a time-based metric of student motivation) will vary across individual learners and, in turn, determine individual levels of student engagement, even in the same classroom with constant allocated time.

As shown in Fig. 31.1, scheduled time can be further broken down into instructional and noninstructional time. Instructional time is the amount

```
┌─────────────────────────────────────────┐
│         Available Instructional Time    │
│  ┌───────────────────────────────────┐  │
│  │ Determined by State and School District Policy │  │
│  └───────────────────────────────────┘  │
└─────────────────────────────────────────┘
                    ▽
┌─────────────────────────────────────────┐
│    Scheduled or Allocated Instructional Time │
│  ┌───────────────────────────────────┐  │
│  │ Determined by Individual Classroom Teachers │  │
│  └───────────────────────────────────┘  │
└─────────────────────────────────────────┘
                    ▽
┌─────────────────────────────────────────┐
│            Instructional Time           │
│  ┌───────────────────────────────────┐  │
│  │ Determined by Amount of Non-Instructional Time │  │
│  └───────────────────────────────────┘  │
└─────────────────────────────────────────┘
                    ▽
┌─────────────────────────────────────────┐
│              Engaged Time               │
│  ┌───────────────────────────────────┐  │
│  │ Determined by Instructional Quality and Student Mortivation │  │
│  └───────────────────────────────────┘  │
└─────────────────────────────────────────┘
                    ▽
         ┌──────────────────────┐
         │   Academic Engaged   │
         │        Time          │
         └──────────────────────┘
```

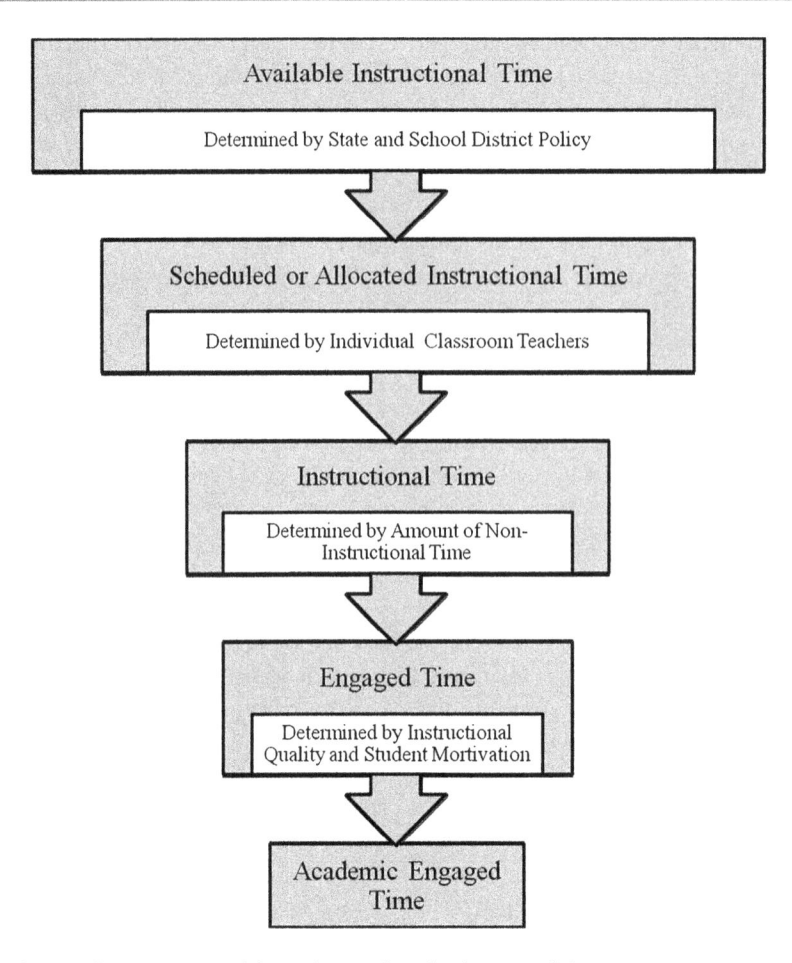

Fig. 31.1 Continuum of components and determinants of academic engaged time

of scheduled time directly devoted to learning and instruction. Noninstructional time, by contrast, is the portion of scheduled time that is spent in nonlearning activities, for example, lunch, recess, or transitions. Research shows that a vast portion of instruction is often eroded by factors such as time spent in maintaining discipline, such that only 38% of a school day is typically spent engaged in learning activities (Aronson, Zimmerman, & Carlos, 1999). Multiple events occur in classrooms that may reduce the amount of scheduled time that is converted to actual instructional time (Caldwell, Huitt, & Graeber, 1982; Hollywood et al., 1995; Kubitschek, Hallinan, Arnett, & Galipeau, 2005; NECTL, 1994). According to Kubitschek et al. (2005), the two primary sources of lost instructional time are transition time and wait time. Transition time is noninstructional time that occurs before (e.g., teacher gives back homework at the start of an instructional activity) and after (e.g., children put away materials after a science lesson) instruction. Whereas transition time is usually a constant time variable for all students, wait time is the amount of time an individual student must wait to receive instructional help, for example, waiting for the teacher's attention after raising one's hand. Although a 60-min period may be scheduled for instruction, some portion of that time is inevitably consumed by noninstructional activities having little to do with learning. The NECTL analysis of how time is used in American schools makes it clear that "reclaiming" the academic day (i.e., protecting and preserving scheduled time for academic content) could nearly double the amount of instructional time students receive.

Engaged time is the proportion of instructional time during which students are cognitively and behaviorally on task or engaged in learning, as evidenced by paying attention, completing work, listening, or participating in relevant discussion. Engaged time includes both passive attending and active responding. Time on task is engaged time on particular learning tasks. Because time on task reflects engaged time on specific learning tasks, it carries a more restricted meaning than engaged time. In terms of learning outcomes, engaged time among students is a necessary, but not sufficient condition for achievement. Time on task reflects engaged time spent on targeted tasks that have clear instructional or learning goals. For example, engagement may be coded as occurring when a student is involved in completing math problems or when reading a book during an instructional time period allocated to science. On-task behavior, however, would not be coded in either situation because the task in which students are engaged is not science. As Carroll (1989) noted, learning time must be filled with activities that are appropriate and relevant. In observational research, time on task is measured in the same way as engaged time; however, the curriculum, instructional activities, or tasks in which the student is engaged, all of which may account for student motivation, are also recorded and enter into the determination of total time on task.

Integral to overall engaged time is what Carroll termed perseverance, or the amount of time a student is willing to spend on learning a task or unit of instruction. Based on Carroll's original conceptualization, the construct of motivation is transformed into a time-based and measurable concept. That is, perseverance is viewed as a time-determined motivational construct. Thus, when measured as the amount of time on task that a student willingly devotes to learning, motivation is a variable that can also be measured in time.

Finally, a certain percentage of engaged time, or time on task, represents the amount of time during which learning actually occurs; this represents academic engaged time. AET is the most carefully delineated conception of time in the literature; it is the portion of time students are actively engaged in relevant academic instruction that leads directly to demonstrated learning. An index of AET is derived by subtracting from the total instructional time not only the amount of time spent on classroom management tasks but also time spent on instructional activities that do not successfully translate into learning. The qualities of both relevance and success are critical for discerning AET. Neither succeeding at irrelevant tasks nor failing at relevant and worthwhile tasks contributes to effective learning. Students gain the most from learning time when they experience a balance of high and medium success on meaningful learning activities. Thus, accurately measuring and ensuring success (e.g., through ongoing progress monitoring) is critical for increasing students' AET.

In sum, a high level of academic engaged time exists when: (a) students are covering content that holds their interest and is viewed as being important and relevant, (b) they are paying attention or on task for most of the class period, and (c) they are experiencing a high level of success or accuracy with most of the assignments they complete. The nexus between student engagement and student motivation is evident in this conceptualization of AET. Students are motivated when they are interested in and understand the purpose of what they are learning, when there are environmental factors to keep them on task (e.g., teacher praise), and when they experience success in learning (Guthrie & Wigfield, 2000). Each variable that contributes to motivation results in high engagement. Whereas learning time components demonstrate varying levels of relationship with student outcomes, AET, determined by both motivation and engagement, has been shown to have the strongest link with school learning and achievement (Gettinger & Ball, 2007).

Practices for Maximizing Academic Engaged Time

Current knowledge about evidence-based approaches to maximize AET derives from effective teaching research which has identified strategies to actively involve students in learning (Gettinger & Stoiber, 2009). As research sug-

Table 31.1 Practices for maximizing academic engaged time

Managerial strategies	Instructional strategies	Student-mediated strategies
• Monitor student behavior • Minimize classroom disruptions and off-task behavior • Reduce transition time • Establish consistent and efficient classroom routines • Decrease class size and learning group sizes	Interactive teaching • Focus on explicit learning objectives • Facilitate active student responding • Provide frequent feedback Instructional design • Match instruction with students' abilities • Use multiple teaching methods • Deliver instruction at a quick, smooth, and efficient pace • Ensure that students understand directions	• Teach students to employ metacognitive and study strategies • Incorporate self-monitoring procedures into the classroom • Support students' self-management skills • Establish consistent classroom routines and structure • Have students set their own goals for learning • Use homework effectively to enhance student learning

gests, rather than simply increasing available instructional time, schools should make better use of existing time and find ways to increase the proportion of time students are engaged in instructional activities (NECTL, 1994). This means ensuring, first, that adequate allocated time is devoted to instruction and, second, that activities which reduce engaged time are minimized. Creating more engaged time, despite its importance, does nothing to advance achievement unless the instructional activities in which students are engaged are appropriate (Prater, 1992). Thus, quality of teaching is the key to enhancing AET. Research demonstrates that when coupled with effective teaching, increased time has a significant impact on student achievement. In effect, providing more instructional time alone cannot be expected to have a significant effect on student learning unless the additional time is devoted to instruction, with students being engaged in well-designed and appropriate learning activities. The purpose of the following sections is to address strategies supported by research that increase AET. The literature points to three factors that, in conjunction with time, contribute to student learning. Two factors (classroom management and appropriateness of instruction) rest primarily with teachers; the third (self-management) rests more with students (see Table 31.1).

Managerial Strategies

Effective classroom management strategies comprise one factor that maximizes AET and contributes to student learning. Research has shown that poor classroom management can erode instructional time and decrease opportunities for students to learn (Smith, 2000). Therefore, it is imperative that teachers implement management strategies to reduce the amount of instructional time that may be lost to noninstructional activities. Several managerial strategies have been shown to promote AET, including closely monitoring student behavior, minimizing classroom disruptions and off-task behavior, reducing transition time, establishing consistent and efficient classroom routines, and decreasing class size or learning group size.

When teachers consistently monitor the behavior of their students during learning activities, AET is maximized. There are myriad ways to facilitate close monitoring, such as planning seating arrangements that enable teachers to view student behavior from anywhere in the classroom, decreasing the amount of time spent at the teacher's desk by frequently circulating the room, going to students when they have questions rather than requiring students to come to the teacher, utilizing student volunteers for handling classroom materials, and acknowledging and responding to appropriate engagement behaviors (Gettinger & Ball, 2007). Teachers can systematically provide reinforcement for student engagement by implementing a token economy in their classrooms. There is strong evidence supporting the effectiveness of token economy interventions for a range of classroom behaviors, including student engagement (DuPaul & Stoner, 2003). Token economies involve the use of secondary reinforcers, or tokens, which are delivered to students to produce positive behavioral change.

Tokens (e.g., poker chips, coins, check marks, points, stickers) can be tailored to the developmental level and individual preferences of children in a classroom. In the case of student engagement, for example, tokens may be dispensed when students are on task and involved in relevant work for a clearly specified amount of time. Token economy interventions typically utilize group contingencies that may be independent, interdependent, or dependent. Independent contingencies involve providing reinforcement to individual students contingent on their behavior; an interdependent contingency requires all students in the classroom to be engaged in order for any single student to receive the reinforcer; and, finally, dependent contingencies involve targeting specific students or a group of students who must meet the engagement criterion level for all students to receive the reinforcer (Litow & Pumroy, 1975). Although research supports the overall effectiveness of group-oriented contingencies, studies comparing the relative benefits of different group contingency procedures have yielded mixed results, indicating that group procedures should be developed and implemented based on the unique characteristics and structure of each classroom (Kelshaw-Levering, Sterling-Turner, Henry, & Skinner, 2000).

Other managerial strategies that minimize disruptions, off-task behavior, and long transitions also contribute to AET. Instructional time that is lost to nonlearning activities, such as disruptions, disciplinary issues, or transitions, can be quite substantial in some schools and classrooms (Aronson et al., 1999). Research has shown that the proportion of noninstructional time may be even greater in schools or classrooms with high percentages of at-risk students. A study by Stichter, Stormont, and Lewis (2008), for example, investigated the amount of scheduled instructional time lost to noninstructional activities in Title I versus non-Title I elementary schools. Results showed that teachers in Title I schools spent more time in noninstructional activities (e.g., transitions, disciplining students) than did teachers in non-Title I schools. In addition, in Title I schools, there was a higher occurrence of students entering and leaving classrooms during periods of academic instruction, such as literacy periods or math instruction. To decrease time spent in transitions, the authors recommended that teachers develop specific entrance and exit routines for students who must leave the classroom for related services. Moreover, the authors recommended that these routines be explicitly taught and practiced to maximize the amount of time students are actively engaged in instruction-related activities (Stichter et al., 2008).

Another strategy to minimize time spent in transitions involves using verbal or nonverbal transition cues when the entire class is making a noninstructional transition, such as going from the classroom to the music room (Kauchak & Eggen, 2003). Procedures for executing transitions should be explicitly communicated and actively taught not only at the beginning of the year but throughout the year as necessary. Teachers can also provide class-wide incentives for following transition routines quickly and accurately. Although the type of effective transition cues varies across classrooms (e.g., flickering lights, using key signal words or phrases), what is most critical is that all students are able to recognize and interpret the cue. If a transition is requiring too much time, teachers can establish a time limit for the transition and provide reinforcement for students who complete the transition within the limit. After students are able to complete transitions quickly, a goal can be set to gradually reduce the time until the targeted transition time is achieved (Ostrosky, Jung, Hemmeter, & Thomas, 2003).

Other managerial strategies to increase AET include having clearly defined and taught rules, expectations for being engaged during learning activities, and consistent routines. Rules and expectations are most effective when they are clearly posted in the classroom to support students' awareness and knowledge of them. In addition to rules being understood by students, appropriate behavior in accordance with rules and expectations should be positively reinforced, whereas failure to comply should receive consistent, immediate, and effective consequences. To the extent possible, teachers can also preserve engaged learning time through implementing consistent routines for noninstructional activities (Odden & Archibald, 2009). Doing so involves handling noninstructional obligations (e.g., taking attendance) after students have begun working on their tasks or by completing all noninstructional activities during a predetermined time of day set aside for such activities (Harmin & Toth, 2006). Soliciting assistance from the administration to minimize external interruptions (e.g., intercom announcements, unscheduled visitations) is another effective way to protect instructional time and increase students' engaged learning time (Odden & Archibald).

Finally, there is clear evidence that the size of a class or learning group can significantly impact AET (Fowler, 1995). Research has demonstrated that small class sizes, particularly in the primary grades, allow teachers to use time more efficiently to increase AET and promote student achievement (Odden & Archibald, 2009). Blatchford, Russell, Bassett, Brown, and Martin (2007) documented more positive learning and social outcomes in schools with class sizes less than 15 students compared to schools with larger class sizes. Using a multimethod approach, these researchers found that small class sizes allowed students to receive a higher degree of teacher attention and take a more active, engaged role in their learning (Blatchford et al., 2007). Because manipulating class size may not be an option in all schools, teachers can also minimize the size of learning groups in their classrooms. Smaller learning groups, especially when teacher-directed, have been shown to promote a higher level of student engagement in learning (Gettinger & Ball, 2007).

Instructional Strategies

Effective instructional practices comprise the second factor related to students' academic engaged time (see Table 31.1). Effective teaching research, conceptualized within a process-outcome perspective, has identified several instructional variables that are positively correlated with AET (Gettinger & Kohler, 2006; Gettinger & Stoiber, 2009). Generally, strategies related to how teachers deliver instruction (i.e., interactive teaching behaviors) and how they design or structure their teaching have been shown to have a significant impact on AET (Rosenshine, 1995).

Interactive Teaching

Teaching behaviors that actively engage in students in learning are collectively referred to as interactive teaching. Interactive teaching strategies involve (a) focusing on explicit learning objectives, (b) facilitating active student responding, and (c) providing frequent feedback (Good & Brophy, 2003).

To maximize AET, it is critical for teaching to incorporate a strong focus on academic content and learning objectives. Academic focus is determined by the amount of time devoted to academic activities as well as by the extent to which instruction is linked with learning goals and student accountability for reaching those goals. Preplanning is necessary to ensure that instruction incorporates a strong academic focus. Effective planning involves, first, developing clear learning goals and objectives for the lesson. Next, learning activities are designed to help students achieve the goals and objectives. According to Kauchek and Eggen (2003), designing effective learning activities with an academic focus requires determination of the instructional format (e.g., whole group, small group), specification of lesson materials, and establishment of assessment procedure to measure student learning and attainment of goals.

In addition to an explicit academic focus, interactive teaching involves promoting high levels of active student responding or engagement. One mechanism to ensure that all students remain engaged in class discussion is the use of effective questioning techniques (Good & Brophy, 2003). "Good questions" that promote engagement are clear, purposeful, brief, sequenced, and focused on extending students' thinking (Gall, 1984). An effective questioning strategy that has been shown to increase engagement among all students follows three sequential steps (Chuska, 1995). Teachers, first, pose a question to the entire class. Then they give students wait time to think about the question. After a sufficient amount of wait time, they call on an individual student to respond. Using this method requires all students to be responsible for carefully considering an answer to the question because the teacher may call on any student. In contrast, when teachers pose a question to a specific student, only that student has the responsibility for answering, and others may be less likely to contribute their thoughts. To heighten engagement among all learners, it is important for teachers to distribute questions evenly to a range of students in their classrooms and not allow a select group of students to answer the majority of the questions (Good & Brophy). Other strategies for promoting active responding include using choral responding, peer tutoring, and cooperative learning groups. Many existing assignments and activities can be easily adapted to involve a higher degree of active student responding, such as having students work in pairs rather than individually on projects or assigned work (Gettinger & Ball, 2007).

Providing frequent feedback is another key element of interactive teaching that fosters student engagement (Bangert-Drowns, Kulik, Kulik, & Morgan, 1991). Effective feedback is characterized as being detailed, accurate, and immediate, as well as encouraging and supportive. Effective feedback acknowledges the accomplishments students have made and contributes to students' self-efficacy, confidence they can attain goals, and motivation to work toward their goals (Butler & Winne, 1995; Kluger & DeNisi, 1996). Self-evaluation is a skill that can be taught to students as a means of providing immediate feedback about performance (Bandura, Martinez-Pons, & Zimmerman, 1992). Although strategies may vary, providing feedback to students that is frequent, specific, and relevant has strong research support as effective means of enhancing AET (Gettinger & Ball, 2007; Kluger & DeNisi, 1996; Mory, 1992).

Instructional Design

In addition to interactive teaching, several instructional design features have been shown to increase students' academic engaged time (Frieberg & Driscoll, 2000). The first design feature is the degree to which instruction is appropriately matched with students' ability. To be academically engaged, students must be both challenged and able to experience a high rate of success. Students differ in the amount of time, exposure, practice, and instruction needed to learn. Therefore, being able to differentiate instruction based on individual student needs is an instructional practice that will promote AET (Tomlinson, 2003). Using collaborative planning with students; assigning students to work with peer tutors, volunteers, or aides; and monitoring student understanding are examples of ways to accommodate the diverse needs of children in a classroom and ensure that all students are academically engaged (Freiberg & Driscoll).

Along with employing strategies to increase academic engagement, it is important for teachers to foster students' motivation for learning, a key determinant of student engagement. According to self-determination theory (SDT; Ryan & Deci, 2000), students will be engaged versus disengaged in learning, in large part, as a function of motivation. Specifically, students initiate and maintain involvement in learning activities to the extent that they believe sustained engagement will lead to desired outcomes or goals. Thus, within SDT, engagement is viewed as a goal-directed or motivated behavior. Research on students' goal-directed behavior has distinguished among different types of goals which, in turn, lead to different long-term behavioral consequences, such as level of engagement (Deci & Ryan, 2000). According to SDT, students experience two types of motivation, autonomous motivation and controlled motivation (Deci & Ryan). Autonomous motivation involves students' intrinsic motivation as well as extrinsic motivation in which students have integrated external values (e.g., the importance of academic engagement) into their own personal value system. Conversely, controlled motivation involves external regulation (e.g., by a teacher) that controls students to behave in a certain way. For example, students could be motivated to engage in learning new skills because they are interested in the content or understand its value. Conversely, students' motivation for engagement in learning might be to get a good grade or to avoid punishment. In these examples, the amount of motivation may not vary, but the nature and focus of motivation does.

Research has demonstrated that autonomous motivation, as illustrated in the first scenario, contributes to higher levels of self-determined engagement in learning and, more importantly, better long-term learning outcomes (Deci & Ryan, 2008; Ryan & Deci, 2000). Therefore, teachers should seek to promote students' autonomous motivation for learning (e.g., through providing student choice, incorporating adequate challenge into learning tasks, establishing meaningful learning goals) to achieve high levels of academic engagement over time.

Using multiple and diverse teachings methods is another aspect of instructional design to increase AET. Students often become disengaged if the same format (e.g., teacher lecture) is always used. Because students learn differently, not all students may be able to benefit from a strict lecture format. Therefore, blending lecture formats with other teaching strategies (e.g., questioning, discussions) will promote active learning and engagement for a greater proportion of students (Freiberg & Driscoll, 2000). It is also important that the instructional sequence is effective and appropriative given students' developmental level. Using a variety of teaching methods is particularly critical when reteaching material to low-achieving students; reteaching content will be effective only if the instruction is delivered in a different format and with different examples than the first time when instruction was given (Gettinger & Ball, 2007).

Considering the pace of the lesson is another feature of instructional design that promotes AET. A quick, smooth, and efficient instructional pace increases the amount of content covered as well as the amount of active learning time available during a class period or school day (Gettinger & Ball, 2007). Breaking lessons into small steps, changing the topic or procedure when the teacher notices a decline in student engagement, and maintaining high expectations for student involvement are all examples of effective strategies for delivering fast-paced instruction (Harmin & Toth, 2006).

Finally, instructional time and AET is often lost when students fail to understand directions for an assignment or task. This underscores the importance of having instructions and expectations that are clearly explained and understood by all students. Research has identified several methods for maximizing the likelihood that students understand directions, including (a) having students paraphrase directions, (b) having them write the directions down, (c) visually displaying directions in the classroom, (d) keeping directions simple, (e) obtaining all students' attention before giving directions, (f) modeling steps of the directions, and (g) allowing students to begin only after all directions have been delivered (Frieberg & Driscoll, 2000; Gettinger & Ball, 2007; Marzano, Pickering, & Pollock, 2001). Research has consistently demonstrated that clear directions and expectations increase students' understanding of learning tasks as well as the amount of time they spend in learning (Marzano et al., 2001).

Student-Mediated Strategies

Consistent with Carroll's model, the amount of time students spend engaged in learning is, to some extent, self-determined and indicative of their level of motivation for learning. Although there are many instructional and managerial strategies teachers can employ to promote AET and increase students' motivation, students ultimately play a major role in determining their own learning and levels of engagement in learning. Factors such as low self-efficacy or limited self-monitoring skills are important to consider as they typically function to decrease the amount of time students spend engaged in learning (Bandura et al., 1992). Student-mediated strategies focus on supporting cognitive engagement, autonomous motivation, and self-regulation among students. Specifically, these strategies include teaching students to employ metacognitive and study strategies, self-monitoring procedures, and self-management skills (Borkowski & Muthukrishna, 1992; Shapiro & Cole, 1994; Zimmerman, Greenberg, & Weinstein, 1994).

According to a metacognitive perspective, the amount of time students are academically engaged is influenced by their learning and studying skills, such as their ability to plan and organize study time or their approach to taking tests (Borkowski & Muthukrishna, 1992; Butler & Winne, 1995; Zimmerman et al., 1994). Providing instruction to develop these cognitive strategies can enhance student's academic engaged time as it enables them to be organized and efficient in their learning. Learning strategies also support active engagement during independent work because students are better equipped to approach the material and plan their studying. Furthermore, these strategies may lead to increased student motivation for learning, which in turn may foster a greater level of engagement. Effective learning strategies include note-taking skills, time management skills, test-taking skills, and accessing resources that support students' understanding and interactions with text, such as story maps or outlines (Gettinger & Ball, 2007; Marzano et al., 2001).

Another student-mediated method for increasing academic engaged time is self-monitoring (Cole & Bambara, 2000; Cole, Marder, & McCann, 2000). Students must be able to self-monitor when they are learning so they can plan and adjust time use according to their learning needs. Even highly motivated students may fail to appropriately monitor their own learning or use of time (Gettinger, 1985; Zimmerman et al., 1994). Self-monitoring alone can be a highly effective intervention to increase AET among students (Levendoski & Cartledge, 2000). In addition to contributing to AET, self-monitoring strategies have several documented benefits, including promoting positive classroom behavior; increasing student motivation for learning, especially when students are able to exercise choice in selecting the self-recording method or target behavior; and providing immediate feedback to students about their behavior and learning (Carr & Punzo, 1993; Moxley, 1998; Trammel, Schloss, & Alper, 1994).

Several approaches for self-monitoring in classrooms have been documented as being effective in promoting students' engagement in learning, such as keeping a tally count on a paper taped to the child's desk or the inside of a notebook (Reid, 1996; Rock, 2005; Shimabukuro, Prater, Jenkins, & Edelen-Smith, 1999). Regardless of the recording method, the process of self-monitoring involves having students self-observe and record predetermined behaviors or outcomes at signaled intervals, such as the duration of engaged time, frequency of engagement behaviors, task completion, or overall accuracy. Evidence-based resources are also available to individualize the self-monitoring procedure to match children's needs and preferences. For younger children or children with disabilities, for example, a self-monitoring tool called "Countoons" has been developed and evaluated (Daly & Ranalli, 2003). Countoons are cartoon illustrations of students' appropriate and inappropriate behaviors, paired with a contingency for meeting an established criterion of appropriate behaviors. The drawings also contain space for children to record the frequency of their own behaviors. This tool is particularly appealing because it enables very young students to monitor their own behavior even when they cannot read. Moreover, by allowing students to draw the cartoons themselves, they may be more motivated to take an active role in their learning and engagement. For example, when the goal is for students to increase their engaged learning time, they can draw a picture of themselves reading at their desk and circle the number of times they perform the behavior at designated intervals (Daly & Ranalli).

Self-monitoring methods are part of the broader set of student-mediated or self-management skills (Cole & Bambara, 2000; Shapiro & Cole, 1994). Self-management skills enable children to self-direct their learning behaviors, experience a greater degree of autonomy in the classroom, and maximize their academic engaged time (Shapiro & Cole, 1994; Wehmeyer et al., 2007; Zimmerman et al., 1994). Research has shown that self-management skills are associated with positive educational outcomes, including higher student engagement, academic performance, and work productivity (Wehmeyer et al.). There are many strategies teachers can use to promote students' self-management skills, such as using guided questioning to teach students a systematic way of approaching tasks. Questions may be used to cue or prompt students to gather necessary materials, review the instructions, approximate the amount of time needed for the assignment, and consider whether they are equipped with the skills and knowledge required for the task. This strategy has been used effectively with individual students or posted in the classroom for all students to use (Rock, 2005).

Structure and routines in the classroom also promote self-management skills and, in turn, function to increase AET. When routines are consistent and explicit, students are able to follow them independently, requiring less assistance from the teacher. For example, if a teacher always has her students do a warm-up activity at the beginning of class, if students understand instructions for the warm-up activity, and if they know where to access the appropriate materials, they will be able to begin working on the task immediately upon arrival to the classroom and minimize the loss of instructional time. Conversely, without consistent expectations, students are not able to direct their own learning and will likely spend less time academically engaged.

Another student-mediated approach to increase AET involves having students set their own goals for engagement and learning (Bandura et al., 1992). Goal-setting strategies provide opportunities for students to establish and monitor a personal learning goal for each day. By allowing students to set their own goals for learning, they can become empowered and may experience greater motivation to work toward their goals. Harmin and Toth (2006) described a goal-setting procedure in which at the beginning of the day, the teacher invites students to identify one goal for themselves and record it in an individualized log book. At the end of the day, students reflect on how successful they were at reaching their goals and share this with the class. Establishing daily goals has been shown to maintain students' engagement in learning activities throughout the day (Rock, 2005).

Self-management skills, particularly self-monitoring and goal setting, are also effective for increasing the degree to which students complete homework assignments (Cooper, Robinson, & Patall, 2006; Dawson, 2007). Effective use of homework in itself is a way to maximize academic engaged time because it extends learning time beyond the typical school day (Cooper et al., 2006). To ensure that homework is being used most effectively, teachers should assign work that is relevant to current learning objectives, matched to students' abilities, motivating, assigned in consistent amounts, and reviewed the following day. Other effective homework strategies may include (a) communicating with parents and families about homework expectations, (b) providing frequent progress reports when needed, (c) clearly explaining homework assignments to students, (d) establishing classroom homework routines and a system for helping students with homework, (e) teaching effective study skills, and, when possible, (f) incorporating student or creating a menu of homework assignments (Dawson).

Concluding Remarks

The link between time and learning remains well documented in educational research. The relationship between time and learning, however, depends on the degree to which available time is devoted to high-quality instruction and the extent to which students are motivated to invest time in learning. Any addition to allocated time will improve achievement to the extent that it is actually used for instruction and, in turn, converted to academic engaged time for learners. Simply assigning more study time to a topic will not automatically increase the student's learning. When instructional quality, appropriateness of instruction relative to student abilities, and incentives for learning, however, are all high, then more time will pay off in greater learning. The key is to maximize students' academic engaged time.

In one form or another, learning time plays an important role in understanding, predicting, and controlling instructional processes across a range of activities. Indeed, AET has the potential to capture critical aspects of the teaching-learning process, including student motivation. For researchers, AET is not only an instructional time variable, it is actually a measure or quantifiable index of quality of instruction. The assumption is that as AET is accrued, quality instruction is taking place.

To the extent that research underscores the need to maximize AET, investigators must continue to address what can be done to enhance or increase AET for all learners, particularly learners who may be at risk for school failure (Goodman, 1990; Woelfel, 2005). Making good use of existing time, whereby students experience high success on meaningful tasks, is more likely to substantially increase both AET and student achievement than simply allocating more instructional time (e.g., lengthening the school day or year). It is only when instructional time is used efficiently and effectively, when student motivation for engagement is high, and when AET is maximized that more time will result in improved academic outcomes for all learners.

References

Adelman, N. E., Haslam, M. B., & Pringle, B. A. (1996). *The uses of time for teaching and learning* (Vol. 1). Washington, DC: Policy Studies Associates, Inc.

Anderson, L. W. (Ed.). (1984). *Time and school learning: Theory, research and practice*. New York: St. Martin's Press.

Anderson, L. W. (Ed.). (1985). *Perspectives on school learning: Selected writings of John B. Carroll*. Hillsdale, NJ: Lawrence Erlbaum.

Aronson, J., Zimmerman, J., & Carlos, L. (1999). *Improving student achievement by extending school: Is it just a matter of time?* San Francisco: WestEd.

Bandura, A., Martinez-Pons, M., & Zimmerman, B. J. (1992). Self-motivation for academic attainment: The role of self-efficacy beliefs and personal goal setting. *American Educational Research Journal, 29*, 663–674.

Bangert-Drowns, R. L., Kulik, C. C., Kulik, J. A., & Morgan, M. (1991). The instructional effects of feedback in test-like events. *Review of Educational Research, 61*, 213–238.

Ben-Peretz, M., & Bromme, R. (Eds.). (1990). *The nature of time in schools: Theoretical concepts, practitioner perceptions*. New York: Teachers College Press.

Berliner, D. (1990a). What's all the fuss about instructional time? In M. Ben-Peretz & R. Bromme (Eds.), *The nature of time in schools: Theoretical concepts, practitioner perceptions* (pp. 3–35). New York: Teachers College Press.

Berliner, D. (1990b). The place of process-product research in developing the agenda for research on teaching thinking. *Educational Psychologist, 24*, 325–344.

Black, S. (2002). Time for learning. *American School Board Journal, 189*, 58–62.

Blatchford, P., Russell, A., Bassett, P., Brown, P., & Martin, C. (2007). The effect of class size on the teaching of pupils aged 7–11 years. *School Effectiveness and School Improvement, 18*(2), 147–172.

Block, J. H. (Ed.). (1971). *Mastery learning: Theory and practice*. New York: Holt, Rinehart, & Winston.

Block, J. H. (1983). Learning rates and mastery learning. *Outcomes, 2*(3), 18–23.

Block, J. H., & Anderson, L. W. (1975). *Mastery learning in classroom instruction*. New York: Macmillan.

Bloom, B. S. (1974). Time and learning. *American Psychologist, 29*, 682–688.

Borkowski, J. G., & Muthukrishna, N. (1992). Moving metacognition into the classroom: "Working models" and effective strategy teaching. In M. Pressley, K. R. Harris, & J. T. Guthrie (Eds.), *Promoting academic competence and literacy in school* (pp. 477–501). San Diego, CA: Academic.

Butler, D. L., & Winne, P. H. (1995). Feedback and self-regulated learning: A theoretical synthesis. *Review of Educational Research, 65*, 245–281.

Caldwell, J. H., Huitt, W. G., & Graeber, A. O. (1982). Time spent in learning: Implications from research. *The Elementary School Journal, 82*, 471–480.

Carr, S. C., & Punzo, R. P. (1993). The effects of self-monitoring of academic accuracy and productivity on the performance of students with behavioral disorders. *Behavior Disorders, 18*, 241–250.

Carroll, J. B. (1963). A model of school learning. *Teachers College Record, 64*, 723–733.

Carroll, J. B. (1984). The model of school learning: Progress of an idea. In L. W. Anderson (Ed.), *Time and school learning: Theory, research and practice* (pp. 15–46). New York: St. Martin's Press.

Carroll, J. B. (1989). The Carroll model: A 25-year retrospective and prospective view. *Educational Researcher, 18*, 26–31.

Chuska, K. (1995). *Improving classroom questions: A teacher's guide to increasing student motivation, participation, and higher level thinking*. Bloomington, IN: Phi Delta Kappa Educational Foundation.

Cole, C. L., & Bambara, L. M. (2000). Self-monitoring: Theory and practice. In E. S. Shapiro & T. R. Kratochwill (Eds.), *Behavioral assessment in schools: Theory, research, and clinical foundations* (2nd ed., pp. 202–232). New York: Guilford Press.

Cole, C. L., Marder, T., & McCann, L. (2000). Self-monitoring. In E. S. Shapiro & T. R. Kratochwill (Eds.), *Conducting school-based assessments of child and adolescent behavior* (pp. 121–149). New York: Guilford Press.

Cooley, W. W., & Leinhardt, G. (1976). *The application of a model for investigating classroom processes*. Pittsburgh, PA: University of Pittsburgh, Learning Research & Development Center.

Cooley, W. W., & Leinhardt, G. (1980). The instructional dimensions study. *Educational Evaluation and Policy Analysis, 2*, 7–26.

Cooper, H., Robinson, J. C., & Patall, A. (2006). Does homework improve academic achievement? A synthesis of research, 1987–2003. *Review of Educational Research, 76*, 1–62.

Daly, P. M., & Ranalli, P. (2003). Using Countoons to teach self-monitoring skills. *Teaching Exceptional Children, 35*(5), 30–35.

Dawson, P. (2007). Best practices in managing homework. In A. Thomas & J. Grimes (Eds.), *Best practices in school psychology V* (pp. 1073–1084). Bethesda, MD: National Association of School Psychologists.

Deci, E., & Ryan, R. (2000). Intrinsic and extrinsic motivations: Classic definitions and new directions. *Contemporary Educational Psychology, 25*, 54–67.

Deci, E., & Ryan, R. (2008). Self-determination theory: A macrotheory of human motivation, development and health. *Canadian Psychology, 49*(3), 182–185.

Denham, C., & Lieberman, A. (Eds.). (1980). *Time to learn.* Washington, DC: U.S. Department of Education.

DuPaul, G. J., & Stoner, G. (2003). *ADHD in the schools: Assessment and intervention strategies.* New York: Guilford Press.

Fisher, C. W., & Berliner, D. C. (1985). *Perspectives on instructional time.* New York: Longman.

Fisher, D. (2009). The use of instructional time in the typical high school classroom. *The Educational Forum, 73*, 168–173.

Fowler, W. (1995). School size and student outcomes. *Advances in Educational Productivity, 5*, 3–26.

Fredrick, W. C., & Walberg, H. J. (1980). Learning as a function of time. *The Journal of Educational Research, 73*, 183–194.

Frieberg, H. J., & Driscoll, A. (2000). *Universal teaching strategies* (3rd ed.). Boston: Allyn & Bacon.

Gall, M. (1984). Synthesis of research on teachers' questioning. *Educational Leadership, 42*, 40–47.

Gettinger, M. (1984). Individual differences in time needed for learning: A review of the literature. *Educational Psychologist, 19*, 15–29.

Gettinger, M. (1985). Time allocated and time spent relative to time needed for learning as determinants of achievement. *Journal of Educational Psychology, 77*, 3–11.

Gettinger, M. (1989). Effects of maximizing time spent and minimizing time needed on pupil achievement. *American Educational Research Journal, 26*, 73–91.

Gettinger, M., & Ball, C. (2007). Best practices in increasing academic engaged time. In A. Thomas & J. Grimes (Eds.), *Best practices in school psychology V* (pp. 1043–1075). Bethesda, MD: National Association of School Psychologists.

Gettinger, M., & Kohler, K. (2006). Process-outcome approaches to classroom management and effective teaching. In C. M. Evertson & C. S. Weinstein (Eds.), *Handbook of classroom management: Research, practice, and contemporary issues* (pp. 73–96). Mahwah, NJ: Lawrence Erlbaum.

Gettinger, M., & Stoiber, K. (2009). Effective teaching and effective schools. In T. B. Gutkin & C. R. Reynolds (Eds.), *The handbook of school psychology* (4th ed., pp. 769–790). Hoboken, NJ: John Wiley.

Gijselaers, W. H., & Schmidt, H. G. (1995). Effects of quantity of instruction on time spent on learning and achievement. *Educational Research and Evaluation, 1*, 183–201.

Good, T. L., & Brophy, J. E. (2003). *Looking in classrooms* (9th ed.). Boston: Allyn & Bacon.

Goodman, L. (1990). *Time and learning in the special education classroom.* Albany, NY: State University of New York Press.

Guskey, T. R. (2001). Mastery learning. In N. J. Smelser & P. B. Baltes (Eds.), *International encyclopedia of social and behavioral sciences* (pp. 9372–9377). Oxford, UK: Elsevier Science.

Guthrie, J. T., & Wigfield, A. (2000). Engagement and motivation in reading. In M. L. Kamil, P. B. Mosenthal, P. D. Pearson, & R. Barr (Eds.), *Handbook of reading research* (Vol. 3, pp. 403–424). Mahwah, NJ: Lawrence Erlbaum.

Haertel, G. D., Walberg, H. F., & Weinstein, T. (1983). Psychological models of educational performance: A theoretical synthesis of constructs. *Review of Educational Research, 53*, 75–91.

Harmin, M., & Toth, M. (2006). *Inspiring active learning: A complete handbook for today's teachers.* Alexandria, VA: Association of Supervision and Curriculum Development.

Harnishfeger, A., & Wiley, D. (1976). The teaching-learning process in elementary schools: A synoptic view. *Curriculum Inquiry, 6*, 5–43.

Harnishfeger, A., & Wiley, D. (1985). Origins of active learning time. In C. W. Fisher & D. C. Berliner (Eds.), *Perspectives on instructional time* (pp. 133–156). New York: Longman.

Hollywood, T. M., Salisbury, C. I., Rainforth, B., & Palombaro, M. (1995). Use of instructional time in classrooms serving students with and without severe disabilities. *Exceptional Children, 61*, 242–254.

Huitt, W. (1995). A systems model of the teaching/learning process. *Educational Psychology Interactive.* Valdosta, GA: College of Education, Valdosta State University. Retrieved March, 2010, from http://teach.valdosta.edu/whuitt/materials/tchlrnmd.html

Karweit, N. (1989). Time and learning: A review. In R. E. Slavin (Ed.), *School and classroom organization* (pp. 69–95). Hillsdale, NJ: Lawrence Erlbaum.

Karweit, N., & Slavin, R. E. (1981). Measurement and modeling choices in studies of time and learning. *American Educational Research Journal, 18*, 151–171.

Kauchak, D. P., & Eggen, P. D. (2003). *Learning and teaching: Research-based methods* (4th ed.). Boston: Allyn & Bacon.

Kelshaw-Levering, K., Sterling-Turner, H. E., Henry, J. R., & Skinner, C. H. (2000). Randomized interdependent group contingencies. *Psychology in the Schools, 37*, 523–534.

Kluger, A. N., & DeNisi, A. (1996). The effects of feedback interventions on performance: A historical review, a meta-analysis, and a preliminary feedback intervention theory. *Psychological Bulletin, 119*, 254–284.

Kubitschek, W. N., Hallinan, M. T., Arnett, S. M., & Galipeau, K. S. (2005). High school schedule changes and the effect of lost instructional time on achievement. *High School Journal, 89*, 63–71.

Leinhardt, G. (1978). Applying a classroom process model to instructional evaluation. *Curriculum Inquiry, 8*, 155–176.

Levendoski, L. S., & Cartledge, G. (2000). Self-monitoring for elementary school children with emotional disturbances: Classroom application for increased academic responding. *Behavioral Disorders, 25*, 211–224.

Litow, L., & Pumroy, D. (1975). A brief review of classroom group-oriented contingencies. *Journal of Applied Behavior Analysis, 8*, 341–347.

Marks, H. M. (2000). Student engagement in instructional activity: Patterns in the elementary, middle, and high school years. *American Educational Research Journal, 37*, 153–184.

Marzano, R. J., Pickering, D. J., & Pollock, J. E. (2001). *Classroom instruction that works: Research-based strategies for increasing student achievement.* Alexandria, VA: Association for Supervision and Curriculum Development.

Mory, E. H. (1992). The use of informational feedback in instruction: Implications for future research. *Educational Technology Research and Development, 40*, 5–20.

Moxley, R. A. (1998). Treatment-only designs and student self-recording as strategies for public school teachers. *Education and Treatment of Children, 21*, 37–61.

Mulholland, R., & Cepello, M. (2006). What teacher candidates need to know about academic learning time. *International Journal of Special Education, 21*, 63–73.

National Education Commission on Time and Learning (NECTL). (1994). *Prisoners of time: Report of the National Commission on Time and Learning.* Washington, DC: U.S. Government Printing Office. (reprinted in 2005).

Odden, A. R., & Archibald, S. J. (2009). *Doubling student performance…and finding the resources to do it.* Thousand Oaks, CA: Corwin.

Ostrosky, M. M., Jung, E. Y., Hemmeter, M. L., & Thomas, D. (2003). *Helping children make transitions between activities.* Washington, DC: Center on the Social and Emotional Foundations for Early Learning.

Prater, M. A. (1992). Increasing time-on-task in the classroom: Suggestions for improving the amount of time learners spend in on-task behaviors. *Intervention in School and Clinic, 28*, 22–27.

Rangel, E. S. (2007). Time to learn. *Research Points, 5*(2), 104.

Reid, R. (1996). Research in self-monitoring with students with learning disabilities. *Journal of Learning Disabilities, 29*, 317–331.

Rock, M. L. (2005). Use of strategic self-monitoring to enhance academic engagement, productivity, and accuracy of students with and without disabilities. *Journal of Positive Behavior Interventions, 7*, 3–17.

Rosenshine, B. (1995). Advances in research on instruction. *The Journal of Educational Research, 88*, 262–268.

Ryan, R. M., & Deci, E. L. (2000). Self-determination theory and the facilitation of intrinsic motivation, social development, and well-being. *American Psychologist, 55*, 68–78.

Shapiro, E. S., & Cole, C. L. (1994). *Behavior change in the classroom: Self-management interventions.* New York: Guilford Press.

Shimabukuro, S. M., Prater, M. A., Jenkins, A., & Edelen-Smith, P. (1999). The effects of self-monitoring of academic performance on students with learning disabilities and ADD/ADHD. *Education and Treatment of Children, 22*, 397–414.

Smith, B. A. (2000). Quantity matters: Annual instruction time in an urban school system. *Educational Administration Quarterly, 36*, 652–682.

Squires, D., Huitt, W., & Segars, J. (1983). *Effective classrooms and schools: A research-based perspective.* Washington, DC: Association for Supervision and Curriculum Development.

Stanley, S. O., & Greenwood, C. R. (1981). *CISSAR: Code for instructional structure and student academic response. Observer's manual.* Kansas City, KS: University of Kansas, Bureau of Child Research, Juniper Gardens Children's Project.

Stichter, J. P., Stormont, M., & Lewis, T. J. (2008). Instructional practices and behavior during reading: A descriptive summary and comparison of practices in Title I and non-Title I elementary schools. *Psychology in the Schools, 46*, 172–183.

Tomlinson, C. A. (2003). Differentiating instruction for academic diversity. In M. Cooper (Ed.), *Classroom teaching skills* (7th ed., pp. 134–165). New York: Houghton Mifflin.

Trammel, D. L., Schloss, P. T., & Alper, S. (1994). Using self-recording, evaluation, and graphing to increase completion of homework assignments. *Journal of Learning Disabilities, 27*, 75–81.

van den Hurk, M., Wolfhagen, H., Dolmans, D., & van der Vleuten, C. (1998). The relation between time spent on individual study and academic achievement in a problem-based curriculum. *Advances in Health Sciences Education, 3*, 43–49.

Wang, M. C., Haertel, G. D., & Walberg, H. J. (1993). Toward a knowledge base for school learning. *Review of Educational Research, 63*, 249–294.

Wehmeyer, M. L., Agran, M., Hughes, C., Martin, J. E., Mithaug, D. E., & Palmer, S. B. (2007). *Promoting self-determination in students with developmental disabilities.* New York: Guilford Press.

Wiley, D. E., & Harnishfeger, A. (1974). Explosion of a myth: Quantity of schooling and exposure to instruction: Major educational vehicles. *Educational Researcher, 3*, 7–11.

Woelfel, K. (2005). Learning takes time for at-risk students. *Education Digest, 71*(4), 28–30.

Wyne, M., & Stuck, G. (1982). Time and learning: Implications for the classroom teacher. *The Elementary School Journal, 83*, 67–75.

Zimmerman, B., Greenberg, D., & Weinstein, C. (1994). Self-regulating academic study time: A strategy approach. In D. H. Schunk & B. J. Zimmerman (Eds.), *Self-regulation of learning and performance: Issues and educational applications* (pp. 181–199). Hillsdale, NJ: Lawrence Erlbaum.

Deep Engagement as a Complex System: Identity, Learning Power and Authentic Enquiry

32

Ruth Deakin Crick

Abstract

This chapter develops a definition of engagement which is underpinned by a participatory enquiry paradigm and invites an exploration of patterns and relationships between variables rather than a focus on a single variable. It suggests that engagement is best understood as a complex system including a range of interrelated factors internal and external to the learner, in place and in time, which shape his or her engagement with learning opportunities. The implications of this approach are explored first in terms of student identity, learning power and competences and second in terms of student participation in the construction of knowledge through authentic enquiry. Examples are used to illustrate the arguments which have been generated from research into the theory and practice of Learning Power and from the Learning Futures programme in the UK and Australia. The chapter argues that what is necessary for deep engagement in the twenty-first century is a pedagogy and an assessment system which empower individuals to become aware of their identity as learners through making choices about what, where and how they learn and to make meaningful connections with their life stories and aspirations in authentic pedagogy. In this context, the teacher is a facilitator or coach for learning rather than a purveyor of expert knowledge.

Introduction

The focus in education policy in the last two decades on measuring and raising academic standards has increased the attention of policy makers and leaders on teaching and the acquisition of knowledge, skills and understanding predetermined by national curricula and assessed against 'standards'. Essentially the process is 'top down' – students are recipients of predetermined knowledge sets and the task of teachers is to make the experience as engaging as possible for young people. Whilst this 'delivery' model works for some, particularly students whose social and cultural capital enables them to 'buy in' to this agenda, for too many there is increasing disengagement which

R.D. Crick (✉)
Graduate School of Education,
University of Bristol, Bristol, UK
e-mail: Ruth.Deakin-Crick@bristol.ac.uk

manifests as either passive compliance or more active rejection of the status quo (Wehlage & Rutter, 1986). The compliant disengaged may not be noticed unless they are at a critical borderline in terms of the school's target outcomes, but active rejecters of the status quo vote with their feet, causing considerable political concern. The focus on outcomes concentrates pedagogical attention on the public and measurable aspects of learning. Whilst this is important, if it is at the expense of the personal and less easily measurable aspects of learning, such as learning identity and the dispositions, values and attitudes necessary for students to be able to take advantage of particular learning opportunities, then there is an impact on the quality of student engagement. Engagement in the form of compliance with a particular school and family culture may yield learning that is fragile and dependent, with a passive acceptance and memorisation of rules, concepts and information and ways of doing things transmitted in traditional ways. Such 'passive' engagement does not equip the learner to cope when things go wrong, or are no longer straightforward, or when knowledge needs to be applied in complex situations or integrated into a personal narrative. In contrast to this, deep engagement in learning requires personal investment and commitment – learning has to be meaningful and purposeful in the life of the learner and this is not procured simply by external demands (Haste, 2001).

Worldview Challenges

Underpinning these issues of student engagement are two key 'taken for granted' worldview issues. The first is an epistemological one, to do with the nature of knowledge and how human beings come to know – that is, to encounter and appropriate existing funds of knowledge and to generate and re-formulate knowledge in new contexts. The second is anthropological, to do with the nature of the person who is learning – and how he or she develops a sense of self, learning, identity and purpose in different sociocultural contexts. Educational practices are shaped by paradigmatic views of both knowledge and what it means to be human – and thus contemporary approaches to student engagement in learning reflect these worldviews. Bottery's (1992) analysis of four major Western educational ideologies demonstrates how each has a differing view of the child, the teacher, the nature of knowledge, assessment and purpose of schooling. In the intervening two decades since Bottery's analysis, a dominant ideology influencing approaches to the reform of education combines managerialism (or the 'new public management') and public choice theory (Aucoin, 1990; Self, 2000). For Goldspink (2007b, p. 77), managerialism is an application of managerial method to public institutions and public choice theory is an extension of the logic of economic markets to administrative and political exchange (Stretton & Orchard, 1994; Udehn, 1996). This ideology, combined with curricula shaped by traditional subjects, with underlying assumptions of scientific reductionism, leads to a tendency towards what Perkins (2010) describes as 'elementitis'. This is a way of approaching complexity by focusing on the elements rather than the whole, or what Darling-Hammond (1997) described as a 'piecemeal curriculum', or Langer (1989) as 'mindless' education.

It is perhaps not surprising in this context that studies of engagement in learning have often focused on elements rather than the whole. Fredricks, Blumenfeld, and Paris (2004) summarise their review of engagement by suggesting that the individual types of engagement (behavioural, cognitive, emotional) have 'not been studied in combination, either as results of antecedents nor as influences on outcomes' and that research has tended to use variable-centred rather than pattern-centred techniques, cross-sectional rather than longitudinal. In other words, studies have focused on particular elements of engagement, and few, if any, have attempted to look at engagement from the perspective of all the relevant elements and the patterns and relationships between them. The result is that we have little information about the interactions between different aspects of engagement and little information about the development and malleability of engagement over time (Fredricks et al., 2004, p. 87). If engagement is a multidimensional construct, influenced by place,

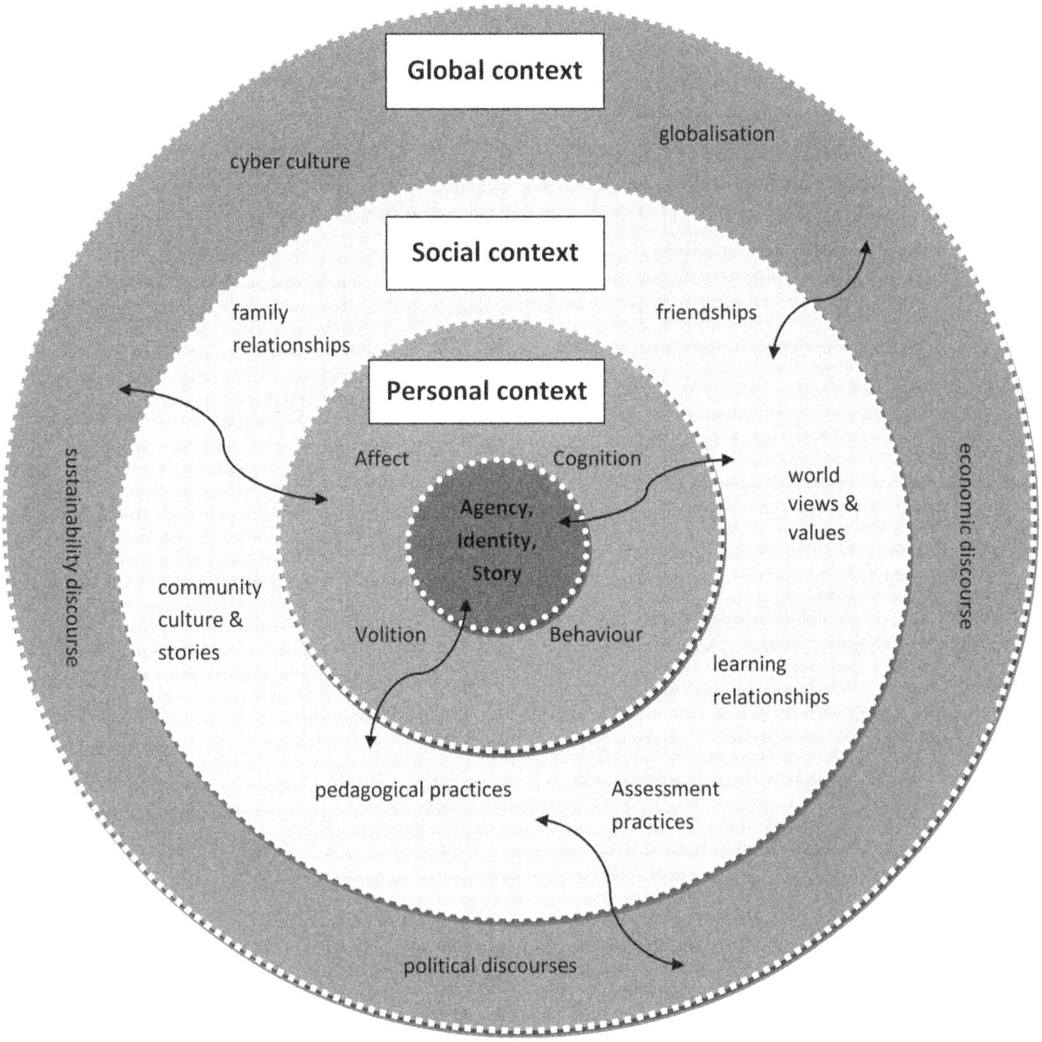

Fig. 32.1 Understanding engagement in learning as a system of systems

time, cultural and social context, as well as factors internal to the person, then it follows that it is important to understand the complex and dialectical relationships between the relevant aspects and to understand engagement as a complex system of systems, including systems internal to the student (such as motivation, agency, meaning making and identity) and in the environment (such as pedagogy, management of learning and culture). Figure 32.1 sets this out in diagrammatic form.

In this chapter, I first explore a definition of engagement which is underpinned by a participatory enquiry paradigm which invites an exploration of patterns and relationships between variables (such as assessment practices and motivation for learning) rather than a focus on a single variable (such as *only* cognitive engagement). Next I explore the implications of this in two ways: first for learning – in terms of student identity, learning power and competences; and second for curriculum – in terms of student participation in the construction of knowledge. I will illustrate my argument with empirical resources generated from two sources. First is the 10-year 'ELLI' research programme (www.vitalpartnerships.com), which has explored and examined the development of engaged learners who understand and are able to deploy their own learning power and the implications for pedagogy, using the Effective Lifelong Learning Inventory (ELLI), a self-report inventory designed to assess a person's learning power. The more recent Learning Futures programme in the UK with its innovative school level practices aimed at increasing student engagement in learning is the second source. The Learning Futures programme was funded by the Paul Hamlyn Foundation, in partnership with the Innovation Unit and worked with a cluster of 15 schools to develop a model of deep engagement in learning (Innovation Unit 2008).

These two programmes of professional development and research, generated from different sources, have involved several hundred teachers and tutors and several thousand learners. The focus of the ELLI programme has been on the dynamic assessment of learning power and ways in which teachers and schools can progressively hand over responsibility for learning to students (e.g., Deakin Crick, 2009a; Deakin Crick & Grushka, 2010; Deakin Crick & Yu, 2008; Goodson & Deakin Crick, 2009; Jaros & Deakin Crick, 2007). The focus of the Learning Futures programme has been on the organizational conditions in schools which support engagement, including enquiry-based learning, coaching and mentoring, school as base camp and school as learning commons (Deakin Crick, Jelfs, Ren, & Symonds, 2010; Paul Hamlyn Foundation & Innovation Unit, 2010).

Deep Engagement

Within the literature, it is common to distinguish between engagement measured by conformance or compliance (e.g., attendance), academic engagement (e.g., commitment to a limited range of academic performance criteria or passing the tests) and intellectual engagement. The former is concerned with whether students conform to the rules of an institution – it has little to say about processes or outcomes of learning. The second concentrates on a very limited subset of outcomes of schooling, whilst the last implies a more complete concern with learning process and outcomes at the whole person level. This last approach is reflected in current policy goals for education in many countries and is the approach advocated here because it enables a fuller theorisation about the person who is learning, his or her development as a person in the community and the ways in which proximal and distal social environments influence that learning, which is important for understanding deep engagement.

Deep engagement in learning is particularly important in the fluid, networked and global twenty-first century world for two reasons, as Bauman eloquently argues. First, the contemporary search for identity is 'the side-effect and by-product of the combination of globalising and individualising pressures and the tensions they spawn' (Bauman, 2001, p. 52) and, second, 'educational philosophy and theory face the unfamiliar and challenging task of theorising a formative process which is not guided from the start by the target form designed in advance' (Bauman, 2001, p. 139). We need a theory and practice of engagement in learning which facilitates the formation of identity and combines this with processes for scaffolding and supporting the processes of knowledge creation in a world where relevant outcomes can no longer be predetermined.

When a learner is deeply engaged in learning, he or she is an intentional participant in a social process which is taking place over time. Seely Brown and Thomas (2009, p. 1) argue that we need to embrace a theory of 'learning to become' in contrast to theories of learning which see learning as a process of becoming *something*. They say that the twentieth century worldview shift from learning as transmission to learning as interpretation is now being replaced by learning as participation – fuelled by structural changes in the way communication happens through new technologies and media. Participation is embodied and experienced – and embraces tacit as well as explicit knowledge (Polanyi, 1967).

> The potential revolution for learning that the networked world provides is the ability to create scalable environments for learning that engages the tacit as well as the explicit dimensions of knowledge. The term we have been using for this, borrowed from Polanyi is indwelling. Understanding this notion requires us to think about the connection between experience, embodiment and learning. (Thomas & Seeley Brown, 2009, p. 10).

This way of knowing is fundamentally experiential (Heron & Reason, 1997; Reason, 2005) and positions the person, as learner, as part of a whole in relation to fellow humans and the natural world. Experiential knowing – through direct encounter – is the distinguishing feature of a participatory enquiry paradigm and is the foundation for the development of critical subjectivity (Heron & Reason, 1997).

The experience of deep engagement then is multidimensional and implies participation and experience which leads to personal commitment and investment in learning over time (Fredricks et al., 2004, p. 82). This form of engagement can be understood as 'deep' in that it is prolonged, purposeful and enacted in a sociohistorical trajectory. It inevitably includes an ethical dimension because it is about how a person embodies and enacts their learning in the world. The first part of a working definition of deep engagement in learning, or our way of recognising it when it happens, is when a learner becomes personally absorbed in and committed to participation in the processes of learning and the mastery of a (chosen) topic, or task, to the highest level of which they are capable. This means that he or she will be aware of, and attend to, the processes of learning, rather than just the outcome, and will utilise his or her own power to learn to serve his or her chosen purpose – developing his or her learning identity and mindfully using the scaffolding provided to pursue the journey towards his or her chosen outcome. He or she will increasingly take responsibility for his or her own learning trajectory, and his or her learning will be meaningful to him or her, both in his or her life beyond the classroom and in the trajectory of his or her particular life story.

This definition of engagement goes beyond the more recent consensus which has emerged around the integration of the cognitive, affective and behavioural elements of engagement (Fredricks et al., 2004; Guthrie & Wigfield, 2000) because it assumes a critical sociocultural context in which students identify value and purpose in their learning and take responsibility as agents of their learning, embodied in a particular context in place and over time (Goodson, 2009; Goodson & Beista, 2010; Goodson & Deakin Crick, 2009). It is critical because it involves 'humanisation' (Freire, 1972) and emancipatory rationality (Habermas, 1973) and is embodied and located within the personal and communal narratives through which human beings seek and make meaning; thus, it is also ethical. Deep engagement leads to what Bateson (1972) describes as third-level learning, which involves personal transformation – rather than only repetition (primary learning) or learning to learn (secondary learning).

Engagement and Motivation for Learning

It is a sine qua non that in order to be engaged in learning, a person needs to be motivated to learn – to have a 'desire to engage' of sufficient quality that it drives the individual to take advantage of particular learning opportunities. Motivation thus precedes engagement. In a systematic review of the impact of testing and assessment on students' motivation for learning, Harlen and Deakin Crick (2003a, 2003b) identified 19 studies from a total collection of 183 which explored, through different research designs, the impact of assessment on students' motivation for learning. Overall, the review suggested that summative testing and assessment can unwittingly depress motivation for learning and that motivation itself is a complex construct which should be an outcome of education as well as a precedent. The study argued that motivation for learning is influenced by a range of psychosocial factors both internal to the learner and present in the learner's social and natural environment. The American Psychological Association's Learner Centred Principles (1997) focus on factors that are internal to and under the control of the learner, as well as taking account of the environmental and contextual factors which interact with those internal factors (McCombs & Lauer, 1997). Of these 14 principles, three deal directly with motivation for learning. The first of these has to do with the motivational and emotional influences on learning, which are affected by the learner's emotional state, beliefs, interests, goals and habits of thinking. The second refers to the learner's creativity, higher-order thinking and natural curiosity that contribute to intrinsic motivation to learn. Intrinsic motivation for learning is stimulated by tasks of optimal novelty and difficulty, relevant to personal interests and providing for personal choice and control. The third principle has to do with the effect of motivation on extended learner effort and guided practice – without motivation to learn, the willingness to exert this effort is unlikely without coercion. These three broad principles indicate the range of factors that have to be taken into account when considering motivation for learning. They have to do with the learner's sense of self, expressed through values and attitudes; with the learner's engagement with learning, including their sense of control and efficacy; and with the learner's willingness to exert effort to achieve a learning goal.

None of the studies in this review dealt with all the variables included in the concept of motivation for learning, but the reviewers grouped them according to the particular outcomes that were investigated in terms of motivation for learning. Expressed from a learner's perspective, these three groups were as follows:
1. What I feel and think about myself as a learner
2. The energy I have for the task
3. How I perceive my capacity to undertake the task.

This tripartite construction of the term motivation for learning was developed in response to the range of empirical studies on aspects of motivation for learning drawn from around the world. It goes beyond a behavioural definition and draws attention to the 'personhood' and the identity of the learner. This attention to the self of the learner is important because the capacity of the individual to become the 'author' of their own learning is another defining feature of both motivation for and deep engagement in learning. The 'author' metaphor implies intentional self-direction (Black, McCormick, James, & Pedder, 2006) and the creation of a unique story. However, beyond this, and relevant to engagement, are the lateral and temporal connectivities which shape a person's sense of self, particularly personal and communal stories and networks of relationships (Bloomer, 2001; Bloomer & Hodkinson, 2000). Attending to the self raises challenges for contemporary pedagogy, particularly within a high accountability, outcomes-focused framework; the theoretical and practical implications are significant. Finding ways of enabling learners to make meaningful connections between their own life story, the world in which they live, their particular community and tradition and the processes and content of their learning in school requires a personalised and local approach and learning and assessment strategies which can move easily between personal and public domains. In the following sections, I begin to explore some of the aspects of learning which are relevant to engagement, using the metaphor of learners as 'authors' heuristically. To be an 'author' of one's own learning suggests that (a) there is an agentic self who is producing the 'texts' of learning, (b) there is a coherent story to be told and (c) there is a context in time and place within which the learning is taking place.

Elements of Deep Engagement in Learning

Perezhivanie: Resources of the Self

An author does not arrive at the creation of a story empty handed. Rather he or she has already an idea to pursue, drawn from his or her experience and interest. In the same way, the learner arrives at a learning opportunity already possessing a way of knowing and being in the world which is the sum of their experience to date. Vygotsky (1962/1934, 1978) described this as 'Perezhivanie', the term used for accumulated lived emotional experience, including values, attitudes, beliefs, schemas and affect. For Vygotsky, Perezhivanie is the process through which interactions in the 'zone of proximal development' are perceived by the learner. The 'zone of proximal development' is entered when a learner and a more experienced other participate in a relationship of 'cognitive scaffolding' through which the learner becomes more capable of achieving particular learning outcomes through

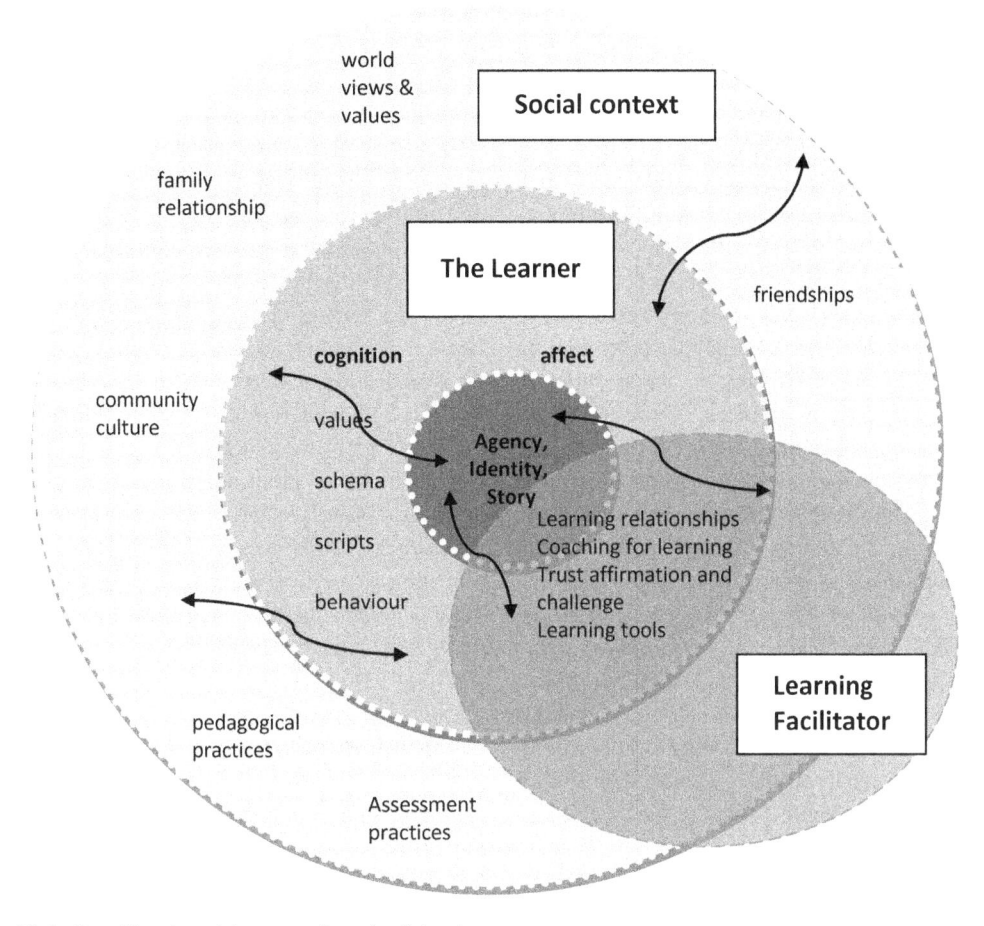

Fig. 32.2 Perezhivanie and the zone of proximal development

modelling, imitation and repetition. What a learner brings to learning in this context is deeply personal and unique, although necessarily experienced and accumulated over time in the context of relationship, community and tradition. Mahn and John-Steiner (2002) argued that by expanding the scope of the examination of the zone of proximal development, we can understand it as a complex whole, a system of systems which includes the interrelated and interdependent elements of participants, environments, artefacts (such as computers or tools) and context. In order to develop a theoretical purchase on this concept of 'Perezhivanie' and explore further its implications for engagement in learning, we will break it down into 'identity', 'story' and 'values, attitudes and dispositions' (see Fig. 32.2).

Identity: The Missing Link

Sfard and Prusak (2005) suggest that the notion of identity is the missing link between learning and its sociocultural context.

> We believe that the notion of identity is a perfect candidate for the role of "the missing link" in the researchers' story of the complex dialectic between learning and its socio-cultural context. We thus concur with the increasingly popular idea of replacing the traditional discourse on schooling with the talk about "construction of identities" (Lave & Wenger, 1991, p. 53) or about the "longer-term agenda of identity building" (Lemke, 2000; Nasir & Saxe, 2003). (Sfard & Prusak, 2005, p. 15).

For Sfard and Prusak, identities are stories about persons. They define identities as 'collections of stories about persons that are 'reifying, endorsable by others and significant' and argue that a person's stories about themselves are profoundly influenced by the stories that important others tell about that person. Identities are discursive counterparts of one's lived experiences – they are stories which are told and re-told and which are open and susceptible to change. The importance of this for understanding engagement in learning is that positive identity talk – that is, reifying statements such as 'I am resilient', or 'You are creative' – makes people more able to engage with new challenges or opportunities in terms of their past experiences. Identity as a discursive activity becomes an important bridge between the lived experience a person brings to the learning encounter and the movement forwards towards the construction of a new identity. Since all learning includes a knowledge content – learning is always about some new knowledge of some sort – it follows that the process of knowledge construction can also scaffold identify formation.

Sfard and Prusak go on to operationalise their definition of identity for learning by describing the gap between a person's actual identity and their designated identity:

> The reifying, significant narratives about a person can be split into two subsets: actual identity, consisting of stories about the actual state of affairs, and designated identity, consisting of narratives presenting a state of affairs which, for one reason or another, is expected to be the case, if not now then in the future (2005, p. 18).

For the learner as 'author', the space between the 'actual' and the 'designated' is a powerful site for engagement and another way of conceptualising the zone of proximal development. Pedagogy for engagement must first acknowledge this space and second facilitate the learner in actively and critically narrating the terrain it represents. Such pedagogical skills of facilitation are more akin to coaching than to traditional teaching or mentoring because the purpose is to facilitate the learner to become the author of his or her own learning journey rather than to transmit information or know-how from an expert to a novice. Where a person is severely disengaged from learning – for example, a young offender in prison for violent crime who may be 'stuck' with their actual identity – then the facilitation task begins to look more like counselling because the task will be to explore those factors in a person's story which block movement forwards and to help them to re-imagine a designated identity: who they want to become. This relates to knowledge construction in that the starting point for engagement is interest in *something* such as an object, or artefact, or event or place. To be interested in something, that something has to have meaning to the 'learner' to connect to their life story in a particular way. Building on that interest (which is personal and idiosyncratic) are certain thinking and learning capabilities such as observing, generating questions or more sophisticated knowledge mapping. These are all activities undertaken by the learner in the process of knowledge construction about something and engagement in the task of knowledge construction is fuelled by its meaningfulness to the learner.

Personal and Community Stories

Within this participatory framing of learning, the individual learner is not a 'monad' or an 'island' but is defined and realised in relation to other people. He or she constructs meaning through time in the form of stories which are developed in the context of relationships, through telling, witnessing and retelling. A person's 'reifying, endorsable and significant stories', which constitute his or her identity, are developed discursively in relationships and community. This discursive process inevitably draws on the wider community stories and worldviews that shape the 'oughts and permissions', the symbols and values and power structures in a particular community. Such stories are particular to time and place, embodied, told and re-told locally. They shape the habits, traditions and rituals of learning – the dispositions, values and attitudes which a learner brings to each encounter with new learning opportunities. For example, in a community where unemployment is historical and widespread, young people growing up are likely to imbibe the wider community story of resignation and low aspiration and internalise it as part of their own actual and designated identity. Their identity as learners – that is, their sense of confidence to learn and change and their awareness of their own power to learn – is therefore a key vehicle for self-directed change, aspiration and movement towards designated identity.

Personal Qualities: Values, Attitudes and Dispositions for Learning

The process of moving from a particular identity towards a designated one is a discursive activity. In Vygotskian terms, it is also scaffolded – the quality of relationships and the language used within this discursive activity are of crucial importance. As well as language about the content of learning, it is the language of the values, attitudes and dispositions for learning which the learner needs in order to engage with the task of change. The term 'disposition' is not sufficient to describe this because although it is in part a rich progeny of Aristotelian 'hexus' and connects with Bourdiuesian 'habitus', it is all too often reduced simply to a 'tendency to behave in a certain way'. What is being described here is a set of personal qualities or orientations towards learning which are understood and manifested in thought, feeling and action and derived from values and attitudes – sets of beliefs with affective loading. The term 'learning power' is more appropriate because it incorporates values, attitudes and dispositions and in addition invokes the important concept of agency and use.

For example, say a learner has chosen to engage with learning about volcanoes. His or her designated identity is to become 'someone who knows a lot about volcanoes'. To become that designated person, he or she will need to utilise his or her *curiosity* in uncovering information, he or she will need to be *creative* in order to devise ways of understanding how volcanoes work and *resilient* in the face of challenge. He or she will need to map new knowledge to what he or she already knows (*meaning making*) and have a sense of the extent and purpose of the task and what resources he or she needs to deploy (*strategic awareness*). He or she will need a level of confidence in his or her capacity to move towards his or her designated identity (*changing and learning*) and to utilise his or her social resources to optimise his or her learning (*learning relationships*). Such personal qualities constitute *learning power* – empirically derived clusters of values, attitudes and dispositions which are necessary for an individual's engagement with learning opportunities.

These seven dimensions emerged from successive factor analytic studies (Deakin Crick, 2004; Deakin Crick, Broadfoot, & Claxton, 2004; Deakin Crick & Yu, 2008). They have been constituted into the ELLI, a self-report questionnaire designed both to measure a person's learning power at any moment in time and to stimulate personal change through providing a framework for a coaching conversation between a learner and teacher/facilitator. The online questionnaire produces a spider diagram, with no numbers, which represents what the individual says about themselves in terms of the seven dimensions of learning power. Ten years of studies with school-age children, students in further and higher education and adults in the workplace have demonstrated the value of awareness of these dimensions of learning power in stimulating engagement in learning.

Learning Power and Engagement at Work: An Illustration

The importance of the relationship between personal learning power and engagement is particularly stark in remote indigenous communities in northern Australia where there is a powerful legacy of marginalisation and the systematic disenfranchisement over 200 years of a particular way of life with its unique ways of knowing, being and relating, traditions and rituals. As an extreme example (alas not the only one), it has explanatory power for mainstream pedagogy. What follows is an explanation of how learning power can form a bridge between individual and community identity and engagement in formal learning opportunities and then a particular example of their application.

In order for young people in these communities to become authors of their own learning, and to articulate positive designated identities, there is a pedagogical imperative for the facilitation of authentic connections between these *particular* ways of knowing, being and doing in *particular* communities and the discursive tasks of identity formation and the generation of learning power. Metaphor, symbol, image and narrative are powerful ways of forming a bridge between two worlds, between a particular culture and learning power (Deakin Crick & Grushka, 2010; Grushka, 2009). They are epistemologically rich because they form a link between two worlds – the experience and 'Perezhivanie' of the learner and his or her community and ideas and practices for learning and (re) engagement in public 'curricula'. Metaphor, image and story can create conditions for the development of deep learning which carries the qualities of the development of critical subjectivity (Heron & Reason, 1997) through generating and linking experiential, presentational, narrative and propositional knowledge.

In the twenty-first century, even the most remote communities are both local and global – cyberspace is ubiquitous. Remote and relatively underdeveloped communities are connected to cyberculture through mobile technologies. The shaping power of cyberspace creates both challenges and opportunities for identity construction and engagement in learning. The sheer complexity and volume of communication and information overwhelm traditional ways of organising and communicating knowledge whilst opening up new opportunities and necessities. Cyberspace challenges traditional ways of living and learning whilst at the same time enabling their reconstruction and reformulation because it makes knowledge and information widely available and provides new tools and artefacts for participation which can transgress geographical and economic boundaries. For example, the ELLI tool is stored online on cloud servers, in a secure repository called 'The Learning Warehouse' and local organisations use a 'portal' to access the tools and ideas, whilst a 'trade entrance' enables researchers with appropriate permissions to access anonymised data for analysis.

Learning Power and Engagement in Indigenous Australian Communities

The following example, drawn from research and development projects in Northern Territory, Australia, provides a graphic illustration of the power of cyberspace to enable a remote indigenous community to connect their traditional culture with the ideas and practices of learning power drawn from research. Damien is a teacher in Gapuwiyak School who has led the community in identifying six birds from the Yolongu sacred songlines, and a seventh bird, which is not sacred, which function as metaphors and symbols for the seven dimensions of learning power. For example, the Sea Eagle, or Djert, was chosen to represent the quality of critical curiosity, and the Emu, or Wurrpan, was chosen to represent the quality of strategic awareness. After long discussions with the whole community, these seven birds were ratified by the elders, painted in original indigenous art forms and used to communicate about learning power with the community. In this picture, Damian has copied his own learning power profile from the computer onto a whiteboard and attached the original paintings of the seven birds at the relevant points of his own spider diagram. He is facilitating his community in understanding learning power as part of the discursive act of identity formation – and giving an invitation to the community to participate in learning, to re-create constructive learning identities, which will facilitate the construction of new designated identities (Deakin Crick, Grushka, Heitmeyer, & Nicholson, 2010) (Fig. 32.3).

The Relationship Between Learning Power and Engagement

The model of deep engagement described in this chapter is one which connects the learner's sense of identity and agency with their personal learning power, and these are utilised by the learner in a meaningful process of knowledge construction which leads to active engagement in the world. These have been referred to elsewhere as four stations in the learning journey (Deakin Crick, 2009b).

Fig. 32.3 Identity formation as a discursive community activity

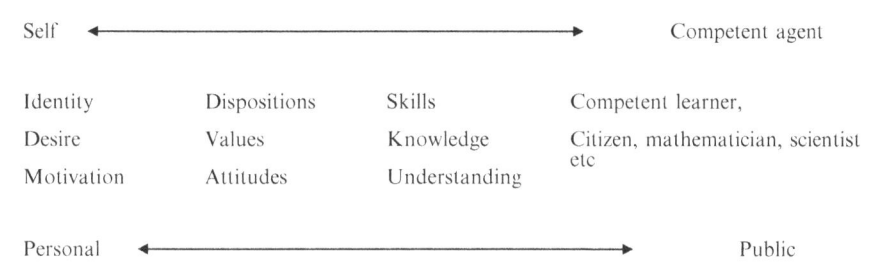

```
Self  ◄──────────────────────────────────►  Competent agent

Identity      Dispositions    Skills          Competent learner,
Desire        Values          Knowledge       Citizen, mathematician, scientist
Motivation    Attitudes       Understanding   etc

Personal  ◄──────────────────────────────────►  Public
```

Fig. 32.4 Four pedagogical moments for deep engagement

They represent four pedagogical moments which require attention for deep engagement in learning (Fig. 32.4).

Research into learning power suggests that its pedagogical value is important for engagement because self-assessment of values, attitudes and dispositions for learning (learning power) provides a framework for a coaching conversation which both reflects 'backward' to the individual's learning identity whilst also providing a framework for scaffolding the journey forwards towards the construction of new knowledge and its meaningful application. This is a pathway for the development of critical subjectivity since it engages experiential, presentational, propositional and practical ways of knowing as a pathway towards intelligent and principled participation in the world (Heron & Reason, 1997). The following sections address key pedagogical themes which are important in this process: language and place, coaching relationships and conversations and scaffolding the process of knowledge construction.

Language and Place

The research into learning power provides a language which can be appropriated differently in diverse communities, in diverse places, and can be used to conduct 'identity talk' about learning and about how a person might choose to engage with learning opportunities. If identity formation is a discursive activity, then it follows that language is

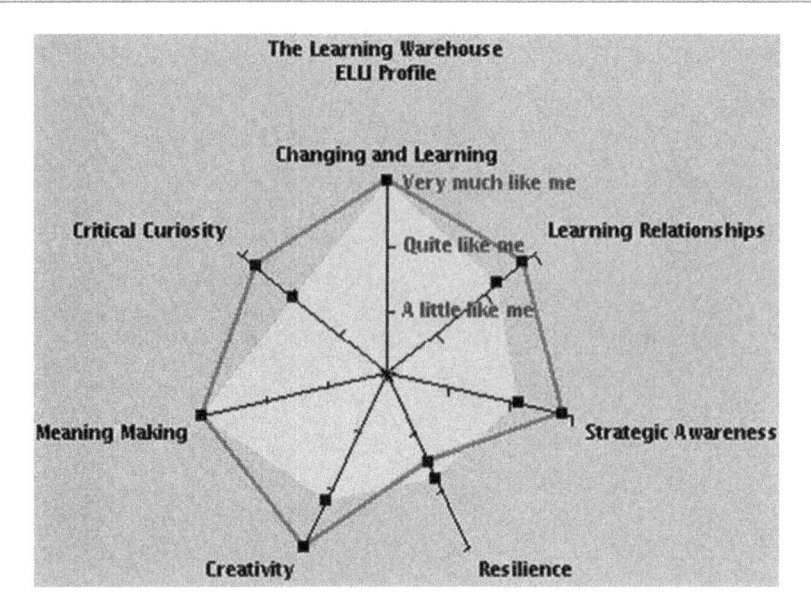

Fig. 32.5 An individual learning power profile with pre- and post-measures

required as a medium for that discourse. The richer the language and the more it reflects, harmonises and critiques the community's stories, which shape the individual's, the more useful it is in creating the conditions for engagement. What Damien was doing in the picture, extending the verbal language of learning power through art, was creating a visual language which connects the deep experiential knowledge of his people with the concepts and ideas of learning power. Engagement in learning is always placed and particular (Deakin Crick & Grushka, 2010; Deakin Crick, Grushka et al., 2010; Goodson & Deakin Crick, 2009). In this example, it was significant simply to be having these conversations with people who have been traditionally disenfranchised from formal western schooling traditions. The first stage is to open up the possibility of learning and change – the next step is to utilise that hopefulness, through coaching conversations in the context of trustful relationships so that the individual can begin to identify and appropriate more formal learning opportunities.

Framework for a Coaching Conversation

A learning power profile provides a framework for such coaching conversations which move in the zone between the identity of the learner and a particular negotiated learning outcome. The fact that the assessment is based on a measurement derived from a self-report questionnaire is important because it reflects back to the individual what they have said about themselves. The feedback (Fig. 32.5) is in the form of a spider diagram without numbers, and the purpose is for the learner and a coach or facilitator to reflect on the shape, how it connects to lived experience and how it might be changed, or on the changes to the shape after a second assessment event. The shaded inner spider diagram represents the pre-test measure from the self-report questionnaire, and the post-test measure is the single, outer line. In this case, the individual's second self-assessment shows an increase in critical curiosity, creativity, learning relationships and strategic awareness. This was a young person in higher education in Bahrain, who had experienced coaching conversations with a tutor about her spider diagram, which included the formulations of targets – what the individual wanted to change and why and how she could achieve that change in the highly academic context in which she was learning.

Feedback alone is not sufficient for deep engagement. For deep engagement, the assessment event needs to be located within a pedagogy which attends to 'identity' and 'authorship' in learning, in a community which operationalises both a shared language with which to describe learning power and pedagogical skill in coaching as well as teaching. What is necessary is a pedagogy and an assessment system which empowers individuals to become aware of their identity as learners through making choices about both what, where and how they learn, and to make meaningful connections with their life stories and aspirations in authentic pedagogy. In this context, the teacher is a facilitator or coach for learning, rather than a purveyor of expert knowledge. The quality of trust is a core resource for such coaching (Bryk & Schneider, 2002).

Scaffolding the Process of Knowledge Construction

The third theme is that the dimensions of learning power provide a framework for the journey from a chosen starting point, where the self is engaged, towards a negotiated learning outcome. The most powerful engagement for learning occurs where learning is authentic, active and enquiry led (Newmann, 1996; Newmann, Marks & Gamoran, 1996). The first condition for this is when the learner is personally involved in selecting the focus for their enquiry which has meaning and relevance to them in their lives beyond the classroom and where the learner is the 'author' of their own learning journey. The second is where learning is designed as enquiry: the co-construction of knowledge through disciplined enquiry which involves building on a prior knowledge base, striving for in-depth understanding and expressing findings through elaborated communication. The third is when the learner is actively engaged in the production of discourse, products or performances that have relevance to learners beyond school and require more active engagement than simply repetition, retrieving information and memorisation of facts or rules (Deakin Crick, Jelfs et al., 2010). These findings from the Learning Futures project, drawing on both quantitative and qualitative data, are consistent with the research in authentic pedagogy developed in Chicago by Newman and colleagues (Newmann, 1996; Newmann & Wehlage, 1995; Newmann et al., 1996) and the related research in Australia into quality teaching (Goldspink, 2007a, 2007b, 2008; Ladwig & Gore, 2004; Ladwig & King, 1991, 2003).

The dimensions of learning power contribute to approaches to enquiry which are authentic and active because they bring a structure to learning which is assessable at key stages in the process and facilitates the process of identity construction. Research and development studies focusing on the learning power dimensions and enquiry identified eight distinct stages in a sequential but iterative and cumulative enquiry pathway which map onto four key aspects of pedagogy for engagement: the self who is learning, the personal learning power necessary for engaging with learning opportunities; the construction of knowledge and its application in the real world (Deakin Crick et al., 2007; Jaros & Deakin Crick, 2007). These begin with the personal, local and experiential choice of the learner and move from there, invoking an increasingly complex sequence of thinking and learning capabilities, to an encounter with pre-existing funds of knowledge which constitute the formal curriculum. The learner is coached in that journey by a facilitator/coach who supports him and provides prompts, guidance and resources at key points. The sequence begins with the person of the learner and her choice. It is described in Fig. 32.6 in table form, then in narrative.

First: Choosing: The student is encouraged to choose an object or place that fascinates them. Careful, 'hands-off' prompting and guidance may be needed from the facilitator/coach to ensure that personal interest is strong and authentic. The rest of the process will be highly influenced by the integrity of this choosing process. Sometimes the 'object' turns out to be a person or event – it is its susceptibility to observation and the strength of the student's interest and engagement that are important.

Second: Observing/describing: The learner observes and describes the chosen object/place,

Fig. 32.6 Sequence of stages in personalised enquiry

Thinking and Learning Capabilities	Eight steps-for framing pedagogy
Choosing and deciding	PERSONAL CHOICE
Observing and describing	OBSERVE AND DESCRIBE
Questioning	GENERATE QUESTIONS
Storying	UNCOVER NARRATIVES
Mapping	CREATE KNOWLEDGE MAP
Connecting	CONNECT TO EXISTING KNOWLEDGE
Reconciling	RECONCILE WITH ASSESSMENT PURPOSE
Validating	CONDUCT ASSESSMENT EVENT
Applying	APPLY NEW KNOWLEDGE

both as a separate, objective entity and in relation to their own interest and reasons for choosing it. In this, the learner is developing their sense of personal responsibility. This initiates the cycles of a personal development process which is recorded in a *workbook* and in which the student, tutor and later others participate. It requires the student to develop the critical curiosity and strategic awareness necessary for independent learning, in the context of learning relationships. The student is also developing a sense of himself or herself as a learner who can change and grow over time.

Third: Questioning: The learner starts asking questions: obvious, but open ones, such as *How did it get there? What was there before? Why is it how it is? Who uses it? How and why did they get involved?* He or she is initiating and conducting a process of inquiry and investigation, driven by personal interest and shaped in turn by the answers to his or her own questions. The learner is exercising and developing critical curiosity. All the time, the student is encouraged to reflect on their motivation, reasoning and identity as a motivator of their own learning.

Fourth: Storying: The questioning leads to a sense of narrative, both around the chosen object and in the unfolding of new learning. Historical and present realities lead to a sense of 'what might be' both for the object/place and for the learner and their learning. She or he is becoming the author of his or her own 'learning story' or journey.

Fifth: Mapping: The learner begins to discern that this 'ad hoc' narrative leads in turn to new concepts, propositions and knowledge. Self-referenced learning starts to be related to a wider awareness of the 'other'. The learning becomes a 'knowledge map' which can be used to make sense of the journey and of new learning as it comes into view. The student is 'making meaning' by connecting new learning to the 'story so far'.

Sixth: Connecting: With informed guidance and support from the teacher, the student's widening 'map' of knowledge can be related to existing maps or models of the world: scientific, historical, social, psychological, theological, philosophical… This is where awareness of the diversity of possible 'avenues of learning' becomes useful. It requires the tutor or teacher to act as supporter, encourager and 'tour guide' in the student's encounter with established and specialist sources and forms of knowledge.

Seventh: Reconciling: The student arrives at the interface between their personal inquiry and the specialist requirements of curriculum, course, examination or accreditation. The student's development as learner enables them to encounter specialist knowledge and make sense of it, in relation to what they already know and in the way they already learn, interrogating it and interacting with it, instead of simply 'receiving' it, using the model of learning and 'knowledge mapping' skills they have developed through the inquiry. This is where the resilience will be tested, that will have started to grow through the responsibility and challenge of a self-motivated inquiry.

Eighth: Validating: The student can forge links between what he or she now knows and institutional and social structures receptive to it: qualifications, job opportunities, learning opportunities, needs, initiatives, outlets, relationships, accreditation, publication.... This may take the form of a portfolio, presentation or written essay, based on the *workbook*, making explicit both process and outcomes of the inquiry. The learning has met its communicative purpose. The learner has created a pathway from subjective response and observation towards the interface with established knowledge. In doing so, he or she has also achieved life-enhancing personal development by asking and answering such questions as: *Who am I? What is my pathway? How did I get there? Where does it lead me? What were the alternatives? Who helped me and how?*

Ninth: Applying: The student has completed an authentic enquiry about an issue of significance and meaning in his or her life. This might be the solution to a problem, which can now be prototyped and tested, or it might have identified an unfolding employment trajectory or niche or raised citizenship issues which can be addressed in the community. At this stage, the question is: *How do I build on and consolidate this knowledge that I have acquired?* The enquiry is authentic and useful in terms of both content and process.

These sequential but iterative stages of authentic enquiry frame a pedagogy which integrates the identity and personhood of the learner with the process of knowledge construction. Although in practice, they are not linear or strictly sequential – each stage may be revisited in a spiral formation throughout the enquiry project – these are nevertheless key aspects of knowledge construction which frame enquiry from the 'bottom up', that is, from the lived experience of the learner in the real world to an outcome which can demonstrate higher-order creative and critical thinking, in contrast to traditional pedagogy which is 'top down' and begins with the (prescribed) knowledge itself, where the teacher's job is to make the experience of acquiring that knowledge as meaningful as possible to the learner. In authentic enquiry, the problems are formulated by the learners themselves – they are seeking to answer questions which they own, rather than find solutions to other people's problems or questions.

For deep engagement, it is this connection between 'experiential knowing' and a 'knowledge product' which is crucial. Even where a completely free choice of starting points in enquiry projects is not possible, for example, in some formal educational contexts where 'coverage of content' is a political necessity, these stepped processes of enquiry ground and engage the learner in an authentic and active process of learning. Even in these circumstances, teachers can facilitate the sort of authentic choice which connects with students' experiential knowledge, even though that choice may be boundaried by curricular demands. Stepped processes of enquiry can provide a form of *structured freedom* which enables learners to connect their learning with their own identity, story and purpose and thus experience deep engagement. Without authentic choice on the part of the student, there is less likelihood of making these deep connections – and students may not get the opportunity to frame their own questions and formulate authentic problems. Indeed, some forms of project-based learning do not allow for this sort of enquiry at all if they begin with predetermined problems or questions which already have predetermined answers. The danger then is that the learner is more concerned with finding the right answer than formulating a solution.

The key role of the seven dimensions of learning power is that where the learner is aware of their own learning power profile and chooses to take responsibility for developing himself or herself as a learner, then the dimensions of learning power provide scaffolding for negotiating these steps. For example, good choosing requires creativity and questioning requires critical curiosity. Knowledge mapping requires meaning making and strategic awareness and reconciling requires resilience and so on. Reciprocally, the enquiry process provides salient opportunities for building strengths in selected learning power dimensions. There is thus an intimate relationship between learning power (dispositions, values and attitudes) and authentic enquiry-based learning.

Research in the Learning Futures project suggests that this approach represents a substantively different paradigm for learning and schooling from conventional models. In order to realise the potential of engagement in learning that this vision represents, schools have needed to engage in processes of profound change. Authentic learning has been modelled at all levels in the system: student, teacher, school and networks. Such a school is personified by teachers, leaders and a community who take collective responsibility for student learning and work together in professional enquiry which is aligned to schools' authentic goals. The school is characterised by people's openness to learn, willingness to change, professional courage, engagement in disciplined professional enquiry and a shared commitment to a locally owned and defined language for organizational, professional and personal learning (Deakin Crick, Jelfs, et al., 2010, p. 185).

A Narrative Example from Practice

In order to ground these ideas in student language and practice, I shall draw on a piece of narrative data from the Learning Futures project in the UK in which we compiled over 180 hours of student talk about learning in schools which were seeking to be radical in their approach to engagement. This example is particularly useful for illustration and representative of many other students who were successfully and deeply engaging in their own learning. The school serves an economically deprived community, and 'Craig' himself faced many challenges arising from these conditions. He was 12 and he and his year group were working in a specially framed curriculum slot (of about 7 hours per week) called 'My World', free of prescribed content and framed by authentic enquiry projects. Within this space, the class selected their own focus for their enquiry, using learning power language as scaffolding. In this case, the teacher had used the metaphor of an island where the class were marooned and had to survive on their own, without their teacher. The focus in this project in terms of content was on 'taking responsibility for my own life and learning'. The teacher framed the project, deliberately gave the students responsibility for the selection of content and process and was available to coach and mentor them individually. The project concluded with an authentic assessment event in which groups of students presented their work to each other and community members. In the following excerpt, Craig was being asked what he had learned in his My World project:

Craig: Well .. when we was in our groups, something I learnt really well is my learning relationships and my changing and learning……..Just sometimes …I used just to go off task. Then something happened, like a spark in my brain or something and all of a sudden I thought I may as well get a good education and do like stuff, don't talk about something I'm not meant to.

Craig: It's just like … it's given me an experience of like the future. Like if I keep acting like a free child in the future, I'm never going to get anywhere….I think it's kind of a gift like that I can actually develop new skills without acting up or nothing. I reckon yeah, it's a gift.

Interviewer: So if I looked at your map would I see this journey on your map?

Craig: In the forest there's a waterfall and I can't get past it… God gives

	Mr M the helicopter, helps me over the waterfall – drops me down to a place I need to be.
Interviewer:	If you had to think of the one best thing about My World what would it be? The single most important thing that you value the most.
Craig:	The ELLI dimensions
Interviewer:	Why is that then?
Craig:	It's helped me get a long life.
Interviewer:	Helped you?
Craig:	Get a long life.
Interviewer:	Say a bit more?
Craig:	Like I never used to know like all this stuff, like (inaudible) I never knew it existed, like changing and learning and resilience. And as soon as I got it all into my head, I've never ever gave up on stuff I need to reach my goal.
Interviewer:	So that's the best thing, because it's given you …
Craig:	Strength to develop skills and get along life easier.
Interviewer:	And what … how does it differ from your other classes then?
Craig:	Like French and all that?
Interviewer:	Like French and History and …
Craig	It's like [French and History] just given me reams and reams of facts, but like this has given me like tips, hints and helping me to get a long life easier.
Interviewer:	But do you think the facts are important?
Craig:	Yes, sometimes I need them.
Interviewer:	Does My World help you with the French and stuff?
Craig:	Yeah.
Interviewer:	Yeah how does it help you with the other stuff then?
Craig:	Like French and all that? …… It helps me with my French to never give up. Helps me to like develop skills with other people – critical curiosity, like to tell … if they say something and they want you to think it's true, you can actually say it's not …

This excerpt demonstrates Craig's sense of identity and a movement towards a designated identity. He is moving from someone who was not engaged or focused on learning in school to someone with an emerging vision of himself with a different future. In a previous interview, he talked about seeing people on the streets asking for money and not wanting to end up like that. In this same interview, he talks about himself going to sixth form and getting a good job. It also shows how the language of learning power has enabled him to understand himself and to project forwards towards a particular outcome. His perceptions of the difference between the enquiry approach and the more traditional 'top down' pedagogy are insightful and demonstrate the beginnings of critical subjectivity. He is using experiential and presentational knowing when he describes being stuck on the island by a waterfall that he could not get past, until God gave his teacher a helicopter to help him get to the place he needed to be. This was describing the profound change he has experienced in his engagement in learning in school. He instinctively knows that this level of engagement in own learning enables him to critique what he experiences around him and what he is told. He is able to evaluate these capabilities in terms of a newly acquired strategic awareness of their value to his lifelong journey. He has seen, for himself it seems, the limitations of the 'free child' which 'used just to go off task' and was 'never going to get anywhere' and has accepted as 'a gift' his newfound idea of himself (designated identity) as someone who is changing and learning and never giving up. He has become engaged in his learning and its story and the effect on his life is transformative.

Conclusions

The ideas discussed in this chapter are in many ways in their infancy, based on only 10 years of research and development, within a growing, but nonetheless still limited, professional community. At the heart of this work is the imperative to find and develop forms of pedagogy which apportion equal significance to the formation of identity and the development of personal learning power, as to the traditional acquisition of knowledge, skills and understanding beloved of conventional curricula. For learners to be deeply engaged in learning over a life time, the learning needs to be personally significant and meaningful to the learner, who also needs to develop the necessary values, attitudes, and dispositions – learning power – to engage with new learning opportunities and to forge their own purpose for learning and acting in the world.

There are many limitations of this research programme – much of it is small scale and mixed methodologically which brings its own challenges. Much of it has been practitioner led, and Western contemporary structures of schooling are not hospitable to it. There is scope for large impact studies, to explore the impact of this approach to learning on both engagement over time and standard achievement outcomes; the subject matter calls for new methods of educational enquiry that can do justice to narrative, qualitative and quantitative evidence as attention moves between the personal (ipsative) and the public (standardised) assessment outcomes of education, only some of which can be measured quantitatively. When all is said and done, the light in a learner's eye that denotes engagement may be recognised in practice but is much more challenging to investigate through traditional research methods.

What also becomes clear is the importance of particular concepts of place and time, which have not been traditionally theorised in pedagogy: a learner is always embedded and embodied in a particular place at a particular time and his or her learning is a journey of which he or she must progressively become the author. The language and assessment practices of learning power provide a way of connecting the deeply personal with the public and scaffolding the journey of learning as enquiry rather than only as received transmission.

Exploring the concept of engagement from the perspective of a participatory paradigm allows us to see it as a complex system of systems which better reflects the reality of learners, classrooms, schools and communities. A complex systems lens may be particularly valuable for understanding the ways in which the development of learning identities and deep engagement is history and community dependent. By accounting for complexity, it becomes clear that there are many factors which influence the level of a student's engagement in learning in school. These range from the deeply personal (such as identity) to the public (such as encounters with existing funds of knowledge and assessment events). In a world of almost infinite complexity, endless change and multiple possibilities, our approach to engagement in learning needs to be as complex and rich as the challenges we face. Understanding deep engagement as participatory enquiry, with a set of pedagogical design principles, which integrate the personal with the public, the process with the outcome, the local with the global, means that we can move beyond the confines of the 'classroom' and 'one size fits all' solutions towards a more flexible, imaginative and professionally rewarding way of designing and managing learning that is deep and engaging.

References

American Psychological Association. (1997). *Learner centred principles: A framework for school reform and redesign.* Washington, DC: American Psychological Association.

Aucoin, P. (1990). Administrative reform in public management: Paradigms, principles, paradoxes and pendulums. *Governance, 3*(2), 115–137.

Bateson, G. (1972). *Steps to an ecology of mind.* San Francisco: Chandler.

Bauman, Z. (2001). *Community seeking safety in an insecure world.* Cambridge, MA: Polity Press.

Black, P., McCormick, R., James, M., & Pedder, D. (2006). Assessment for learning and learning how to learn: A theoretical enquiry. *Research Papers in Education, 21*(2), 119–132.

Bloomer, M. (2001). Young lives, learning & transformation: Some theoretical considerations. *Oxford Review of Education, 27*(3), 429–447.

Bloomer, M., & Hodkinson, P. (2000). Learning careers: Continuity and change in young people's dispositions to learning. *British Educational Research Journal, 26*(5), 583–597.

Bottery, M. (1992). *The ethics of educational management.* London: Cassell Educational Ltd.

Bryk, A., & Schneider, B. (2002). *Trust in schools: A core resource for improvement.* New York: Russell Sage.

Darling-Hammond, L. (1997). *The right to learn: A blueprint for creating schools that work.* San Francisco: Jossey Bass.

Deakin Crick, R. (2004). *The ecology of learning.* Paper presented at the ESRC Knowledge and Skills for Learning to Learn Seminar Series, University of Newcastle, Newcastle Upon Tyne, UK.

Deakin Crick, R. (2009a). Inquiry-based learning: Reconciling the personal with the public in a democratic and archaeological pedagogy. *Curriculum Journal, 20*(1), 73–92.

Deakin Crick, R. (2009b). Assessment in schools – dispositions. In B. McGaw, P. Peterson, & E. Baker (Eds.), *The international encyclopedia of education* (3rd ed.). Amsterdam: Elsevier.

Deakin Crick, R. (2009c). Pedagogical challenges for personalisation: Integrating the personal with the public through context-driven enquiry. *Curriculum Journal, 20*(3), 185–189.

Deakin Crick, R., Broadfoot, P., & Claxton, G. (2004). Developing an effective lifelong learning inventory: The ELLI Project. *Assessment in Education, 11*(3), 248–272.

Deakin Crick, R., & Grushka, K. (2010). Signs, symbols and metaphor: Linking self with text in inquiry based learning. *Curriculum Journal, 21*(1).

Deakin Crick, R., Grushka, K., Heitmeyer, D., & Nicholson, M. (2010). *Learning, place and identity: An exploration of the affordances of a pedagogy of place amongst Indigenous Australian students*. Bristol, UK: University of Bristol.

Deakin Crick, R., Jelfs, H., Ren, K., & Symonds, J. (2010). *Learning futures*. London: Paul Hamlyn Foundation.

Deakin Crick, R., Small, T., Jaros, M., Pollard, K., Leo, E., Hearne, P., et al. (2007). *Inquiring minds: Transforming potential through personalised learning*. London: Royal Society of Arts.

Deakin Crick, R., & Yu, G. (2008). The effective lifelong learning inventory (ELLI): Is it valid and reliable as a measurement tool? *Education Research, 50*(4), 387–402.

Fredricks, J. A., Blumenfeld, P. C., & Paris, A. H. (2004). School engagement: Potential of the concept, state of the evidence. *Review of Educational Research, 74*(1), 59–109.

Freire, P. (1972). *Pedagogy of the oppressed*. Harmondsworth, UK: Penguin.

Goldspink, C. (2007a). Rethinking educational reform – A loosely coupled and complex systems perspective. *International Journal of Educational Management, Administration and Leadership, 35*(1), 27–50.

Goldspink, C. (2007b). Transforming education: Evidential support for a complex systems approach. *Emergence: Complexity and Organisation, 9*(1–2), 77–92.

Goldspink, C. (2008). *Student engagement and quality pedagogy*. Paper presented at the European Education Research Conference, Gottenburg, Sweden.

Goodson, I. (2009). Listening to professional life stories: Some cross-professional perspectives. In M. Bayer, U. Brinkkjær, H. Plauborg, & S. Rolls (Eds.), *Teachers' career trajectories and work lives* (Vol. 3, pp. 203–210). Dordrecht, The Netherlands: Springer.

Goodson, I., & Beista, G. (2010). *Narrative learning*. London/New York: Routledge.

Goodson, I., & Deakin Crick, R. (2009). Curriculum as narration: Tales from the children of the colonised. *Curriculum Journal, 20*(3), 225–236.

Grushka, K. (2009). Meaning and identities: A visual performative pedagogy for socio-cultural learning. *Curriculum Journal, 20*(3), 237–251.

Guthrie, J., & Wigfield, A. (2000). Engagement and motivation in reading. In M. Kamil & P. Mosenthal (Eds.), *Handbook of reading research* (Vol. 3, pp. 403–422). Mahwah, NJ: Lawrence Erlbaum.

Habermas, J. (1973). *Knowledge and human interests*. Cambridge, MA: Cambridge University Press.

Harlen, W., & Deakin Crick, R. (2003a). *A systematic review of the impact of summative assessment and testing on pupils' motivation for learning*. London: Evidence for Policy and Practice Co-ordinating Centre Department for Education and Skills.

Harlen, W., & Deakin Crick, R. (2003b). Testing and motivation for learning. *Assessment in Education, 10*(2), 169–207.

Haste, H. (2001). Ambiguity, autonomy and agency. In D. Rychen & L. Salganik (Eds.), *Definition and selection of competencies: Theoretical and conceptual foundations*. Seattle, WA: OECD/Hogreffe/Huber.

Heron, J., & Reason, P. (1997). A participatory inquiry paradigm. *Qualitative Inquiry, 3*(3), 274–294.

Innovation Unit. (2008). *Learning futures: Next practice in learning and teaching*. London: Innovation Unit.

Jaros, M., & Deakin Crick, R. (2007). Personalised learning in the post mechanical age. *Journal of Curriculum Studies, 39*(4), 423–440.

Ladwig, J., & Gore, J. (2004). *Quality teaching in NSW public schools: An assessment practice guide*. Sydney, Australia: Professional Support and Curriculum Directorate, NSW Department of Education and Training.

Ladwig, J., & King, M. (1991). *Restructuring secondary social studies: The association of organizational features and classroom thoughtfulness*. Madison, WI: National Center on Effective Secondary Schools [BBB24601].

Ladwig, J., & King, M. (2003). *Quality teaching in NSW public schools: An annotated bibliography*. Sydney, Australia: NSW Department of Education and Training.

Langer, E. (1989). *Mindfulness*. Reading, MA: Addison-Wesley.

Lave, J., & Wenger, E. (1991). *Situated learning: Legitimate peripheral participation*. Cambridge, UK: Cambridge University Press.

Lemke, J. (2000). Across the scales of time: Artifacts, activities, and meanings in ecosocial systems. *Mind, Culture, and Activity, 7*, 273–290.

Mahn, H., & John-Steiner, V. (2002). Developing the affective zone of proximal development. In G. Wells & C. Claxton (Eds.), *Learning for life in the 21st century: Socio-cultural perspectives on the future of education* (pp. 46–58). Oxford, UK: Blackwell.

McCombs, B., & Lauer, P. (1997). Development and validation of the learner-centred battery: Self assessment tools for teacher reflection and professional development. *Professional Educator, 20*(1), 1–20.

Nasir, N., & Saxe, G. (2003). Ethnic and academic identities: A cultural practice perspective on emerging tensions and their management in the lives of minority students. *Educational Researcher, 32*(5), 14–18.

Newmann, F. (1996). *Authentic achievement: Restructuring schools for intellectual quality* (1st ed.). San Francisco: Jossey-Bass.

Newmann, F., Marks, H., & Gamoran, A. (1996). Authentic pedagogy and student performance. *American Journal of Education, 104*(4), 280–312.

Newmann, F., & Wehlage, G. (1995). *Successful school restructuring*. Madison, WI: Center on Organisation and Restructuring of Schools.

Paul Hamlyn Foundation, & Innovation Unit. (2010). *Learning futures engaging schools: Principles and practice*. London: Paul Hamlyn Foundation.

Perkins, D. (2010). *Making learning whole: How seven principles of teaching can transform learning*. San Francisco: Jossey-Bass.

Polanyi, M. (1967). *The tacit dimension*. New York: Anchor/Doubleday.

Reason, P. (2005). Living as part of the whole: The implications of participation. *Journal of Curriculum and Pedagogy, 2*(2), 35–41.

Seely Brown, J., & Thomas, D. (2009). *Learning for a world of constant change*. Paper presented at the 7th Gillon Colloquium, University of Southern California, Los Angeles, CA.

Self, P. (2000). *Rolling back the market*. New York: St Martin's Press.

Sfard, A., & Prusak, A. (2005). Telling identities: In search of an analytic tool for investigating learning as a culturally shaped activity. *Educational Researcher, 34*(4), 14–22.

Stretton, H., & Orchard, L. (1994). *Public goods, public enterprise, public choice: Theoretical foundations of the contemporary attack on government*. Basingstoke, UK: Palgrave Macmillan.

Udehn, L. (1996). *The limits of public choice: A sociological critique of the economic theory of politics*. London: Routledge.

Vygotsky, L. (1962/1934). *Thought and language* (E. Hanfmann & G. Vakar, Trans.). Cambridge, MA: MIT Press.

Vygotsky, L. (1978). *Mind in society: The development of higher psychological processes*. Cambridge, MA: Harvard University Press.

Wehlage, G., & Rutter, R. (1986). Dropping out: How much do schools contribute to the problem? *Teachers College Record, 87*, 374–392.

Part IV Commentary: Outcomes of Engagement and Engagement as an Outcome: Some Consensus, Divergences, and Unanswered Questions

33

Michel Janosz

Abstract

The well-respected engagement scholar, Michel Janosz, shared his thoughts on the chapters in Part IV of this volume. His commentary articulated the areas of agreement and disagreement across scholars regarding the conceptualization of engagement and views on engagement as a process or outcome. He argued for the consideration of (1) the contexts of engagement and understanding the relations between engagement in the classroom and engagement in school; (2) systematic study of the roles of emotional, cognitive, and behavioral engagement; (3) investigation of the relation of engagement with other aspects of psychosocial and neurobiological development; and (4) exploration of engagement within a categorical and person-centered approach in addition to the predominant dimensional and variable-oriented perspective.

Introduction

One extraordinary evolutionary skill of mankind is its capacity to learn. If, at one time, learning was a matter of basic survival, we can still be struck by the fact that knowledge and skills acquisition continues to be, nowadays, one of the most powerful determinants of health and well-being (Heckman, 2006; Muennig, 2007). The benefits of learning are indisputable, but they come with a price: effort. To develop new skills and acquire new knowledge, individuals must consciously mobilize and devote some of their physical and psychological (cognitive, emotional) energy; they must *engage* themselves in the learning situation.

The amount and the quality of the effort put into school learning activities vary between students. Some students are less engaged than others. How important is that? Is there a *price* to pay for disengaging from school? This is one of the two fundamental questions eminent scholars have been invited to address in this chapter of the book. The second is about influencing student engagement. What organizational and educational actions affect student engagement? In deciding to tackle this question, the authors shared their understanding of what are the determinants of engagement and how we can influence them.

M. Janosz (✉)
School Environment Research Group
and School of Psychoeducation, University of Montreal,
Montreal, Canada
e-mail: Michel.janosz@umontreal.ca

Hence, while the first issue refers to the outcomes of engagement, the second concentrates on engagement as an outcome.

In this chapter, I highlight some major convergences and divergences in authors' responses to these questions and share some of the thoughts they inspire. As this book illustrates, the recent mobilization of the scientific community over the construct of engagement has led to the emergence of fundamental theoretical and methodological debates (e.g., definition of engagement, difference between engagement and motivation, measures of engagement). Although most authors of this chapter have shared their views on these important topics, I will only briefly comment on those since others have been specifically invited to do so. I propose instead to underline some conceptual and methodological issues that emerged from the reading of these enlightening texts. Because the systematic study of student engagement is still young, it is easier to identify the unexplored territories, the unanswered questions. This task is also made much easier and stimulating when authors do a superb job of reviewing the state of the knowledge in their area. Thus, in revisiting the chapters in this book, I will argue that our comprehension of the relations between the determinants and outcomes of engagement would benefit from (1) taking into account the contexts of engagement and understanding the relations between engagement in the classroom and engagement in school; (2) studying more systematically the specific roles of emotional, cognitive, and behavioral engagement; (3) investigating the relation of engagement with other aspects of psychosocial and neurobiological development; and (4) exploring engagement within a categorical and person-centered approach in addition to the predominant dimensional and variable-oriented perspective.

Engagement in Learning Activities and Engagement in School

Some researchers study student engagement in relation to learning activities in the classroom. Others address engagement within the broader context of school. Engagement in *both* contexts has been shown to predict different aspects of school success. Nevertheless, we think that student engagement in school is not merely an aggregate version of classroom engagement. Not only is the operationalization of engagement changing according to the context, but I believe that engagement in school encompasses a different reality than engagement in the classroom or, even more circumscribed, in learning activities. For that reason, I think we can expect differences in the outcomes and determinants of engagement, which in turn, can have implications for intervention.

Outcomes and Contexts of Engagement

Some authors address student engagement in the context of the classroom and learning activities (Gettinger & Walter, 2012; Guthrie, Wigfield, & You, 2012; Wolters & Taylor, 2012). For example, Gettinger and Walter referred to engagement as the time a student is involved or participates in the classroom. With a similar definition, Guthrie et al. (2012) restricted their analysis of engagement to reading activities. Interestingly, these authors tend to concentrate on the role of behavioral and cognitive dimensions of engagement while recognizing the emotional component of it (see also Wolters & Taylor). In any case, they all demonstrate that behavioral and cognitive engagement in learning activities strongly predicts achievement and learning competencies.

Other authors tackle engagement at the school level. Behavioral (attendance, participation in extracurricular activities, misbehavior, mobility) and emotional engagement (identification to school, belongingness, student-teachers and peer relations, emotions accompanying learning tasks) seem to be the most frequent aspects studied in regard to school engagement (Brooks, Brooks, & Goldstein, 2012; Griffiths, Lilles, Furlong, & Sidwha, 2012; Rumberger & Rotermund, 2012). A recent overview of longitudinal studies (Rumberger & Lim, 2008) indicated that student engagement, and especially behavioral engagement, is one of the strongest predictors of persistence and school dropout. Longitudinal studies show that academic achievement and engagement are among the strongest predictors of school dropout (Alexander, Entwisle & Kabbini, 2001; Battin-Pearson et al., 2000; Janosz, LeBlanc, Boulerice, & Tremblay 2000; Rumberger & Rotermund, 2012).

In sum, being engaged during learning activities makes a significant difference in how much is learned and how well intellectual skills are developed. Being engaged or not in school makes a difference in how long a student will persist in their schooling career.

Nevertheless, the specific contribution of the different dimensions of engagement is much less known and demonstrated empirically. It is my contention that in order to advance our comprehension of student engagement, we need to better understand to what extent emotional, cognitive, and behavioral engagement have separate and cumulative impacts on student outcomes and the potential meditational or transactional processes involved. In fact, theoretical elaboration and empirical demonstration of the relations between emotional, cognitive, and behavioral engagement are still lacking. For example, in a recent longitudinal study on engagement in school, Archambault, Janosz, Morizot, and Pagani (2009) demonstrated that cognitive and emotional engagement tended to evolve in synchronicity while behavioral engagement seemed to evolve differently, especially for students with low and unstable overall engagement (which are the students more at risk of dropping out; see Janosz, Archambault, Morizot, & Pagani, 2008). Furthermore, some recent studies propose that academic achievement and engagement mediate the influence of emotional and cognitive engagement on dropout (Archambault, Janosz, Fallu, & Pagani, 2009; Rotermund, 2010). Thus, while we can affirm that student engagement is a major determinant of school success, we have still a lot to learn on how the different dimensions are related to it.

The Nature of Engagement According to the Context

There appears to be a shared consensus about the fact that engagement is multidimensional and comprises a behavioral, cognitive, and emotional component (Fredricks, Blumenfeld, & Paris, 2004). Some researchers have proposed a fourth dimension labeled *academic engagement*, referring to things like time on task, credits earned, and homework completion (Appleton, Christenson, Kim, & Reschly, 2006; Reschly & Christenson, 2006). Although fundamental, we do not think that academic engagement should be considered along the same taxonomy since emotions, cognitions, and behaviors all refer to developmental aspects, while academic engagement refers the context to which engagement is linked (e.g., behavioral engagement in the classroom).

Defining and measuring engagement with rigor and tracing the boundaries of this construct with related concepts like motivation, grit (Duckworth, Peterson, Matthews, & Kelly, 2007), and self-regulation (see the challenging and critical thoughts of Wolters & Taylor, 2012) are undisputable critical issues (Appleton, Christenson, & Furlong, 2008). As the frontiers of student engagement are still a matter of scientific discussion, we would plead for the integration of an additional vector in the actual debate: the context of engagement. We can think of engagement (a) in the context of a specific academic learning activity (i.e., reading lesson); (b) in the context of the classroom, a setting strongly oriented toward academic learning but also providing socioemotional learning opportunities (in a more or less systematic way according to teachers' practices); and (c) in the context of school, which can be conceptualized as a more global educational environment providing many social learning opportunities in addition to stimulating intellectual development (Eccles & Roeser, 2011). We could even extend this nested conceptualization to engagement in learning activities in the community (see Wylie & Hodgen, 2012). As we move from specific learning activities to a more global educational environment, the educational setting (structure, practices) becomes less specific and constraining (in space and time) with regard to the learning it provides.

I think that the multidimensionality of engagement is invariant, cross-sectional to the contexts, that there are always some emotions, cognitions, and behaviors involved when one is making efforts to learn. This does not imply, however, that the expression of engagement is invariant. To the contrary, what can be considered as the expression of emotional, cognitive, and behavioral engagement may be quite context specific and, by extension, lead to the identification of different determinants and outcomes. Consider the example of belongingness. For many, belongingness (or bonding for social development researchers and criminologists) is an indicator of emotional/psychological engagement (Appleton et al., 2006; Finn, 1989; Fredricks et al., 2004; Griffiths et al., 2012). For others, belongingness is more a basic psychological need that must be fulfilled in order to be motivated (Baumeister & Leary, 1995; Ryan & Deci, 2009). Thus, the sense of belongingness is conceptualized by some as a determinant and by others as a manifestation (or even an outcome) of engagement.

Especially for those studying engagement at a more molecular level (e.g., learning activity) (Gettinger & Walter, 2012; Guthrie et al., 2012), motivation is perceived as a determinant of engagement as it expresses, at least in part, the extent to which the learning situation (context, content) responds to the need for belongingness. Thus, sense of belongingness appears to be a determinant of engagement rather than an outcome. Emotional engagement in learning situations may reflect the affects involved during the activity (interest, boredom, happiness, sadness, anxiety). However, in the context of school, the sense of being related to others may be more than just a determinant. School is more than just an academic learning setting; it is a social learning environment, a life environment, and a socialization agent (Wentzel & Looney, 2007). School is also about social learning experiences occurring outside the classroom and between academic activities. In that sense, how one feels about others can be more easily conceived as part of the emotions elicited by being and going to school. This representation is echoed in theories of school dropout, where social integration or bonding is perceived as important determinants of school dropout rather than academic engagement (Tinto, 1994; Wehlage, Rutter, Smith, Lesko, & Fernandez, 1989). Participation in extracurricular activities is another example. Such conduct, by definition, can hardly be used as an indicator of behavioral engagement in the classroom. However, if school is viewed as a social learning environment as well as a setting for intellectual growth, using participation in extracurricular activities as an indicator of engagement seems more than appropriate.

In addition to distinguishing contexts of engagement, we also call for a better understanding of the relations between engagement in different settings. In Finn's model of engagement (1989), participation in extracurricular activities represents a deeper manifestation of engagement. This interesting stage-developmental approach has yet to be empirically tested however. Furthermore, there may be no necessary equivalence between engagement in school and engagement in specific learning activities (Davis & McPartland, 2012). For example, we can easily think of a student highly engaged in extracurricular activities without being deeply engaged in the classroom or in reading activities. Nonetheless, it would also be improbable for a student to be highly engaged in the classroom and not be engaged in school. Is student engagement in the classroom (partially) determined by their engagement in learning activities? Is engagement in school dependent on the level of engagement in the classroom and in learning activities? Conversely, can increased engagement at a broader level (school) have a positive impact on classroom engagement? Wylie and Hodgen (2012) expand even more the complexity of this issue by drawing our attention on the stability (depth and manner) of engagement in and out of school. Their results raise interesting questions about the transactional nature of engagement and the relative contribution of the individual and its educational environments (school, but also the family, peer group, community). This stability across contexts introduces also the possibility that student engagement is, in part at least, the manifestation of more stable personality traits.

Determinants, Intervention, and Contexts of Engagement

Although researchers address student engagement in several contexts, most of them share the idea that motivation, understood as a set of affects, attitudes, and intentions toward learning (values, aspirations, perceived competence/control, goals, etc.) (Wentzel & Wigfield, 2009), is the proximal determinant of engagement. There appears to be a consensus that motivation *precedes* engagement in the sense that the intensity and the quality of student self-mobilization (action) depends directly upon their values, goals, perceived competency/control, and expectancies regarding the learning activity or environment (school). This is not to say however that motivation ceases to exist when the action begins or that engagement does not impact on later motivation. This is presumably why some authors like Guthrie et al. (2012) prefer to talk of the relation between motivation and engagement as *engagement processes*.

This shared perspective introduces another important point of convergence with regard to intervention: (1) to increase student school success (e.g., competencies, achievement, graduation), we must increase engagement; (2) to increase engagement, we must increase motivation; and (3) to increase motivation, we must provide the organizational conditions and educational practices known to sustain or increase student's motivation. The paper from Guthrie et al. (2012) is particularly exemplary of that perspective and offers a substantial demonstration of the validity of this pathway of change at the classroom. To these principles, Gettinger and Walter (2012) bring to our attention that the quantity of engaged time is determinant for success; that engagement is not only determined by individual motivation and learning skills but also by organizational and educational practices (e.g., classroom management and instructional strategies) that maximize the quantity of quality time for learning (time effectively used for learning). For her part, Deakin Crick (2012) focuses on the other side of the coin: the quality of engagement. She argues convincingly that deep engagement generates better and sustained student outcomes, and that it is closely linked to the foundation of identity. Brooks et al. (2012) further develop the social-constructivist view, partially introduced by Deakin Crick, by showing how motivation and engagement are profoundly influenced by the feedback the student receives and interprets from their schooling experience. This perspective also recognizes the active role the student has and must have to become and be engaged, a point of view insufficiently shared in the engagement research field according to Wolter and Taylors (2012). Nonetheless, in my opinion, the most powerful and challenging implication of this latter perspective is to be more critical about the dominant vision of teachers as transmitters of knowledge and students as receptacles of the teachers' words. The benefits of asking teachers to become supportive guides of responsible and active learners should certainly be tested empirically and more systematically.

In sum, whatever specific theoretical background researchers adhere to, most of them recognize that to increase motivation and engagement, we must privilege age-appropriate interventions, educational environments, and learning situations that respond to fundamental individual needs: to feel secure and respected, be active and autonomous, experience success, feel competent and have control over the outcome (success) of a learning task or situation, be related to others, understand the meaning and value of the effort demanded, etc. (Deci & Ryan, 2002; Eccles & Roeser, 2010).

To complete this commentary, I would like to highlight two aspects I think have received insufficient attention and that may provide new insights on the determinants/outcomes of engagement and for intervention: understanding the relation of engagement with other aspects of the biopsychosocial development and tackling engagement within a more person-oriented approach.

Student Engagement and Biopsychosocial Development

As there is a necessity to clarify the definition and conceptual boundaries of student engagement, I also think we should move toward understanding how it is linked to other aspects of children and adolescent development. Manifestations of lack of engagement could express difficulties in other spheres of development and not be the direct or sole consequence of lack of motivation. Rumberger and Rotermund (2012) remind us that

40 years ago, Bachman and his colleagues asked themselves whether school dropout was a symptom of social maladjustment or a problem of its own (Bachman, Green, & Wirtanen, 1971). They showed that many young people who dropped out of school had problems in several other spheres of their development, as part of a general deviance syndrome (Jessor & Jessor, 1977). Student lack of engagement may also be the manifestation of other causes than lack of motivation. For example, taken individually, behaviors used to measure school behavioral (dis)engagement (skipping school, not responding to teachers, not doing homework, etc.) could likewise be used as indicator of externalizing problem behaviors or even delinquency. Griffiths et al. (2012) do a very good job of reminding us of the correlates of engagement with other types of difficulties in adolescence (e.g., substance use, mental health). We should also think of students with attention deficit disorder or with executive functions vulnerabilities (Blair, 2002). These students most probably manifest symptoms (lack of attention, poor self-regulation) that could be easily interpreted as cognitive disengagement. What about students with depression or drug abuse problems?

Thus, many scenarios of relationships are plausible and not mutually exclusive: disengagement could be a cause or a risk factor for psychosocial maladjustment; disengagement and concurrent psychosocial difficulties could be the consequence of the same underlying cause (e.g., ADHD); school motivation may (partially) mediate the influence of socioemotional or neurobiological problems on engagement; and moreover, we could explore the potential moderating influence (protective role) of engagement over the relationship between biopsychosocial early difficulties and later adjustment problems like dropout, criminality, etc.

Underlining the importance of these issues without referring to the recent work of Skinner, Kinderman, and Furrer (2009) would be an incomplete comment. Throughout this chapter, we have used the expressions *engagement* and *disengagement* interchangeably, as if one was the contrary of the other. This polarized or dimensional view is certainly widely shared in the present literature on student engagement. Recently however, Skinner et al. (2009) challenged this vision and demonstrated that disengagement, or what they prefer to call *disaffection*, is best measured and conceived as a related but separate construct. This perspective suggests, for example, that (very) low engagement is not exactly the same thing as being disengaged (see also Griffiths et al., 2012). This proposition reminds how positive and warm student-teachers relations are not the opposite of negative and conflicting relations (Jerome, Hamre, & Pianta, 2009). One implication of this finding is that we should verify to what extent (emotional, cognitive, behavioral) engagement is related to the same determinants and outcomes as disengagement/disaffection.

Unraveling the existence and strength between engagement and psychosocial adjustment is important for intervention and targeted prevention efforts. If motivational and engagement difficulties are not so much affected by weaknesses in the educational environment than by other determinants (family, peers, community, neurobiological development), then interventions should focus on these other targets as well. For example, we could easily assume that the intervention plan should not be the same for a student with a lack of cognitive engagement that has, or not, an attention deficit disorder or for a student with a lack of behavioral engagement that has, or not, a drug abuse problem.

We are certainly in need of more comprehensive longitudinal studies, beginning in early childhood, to help us disentangle the relations between engagement, motivation, and other biopsychosocial aspects of the child and adolescent development. This can be done by examining the potential direct and indirect (mediating and moderating) relations between variables, including all the appropriate controls. Well-designed intervention studies can also be very instructive of the relative importance of different factors and meditational processes involved (Lacourse et al., 2002). Another approach would be to adopt a person-centered perspective.

A Person-Centered Approach in the Study of Engagement

The vast majority of studies of student engagement examine how isolated aspects of human experience are related (e.g., the relation between self-efficacy and engagement or student-teachers relations and engagement). These studies provide us with extremely valuable information, especially when having a longitudinal design. Nonetheless, a complementary approach to the study of human development is trying not to isolate specific aspects but rather to better capture its multidimensionality and diversity (see Bergman & Trost, 2006; Cairns, Bergman, & Kagan, 1998). For example, in a longitudinal and replication study using cluster analyses, Janosz et al. (2000) showed that the dropout population was quite heterogeneous. In both longitudinal samples, approximately 40% of high school dropouts previously reported high levels of school motivation and showed similar, and sometimes even better, behavioral and psychological profiles than the average graduate (labeled *quiet dropouts*). Another 40% (*maladjusted* dropouts) had experienced severe levels of school and psychosocial difficulties. Two other interesting profiles emerged: the *disengaged* dropout (10%), strongly unmotivated while in school yet showing no socioemotional difficulties and getting average grades; and the *low-achiever* dropout (10%), disengaged in addition to experiencing academic failure yet not showing any externalizing problem behaviors. This study illustrates that by looking at profiles of individuals, we may more easily identify how engagement and other aspects of development tend to associate and the prevalence of such interactions. A typological and person-oriented approach may also be very useful to plan differential interventions and programs, more closely suited to student needs, to the extent that actions are taken to prevent the potential iatrogenic effects of labeling or, paraphrasing Brooks et al. (2012), *mindsetting* negatively the educators.

Some recent studies of student engagement, like the one of Wylie and Hodgen (2012), are now combining person-oriented and longitudinal approaches (Archambault, Janosz, et al., 2009; Janosz et al., 2008). Indeed, recent statistical developments, stimulated by the power increase of personal computers, now permit researchers to examine how different groups of students, characterized by different levels or types of engagement and other concomitant individual or contextual characteristics, evolve over time (Muthén, 2004; Muthén & Muthén, 2008). This method increases our capacity to study quantitative and qualitative differences in the development of student engagement, integrating a person-oriented perspective.

Conclusion

With the growing recognition that engagement is a multidimensional construct comes the scientific duty of verifying more systematically if the dimensions of engagement share the same determinants or lead to the same outcomes. This task is only beginning. Reviewing the authoritative chapters of this book, I have first come to suggest that, since the nature of engagement is not independent of the context to which it refers, we should try to answer the causes and consequences questions by distinguishing the distinct however nested contexts of engagement: the learning activity, the classroom, and the school environments. Second, because of the importance of schooling in social development and the multiple nonschool factors that may interfere or facilitate student engagement, I proposed that we expand our understanding of determinants and outcomes of engagement to biopsychosocial aspects of development. Third, as the study of engagement is largely dominated by a dimensional and variable-centered perspective, which tends to mask the heterogeneity of trajectories toward engagement/disengagement, I suggested we approach more often the study of engagement within a person-centered perspective.

The quality and quantity of effort a student put in school greatly influence the benefits of schooling. Learning will be better, and the probabilities of pursuing higher education or integrating the workforce with success will be higher. As a whole, the quality of life will be superior. Increasing our understanding of the modifiable precursors of engagement is thus a key issue toward increasing the education level of the population, especially for the most vulnerable children of the society.

References

Alexander, K. L., Entwisle, D. R., & Kabbini, N. S. (2001). The dropout process in life course perspective: Early risk factors at home and school. *Teachers College Record, 103*, 760–882.

Appleton, J. J., Christenson, S. L., & Furlong, M. J. (2008). Student engagement with school: Critical conceptual and methodological issues of the construct. *Psychology in the Schools, 45*, 369–386.

Appleton, J. J., Christenson, S. L., Kim, D., & Reschly, A. L. (2006). Measuring cognitive and psychological engagement: Validation of the student engagement instrument. *Journal of School Psychology, 44*, 427–445.

Archambault, I., Janosz, M., Fallu, J.-S., & Pagani, L. S. (2009). Student engagement and its relationship with early high school dropout. *Journal of Adolescence, 32*, 651–670.

Archambault, I., Janosz, M., Morizot, J., & Pagani, L. (2009). Adolescent behavioral, affective, and cognitive engagement in school: Relationship to dropout. *Journal of School Health, 79*, 408–415.

Bachman, J. G., Green, S., & Wirtanen, I. D. (1971). *Youth in transition, vol. III: Dropping out: Problem or symptom?* Ann Arbor, MI: Institute for Social Research, The University of Michigan.

Battin-Pearson, S., Newcomb, M. D., Abbott, R. D., Hill, K. G., Catalano, R. F., & Hawkins, J. D. (2000). Predictors of early high school dropout: A test of five theories. *Journal of Educational Psychology, 92*, 568–582.

Baumeister, R. F., & Leary, M. R. (1995). The need to belong: Desire for interpersonal attachments as a fundamental human motivation. *Psychological Bulletin, 117*, 497–529.

Bergman, L. R., & Trost, K. (2006). The person-oriented versus variable-oriented approach: Are they complementary, opposites, or exploring different worlds? *Merrill-Palmer Quarterly, 52*, 601–632.

Blair, C. (2002). School readiness: Integrating cognition and emotion in a neurobiological conceptualization of children's functioning at school entry. *American Psychologist, 57*, 111–127.

Brooks, R., Brooks, S., & Goldstein, S. (2012). The power of mindsets: Nurturing engagement, motivation, and resilience in students. In S. L. Christenson, A. L. Reschly, & C. Wylie (Eds.), *Handbook of research on student engagement* (pp. 541–562). New York: Springer.

Cairns, R. B., Bergman, L. R., & Kagan, J. (Eds.). (1998). *Methods and models for studying the individual.* Thousand Oaks, CA: Sage.

Davis, M. H., & McPartland, J. M. (2012). High school reform and student engagement. In S. L. Christenson, A. L. Reschly, & C. Wylie (Eds.), *Handbook of research on student engagement* (pp. 515–539). New York: Springer.

Deakin Crick, R. (2012). Deep engagement as a complex system: Identity, learning power and authentic enquiry. In S. L. Christenson, A. L. Reschly, & C. Wylie (Eds.), *Handbook of research on student engagement* (pp. 675–694). New York: Springer.

Deci, E. L., & Ryan, R. M. (Eds.). (2002). *Handbook of self determination theory research.* Rochester, NY: University of Rochester Press.

Duckworth, A. L., Peterson, C., Matthews, M., & Kelly, D. (2007). Grit: Perseverance and passion for long-term goals. *Journal of Personality and Social Psychology, 92*, 1087–1101.

Eccles, J. S., & Roeser, R. W. (2010). An ecological view of schools and development. In J. L. Meece & J. S. Eccles (Eds.), *Handbook of research on schools, schooling, and human development* (pp. 6–22). New York: Routledge.

Eccles, J. S., & Roeser, R. W. (2011). Schools as developmental contexts during adolescence. *Journal of Research on Adolescence, 21*, 225–241.

Finn, J. D. (1989). Withdrawing from school. *Review of Educational Research, 59*, 117–142.

Fredricks, J. A., Blumenfeld, P. C., & Paris, A. H. (2004). School engagement: Potential of the concept, state of the evidence. *Review of Educational Research, 74*, 59–109.

Gettinger, M., & Walter, M. J. (2012). Classroom strategies to enhance academic engaged time. In S. L. Christenson, A. L. Reschly, & C. Wylie (Eds.), *Handbook of research on student engagement* (pp. 653–673). New York: Springer.

Griffiths, A.-J., Lilles, E., Furlong, M., & Sidwha, J. (2012). The relations of adolescent student engagement with troubling and high-risk behaviors. In S. L. Christenson, A. L. Reschly, & C. Wylie (Eds.), *Handbook of research on student engagement* (pp. 563–584). New York: Springer.

Guthrie, J. T., Wigfield, A., & You, W. (2012). Instructional contexts for engagement and achievement in reading. In S. L. Christenson, A. L. Reschly, & C. Wylie (Eds.), *Handbook of research on student engagement* (pp. 601–634). New York: Springer.

Heckman, J. J. (2006). Skill formation and the economics of investing in disadvantaged children. *Science, 312*, 1900–1902.

Janosz, M., Archambault, I., Morizot, J., & Pagani, L. (2008). School engagement trajectories and their differential predictive relations to dropout. *Journal of Social Issues, 64*, 21–40.

Janosz, M., LeBlanc, M., Boulerice, B., & Tremblay, R. E. (2000). Predicting types of school dropouts: A typological approach with two longitudinal samples. *Journal of Educational Psychology, 92*, 171–190.

Jerome, E. M., Hamre, B. K., & Pianta, R. C. (2009). Teacher—child relationships from kindergarten to sixth grade: Early childhood predictors of teacher-perceived conflict and closeness. *Social Development, 18*, 915–945.

Jessor, R., & Jessor, S. L. (1977). *Problem behavior and psychosocial development: A longitudinal study of youth*. New York: Academic.

Lacourse, E., Côté, S., Nagin, D. S., Vitaro, F., Brendgen, M., & Tremblay, R. E. (2002). A longitudinal-experimental approach to testing theories of antisocial behavior development. *Development and Psychopathology, 14*, 909–924.

Muennig, P. (2007). How education produces health: A hypothetical framework. *Teachers College Record, 109*, 1–17.

Muthén, B. (2004). Latent variable analysis: Growth mixture modeling and related techniques for longitudinal data. In D. Kaplan (Ed.), *Handbook of quantitative methodology for the social sciences* (pp. 345–368). Newbury Park, CA: Sage.

Muthén, L. K., & Muthén, B. O. (2008). *Mplus user's guide*. Los Angeles, CA: Muthén & Muthén.

Reschly, A., & Christenson, S. L. (2006). Research leading to a predictive model of dropout and completion among students with mild disabilities and the role of student engagement. *Remedial and Special Education, 27*, 276–292.

Rotermund, S. L. (2010). *The role of psychological antecedents and student engagement in a process model of high school dropout*. Doctoral dissertation. Gevirtz Graduate School of Education, University of California, Santa Barbara, CA.

Rumberger, R. W., & Lim, S. A. (2008). *Why students drop out of school: A review of 25 years of research*. Santa Barbara, CA: California Dropout Research Project. Retrieved December 20, 2010, from, http://cdrp.ucsb.edu/dropouts/pubs_reports.htm#15

Rumberger, R. W., & Rotermund, S. (2012). The relation between engagement and high school dropout. In S. L. Christenson, A. L. Reschly, & C. Wylie (Eds.), *Handbook of research on student engagement* (pp. 491–513). New York: Springer.

Ryan, R. M., & Deci, E. L. (2009). Promoting self-determined school engagement: Motivation, learning, and well-being. In K. Wenzel & A. Wigfield (Eds.), *Handbook of motivation at school* (pp. 171–195). New York: Routledge/Taylor & Francis Group.

Skinner, E., Kinderman, T., & Furrer, C. (2009). A motivational perspective on engagement and disaffection: Conceptualization and assessment of children's behavioral and emotional participation in academic activities in the classroom. *Educational and Psychological Measurement, 69*, 493–525.

Tinto, V. (1994). *Leaving college: Rethinking the causes and cures for student attrition* (2nd ed.). Chicago: University of Chicago Press.

Wehlage, G. G., Rutter, R. A., Smith, G. A., Lesko, N., & Fernandez, R. R. (1989). *Reducing the risk: Schools as communities of support*. New York: Falmer Press.

Wentzel, K. R., & Looney, L. (2007). Socialization in school settings. In J. E Grusec, & P. D. Hastings (Eds.), *Handbook of socialization: Theory and research* (pp. 382–403). New York: Guilford Press.

Wentzel, K. R., & Wigfield, A. (Eds.). (2009). *Handbook of motivation at school*. New York: Routledge.

Wolters, C. A., & Taylor, D. J. (2012). A self-regulated learning perspective on student engagement. In S. L. Christenson, A. L. Reschly, & C. Wylie (Eds.), *Handbook of research on student engagement* (pp. 635–651). New York: Springer.

Wylie, C., & Hodgen, E. (2012). Trajectories and patterns of student engagement: Evidences form a longitudinal study. In S. L. Christenson, A. L. Reschly, & C. Wylie (Eds.), *Handbook of research on student engagement* (pp. 585–599). New York: Springer.

Part V

Measurement Issues, Instruments, and Approaches

Measuring Student Engagement: The Development of a Scale for Formative Use

34

Charles W. Darr

Abstract

An important part of the short history of student engagement has been the development of self-report instruments designed to measure engagement. This chapter describes the development of a self-report tool designed for Year 7–10 students (11- to 15-year olds) in New Zealand schools. A feature of the development was the use of Rasch Measurement, which allows raw survey scores to be transformed to locations on a described equal-interval scale. Once located on the scale, students' scores can be compared with the scores of nationally representative reference groups and interpreted using the scale descriptors. The chapter begins by describing the development of the survey instrument, including how researchers used a multi-faceted definition of engagement to select and develop items. It then goes on to describe findings from the national trial of the instrument. The last part of the chapter looks at possible future directions for the survey.

Introduction

Interest in the construct of student engagement has been growing for the last 25 years or so (Appleton, Christenson, & Furlong, 2008). As a construct, it appeals to a range of educational stake holders, particularly because of its association with positive outcomes and its relevance to all students. An important part of the short history of student engagement has included the development of self-report instruments designed to measure engagement (Appleton, Christenson, Kim, & Reschly, 2006; Finn, 1989; Martin, 2009; Yazzie-Mintz, 2007). Although varied in their approaches, these tools represent attempts to provide an operational definition of engagement that can be used to explore important issues in the field in a consistent and psychometrically sound manner.

In recent years, New Zealand schools have invested an increasing amount of time and resources collecting achievement data for formative use in core learning areas. To assist them to do this, several new sophisticated assessment tools have been developed that are capable of tracking achievement over time and supported by online administration and analysis options. When it comes to measuring student engagement,

C.W. Darr, B.Sc., M.Ed. (Dist), Dip. Tchng (✉)
New Zealand Council for Educational Research (NZCER),
Te Aro, Wellington, New Zealand
e-mail: Charles.darr@nzcer.org.nz

schools have not been so well supported. For the most part, when motivated to collect data around engagement, schools have used more ad hoc indicators. Most often these are not comparable across schools and are not supported by national reference data.

This chapter describes the development of a new survey tool for New Zealand schools designed to measure self-perceived levels of engagement. Called *Me and My School* and developed by researchers at the New Zealand Council for Educational Research (NZCER), the survey reports levels of engagement on a described interval scale. Once located on the scale, engagement scores can be compared with descriptors that illustrate the types of survey responses typical at different levels of the scale and the engagement scores of nationally representative groups of students at each of Years 7–10.

At the heart of *Me and My School* is a belief that student engagement matters, that students' voices provide an essential perspective on engagement, and that schools should have access to tools that they can use to investigate engagement. This chapter describes the development of the survey from the pilot stage through to a national standardisation exercise involving over 8,000 students. It also includes an exploration of some of the patterns found in the national data.

Measuring Student Engagement in New Zealand

The term 'student engagement' is widely used in New Zealand, albeit with a range of meanings. For instance, a series of official reports on student engagement published since 2001 has used it in a relatively narrow sense to describe patterns of attendance at school (see Lane [2008] for an example). Somewhat ironically, the reports provide statistics on indicators of *dis*engagement such as stand-downs (formal removal from school for up to 5 days), suspensions (formal removal from the school until a formal hearing takes place), exclusions (formal exclusion from a school with the requirement that the student enrols elsewhere), expulsions (formal exclusion for over 16-year olds with no requirement for enrolment at another school) and early-leaving exemptions (formal permission to leave school before the age of 16).

Elsewhere, a richer concept of engagement has been adopted, for instance, in significant research projects (see Wylie & Hodgen this edition) and in professional development programmes. The Te Kōtahitanga initiative (Bishop, Berryman, Cavanagh, & Teddy, 2007) is an example of the later. Te Kōtahitanga emphasised the development of connectedness between teachers and students to raise the engagement levels of the indigenous Māori students to improve their school achievement.

Prior to the development of *Me and My School* and despite the general interest in student engagement, there were no standardized tools that New Zealand schools could use to measure student engagement. This lack of a standardized instrument was one motivator for the development of *Me and My School*. Other motivators included evidence in the research literature that:

- High levels of engagement are associated with positive educational and health outcomes (National Research Council and the Institute of Measurement, 2004).
- Unlike some educational variables, for instance, socioeconomic status or previous academic success, student engagement can be influenced by the ways we teach and the ways we organise our schools (Appleton et al., 2008).
- The middle school years (Years 7–10) are pivotal years for students, marked by school transitions, emotional and physical changes and increased rates of suspensions and stand-downs (Dinahm & Rowe, 2007; Ng, 2006).

The overall intention in developing the survey then was to create a set of survey items and associated reporting functions with sound psychometric credentials that New Zealand schools could use to inform their understanding of how students perceived their own engagement.

Defining Student Engagement

The development of *Me and My School* began with discussion regarding how the survey would define student engagement. Student engagement is an abstract idea—it does not exist as a physical entity that can be poked, prodded or contained in a vial. However, most educators would feel that they can sense when it is present and believe that they themselves have an important role in creating the conditions where high levels of engagement can occur.

In the research literature, student engagement is defined in various ways and, at times, used interchangeably with terms such as school bonding, school attachment, school engagement and school connectedness (Libbey, 2004). In a major review of the literature, Fredricks, Blumenfeld, and Paris (2004) recognised three definitions of engagement. The first of these is behavioral engagement and refers to students' actual participation in school and learning. This includes observable behaviours such as positive conduct, persistence in learning and involvement in school life. Behavioral engagement is seen as crucial to academic achievement and the prevention of dropping out of school. The second definition is emotional engagement and refers to students' emotional responses to teachers, peers, learning and school. Emotional engagement is seen as creating connections with school and influencing willingness to do the work. Finally, cognitive engagement stresses investment in learning, seeking challenge and going beyond the requirements. It also includes employing self-regulation strategies to control and monitor learning.

The distinctions between these definitions are blurred. In research studies, similar survey items are often used to assess the different types of engagement (Jimerson, Campos, & Greif, 2003). The multifaceted nature of engagement led Fredricks et al. (2004, p. 60) to describe engagement as a 'meta' construct. They noted that:

> The fusion of behaviour, emotion and cognition under the idea of engagement is valuable because it may provide a richer characterisation of children than is possible in research on single components. Defining and examining the components of engagement individually separates students' behaviour and cognition. In reality these factors are dynamically interrelated within the individual; they are not isolated processes (Fredricks et al., 2004, p. 61).

The terms engagement and motivation are sometimes used interchangeably. However, they can be distinguished, with motivation understood as the 'why' or reasoning behind a given behaviour, and engagement as the actual patterns of action and involvement a person displays in tasks and activities (Appleton et al., 2008). These patterns can involve physical, cognitive and emotional responses and commitments.

The researchers involved in the development of the *Me and My School* survey decided to develop an item set that spanned the three definitions of engagements described above. This broad approach reflected the national curriculum in New Zealand, which outlined a comprehensive agenda for education involving a range of competencies, values and attitudes. In a vision statement, it described young people '… who in their school years, will continue to develop the values knowledge, and competencies that will enable them to live full and satisfying lives' (Ministry of Education, 2007, p. 8). It was thought important not to narrow the idea of engagement to a set of behaviours and attitudes sometimes associated with academic success, such as following routines and spending time on task. It was also decided to take a global perspective on engagement, focusing on students' overall perceptions of their connection with school and involvement in learning, rather than their engagement in a specific classroom context or learning area. Particular value was placed on items that indicated:

- Positive, trusting, active relationships with teachers and peers
- Feelings of personal safety and belonging
- Positive beliefs and commitments involving the purpose, relevancy and efficacy of school
- Active involvement in learning situations and a preparedness to persist

In terms of response format, it was decided to use Likert-type items with four response categories: strongly disagree, disagree, agree and strongly agree. Some of the item stems were sourced from the research literature, for instance: 'Most mornings I look forward to going to school', which points towards the emotional definition of engagement (Battin Pearson et al., as cited in Jimerson et al., 2003, p. 16). Others had been used in previous survey work done by NZCER or were written specifically for the instrument, for example: 'There is just the right amount of challenge at school for me', which links to the cognitive definition. As part of the development process, researchers from both inside and outside NZCER reviewed the item choices.

An effort was made to use item stems that were expressed in terms of beliefs, attitudes and behaviours that the students responding held or exhibited themselves, rather than as observations or judgments they made of the school, their teachers or their peers in general. For instance, 'I feel safe', rather than 'This school is a safe place', and 'I pay attention in class', rather than 'Students in our school pay attention'. Only one item in the final survey was of an observational nature ('People care about others at this school').

Rasch Measurement and Me and My School

A fundamental aspect of the development of *Me and My School* was the application of Rasch Measurement (Bond & Fox, 2007). Rasch Measurement is a probabilistic approach to measurement in the social sciences built around a mathematical model that transforms raw survey scores into locations on an equal-interval scale. High scores on the survey indicate higher levels of the trait being investigated and are transformed to higher locations on the scale. Low survey scores on the other hand indicate lower levels of the trait and are transformed to lower locations on the scale. Unlike scales that are based on raw scores or percentiles, each unit on an equal-interval scale indicates the same amount of the construct or trait being measured. The unit of measurement used by the Rasch model is called the logit.

When transforming a raw survey score to a location on the scale, the model takes into account that some survey items are harder to agree with (involve higher levels of the trait) than others. It also takes into account that the differences, or changes in the level of agreement indicated by the response categories for an item (strongly disagree to strongly agree), are not necessarily constant within the item or between items. For instance, on one item selecting strongly agree rather than agree might represent only a small difference in the underlying trait, while for another this could be an indication of a much greater trait level.

Constructing a survey using Rasch Measurement begins with a theory regarding the trait to be measured. The theory anticipates the kinds of questions and responses that will be associated with higher and lower points on the scale. The theory is then operationalised in the form of survey items (indicators of the latent trait under consideration). Sets of items are trialled and the responses analysed to see how well they fit the measurement model.

A basic assumption of the Rasch model is that the survey is measuring one dominant trait. Good model fit indicates that this assumption has been met well enough for most practical purposes—the survey items are discriminating in a uniform way to measure the same trait. When responses for a survey item show poor fit to the model, evidence exists that the item could be measuring something different from the other items, or that it is causing confusion for respondents. When this happens, the item becomes a candidate for exclusion from the final instrument.

Fit to the model is investigated using a number of different statistical and graphical indicators. Figure 34.1 shows an example of a graph used to check the fit of the *Me and My School* item 'Most mornings I look forward to going to school'. The horizontal axis is used to show the measurement scale, while the vertical axis shows the range of raw scores possible for this item (0–3). The black curve is used to plot the expected response score (agreement level) calculated using the Rasch model for respondents at different locations along

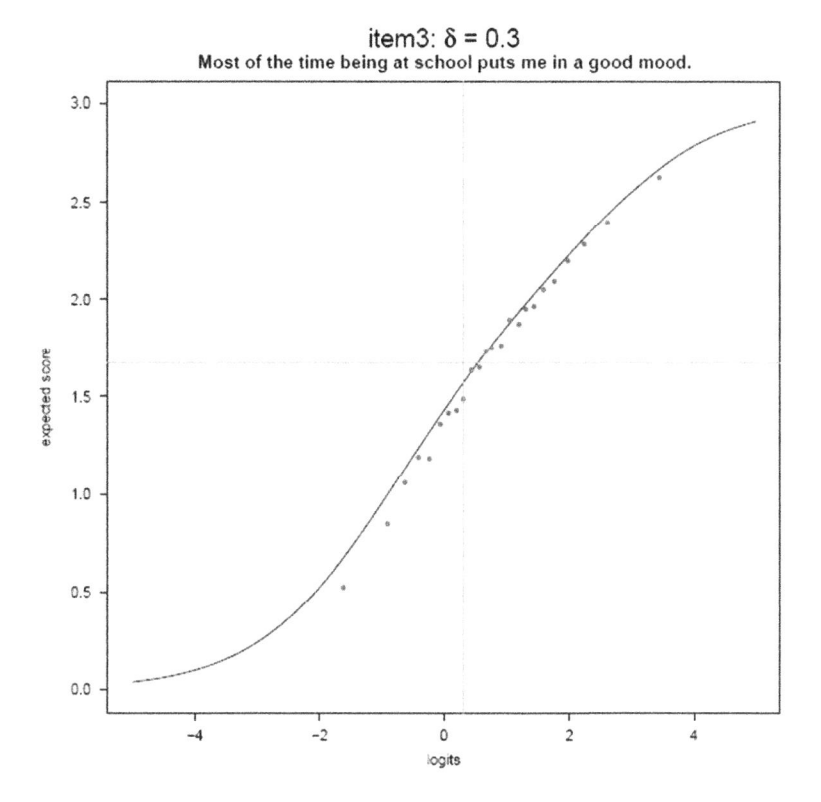

Fig. 34.1 An example of an expected score curve used to investigate model fit

the scale. As the scale score shown on the horizontal axis increases, the expected score on the item goes up. The black dots show the average item scores for groups of actual respondents located at different points along the scale. As can be seen, the average scores are very close to the expected scores; in other words, responses to this item show good fit to the model.

The outcome of the item calibration process is a set of threshold locations for each item on the scale. A threshold locates the point on the scale where the probabilities of choosing two adjacent response categories for a particular item (for instance, agree and strongly agree) are equally likely. Figure 34.2 illustrates this using the response categories for the statement 'Most mornings I look forward to going to school'. Each response category is associated with the region or part of the scale (shown by the vertical line) where it is the most probable response to the item stem. The dotted lines between these regions are used to show the thresholds, where choosing either of the adjacent response categories is equally likely.

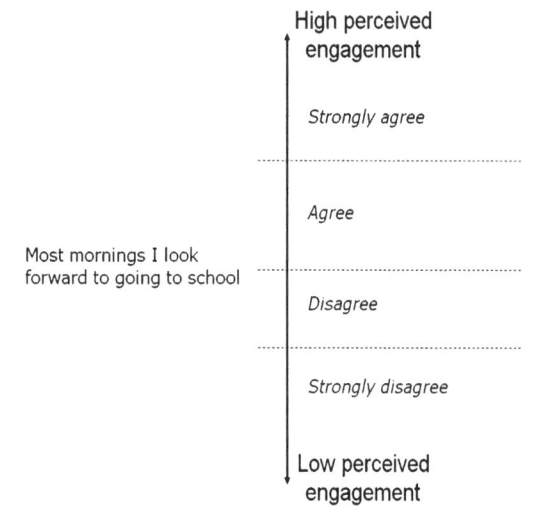

Fig. 34.2 Locating a survey item on the scale

Piloting

The large pool of items was trialled in two pilot studies. The first pilot used a survey form consisting of 64 items. Responses were collected from approximately 1,200 Year 7 and 8 students at a large multi-ethnic North Island school. An analysis of the data was carried out using a polytomous form of the Rasch model called the Partial Credit Model (Wright & Masters, 1982). The Quest software (Adams & Khoo, 1999) was used to perform the analysis.

Statistical fit indicators from Quest and graphical fit indicators generated using the open source statistical package R suggested that overall the response data fitted the measurement model well. Although the items had been purposefully chosen to represent the three different definitions of student engagement described by Fredricks et al. (2004), the strength of the overall fit suggested a single underlying dimension made up of three aspects.

We also investigated the dimensionality of response data using factor analysis. A three-factor model generated three highly correlated factors, and a single-factor model showed that one predominant factor explained most of the variance. It was decided therefore to produce one measurement scale.

The analysis of data from the first pilot was used to help inform the development of a more concise instrument. We carried out a careful 'weeding' process, examining each item's ability to represent one or more of the engagement aspects, demonstrate a level of uniqueness when compared to other items, and show satisfactory fit to the measurement model. As a result of this work, the original instrument was reduced from 64 to 36 items. A subsequent analysis using data from the remaining items suggested negligible changes in overall reliability.

The shorter instrument was used in the second pilot trial involving approximately 1,800 Year 7–10 students from four schools chosen for their contrasting student populations. For instance, one of the schools was a girls' high school with a student population of predominantly European descent and a high decile rating (the New Zealand government's index indicating the socioeconomic status of the school community). The other high school was coeducational, had a diverse ethnic mix and a much lower socioeconomic rating.

Data from the second pilot were first analysed school by school and then for all of the schools together, again using the Partial Credit Model. The analyses showed that overall the data fitted the measurement model well, and the items functioned consistently across the different schools. Once more, the analysis was used to inform the construction of a subsequent survey form, which was used in a much larger national trial.

The National Trial

In August 2007, data were collected from approximately 8,500 students in Years 7–10 (11- to 15-year olds). Two nationally representative samples of schools were used, one based on schools with Year 7 and 8 students and the other on schools with students in Years 9 and 10. Both samples were stratified according to decile and school size. Schools were invited to involve 1, 2 or 3 classes at each year level depending on the size of the school. Each school was asked to select classes of students within each year level that they believed were representative of the range of engagement levels in the school. Some schools asked if they could involve more than three classes. This was allowed, and a later sub-sampling procedure was used to remove any potential bias from school types that were over-represented.

As had happened in the pilot trials, students completed the survey anonymously. We felt that anonymity would lead to more valid engagement with the survey, particularly as some of the survey items related directly to teachers. Teachers were asked to read a short introduction regarding the survey to the students, which included some general instructions. The students then read and completed the survey independently. Teachers were instructed that they could read a question to any students struggling to read the survey but that this should be done on an individual basis rather than to the whole group. Once the students had completed the survey, a class member was selected to collect the forms and return them in a sealed envelope to the school office. When all classes had completed the survey, they were returned to NZCER for analysis.

Analysis of National Trial Data

Data from the national trial were analysed using the Partial Credit Model. Graphical and statistical fit indicators were used to show how well the data fitted the measurement model. The overall fit was very good. Three items, however, persisted in showing poor fit, and after some deliberation, it was decided to discard these items from further analysis. In addition, a number of items exhibited little or no separation between at least two adjacent response categories. In these cases, we merged (collapsed) the adjoining response categories. For instance, for some items, strongly disagree and disagree were merged into one disagreement category. Subsequent analyses indicated improved fit to the model.

Table 34.1 shows the final threshold calibrations for the 33 remaining items. Often referred to as deltas, these are provided in the columns

Table 34.1 Item calibrations for the student engagement scale

Q	Aspect[a]	Item stem	d_{01}	d_{12}	d_{23}	Infit
1	E	Most mornings I look forward to going to school	−1.25	0.34	2.83	0.97
2	E	I am proud to be at this school	−2.13	−0.71	1.55	0.97
3	E	Most of the time being at school puts me in a good mood	−1.74	0.00	2.64	0.97
4	B	I think it is important for me to behave well at school	−1.54	0.42		0.88
5	E (R)	School often feels like a waste of time to me	−1.47	−0.51	0.99	1.15
6	B	I respect other students' space and property at this school	−1.92	0.34		1.16
7	E	I feel safe at school	−0.78	1.10		1.18
8	E	People care about each other in this school	0.03	2.55		1.22
10	E/B	I have a lot of respect for my teachers	−2.19	−1.17	1.11	0.81
11	E	My family's culture is treated with respect by the teachers	−1.65	−0.05		1.13
12	E	I am comfortable talking to the teachers at this school about problems	−0.76	0.34	2.07	1.20
13	E	I care a lot about what my teachers think of me	−1.03	−0.23	1.33	1.09
14	E	Most of my teachers like me	−0.67	1.71		0.92
15	E/B	It is easy for me to talk about my schoolwork with most of my teachers	−1.79	−0.82	1.23	1.05
16	E	I feel my teachers help me learn	−1.24	0.74		0.81
17	C	I feel like I am making progress at school	−1.17	0.89		0.84
18	C	There is just the right amount of challenge for me at school	−0.63	1.41		1.13
19	C	I pay attention in class	−2.00	−0.52	2.22	0.87
20	B/C	I take school seriously	−1.88	−0.73	1.47	0.77
22	B/C (R)	I do as little work as possible; I just want to get by	−0.49			1.09
23	C	I am interested in what I am learning at school	−1.81	−0.62	1.85	0.81
24	C	I look for ways to improve my school work	−2.05	−0.46	1.68	0.93
25	B/C (R)	When schoolwork is difficult I stop trying	−0.55			1.07
26	C	I like learning new things in school	−1.32	0.72		0.90
27	B/C	I take care that my homework is done properly	−1.14	−0.08	1.58	0.97
28	C	I find it easy to concentrate on what I am doing in class	−1.49	−0.04	2.61	1.00
29	C	I take notice of the comments my teachers make about my work	−0.57	1.07		0.90
30	C	At school I really care that I do my best work	−2.06	−0.68	1.30	0.77
31	C	My schoolwork helps in things I do outside of school	−1.19	−0.18	1.68	1.09
33	B (R)	I think most of my classes are a waste of time	−0.37	0.55		0.94
34	B (R)	I often feel bored in class	−0.30	0.78	2.34	1.13
35	E	My friends think school is important	−1.05	0.03	2.25	1.24
36	C	I talk to other people about what I am learning at school.	0.49	1.93		1.07

[a]*E* emotional, *B* behavioral, *C* cognitive, (*R*) reversed

labelled d_{01}, d_{12} and d_{23}. For instance, d_{01} is the scale location of the threshold between category 0 (usually strongly disagree) and category 1 (usually disagree).

Response categories were merged for the 15 items shown with fewer than three deltas. In most cases, this merging has involved the two lowest categories (strongly disagree and disagree). For two items however, the two lowest and two highest categories have been collapsed, resulting in a dichotomous item with disagree and agree categories. The final column in the table is used to display the Infit statistic for each item. The Infit statistic provides an overall indication of how well the item fits the measurement model. Values that are less than or greater than indicate deviation from the model. Although there is no set cut off, items with Infit statistics greater than 1.2 or less than 0.8 are often examined further to see whether they should be excluded.

Figure 34.3 locates both the item thresholds and the national distribution of engagement scores on the scale. In the figure, each 'X' is used to represent 31 student scores. The thresholds are represented by number labels. For instance, '19.1' is used to plot the threshold between categories 0 and 1 (strongly disagree and disagree) for item 19 in the survey. As can be seen, the items target (match) the range of engagement scores well.

Describing the Student Engagement Scale

Rasch measurement scales can be described to provide qualitative information regarding different parts of the scale. To do this, item descriptors must be developed and a decision made regarding the best way to associate the descriptors with locations on the scale. Once this has been decided, descriptors that cluster around a given point on the scale can be used to describe the typical types of responses for respondents located at that part of the scale.

In order to describe the *Me and My School* scale, descriptors for each response category within an item were generated by combining the item stem with the different levels of agreement (strongly disagree to strongly agree). For example, with a stem such as 'Most mornings I look forward to going to school', the different categories where described as:

- Strongly disagrees that they look forward to going to school each day
- Disagrees that they look forward to going to school each day
- Agrees that they look forward to going to school each day
- Strongly agrees that they look forward to going to school each day

Descriptors were not generated for response categories that had been merged with adjacent response categories during the analysis.

There are several ways to demarcate a scale according to response categories. For the purposes of describing the student engagement scale, a descriptor for each response category was associated with the location on the scale where the category has the greatest modelled probability of being selected. The descriptor can then be said to signal a behaviour or belief most likely to be associated with respondents scoring at this scale location.

For middle response categories, for example, the 'agree' and 'disagree' categories, finding the point of maximum probability is relatively straightforward. These points for inner categories occur around about the halfway point between adjacent category thresholds. Using the halfway point as the most probable location for a response category is precise enough for the purposes of describing the scale.

Outer response categories, on the other hand, do not have these points of maximum probability; the probability of choosing the 'strongly disagree' or 'strongly agree' categories reaches a maximum at minus and plus infinity, respectively. For the purposes of describing the scale, points must be selected where it is reasonable and consistent to attach the description for these outside categories. Locating the descriptors for these categories half a logit below the lowest threshold and half a logit above the highest threshold achieves this. In each case, this is clearly the most probable category at the chosen scale location.

Figure 34.4 illustrates this by showing the category probability curves for item 3: 'Most of the time being at school puts me in a good mood'. Each

```
ENGAGEMENT SURVEY - NATIONAL TRIAL SEPTEMBER 2007
---------------------------------------------------------------------------------
Item Estimates (Thresholds)
all on all (N = 8641 L = 33 Probability Level=0.50)
---------------------------------------------------------------------------------
  6.0                                    |
                                         |
                                         |
                                         |
  5.0                                    |
                                         |
                                         |
                             X           |
                                         |
  4.0                        X           |
                                         |
                             X           |
                            XX           |
                            XX           |
  3.0                       XX           |  Q1.  3
                           XXX           |  Q3   .3
                         XXXXXX          |  Q8   .2 Q28 .3
                          XXXX           |  Q34  .3 Q35 .3
                        XXXXXXXX         |  Q12  .3 Q19 .3 Q36 .2
  2.0                  XXXXXXXXXX        |  Q23  .3
                       XXXXXXXXXX        |  Q14  .2 Q24 .3 Q27 .3 Q31 .3
                       XXXXXXXXXXX       |  Q2   .3 Q13 .3 Q18 .2 Q20 .3
                       XXXXXXXXXXXX      |  Q15  .3 Q30 .3
                   XXXXXXXXXXXXXXXXXX    |  Q5   .3 Q7  .2 Q10 .3 Q29 .2
  1.0                 XXXXXXXXXXXXX      |  Q17  .2
                   XXXXXXXXXXXXXXXXX     |  Q16  .2 Q26 .2 Q33 .2 Q34 .2
                XXXXXXXXXXXXXXXXXXXX     |  Q4   .2
                  XXXXXXXXXXXXXXXXXX     |  Q1   .2 Q6  .2 Q12 .2 Q36 .1
                 XXXXXXXXXXXXXXXXXXX     |  Q11  .2 Q35 .2
  0.0             XXXXXXXXXXXXXXXXXX     |  Q3   .2 Q8  .1 Q27 .2 Q28 .2 Q31 .2
                     XXXXXXXXXXXXXX      |  Q13  .2
                   XXXXXXXXXXXXXXXXX     |  Q5   .2 Q19 .2 Q22    Q23 .2 Q24 .2
                      XXXXXXXXXXX        |  Q2   .2 Q15 .2 Q20 .2 Q25 .1  Q30 .2 Q33 .1 Q34 .1
                        XXXXXXXX         |  Q14  .1 Q18 .1 Q29 .1
 -1.0                   XXXXXXXX         |  Q7   .1 Q10 .2 Q12 .1
                         XXXXXX          |  Q17  .1 Q35 .1
                           XXX           |  Q1   .1 Q13 .1 Q16 .1 Q26 .1 Q27 .1 Q31 .1
                           XXX           |  Q4   .1 Q28 .1
                             X           |  Q3   .1 Q5  .1 Q11 .1
 -2.0                        X           |  Q6   .1 Q15 .1 Q20 .1 Q23 .1
                             X           |  Q19  .1 Q24 .1 Q30 .1
                             X           |  Q2   .1 Q10 .1
                             X           |
                                         |
 -3.0                                    |
                                         |
                                         |
                                         |
                                         |
 -4.0                                    |
                                         |
                                         |
                                         |
                                         |
 -5.0                                    |
---------------------------------------------------------------------------------
 Each X represents    31 students
=================================================================================
```

Fig. 34.3 Item calibration on the student engagement scale

curve, from left to right plots the modelled probability of selecting a particular response category (strongly disagree to strongly agree). The points of maximum probability for the two middle categories are indicated by the vertical lines, along with the locations on the scale chosen to represent the outer categories (one-half logit below and above the lowest and highest category thresholds, respectively).

Item: 3
Most of the time being at school puts me in a good mood.

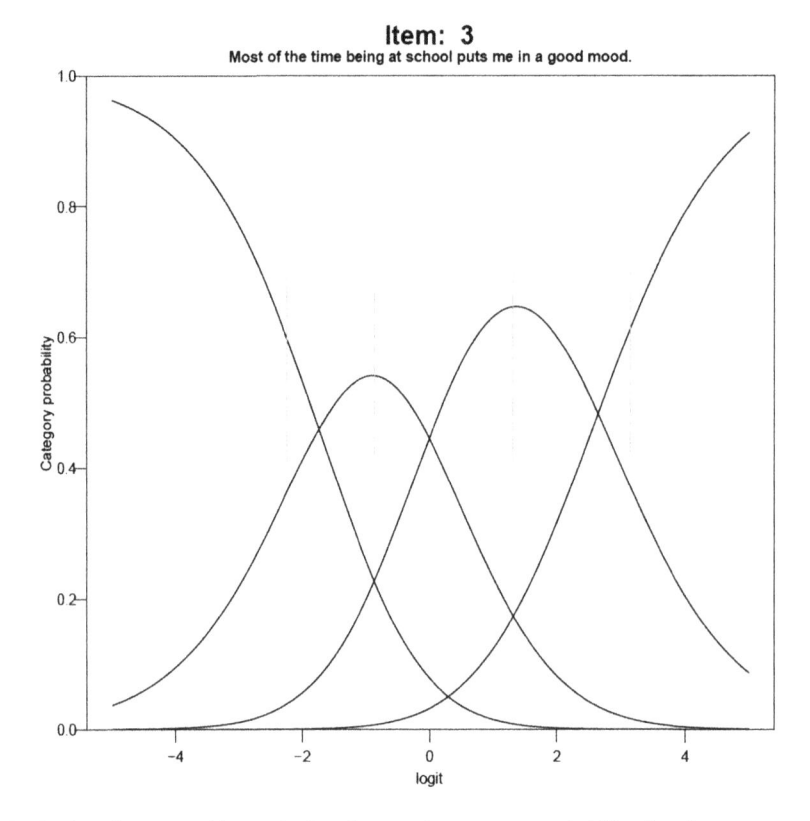

Fig. 34.4 Selecting locations to position scale descriptors using category probability functions

The Described Scale

Figure 34.5 shows the described engagement scale numbered from 20 to 105 'es' (engagement scale) units. The numbers themselves are simply markers and indicate increasing scale locations. The 'es' unit is a linear transformation of the original logit unit used in the scale construction: Student Engagement Scale Score (es) = (logit + 5) × 10. It follows that the mean category threshold is set to 50 es units, and 10 es units is the equivalent of 1 logit. Scale descriptors, each covering a specific section of the scale, are presented to the right of the scale. As can be seen, high locations on the scale are associated with strong positive responses to the survey items and low scale locations with strongly negative responses.

There are some interesting observations that can be made using the scale description. First, it is interesting to note which statements are associated with high locations on the scale. For these statements, strong agreement only becomes most probable when students' overall survey scores are very high. Statements at this high level include: 'I find it easy to concentrate on what I am doing in class'; 'People care about each other in this school'; and 'Most of the time being at school puts me in a good mood'. Strong disagreement with the statement 'I often feel bored in class' is also located high on the scale.

Conversely, some statements are relatively much easier to agree with than others. These occur at lower levels on the scale and include items such as: 'I respect other students' space and property at this school'; 'I think it is important for me to behave well at school'; and 'My family's culture is treated with respect by the teacher'. These latter statements could be seen to represent an interesting pivot or tipping point. Their location on the scale indicates that they are generally

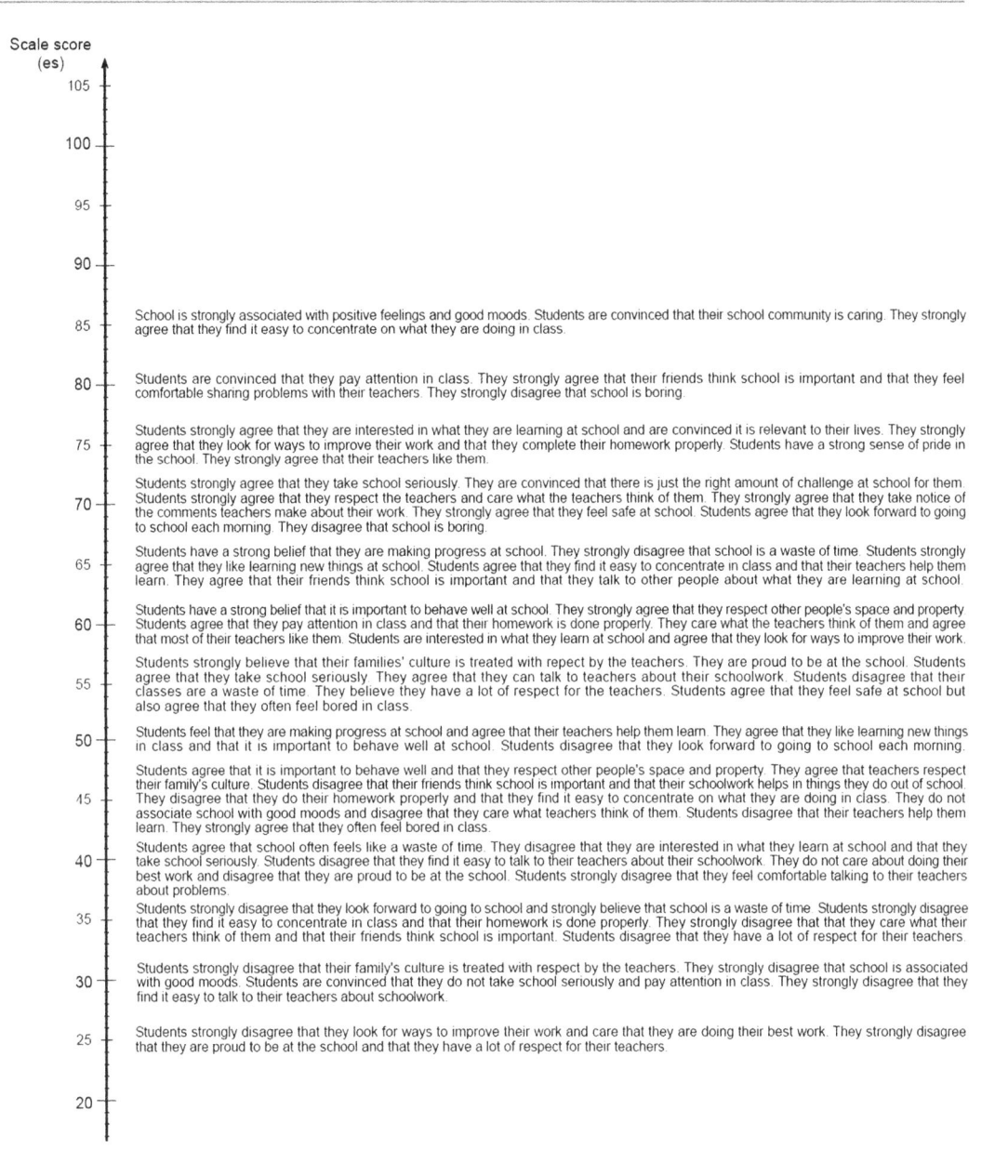

Fig. 34.5 The described student engagement scale

the first positive indicators to 'turn on' as perceived engagement increases and the last to 'turn off' as it decreases. In other words, a person who cannot agree with these statements is generally unlikely to agree with other positive statements about engagement. It is also interesting to note the negative responses associated with this part of the scale. These could be seen as either some of the first negative statements to appear as we go down the scale or some of the last negative responses to disappear as we go up the scale. The negative responses at this level include disagreeing with the statements: 'Most mornings I look forward to going to school'; 'I am comfortable talking to the teachers about problems'; 'I take care that my homework is done properly'; and agreeing with the statement 'I often feel bored in class'.

National Patterns of Perceived Engagement

Once the scale was finalised, it became possible to estimate students' survey scores on the scale and obtain the distribution of student engagement by year level. As previously noted, to ameliorate against the effect of some schools being over represented, an iterative sub-sampling procedure was used to see if any adjustments should be made to the initial estimate of national norms. The procedure involved repeatedly sub-sampling the student data according to national proportions in relation to decile group and gender. The estimates from each of the 200 subsamples provided a sample of means and standard deviations from which to estimate national norms accurately and precisely. The national data exposed some interesting patterns. These include differences by year level, gender, ethnicity, school and class.

Perceived Engagement by Year Level and Gender

Figure 34.6 shows that overall the level of perceived engagement recorded by the national New Zealand sample decreases from Years 7–10. At the median level, scores drop from 68 units

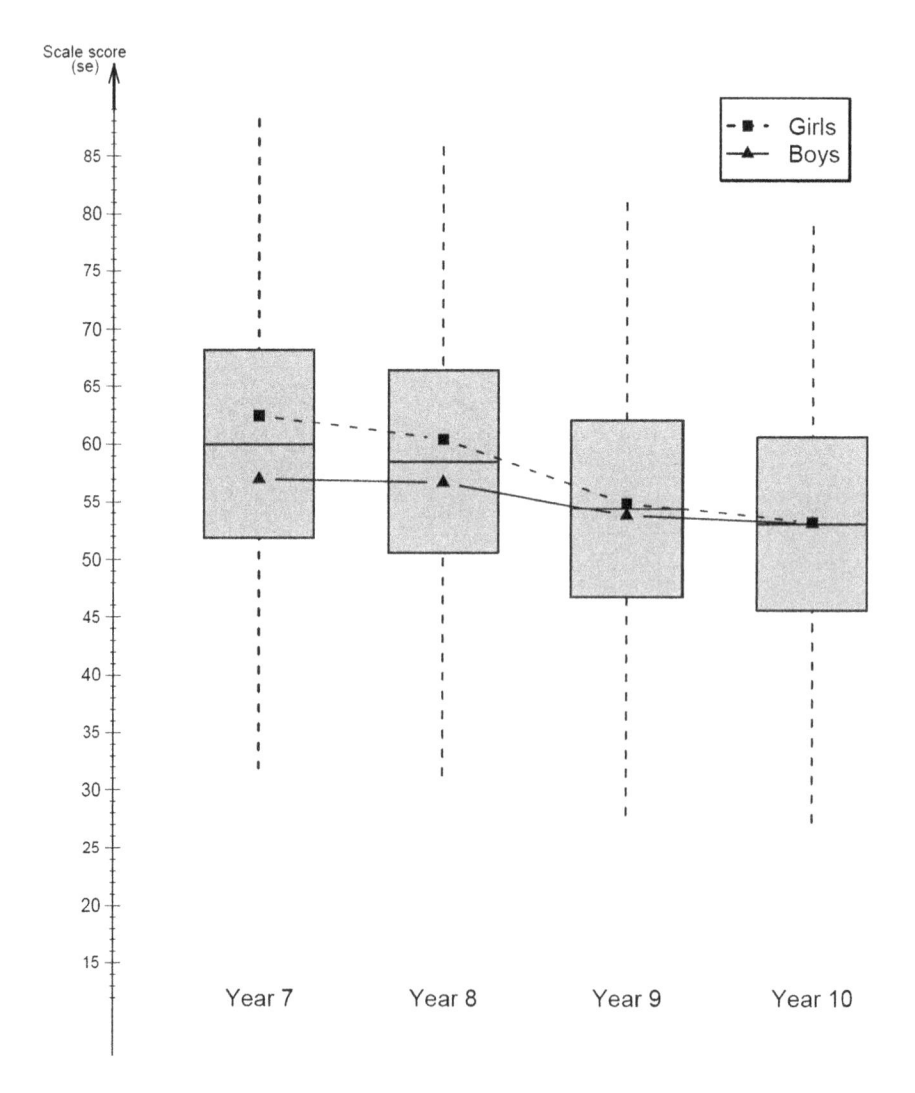

Fig. 34.6 Perceived engagement by year level

Table 34.2 Comparison of the scale descriptors for students scoring at the 25th and 75th percentile for Year 10

Scale description for 25th percentile	Scale description for 75th percentile
Students agree that it is important to behave well and that they respect other people's space and property. They agree that teachers respect their family's culture. Students disagree that their friends think school is important and that their schoolwork helps in things they do out of school. They disagree that they do their homework properly and that they find it easy to concentrate on what they are doing in class. They do not associate school with good moods and disagree that they care what teachers think of them. Students disagree that their teachers help them learn. They strongly agree that they often feel bored in class	Students have a strong belief that it is important to behave well at school. They strongly agree that they respect other people's space and property. Students agree that they pay attention in class and that their homework is done properly. They care what the teachers think of them and agree that most of their teachers like them. Students are interested in what they learn at school and agree that they look for ways to improve their work

on the scale in Year 7–53 units in Year 10. This pattern of decline in engagement scores mirrors findings from studies of engagement in the United States (National Research Council and the Institute of Measurement, 2004). A very noticeable feature of this decline is the steeper drop that occurs between Years 8 and 9. This is a transition point for most students in New Zealand when they will often change to a much larger school, usually with very different organizational structures and patterns.

Figure 34.6 uses triangles and squares to indicate the median scale scores for boys and girls, respectively. As can be seen, at the median level Year 7, female students tend to report higher levels of perceived engagement than their male counterparts. What is interesting, however, is that while overall engagement for both boys and girls declines from Years 7 to 10, the downward trajectory for females is much greater than that for males. By Year 10, the median engagement scores for both genders are almost exactly the same.

As an example of how the scale description can provide an interpretation of the scale scores, it is interesting to observe how the most probable responses for students scoring at the 25th percentile for Year 10 differ from those scoring at the 75th percentile. These are juxtaposed in Table 34.2 and suggest a readiness on the part of the lower scoring Year 10 to nominate some negative responses.

Perceived Engagement by Ethnicity

When *Me and My School* is administered, students are asked to indicate their ethnicity by choosing from New Zealand European, Mäori, Pacific, Asian and Other. If they choose to, they can select more than one ethnic group. Figure 34.7 shows the median scale score by year level for New Zealand European, Mäori, Pacific and Asian students. At Years 7 and 8, the median scale score for Mäori students is slightly lower than the medians for other ethnic groups but only slightly. At Year 9, however, there is a much larger drop for Mäori than for any other ethnic group. The result is a fairly large difference at the median for Mäori in their overall perception of engagement at Years 9 and 10. As has already been noted, most students in Year 9 are in their first year of high school.

Interestingly, students who choose Pacific as their ethnicity are generally more positive than students who choose other ethnicities. Figure 34.7 shows them as recording higher median levels at Years 7, 8 and 9 on the scale than students of all other ethnicities. However, the drop that occurs between Years 8 and 9 is as steep as that recorded by Mäori students.

Perceived Engagement by School and by Class

The national survey results also show that there are differences between schools. Figure 34.8 shows a range of schools with Year 8 students. As can be seen, students at some schools have responded much more positively overall than students at other schools.

Within a school, there can be a large amount of variance at the class level. Figure 34.9 plots the scale scores by class for a large intermediate school. As shown, some students in particular

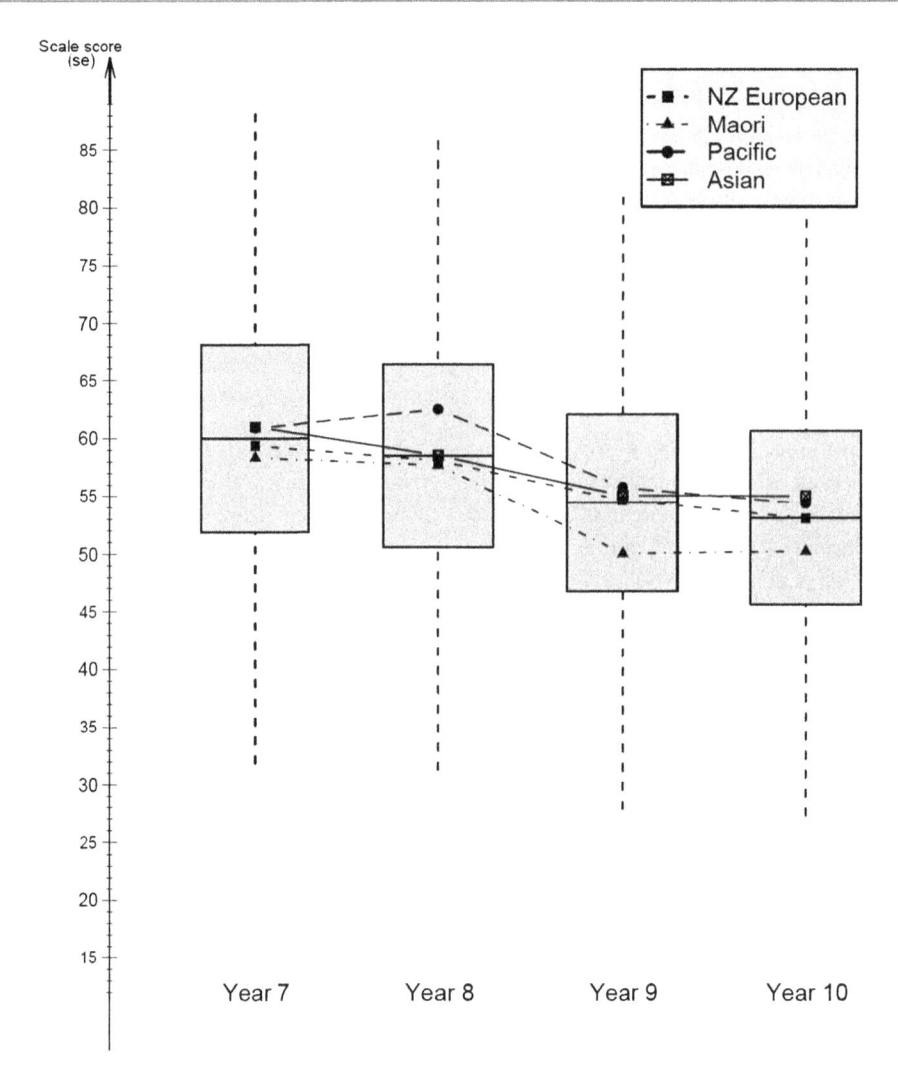

Fig. 34.7 Perceived engagement by ethnic group

classes tend to respond much more positively than students in other classes. This might be explained by differences in the class context, for instance, differences in teaching style, or because the class contains a particular group of students or both. It is interesting to note that even when a class or school has higher overall perceived engagement, there is still a spread of results indicating different experiences for different individual students.

Future Directions and Final Thoughts

The *Me and My School* survey is available for use by New Zealand schools on a subscription basis. As well as the paper and pencil version, an online version of the survey has been developed. NZCER supports the survey with data entry and reporting services. Over the last 3 years, more than 200 schools have subscribed to use the

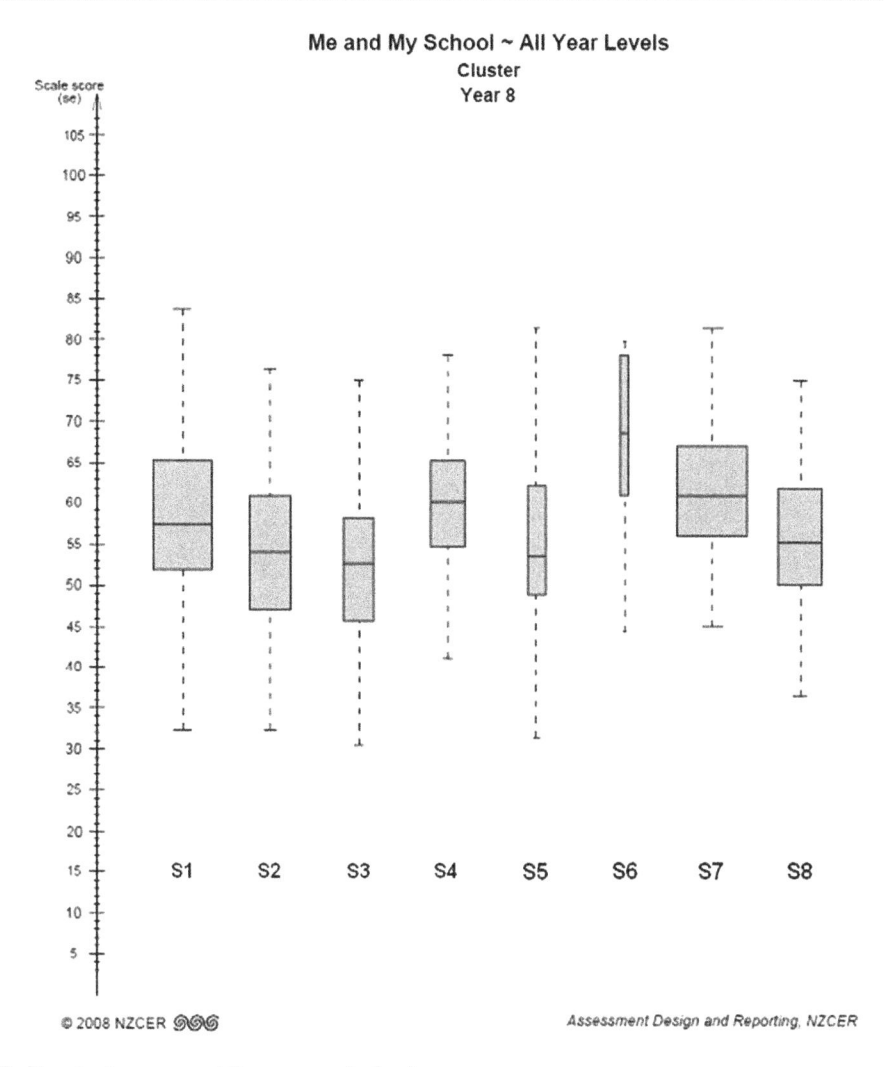

Fig. 34.8 Perceived engagement for a group of schools

survey, some of them multiple times. Reactions have been favourable with schools describing it as a catalyst for deeper involvement and interest in student engagement issues. The survey has also been used outside of New Zealand. In these cases, NZCER has worked with interested organisations and researchers to provide support with analysis.

A number of avenues for future directions have begun to be explored. One of these involves the extension of the survey to other year levels. Recently, national trials occurred for a version of the survey aimed at students in Years 4–6 (8- to 11-year olds). This version of the survey used a subset of the items contained in the Year 7–10 version. Many of the items were reworded to make them more age appropriate. To administer the survey, the questions were read to the students, rather than being read independently. The work carried out so far has suggested that there are developmental differences that need to be taken into account when measuring engagement at different year levels. It is plausible that the nature of engagement changes over time and that indicators of engagement can be more or less relevant at different ages. A Rasch analysis of the two surveys, linked through common items, suggests that there are differences in item functioning between the two levels.

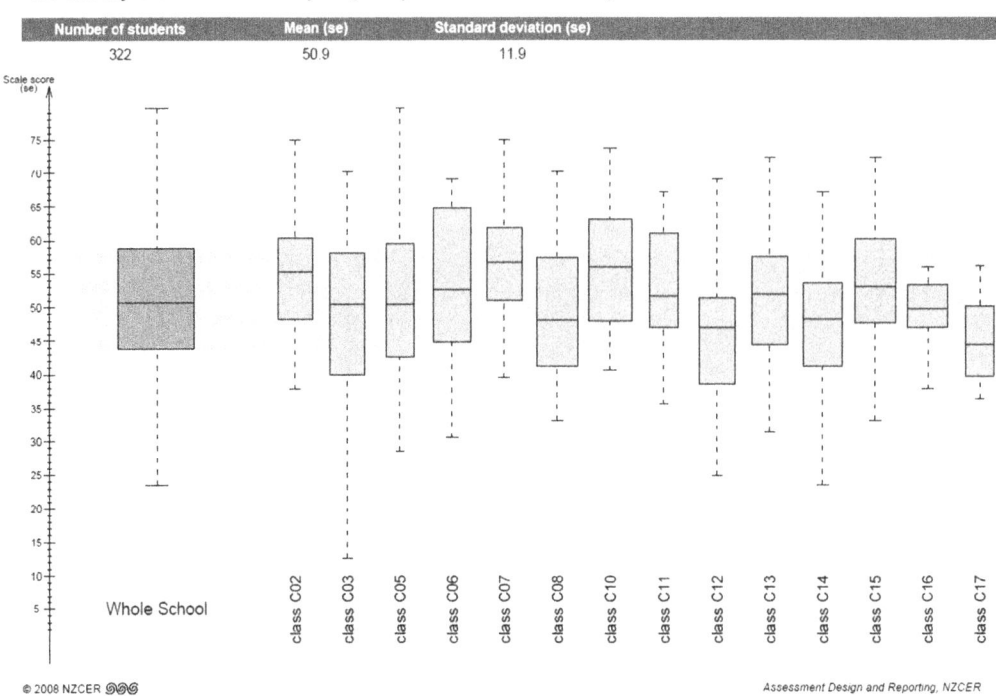

Fig. 34.9 Perceived engagement for a group of classes within a school

Another avenue for future research involves exploring how the survey can better recognise aspects of engagement that are pertinent to Māori students. Recently the Ministry of Education's Māori Education Strategy, Ka Hikitia—Managing for Success: The Māori Education Strategy 2008–2012 (Ministry of Education, 2009) has placed an emphasis on developing educational contexts that engage Māori students by recognising the importance of language, identity and culture, and which develop a reciprocal learning relationship between teachers and students. It has been suggested that an engagement survey for Māori students should include items which are sensitive to this type of engagement. Future work in this direction could involve the development of additional items for the *Me and My School* survey or the development of a stand-alone instrument.

The *Me and My School* survey provides a standardized mechanism that students can use anonymously to make judgements on a series of indicators related to their own level of engagement. As such, it brings an important voice to the table—student voice. As a mechanism for providing student voice, it is systematic and has been developed with some rigour. However, it is not necessarily a strong example of student voice—it is, at best, a starting point, or as schools describe it, a catalyst for something deeper and more real.

A voice requires a listener.

Brent Davis (1996) explained listening as a coming together, a kind of touching from a distance. He argued that the most powerful type of listening involves a conversation where, rather than trying to impose or provide a viewpoint to another—as in a discussion—we work together to reach a joint understanding. This type of listening means that:

> There is no winner, no gaining of the upper hand, no final word, no compulsion to stick with the topic. Rather, the conversation allows us to move freely and interactively towards those questions that animate us while enabling us to explore not just the topics that emerge, but why such topics capture our interest in the first place (p. 40).

For Davis, 'A goal of the conversation is to deepen understanding and, in that deepening, to create knowledge' (p. 40).

Perhaps the real secret of engagement is to develop our ability to listen to students' voices and to involve them in conversations. Conversations will sometimes be about learning areas like mathematics, science, English and history and/or about the students themselves, their heritage, culture, intuitions and experiences, and their emerging place in the world. If *Me and My School* helps us listen, then it will have served its purpose.

References

Adams, R. J., & Khoo, S. T. (1999). *ACER QUEST: The interactive test analysis system*. Melbourne, Australia: Australian Council for Educational Research.

Appleton, J., Christenson, S., & Furlong, M. (2008). Student engagement with school: Critical conceptual and methodological issues of the construct. *Psychology in the Schools, 45*(5), 369–386.

Appleton, J. J., Christenson, S. L., Kim, D., & Reschly, A. L. (2006). Measuring cognitive and psychological engagement: Validation of the Student Engagement Instrument. *Journal of School Psychology, 44*, 427–445.

Bishop, R., Berryman, M., Cavanagh, T., & Teddy, L. (2007). *Te Kōtahitanga Phase 3 Whanaungatanga: Establishing a culturally responsive pedagogy of relations in mainstream secondary school classrooms*. Wellington, New Zealand: Ministry of Education.

Bond, T. G., & Fox, C. M. (2007). *Applying the Rasch Model: Fundamental measurement in the human sciences* (2nd ed.). Mahwah, NJ: Lawrence Erlbaum.

Davis, B. (1996). *Teaching mathematics: Toward a sound alternative*. New York: Garland Publishing.

Dinahm, S., & Rowe, K. (2007). *Teaching and learning in middle schooling: A review of the literature*. A report prepared for the Ministry of Education. Wellington, New Zealand: Australian Council for Educational Research.

Finn, J. D. (1989). Withdrawing from school. *Review of Educational Research, 59*, 117–142.

Fredricks, J. A., Blumenfeld, P. C., & Paris, A. H. (2004). School engagement: Potential of the concept, state of the evidence. *Review of Educational Research, 74*(1), 59–109.

Jimerson, S., Campos, E., & Greif, J. (2003). Towards an understanding of definitions and measures of school engagement and related terms. *The California School Psychologist, 8*, 7–27.

Lane, R. (2008). *A report to schools on New Zealand student engagement 2007*. Wellington, New Zealand: Ministry of Education. Retrieved from http://www.educationcounts.govt.nz/publications/series/2303/28883/28884

Libbey, H. (2004). Measuring student relationships to school: Attachment, bonding, connectedness, and engagement. *Journal of School Health, 74*, 7.

Martin, A. J. (2009). *The motivation and engagement scale*. Sydney, Australia: Lifelong Achievement Group. Retrieved from http://www.lifelongachievement.com

Ministry of Education. (2007). *The New Zealand curriculum for English-medium teaching and learning in years 1–13*. Wellington, New Zealand: Learning Media.

Ministry of Education. (2009). *Ka Hikitia—Managing for success: The Māori education strategy 2008–2012*. Wellington, New Zealand: Ministry of Education. Retrieved from http://www.minedu.govt.nz/theMinistry/PolicyAndStrategy/KaHikitia/PublicationsAndResources-EnglishLanguageVersions.aspx

National Research Council and the Institute of Measurement. (2004). *Engaging schools: Fostering high school students' motivation to learn. Committee on increasing high school students' engagement and motivation to learn*. Board on Children, Youth, and Families, Division of Behavioural and Social Science and Education. Washington, DC: The National Academy Press.

Ng, L. (2006). *Attendance, absence and truancy in New Zealand schools in 2006*. Wellington, New Zealand: Ministry of Education.

Wright, B., & Masters, G. (1982). *Rating scale analysis. Rasch measurement*. Chicago: MESA Press.

Yazzie-Mintz, E. (2007). *Voices of students on engagement. A report on the 2006 High School Survey of Student Engagement*. Bloomington, IN: Center for Evaluation & Education Policy, Indiana University. Retrieved from http://www.indiana.edu/~ceep/hssse/reports.html

Systems Consultation: Developing the Assessment-to-Intervention Link with the Student Engagement Instrument

James J. Appleton

Abstract

Schools and districts encounter many challenges when attempting to support systems-level use of engagement data. These challenges range from integrating disparate sources of data to collecting (and ensuring the meaningfulness of) data on the less observable cognitive and affective subtypes of engagement, to increasing the frequency with which data can be updated and disseminated, and to implementing appropriate interventions based upon assessed engagement. Acknowledging the need for further study on school systems' empirically guided efforts to effectively use engagement data, this chapter details one, large, urban-fringe district's effort to use these types of data. The delineation is intended as a tangible example with sufficient detail to support commentary, suggestions for improvements, and calls for relevant further research. The example should also provide guidance sufficient for other school systems to consider and select types of information and methods of dissemination useful within their efforts to promote student engagement and outcomes related to it. Suggestions for further research and visions of future use of engagement data are also provided.

Student engagement has emerged as a desirable target for intervention efforts due to perceptions of its value as an outcome, critical contributions to authentic and continued learning, and malleability (Fredricks, Blumenfeld, & Paris, 2004). School and district efforts to focus upon engagement have the potential to not only impact valued student outcomes but also to underscore the importance of engaged learners themselves. At the intersection of theory and practical application stand many challenges, decisions, and lessons learned. This chapter focuses on the experiences of a single, large district in addressing the challenges, explicating the decisions, and sharing the resulting successes and shortcomings of an effort to systematically analyze, disseminate, and utilize student engagement data. The intent is to offer a forthright example that can serve as a beginning point for further conversations and research on how engagement theory can practically influence district-wide data use and intervention efforts.

J.J. Appleton, Ph.D. (✉)
Office of Research and Evaluation, Gwinnett County
Public Schools, Suwanee, GA, USA
e-mail: Jim_Appleton@gwinnett.k12.ga.us

Definition of Student Engagement

This chapter adopts a perspective of engagement that is closely aligned with Newmann and colleagues' (Newmann, Wehlage, & Lamborn, 1992) definition as the "…student's psychological [mental, cognitive, emotional] investment in and effort [behaviors] directed toward learning, understanding, or mastering the knowledge, skills, or crafts that academic work is intended to promote" (p. 12). Key in this perspective is the multidimensional nature implied by psychological as well as behavioral components and the importance of a persistent focus on educational outcomes. The adherence to a multidimensional view of the engagement construct is consistent with seminal theoretical and empirical work in the field (e.g., Finn, 1989; Fredricks et al., 2004; National Research Council and Institute of Medicine, 2004). Specifically, the definition adopted here considers four subtypes of engagement: academic, behavioral, cognitive, and affective/emotional. Academic engagement is defined by behaviors that have, as their purpose, the high-quality accomplishment of the academic tasks of schooling and can be indexed by student data such as asking questions on content in class, completing assigned class work, and accruing credits toward graduation. Behavioral engagement is defined as additional school supportive behaviors that demonstrate an allegiance or adherence to the school and/or its staff and can be observed in actions such as prompt and persistent school attendance, involvement in extracurricular activities, and the avoidance of deviant behaviors. Cognitive engagement is defined as investment in the work of learning as well as the refinement and deployment of strategic thinking (Fredricks et al.). Affective/emotional engagement is defined as affiliation/identification with school (e.g., Finn), including the staff and students that populate it and the emotions experienced during the tasks of schooling. Cognitive and affective/emotional subtypes of engagement are frequently assessed via student perceptions and considered less observable than academic or behavioral subtypes (Appleton, Christenson, & Furlong, 2008). This definition honors the traditional theoretical adherence to three subtypes while acknowledging the practical concern that aggregation of data across academic and behavioral subtypes may provide similar profiles for socially but not academically active students and those involved academically but not socially.

Student Engagement Versus Motivation

Discussions of student engagement often raise questions concerning the construct's relationship to motivation. From the perspective of this chapter, motivation is perceived to be necessary, but not sufficient for engagement (Appleton et al., 2008). Engagement operates within a motivational framework (Connell & Wellborn, 1991) and is dependent upon psychological processes such as autonomy (Skinner, Wellborn, & Connell, 1990), relatedness/belonging (Goodenow & Grady, 1993), and competence (Baumeister & Leary, 1995; Schunk, 1991). Yet, engagement represents action taken upon that motivation or "*energy in action*, the connection between person and activity" (Russell, Ainley, & Frydenberg, 2005, p. 1) that is dependent upon the fit between student and context (Reschly & Christenson, 2006a, 2006b). A comparison between the breadth of motivational constructs (Maehr & Meyer, 1997) and efforts to sample aspects of these constructs to predict engagement quickly demonstrates the minimalist nature of the engagement construct. Engagement represents a pragmatic effort to reduce queries of motivation to fewer items across constructs in order to predict directed energy/action.

Context

Gwinnett County Public Schools (GCPS) is a large, urban-fringe district northeast of Atlanta with nearly 161,000 students, 130 facilities, and a fiscal year 2011 annual budget of 1.76 billion dollars. The student demographic characteristics, as of spring 2010, included 0.4% American

Indian, 28.6% African American, 10.3% Asian American, 25.3% Hispanic, 3.8% multiracial, and 31.6% White. Additionally, 12% of students were served in special education, 16% were designated as English language learners (ELLs), and 50% were eligible for free or reduced-price school lunch (GCPS, 2010).

In many respects, GCPS could be considered a near best-case scenario for a district attempt to systematically analyze and utilize engagement data. First, the importance of promoting engagement, as a critical component of student learning, is recognized and supported by the CEO/superintendent. This support is demonstrated within discussions of teaching and learning, advocacy for a district-wide Student Advisement Program (SAP), fall and spring semester surveying of student perspectives of engagement, and the implementation of several smaller, complementary engagement-supportive programs. Schools are required to provide an advisement program with every student assigned to an advisor. Research-based optimal and minimal parameters are provided for the frequency and duration of advisement group meetings, size of advisement groups, and duration of advisor-advisee relationships. Secondly, the diversity and size of the student population of GCPS increased the likelihood of a rich dataset for examining baseline characteristics of engagement as well as trends not only over time but also across and within students of differing demographic backgrounds. Thirdly, the district focus on data-based decision-making and an engagement-based logic model ensured the need for several years of engagement data to properly evaluate the effectiveness of the SAP. Finally, many of the challenges of scale were mitigated, and often outweighed, by the data-processing infrastructure (e.g., survey scanning, data integration, data-querying capacity) of GCPS' Information Management Division (IMD).

Despite the existing facilitative components, several challenges also confronted this effort to make wider use of engagement data. These challenges included logistical issues with integrating existing academic and behavioral data as well as reporting in a format considered relevant and meaningful to report to consumers. Statistical concerns also surfaced in comparing engagement factors consisting of different numbers of items and attempting to link engagement to meaningful district-, school-, and student-level outcomes. Data privacy issues and database limitations occurred during efforts to quickly and widely disseminate reports only to those staff with a need for the information. The sections that follow detail the efforts and processes undertaken to implement a systems-level use of student engagement data as well as the vision these efforts engendered for an improved set of future processes. The current implementation and vision of future implementations are offered in a manner as transparent and thorough as possible. The belief is that transparency and thoroughness will support detailed conversations and research agendas for furthering the effectiveness of using engagement data within districts.

Implementation

Data Integration

As documented by many, data indicating the academic and behavioral engagement of students typically exist within district current electronic collections (Appleton et al., 2008; Fredricks et al., 2004). The decision within GCPS to begin to gather data on the cognitive and affective subtypes of engagement was mainly the result of the need to evaluate the SAP. The conceived purpose for these data was to represent a mediating or moderating variable linking or attenuating the relationship between implementation of the SAP and academic outcomes of interest. Beginning in the fall of the 2007–2008 school year, the Student Engagement Instrument (SEI) (Appleton, Christenson, Kim, & Reschly, 2006; Betts, Appleton, Reschly, Christenson, & Huebner, 2010) was administered, each fall and spring semester, as the means for collecting cognitive and affective engagement data on nearly all 6th–12th grade GCPS students. To date, SEI data have been collected each fall and spring semester. Moreover, as school and district staff learned of the plan to gather data on student perceptions of

Gwinnett County Public Schools
Student Advisement Program
STUDENT ENGAGEMENT INSTRUMENT
Used by permission

Your honest answers to this questionnaire will be used to improve your school's climate for teaching and learning. Your responses will be <u>confidential</u>: your advisor and teachers will not see your individual answers, but will be given summarized data reports to let them know how they can serve you and other students better.

Fig. 35.1 SEI introductory text

engagement, they requested reports and data, and the initial purpose for the results expanded into other potential uses.

Given this expansion, appropriate language for conveying the importance of forthright answers, informing students that their data would be merged with other student-level data, and guaranteeing the confidentiality of their responses was an important initial challenge. The selected introductory text (see Fig. 35.1) highlighted the lack of access of any school staff member to individual student responses while informing students of staff access to aggregations of their responses at the factor/theme[1] level. An additional goal of the introductory text on the GCPS SEI was to convey the intended use of the results for modifying the school climate and improving the experiences of those less engaged students. The intent was to increase student perceptions of the value of providing forthright responses. Also, a GCPS version of the standardization procedures used in the piloting of the SEI was provided to staff administering the engagement instrument (see Fig. 35.2). Subsequent presentations to advisors on the role of student engagement, plan to survey cognitive and affective engagement, and intent to report results provided rich qualitative data on advisor concerns and opportunities for clarification of processes. Advisors provided comments to clarify the introductory text on the GCPS SEI. Moreover, they preferred "affective" to "psychological" engagement to avoid confusion with psychopathology and expressed the desire to receive student-level engagement datasets in addition to reports.

SEIs were administered during SAP group meetings using paper surveys with results scanned into a data file by the IMD. IMD and Office of Research and Evaluation (ORE) staff spent time clarifying several critical aspects of the data. Since students were responsible for entering their unique GCPS student ID on the SEI, a convention was needed to ensure engagement responses were used only when one could have great confidence that the student was correctly identified. Also, a decision on whether to include the multiple SEI completions of concurrently enrolled students (e.g., a survey response at both their home high school and at a district technological charter school) was needed. IMD and ORE staff decided that an exact match from the provided student ID (PSID) and location code from the school at which the SEI was completed (CLC) to the GCPS data systems student ID (DSID) and enrolled location code (ELC) would indicate a correct identification. Moreover, to avoid losing mobile students from the datasets, the PSID and CLC would be considered a correct identification if they matched the DSID and the former location code of a student (FLC). ORE staff decided that the SEI's focus upon the school at which the student responded supported the relevance of including responses from both schools of a concurrently enrolled student. Finally, the inability to differentiate the true response (or even if both responses originated from the same student given that a one-digit change in a PSID can be an exact match with another student's DSID), multiple responses with the same PSID and CLC were deleted from the datasets.

---

[1] "Theme" is the term used in descriptions of results to consumers of these reports in our district.

What to Say to Students:

1) "Today we have a questionnaire to learn about your experiences while attending this school. Your responses will be <u>confidential</u>: no one at this school will see your individual answers. To keep them confidential, I will select a student to collect the questionnaires and seal them inside an envelope before sending them to the central office. Reports of the survey results will show only summarized data. Your honest answers will be used to help me and the school serve you and other students better."

2) "Do not begin marking answers until we discuss the directions and I begin to read the questionnaire items aloud."

3) "First, use a pencil to fill in your student number in the boxes in the upper right corner of the form. Then darken the circles corresponding to each digit of your student number."

4) "For most of the questionnaire items you will be choosing how much you agree with the statement by selecting from 'strongly agree,' 'agree,' 'disagree,' or 'strongly disagree.' The last two items of the questionnaire are different, and require you to fill in two-digit numbers."

5) "For each item mark only one answer by filling in the circle completely with a pencil. If you make a mistake or change your mind, erase your old answer entirely and fill in your new answer."

6) "I'll be reading the items so that I can respond to any questions you might have right away."

7) "If you have any questions about the items I'm reading or if you need a bit more time with an item be sure to let me know." *[Read items as directed in the right column 'Administration Procedures.']*

8) "Thank you for your time and opinions."

Administration Procedures:

- <u>Read questionnaire items aloud</u> with 3- to 5-second pauses between items depending on the reading levels within the class
- Items should be read with brief pauses between the general text and parenthetical sections to aid in understanding, e.g., "extracurricular (after school) activities"
- Plural versions should be used for items with a plural option, e.g., "parent/guardian(s)".
- Choices (i.e., "strongly agree" to "strongly disagree") are described during the introduction. Following the introduction, the questions can be read without the choices.

Note:

- If students ask, they may work ahead on items if the Advisor's pace of reading is too slow for them.

Collection:

- Give the questionnaire collection envelope to a student and ask that student to:
  o collect all of the completed questionnaires,
  o arrange them so they all face the same way,
  o place them in the envelope, and
  o seal the envelope closed.
- Return the sealed envelope as directed by your school's advisement program coordinator.

Fig. 35.2 SEI administration standardization procedures

After distilling all responses to those matched, with great confidence, to GCPS students, the IMD merged several other data identifiers of engagement including days enrolled, days tardy, days absent, disciplinary incidents, in-school suspension days, out-of-school suspension days, credits accrued, as well as demographic data and each student's advisor's name. This data file was used to generate all reports and datasets provided to advisors and schools. The proportion of cognitive and affective engagement data that matched district student data records ranged from around 65–75% of all GCPS middle and high school students across the years of administrations.

The provision of engagement results could be grouped into two main categories: student-focused and aggregated. Student-focused reports and datasets were those whose primary purpose was juxtaposing data on individual students with the goal of identifying students demonstrating disengagement from school. Aggregated results were summary reports whose purpose was providing schools and the district with information on the general engagement of students across meaningful subgroups and for assisting in detecting engagement changes that may be associated with group intervention efforts.

Student-Focused Results

The information provided and the dissemination formats of results were the outgrowth of iterative processes of reporting, eliciting responses, and issuing modified reports for further response. Additionally, the information reported was influenced by large dataset analyses attempting to link student engagement to district-valued outcomes. Through this process, several reports and datasets were settled upon for routine distribution. Student-focused information included the advisor-advisee report and the engagement pattern dataset. The advisor-advisee reports contained a stacked horizontal bar graph with each of the six SEI factors contributing a portion (i.e., one sixth) to the total bar length. Each of the SEI factors was represented by an average of the respective items which were scaled from one to four (responses are reversed to 1 (strongly disagree) to 4 (strongly agree)). Currently, averages are calculated from the unweighted response values of one to four. Another approach would be to present the value of an item according to its contribution to the factors estimated in factor analyses of the SEI (see Appleton et al., 2006; Betts et al., 2010). The six factors, teacher-student relationships (TSR), control and relevance of schoolwork (CRSW), peer support at school (PSS), future aspirations and goals (FG), family support for learning (FSL), and intrinsic motivation (IM), are composed of two to nine items each. To ensure that factor means contained a meaningful portion of the items composing them, means were only computed if respondents answered 50% or more of the items (except the IM factor for which the completion of both items was required). In this report, a stacked horizontal bar was presented for each advisee in an advisor's group along with a single lower stacked horizontal bar indicating the averages for the group of advisees (see Fig. 35.3). Since each factor is scaled from one to four, the stacked bar for a student with responses sufficient to calculate a mean for each factor ranged from 6 to 24.

The distinction between *level* of engagement and *change* in engagement is critical for understanding the meaning and potential uses of the advisor-advisee reports produced in the fall and spring of the academic year. After each administration (fall and spring of each academic year), advisor-advisee engagement *level* reports were prepared to detail the average of each student, at that administration, within each SEI factor. These reports were intended to enable advisors to compare the overall cognitive and affective engagement of each advisee to the group as a whole as well as discern student areas of relatively higher and lower engagement among the SEI factors. When compared with aggregated reports of school and district results, these reports could be used to situate students within typical school and district levels of engagement. In addition, means that were relatively low could be considered along with available academic and behavioral engagement data sources to note potential students in need of intervention as well as the relative strengths and weaknesses that might be consulted in implementing an intervention.

In the spring of each academic year, advisor-advisee engagement *change* reports were produced. These reports again used stacked bar graphs but displayed the differences between the spring and fall means for each SEI factor. Differences were reported for all students completing an SEI at both the fall and spring administrations. Since the fall mean was subtracted from the spring mean, values were positive only when student reports of cognitive and affective engagement increased from fall to spring on a particular SEI factor. Also, rather than the values from 6 to 24 (the typical range of scores on the level reports), the focus in these reports was zero on the change scale. Zero represented a student who maintained the same level of engagement from fall to spring. While bars to the positive side (right) of zero suggested improvements in engagement, bars to the negative side (left) of zero suggested declines in engagement (see Fig. 35.4). The values in these reports were weighted as described below and enabled advisors to compare engagement changes among their individual advisees and in reference to district change values. Also, the interpretation of

Gwinnett County Public Schools: Office of Research and Evaluation
*Scale is 1-4 for each theme: 1 = scale floor; 4 = scale ceiling   *Scores from only one administration; use accordingly

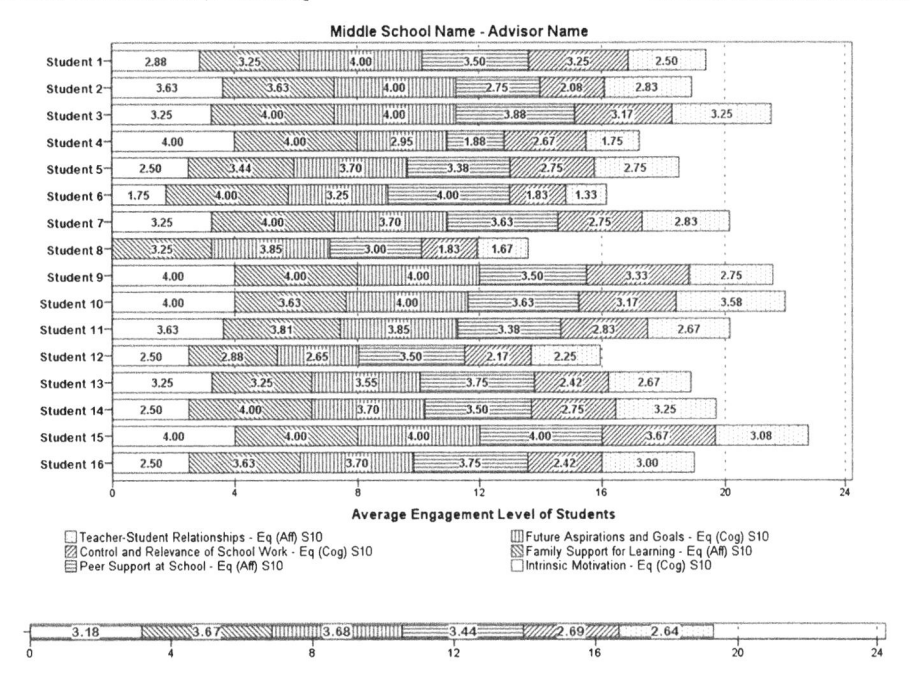

Middle School Name - Advisor Name

Student	Teacher-Student Relationships	Control and Relevance of School Work	Peer Support at School	Future Aspirations and Goals	Family Support for Learning	Intrinsic Motivation
Student 1	2.88	3.25	4.00	3.50	3.25	2.50
Student 2	3.63	3.63	4.00	2.75	2.08	2.83
Student 3	3.25	4.00	4.00	3.88	3.17	3.25
Student 4	4.00	4.00	2.95	1.88	2.67	1.75
Student 5	2.50	3.44	3.70	3.38	2.75	2.75
Student 6	1.75	4.00	3.25	4.00	1.83	1.33
Student 7	3.25	4.00	3.70	3.63	2.75	2.83
Student 8	3.25	3.85	3.00	1.83	1.67	
Student 9	4.00	4.00	4.00	3.50	3.33	2.75
Student 10	4.00	3.63	4.00	3.63	3.17	3.58
Student 11	3.63	3.81	3.85	3.38	2.83	2.67
Student 12	2.50	2.88	2.65	3.50	2.17	2.25
Student 13	3.25	3.25	3.55	3.75	2.42	2.67
Student 14	2.50	4.00	3.70	3.50	2.75	3.25
Student 15	4.00	4.00	4.00	4.00	3.67	3.08
Student 16	2.50	3.63	3.70	3.75	2.42	3.00

Average Engagement Level of Students

- ☐ Teacher-Student Relationships - Eq (Aff) S10
- ▨ Control and Relevance of School Work - Eq (Cog) S10
- ☰ Peer Support at School - Eq (Aff) S10
- ▥ Future Aspirations and Goals - Eq (Cog) S10
- ▧ Family Support for Learning - Eq (Aff) S10
- ☐ Intrinsic Motivation - Eq (Cog) S10

| 3.18 | 3.67 | 3.68 | 3.44 | 2.69 | 2.64 |

**Separate lower bar depicts the average of this group

Spring 2010 Report

Fig. 35.3 Spring student-focused SEI-based advisor-advisee level report

change within the context of the level data of fall or spring was important. The use of these two types of reports together (see Figs. 35.3 and 35.4) enabled an advisor to not only evaluate the meaningfulness of the change of a student (relative to the district) but also to determine whether the amount of change resulted in a satisfactory concluding position or, alternatively, represented the influence of a floor or ceiling effect. That is, how much change occurred given the "change space" (i.e., room for change) and did that change result in a final level that (relative to district data) seems to position the student well among his or her peers?

In striving to ensure student-focused change reports were meaningful, an important issue surfaced. This issue involved the divisibility of factors and arose as a result of the varying number of items across SEI factors. Consider that the TSR factor contained nine items while the FSL factor contained four. For a student completing all of the items for each of these factors, the TSR factor would result in a mean with eight potential non-zero decimal suffixes while the FSL factor produced a resulting mean with the potential for only three. That is, the mean for the TSR factor was calculated with division by nine enabling a decimal suffix the same as that of any integer multiple of 1/9 (or approximately .11) while the mean of the FSL factor resulted from division by four allowing for a suffix the same as integer multiples of 1/4 (or .25). Further, fall-to-spring differences on these factors would be constrained to differences containing these same suffixes. The critical issue arose upon examination, across SEI factors, of the size of student changes from fall to spring. Inevitably, the change of a single response to a single item by a one-unit move upward or downward on the (1 = strongly disagree (SD) to 4 = strongly agree (SA)) scale would produce a change of 1/9 on the

Gwinnett County Public Schools (GCPS): Office of Research and Evaluation

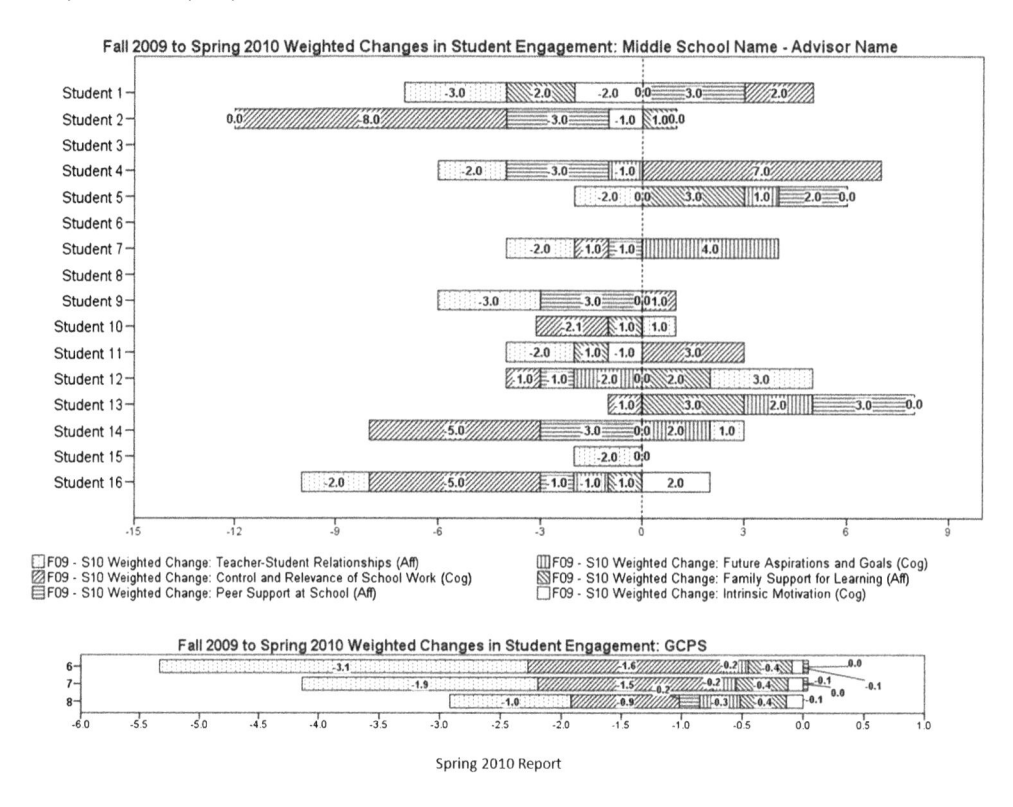

Fig. 35.4 Spring student-focused SEI-based advisor-advisee change report

TSR factor but 1/4 on the FSL factor. Essentially, a change of approximately .11 could be misconstrued as smaller than a change of .25 when, in fact, both represented a change of the smallest unit possible on that factor.

To offset this issue and produce reports that better-supported comparisons of change across SEI factors, the difference in means was multiplied by the number of items composing that factor. For instance, the one-item, one-unit change on the TSR of 1/9 was multiplied by 9, and that same change of 1/4 on the FSL was multiplied by 4. This standardization would produce a value of 1 for each of these changes. The interpretation of the value, for these weighted change factors, then became the number of smallest changes possible that were made from fall to spring. Implicitly, this standardization elevated the importance of focusing upon the smallest unit of change and considered these changes equal across factors.

This standardization also limits the total amount of change on a factor to be a function of the number of items. For instance, the maximal change on a nine-item factor is between 9 (all SDs) and 36 (all SAs) or 27 units of change, while for a four-item factor, it is between 4 and 16 or 12 units of change. Nearly all fall-to-spring changes on the SEI were not extreme enough to use all (or even most) units of change, but the difference in change units available due to factor size does deserve mention.

Beyond the reports, student-focused datasets have also been generated for use by schools. These datasets evolved as student-reported engagement was statistically related to academic and behavioral outcomes of interest. At both the middle and high school levels, SEI-reported cognitive and affective engagement *level* was related to significant and substantive differences in state test performance as well as the frequency

SEI All Items Mean	Teacher-Student Relationships	Control and Relevance of Schoolwork	Peer Support at School	Future Aspirations and Goals	Family Support for Learning	Intrinsic Motivation	SEI All Items Category (Relative to GCPS)	(Distance from GCPS Mean) Teacher-Student Relationships	(Distance from GCPS Mean) Control and Relevance of Schoolwork	(Distance from GCPS Mean) Peer Support at School	(Distance from GCPS Mean) Future Aspirations and Goals	(Distance from GCPS Mean) Family Support for Learning	(Distance from GCPS Mean) Intrinsic Motivation
2.82	2.75	2.50	2.88	3.25	2.88	3.25	Lowest 10%	-0.45	-1.56	-0.79	-1.33	-1.63	0.23
3.59	3.50	3.42	3.75	3.85	3.81	3.25	Middle 80%	0.85	0.47	0.96	0.32	0.46	0.23
3.64	3.83	3.75	3.13	4.00	4.00	2.13	Middle 80%	1.43	1.22	-0.29	0.73	0.88	-1.10
3.40	3.50	3.00	2.75	4.00	4.00	4.00	Middle 80%	0.85	-0.45	-1.04	0.73	0.88	1.12
2.48	3.00	2.08	1.88	3.55	1.19	3.63	Lowest 10%	-0.02	-2.19	-2.79	-0.51	-5.39	0.68
3.31	3.33	2.92	3.75	3.55	3.25	3.25	Middle 80%	0.56	-0.64	0.96	-0.51	-0.79	0.23
3.27	3.08	3.25	3.25	3.85	3.81	1.75	Middle 80%	0.13	0.10	-0.04	0.32	0.46	1.58
3.61	3.50	3.50	3.25	4.00	4.00	4.00	Middle 80%	0.85	0.66	-0.04	0.73	0.88	1.12
3.44	3.17	3.25	3.13	4.00	4.00	4.00	Middle 80%	0.27	0.10	-0.29	0.73	0.88	1.12
3.38	3.08	3.00	3.63	3.85	4.00	3.25	Middle 80%	0.13	-0.45	0.71	0.32	0.88	0.23
3.29	3.00	3.42	2.75	4.00	4.00	2.50	Middle 80%	-0.02	0.47	-1.04	0.73	0.88	-0.65
3.64	3.08	3.58	4.00	4.00	4.00	3.63	Middle 80%	0.13	0.84	1.46	0.73	0.88	0.68
2.74	2.67	1.75	3.38	3.70	2.88	2.88	Lowest 10%	-0.60	-3.23	0.21	-0.10	-1.63	-0.21
2.69	2.08	2.25	3.00	3.85	3.25	2.50	Lowest 10%	-1.63	-2.12	-0.54	0.32	-0.79	-0.65
3.49	3.25	3.25	3.63	4.00	3.81	3.25	Middle 80%	0.42	0.10	0.71	0.73	0.46	0.23
3.25	3.17	2.83	3.38	3.85	3.81	2.50	Middle 80%	0.27	-0.82	0.21	0.32	0.46	-0.65
3.91	4.00	4.00	4.00	4.00	4.00	2.50	Highest 10%	1.72	1.77	1.46	0.73	0.88	-0.65

Fig. 35.5 Fall SEI portion of student-focused dataset

and severity of disciplinary infractions and attendance (see Appleton, Reschly, & Martin, 2011). These differences in outcomes were pronounced between reported cognitive and affective engagement values in the percentiles of top 10%, middle 80%, and lowest 10% for the district. Moreover, these relationships persisted, at substantive levels, across 3 years of data (2007–2008, 2008–2009, and 2009–2010). Therefore, separately for middle and high school levels, SEI all items (SEI total) response averages at or above the 90th percentile, between the 90th and 10th percentiles, and at the 10th percentile or lower were differentiated in the school-provided datasets. In the dataset, each student provided a unique case with a single value for the SEI total mean and percentile category. In addition to these values based upon the SEI total, student means on each of the SEI factors were expressed in standard deviation units from the GCPS mean (i.e., standardized). To assist users, Excel cells were modified (conditionally formatted) to automatically set background color and font such that percentile category values of "lowest 10%" would be highlighted among the values of "middle 80%" and "highest 10%" (see Fig. 35.5). In the reports provided to district staff, an automatic formatting color scheme was also adopted for the standardized SEI factor means with those greater than or equal to 1.0 changed to green, between −1.5 and −2.5 to yellow, and those less than or equal to −2.5 to red.[2]

The intent of the formatting was to enable staff to differentiate the intensity of intervention needed across groups of students. Staff were advised to first examine the percentile category value since it related most closely to district-level analyses relating engagement to desired outcomes. Suggested subsequent examinations were to consider the standardized SEI factor values as well as other academic and behavioral engagement data included in the dataset. Guidance was also provided that staff should consult daily updated web-accessible sources of attendance and disciplinary data and, potentially, stand-alone databases containing current course performance data. The simple goal of the guidance was to encourage consideration of the total and factor-level cognitive and affective engagement data within the context of current information offered by more dynamic academic and behavioral engagement data. As an example, one school may have several students within the "lowest 10%" category of the district while another may have few. The first school may exhaust their resources attending solely to their large number of students

---

[2] The category-driven methods used to convey student-level information to school staff within these datasets are an improvement upon the single values provided in the advisor-advisee reports, but the concern with measurement error is one which requires consideration in future research and report production efforts.

in the lowest percentile category while the second may also be able to add students with moderate percentile category (e.g., "middle 80%") values but some (or several) low standardized SEI factor values. In either case, upon identifying the students at greatest risk based upon SEI results, both schools would then consult current academic and behavioral data to triangulate information and confirm the students most in need of intervention at that specific point in time.

Logistically, these student-level reports required numerous iterations with the dataset as well as an efficient method for outputting the results into a format accessible to the users. To provide an understanding of the scale of the project in GCPS, there are approximately 3,500 advisors with spring reports including four graphs per advisor resulting in the need to generate, and efficiently output, around 14,000 graphs. Fortunately, several relatively common software applications enabled the systematic and efficient generation of these graphs.[3] The main application was SPSS 15.0 for formatting and cleaning the data as well as generating the graphs. SPSS provides the ability to use menu-driven options to filter and create the desired graphs and then to be able to paste the syntax into the editor. Using an export of the frequency table of school names merged with advisor names (e.g., "Gwinnett High – John Advisor") to MS Excel, one can paste the SPSS syntax into MS Word and then merge all school-advisor combinations into the syntax using a common Word feature. The frequency table was also used to find advisor-advisee groups too large for all advisee stacked bars to fit within single-page graphs. These groups were reduced to alphabetized subgroups (about 32–34 students per graph) using an algorithm and the "compute" option within SPSS. The Word feature used to combine the Excel data and SPSS syntax was "mail merge" which is often used to integrate names and addresses within the context of a Word-created letter. In this case, the components of the SPSS syntax that changed from one group of advisees to the next were merged from the Excel file into the SPSS syntax contained in Word. Following the generation of the merged syntax within Word, the syntax was copied and pasted into Notepad to remove most formatting and then back into the SPSS syntax editor for generating the reports. The created SPSS syntax iteratively filtered out all but the advisees for a particular advisor, generated the graphs for that advisor, and then applied that school-advisor title before moving onto the next advisor.

In many cases, looping commands are able to be used directly within the syntax to avoid the merging process. The looping command would direct the processor to iterate graphs between a specified beginning and end point. In this case, the graphing function called was not able to be combined with a looping command. In the process used, graphs were generated with menu-driven options until generating as expected and until the page setup specifications ensured graphs required minimal additional formatting before exporting. Then syntax was pasted, and the merge process was conducted and tested until also generating graphs as expected. Then as many graphs as possible were generated with a single section of syntax[4] with the graphs of each SPSS output file exported to individual PDFs named according to the first and last school and advisor name contained within the graphs. These individual files were merged into a single PDF, and the large PDF was updated to contain any information considered important to convey to users. A confidentiality warning, interpretive guide, and commentary on the scale values and date of assessment were all added to the single PDF (see Figs. 35.3 and 35.6). Finally, the comprehensive PDF was split by school and pasted to the Lotus Notes database used to provide information to the leadership of individual schools.

---

[3] District-owned software specific to GCPS' method of generating graphs are highlighted, but freeware such as R (see http://www.r-project.org/) and Open Office (see http://www.openoffice.org/) may be suitable alternatives.

[4] Memory limitations of the computer used will dictate the maximum able to be generated at once.

Student Engagement Instrument (SEI)
INTERPRETIVE GUIDE

Dear Advisor:

Students show their engagement with school through their behavior and their academic performance, but these outward signs of engagement reflect inner attitudes and beliefs. Feelings of connectedness with other students, teachers and family members strongly influence school engagement, as do attitudes about the importance of school for achieving personal goals.

This report of your advisee's SEI Theme scores was created to provide you with insights about your students' feelings about school (Affective Engagement) and beliefs about school (Cognitive Engagement). The items are categorized by three Affective Engagement Themes and three Cognitive Engagement Themes as listed in the color-coded headings of the table on the right side of this page. Actual items from the instrument are listed below each Theme heading.

The colored bar graphs show how strongly students tended to agree with the statements. Responses to the items were coded 1 for Strongly Disagree through 4 for Strongly Agree, and these values were averaged to provide the six Theme scores represented by the color-coded bar segments on the graph. A bar segment of 4.0 represents responses of Strongly Agree for every item to which the student responded in the Theme, whereas a bar segment of 1.0 represents responses of Strongly Disagree for every responded to item of the Theme.

An overall measure of a student's Affective and Cognitive Engagement is provided by the total length of the stacked Theme bar segments such that a longer set of bars represent stronger engagement than a shorter set of bars.

Use this report in conjunction with your observations and intuition about your students. When the report either confirms or leads you to suspect more serious problems with school engagement, find opportunities to be the Advisor advocate that the student needs. Your school counselors and Advisement Program Coordinator can assist you in this role.

Please protect the confidentiality of this information; do not share individual student results with students. As promised to the students, we are not providing you with individual item responses, but we are providing the Theme-aggregated information that might assist you as the Advisor for each one of your advisement students.

We know that your dedication to teaching is an expression of your care and concern for kids. Thank you for turning your dedication into the teaching, learning, and caring that our students need for success.

The Advisement Program Planning Team

Not Your Advisees?
This report was prepared by linking student IDs with Advisors based on the staff member listed in "Stu.Adv#" of the student's SASI record. Updating the data in the "Stu.Adv#" field will improve the linking of Advisees to Advisors in future reports. For now, please share these results with the Advisors of the students who are not in your Advisement section.

Item #	SEI Themes and Item Text
	Teacher-Student Relationships (Affective Engagement)
3	My teachers are there for me when I need them.
5	Adults at my school listen to the students.
10	The school rules are fair.
13	Most teachers at my school are interested in me as a person, not just as a student.
16	Overall, my teachers are open and honest with me.
21	Overall, adults at my school treat students fairly.
22	I enjoy talking to the teachers here.
27	I feel safe at school.
31	At my school, teachers care about students.
	Control and Relevance of School Work (Cognitive Engagement)
2	After finishing my schoolwork I check it over to see if it's correct.
9	Most of what is important to know you learn in school.
15	When I do schoolwork I check to see whether I understand what I'm doing.
25	When I do well in school it's because I work hard.
26	The tests in my classes do a good job of measuring what I'm able to do.
28	I feel like I have a say about what happens to me at school.
33	Learning is fun because I get better at something.
34	What I'm learning in my classes will be important in my future.
35	The grades in my classes do a good job of measuring what I'm able to do.
	Peer Support at School (Affective Engagement)
4	Other students here like me the way I am.
6	Other students here care about me.
7	Students at my school are there for me when I need them.
14	Students here respect what I have to say.
23	I enjoy talking to the students here.
24	I have some friends at school.
	Future Aspirations and Goals (Cognitive Engagement)
8	My education will create many future opportunities for me.
11	Going to school after high school is important.
17	I plan to continue my education following high school.
19	School is important for achieving my future goals.
30	I am hopeful about my future.
	Family Support for Learning (Affective Engagement)
1	My family/guardian(s) are there for me when I need them.
12	When something good happens at school, my family/guardian(s) want to know about it.
20	When I have problems at school, my family/guardian(s) are willing to help me.
29	My family/guardian(s) want me to keep trying when things are tough at school.
	Intrinsic Motivation (Cognitive Engagement)
18	I'll learn, but only if the teacher gives me a reward. *(Reversed)*
32	I'll learn, but only if my family/guardian(s) give me a reward. *(Reversed)*

Fig. 35.6 SEI data interpretive guide including item and factor descriptions

Aggregated Results

In addition to student-level results, school and district-level results were also generated. These types of aggregated results, whether stand-alone or embedded within advisor-advisee reports, are critical for supporting appropriate and useful comparisons. For instance, given that previous research has suggested that student levels of engagement tended to decrease across time in secondary schools (Eccles et al., 1993), how should one interpret decreases in engagement among their group of advisees or at their particular school? Deferring to previous research suggesting differences in engagement for students at higher secondary grade levels, school and district SEI data were differentiated by grade level (see Fig. 35.7). Given the usefulness of evaluating both level and change results, these data were combined in a single report. Also, the issue of divisibility across factors with differing numbers of items, discussed above, was able to be addressed using a more common method. It was believed that larger increments in terms of divisibility would result in larger standard deviations. Therefore, the change values for both school- and district-grade levels were subjected to paired-samples t-tests as well as reported as effect sizes in terms of Cohen's d. These steps were taken to increase the likelihood that differences represented as meaningful changes would be so. The use of Cohen's d also supported the reference to common effect size differences for interpreting the meaning of small, moderate, and large changes (i.e., .20, .50, and .80, respectively). Though some have recommended the development of empirical benchmark rather than rules of thumb (e.g., see Hill, Bloom, Black, & Lipsey, 2008), and alternatives are being considered for future reports.

Gwinnett County Public Schools: Office of Research and Evaluation
*System data include 24 of 25 regular middle schools or 17 of 18 regular high schools
*LEVEL scores range from 1=Strongly Disagree to 4=Strongly Agree

Spring 2010 LEVELS of Student Engagement: Middle School and System

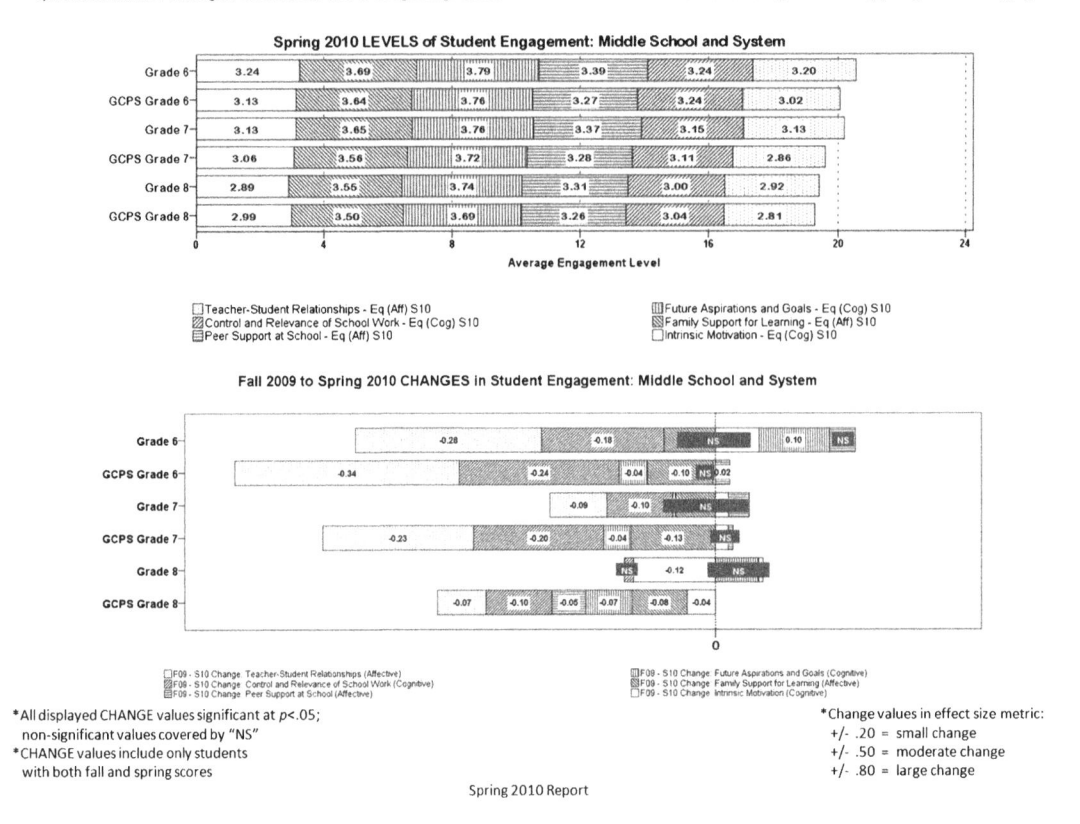

Fall 2009 to Spring 2010 CHANGES in Student Engagement: Middle School and System

*All displayed CHANGE values significant at p<.05; non-significant values covered by "NS"
*CHANGE values include only students with both fall and spring scores

*Change values in effect size metric:
+/- .20 = small change
+/- .50 = moderate change
+/- .80 = large change

Spring 2010 Report

Fig. 35.7 Spring aggregated SEI-based school and district report

Ad Hoc Results

Beyond the data produced routinely following each SEI administration, requests have also been received for specialized analyses. Examples included the use of SEI data in the evaluation of both the effect of the graduation coach (GC) and of the community-based mentoring (CBM) programs. The GC program assigned a school adult to monitor, coordinate resources, and intervene with middle and high students at-risk for dropping out based upon state-provided risk ratios and ongoing school-retrieved student data. The CBM program matched community mentors with at-risk, male, middle school students to provide support for academic and social development. The analyses conceptualized student cognitive and affective engagement as variables moderating the relationships between the influence of these programs and desired academic and behavioral outcomes.

Future Directions

The sections above describe efforts to attend to aspects of engagement beyond the academic and behavioral subtypes that are generally either easily accessible from district web-based data systems or extractable, with more effort, from separate data systems. The vision for the future focuses on the results of further analyses with newly acquired outcome data as well as advancing the delivery methods of timely engagement data.

Vision

Effectively monitoring student engagement requires dynamic data converted to useful information and delivered routinely across those adults interacting with the student. To date, SEI data provide values on subtypes of engagement

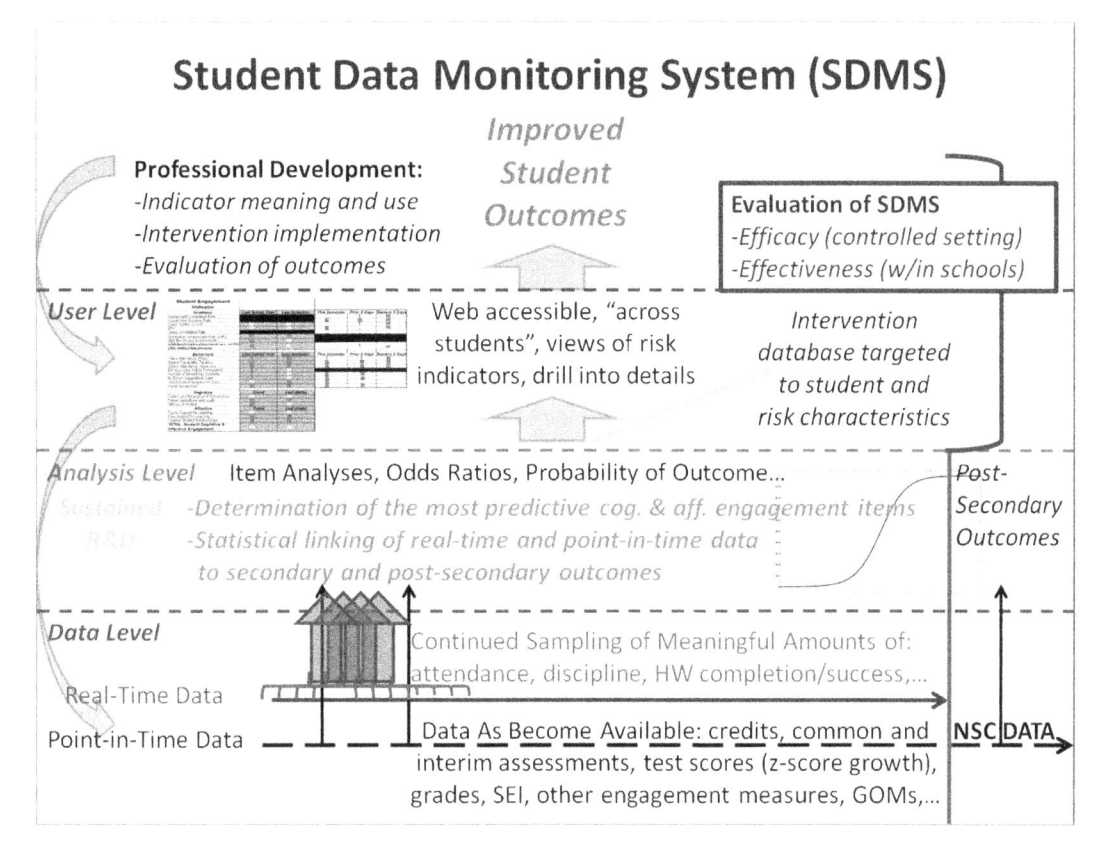

Fig. 35.8 Model for building, evaluating, and refining a dynamic, engagement-based assessment-to-intervention report

previously not assessed or monitored. Yet, the current sources of information are difficult to act upon at times (especially the farther from the administration date the reports and datasets are utilized). Also, a comprehensive view of a student's engagement currently requires the juxtaposition of a number of different resources. Moreover, the resources, once assembled, are not easily shared between the adults interacting with the students examined. Ideally, the most important engagement data would be provided across the contexts interacting with the student (e.g., school staff, family, community mentors). Moreover, the engagement data would have been statistically related to valued outcomes and therefore provide meaningful cut scores on engagement variables to facilitate efficient intervention efforts. Additionally, all values with data accruing across the academic year would be updated as frequently as relevant and meaningful.

Figures 35.8 and 35.9 provide a graphical representation of the vision for future systems-level uses of student engagement data. Through a partnership with the National Student Clearinghouse (NSC), data were able to be acquired on the postsecondary education outcomes of several years of the district's students. These data include enrollment and persistence within, as well as graduation from, over 92% of the nation's institutions of higher education (including 2–4-year, trade, and vocational schools). As depicted in Fig. 35.8, the NSC data provide objective valued outcomes to which earlier benchmarks can be statistically linked. These efforts at linking will have to heed the advice of researchers such as Gleason and Dynarski (2002) and Hintze and Silberglitt (2005) to attend to the properties of predictors. Predictive power (PP), both in terms of the percentage of those predicted to fall short of some valued outcome that actually do and those predicted to achieve an outcome that actually do, will be important. The important role of the first aspect of PP is ensuring that those designated for an intervention truly are in need of it.

Student Engagement Indicator	Historical Data		Formative Data		
Academic	Last School Year	Last Semester	This Semester	Prior 5 Days	Recent 5 Days
Assignment Completion Rate				!	
Assignment Success Rate					
Class Grades (Count)				!	
GPA					
Class Completing Rate					
Graduation Achievement Rate (GAR)[1]					
AKS Benchmark Assessments					
GOM Benchmark Assessments (e.g., CBM, DIBELS Benchmarks)				!	
Behavioral	Last School Year	Last Semester	This Semester	Prior 5 Days	Recent 5 Days
Class Attendance (Skips)	!		!	!	
School Punctuality (Tardies)					
School Attendance (Absences)					
Extracurricular Activity Participation	!				
Semester Discipline Mark	!				
Disciplinary Incidents Per Enrolled Day	!				
Most Severe Disciplinary Disposition					
Typical Severity of Dispositions (Mean)					
Cognitive	Trend	Last (Date)			
SEI: Control and Relevance of School Work					
SEI: Future Aspirations and Goals					
SEI: Intrinsic Motivation					
Affective	Trend	Last (Date)			
SEI: Family Support for Learning					
SEI: Peer Support for Learning					
SEI: Teacher Student Relationships					
SEI TOTAL: Student Cognitive & Affective Engagement					

Legend: ■ Low Risk, — Moderate Risk, ! High Risk

Fig. 35.9 Vision for types and format for reporting engagement indicators to staff

Additional properties include sensitivity (yield) and specificity which examine the percentage of all those falling short of an outcome that are flagged by the cut score on the predictor as well as those achieving the outcome that are also above the cut score, respectively. Perhaps most critical are the first aspect of PP (also called efficiency) which represents a loss of efficient use of resources if students are incorrectly designated at-risk (see Gleason & Dynarski) and sensitivity which represents those students truly at-risk but missing out on interventions due to their classification.

Cut scores will be generated on predictors across the subtypes of engagement as well as primary and secondary grades and then refined as their properties are examined. Initial efforts will involve a chain of predictors extending from the final valued outcome with most connected via their prediction of a subsequent predictor. As the longitudinal dataset extends over time, more intermediary predictors will be examined for utility in predicting the final valued outcome.

Additionally, the intent will be to continue to add even more formative predictors, each reducing the time between cut scores to assess a given student's trajectory. In Fig. 35.8, these ideas are illustrated in the "Analysis Level" with the results arriving for consumption in the "User Level" and a more detailed report illustrated in Fig. 35.9. The report displayed will be the level below a single icon representing cumulative risk and the level above more detailed information specifying the exact source responsible for the color and shape change of an icon (e.g., the specific subject and assignments missed that resulted in the "Assignment Completion Rate" indicator changing from a green square to yellow triangle or red exclamation point).

Also, the student engagement indicators are separated by subtype to facilitate intervention, and the values of indicators are separated based upon whether they provide context (and are fixed) or represent the accruing reality of the present. Some indicators are relevant both when fixed and as they accrue (e.g., actual GPA and an approximation of GPA). Others are relevant as approximations (e.g., Assignment Success Rate and Assignment Completion Rate) for other semester and year values (i.e., class grade count of Ds or Fs) as well as informative for intervention (i.e., "can't do" or "won't do"). The idea is akin to that of a limit in calculus. Information can be gleaned from a function predictably approaching a value, so much so, that as it gets close enough to the value, it is considered to be that value. Accordingly, it is not enough to wait for a student to fail a core class and then decide that risk is certain enough to intervene; it is better to use approximations of that failure, when reliable enough, to establish risk and intervention efforts earlier.

Additional aspects of Fig. 35.8 focus on the link between assessment of risk and intervention as well as the difference between the *efficacy* of intervention using these types of electronic risk reports and its *effectiveness*. Given the tremendous technological advances in linking data sources via data warehouses, the characteristics of a student displaying risks on the engagement report should be able to be linked to database-housed intervention characteristics such as those contained within the What Works Clearinghouse (WWC). If student characteristics are contained within our district systems, then these, as well as specific aspects of risk, should be utilized in matching the details of the most appropriate intervention for a student displaying risks. Finally, Fig. 35.8 also displays the iterative process of examining the results of report-guided interventions implemented under best-case scenarios (i.e., efficacy) and when implemented in the typical setting in which they will customarily be used (i.e., effectiveness). Admittedly, guidance for staff, family, and community users of data will necessarily be ongoing and iterative based upon information gained from use.

Progress

To date, we have cleaned and merged our NSC data into a format able to be used for longitudinal analyses. Also, we have initially examined the research literature for robust engagement-based predictors and then commissioned and received a literature review documenting the extent of these types of predictors. Moreover, our district has transitioned from several stand-alone databases to an operational data store (ODS) that will be updated nightly and integrate numerous previously disconnected academic and behavioral engagement data elements. The ODS supports a reporting tool that utilizes established cut scores to act upon virtually live data. Further, we have been refining our analyses of disciplinary data (an aspect of behavioral engagement) to the point where our metrics are producing useful approximations of frequency, average severity, and maximum severity of disciplinary infractions. We are in contact with districts also embarking on these types of predictive efforts and continue to gain useful information through these collaborations. Finally, the long-term negative outcomes of students that do not receive interventions at critical points in their tenure in our schools are often not witnessed by those tasked with providing those interventions, and the standardization of the monitoring and intervention process is often not as rigorous as could be beneficial. Perhaps, if cut scores and trajectories are sufficiently predictive, likely negative outcomes could be rendered in a more tangible manner to the user. Also, the checklist approach whereby communication is improved and the consistency of key aspects of monitoring and intervention could be increased across contexts may be a useful one (Gawande, 2009).

Limitations

A systems-level use of engagement data requires well-trained personnel acting upon accessible, timely, and relevant information in order to monitor all students and intervene more intensively as the information indicates. Yet, limitations of adult (e.g., teachers, advisors, or parents/guardians) time and training on using engagement data within an assessment-to-intervention paradigm would seem to be commonalities across many districts. Moreover, the benefits of engagement-focused efforts as well as a thorough understanding of the engagement reports and data are not as prevalent as necessary for systems-level decision-making. Given the many worthwhile endeavors vying for staff time, greater efforts and increasingly convincing evidence of relationships to valued outcomes need to be provided to facilitate school-wide support in engaging students. Additionally, many concepts common to research personnel, included in reports and datasets of engagement information (e.g., significance tests, effect sizes), are often not as familiar across school staff. Also, research personnel may lack familiarity with the training required of skilled classroom teachers and other school staff and would benefit from collaborations with these staff to determine the timeliest opportunities for intervention. Thus, careful thought and planning as well as additional time will need to be part of any presentations that aim for staff to walk away prepared to effectively use engagement information to guide intervention.

Beyond the above general limitation, several specific limitations of the approach specified in this chapter should be mentioned. Advisor-advisee level reports juxtapose the means of SEI factors meaningfully among school and district values and even among other relevant student data. Yet, report users are left to decide when values are meaningfully above or below scores on other SEI factors or school and district values. The advisor-advisee change reports address this somewhat by standardizing differences by the smallest unit of change possible. Nevertheless, a more empirical method for comparing engagement levels would be beneficial. Such a method is not viewed as a replacement for sound judgment; rather it is meant to provide increased information and improved guidance to complement the best practice efforts of clinicians, school staff, and parents/guardians alike.

Questions have been raised about the usefulness of the intrinsic motivation factor of the SEI (see Betts et al., 2010). Given that the item is composed of two items, both negatively worded, suggestions have been made to remove that factor from the SEI and subsequent reports.

The current student-focused reports of academic year changes in engagement did not account for measurement error, and further development is needed to include that consideration. However, issues of meaningful differences and changes have been more thoroughly addressed in the student-focused engagement pattern datasets as well as in the school and district aggregated reports.

Some of the formatting on the reports is not as refined as desired due to limitations of the mass production process (e.g., reduction of numbers to "…" when value space is limited on the bar and font colors set to match bar color not retained on change graphs). In addition, delivery is currently limited to a Lotus Notes database that is dependent upon leadership for dissemination to most advisors, counselors, graduation coaches, etc. Also, PDFs of advisor-advisee reports are not yet able to be efficiently split into single page documents named for the title atop the graph in them.

Logistic functions and item response theory models have not yet been created for SEI responses. Increased information on item characteristics and item functioning across important demographic characteristics and ethnic and poverty subgroups would increase understanding of the strengths and limitations of the SEI.

Conclusion

While the efforts and ideas described in this chapter are fraught with shortcomings and riddled with opportunities for improvement, they are offered as an exciting, forthright documentation of one large and diverse district's effort to make meaning of a construct considered important, even critical, by the authors in this handbook. The intent is to provide a tangible example of systematic utilization of engagement data across subtypes and to offer a forum for the necessary commentary and research agendas to further understanding and improve school and district use of engagement data.

Future research could consider robust engagement-subtype predictors of valued outcomes as well as reliable and meaningful cut scores on these predictors. Examinations of the efficiency and yield of these scores remain critical. Also important will be continued evaluation of stakeholder uses of dynamic engagement reports in order to isolate the training and presentation of information most closely related to positive outcomes. Within the context of increased knowledge on the meaning of specific values on predictors paired with a committed district effort to promote engagement, the implementation of a coherent systems-level assessment-to-intervention paradigm is well within reach.

Acknowledgments The author would like to express sincere gratitude to his colleagues within the offices of Research and Evaluation, Advisement and Counseling, the Information Management Division, as well as within the advisement programs at the schools for the many contributions that furthered the efforts described within this chapter.

References

Appleton, J. J., Christenson, S. L., & Furlong, M. J. (2008). Student engagement with school: Critical conceptual and methodological issues of the construct. *Psychology in the Schools, 45*(5), 369–386.

Appleton, J. J., Christenson, S. L., Kim, D., & Reschly, A. L. (2006). Measuring cognitive and psychological engagement: Validation of the Student Engagement Instrument. *Journal of School Psychology, 44*, 427–445.

Appleton, J. J., Reschly, A. L., & Martin, C. (2011). *Research to practice: Measurement and reporting of student engagement data in applied settings.* Manuscript submitted for publication.

Baumeister, R. F., & Leary, M. R. (1995). The need to belong: Desire for interpersonal attachments as a fundamental human motivation. *Psychological Bulletin, 117*, 497–529.

Betts, J., Appleton, J. J., Reschly, A. L., Christenson, S. L., & Huebner, S. (2010). A study of the factorial invariance of the Student Engagement Instrument (SEI): Results from middle and high school students. *School Psychology Quarterly, 25*(2), 84–93.

Connell, J. P., & Wellborn, J. G. (1991). Competence, autonomy, and relatedness: A motivational analysis of self-system processes. In M. R. Gunnar & L. A. Sroufe (Eds.), *Self processes and development* (Vol. 23, pp. 43–77). Hillsdale, NJ: Lawrence Erlbaum.

Eccles, J. S., Midgley, C., Wigfield, A., Buchanan, C. M., Reuman, D., Flanagan, C., et al. (1993). Development during adolescence: The impact of stage-environment fit on young adolescents' experiences in schools and families. *American Psychologist, 48*, 90–101.

Finn, J. D. (1989). Withdrawing from school. *Review of Educational Research, 59*, 117–142.

Fredricks, J. A., Blumenfeld, P. C., & Paris, A. H. (2004). School engagement: Potential of the concept, state of the evidence. *Review of Educational Research, 74*, 59–109.

Gawande, A. (2009). *The checklist manifesto: How to get things right.* New York: Henry Holt and Company, LLC.

GCPS. (2010). *2010–11 Fast facts.* Retrieved December 12, 2010, from http://www.gwinnett.k12.ga.us/gcps-mainweb01.nsf/7b206fefc3472ddf85257523004bcb46/7b6e15e7f04b0bae852577670052026d?OpenDocument&1~QuickLinks

Gleason, P., & Dynarski, M. (2002). Do we know whom to serve? Issues in using risk factors to identify dropouts. *Journal of Education for Students Placed at Risk, 7*, 25–41.

Goodenow, C., & Grady, K. E. (1993). The relationship of school belonging and friends' values to academic motivation among urban adolescent students. *The Journal of Experimental Education, 62*, 60–71.

Hill, C. J., Bloom, H. S., Black, A. R., & Lipsey, M. W. (2008). Empirical benchmarks for interpreting effect sizes in research. *Child Development Perspectives, 2*(3), 172–177.

Hintze, J. M., & Silberglitt, B. (2005). A longitudinal examination of the diagnostic accuracy and predictive validity of R-CBM and high-stakes testing. *School Psychology Review, 34*(3), 372–386.

Maehr, M. L., & Meyer, H. A. (1997). Understanding motivation and schooling: Where we've been, where we are, and where we need to go. *Educational Psychology Review, 9*, 371–408.

National Research Council and Institute of Medicine. (2004). *Engaging schools: Fostering high school students' motivation to learn.* Washington, DC: The National Academies Press.

Newmann, F. M., Wehlage, G. G., & Lamborn, S. D. (1992). The significance and sources of student engagement. In F. M. Newmann (Ed.), *Student engagement and achievement in American secondary schools* (pp. 11–39). New York: Teachers College Press.

Reschly, A., & Christenson, S. L. (2006a). Promoting successful school completion. In G. Bear & K. Minke (Eds.), *Children's needs III: Development, prevention, and intervention* (pp. 103–113). Bethesda, MD: National Association of School Psychologists.

Reschly, A., & Christenson, S. L. (2006b). Research leading to a predictive model of dropout and completion among students with mild disabilities and the role of student engagement. *Remedial and Special Education, 27*, 276–292.

Russell, V. J., Ainley, M., & Frydenberg, E. (2005). *Schooling issues digest: Student motivation and engagement.* Retrieved November 9, 2005, from http://www.dest.gov.au/sectors/schooleducation/publications resources/schooling issues digest/schooling issues digest motivation engagement.htm

Schunk, D. H. (1991). Self-efficacy and academic motivation. *Educational Psychologist, 26*, 207–231.

Skinner, E. A., Wellborn, J. G., & Connell, J. P. (1990). What it takes to do well in school and whether I've got it: A process model of perceived control and children's engagement and achievement in school. *Journal of Educational Psychology, 82*, 22–32.

Finding the Humanity in the Data: Understanding, Measuring, and Strengthening Student Engagement

36

Ethan Yazzie-Mintz and Kim McCormick

Abstract

Within the emerging field of research on student engagement, there exists a wide variety of work in terms of definitions, constructs, and methodologies. In this chapter, we argue for the importance of "finding the humanity in the data," understanding and investigating student engagement and disengagement as a function of the perceptions of students about their experiences in the learning environment. After setting out a conceptualization of engagement, we examine data from the High School Survey of Student Engagement (HSSSE), a self-report survey containing both multiple-option and open-response questions. Our analysis is focused on the words and school experiences of students as a way of understanding levels and dimensions of student engagement in school. Using examples from the field, we describe ways in which schools use student perception data to understand and strengthen student engagement. We conclude by setting out challenges for research, policy, and practice in the field of student engagement.

My school is a good school, but I feel the only thing they care about are scores on standardized tests, not us students as individuals.

– Student respondent on the High School Survey of Student Engagement (HSSSE),
Spring 2010

E. Yazzie-Mintz, Ed.D. (✉)
First Light Education Project, Denver, CO, USA
e-mail: e@post.harvard.edu

K. McCormick, M.A.
Department of Counseling and Educational Psychology,
Indiana University School of Education,
Bloomington, IN, USA
e-mail: mccormkm@indiana.edu

Introduction

In this age of accountability as defined by standardized measures of achievement and rigorous research on schooling as defined by the utilization of highly controlled input-output models, data – as in "data-driven instruction" and "data-driven decision-making" – are invariably comprised of those measures that can be counted, standardized, replicated, and predictive of an academic outcome. The resulting focus on scores and outcomes, incentivized and dictated by state and federal policy, leaves many students feeling like the student quoted above, in which their value to the school community, particularly to the adults, is not based on who they are as developing adolescents, their potential for learning and growing, or their emerging passions and curiosity, but rather on their performance on standardized assessments.

These student perceptions cut across student demographics: race/ethnicity, gender, socioeconomic status, grade level, academic track, and level of academic achievement. The High School Survey of Student Engagement (HSSSE) is one instrument that serves to measure student engagement through self-reported perceptions of the students themselves. Schools use the data from HSSSE in a variety of ways; effective school uses of these data include understanding the experience of students in the school, investigating particular interventions, and improving a particular aspect of students' connection to school (academic, social, emotional).

Several years ago, a school that participated in HSSSE, after receiving their data report, was particularly interested in and baffled by their data, asking: *Why are our kids just as bored as the rest of the country?* This high school, which we will call "Tech High School," was a well-resourced school located in a wealthy suburb of a large urban center in the USA. There was little poverty or concern about resources in this community – "all of the students' basic needs are met," according to a school staff member – and academic achievement was high in the school based on standard measures such as standardized tests and graduation rates.

Amid such economic advantage and high achievement, the school administrators expected that the students would be more engaged in work and learning at school. Their surprise at the results of the student survey was compounded by the fact that the school had recently spent a large amount of money getting the building "wired up": installing high-tech equipment in every classroom, including advanced projectors, interactive whiteboards, and laptops – all technologies purported to engage students more intensely in classroom learning. However, on the survey, the students' data looked very similar to data from students across the country who had participated in HSSSE; students were no more engaged at "Tech High School" than students at other high schools.

Rather than investigate more deeply the source of the students' perceptions or evaluate more closely why the technological improvements to the building had not generated greater engagement in learning among students, the principal, on seeing the results of the survey, proclaimed, "They're making that up…They just want to make us look bad." The first reaction of the principal was to distrust the students' perceptions, create an us (school) versus them (students) demarcation, and imply that the students completed the surveys with a group intent to tarnish the image of the school.

We pointed the school team toward the open-response question at the end of the survey, which asks students: *Would you like to say more about any of your answers to these survey questions?* Students at "Tech High School" gave these answers:

- I feel like administrators put too much emphasis on making the school look good, not the students' best interest. High school years are supposed to be a prime time of growing in all ways but ridiculous busy work prevents personal growth outside of school.
- I am not engaged in any classes and think there is too much emphasis on TESTS.
- I often feel that we are pushed to learn answers instead of material, or to do well on a test instead of understand the concept.
- I just wished the school cared more about what the student wants, not just how they can make the school look good.
- I personally feel that too much time is spent in preparation for standardized tests, not enough time is spent learning relevant information.
- [This school] cares a lot about its image. Maybe too much!

Many of these students described their perception of a school that put a heavy focus on the image that the school presented to the outside world. Despite the advanced technology, the students described a school that was focused on test scores and image, but not as much on deep understanding of concepts, relevance of learning, and students' growth and development. These open responses, in combination with students' responses to the multiple-option questions on the survey, present a picture of "Tech High School" as a school that, though possessing the resources to provide more materials and structures, was both facing the same challenges of engagement as other schools across the country and failing to use their resources to deepen learning or engagement. Further, the principal's assertion that the students were "trying to make the school look bad" through their survey responses – that is, they weren't really giving honest answers, but were using the survey to create a negative image of the school – was picked up by the students and highlighted by their written perceptions on the survey that the school is more focused on its image than on teaching, learning, and development. In a similar way as the student quoted at the top of this chapter, these students of "Tech High School" see themselves as data points in service of a particular school agenda revolving around accountability to the outside world, and not as individuals experiencing a place and time to learn, grow, and develop curiosity about the world.

This discrepancy between adult and student perceptions of the student experience in school raises several questions regarding student engagement that will be examined in this chapter:

- What is student engagement, and how is it conceptualized and measured?
- What do students say about their learning experiences and environments?
- Why does student engagement matter for research and practice?

In this chapter, we argue for the importance of "finding the humanity in the data," understanding and investigating student engagement and disengagement as a function of the perceptions of students about their experiences in the learning environment. The culture of schools is too often focused on the needs of adults in the school environment, preventing deep reforms and improvements; students are expected to function effectively and productively within learning environments from which they feel alienated and within which they feel unimportant. Strengthening student engagement by first understanding the learning environment from the perspectives of students and then implementing changes that address the academic, social, and emotional needs of students can have an enormous impact on both school processes and outcomes.

What Is Student Engagement?

The question, "What is student engagement?," is deceptively complex. An informal poll of teachers, principals, researchers, and policymakers yields a range of responses to this question: one-word definitions including "involvement," "participation," and "investment"; more expansive answers, such as "deep connection to learning" and "interest in the subject matter"; articulation of ways to measure engagement, such as "amount of time students spend on tasks" and "students asking and answering questions in class"; and metaphors – "I see students huddled together literally digging in." The wide spectrum of understandings about engagement present a picture of a concept that has lent itself better to identification by observation – "I know it when I see it" – than to a commonly accepted definition in research and practice, leaving the question "How do we measure student engagement?" up for debate.

This complexity is reflected in the multiple and evolving definitions, indicators, and conceptions of engagement guiding research and practice. Despite the complexity, the thrust of applied research focuses heavily on discrete predictors and indicators of engagement, primarily student behaviors and school structures. For example, schools such as "Tech High School" are driven by a body of current research that links the use of technology with higher student engagement. The prevailing philosophy is that students in K-12 institutions today have grown up with a burgeoning array of visual media options and advanced technology (e.g., laptops, social networking websites, cell phones); hence, the thinking goes, these students will learn best if these technologies are brought into the classroom. However, just as with any school structure or pedagogical strategy, the "how" is even more important than the "what." Technology in and of itself is not engaging, though it can provide opportunities to engage students in learning. A recent study of math teaching and learning in Australia provides insight into the relationship between engagement and learning as mediated by structures such as technology (Attard, 2009, 2010). Students, transitioning from primary school to secondary school, experienced as well a transition in pedagogy – from a hands-on, active style of math teaching to a computer-based pedagogy that involved less interaction with the teacher. The effect of this change in pedagogy was a weakening of teacher-student relationships and a lowering of student engagement in math. The further danger is the possibility that such changes in student engagement can precipitate decreases in student achievement.

In its most fundamental sense, engagement is about relationships (Yazzie-Mintz, 2007). Whether two people choose to become "engaged" by embarking on a permanent and intimate relationship, or two forces "engage" in battle by entering a violent and confrontational relationship, the necessary component of "engagement" is a relationship; engagement cannot be achieved or accomplished by oneself.

Engagement is often misunderstood as synonymous with *motivation*. For the purposes of this chapter, the authors view motivation as one component of what makes a student engaged in their learning and school. Motivation describes the *processes* and *factors* that drive or move a student to take action. These processes and factors are not generally defined in relationship, but as a function of the individual student in response to a set of internal or external stimuli. What hinders or supports motivation can be contingent on the context or environment.

Extrinsic motivation describes an external reward as the stimulus for action; for example, a student will engage in a behavior to receive a positive reward or consequence, such as a grade, that is separate from the behavior (deCharms, 1968; Lepper & Greene, 1978). *Intrinsic motivation* describes an internal stimulus – for example, enjoyment of the task or project – that drives action; the reward is the behavior itself, which brings enjoyment to the individual student. Students who are intrinsically motivated to work and learn tend to be curious, persistent, and eager for challenging tasks; these are students who want to build a body of knowledge instead of learning something solely for a reward or other outcome (Gottfried, Fleming, & Gottfried, 1994; Gottfried & Gottfried, 1996). While these students need little more than an appropriate task to stimulate them to work, research shows that intrinsic motivation lessens as students move from elementary to middle to high school (Lepper, Corpus, & Lyengar, 2005; Lepper, Sethi, Dialdin, & Drake, 1997). As time in school increases, students' interest and curiosity in learning lessens, and many seek tasks that are not challenging (Harter, 1992; Harter & Jackson, 1992).

Focusing on students' motivation to work and learn, then, may lead to a classroom trap: create rewards that activate extrinsically motivated students, leading to a focus on the reward rather than the project or related learning, or create appropriate tasks that activate the intrinsically motivated students, though the number of these types of students decreases as students move through the K-12 system (perhaps as a result of the system itself). Often, adults expect students who are motivated to be engaged in school. In fact, those students who are motivated intrinsically may be more likely to seek opportunities for learning and engagement outside of school, if school does not provide such opportunities (Jordan & Nettles, 1999). Students who are motivated by external rewards may participate in schooling to the extent they receive the rewards they seek, but not engage deeply in learning or work. Further, adults in school tend to give up on students who are not motivated in traditionally understood ways (either intrinsically or through an external rewards system). Focusing on engagement provides both an opportunity and a responsibility for school communities – adults and students – to work collectively and systemically toward greater learning for all.

We approach this research from an engagement perspective in which motivation is one aspect of the larger engagement construct. In the case of students and schools, engagement is about the student's relationship to the school and learning community: the people (including adults and peers), the structures (including rules, schedules, and the organization of the school), the instruction, the curriculum and content, and the opportunities for participation in this community (including curricular, cocurricular, and extracurricular). Researching student engagement is essentially about investigating the dimensions and depth of the relationship between the student and the school community, and the ways in which this relationship is enacted. The HSSSE focuses on investigating and understanding, from the students' perspectives, the relationship between the student and the learning community and utilizing research and professional development to strengthen this relationship.

Research on Student Engagement

As a result of efforts to study and formalize thinking and research on student engagement, multiple models of engagement have been developed. Within the research literature, a complex, multidimensional definition of "student engagement" is drawn (Fredricks, Blumenfeld, & Paris, 2004), though understandings of student engagement continue to evolve. The concept of student engagement as an area of study has emerged relatively recently in education research, becoming increasingly prevalent over the last 20 years (Appleton, Christenson, & Furlong, 2008), though the notion of students being engaged and involved in learning is a foundational concept in the history of education and schooling. Given that student engagement is often associated with student choice (i.e., students choosing classes, schools, how to spend their time, etc.), compulsory schooling at the K-12 level in the USA has made student engagement less widely studied (particularly at the systemic level) than at the postsecondary level, where student engagement often falls under the purview of offices of institutional research as well as student services. From a policy perspective, schooling at the K-12 level is predominantly viewed as something that students have to do, as a matter of law and as an entry into the world of work or further schooling; whether students are involved or engaged in their learning is less consequential than the outcomes of their schooling (achievement, persistence, and graduation).

In the course of the short history of the study of student engagement and the growing understanding of the importance of the concept, many different definitions and models have been created. The most common definition of student engagement consists of two components: a behavioral component associated with positive behavior, effort, and participation, and an emotional/affective component that includes interest, identification with school, a sense of belonging, and a positive attitude about learning (Finn, 1989; Marks, 2000; Newmann, Wehlage, & Lamborn, 1992; Willms, 2003). Some researchers have added a third cognitive component to the definition of student engagement, which includes self-regulation, learning goals, and a measure of students' investment in their learning (Fredricks et al., 2004; Jimerson, Campos, & Greif, 2003; Linnenbrink & Pintrich, 2003).

Behavioral engagement typically describes student actions that can easily be observed inside the classroom – for example, students actively participating in classroom activities, assignments, and projects. This type of engagement focuses on the degree to which students take an active role in school-related activities, both inside the classroom and across all school areas (Fredricks et al., 2004; Munns & Woodward, 2006). Cognitive engagement describes students' investment in the actual learning process – not just demonstration of involvement through external behaviors but internal investment, where the mind is engaged in classroom work. For example, cognitive engagement can be demonstrated by a student's mastery of the full meaning of curricular material, taking a position more of an expert than that of a novice (Linnenbrink & Pintrich, 2003; Munns & Woodward, 2006). Motivational/emotional engagement describes the degree to which students see the value of what they are doing in school. Students engaged in this way are not just going through the motions of the academic experience but are self-reflective about their learning and feel connections between their lives and their work (Linnenbrink & Pintrich, 2003; Munns & Woodward, 2006).

This three-component model of student engagement continues to evolve (Appleton et al., 2008). The behavioral component of engagement has been split into two more specific subtypes to include *academic engagement*, encompassing measures, such as time on task, credit hours, and homework completion, and *behavioral engagement*, which includes attendance, voluntary classroom participation, and extracurricular participation. The expansion of the model also includes the varying contexts that influence student engagement (e.g., family, peers, and school), students' interactions within these contexts, and the degree to which students' interactions within these contexts help students meet fundamental needs of autonomy, competence, and relatedness (Appleton, Christenson, Kim, & Reschly, 2006; Appleton et al., 2008).

A number of studies have asserted a connection between engagement and school processes or outcomes. For example, engagement has been associated with *student achievement* (Appleton et al., 2008; Finn, 1993, Furrer & Skinner, 2003; Klem & Connell, 2004), *positive classroom and school climate* (Appleton et al., 2006; Cohen, McCabe, Michelli, & Pickeral, 2009; Newmann et al., 1992), and *effective instructional practices* (Mant, Wilson, & Coates, 2007; Shernoff, Csikszentmihalyi, Schneider, & Shernoff, 2003).

In the policy climate heavily dependent on academic outcomes, it is important to note that a number of studies have asserted a relationship between student engagement and student academic outcomes (Yazzie-Mintz, 2010). However, much of the research literature on engagement and achievement focuses on two primary areas: student behaviors (e.g., self-efficacy, self-regulation, and motivation; see, for example, Furrer & Skinner, 2003; Linnenbrink & Pintrich, 2003; Skinner, Wellborn, & Connell, 1990) and school structures (e.g., class scheduling, school and class size, attendance, use of technology). Few studies focus on all the parts of the school system simultaneously, including the interaction among the various relationships, structures, and stakeholders in schools in connection with student engagement and its association with student achievement (Johnson, Crosnoe, & Elder, 2001).

The Culture of Schools and Student Engagement

How can we conceptualize student engagement in a systemic way? Given the focus on motivation and the current research imperative to give primacy to "countable" measures, student engagement is largely understood as an individual student behavioral issue. However, this narrow focus generates only a partial picture. Conceptualizing student engagement as a cultural issue in schools rather than a policy, behavioral, or structural issue provides a window through which the student experience can be understood.

In "Thick Description: Toward an Interpretive Theory of Culture," Clifford Geertz (1973) described the individual as "an animal suspended in webs of significance he himself has spun," and "culture" as these "webs of significance." Culture is a set of relationships that are interrelated, overlapping, nonlinear, and rarely compartmentalized; when looked at all together and from a distance, the picture is that of a web or a set of webs. Understanding the student experience in schools as a set of "webs of significance" provides the opportunity to explore the complexity of student engagement and highlights the traps inherent in parsing out the various pieces of school so common to the input-output models. This conception illuminates why implementing a structure does not necessarily have a direct and uniform impact on student outcomes. For example, though block scheduling (longer class times for key subject areas than traditional class periods) is often asserted to increase student learning and achievement, implementing block scheduling, absent other changes, does not necessarily accomplish this purpose due to the need to change styles of teaching to adapt to the longer class periods; the importance of making effective use of the increased time for interaction between teachers and students, students and peers, and students and subject matter; and the resistance members of the school community will have to a change in established routine. As a structural issue, longer classes are theorized to have a positive impact on learning and achievement; however, failure of the structure is a near certainty unless the ways in which a structural change has an impact on the culture of the school – the various and multiple "webs of significance" – are investigated, understood, and addressed.

In attempting to investigate and measure student engagement, the importance of understanding student engagement as a culture is further highlighted. Geertz (1973) described the process of studying culture (through ethnography) as much more than just a set of "techniques" and "procedures"; the focus must be the "intellectual effort" and creation of "thick description" that lights the way toward understanding the culture rather than just observing and counting it. Applying these insights to research on student engagement, we are compelled to look beyond just countable and observable measures – time on task, attendance/truancy, and lateness – to gain an understanding of the relationships, connections, and multiple pathways that lead to student engagement with work and learning.

Frequently left out of the conversations and research on student engagement are the experiences of the students from the perspectives of the students themselves. Students are in a unique position where they not only see and feel what is going on in their schools, but they have the voices to let people know what they think. Giving power to student perspectives can directly improve education practice because when teachers and school officials listen to and learn from students, they can begin to see the world from those students' perspectives (Cook-Sather, 2001). Why would these important and relevant voices be so often excluded? First, as we have heard from numerous school leaders and other school adults, including the principal of "Tech High School" cited earlier, adults do not trust what students say. Second, school adults often believe they are charged with creating, organizing, and directing the teaching, learning, and school structures; what students say or believe does not matter to them or they assume they know what the student perspective is. Finally, researchers often avoid studying students directly due to the increased requirements – including consent forms, parent/guardian permission, and scrutiny from Institutional Review Boards – for doing research with (or *on*, as is frequently the case) minors.

Though it is easier to do research with school adults, on externally observable behavior, and using countable data and records, students' perspectives on their own experiences are critical in understanding student engagement. The school is not a set of isolated pieces that function in their own realms, but rather a "social organism," in which "the life of the whole is in all its parts, yet the whole could not exist without any of its parts" (Waller, 1932). To understand how, why, and to what degree students engage in or disengage from the life and work of the school, it is necessary to understand the ways in which all of these different parts function and interact as part of the whole. As in any social system, an understanding of the complexities of the system does not necessarily reside in those at the top of the system, who only have a narrow understanding and perspective on the ways in which the system operates; those at the bottom of the social hierarchy within a system often have the greatest insights into the whole system. Within schools, those at the bottom of the social hierarchy are the students; understanding a complex process such as student engagement necessitates understanding the student experience from the perspective of the students themselves. As Senge (2000) wrote, "Students are the only players who see all sides of the nested systems of education, yet they are typically the people who have the least influence on its design."

The High School Survey of Student Engagement

The HSSSE is designed to both help schools ascertain students' beliefs about their school experience and provide assistance to schools in translating data into action. HSSSE investigates deeply the attitudes, perceptions, and beliefs of students about their work, the school learning environment, and their interaction with the school community. Survey questions investigate the levels and dimensions of student engagement in the life and work of high schools, providing schools with rich and valuable data on students' beliefs, attitudes, and behaviors. The data from the survey help schools explore the causes and conditions that lead to student success or failure, engagement or "disengagement," and persistence or dropping out.

Built on the foundation of the National Survey of Student Engagement (NSSE) for postsecondary students, the HSSSE survey originally measured similar constructs of engagement (Kuh, 2003). More recently, HSSSE has been a research and professional development project directed by the Center for Evaluation and Education Policy (CEEP) at Indiana University in Bloomington. From 2006 through 2010, more than 350,000 students in over 40 states took the survey.

There are 35 major items on the survey; including sub-questions, there are over 100 items to which students respond. Survey questions cover a wide range of aspects of engagement, including how students spend their time, the importance they place on particular activities, the rigor and challenge of classes, reasons for going to school, tendency toward boredom in school, potential for dropping out, and types of teaching they find engaging. The last question on the survey is an open-response question, to which students can provide longer-form thoughts on their school experience.

HSSSE is built on a three-component framework of engagement, taking into account both the demands of research and the utility of the construct to schools and other learning organizations. As such, the High School Survey of Student Engagement utilizes three dimensions of engagement for analysis of data (Yazzie-Mintz, 2007, 2009, 2010): *cognitive/intellectual/academic engagement*, *social/behavioral/participatory engagement*, and *emotional engagement*. A recent psychometric study of these scales found the three-dimension construct to be valid and reliable (Johnson & Dean, 2011).

Cognitive/intellectual/academic engagement captures students' effort, investment in work, and strategies for learning: the work students do and the ways students go about their work. This dimension, focusing primarily on engagement during instructional time and with instruction-related activities, can be described as *engagement of the mind*. Survey questions that are grouped within this dimension of engagement include questions about homework, preparation for class, classroom discussions and assignments, and the level of academic challenge that students report. Cronbach's alpha for this dimension is 0.943 (Johnson & Dean, 2011).

Social/behavioral/participatory engagement emphasizes students' actions and participation within the school outside of instructional time, including nonacademic school-based activities, social and extracurricular activities, and interactions with other students – the ways in which students interact within the school community beyond the classroom. This dimension, with its focus on student actions, interactions, and participation within the school community, can be described as *engagement in the life of the school*. Survey questions that are grouped within this dimension of engagement include questions about extracurricular activities, students' interactions with other students, and students' connections to the community within and around the school. Cronbach's alpha for this dimension is 0.760 (Johnson & Dean, 2011).

Emotional engagement encompasses students' feelings of connection to (or disconnection from) their school – how students feel about where they are in school, the ways and workings of the school, and the people within the school. This dimension, focusing largely on students' internal lives not frequently expressed explicitly in observable behavior and actions, can be described as *engagement of the heart*. Survey questions that are grouped within this dimension include questions about general feelings regarding the school, level of support students perceive from members of the school community, and students' place in the school community. Cronbach's alpha for this dimension is 0.937 (Johnson & Dean, 2011).

Data Sample

In this chapter, we examine data from HSSSE 2009 to provide examples of the kinds of school-wide perspectives that can be gathered through HSSSE. In 2009, 42,754 students participated in HSSSE, representing a response rate of 74%. These students came from 103 high schools across 27 different states within the USA. Schools came from all five regions of the country (Northeast, Southeast, Midwest, Southwest, and West), with 63% of the participating schools located in the West and Midwest. The smallest participating school enrolled 20 students, and the largest participating school enrolled 3,143 students; average student enrollment was 787. By grade level, 30% of respondents were in grade 9, 27% in grade 10, 23% in grade 11, and 20% in grade 12. Respondents were 52% female and 48% male. Of the sample, 25% reported being eligible for free and reduced-price lunch, 54% reported not being eligible, and 21% did not know or preferred not to respond to the question of eligibility. By race/ethnicity, 49.9% of the respondents categorized themselves as White, 12.5% as Black or African American, 6.5% as Latino or Hispanic, 5.9% as Asian, 1.8% as Native American (including Native Alaskan or Hawaiian), and 1.0% as Middle Eastern; 9.3% identified themselves as more than one race (multiracial), and 13.1% preferred not to respond to the question (Yazzie-Mintz, 2010).

Data Analysis

Why is it important to understand the school experience from the perspective of students? There is the notion that for students to be full participating members of a school community, their voices and beliefs must be a part of conversations and decisions on school policies, structures, and teaching and learning. In addition, there are academic and policy considerations. There is a real and serious gap between student aspirations and rates of student graduation. Data from the US Department of Education indicate that for the class of 2008 in public high schools in the USA, 25% of students did not graduate within 4 years of entering high school, considered "on time" graduation (Stillwell, 2010).

In 2009, only 1.5% of HSSSE respondents expected to leave high school without a diploma; from 2006 to 2010, only 3% of student respondents on the High School Survey of Student Engagement ($n=352,140$) expected not to finish high school. Even looking at the rates within schools, and across grade levels, the aspirations outpace the actual graduation numbers. What happens between aspiration and graduation? Student perspectives provide insight.

Several questions in particular are highlighted here as describing students' perspectives on their school experiences:
- Why do you go to school?
- Have you ever been bored in class in high school?
- If you have been bored in class, why?
- Have you ever considered dropping out of high school?
- If you have thought about dropping out of high school, why?
- To what degree does each of the following types of work in class excite and/or engage you?

These questions were selected for analysis in this chapter for several reasons: (1) these items represent important cornerstones in understanding students' thinking in terms of their school attendance, daily school and classroom experience, and possibility of exiting school prior to graduation, and (2) these items provide rich data for schools in several critical areas and are especially useful for schools beginning the process of using student perspectives as a starting point for analysis and school improvement.

Reasons for Going to School

As a first step in the process of understanding student perspectives, it is critical to know why students attend school. While K-12 schooling in the USA is compulsory, compliance with the law is only the fifth most reported reason for why students attend high school. In fact, there are three primary purposes students have for attending school: an academic purpose, a social purpose, and a family related purpose (Yazzie-Mintz, 2010).

On the survey, students were asked, "Why do you go to school?" Students could provide as many responses to this question as they wanted. As can be seen in Table 36.1, the most-reported reason for attending school was "Because I want to get a degree and go to college" (73.1%).

Table 36.1 HSSSE Spring 2009 aggregate

Why do you go to school?	
I enjoy being in school	35.8%
What I learn in classes	40.5%
My teacher(s)	23.1%
My parents/guardians	64.0%
My peers/friends	66.1%
It's the law	55.7%
I want to get a degree and go to college	73.1%
I want to acquire skills for the workplace	44.8%
There's nothing else to do	17.2%
I want to get a good job	66.8%
To stay out of trouble	21.5%
Other	10.3%

Table 36.2 HSSSE Spring 2009 aggregate

Have you ever been bored in class in high school?	
Never	2.5%
Once or twice	4.2%
Once in a while	27.6%
Every day	48.7%
Every class	17.0%

Table 36.3 HSSSE Spring 2009 aggregate

If you have been bored in class, why?	
Work wasn't challenging enough	32.8%
Work was too difficult	26.3%
Material wasn't interesting	81.3%
Material wasn't relevant to me	41.6%
No interaction with teacher	34.5%
Other	16.4%

Close behind were "Because I want to get a good job" (66.8%), "Because of my peers/friends" (66.1%), and "Because of my parents/guardians" (64.0%). These reasons can be understood as focused on the future, on the people with whom the students attend school, and on family.

By contrast, students' experiences inside the school and inside the classroom were reasons for going to school for fewer than half of respondents: "Because of what I learn in classes" (40.5%), "Because I enjoy being in school" (35.8%), and "Because of my teachers" (23.1%). Schools can use these student responses to dig deeper into why the essential functions of schools (teaching and learning) are not the reasons most of their students are attending their schools on a daily basis.

Boredom

Student boredom is an important variable to investigate in understanding engagement and disengagement. On the survey, students were asked two specific questions related to boredom: "Have you ever been bored in class in high school?" and "If you have been bored in class, why?"

Table 36.2 presents results from student responses to the first question. Predictable as it may be, two-thirds of student respondents report being bored in class at least every day, if not in every class: 17.0% of students report being bored in every class, and 48.7% of students report being bored every day. In addition, 27.6% of students report being bored "once in a while." Only 4.2% report being bored "once or twice," and only 2.5% report "never" being bored in class in high school.

While there is widespread boredom among students in high school, even more important than the frequency of boredom is why students are bored. Students could provide as many answers as applicable to the second question, with results presented in Table 36.3. The most frequent reason cited is "Material wasn't interesting" (81.3%), followed by "Material wasn't relevant to me" (41.6%). These responses provide a foundation for understanding the challenges schools face in creating engaging curriculum and instruction; while schools are often focused on outcome measures and assessments, most students are reporting that they do not find the content engaging enough, and many report that they do not understand the importance of what they are learning, and the connection between what they are learning and other content or their lives outside of school. Further, 34.5% of the students report that they are bored because they have "No interaction" with their teachers; given the importance of interaction to the instructional process, it is important to look at why more than one-third of this sample of students report that a key source of their boredom lies in a lack of teacher-student interaction.

Table 36.4 HSSSE Spring 2009 aggregate

Have you ever considered dropping out of high school?	
Never	79.0%
Once or twice	14.3%
Many times	6.7%

Table 36.5 HSSSE Spring 2009 aggregate

If you have thought about dropping out of high school, why?	
The work was too hard	35.0%
The work was too easy	12.9%
I didn't like the school	49.8%
I didn't like the teachers	38.5%
I didn't see the value in the work I was being asked to do	42.3%
I was picked on or bullied	16.3%
I needed to work for money	20.0%
No adults in the school cared about me	16.0%
Family issues	29.2%
I felt I was too far behind in credits to graduate	21.5%
I failed required standardized tests for graduation	8.5%
Adults in school encouraged me to drop out	9.4%
Other	22.2%

Potential for Dropping Out

Bridgeland, DiIulio, and Morison (2006) have described the process of dropping out of school as a "slow process of disengagement." Schools across the USA struggle with keeping students in school through completion of the diploma, reducing dropout rates and raising graduation rates. As a policy issue, the debate between encouragement and punishment as a means of dealing with students who drop out remains active, and the costs to individuals and society of dropping out are significant (Sum, Khatiwada, McLaughlin, with Palma, 2009).

Table 36.4 presents data from student responses to the survey question "Have you ever considered dropping out of high school?" Though 79% of the students have never considered dropping out of high school, 21% have considered dropping out either "once or twice" (14.3%) or "many times" (6.7%).

As with the question on boredom, the reasons students give for considering dropping out are instructive in addressing the issue. Table 36.5 presents the reasons students provide for considering dropping out; students could give as many reasons as were applicable. Of the students who have considered dropping out, the most frequently indicated reasons are: "I didn't like the school" (49.8%), "I didn't see the value in the work I was being asked to do" (42.3%), and "I didn't like the teachers" (38.5%). It is interesting and important to note that students' experiences in school and in class were reported as reasons for going to school by fewer than half of the respondents, as reported above; these experiences in school and in class were also reported most frequently by students as the reasons why they consider dropping out of school. While there are other factors that students report as moving them to consider dropping out, including family issues (29.2%), schools can have great influence over the in-school and in-class factors and can look to these data for guidance in addressing the dropout issue.

Pedagogy

Looking inside the classroom, it is important to investigate the kinds of instruction that engage students and activate their interest in learning. Table 36.6 presents students' responses to the question "To what degree does each of the following types of work in class excite and/or engage you?"

"Teacher lecture" is the least-preferred type of teaching; 44.2% of students report liking teacher lecture "not at all" and 29.8% of students report liking teacher lecture "a little," while only 6.0% of students like it "very much." By contrast, 60.9% of students reported that "Discussion and debate" excited and/or engaged them "some" or "very much," while only 15.8% reported liking this type of work "not at all"; similarly, 60.1% of students reported that "Group projects" excited and/or engaged them "some" or "very much," while only 16.4% reported liking this type of work "not at all." Both "Discussion and debate" and "Group projects" provide learning forums in which students are interacting with their peers and the teacher and working collaboratively to learn and generate knowledge.

Data from this question can be instructive for schools, as they work to examine and improve the learning experiences of students in class.

Table 36.6 HSSSE Spring 2009 aggregate

To what degree does each of the following types of work in class excite and/or engage you?

	Not at all (%)	A little (%)	Some (%)	Very much (%)
Teacher lecture	44.2	29.8	20.0	6.0
Discussion and debate	15.8	23.3	32.3	28.6
Individual reading	33.6	29.7	26.3	10.4
Writing projects	37.0	29.6	24.4	9.0
Research projects	33.0	29.7	27.9	9.4
Group projects	16.4	23.5	37.9	22.2
Presentations	27.5	26.9	31.2	14.4
Role plays	31.3	25.9	25.6	17.1
Art and drama activities	27.8	22.7	25.2	24.3
Projects and lessons involving technology	19.2	25.8	34.1	21.0

Students are less likely to be engaged by work in which they are passively receiving knowledge, such as teacher lecture, but will be more engaged by instructional methods in which they are working and learning with the teacher and peers and/or where they are active participants in their learning (such as presentations, which 45.6% of students report liking "some" or "very much"; role plays, which 42.7% of students report liking "some" or "very much"; and art and drama activities, which 49.5% of students report liking "some" or "very much"). In addition, schools can explore effective uses of technology within the curriculum, as 55.1% of students report being engaged by "Projects and lessons involving technology."

Student Engagement in Students' Words

The last question on the survey is an open-response question asking respondents "Would you like to say more about your answers to these survey questions?" This question provides a space for students to give longer-form, narrative thoughts on their school experiences and school engagement. Students are in a unique position within the social hierarchies of schools, seeing the school from a perspective that adults cannot access easily. For this reason, the open-response statements that students share on the High School Survey of Student Engagement offer myriad insights into what students think about their experiences and what improvements can be made. Schools, for their part, must be prepared to hear and act on the perspectives of students. Commonly, of all stakeholders in the school community, it is the student who has the least amount of say about what goes into the policies and practices of the school; it is the adults who determine what happens in schools and what changes are made. It is more than ironic that the very people who everyone wants to better serve typically are not consulted (Cook-Sather, 2002).

The student responses to this open-response question expand on and enlighten the responses students give to the multiple-option questions. For researchers, these responses provide another check on the interpretation of the multiple-option survey responses. For schools, these responses provide deeper insight into student thinking about their school experience, in a way that schools might otherwise not be able to access. In 2009, 8,150 students provided a response to the open-response question on the survey. From 2006 through 2010, more than 50,000 students provided responses to this question.

Several themes that emerge in students' open responses highlight important issues in the student experience. One common theme, frequently expressed by students, is that what they have to say does not matter within the school community and that no change will come about as a result of their participation in this survey. One student respondent expressed this thought in this way: *These surveys are pointless because no matter what we say, none of the supervisors will listen to us.* Over several years, this theme has come up among students from across the spectrum of schools and demographics, expressed as some variation of this student's response.

All of the students who respond in this way have actually completed this survey and then noted that they do not believe their words and ideas will be taken seriously in any meaningful, action-resulting way. It will be important for further research to examine those students who also feel this way but did not complete a survey, and for schools to find a way to solicit those students' ideas. This body of students is sending the message that schools need to be places that actually listen and respond to what students have to say, particularly when they ask for students' viewpoints through surveys such as HSSSE. Schools need to demonstrate to students that they use the data in meaningful ways; students feeling disconnected from the workings of the school may be prone to be disconnected from the learning as well.

Another theme that emerges is the power of teachers in the lives of students, expressed by a student in this way: *I always wished at least one teacher would see a skill in me that seemed extraordinary, or help to encourage its growth.* While the current policy debates in state legislatures across the country often focus on the ineffectiveness of teachers, students in their open responses on the survey identify teachers as the possible link to engagement with school and learning. On the multiple-option questions on the survey cited above, students point to their in-class experiences as being low on the list of reasons they go to school and high on the list of reasons why they have considered dropping out; however, on the open-response questions, students often identify individual teachers and other adults who have created engaging learning environments for them. Teachers are most often and publicly judged on their progress with students based on standardized outcome measures; students most often look to teachers for supportive and meaningful relationships. Through both positive and negative student responses regarding teachers, schools can identify ways to strengthen the student learning experience in the classroom.

One student's response – *I wish school could be intellectually challenging as well as academically challenging* – raises another common issue, the distinction between tasks to complete and assignments that provide opportunities to pursue knowledge. Students look for challenge and meaning in their work, not just memorization of facts and figures and tasks out of context. Students distinguish between work that is necessary to complete for academic reasons and work that challenges them to think and learn. Engagement can be pursued and sustained through intellectually challenging work.

Instructional methods play a role in engagement and disengagement within the classroom, as evidenced by data cited from the multiple-option survey question on pedagogy. Students follow through on this theme on the open-response question in which they frequently assert the need for more hands-on, interactive learning. One student captured this idea by writing out this question: *Why won't they bring what we are learning to life?* Interaction is high on the list of students' desires for engaging methods of teaching and learning. Both on the multiple-option question and on the open-response question, students cite those methods in which they are interacting with the teacher, peers, and the material – group projects, discussion, and debate – as the most engaging. Students do not want to be told what to know, but instead want to discover knowledge, see how information is related to them, and how it can be beneficial for their future. Teachers can accomplish this by using a variety of hands-on, active instructional practices that elicit interaction and, ultimately, engagement.

Schools are most frequently assessed on outcomes, which raises the question of the purpose of teaching and learning in schools: Is it just to get students to the finish line and earn the diploma? Or is it to produce students who are lifelong learners actively in pursuit of knowledge? Students ask this question as well, as they identify the limits of their schooling experience: *School does not determine how smart a student is. A "smart" student is one who absorbs everything they are told. I hate school because it limits students to one kind of smart.* Students who are highly engaged in their school experience have higher achievement, better images of themselves as students and learners, and better overall attitudes about school and learning. The data from the open-response question indicate that, while adults (teachers, administrators, policymakers, researchers, etc.) are focused on achievement and outcomes, students are overwhelmingly looking for engaging learning experiences: *I hate learning for tests. I want to learn for the joy of learning.*

Often because adult perspectives are at the forefront of policy and structural decisions in high schools, there is a mismatch between what is being implemented and how the needs of the actual students are being met. Expressing both consciousness that the popular image of students is that they do not want to learn in schools and a critique that the school is not focused on learning, one student wrote: *I can't stress enough that we want to learn, but the focus at our school is not on knowledge nearly as much as it is on letter grades.* Students feel and resist the intense focus on measurement and outcomes at the expense of learning and knowledge: *I hate school because I love learning. All they ever want is work. They don't care if you learn…Just get good grades and make the school look good.* These perspectives on the purpose of going to school and the kinds of work that students experience are expressed often within students' responses to this question on the survey.

When students feel that they are being taken seriously and are included in conversations where they are viewed as knowledgeable stakeholders in their school, they feel empowered (Hudson-Ross, Cleary, & Casey, 1993). This empowerment can be achieved by listening and responding to what students have to share about their high school experiences. For example, a school could begin by looking at an actual open-response statement such as: *I find that some of my teachers do the same exact thing every day. This makes class very boring. School needs to be more interesting.* This could begin school conversations about what makes school "boring" and what would make school more "interesting" to students. The school could then look at the overall results from the question about how often in the last school year students have "made a class presentation" or "discussed questions in class that have no clear answers." Schools could also examine the pedagogy questions regarding what kinds of work excite and/or engage students. Data from both the multiple-option and open-response questions provide opportunities for schools to begin an examination of what engaged learning means to students and what students are looking for in their school experience. The data open up the possibility for transformation and genuine improvement of teaching, learning, and school culture.

Strengthening Student Engagement: The Importance of Context

Student engagement in school work and learning is often viewed as a psychological or behavioral issue (Fredricks et al., 2004), with the responsibility for engagement resting solely on the individual student. However, research focused on student perspectives indicates that the school and the school community – including the people, programs, and practices – play important roles in engaging or disengaging students. For example, while school leaders often point to factors external to the school when identifying reasons why students disengage (Bridgeland, DiIulio, & Balfanz, 2009), dropout research finds that, from the student perspective, many of the factors that lead students to disengage from school, either temporarily or permanently, are within the purview of the school leader (Bridgeland et al., 2006).

The placement of responsibility for engagement on individual students has limited the opportunities for understanding and strengthening student engagement, in large part by focusing on student behaviors separate and apart from student experience or school factors. While narrowing the focus creates a manageable body of data, many school-based variables associated with engagement – such as the structural and regulatory environment of the school (Finn & Voelkl, 1993), the role of teachers (Reeve, Jang, Carrell, Jeon, & Barch, 2004), and the interaction among school people, structures, and relationships (Johnson et al., 2001) – tend to be overlooked.

Schools address student engagement, and use data from the HSSSE, in a variety of ways based on their purpose, needs, and context (Yazzie-Mintz, 2010). For example, the Chesterfield County Public Schools is a high-achieving district in Virginia (a "banner district" in the state) that has recently incorporated student engagement and HSSSE into their 6-year strategic plan for improvement. The district asserts a connection between engaging students and improving achievement, identifying students who are struggling academically to provide support and working to make students feel part of more individualized learning environments. One of the high schools in the district, James River High School, has been particularly aggressive about using their HSSSE data. The staff, through analysis of their data, identified two specific issues: (1) providing individual support to students who were struggling academically and (2) reaching out to make stronger connections with students of color, who were a minority in the school and were thought to be largely disengaged. The school, rather than put the responsibility on the students to address these issues of engagement, put into place a set of mentoring and remediation programs built on the idea that relationships and academics work together. The results are that students previously struggling at James River are now getting back to the level of their original classes, and, on the HSSSE survey, students are reporting greater levels of engagement and connection to the school community.

At Yorkville High School in Illinois, high graduation and college-going rates masked some internal signs of academic concern for the school – in particular, course failure rates among ninth graders and stagnant ACT scores. The principal, familiar with HSSSE from another high school, decided to investigate student engagement within the school, though it was entirely unclear to him what they would discover from the data relative to the academic issues they were facing. Getting students' perspectives about their experiences from the HSSSE survey – including their beliefs about support, challenge, priorities, and structures – led to a shift in thinking at Yorkville. As is the case within many high schools, adult needs drove policy and structure decisions at Yorkville: scheduling, space, professional development, and discipline. For example, scheduling decisions – including whether or not to move to some form of block scheduling – were driven by issues of space availability, growth in the district, and research on the connection between time and achievement. However, what was not accounted for was how the students experienced the outcomes of these decisions. In fact, what worked structurally for the adults was actually disengaging for the students.

The principal, as a result of analysis of HSSSE data, now asserts that "engagement will drive structures." Yorkville is moving to a process of decision-making that includes the perspectives of students, transitioning from a philosophy of "If we teach it, they will learn it" to a process of asking questions such as: "Are the students learning it?" "How are we teaching it?" "How are students experiencing what we are teaching?" Yorkville, in exploring academic issues, has decided that engagement is the area where they will focus their most intense efforts; they have discovered that strengthening student engagement is their path to making a school with high graduation rates into a school where students are engaged in learning all the way through and in which the students are participating members of the school community in both words and actuality.

A rough sketch of a continuum can be drawn, in which schools are situated based on how they use student viewpoints, from not listening to students, to listening but not taking action, to listening and taking action to change and improve schools. "Tech High School" has solicited students' perspectives but is not yet at the point to believe students enough to analyze the data and take action. Both James River High School and Yorkville High School have moved across the continuum to a place where they are listening to students and taking action, and seeing the resulting positive changes.

Finding the Humanity in the Data

Listening to students about their schooling experiences is not a new concept, just an infrequently invoked one. The importance of student data in investigating and evaluating schooling is, in fact, a cornerstone of research, policy, and practice today. However, the kinds of data that researchers, policymakers, and school administrators are interested in for analysis and evaluation represent a very narrow band of the student experience in school.

The current input–output model of schooling – largely analogous to assembly line production in which materials and parts are assembled to produce identical products over and over again – puts the focus on only those factors that are directly associated with a countable output measure of achievement (standardized test scores, graduation rates, etc.). What about the processes, interactions, and relationships that are important parts of students' schooling experiences as students move from being "inputs" to "outputs"? What about the consideration of other measures of achievement, success, and output? What about the differential ways in which students experience schooling? Unlike the assembly line, identical schooling processes can create very different products, given the human factor: students experience the same processes differently, adults do not mechanically teach and interact with every student in exactly the same way, and engagement is a complex process that does not happen the same way every time and with every person. Contrary to much popular criticism of schooling today, this is a good thing.

The input-output model attempts to create identical products quantitatively described: that is, students who have achieved a certain score on a standardized test or set of tests, students who have achieved an agreed-upon number of course credits, and/or students who have acquired a particular grade point average. The data required to measure these types of achievement do not provide information on how much students have learned or the kinds of learning they have done, the depth with which students have engaged in their learning, the causes of or processes by which students have come to reach or not reach particular levels of achievement, or what adults might do differently to help students learn more, achieve greater, or experience school in a more engaged way. Though these data are used to declare whether or not a student is academically ready to leave one level of schooling and move to the next, these data do not provide any indication of what the student is actually taking – cognitively, intellectually, substantively, or in terms of work habits and processes – to the next stage of schooling or work.

One of the critiques of student perception data, raised often in the form of a question, is: *Can we really trust the students?* In truth, researchers, policymakers, and administrators trust students all the time – as long as the data come from a standardized test, a transcript, or another "verifiable" quantitative measure. When the data exist in the form of student perceptions or student perspectives, even if the instrument or method used to gather the data is "valid" and "reliable," adults do not often trust what students say. Why do adults trust student performance on assessments but not their perspectives on their own school experiences? In fact, understanding student perspectives on their school experiences can lead to changes in school processes (including teaching and learning) that may ultimately have a positive effect on the holy grail of success in today's schooling context: quantifiably measured student achievement.

The data that are given primacy in the current policy and evaluation context have three basic characteristics: the data are quantitative, the data are standardized across populations, and the data describe only a very narrow slice of students' schooling experiences. And students know this. The student quoted at the beginning of this chapter echoes the views of many other students: *I feel the only thing they care about are scores on standardized tests, not us students as individuals.* In a system guided by a policy titled *No Child Left Behind*, a phrase focused on individual students, these students are pointing out a serious contradiction at the root of the system.

This chapter argues for finding the humanity in the data, focusing on who the students are who constitute the quantitative data that dominate the policy and popular conversation around schooling in the USA today. While quantifiable data (including data on student engagement) describe a particular slice of the student experience, we argue for understanding and investigating student engagement and disengagement as a function of the perceptions of students about their experiences in the learning environment. Student perspectives provide a different view of schools from what other data show, and a variety of types of data on student perspectives – including traditional multiple-option survey questions and open-response questions – deepen our understanding of the student experience. As Yorkville High School came to realize, the key question was not just focused on whether teachers were teaching the content, but whether the students were learning the content and how the students were experiencing the instruction; the way to collect data on these questions is to target the students as research participants.

Finding the humanity in the data presents challenges for research, policy, and practice. The challenges for research include expanding the definitions and understandings of student engagement, moving beyond traditional indicators and measures of engagement (including time on task, internal motivation, and attendance/truancy), and investigating student engagement from the perspective of students themselves. The current model of research that narrowly draws a direct line from input to output needs to be altered and expanded. For example, lower attendance in school is associated with low student engagement and low student achievement (Morse, Anderson, Christenson, & Lehr, 2004; Willms, 2003). By logic and analysis, data indicate that an important intervention will be one that gets students to attend school more frequently; however, if the *only* goal is to get students into school, then the effect of the intervention may be marginal at best. Finding the humanity in the data involves digging deeper into the data: finding out from students what causes them to attend school infrequently if at all, addressing those factors through school-based programs and relationships, examining and improving in-school factors that may lead to low student attendance, and following up to see if the inputs (attendance) have been accompanied by strengthening of the school factors and processes. Focusing solely on the direct line from input to output may create higher student attendance but no greater engagement or achievement.

The challenges for policy are related to those for research. Policy creation and implementation is designed to create structures and directives that accomplish specified goals. Student engagement, though, as we argued earlier, is a cultural aspect of schools, rather than an issue that can be adequately addressed solely through policy or structures. For example, raising high school graduation rates and lowering dropout rates have been dominant issues in education policy in recent years. Policymakers and implementers have most frequently attempted to deal with this problem through structures and directives: punishment for dropouts (such as preventing dropouts from obtaining driver licenses), programs (such as credit recovery, alternative paths to attaining a high school diploma, or reducing the number of credits needed to graduate), and new organizations of schooling (early college and dual high school/college credit programs). While implementation of these policies may have the effect of getting some more students to graduate, thus accomplishing the paired goals of raising graduation rates and lowering dropout rates, by and large, they do not take into account or address the reasons that students opt to disengage from school in the first place; they attempt to change an outcome rather than address what is often a very individual – and human – decision on the part of students. Finding the humanity in the data means that policy will need to understand why students disengage and focus on the culture of engagement instead of creating policies and structures designed merely to drag students across the high school graduation line. Addressing students' reasons for disengagement, including relevance, interest, challenge, and instructional method – and the processes by which students disengage – is likely to have a greater impact on the graduation/dropout problem than any isolated policy or structure.

The challenges for practice are illuminated by the varying degrees of effort and success of the three high schools highlighted in this chapter – "Tech High School," Yorkville High School, and James River High School – in hearing, understanding, and acting on students' perspectives as part of school improvement initiatives. Whether by design or evolution, schools have been created largely as a culture of adult needs: adult expertise, adult schedules, adult structures and programs.

The greatest shift for schools to make in finding the humanity in the data is to view schools through the culture and perspectives of students. Yorkville High School, for example, as a result of focusing on engagement and data in this way, has shifted the foundation and purpose of their work. A productive way of understanding the challenges for practice of finding the humanity in the data is to view schools as sitting along a continuum of the ways in which they look for and incorporate student perspectives into the work of the school, from fully adult-focused on one end, to listening to students but not taking action in the middle, to listening to students and acting on student perspectives on the other end.

What is the *truth* about the student experience? Ultimately, data from the HSSSE– both the multiple-option questions and the open responses – indicate that students want to be interacted with, challenged, cared for, and valued. The challenge for us adults – researchers, policymakers and policy implementers, teachers, administrators, youth-serving workers – is to create learning environments in which students experience exactly those four things. That will provide the foundation for engagement and point the way toward all types of stronger outcome measures. The first step is to look for and find the humanity in the data.

References

Appleton, J. A., Christenson, S. L., & Furlong, M. J. (2008). Student engagement with school: Critical conceptual and methodological issues of the construct. *Psychology in the Schools, 45*(5), 369–386.

Appleton, J. A., Christenson, S. L., Kim, D., & Reschly, A. L. (2006). Measuring cognitive and psychological engagement: Validation of the Student Engagement Instrument. *Journal of School Psychology, 44*, 427–445.

Attard, C. (2009, November). *Student perspectives of mathematics teaching and learning in the upper primary classroom.* Paper presented at the annual meeting of the International Conference on Science and Mathematics Education, Penang, Malaysia.

Attard, C. (2010, July). *Students' experiences of mathematics during the transition from primary to secondary school.* Paper presented at the annual meeting of the Mathematics Education Research Group of Australasia, Fremantle, Western Australia.

Bridgeland, J. M., DiIulio, J. J., Jr., & Balfanz, R. (2009). *On the frontlines of schools: Perspectives of teachers and principals on the high school dropout problem.* Washington, DC: Civic Enterprises.

Bridgeland, J. M., DiIulio, J. J., Jr., & Morison, K. B. (2006). *The silent epidemic: Perspectives of high school dropouts.* Washington, DC: Civic Enterprises.

Cohen, J., McCabe, M. E., Michelli, N. M., & Pickeral, T. (2009). School climate: Research, policy, practice, and teacher education. *Teachers College Record, 111*(1), 180–213.

Cook-Sather, A., & Shultz, J. (2001). Starting where the learner is: Listening to students. In J. Shultz & A. Cook-Sather (Eds.), *In our own words: Students' perspectives on school* (pp. 1–17). Lanham, MD: Rowman & Littlefield.

Cook-Sather, A. (2002). Authorizing students' perspectives: Toward trust, dialogue, and changes in education. *Educational Researcher, 31*(4), 3–14.

DeCharms, R. (1968). *Personal causation: The internal affective determinants of behavior.* New York: Academic Press.

Finn, J. D. (1989). Withdrawing from school. *Review of Educational Research, 59*(2), 117–142.

Finn, J. D. (1993). *School engagement and students at risk.* Washington, DC: National Center for Educational Statistics, U.S. Department of Education (NCES 93 470).

Finn, J. D., & Voelkl, K. E. (1993). Social characteristics related to school engagement. *The Journal of Negro Education, 62*, 249–268.

Fredricks, J. A., Blumenfeld, P. C., & Paris, A. H. (2004). School engagement: Potential of the concept, state of the evidence. *Review of Educational Research, 74*(1), 59–109.

Furrer, C., & Skinner, E. (2003). Sense of relatedness as a factor in children's academic engagement and performance. *Journal of Educational Psychology, 95*(1), 148–162.

Geertz, C. (1973). *Thick description: Toward an interpretive theory of culture.* New York: Basic Books.

Gottfried, A. E., Fleming, J. S., & Gottfried, A. W. (1994). Role of parental motivational practices in children's academic intrinsic motivation and achievement. *Journal of Educational Psychology, 86*, 104–113.

Gottfried, A. E., & Gottfried, A. W. (1996). A longitudinal study of academic intrinsic motivation in intellectually gifted children: Childhood through early adolescence. *Gifted Child Quarterly, 40*, 179–183.

Harter, S. (1992). The relationship between perceived competence, affect, and motivational orientation within the classroom: Process and patterns of change. In A. Boggiano & T. Pittman (Eds.), *Achievement and motivation: A social-developmental perspective* (pp. 77–114). New York: Cambridge University Press.

Harter, S., & Jackson, B. K. (1992). Trait vs. nontrait conceptualizations of intrinsic/extrinsic motivational orientation. *Motivation and Emotion, 16*, 209–230.

Hudson-Ross, S., Cleary, L. M., & Casey, M. (Eds.). (1993). *Children's voices: Children talk about literacy.* Portsmouth, NH: Heinemann.

Jimerson, S. R., Campos, E., & Greif, J. L. (2003). Toward an understanding of definitions and measures of school engagement and related terms. *California School Psychologist, 8*, 7–27.

Johnson, M. K., Crosnoe, R., & Elder, G. H. (2001). Students' attachment and engagement: The role of race and ethnicity. *Sociology of Education, 74*, 318–340.

Johnson, M. S., & Dean, M. (2011). *Student engagement and International Baccalaureate: Measuring the social, emotional, and academic engagement of IB students*. Paper presented at the annual meeting of the American Educational Research Association. New Orleans, LA.

Jordan, W., & Nettles, S. (1999). *How students invest their time out of school: Effects on school engagement, perceptions of life chances, and achievement* (Report No. 29). Baltimore, MD: Center for Research on the Education of Students Placed At Risk (ERIC Document Reproduction Service No. ED 428 174).

Klem, A. M., & Connell, J. P. (2004). Relationships matter: Linking teacher support to student engagement and achievement. *Journal of School Health, 74*(7), 262–273.

Kuh, G. (2003). *The National Survey of Student Engagement: Conceptual framework and overview of psychometric properties*. Bloomington, IN: Center for Postsecondary Research.

Lepper, M. R., Corpus, J. H., & Lyengar, S. S. (2005). Intrinsic and extrinsic motivational orientations in the classroom: Age differences and academic correlates. *Journal of Educational Psychology, 97*(2), 184–196.

Lepper, M. R., & Green, D. (1978). *The hidden costs of reward*. Hillsdale, NJ: Erlbaum.

Lepper, M. R., Sethi, S., Dialdin, D., & Drake, M. (1997). Intrinsic and extrinsic motivation: A developmental perspective. In S. S. Luthar, J. A. Burack, D. Cicchetti, & J. R. Weisz (Eds.), *Developmental psychopathology: Perspectives on adjustment, risk, and disorder* (pp. 23–50). New York: Cambridge University Press.

Linnenbrink, E. A., & Pintrich, P. R. (2003). The role of self-efficacy beliefs in student engagement and learning in the classroom. *Reading and Writing Quarterly: Overcoming Learning Difficulties, 19*, 119–137.

Mant, J., Wilson, H., & Coates, D. (2007, July). The effect of increasing conceptual challenge in primary science lessons on pupils' achievement and engagement. *International Journal of Science Education, 29*(14), 1707–1719.

Marks, H. M. (2000). Student engagement in instructional activity: Patterns in the elementary, middle, and high school years. *American Educational Research Journal, 37*(1), 153–184.

Morse, A. B., Anderson, A. R., Christenson, S. L., & Lehr, C. A. (2004, February). Promoting school completion. *Principal Leadership Magazine, 4*(5), 9–13.

Munns, G., & Woodward, H. (2006). Student engagement and student self-assessment: The REAL framework. *Assessment in Education: Principles, Policy and Practice, 13*(2), 193–213.

Newmann, F. M., Wehlage, G. G., & Lamborn, S. D. (1992). The significance and sources of student engagement. In F. M. Newmann (Ed.), *Student engagement and achievement in American secondary schools* (pp. 11–39). New York: Teachers College Press.

Reeve, J., Jang, H., Carrell, D., Jeon, S., & Barch, J. (2004). Enhancing student's engagement by increasing teacher's autonomy support. *Motivation and Emotion, 28*(2), 147–169.

Senge, P. M. (2000). Systems change in education. *Reflections, 1*(3), 52–60.

Shernoff, D. J., Csikszentmihalyi, M., Schneider, B., & Shernoff, E. S. (2003). Student engagement in high school classrooms from the perspective of flow theory. *School Psychology Quarterly, 18*(2), 158–176.

Skinner, E. A., Wellborn, J. G., & Connell, J. P. (1990). What it takes to do well in school and whether I've got it: A process model of perceived control and children's engagement and achievement in school. *Journal of Educational Psychology, 82*(1), 22–32.

Stillwell, R. (2010). *Public school graduates and dropouts from the common core of data: School year 2007–08* (NCES 2010–341). Washington, DC: National Center for Education Statistics, Institute of Education Sciences, U.S. Department of Education. Retrieved June 4, 2010, from http://nces.ed.gov/pubsearch/pubsinfo.asp?pubid=2010341

Sum, A., Khatiwada, I., McLaughlin, J., with Palma, S. (2009). *The consequences of dropping out of high school: Joblessness and jailing for high school dropouts and the high cost for taxpayers*. Boston, MA: Center for Labor Market Studies, Northeastern University.

Waller, W. (1932). *The sociology of teaching*. New York: Russell & Russell.

Willms, J. D. (2003). *Student engagement at school: A sense of belonging and participation*. Paris, France: Organisation for Economic Co-Operation and Development.

Yazzie-Mintz, E. (2007). *Voices of students on engagement: A report on the 2006 High School Survey of Student Engagement*. Bloomington, IN: Center for Evaluation & Education Policy.

Yazzie-Mintz, E. (2009). *Engaging the voices of students: A report on the 2007 & 2008 High School Survey of Student Engagement*. Bloomington, IN: Center for Evaluation & Education Policy.

Yazzie-Mintz, E. (2010). *Charting the path from engagement to achievement: A report on the 2009 High School Survey of Student Engagement*. Bloomington, IN: Center for Evaluation & Education Policy.

The Measurement of Student Engagement: A Comparative Analysis of Various Methods and Student Self-report Instruments

Jennifer A. Fredricks and Wendy McColskey

Abstract

One of the challenges with research on student engagement is the large variation in the measurement of this construct, which has made it challenging to compare findings across studies. This chapter contributes to our understanding of the measurement of student in engagement in three ways. First, we describe strengths and limitations of different methods for assessing student engagement (i.e., self-report measures, experience sampling techniques, teacher ratings, interviews, and observations). Second, we compare and contrast 11 self-report survey measures of student engagement that have been used in prior research. Across these 11 measures, we describe what is measured (scale name and items), use of measure, samples, and the extent of reliability and validity information available on each measure. Finally, we outline limitations with current approaches to measurement and promising future directions.

Researchers, educators, and policymakers are increasingly focused on student engagement as the key to addressing problems of low achievement, high levels of student boredom, alienation, and high dropout rates (Fredricks, Blumenfeld, & Paris, 2004). Students become more disengaged as they progress from elementary to middle school, with some estimates that 25–40% of youth are showing signs of disengagement (i.e., uninvolved, apathetic, not trying very hard, and not paying attention) (Steinberg, Brown, & Dornbush, 1996; Yazzie-Mintz, 2007). The consequences of disengagement for middle and high school youth from disadvantaged backgrounds are especially severe; these youth are less likely to graduate from high school and face limited employment prospects, increasing their risk for poverty, poorer health, and involvement in the criminal justice system (National Research Council and the Institute of Medicine, 2004).

Although there is growing interest in student engagement, there has been considerable variation in how this construct has been conceptualized over time (Appleton, Christenson, & Furlong, 2008; Fredricks et al., 2004; Jimerson, Campos, & Grief, 2003). Scholars have used a broad range

J.A. Fredricks, Ph.D.(✉)
Human Development, Connecticut College,
New London, CT, USA
e-mail: jfred@conncoll.edu

W. McColskey, Ph.D.
SERVE Center, University of North Carolina,
Greensboro, NC, USA
e-mail: wmccolsk@serve.org

of terms including student engagement, school engagement, student engagement in school, academic engagement, engagement in class, and engagement in schoolwork. In addition, there has been variation in the number of subcomponents of engagement including different conceptualizations. Some scholars have proposed a two-dimensional model of engagement which includes behavior (e.g., participation, effort, and positive conduct) and emotion (e.g., interest, belonging, value, and positive emotions) (Finn, 1989; Marks, 2000; Skinner, Kindermann, & Furrer, 2009b). More recently, others have outlined a three-component model of engagement that includes behavior, emotion, and a cognitive dimension (i.e., self-regulation, investment in learning, and strategy use) (e.g., Archaumbault, 2009; Fredricks et al., 2004; Jimerson et al., 2003; Wigfield et al., 2008). Finally, Christenson and her colleagues (Appleton, Christenson, Kim, & Reschly, 2006; Reschly & Christenson, 2006) conceptualized engagement as having four dimensions: academic, behavioral, cognitive, and psychological (subsequently referred to as affective) engagement. In this model, aspects of behavior are separated into two different components: academics, which includes time on task, credits earned, and homework completion, and behavior, which includes attendance, class participation, and extracurricular participation. One commonality across the myriad of conceptualizations is that engagement is multidimensional. However, further theoretical and empirical work is needed to determine the extent to which these different dimensions are unique constructs and whether a three or four component model more accurately describes the construct of student engagement.

Even when scholars have similar conceptualizations of engagement, there has been considerable variability in the content of items used in instruments. This has made it challenging to compare findings from different studies. This chapter expands on our understanding of the measurement of student engagement in three ways. First, the strengths and limitations of different methods for assessing student engagement are described. Second, 11 self-report survey measures of student engagement that have been used in prior research are compared and contrasted on several dimensions (i.e., what is measured, purposes and uses, samples, and psychometric properties). Finally, we discuss limitations with current approaches to measurement.

What is Student Engagement

We define student engagement as a meta-construct that includes behavioral, emotional, and cognitive engagement (Fredricks et al., 2004). Although there are large individual bodies of literature on behavioral (i.e., time on task), emotional (i.e., interest and value), and cognitive engagement (i.e., self-regulation and learning strategies), what makes engagement unique is its potential as a multidimensional or "meta"-construct that includes these three dimensions. Behavioral engagement draws on the idea of participation and includes involvement in academic, social, or extracurricular activities and is considered crucial for achieving positive academic outcomes and preventing dropping out (Connell & Wellborn, 1991; Finn, 1989). Other scholars define behavioral engagement in terms of positive conduct, such as following the rules, adhering to classroom norms, and the absence of disruptive behavior such as skipping school or getting into trouble (Finn, Pannozzo, & Voelkl, 1995; Finn & Rock, 1997). Emotional engagement focuses on the extent of positive (and negative) reactions to teachers, classmates, academics, or school. Others conceptualize emotional engagement as identification with the school, which includes belonging, or a feeling of being important to the school, and valuing, or an appreciation of success in school-related outcomes (Finn, 1989; Voelkl, 1997). Positive emotional engagement is presumed to create student ties to the institution and influence their willingness to do the work (Connell & Wellborn, 1991; Finn, 1989). Finally, cognitive engagement is defined as student's level of investment in learning. It includes being thoughtful, strategic, and willing to exert the necessary effort for comprehension of complex ideas or mastery of difficult skills (Corno & Mandinach, 1983; Fredricks et al., 2004; Meece, Blumenfeld, & Hoyle, 1988).

An important question is how engagement differs from motivation. Although the terms are used interchangeably by some, they are different and the distinctions between them are important. Motivation refers to the underlying reasons for a given behavior and can be conceptualized in terms of the direction, intensity, quality, and persistence of one's energies (Maehr & Meyer, 1997). A proliferation of motivational constructs (e.g., intrinsic motivation, goal theory, and expectancy-value models) have been developed to answer two broad questions "Can I do this task" and "Do I want to do this task and why?" (Eccles, Wigfield, & Schiefele, 1998). One commonality across these different motivational constructs is an emphasis on individual differences and underlying psychological processes. In contrast, engagement tends to be thought of in terms of action, or the behavioral, emotional, and cognitive manifestations of motivation (Skinner, Kindermann, Connell, & Wellborn, 2009a). An additional difference is that engagement reflects an individual's interaction with context (Fredricks et al., 2004; Russell, Ainsley, & Frydenberg, 2005). In other words, an individual is engaged in something (i.e., task, activity, and relationship), and their engagement cannot be separated from their environment. This means that engagement is malleable and is responsive to variations in the context that schools can target in interventions (Fredricks et al., 2004; Newmann, Wehlage, & Lamborn, 1992).

The self-system model of motivational development (Connell, 1990; Connell & Wellborn, 1991; Deci & Ryan, 1985) provides one theoretical model for studying motivation and engagement. This model is based on the assumption that individuals have three fundamental motivational needs: autonomy, competence, and relatedness. If schools provide children with opportunities to meet these three needs, students will be more engaged. Students' need for relatedness is more likely to occur in classrooms where teachers and peers create a caring and supportive environment; their need for autonomy is met when they feel like they have a choice and when they are motivated by internal rather than external factors; and their need for competence is met when they experience the classroom as optimal in structure and feel like they can achieve desired ends (Fredricks et al., 2004). In contrast, if students experience schools as uncaring, coercive, and unfair, they will become disengaged or disaffected (Skinner et al., 2009a, 2009b). This model assumes that motivation is a necessary but not sufficient precursor to engagement (Appleton et al., 2008; Connell & Wellborn, 1991).

Methods for Studying Engagement

Student Self-report

Self-report survey measures are the most common method for assessing student engagement. In this methodology, students are provided items reflecting various aspects of engagement and select the response that best describes them. The majority of these self-report engagement measures are general and not subject specific, though there are some examples of measures that assess engagement in a specific domain like math (Kong, Wong, & Lam, 2003) or reading (Wigfield et al., 2008). One of the arguments for using self-report methods is that it is critical to collect data on students' subjective perceptions, as opposed to just collecting objective data on behavioral indicators such as attendance or homework completion rates, which are already commonly collected by schools (Appleton et al., 2006; Garcia & Pintrich, 1996). Self-report methods are particularly useful for assessing emotional and cognitive engagement which are not directly observable and need to be inferred from behaviors. In fact, Appleton et al. (2006) argue that self-report methods should only be used to assess emotional and cognitive engagement because collecting data on these subtypes through other methods, such as observations and teacher rating scales, is highly inferential.

Self-report methods are widely used because they are often the most practical and easy to administer in classroom settings. They can be given to large and diverse samples of children at a relatively low cost, making it possible to gather data over several waves and compare results across schools. However, one concern with self-report measures is that students may not answer honestly under some conditions (e.g., if administered by their teacher with no anonymity provided), and thus, self-reports may not reflect their actual behaviors or strategy use (Appleton et al., 2006; Garcia & Pintrich, 1996). Furthermore, these measures generally contain items that are worded broadly (e.g., I work hard in school) rather than worded to reflect engagement in particular tasks and situations. For researchers interested in studying how much engagement varies as a function of contextual factors, the general items may not be appropriate.

Experience Sampling

Experience sampling (ESM) is another technique that has been used to assess student engagement in the classroom (Shernoff, Csikszentmihalyi, Schneider, & Shernoff, 2003; Shernoff & Schmidt, 2008; Uekawa, Borman, & Lee, 2007; Yair, 2000). ESM methods grew out of research on "flow," a high level of engagement where individuals are so deeply absorbed in a task that they lose awareness of time and space (Csikszentmihalyi, 1990). In this methodology, individuals carry electronic pagers or alarm watches for a set time period. In response to ESM signals, students fill out a self-report questionnaire with a series of questions about their location, activities, and cognitive and affective responses (see Hektner, Schmidt, & Csikszentmihalyi, 2007, for more description of ESM methods). This methodology allows researchers to collect detailed data on engagement in the moment rather than retrospectively (as with student self-report), which reduces problems with recall failure and the desire to answer in socially desirable ways (Hektner et al., 2007). This technique can be used to collect information on variations in engagement across time and situations. However, this methodology also has some limitations. ESM methods require a large time investment for respondents, and the success of the method depends largely on participants' ability and willingness to comply. In addition, engagement is a multifaceted construct and may not be adequately captured by the small number of items included in ESM studies.

Teacher Ratings of Students

Another method for assessing student engagement is teacher checklists or rating scales. Teacher ratings of individual students' engagement, when averaged across students in their classrooms, offer an alternative perspective on student engagement from that reported by the students themselves. Some teacher rating scales include items assessing both behavioral and emotional engagement (Skinner & Belmont, 1993), and others reflect a multidimensional model of engagement (i.e., behavioral, emotional, and cognitive) (Wigfield et al., 2008). Researchers have also developed teacher ratings of student participation as indicative of behavioral engagement (Finn, Folger, & Cox, 1991; Finn et al., 1995), and teacher ratings of adjustment to school, as indicative of engagement (Birch & Ladd, 1997; Buhs & Ladd, 2001). This methodology can be particularly useful for studies with younger children who have more difficulty completing self-report instruments due to the reading demands and limited literacy skills. Some studies have included both teacher ratings and students' self-reports of engagement in order to examine the correspondence between the two measurement techniques (Skinner, Marchand, Furrer, & Kindermann, 2008; Skinner et al., 2009b). These studies show a stronger correlation between teacher and student reports of behavioral engagement than teacher and student reports of emotional engagement. This finding is not surprising as behavioral indicators are directly observable. In contrast, emotional indicators need to be inferred from behavior, and it is possible that some students have learned to mask their emotions (Skinner et al., 2008).

Interviews

A few studies have used interview techniques to assess engagement in school (Blumenfeld et al., 2005; Conchas, 2001; Locke Davidson, 1996). Interviews fall on a continuum from structured and semistructured interviews with predesignated questions to interviews where participants are asked to tell their stories in more open-ended and unstructured ways (Turner & Meyer, 2000). One benefit of interview methods is they can provide insight into the reasons for variability in levels of engagement to help understand why some students do engage while others begin to withdraw from school. Interviews can provide a detailed descriptive account of how students construct meaning about their school experiences, which contextual factors are most salient, and how these experiences relate to engagement (Blumenfeld et al.). However, interviews are not without problems. The knowledge, skills, and biases of the interviewer can all impact on the quality, depth, and type of responses. There are also questions about the reliability (stability and consistency) and validity of interview findings (McCaslin & Good, 1996). Finally, concerns about social desirability are an issue with interview techniques.

Observations

Observational methods at both the individual and classroom level have also been used to measure engagement. At the individual level, observational measures have been developed to assess individual students' on and off task behavior as an indicator of academic engagement (Volpe, DiPerna, Hintze, & Shapiro, 2005). Academic engagement refers to a composite of academic behaviors such as reading aloud, writing, answering questions, participating in classroom tasks, and talking about academics (Greenwood, Horton, & Utley, 2002). These measures use a form of momentary time sampling, in which an observer records whether a predetermined category of behavior is present or absent for an individual student during a defined time interval (Salvia & Ysseldyke, 2004). In addition to use in research studies, these techniques have been used by school psychologists to screen individual children in both typical and special needs populations, especially those at risk for disengagement and academic failure (Shapiro, 2004).

One concern with these types of observations is that they can be time consuming to administer, and observers may need to collect data across various types of academic settings (i.e., group work, seatwork) to get an accurate picture of student behavior. There are also concerns about the reliability of observational methods without proper training. Finally, another potential problem with individual observational measures is they provide limited information on the quality of effort, participation, or thinking (Fredricks et al., 2004; Peterson, Swing, Su, & Wass, 1984). For example, Peterson and colleagues found that some students judged to be on-task by observers reported in subsequent interviews that they were not thinking about the material while being observed. In contrast, many of the students who appeared to be off-task reported actually being very highly cognitively engaged.

Rather than assessing engagement with pre-specified coding categories, other studies have used narrative and descriptive techniques to measure this construct. For example, Nystrand and colleagues (Gamoran & Nystrand, 1992; Nystrand & Gamoran, 1991; Nystrand, Wu, Gamaron, Zeiser, & Long, 2001) assessed the quality of instructional discourse in the classroom as an indicator of substantive engagement, defined as a sustained commitment to the content of schooling. In these studies, the frequency of high-level evaluation questions, authentic questions, and uptake (i.e., evidence that teachers incorporate students' answers into subsequent questions) was observed as indicative of substantive engagement. That is, these teacher behaviors were assumed to involve active student engagement. Furthermore, Helme and Clarke (2001) observed math classes for indicators of cognitive engagement such as self-monitoring, exchanging ideas, giving directions, and justifying answers. Finally, Lee and her colleagues used observational techniques to examine the quality of students' task engagement when involved in science activities (Lee & Anderson, 1993; Lee & Brophy, 1996). In these studies, they noted behaviors such as relating the task to prior knowledge, requesting clarification, and using analogies as measures of cognitive engagement.

The prime advantage of using observation techniques to study engagement is that they can provide detailed and descriptive accounts of the contextual factors occurring with higher or lower engagement levels. These descriptions enhance our understanding of unfolding processes within contexts. Observational methods also can be used to verify information about engagement collected from survey and interview techniques. The major disadvantages of observations are that they are labor intensive, and they usually involve only a small number of students and contexts. This raises concerns about the generalizability to other settings. Finally, the quality of descriptive observations depends heavily on the skills of the observer and on his or her ability to capture and make sense of what was observed (Turner & Meyer, 2000).

Comparison of Self-report Measures

In the next section, we describe survey measures that have been developed and used in prior research on student engagement and compare these surveys on several dimensions. This chapter builds on a literature review conducted to identify measures of student engagement available for use in the upper elementary through high school years (Fredricks & McColskey, 2010). We focus on student self-report measures because this is the most common method for assessing engagement and most likely to be of interest to researchers. As a first step toward identifying student engagement instruments, a literature search was conducted by members of the research team using terms that were broad enough to capture both subject-specific and general measures of student engagement. The search was restricted to studies published between 1979 (which was selected to predate the earliest emergence of engagement studies in the early 1980s) and May 2009 and resulted in 1,314 citations.

The research team systematically reviewed the 1,314 citations to identify named instruments used to measure student engagement. A total of 156 instruments were identified from the citations. From this initial list of 156 instruments, we excluded measures for a variety of reasons including (1) developed and used only with college age samples, (2) used only with special education populations, (3) measured a construct other than engagement (e.g., school bonding, attitudes toward school), (4) based on items from a larger national dataset [e.g., National Education Longitudinal Study (NELS), National Survey of American's Families (NSAF)], (5) did not have enough published information on the measure, (6) adapted from other instruments already included in the list, or (7) developed for use in nonacademic subject areas (e.g., physical education). This resulted in a total of 21 measures (14 self-report, 3 teacher report, and 4 observation methods) which had been used with upper elementary to high school years.

By way of describing the substantial variation that exists across engagement measures, in this chapter, we describe 11 of these self-report measures. The 11 self-report measures in this chapter are for illustrative purposes and should not be considered an exhaustive list but rather are included to show the types of self-report instruments available. We compared these 11 self-report surveys on several dimensions including: definition of engagement, usage, samples, and psychometric information. The self-report measures ranged in length from a 4-item scale [School Engagement Scale Questionnaire (SEQ)] to the High School Survey of Student Engagement (HSSSE), a broad 121-item questionnaire. In some cases, the engagement items are a subset of a longer self-report instrument that assesses constructs other than student engagement.

Table 37.1 lists the names of the 11 self-report measures and the availability of the measure (i.e., journal article, website, and contact person). Eight measures are either available in a published source, can be accessed online, or are available by contacting the developer. Three of the instruments have commercially available services for purchase (School Success Profile [SSP], High School Survey of Student Engagement [HSSSE], and the Motivation and Engagement in Schools Scale [MES]). This cost covers questionnaire materials, administration of surveys, data preparation, individual and school reports, and other technical assistance related to the use of the information.

What Is Measured

Table 37.2 lists the student self-report measures, the subscales/domains measured, and sample items for each of the subscales. Some of these survey instruments were explicitly designed to

Table 37.1 Overview of 11 instruments

Instrument name	Availability
Attitudes Toward Mathematics Survey (ATM)	Miller, Greene, Montalvo, Ravindran, and Nichols (1996)
Engagement vs. Disaffection with Learning – Student Report (EvsD)	Skinner, Kindermann, and Furrer (2009b) or www.pdx.edu/psy/ellen-skinner-1
High School Survey of Student Engagement (HSSSE)	www.indiana.edu/~ceep/hssse/
Identification with School Questionnaire (ISQ)	Voelkl (1996)
Motivated Strategies for Learning Questionnaire (MSLQ)	Pintrich and DeGroot (1990)
Motivation and Engagement Scale (MES)	www.lifelongachievement.com
Research Assessment Package for Schools (RAPS)	irre.org/sites/default/files/publication_pdfs/RAPS_manual_entire_1998.pdf
School Engagement Measure (SEM) – MacArthur	Fredricks, Blumenfeld, Friedel, and Paris (2005)
School Engagement Scale/Questionnaire (SEQ)	Available by contacting Dr. Steinberg at Temple University
School Success Profile (SSP)	www.schoolsuccessprofile.org
Student Engagement Instrument (SEI)	Appleton et al. (2006)

assess engagement, while other measures were designed to assess constructs such as identification with school, motivation, and self-regulation and strategy use, but have been used in subsequent studies as measures of engagement. For example, the Motivated Strategies for Learning Questionnaire (MSLQ) was initially designed to measure self-regulation and strategy use but has been used in some studies as an indicator of cognitive engagement (Pintrich & DeGroot, 1990). Similarly, the Identification with School questionnaire has been used in some studies as a measure of student identification with school and in other studies as a measure of emotional engagement.

There are a variety of ways to compare these measures. First, the surveys differ in terms of whether they focus on general engagement or subject- or class-specific engagement. Seven of the measures have items worded to reflect general engagement in school, while 4 of the self-report instruments are worded for use at the class level, in particular classes, or in particular skill areas [Attitudes Toward Math (ATM), Engagement vs. Disaffection with Learning (EvsD), Motivated Strategies for Learning Questionnaire (MSLQ), and School Engagement Questionnaire (SEQ)]. The self-report measures also differ in whether and how they conceptualize disengagement. Some of the measures include subscales that assess the opposite of engagement, which has been referred to as disengagement, disaffection, and alienation (Skinner et al., 2009a, 2009b). For example, three instruments have subscales measuring the extent of negative engagement (disengagement in the MES, trouble avoidance in the SSP, and behavioral disaffection and emotional disaffection in Engagement vs. Disaffection with Learning). Other measures imply that negative engagement is simply a low engagement score indicating a lack of engagement (Appleton et al., 2006). Finally, some of the measures blur the lines between engagement and contextual precursors (e.g., quality of students' social relationships). For example, the three Student Engagement Instrument (SEI) "psychological engagement" subscales include items about students' relationships with teachers and peers and support for learning from families that are not direct measures of engagement but indirect measures. Other self-report measures include separate scales for the aspects of classroom or school context that are assumed to influence or be related to engagement (e.g., Research Assessment Package for Schools).

Another way to compare the self-report survey measures is in terms of the extent to which they represent the multidimensional nature of engagement. Table 37.3 shows the various self-report measures in terms of whether they reflect behavioral, emotional, or cognitive aspects of engagement. In addition to differences in scale names used by developers (see Tables 37.2 and 37.4), there were differences in how the developers aligned similar items within the behavioral, emotional, and cognitive engagement constructs. For example, class participation was used as an indicator of both behavioral and cognitive engagement, and students' valuing of school was used as an indicator of both emotional and cognitive engagement. Below we describe the subscales and items found across the 11 instruments by behavioral, emotional, and cognitive engagement.

Table 37.2 Self-report subscales with sample items

Name of measure	Subscales	Sample items
Attitudes Toward Mathematics Survey (ATM)	Self-regulation (12 items)	"Before a quiz or exam, I plan out how to study the material"
	Deep cognitive strategy use (9 items)	"I work several examples of the same type of problem when studying mathematics so I can understand the problems better"
	Shallow cognitive strategy use (5 items)	"I find reviewing previously solved problems to be a good way to study for a test"
	Persistence (9 items)	"If I have trouble understanding a problem, I go over it again until I understand it"
Engagement vs. Disaffection with Learning (EvsD)	Behavioral engagement (5 items)	"When I am in class, I listen very carefully"
	Behavioral disaffection (5 items)	"When I am in class, I just act like I am working"
	Emotional engagement (5 items)	"I enjoy learning new things in class"
	Emotional disaffection (7 items)	"When we work on something in class, I feel discouraged"
High School Survey of Student Engagement (HSSSE)	Cognitive/intellectual/academic engagement (65 items)	Thinking about this school year, how often have you done each of the following? (A) Asked questions in class; (B) contributed to class discussions; (C) made a class presentation; (D) prepared a draft of a paper or assignment before turning it in; (E) received prompt feedback from teachers on assignments or other class work
	Social/behavioral/participatory engagement (17 items)	Thinking about this school year, how often have you done each of the following? (a) had conversations or worked on a project with at least one student of a race or ethnicity different from your own; (b) picked on or bullied another student
	Emotional engagement (39 items)	How do you feel about the following statements related to your high school? Overall, (a) I feel good about being in this school; (b) I care about this school; (c) I feel safe in this school; (d) I have a voice in classroom and/or school decisions
Identification with School Questionnaire (ISQ)	Belongingness (9 items)	"School is one of my favorite places to be"
	Valuing of school (7 items)	"Most of the things we learn in class are useless"
Motivated Strategy and Learning Use Questionnaire (MSLQ)	Self-regulation (9 items)	"I outline the chapters in my book to help me study"
	Cognitive strategy use (13 items)	"I ask myself questions to make sure I know the material that I have been studying"
Motivation and Engagement Scale (MES)	Self-belief (4 items)	"If I try hard I believe I can do my schoolwork well"
	Learning focus (4 items)	"I feel very happy with myself when I really understand what I am taught at school"
	Valuing school (4 items)	"Learning at school is important"
	Persistence (4 items)	"If I cannot understand my schoolwork, I keep trying until I do"
	Planning (4 items)	"Before I start a project, I plan out how I am going to do it"
	Study management (4 items)	"When I do homework, I usually do it where I can concentrate best"
	Disengagement (4 items)	"I have given up being interested in school"
	Self-sabotage (4 items)	"Sometimes I do not try at school so I can have reason if I do not do well"
	Failure avoidance (4 items)	"The main reason I try at school is because I do not want to disappoint my parents"
	Anxiety (4 items)	"When I have a project to do, I worry a lot about it"
	Uncertain control (4 items)	"When I do not do well at school, I do not know how to stop that happening next time"

(continued)

Table 37.2 (continued)

Name of measure	Subscales	Sample items
Research Assessment Package for Schools (RAPS)	Ongoing engagement (5 items) Reaction to challenge (6 items)	"I work hard on my schoolwork" "When something bad happens to me in school, I say the teacher did not cover the things on the test"
School Engagement Measure (SEM)-MacArthur	Behavioral engagement (5 items) Emotional engagement (6 items) Cognitive engagement (8 items)	"I pay attention in class" "I am interested in the work at school" "When I read a book, I ask myself questions to make sure I understand what it is about"
School Engagement Scale/Questionnaire (SEQ)	School engagement scale (4 items in 3 subject areas)	"How much time do you put into homework each week, including reading assignments?"
School Success Profile (SSP)	School engagement (3 items) Trouble avoidance (11 items)	"I find school fun and exciting" "I turned in a homework assignment late or not at all"
Student Engagement Instrument (SEI)	Affective engagement: teacher-student relationships (9 items) Affective engagement: peer support for learning (6 items) Affective engagement: family support for learning (4 items) Cognitive engagement: control and relevance of schoolwork (9 items) Cognitive engagement: future aspirations and goals (5 items)	"Adults at my school listen to the students" "I have some friends at school" "My family/guardian(s) are there for me when I need them" "The tests in my classes do a good job of measuring what I am able to do" "I am hopeful about my future"

Table 37.3 Dimensions of engagement assessed by instruments

Instrument	Behavioral	Emotional	Cognitive
Multidimensional self-report instruments			
HSSSE	✓	✓	✓
MES	✓	✓	✓
SEM	✓	✓	✓
Bidimensional student self-report instruments			
ATM	✓	✓	✓
EvsD	✓	✓	
RAPS	✓	✓	
SSP	✓		
SEI		✓	✓
Unidimensional student self-report instruments			
ISQ	✓	✓	✓
MSLQ			
SEQ			

Behavioral Engagement

Eight measures have scales that seem to reflect (either by the subscale name or the sample items) aspects of behavioral engagement (see Tables 37.2, 37.3 and 37.4). Two of the behavioral subscales (behavioral disaffection and trouble avoidance) assess the extent of negative behavioral engagement (pretending to work, not turning in homework, and cutting class). A third subscale (disengagement subscale of the MES) includes items assessing both behavioral disengagement (e.g., each day I try less and less) and emotional disengagement (I have given up being interested in school). Across the various behavioral engagement scales/subscales, individual items ask students to report on their attention, attendance, time on homework, preparation for class, class participation, concentration, participation in school-based activities, effort, adherence to classroom rules, and risk behaviors.

Emotional Engagement

Eight subscales, either by subscale name or items, appear to reflect aspects of emotional engagement. Some subscales assess emotional reaction to class or school, while others assess the quality of students' relationships with peers and teachers as an indicator of emotional engagement. Two subscales (emotional disaffection and disengagement)

Table 37.4 Scales and subscales by each engagement dimension[a]

	Behavioral	Emotional	Cognitive
Instrument subscales/ subscale name	Behavioral disaffection Behavioral engagement[c] Disengagement Persistence[b, c] Social/behavioral/participatory engagement School Engagement Questionnaire Trouble avoidance	Anxiety Belonging Emotional engagement[c] Emotional disaffection Failure avoidance Affective engagement – family support for learning Affective engagement – peer support for learning Affective engagement – teacher-student relationships Reaction to challenge School engagement Self-belief Valuing[c] Uncertain control	Cognitive engagement[c] Cognitive/intellectual/academic Cognitive strategy use Deep cognitive strategy use Learning focus Control and relevance of schoolwork Future aspirations and goals Planning Self-regulation[c] Shallow cognitive strategy use Study management

[a] Disengagement could also be listed under the Emotional engagement column, as they contain items reflecting both
[b] Persistence is also considered an aspect of Cognitive engagement
[c] These subscale/scale names were used by more than one instrument

include items assessing the extent of negative emotions (discouragement when working on something, given up being interested in school). Overall, emotional engagement scales include questions about a myriad of topics related to emotional reactions to school such as being happy or anxious; expressing interest and enjoyment; reporting fun and excitement; reacting to failure and challenge; feeling safe; having supportive or positive relationships with teachers and peers; having family support for learning; expressing feelings of belonging; and perceiving school as valuable.

Cognitive Engagement Subscales

Six surveys include subscales measuring cognitive engagement, though there is large variation in how this is defined and measured. Cognitive engagement is used as a broad umbrella term for (1) beliefs about the importance or value of schooling, learning goals, and future aspirations; (2) cognitive strategy use (how deeply students study material); (3) self-regulatory or meta-cognitive strategies (how students manage the learning processes such as planning and seeking information); and (4) doing extra work and going beyond the requirements of school. These measures of cognitive engagement incorporate aspects of motivation, self-regulated learning, and strategy use.

Purposes and Uses

The measures included in this chapter were developed from a range of disciplinary perspectives and for a variety of purposes. A number of the measures were developed by psychologists studying motivation, cognition, and engagement. For example, one widely used measure, the Engagement versus Disaffection with Learning scale, was part of a larger instrument that was initially developed to test the self-system model of student engagement. According to this model, the relation between classroom context (i.e., structure, autonomy support, and involvement) and patterns of action (cognitive, behavioral, and emotional engagement) is mediated through self-system processes (competence, autonomy, and relatedness) (Connell, 1990; Connell & Wellborn, 1991). The Engagement versus Disaffection scale has been most recently used in research by Skinner and her colleagues (see Furrer & Skinner, 2003; Skinner et al., 2008, Skinner et al., 2009b, for examples). In 1998, Connell and others at the Institute for Research and Reform in

Education (www.irre.org) revised the original instruments to provide a shorter set of instruments (RAPS) for use in evaluating school reform efforts based on the same theoretical framework. Two of the survey measures identified in the review (Attitudes Toward Mathematics Survey [ATM] and the Motivated Strategies for Learning Questionnaire [MSLQ]) were developed as part of research exploring the relationships between students' self-regulation, cognitive strategy use, and achievement outcomes. Research in this area examines the use of cognitive, meta-cognitive, and self-regulatory strategies that foster active cognitive engagement in learning (Corno & Mandinach, 1983; Meece et al., 1988).

Other measures were developed by researchers studying the relationship between context and engagement. For example, the Student Engagement Measure (SEM) – MacArthur was developed for a longitudinal study of the relationship between classroom context and engagement in urban minority youth in the upper elementary grades (Fredricks et al., 2005). In addition, the School Engagement Scale/Questionnaire (SEQ) was developed as part of a large study in nine high schools that reported on ways that parents, peers, and communities influence students' commitment to, or engagement with, school (Steinberg et al., 1996). This scale has subsequently been used by researchers trying to understand factors that explain differences in vocational attitudes and career development behaviors among subgroups of high school students (Perry, 2008; Wettersten et al., 2005).

Increasing student engagement is the primary goal of many interventions to reduce dropout rates (Appleton et al., 2008; Finn, 1989). Two measures were developed in the context of this work on dropout prevention [Identification with School Questionnaire (ISQ) and Student Engagement Instrument (SEI)]. For example, the Student Engagement Instrument (SEI) was developed to measure affective (formerly psychological) and cognitive engagement and to expand on the behavioral and academic indicators that were collected as part of Check & Connect, an intervention model designed to improve student engagement at school, reduce dropouts, and increase school completion (Anderson, Christenson, Sinclair, & Lehr, 2004). The Student Engagement Instrument (SEI) is currently being used to evaluate the effectiveness of district initiatives to improve student engagement in the Gwinnett County Public Schools (*this volume*). The Identification with School questionnaire was developed to assess the extent to which students identify with or disengage from school, and was based on the theory that school identification is a crucial factor in the prevention of school dropouts (Finn, 1989).

Other measures have been developed to help schools and districts monitor engagement and to assist schools in identifying areas in need of improvement. For example, the High School Survey of Student Engagement (HSSSE) was developed to provide descriptive and comparative data on high school students' views about their schoolwork, the school learning environment, and interactions with the school community, relative to the responses of other schools (Yazzie-Mintz, 2007). Each school that participates receives a customized report that compares the students' responses to that of other schools. Similarly, the School Success Profile (SSP) was developed to provide insight into how students perceive themselves and their environments and to compare school scores relative to a national sample (Bowen, Rose, & Bowen, 2005).

Finally, one survey measure [the Motivation and Engagement Survey (MES)] was developed to diagnose and identify students who are struggling or at risk for disengagement and academic failure. The MES creates profiles for individual students based on responses to 11 different subscales reflecting a multidimensional model of motivation and engagement. This measure has been used to diagnose students with low motivation and engagement, in studies evaluating the effectiveness of interventions and in studies examining demographic differences in engagement and motivation (Fredricks & McColskey, 2010).

Samples

The surveys included in this chapter have been used with students from the upper elementary school years (third to fifth grades) through the

Table 37.5 Samples

Instrument name	Samples
Attitudes Toward Mathematics Survey (ATM)	Original sample 297 suburban, southeastern high school students in their math courses Versions of the cognitive engagement items also have been used with high school English students in a Midwestern high school and college-level samples (educational psychology students, preservice teachers, and students in statistics classes)
Engagement vs. Disaffection with Learning – Student Report (EvsD)	Sample of 1,018 elementary school students in grades 3–6 in suburban and rural schools The items have also been used with samples of elementary, middle, and high school White and low-income minority youth in urban and suburban districts
High School Survey of Student Engagement (HSSSE)	Original sample 7,200 students from four high schools Survey has been administered to 200,000 students from across the nation. Students are ethnically and economically diverse and attend rural, suburban, and urban schools
Identification with School Questionnaire (ISQ)	Original sample 539 eighth grade students from 163 schools in rural, urban, suburban, and inner-city settings (25% Black, 75% White) Survey has been used with racially diverse samples including Black, Hispanic, Asian, and American Indian students, and with low-income students in the middle and high school grades
Motivated Strategies for Learning Questionnaire (MSLQ)	Original sample 173 primarily White middle and working class seventh graders across 15 classrooms Survey has been used in both English- and non-English-speaking countries across the world
Motivation and Engagement Scale (MES)	The Junior High version normed with 1,249 students in Australia, aged 9–13, across 63 classes in 15 schools. The High School version normed with 21,579 students, aged 12–18, across 58 schools Samples were from urban, rural, and suburban areas of Australia, and predominately middle class students
Research Assessment Package for Schools (RAPS)	Large populations of Black, White, Hispanic, and low-income youth in urban districts engaged in comprehensive school reform
School Engagement Measure (SEM) – MacArthur	Original sample 641 urban, low-income, primarily Black and Hispanic students in grades 3 to 5 attending neighborhood schools Survey also used with other low-income ethnically diverse upper elementary school students
School Engagement Scale/Questionnaire (SEQ)	Original sample 12,000 ethnically and economically diverse students in nine high schools in Wisconsin and Northern California Items also used with racially diverse high school students in rural and urban areas in the Northeast and Midwest
School Success Profile (SSP)	Original sample 805 middle school students in 26 schools in North Carolina totaling approximately 805 students Survey also used with racially diverse and low-income students in middle and high schools
Student Engagement Instrument (SEI)	Original sample 1,931 ninth grade students from an ethnically diverse, majority low income, urban school district Survey also used with students in grades 6 through 12

high school years. Two of the measures were initially developed for use with upper elementary school populations [Engagement vs. Disaffection with Learning and MacArthur (SEM)]. On the other end of the spectrum, the Motivated Strategies for Learning Questionnaire (MSLQ) was originally developed for use with college samples, but a version was adapted for use with middle school students. In addition, the High School Survey of Student Engagement (HSSSE) was modeled after the National Survey of Student Engagement (NSSE), a widely used measure of student engagement at the college level.

Table 37.5 shows that the majority of measures have been used with ethnically and economically diverse samples. In addition, four of the measures have been translated into other languages [MSLQ, MacArthur measure, SSP, and SEI]. For example, the MSLQ has been translated into multiple languages and has been used in English-speaking and non-English-speaking countries all over the world (Garcia-Duncan & McKeachie, 2005). The SSP and the MacArthur measure have been translated into Spanish. Sections of the SSP have also been translated into Hebrew, Lithuanian, Romanian, and Portuguese (Fredricks & McColskey, 2010). Finally, the SEI has been translated into Portuguese and Mandarin (Moreira, Vaz, Dias, & Petracchi, 2009).

Psychometric Information

Technical information on reliability and validity was found on all but one self-report measure, though there were variations in the amount and types of technical information available (see Fredricks & McColskey, 2010, for more detailed information on psychometric properties). The one exception was the High School Survey of Student Engagement (HSSSE) which currently has no published information on the psychometric property of this measure. However, developers of this measure have indicated that a reliability and validity study is currently underway. They also make reference to the reliability and validity reported on the National Survey of School Engagement, a widely used measure of engagement at the college level, from which the HSSSE was adapted.

Reliability

Internal consistency is the extent to which individuals who respond in one way to items tend to respond the same way to other items intended to measure the same construct. A Cronbach's alpha of .70 or higher for a set of items is considered acceptable (Leary, 2004). Cronbach's alpha of the engagement scales/subscales was reported for all but one measure. The HSSSE was originally reported on an item-by-item basis, but recently the developers began grouping the 121 items in the questionnaire by the three aspects of engagement. However, no information on the internal consistency of these subscales is currently available.

The reliabilities of these scales reported by both the developers and other users of the

Table 37.6 Reliability information

Instrument name	Internal consistency	Test-retest interrater
Attitudes Toward Mathematics Survey (ATM)	.63–.81	–
Engagement vs. Disaffection with Learning (EvsD)	.61–.85	.53 –.68
High School Survey of Student Engagement (HSSSE)	–	–
Identification with School Questionnaire (ISQ)	.54–.84	–
Motivated Strategies for Learning Questionnaire (MSLQ)	.63–.88	–
Motivation and Engagement Scale (MES)	.70–.87	.61–.81
Research Assessment package for Schools (RAPS)	.68–.77	–
School Engagement Measure (SEM)-MacArthur	.55–.86	–
School Engagement Scale/ Questionnaire (SEQ)	.74–.86	–
School Success Profile (SSP)	.66–.82	
Student Engagement Instrument (SEI)	.72–.92	.60–.62

Note: Ranges within cells indicate either differing results for individual subscales, differing results based on age groups, or differing results from various researchers

measure ranged from .54 to .93, with most scales in the range of the .70 to .80 (see Table 37.6). Because of the variation in alphas across measures and subscales, it is important to examine the information on reliability more closely in light of the particular sample and intended use.

In addition, three of the measures [Motivation and Engagement Survey (MES), Engagement vs. Disaffection with Learning (EvsD), and the Student Engagement Instrument (SEI)] reported information on test-retest reliability, or the extent to which two different administrations of the measure give the same results.

Validity

In this chapter, we summarize the information available on these measures under the broad umbrella of construct validity (see Fredricks & McColskey, 2010, for more information on validity). One way to investigate construct validity is to examine whether the correlations between the engagement scales and the other related constructs are in the hypothesized direction based on theory and prior empirical work. The following three examples from the surveys illustrate these relations. First, the engagement scales in the School Success Profile (SSP) were positively correlated with teacher, parent, and peer support variables (Bowen, Rose, Powers, & Glennie, 2008). Additionally, the three engagement subscales (i.e., behavioral, emotional, and cognitive) in the MacArthur measure (SEM) were moderately correlated with students' perceptions of aspects of the academic and social context, school value, and school attachment (Fredricks et al., 2005). Finally, the cognitive strategy use and self-regulation scales of the MSLQ were positively correlated with students' self-reports of interest, efficacy, and task value (Pintrich, 1999; Pintrich & DeGroot, 1990).

We also found evidence of criterion-related validity, or the extent to which a measure is associated with a key behavior or outcome (Leary, 2004) on the majority of measures. Eight out of the 11 measures reported positive correlations between engagement and indicators of academic performance. For example, several studies using the MSLQ have documented that cognitive strategy use and self-regulation scales are positively related to course assignments, exams, and grades (Pintrich & DeGroot, 1990; Wolters & Pintrich, 1998; Wolters, Yu, & Pintrich, 1996). Similarly, the two engagement scales of the RAPS were positively correlated with indicators of performance (Institute for Research and Reform in Education, 1998). In addition, Appleton, Reschly, and Martin (under review) documented significant differences between affective and cognitive engagement data and academic performance; students with the lowest reports of engagement had the lowest scores on state tests and the lowest graduation rates. Finally, three of the measures (SSE, ISQ, and SEM) reported correlations between engagement and indicators of participation (i.e., attendance, teacher ratings of participation) (Fredricks & McColskey, 2010).

Another way to assess construct validity is to use exploratory or confirmatory factor analyses techniques to examine how survey items load onto the engagement constructs. Seven of the instruments reported results from either exploratory or confirmatory factor analyses. However, because of large differences in both the number and types of items, it is challenging to compare the resulting scales from these analyses. The following three examples illustrate this variability. Voelkl (1997) used confirmatory factor analysis with 16 items on the Identification with School Questionnaire (ISQ) on a sample of 3,539 urban eighth graders. These analyses confirmed two subscales: belonging and value. Martin (2008, 2009a, 2009b) used confirmatory factor analyses on 44 items of the Motivation and Engagement Survey with large samples of Australian middle and high school students. These analyses resulted in 11 subscales (self-belief, learning focus, valuing of school, persistence, planning, study management, disengagement, self-sabotage, anxiety, failure avoidance, and uncertain control). Finally, Appleton et al. (2006) used confirmatory factor analysis with 56 items from the Student Engagement Instrument on a sample of 1,931 ninth graders. These analyses resulted in six subscales (teacher-student relationships, peer support, family support, control relevance of schoolwork, future aspirations, and extrinsic motivation). A more recent confirmatory factor analysis of the Student Engagement Instrument (SEI) showed evidence of the validity of five subscales, dropping extrinsic motivation as a subscale (Betts, Appleton, Reschly, Christenson, & Huebner, 2010).

Finally, construct validity can be assessed by examining the correlations between engagement measured by different methodological approaches. Three of the measures (EvsD, RAPS, and SEM) reported correlations of scores from student self-report measures with other techniques to assess engagement (teacher ratings, external observers, and interviews). For example, the student and teacher versions of the Engagement versus Disaffection with Learning scale were moderately correlated with each other. In addition, teacher reports of behavioral and emotional engagement correlated with external observations of on and off task behavior, but student self-reports did not correlate with external observations of engagement (Skinner et al., 2008). Similarly, the developers of the SEM-MacArthur measure correlated students' self-reports with teachers' reports of student behavior. In addition, students' responses on the survey were compared to interviews about engagement with the same sample of students. They reported a positive correlation between the three subscales of engagement (behavioral, emotional, and cognitive engagement) and numerical ratings given to interview responses (Blumenfeld et al., 2005; Fredricks et al., 2005).

Overall, the psychometric information on these measures suggests that student engagement can be reliably measured through self-report methods. In addition, the measures of engagement relate to both contextual variables and outcome variables as expected. Moreover, the fact that engagement has been shown to positively correlate with achievement indicates that it could serve as a worthwhile intermediate outcome to monitor. Finally, the results of exploratory and confirmatory factor analyses demonstrate the variability in the different conceptualizations of engagement and challenges in comparing across different survey measures.

Conclusions and Future Directions

As evident from this chapter, there are a variety of methods for assessing engagement, each with strengths and limitations and useful for particular purposes. However, even when researchers use the same methodology (i.e., self-report surveys), there is variation in how engagement is defined and measured. For example, some of the surveys in this chapter focus primarily on behaviors such as effort, homework, and attendance. In contrast, other surveys include items related to emotional dimensions such as relationships with teachers and cognitive dimensions such as strategy use. Below we outline some of the key concerns related to measurement.

Operationalization of Engagement

As outlined in prior reviews (Appleton et al., 2008; Fredricks et al., 2004; Jimerson et al., 2003), there is considerable variation in the definitions of engagement used across studies. Although scholars have used a broad range of terms for engagement, the two most common are *student engagement* and *school engagement*. Differences between the terms were raised in a prior review of the literature (see Appleton et al., 2006, for more discussion). We echo Appleton et al. (2006) point that greater attention needs to be paid to the use of the terms *student engagement* and *school engagement* in future work and potential differences in the meaning of these constructs. Another concern is that many of the definitions of engagement overlap with other educational constructs (i.e., school bonding, belonging, and school climate). It is important that researchers acknowledge this overlap with earlier literatures, many of which have stronger bodies of literature supporting the construct, and be clearer in terms of both research and practice about the "value added" from studying engagement (Fredricks et al., 2004; Jimerson et al., 2003).

Although there is some agreement that engagement is a multidimensional construct, there is variation in both the number (i.e., 2–4) and types (academic, behavioral, emotional, and cognitive) of engagement dimensions. As can be seen in this chapter, different conceptualizations of engagement have resulted in a variation in the content of items used in instruments. Moreover, even within the same dataset, researchers sometimes use different variables to operationalize engagement, often without a strong theoretical or conceptual framework guiding the choice of indicators. For example, researchers have selected different items from large nationally representative datasets like the National Education Longitudinal Study (NELS:88) to create different scales of engagement (Glanville & Wildhasen, 2007). This makes it difficult to compare findings concerning both the predictors and outcomes of engagement. An additional problem is that similar items have sometimes been used to assess different dimensions of engagement. For example, student effort is used by some to describe the degree of psychological investment in learning (i.e., cognitive engagement) and by others to reflect basic compliance with schoolwork (i.e., behavioral engagement). In addition, students' valuing of school has been used as part of both emotional and cognitive engagement scales.

Given the variations in the definitions and measures of student engagement, one of the first steps to improving measurement is for researchers to more clearly describe their particular definition of engagement. It will also be important as a field to come to a stronger consensus on the operationalization of engagement (Appleton et al., 2008; Fredricks et al., 2004). Currently, we believe that the strongest empirical and theoretical support exists for a tripartite conceptualization of student engagement which includes a behavioral, emotional, and cognitive subcomponent. However, further empirical research is needed to determine what are the best indicators of each subtype and the extent to which behavioral, emotional, and cognitive engagement are separate constructs.

Assessing Malleability of Engagement

Several scholars have argued that one of the strengths of engagement is that it represents a shift from the focus on individual characteristics toward an investigation of potentially malleable contextual factors that can be targeted in interventions (Appleton et al., 2008; Fredricks et al., 2004; Sinclair, Christenson, Lehr, & Anderson, 2003). Appleton (Chap. 35) presents an example of how the Student Engagement Instrument (SEI) is being used to guide intervention efforts aimed at improving student engagement and identifying students who are at risk. Unfortunately, many of the current measures make it difficult to test questions of malleability. The majority of engagement measures tend to be general (i.e., I like school), though there are a few examples of domain-specific measures (i.e., Kong et al., 2003; Wigfield et al., 2008). Furthermore, measures are rarely worded to reflect specific situations or tasks, making it difficult to examine the extent to which engagement varies across contexts. In addition, most current survey measures do not adequately address qualitative differences in each of the dimensions of engagement. For example, behavioral engagement can range from basic compliance with school rules to doing more than is required (Finn, 1989). Emotional engagement can range from liking school to a deeper attachment and identification with the institution (Fredricks et al.). Cognitive engagement can range from the use of shallow rote strategies to the use of deep processing strategies that promote deep understanding (Greene, Miller, Crowson, Duke, & Akey, 2004). Future research should explore qualitative differences in engagement across different contexts (i.e., teacher directed as compared to small group work).

Developmental Differences

Another important research area concerns developmental differences in the measurement of engagement. There may be different indicators of engagement depending on the age of the child, and these different types of engagement may change and evolve over time. For example, students might not be cognitively engaged in learning until they are able to self-regulate and become intentional learners (Fredricks et al., 2004). There is a critical need for research that uses confirmatory factor analytic techniques to validate surveys at different ages. One example of this is research using the Motivated Learning and Strategy Use Questionnaire (MSLQ). Exploratory and confirmatory factor analyses with this measure demonstrated different factor structures in college and middle school classrooms. In college samples, analyses resulted in four cognitive strategy factors (rehearsal, elaboration, organization, and meta-cognitive strategy use) (Pintrich, Smith, Garcia, & McKeachie, 1993). In contrast, factor analyses with younger students resulted in one general cognitive strategy use scale and one meta-cognitive strategy use scale, suggesting that younger students do not make as fine of distinctions between types of strategy use as older students (Pintrich & DeGroot, 1990; Wolters, Pintrich, & Karbenick, 2005).

Variation Across Groups

Another important question is whether engagement can be measured similarly for all groups of students. If measures of engagement behave differently by race, SES, gender, and grade, and these differences are not taken into account, comparisons in the level of engagement or effects across groups are invalid (Glanville & Wildhagen, 2007). For example, Glanville and Wildhagen used confirmatory factor analyses to create a measurement model for school engagement using NELS:88 across White, African American, Latino, and Asian youth. They found that this measurement model was invariant across ethnic groups, and it was therefore appropriate to compare the effects of disengagement across these groups. In addition, Betts et al. (2010) used confirmatory factor analysis to test model invariance across gender and grade. They found that the Student Engagement Instrument (SEI) had a similar factor structure across gender and grade-level. Further research should use confirmatory factor analytic techniques to validate existing instruments and factor structures across different groups of students (i.e., age, gender, race, and SES).

Use of Multiple Methods

Finally, we recommend researchers use multiple methods to assess engagement. Qualitative methods can help to supplement our understanding of the contextual factors that are associated with engagement. In depth descriptions of context and engagement are critical for knowing how and where to intervene. Moreover, the measurement of engagement is often related to the affordances in the environment, and it may be difficult to assess cognitive engagement in classrooms where tasks involve only superficial strategy use. Observational methods can be used to better understand variations in engagement across different contexts and how this variation may relate to affordances within the context. Qualitative methods also are a useful method for describing how the different types of engagement evolve and develop to help understand why some youth begin to disengage from school (Fredricks et al., 2004). Finally, most current methods do not adequately capture the dynamic and interactive nature of engagement. One promising approach to assessing the dynamic nature of engagement is experience sampling methods which can track fluctuations in engagement over time.

In sum, although the construct of student engagement has considerable promise, measurement issues should continue to be explored in order to fully realize this promise (Glanville & Wildhagen, 2007). We believe that a more systematic and thoughtful attention to the measurement of student engagement is one of the most pressing and imperative directions for future research. First, it is important that researchers are clearer about their definitions of student engagement and how their conceptualizations of this construct relate to both other scholars' operationalization of student engagement and to other related educational constructs. The field will benefit if researchers spent less time generating slight variations on this construct and spent more time on theory development and integration of the different conceptualizations of engagement. Greater consistency in the use of measures across studies will also make it easier to compare findings about the outcomes and precursors of student engagement. However, as our review has also highlighted, there is large variation in the extent of psychometric evidence available on current measures. Future research testing the psychometric properties of these measures is critical. Finally, we strongly support the use of a wide range of methods to assess engagement including observations, interviews, and experience sampling techniques.

References

Anderson, A. R., Christenson, S. L., Sinclair, M. F., & Lehr, C. A. (2004). Check & Connect: The importance of relationships for promoting engagement with school. *Journal of School Psychology, 42*(2), 95–113. doi:10.1016/j.jsp. 2004.01.002.

Appleton, J. J., Christenson, S. L., & Furlong, M. J. (2008). Student engagement with school: Critical conceptual and methodological issues of the construct. *Psychology in the Schools, 45*, 369–386. doi:10.1002/pits.20303.

Appleton, J. J., Christenson, S. L., Kim, D., & Reschly, A. L. (2006). Measuring cognitive and psychological engagement: Validation of the Student Engagement Instrument. *Journal of School Psychology, 44*, 427–445. doi:10.1016/j.jsp. 2006.04.002.

Appleton, J. J., Reschly, A. L., & Martin, C. (under review). Research to practice: Linking assessment of student cognitive and affective engagement to intervention.

Archambault, I. (2009). Adolescent behavioral, affective, and cognitive engagement in school: Relation to dropout. *Journal of School Health, 79*, 408–415.

Betts, J. E., Appleton, J. J., Reschly, A. L., Christenson, S. L., & Huebner, E. S. (2010). A study of the factor invariance of the Student Engagement Instrument (SEI): Results from middle and high school students. *School Psychology Quarterly, 25*, 84–93. doi:10.1037/a0020259.

Birch, S., & Ladd, G. (1997). The teacher-child relationship and children's early school adjustment. *Journal of School Psychology, 35*, 61–79.

Blumenfeld, P., Modell, J., Bartko, W. T., Secada, W., Fredricks, J., Friedel, J., et al. (2005). School engagement of inner city students during middle childhood. In C. R. Cooper, C. Garcia Coll, W. T. Bartko, H. M. Davis, & C. Chatman (Eds.), *Developmental pathways through middle childhood: Rethinking diversity and contexts as resources* (pp. 145–170). Mahwah, NJ: Lawrence Erlbaum.

Bowen, G. L., Rose, R. A., & Bowen, N. K. (2005). *The reliability and validity of the school success profile*. Blomington, IN: Xlibris Corporation.

Bowen, G. L., Rose, R. A., Powers, J. D., & Glennie, E. J. (2008). The joint effects of neighborhoods, schools, peers, and families on changes in the school success of middle school students. *Family Relations, 57*, 504–516.

Buhs, E. S., & Ladd, G. W. (2001). Peer rejection as an antecedent of young children's school adjustment: An examination of mediating process. *Developmental Psychology, 37*, 550–560. doi:10.1037/0012-1649_37.4.50.

Conchas, G. Q. (2001). Structuring failure and success: Understanding the variability in Latino school engagement. *Harvard Educational Review, 71*, 475–504.

Connell, J. P. (1990). Context, self, and action: A motivational analysis of self-system processes across the life-span. In D. Cicchetti (Ed.), *The self in transition: Infancy to childhood* (pp. 61–97). Chicago: University of Chicago Press.

Connell, J. P., & Wellborn, J. G. (1991). Competence, autonomy, and relatedness: A motivational analysis of self-system processes. In M. R. Gunnar & L. A. Sroufe (Eds.), *Self-processes and development: Minnesota symposium on child psychology* (Vol. 23, pp. 43–77). Chicago: University of Chicago Press.

Corno, L., & Mandinach, E. (1983). The role of cognitive engagement in classroom learning and motivation. *Educational Psychologist, 18*, 88–108.

Csikszentmihalyi, M. (1990). *Flow: The psychology of optimal experience*. New York: Harper Perennial.

Deci, E. L., & Ryan, R. M. (1985). *Intrinsic motivation and self-determination in human behavior*. New York: Plenum Press.

Eccles, J. S., Wigfield, A., & Schiefele, U. (1998). Motivation to succeed. In W. Damon (Series Ed.), & N. Eisenberg (Vol. Ed.), *Handbook of child psychology: Vol. 3. Social, emotional and personality development* (5th ed., pp. 1017–1094). New York: Wiley.

Finn, J. D. (1989). Withdrawing from school. *Review of Educational Research, 59*, 117–142. doi:10.3102/00346543059002117.

Finn, J. D., Folger, J., & Cox, D. (1991). Measuring participation among elementary grade students. *Educational and Psychological Measurement, 51*, 393–402.

Finn, J. D., Pannozzo, G. M., & Voelkl, K. E. (1995). Disruptive and inattentive-withdrawn behavior and achievement among fourth graders. *The Elementary School Journal, 95*, 421–454.

Finn, J. D., & Rock, D. A. (1997). Academic success among students at risk for school failure. *Journal of Applied Psychology, 82*, 221–234.

Fredricks, J. A., Blumenfeld, P. C., Friedel, J., & Paris, A. (2005). School engagement. In K. A. Moore & L. Lippman (Eds.), *Conceptualizing and measuring indicators of positive development: What do children need to flourish* (pp. 305–321). New York: Kluwer Academic/Plenum Press.

Fredricks, J. A., Blumenfeld, P. C., & Paris, A. (2004). School engagement: Potential of the concept: State of the evidence. *Review of Educational Research, 74*, 59–119. doi:10.3102/00346543074001059.

Fredricks, J., & McColskey, W., with Meli, J., Mordica, J., Montrosse, B., and Mooney, K. (2010). *Measuring student engagement in upper elementary through high school: A description of 21 instruments* (Issues & Answers Report, REL 2010–No. 098). Washington, DC: U.S. Department of Education, Institute of Education Sciences, National Center for Education Evaluation and Regional Assistance, Regional Educational Laboratory Southeast. Retrieved from http://ies.ed.gov/ncee/edlabs.

Furrer, C., & Skinner, E. (2003). Sense of relatedness as a factor in children's academic engagement and performance. *Journal of Educational Psychology, 95*, 148–162. doi:10.1037/0022-0663.95.1.148.

Gamoran, A., & Nystrand, M. (1992). Taking students seriously. In M. N. Fred (Ed.), *Student engagement and achievement in American secondary schools* (pp. 40–61). New York: Teachers College Press.

Garcia-Duncan, T. G., & McKeachie, W. J. (2005). The making of the motivated strategies for learning questionnaire. *Educational Psychologist, 40*(2), 117–128.

Garcia, T., & Pintrich, P. (1996). Assessing students' motivation and learning strategies in the classroom context: The motivation and strategies in learning questionnaire. In M. Birenbaum & F. J. Dochy (Eds.), *Alternatives in assessment of achievements, learning processes, and prior knowledge* (pp. 319–339). New York: Kluwer Academic/Plenum Press.

Glanville, L., & Wildhagen, T. (2007). The measurement of school engagement: Assessing dimensionality and measurement in variance across race and ethnicity. *Educational and Psychological Measurement, 6*, 1019–1041. doi:10.1177/0013164406299126.

Greene, B. A., Miller, R. B., Crowson, H. M., Duke, B. L., & Akey, K. L. (2004). Predicting high school students' cognitive engagement and achievement: Contributions of classroom perceptions and motivation. *Contemporary Educational Psychology, 29*(4), 462–482. doi:10.1016/j.cedpsych.2004.01.006.

Greenwood, C. R., Horton, B. T., & Utley, C. A. (2002). Academic engagement: Current perspectives on research and practice. *School Psychology Review, 31*, 328–349.

Hektner, J. M., Schmidt, J. A., & Csikzentmihalyi, M. (2007). *Experience sampling method: Measuring the quality of everyday life*. Thousand Oaks, CA: Sage.

Helme, S., & Clarke, D. (2001). Identifying cognitive engagement in the mathematics classrooms. *Mathematics Educational Journal, 13*, 133–153.

Institute for Research and Reform in Education. (1998). *Research Assessment Package for Schools (RAPS) manual for elementary and middle school assessments*. Retrieved August 1, 2009, from http://www.irre.org/publications/pdfs/RAPS_manual_entire_1998.pdf.

Jimerson, S. R., Campos, E., & Grief, J. L. (2003). Toward an understanding of definitions and measures of school engagement and related terms. *California School Psychologist, 8*, 7–27.

Kong, Q., Wong, N., & Lam, C. (2003). Student engagement in mathematics: Development of instrument and validation of a construct. *Mathematics Education Research Journal, 54*, 4–21.

Leary, M. R. (2004). *Introduction to behavioral research methods* (4th ed.). Boston: Pearson Education, Inc.

Lee, O., & Anderson, C. W. (1993). Task engagement and conceptual change in middle school science classrooms. *American Educational Research Journal, 30*, 585–610.

Lee, O., & Brophy, J. (1996). Motivational patterns observed in sixth-grade science classrooms. *Journal of Research in Science Teaching, 33*, 303–318.

Locke, D. A. (1996). *Making and molding identity in school: Student narratives on race, gender and academic engagement*. Albany, NY: State University Press.

Maehr, M. L., & Meyer, H. A. (1997). Understanding motivation and schooling: Where we've been, where we are, and where we need to go. *Educational Psychology Review, 9*, 371–408.

Marks, H. M. (2000). Student engagement in instructional activity: Patterns in the elementary, middle, and high school years. *American Educational Research Journal, 37*, 153–184. doi:10.3102/00028312037001153.

Martin, A. J. (2008). Motivation and engagement in diverse performance domains: Testing their generality across school, university/college, work, sport, music, and daily life. *Journal of Research in Personality, 42*(6), 1607–1612. doi:10.1016/j.jrp.2008.05.003.

Martin, A. J. (2009a). Motivation and engagement across the academic life span: A developmental construct validity study of elementary school, high school, and university/college students. *Educational and Psychological Measurement, 69*(5), 794–824. doi:10.1177/0013164409332214.

Martin, A. J. (2009b). *The motivation and engagement scale*. Sydney, Australia: Lifelong Achievement Group. Retrieved from http://www.lifelongachievement.com.

McCaslin, M. M., & Good, T. L. (1996). *Listening in classrooms*. New York: HarperCollins.

Meece, J., Blumenfeld, P. C., & Hoyle, R. H. (1988). Students' goal orientation and cognitive engagement in classroom activities. *Journal of Educational Psychology, 80*, 514–523.

Miller, R. B., Greene, B. A., Montalvo, G. P., Ravindran, B., & Nichols, J. D. (1996). Engagement in academic work: The role of learning goals, future consequences, pleasing others, and perceived ability. *Contemporary Educational Psychology, 21*(4), 388–422.

Moreira, P. A. S., Vaz, F. M., Dias, P. C., & Petracchi, P. (2009). Psychometric properties of the Portuguese version of the Student Engagement Instrument. *Canadian Journal of School Psychology, 24*, 303–307. doi:10.1177/0829573509346680.

National Research Council and the Institute of Medicine. (2004). *Engaging schools: Fostering high school students' motivation to learn*. Committee on Increasing High School Students' Engagement and Motivation to Learn. Board on Children, Youth, and Families, Division of Behavioral and Social Science and Education. Washington, DC: The National Academy Press.

Newmann, F., Wehlage, G.G., & Lamborn, S. D. (1992). The significance and sources of student engagement. In F. Newmann (Ed.), *Student engagement and achievement in American secondary schools* (pp. 11–39). New York: Teachers College Press.

Nystrand, M., & Gamoran, A. (1991). Instructional discourse, student engagement, and literature achievement. *Research in the Teaching of English, 25*, 261–290.

Nystrand, M., Wu, L. L., Gamaron, A., Zeiser, S., & Long, D. (2001). *Questions in time: Investigating the structure and dynamics of unfolding classroom discourse*. Albany, NY: National Research Center on English Learning & Achievement.

Perry, J. (2008). School engagement among urban youth of color: Criterion pattern effects of vocational exploration and racial identity. *Journal of Career Development, 34*(4), 397–422. doi:10.1177/0894845308316293.

Peterson, P., Swing, S., Stark, K., & Wass, G. (1984). Students' cognitions and time on task during mathematics instruction. *American Educational Research Journal, 21*, 487–515.

Pintrich, P. R. (1999). The role of motivation in promoting and sustaining self-regulated learning. *International Journal of Educational Research, 31*(6), 459–470.

Pintrich, P. R., & DeGroot, E. (1990). Motivational and self-regulated learning components of classroom academic performance. *Journal of Educational Psychology, 82*, 33–40.

Pintrich, P. R., Smith, D. A. F., Garcia, T., & McKeachie, W. (1993). Reliability and predictive validity of the motivated strategies for learning questionnaire (MSLQ). *Educational and Psychological Measurement, 53*(3), 801–813.

Reschly, A. L., & Christenson, S. L. (2006). Prediction of dropout among students with mild disabilities: A case for inclusion of student engagement variables. *Remedial and Special Education, 27*, 276–292.

Russell, V. J., Ainsley, M., & Frydenberg, E. (2005). *Schooling issues digest: Student motivation and engagement*. Retrieved March 1, 2010, from http://www.dest.gov/au/sectors/school_education/publication_resources/schooling_issues_digest/schooling_issues_digest_motivation_engagement.htm.

Saliva, J., & Ysseldyke, J. E. (2004). *Assessment* (9th ed.). Princeton, NJ: Houghton Mifflin.

Shapiro, E. S. (2004). *Academic skills problems: Direct assessment and intervention* (3rd ed.). New York: Guilford Press.

Shernoff, D. J., Csikszentmihalyi, M., Schneider, B., & Shernoff, E. S. (2003). Student engagement in high school classrooms from the perspective of flow theory. *School Psychology Quarterly, 18*, 158–176.

Shernoff, J. D., & Schmidt, J. A. (2008). Further evidence of the engagement-achievement paradox among U.S. high school students. *Journal of Youth and Adolescence, 5*, 564–580. doi:10.1007/s10964-007-9241-z.

Sinclair, M. F., Christenson, S. L., Lehr, C. A., & Anderson, A. R. (2003). Facilitating student learning and engagement: Lessons from Check & Connect longitudinal studies. *The California School Psychologist, 8*, 29–41.

Skinner, E., & Belmont, M. J. (1993). Motivation in the classroom: Reciprocal effect of teacher behavior and student engagement across the school year. *Journal of Educational Psychology, 85*, 571–581.

Skinner, E. A., Marchand, G., Furrer, C., & Kindermann, T. (2008). Engagement and disaffection in the classroom: Part of a larger motivational dynamic. Journal of Educational Psychology, 100(4), 765–781. doi:10.1037/a0012840.

Steinberg, L. D., Brown, B. B., & Dornbush, S. M. (1996). *Beyond the classroom: Why school reform has failed and what parents need to do*. New York: Simon and Schuster.

Turner, J. C., & Meyer, D. K. (2000). Studying and understanding the instructional context of classroom: Using our past to forge our future. *Educational Psychologist, 35*, 69–85.

Uekawa, K., Borman, K., & Lee, R. (2007). Student engagement in the U.S. urban high school mathematics and science classrooms: Findings on social organization, race, and ethnicity. *Urban Review, 39*, 1–43.

Voelkl, K. E. (1996). Measuring students' identification with school. *Educational and Psychological Measurement, 56*(5), 760–770. doi:10.1177/0013164496056005003.

Voelkl, K. E. (1997). Identification with school. *American Journal of Education, 105*, 204–319. doi:10.1007/s11256-006-0039-1.

Volpe, R. J., DiPerna, J. C., Hintze, J. M., & Shapiro, E. S. (2005). Observing students in classroom settings: A review of seven coding schemes. *School Psychology Review, 34*(4), 454–474.

Wettersten, K. B., Gulmino, A., Herrick, C. G., Hunter, P. J., Kim, G. Y., Jagow, D., et al. (2005). Predicting educational and vocational attitudes among rural high school students. *Journal of Counseling of Psychology, 52*(4), 658–663. doi: 10.1037/0022-0167.52.4.658.

Wigfield, A., Guthrie, J. T., Perencevich, K. C., Taboada, A., Klauda, S. L., McRae, A., et al. (2008). Role of reading engagement in mediating the effects of reading comprehension instruction on reading outcomes. *Psychology in the Schools, 45*, 432–445. doi: 10.10002/pits.20307.

Wolters, C., & Pintrich, P. R. (1998). Contextual differences in student motivation and self-regulated learning in mathematics, English, and social studies classrooms. *Instructional Science, 26*, 27–47.

Wolters, C., Yu, S., & Pintrich, P. R. (1996). The relation between goal orientation and students' motivational beliefs and self-regulated learning and academic learning. *Journal of Educational Psychology, 81*(3), 329–339.

Wolters, C. A., Pintrich, P. R., & Karabenick, S. A. (2005). Assessing academic self-regulated learning. In K. A. Moore & L. H. Lippman (Eds.), *What do children need to flourish: Conceptualizing and measuring indicators of positive development*. New York: Springer.

Yair, G. (2000). Educational battlefields in America: The tug of war over students' engagement with instruction. *Sociology of Education, 73*, 247–269.

Yazzie- Mintz, E. (2007). *Voices of students on engagement: A report on the 2006 High School Survey of Student Engagement*. Bloomington, IN: Center for Evaluation & Educational Policy, Indiana University. Retrieved February 1, 2010, from http://ceep.indiana.edu/pdf/HSSSE_2006_Report.pdf.

Issues and Methods in the Measurement of Student Engagement: Advancing the Construct Through Statistical Modeling

Joseph Betts

Abstract

This chapter will provide an overview of statistical modeling to further the measurement of student engagement. After a discussion of the complexity of defining and therefore measuring engagement, a general introduction and guide to the construction of productive measures of engagement will be provided. Confirmatory factor analysis and item response theory will be elaborated and used to highlight modern methods of evaluating and scoring instruments to measure engagement. Additionally, the bifactor model will be displayed and elaborated upon as a potentially useful model for disentangling some of the intricacies of engagement along with parsing the relationship with motivation. The Student Engagement Instrument (SEI) will be utilized throughout the chapter to highlight the specific methods and provide some guidance on potentially useful applications related to theoretical issues.

Student engagement is an important aspect of an educational milieu. Students must invest considerable time and effort on a daily basis to acquire the knowledge and skills necessary to facilitate ongoing learning and be successful in their educational careers. Additionally, engagement with peers, teachers, and administrators can help to foster prosocial relationships. As engagement is vital to education, it has become an important construct for researchers with quite a broad appeal (Appleton, Christenson, Kim, & Reschly, 2006; Fredricks, Blumenfeld, & Paris, 2004).

However, there are a number of outstanding conceptual and methodological issues to be addressed by the nascent research into student engagement (Appleton, Christenson, & Furlong, 2008; Fredricks et al., 2004).

While the construct of engagement has unique theoretical importance, there is some question about what key elements constitute it. While many issues are yet to be evaluated with respect to how student engagement is intertwined with student outcomes and other psychological/educational variables, a foundational issue that needs to be contended with before any results can be meaningfully interpreted is the appropriate measurement of the construct. Without appropriate measurement, there can be little intriguing or useful research.

J. Betts, MMIS, Ph.D., NCSP (✉)
Center for Cultural Diversity & Minority Education,
Madison, WI, USA
e-mail: Jbetts5118@aol.com

This chapter will discuss the construct of student engagement with an emphasis on measurement and statistical modeling. The chapter will highlight the use of modern techniques of confirmatory factor analysis (CFA; Bartholomew & Knott, 1999) and item response theory (IRT; Crocker & Algina, 1986; Yen & Fitzpatrick, 2006) for evaluating measures of engagement. The Student Engagement Instrument (SEI; Appleton et al., 2006) will be used to exemplify the approaches, but the methodology will be generally extensible for any measurement instrument.

Contemplating and Defining Engagement

One of the first issues when attempting to measure anything is deciding upon a relevant definition of the object of interest and what attributes or properties of that object are most salient (Crocker & Algina, 1986; Downing & Haladyna, 2006; Lord & Novick, 1968; Thorndike, 1982; Wilson, 2005) for one's purposes. In the area of educational and psychological measurement, it is sometimes difficult to conceptualize the object of measurement because it is usually an abstract entity whose attributes of interests for measurement can be arguable and not easily observable (Crocker & Algina). Given that constructs are hypothetical concepts, there can be a great deal of difference in conceptualization, for instance, see the debate concerning IQ, in general, and the existence of g-factor, in particular (Jensen, 1998). Thus, authoritative definitions or widespread acceptance of a specific set of attributes can be difficult to establish in general for psychological variables and student engagement is no different (Appleton et al., 2008).

Presently there are different models of student engagement that accentuate different aspects but also have substantial overlap (Appleton et al., 2006; Finn, 1989; Fredricks et al., 2004). Fredricks et al. propose a multidimensional approach to investigating engagement through the use of three broad types of engagement: behavioral, emotional, and cognitive. Appleton and colleagues have attempted to further this perspective while also situating engagement within a broader contextualization where engagement is seen as a mediating variable between specific contexts and important outcomes.

Appleton et al. (2006) utilize their general theoretical framework to develop an instrument to measure student engagement. Their work can be seen as an instantiation of the previous work by Fredricks et al. (2004) with an understanding of the potential multidimensionality of the construct of engagement but also a broadening as they take the conceptualization and measurement of engagement beyond the general types, that is, cognitive, behavioral, and emotional, to encompass academic engagement and specific aspects or subcomponents of the general type of engagement related to unique contexts. For instance, there is no attempt to simply measure a singular, broad construct called affective/emotional engagement, but care is taken to specify specific aspects where emotional engagement might show itself within different contexts, that is, relationships with teachers, support from peers, and family support. Similarly with cognitive engagement, they define two subcomponents of cognitive engagement that are related to different aspects of cognitive engagement with one focusing on a student's sense of control and relevance of schoolwork and one related to the student's future aspirations and goals.

Fredricks et al. (2004) conceptualization of three broad types will serve as a starting point for an initial definition of student engagement in this paper. Behavioral engagement relates to a student's willingness to become involved in school-related activities in a positive manner. This can take the form of following rules of conduct, participating in school activities, or showing persistence and positive effort in learning tasks. Emotional engagement subsumes students' feelings about the educational milieu within which they find themselves. This can relate to reactions to teachers, peers, or even the school culture, in general. Cognitive engagement generally reflects the student's willingness to invest cognitive facilities into learning and mastering new and potentially difficult skills. This type of engagement can also relate to the setting of learning goals and consciously striving to meet those goals.

These three types of engagement can readily be seen to have a significant level of crossover and overlap with other important areas of study in psychology. For instance, research on cognitive engagement can easily be related to research in other areas of psychology and education, such as setting goals, planning, monitoring, and evaluating progress that are common metacognitive (Blumenfeld, Kempler, & Krajcik, 2006) or self-regulated learning (Cleary & Zimmerman, Chap. 11) themes. Additionally, research in the area of social development models related to such diverse issues as delinquency (Hawkins & Weis, 1985) and drug use (Catalano, Kosterman, Hawkins, Newcomb, & Abbott, 1996; Guo, Hawkins, Hill, & Abbott, 2001) bears directly on the emotional engagement students have with their teachers and social environment. Similarly, research in areas as diverse as internal motivation and reward contingencies (Cameron & Pierce, 1994) has relevance to behavioral engagement. As can be inferred, the area of student engagement has a substantial body of work from which it is able to draw.

Further complicating the elucidation of engagement is the growing relevance of situating engagement within a more complex ecology where specific antecedents and outcomes are conceptualized (Appleton et al., 2006, 2008; Fredricks et al. 2004). Within this conceptualization are important antecedent variables related to such things as school and classroom contexts (subsuming diverse variables such as relationships with teachers or peers to the more overt demands and contingencies of the organizational structure), home contexts (subsuming such domains as relations with family members and their ideations concerning education), and individual level context related to the student's comportment and attitudes. Additionally, there are a number of key outcomes of interest, two of which appear most important are achievement and dropping out of school, as both of these outcomes have lifelong repercussions (Alexander, Entwisle, & Horsey, 1997; Balfanz, Herzog, & Mac Iver, 2007; Christenson et al., 2008; Finn & Rock, 1997).

Disentangling Motivation and Engagement

An outstanding issue in the study of student engagement is the relationship between motivation and engagement (Appleton et al., 2006; Wentzel & Wigfield, 2007). Much of the problem is related to defining the difference between the two constructs and highlighting the potential interactions. This area of study is potentially fecund due both to the dearth of specific research and the vast array of possible theoretical forays. What follows is a brief sortie into some incipient issues with attempted adumbration of research ideas and statistical models to be presented in later sections.

Motivation can be conceived broadly as the cause for a person's action in the world (Franken, 2001; Kleinginna & Kleinginna, 1981). It is that thing which compels us to action. However, motivation also carries within it the connotation of its root, motive, which implies both a cause to act and the implicit goal of the action. Therefore, motivation seems to suggest both the movement to action and the goal associated with that action. This goal-directed action can be elicited either by internal or external/social stimulus. For instance, one can be motivated to play a sport because there is something appealing to the individual or because one's friends are playing. Likewise, one can be motivated to avoid actions due to internal/external stimuli.

Engagement appears to engender a sense of active commitment or participation (Fredricks et al., 2004). However, care should be taken when attempting to equate active commitment and participation, as one might participate in an activity but with little active commitment. This might have some interesting theoretical repercussions for engagement research as there might be different relationships between engagement and outcome variables of interest, such as drop out or achievement, when one measures active commitment to engage in activity as opposed to passive participation. Simply coming to school can be either an active commitment to learning and interacting with others or a passive participation in a socially manifest activity that one feels compelled to do to avoid adverse repercussions. Additionally, different underlying types of motivation could be at play in those situations, with active engagement potentially motivated by an internal stimulus where as passive participation motivated by external/social expectations or punishing consequences for lack of participation.

One possible way to conceptualize the relationship between motivation and engagement is that motivation can be seen as the underlying psychological state that sets the stage for engagement (Blumenfeld et al., 2006). Appleton et al. (2006) suggest that motivation is a necessary but not sufficient condition for engagement. From this perspective, if one is engaged, then one could be seen to have been motivated toward that action. However, one might be motivated to act but not actually initiate an active involvement or participation. That lack of moving from a state of motivation to a state of engagement could derive from personal/individual reasons or from barriers in the environment that act as a bulwark inhibiting engagement.

There can be structural barriers within an educational environment that hinder a student from bridging the gap between being motivated to act and the realization of that act. For instance, a student might be motivated to learn a martial art or piano but not have that option available in school. A student might be motivated to learn about history but have significant peer pressure to not develop erudition in that area or even actively encouraged by peers to "act dumb" or devalue educational attainment in general. Here is where interesting questions within the motivation/engagement research milieu can extend from the study of individuals and individual differences to the study of environments and local ecologies that foster or inhibit active engagement related to education and school.

An interesting scenario arises when considering the interplay of motivation and engagement: To what extent does engagement in an activity increase an individual's motivation to continue with active participation? Additionally, what aspects of being engaged in an activity would continually discourage an individual from participating and potentially lead to disengagement? The relationship becomes more of a recursive type of interplay, where motivation facilitates engagement, which facilitates new learning, experiences, and growing competence in an area, which then facilitates an increase in motivation to continue the learning and discovery process. As research on talent development has also shown (Bloom, 1985), there can be unique dynamics to this interplay at different developmental periods as the child moves from initial exploration to professional development. There is active research in exploring the more dynamic model where engagement acts as a mediator between motivation and achievement (Appleton et al., 2006; Blumenfeld et al., 2006).

The relationship between motivation and engagement is not one that is easily disentangled. However, there are numerous lines of research potential. While the severability of engagement and motivation might not be easily accomplished, the measurements of engagement and motivation are necessary precursors to any research program that will attempt to elucidate the possible relationships and interdependencies. The following sections will outline some important concepts and ideas for extending the present research into engagement by explicitly focusing on issues related to measurement.

Measurement Issues in Student Engagement

Given the complexity of the engagement variable and its potential multidimensionality, developing an instrument to measure engagement could be seen as quite difficult. It is likely that numerous measures would need to be developed for the multitude of potentially salient research questions in the broad field of student engagement. Fredricks et al. (2004) provide an insightful critique of the difficulties in measuring different types of engagement. They also highlight the conceptual issues and inherent problems related to the great deal of overlap between the different types of engagement that could make measurement more complex. Appleton et al. (2006) also provide a perceptive method of organizing the construct of engagement within a structure that accounts for both antecedent and consequent variables.

The three types of engagement, behavioral, cognitive, and emotional, might facilitate the construction of three different measures of engagement with each focused on a single type. However, it would also seem appropriate to identify specific aspects of each general type that could constitute a subcomponent, or subdimension, of the general type. For instance, the conceptualization of a measure of behavioral engagement would need to account for work-related behaviors such as completing school assignments and the level of achievement on that work but might also have to account for the students' behavior with respect to following rules or interfering with others. It is easy to see that a student might have serious problems completing work but have a high regard for following rules, and vice versa. Therefore, the extent to which each of the three engagement types are homogeneous constructs is highly questionable, and therefore, measurement should focus on examining specific aspects of each general type. An example of this can be seen with the SEI, which attempts to measure specific aspects of cognitive engagement relating to both future aspirations and control/relevance of schoolwork. While both of these subcomponents are related to cognitive engagement, it was thought they represented unique and important aspects of cognitive engagement and therefore required distinct measures, for example, independent scales.

Further complicating the measurement of engagement is the extent to which differing contexts of engagement are important. For instance, is it important to measure emotional engagement separately with respect to teachers than to peers, or can they be comprised as an overall measure of engagement within the school context? Moreover, should school level structure variables, such as student beliefs and thoughts about the rules and enforcement of those rules in school or the student sense of the type of work and assessments they are given, be measured within the context of a general engagement construct related to the school environment? These are open issues that can drive the development of appropriate scales for measuring different aspects of engagement and also help to begin to parse out the answers about the interrelated aspects of engagement.

The next section will provide a general overview of the process for constructing measures. This is meant to provide a basis and foundation for future developers of instruments to measure those aspects of engagement that suite their research endeavors. There are a number of good references on test construction (see, for instance, DeVellis, 2003; Downing & Haladyna, 2006; Spector, 1992; or Wilson, 2005) to help guide the specifics of test development. The following section is not meant to be a complete or definitive methodology for test construction, but rather to provide a general outline for moving the measurement of engagement forward.

General Approach to Constructing Appropriate Measures

After a psychological construct, for instance, cognitive engagement or some relevant subcomponent, of interest has been defined, one would attempt to delineate those relevant aspects or attributes that constitute the construct. One might consult the research and find only a single dimension could constitute the construct or that multiple aspects of the construct are important and a multidimensional approach should be considered. If the construct was thought to be multidimensional, then not only would there be a necessity to define each dimension of importance but also a need to identify the possible relationship between those dimensions.

For instance, the SEI identified two important types of engagement, cognitive and affective, from the research literature (Appleton et al., 2006). Furthermore, there was an identification of aspects of those general engagement types that could be thought of as different manifestations, or subcomponents or subtypes, of the general type. For instance, in the emotional/affective type of engagement, the SEI measures distinct types of relationships between the student and teacher, the student and their peers, and the student and their family. In the area of cognitive engagement, subtypes of control and relevance of schoolwork and future aspirations and goals are measured. It was believed that these were unique subcomponents or context within which each general type of engagement would be expressed, but differently enough to constitute measuring them independently.

The next step is to bring the theoretical and abstract construct into a tool to measure the purported construct. The basic idea is to find some manner of eliciting observable responses from individuals that relate to the latent construct and then apply a numerical quantity to those responses. The area of psychometrics in education and psychology is the field that applies the scientific study of the measurement of latent traits and uses a range of test theories and statistical models to help construct a useful instrument for measurement (Crocker & Algina, 1986; Lord & Novick, 1968; Wilson, 2005). There can be numerous methods for obtaining information such as observations, structured interviews, or basic psychological assessments. This chapter will focus on a specific method of obtaining information through the use of a summated rating scale, which will be elaborated in the following sections.

Moving from the Theoretical to the Applied

This step in the process attempts to bring the theoretical aspect of the construct of interest into focus by developing items to measure the construct. We expect to observe the salient aspects of the construct by eliciting student responses to items/questions that are thought to reveal the continuum of the construct. We would like to find out how individuals differ in the amount of a construct they have, so we ask them questions and seek their responses.

Item development is critical to the process of measurement, as the items are the only window we have into the construct for the measurement instrument. The relationship between the item content and the construct of interest is vitally important, as inferences from the scores on the instrument are only generalizable to the extent that the items appear to have been sampled from an appropriate domain. For instance, if we were developing a test for eighth graders' mathematics ability and only sampled items from single-digit addition, there would be legitimate questions about how well we represented the appropriate set of appropriate mathematical problems. Furthermore, there would be legitimate questions about how well the scores from the test generalized to making inferences about the students overall mathematical ability.

After an appropriate number of items have been compiled for which one believes are broad enough to cover the relevant domain of the construct, there are three basic steps that follow: (1) evaluating the extent to which the items measure the intended attribute of the construct, (2) computing a method to score the aggregated responses, and (3) providing evidence that the rating scale is measuring what it was intended to measure and other issues related to score validity, such as measurement invariance and differential item functioning.

The following sections will highlight issues (1) and (2) from above, and later sections will focus on using confirmatory factor analysis (CFA) and item response theory (IRT) to guide item analysis and scale development. Thus, the chapter will provide a more general theoretical overview of the issues (1) and (2), but then provide applicable statistical methods for analyzing data for scale construction. These sections provide a foundation for the development of the underlying measurement model of the instrument. Note that a glossary of terms appears in Appendix A.

Issue (3) is related to the compilation of evidence for validity and will not be directly discussed in this chapter. The reason for this is validity-related research is usually developed within the specific context of the intended inferences of the measurement instrument. Therefore, research design and analytical methodologies are usually more defined by that context than a general approach (see, for instance, Crocker &

Algina, 1986; Kane, 2006; Thorndike, 1982; or Wainer & Braun, 1988 for more comprehensive approaches to the study of test score validity). Also, only after the items can be confirmed to measure a common construct (1) and the aggregation of those items into a single scale justified (2) can research related to validity issues (3) be undertaken. Thus, the following sections seek to provide a basis for the foundational aspects of developing an instrument which would precede issues related to the validity of that score(s) from the instrument, which wouldced to the study of test score validity). Also, only after the items can be confirmed to measure a common construct (1) and the aggregation of those items into a single scale justified (2) can research related to validity issues (3) be undertaken. Thus, the following sections seek to provide a basis for the foundational aspects of developing an instrument which would precede issues related to the validity of that score(s) from the instrument, which would be addressed with an ongoing research program (Crocker & Algina, 1986; Embretson & Reise, 2000; Kane, 2006; McDonald, 1999; Thorndike, 1982).

Evaluating the Items for Appropriateness

It is vital to ensure that all the items are indeed measuring a similar construct and therefore provide the basis for a unified interpretation of an aggregate of those items. Thus, field-testing the items in an appropriate sample of individuals on an intended measurement instrument is crucial to evaluate the functioning of the items themselves. Not only is the sample of items important, so is the sample of students. Just as one wishes to generalize from the item responses to the construct of interest, one would like to generalize from the sample performance to the population of interest.

It is important to evaluate the extent to which each item contributes to the understanding of the construct of interest. Each item needs to contribute to the measurement and should be positively related to the overall construct. As item responses across multiple items will be compiled into a score for the student, each item needs to add significantly to the overall understanding. So not only must the items themselves be positively related, they must also conform to the intended measurement model. In essence, the items must fit to the intended structure of the measurement model.

A few issues should be noted. First of all, as there are a number of items to be aggregated in order to inform the measurement of the construct, we must provide evidence that indeed the items are measuring a common hypothetical construct. This is a basic psychometric consideration related to the homogeneity of items that form the scale (McDonald, 1999; Thorndike, 1982). If the items do not appear to measure a common construct, then it would be difficult to make inferences from scores as to a particular attribute of the construct because measurement would be confounded.

For instance, if an item had little relationship with the construct being measured, all measurements would be useless in measuring the construct. Imagine using a temperature gauge to measure your basement's dimensions or using a student's math scores to make judgments about a student's reading skills. In these situations, if the items are not measuring the intended construct, then they do not give us any useful information about the construct and would be misleading. Additionally, if an item appears to be measuring two or more attributes, for example, measured both cognitive engagement and emotional engagement, then there would be a question as to what we should attribute higher or lower response option by the student. Here, the issue of confounded measurement would be apparent. It would be difficult to understand if the higher response was due to higher levels of cognitive or emotional engagement.

Generally, when constructing a measure, we would like each item to measure only a single attribute. This ensures that higher or lower scores on the items can be referenced to higher or lower levels of the single variable/construct being measured. For instance, we would like to attribute higher scores on cognitive engagement items to something related to cognitive engagement. Item analysis can provide both justification for item use and retention and also help in the nascent theory development.

Issues Related to Scoring the Instrument

One of the common methods of obtaining response information from students is by asking questions in a survey format and eliciting responses on a forced-choice, ordered category scale (McDonald, 1999). We will refer to this method of obtaining information as a rating scale for this chapter; it is generally a method that assigns a series of fixed, ordered categories to the item response options. In general, the respondent is asked a series of questions thought to elicit the attributes of the latent construct of interest, and then the respondent is asked to respond to each question by selecting one of a number of categories which are ordered from one end of the spectrum to the other. A common set of ordered categories could be as follows: strongly agree (SA), agree (A), disagree (D), and strongly disagree (SD). For any question, the respondent simply chooses the level of the ordered category for which they feel best applies.

For scoring the rating scale, a bijective, or one-to-one, relationship is usually established between the qualitative representations, for example, SA, A, D, and SD, and a numerical representation, for example, 3, 2, 1, and 0. For instance, if one were interested in having higher scores correspond to higher levels of positive feelings/beliefs related to the item content, then one could use the following bijective relation: $SA = 3$, $A = 2$, $D = 1$, and $SD = 0$. Thus, higher scores would result in higher levels of agreement. Student scores are then computed by summing the numeric representations of all items in order to obtain a total score and can be referred to as a summated rating scale. Furthermore, to make scores interpretable, a norming process can be undertaken (Thorndike, 1982).

After evaluating the items, settling on a set of items that appear to provide useful measurement of the construct, and deciding on a transformation from the qualitative response format to a quantitative measure, some method of scaling the test must ensue in order to provide score scale with interpretable scores. Scaling basically entails combining the scores across items into a single metric expressing the continuum of the construct. So, after a field test has provided information on actual response patterns from the intended population and some analysis has provided insights into which set of items provide productive measurement for the construct, then one would focus on the most appropriate method of combining item responses into a total score.

Analyzing the Rating Scale and the Intended Measurement Model

The following sections will provide an overview of two complementary models for item analysis and the extent to which the intended measurement model appears to hold. These analyses will help provide evidence for (1) and (2) above. The first model will be an extension of classical test theory (CTT) called the congeneric measurement model. The second will be one of a number of modern item response theory models specifically from the Rasch family of measurement models.

Congeneric Measurement Model and Confirmatory Factor Analysis

One common method of evaluating the intended measurement model of a psychometric instrument is through the use of congeneric measurement theory (Jöreskog, 1971) and confirmatory factor analytic models (CFA; Bartholomew & Knott, 1999; Bollen, 1989; Brown, 2006; Harman, 1967; Jöreskog, 1969; McDonald, 1985, 1999). The congeneric measurement theory can be seen as an extension of the basic classical test theory (Gulliksen, 1950; Lord & Novick, 1968) where items measuring a common construct can have different levels of relationship to that construct; for instance, some items do a better or worse job of measuring that construct. The congeneric measurement model can be expressed as follows:

$$X_i = \alpha_i + \gamma_i T + \varepsilon_i. \qquad (38.1)$$

Here the score, X, on an item i, X_i, is composed of a linear function of the underlying true score T. In the common classical test theory, all items have a similar level of difficult, $\alpha_i = \alpha_j = 0$, and measure the true score with equivalent precision, $\gamma_i = \gamma_j = 1$. Additionally, a strong true score model would presume the error term, ε, was similar across items. The congeneric model can be seen as a more robust model when attempting to measure a common true score factor. The model presented above is the unidimensional model

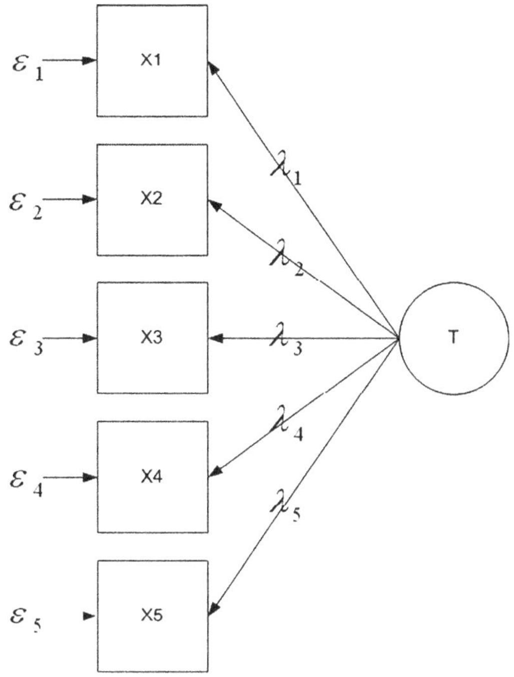

Fig. 38.1 Congeneric measurement model represented within the context of confirmatory factor analysis. *Circle* with "*T*" represents the latent variable, *X*1 to *X*5 represent distinct items measuring "*T*," λ_1 to λ_5 represent the factor loadings, and ε_1 to ε_5 represent the error terms

where a single factor is thought to underlie responses to the items; however, the model can be extended to multidimensional models by adding additional factors into the model.

The congeneric model can be evaluated within the context of CFA (Bollen, 1989; Brown, 2006; Jöreskog, 1969, 1971; McDonald, 1985, 1999). Figure 38.1 shows a pictorial representation of the congeneric measurement model within the context of CFA. The square boxes represent observed responses to items, and the circular variable represents the underlying latent trait of interest that is hypothesized to be producing those responses. The γ_i variables represent the factor loadings on the true score, *T*, and the ε_i represents the error or residual term for each item *i* (please note the mean structure aspect of the model to evaluate the intercept term, α_i, has been left off Fig. 38.1 for simplicity but would be a part of the congeneric model (see Brown, 2006, for a practical example and Jöreskog, 1969, 1971, for the statistical background)). Figure 38.1 represents a 5-item scale measuring a common factor, or a true score representative of a unidimensional latent trait, with each item measuring the common factor with different levels of precision.

CFA provides a unified statistical model procedure to evaluate different aspects of the underlying measurement models. For instance, evaluation of the factor loadings provides evidence of the extent to which an item appears to be related to the underlying latent factor. Thus, evidence can be obtained to evaluate whether or not an item appears to be functioning in the manner expected, given it was expected to contribute significantly to the measurement of the latent factor. Items with small or insignificant factor loadings could be considered for deletion from the instrument or in need of reworking and further field-testing.

Another attribute of CFA that makes it an attractive method for testing measurement models is that it has a number of well-known and highly utilized measures of model fit, for example, Tucker-Lewis Index (TLI) and Root Mean Square Error of Approximation (RMSEA), to gauge the extent to which the intended model comports with the observed data (Bollen, 1989; Brown, 2006; Cheung & Rensvold, 2002; Hu & Bentler, 1999). Additionally, CFA is easily used within the context of structural equation models to help test the interrelations between numerous variables of interest (Bollen, 1989) and to test not only the measurement models of the measuring instruments but hypothesized relationships between variables of interest.

A potentially useful application of CFA is for scoring student responses across items to obtain an overall score on the factor of interest. When items measuring a common factor, or common latent trait, provide different levels of measurement precision then a simple summation of those item scores can result in less than optimal scoring for the common factor (Lord, 1980). Additionally, this would contradict some of the basic assumptions of the classical theory of tests (Lord & Novick, 1968; McDonald, 1999). Obtaining optimal scoring is critically important for making inferences about student scores and can help to reduce the random error associated with statistical tests (Shadish, Cook, & Campbell, 2002), which is important for interpretation of research results. The congeneric model evaluated within the context of CFA can utilize the measurement model to differentially weight items and improve upon simple summation.

Item Response Theory for Modeling Rating Scales

For decades, CTT was the underlying methodology for constructing psychological and educational tests (Crocker & Algina, 1986; Gulliksen, 1950; Lord & Novick, 1968). Recent movement in the field of psychometrics has highlighted some of the inherent problems with CTT and the emerging utility of item response theory (IRT) to overcome those problems (Embretson, 1995; Embretson & Reise, 2000; Fischer & Molenaar, 1995; Hambleton, Swaminathan, & Rogers, 1991; Thorndike, 1982; van der Linden & Hambleton, 1997). IRT addresses many of the same issues as those outlined above with the CFA implementation of the congeneric measurement model.

Analysis of item level data can be facilitated through the use of a particular set of item response models derived from the work of Georg Rasch (Andersen, 1997; Bond & Fox, 2001; Rasch, 1980). Numerous advantages of the Rasch model have been outlined (Keeves & Masters, 1999; Wright & Masters, 1982). A specific model in the family of Rasch models (Wright, 1999) has been developed to address issues with calibrating items structured in an ordered category response manner called the Rating Scale Model (RSM; Andrich, 1978a, 1978b, 1999; Wright & Masters, 1982).

The RSM provides a method for scaling the internal transition from one category response within an item to the subsequent category. Rather than simply providing an integer value to each subsequently higher category, each item has a set of internal thresholds that provides information about the progression from each sequential category, for example, from the Disagree to the Agree categories. The RSM takes the ordered categories and transforms them into a linear scale (Bond & Fox, 2001; Wright & Masters, 1982). One assumption of the model is that the category scores and thus the thresholds are similar across all items in the scale (Andersen, 1997; Wright, 1999; Wright & Masters, 1982).

The RSM is based on a probability model for an individual choosing category k, for example, Strongly Agree (SA), on an item as opposed to choosing the adjacent category, $k - 1$, for example, Agree (A). The RSM is intended to provide a set of threshold parameters within each item that specifies the transition from one category to the adjacent category (see Fig. 38.3 for an example using a single item). The relative values of the thresholds suggest the higher ratings indicate higher levels of agreement with the items. The RSM can be written as follows:

$$\phi_{nik} = \frac{\pi_{n,i,k}}{\pi_{n,i,k-1} + \pi_{n,i,k}} = \frac{e^{[\beta_n - (\delta_i + \tau_k)]}}{1 + e^{[\beta_n - (\delta_i + \tau_k)]}} \quad (38.2)$$

which represents the probability of person n responding to item i with category k is the ratio of that person scoring in category k on item i to the sum of the probability of scoring in category k and $k - 1$. Thus, the resulting form provides a person estimate for their position on the variable being measured, β_n, a scale value for each item, δ_i, and the threshold values for the number of categories of responses minus one, τ_k.

Each item on the scale would provide information about the ease for which a person high on engagement would respond positively to the item. For instance, given two items on the Peer Support at School scale (SEI; Appleton et al., 2006), the item with the higher scale value would indicate that students needed a higher level of feelings of engagement to respond positively. Put another way, if a student were responding to two different items, then they would potentially choose a lower category on the item with the higher scale value than they would on the item with a lower scale value. Thus, the higher the scale value for an item, the more difficult it is to endorse a higher positive rating.

Examples of the Measurement Approaches: Evaluating the SEI

This section will provide an evaluation of the Student Engagement Instrument (SEI; Appleton et al., 2006) to highlight the measurement issues. First of all, CFA will be used to evaluate the intended 5-factor, correlated structure of the SEI using a congeneric measurement model. This will provide cross-validation evidence for support of the intended measurement model underlying the SEI. Next, we will highlight the use of the RSM as a complementary method to the CFA for calibrating the items for the 5-factor model and show some methods of evaluating the item statistics. Finally, we will highlight a potentially valuable measurement model called the bifactor model that could potentially be useful in disentangling the complex issues related to measuring student engagement.

All results were based on the same sample of students ($N=1,796$). The sample was obtained from middle ($N=793$) and high ($N=1,003$) school students attending schools in Upper Midwest. The CFA and bifactor models were analyzed using MPlus 4.1 software (Muthén & Muthén, 1998–2005) and the RSM analysis used WinSteps 3.69 (Linacre, 2007). Common metrics for evaluating CFA models (Bollen, 1989; Brown, 2006; Hu & Bentler, 1999) and RSM models (Bond & Fox, 2001; Fischer & Molenaar, 1995; Linacre, 2007; Wright & Masters, 1982) were used to interpret the empirical fit of the data to the underlying models.

The Student Engagement Instrument

The Student Engagement Instrument (SEI: Appleton et al., 2006) was constructed to measure five important subtypes of student engagement falling within two broad types of student engagement. The SEI measures two unique subtypes of cognitive engagement called Control and Relevance of School Work (Control) and Future Aspirations and Goals (Aspire). The affective type of engagement measures three unique subtypes called Teacher-Student Relationships (Teacher), Peer Support at School (Peer), and Family Support for Learning (Family). The three affective engagement subtypes support the measurement of the sense of belongingness through mutually positive relationships with important groups in the student's life, for example, family, teachers, and peers. Methods of evaluating the sense of belongingness can be done through eliciting a student's sense of the extent to which the important groups have respect and concern/caring for them and their learning performance (Battistich, Solomon, Watson, & Schaps, 1997; Davis, 2003; Wentzel, 1997).

The SEI is comprised of 33 items covering the five subtypes, which we will also refer to as factors in the following analysis. There is no item overlap between the scales. The five subtypes were expected to correlate positively. A visual representation of the SEI is provided in Fig. 38.2 where the circles represent the latent factors, the boxes represent the sets of items for which students respond on the rating scale, and the double-headed arrows represent the correlations between factors. The SEI uses the following ordered categories: Strongly Agree (SA), Agree (A), Disagree (D), and Strongly Disagree (SD). Higher scores represent higher levels of student engagement for each subtype.

Research has provided evidence of good score reliability and validity (Appleton et al., 2006; Betts, Appleton, Reschly, Christenson, & Huebner, 2010; Reschly, Betts, & Appleton, 2011). Additionally, recent research has suggested that the SEI provides invariant measurements across students from 6th to 12th grade and also across genders (Betts et al., 2010). This suggested that the factors being measured by the SEI probably are similar across genders and grades and could be used to follow students across their middle to high school years. Recent research (Reschly et al., 2011) has provided initial evidence of the strong relationship between motivation and cognitive engagement along with evidence for score validity to important outcomes thought to be related to engagement.

Fig. 38.2 Student engagement instrument measurement model with correlated factors. The latent engagement factors are represented by the *circles*, the set of items measuring the latent factors are represented by the *boxes*, and the *double-headed arrows* represent the correlations between factors

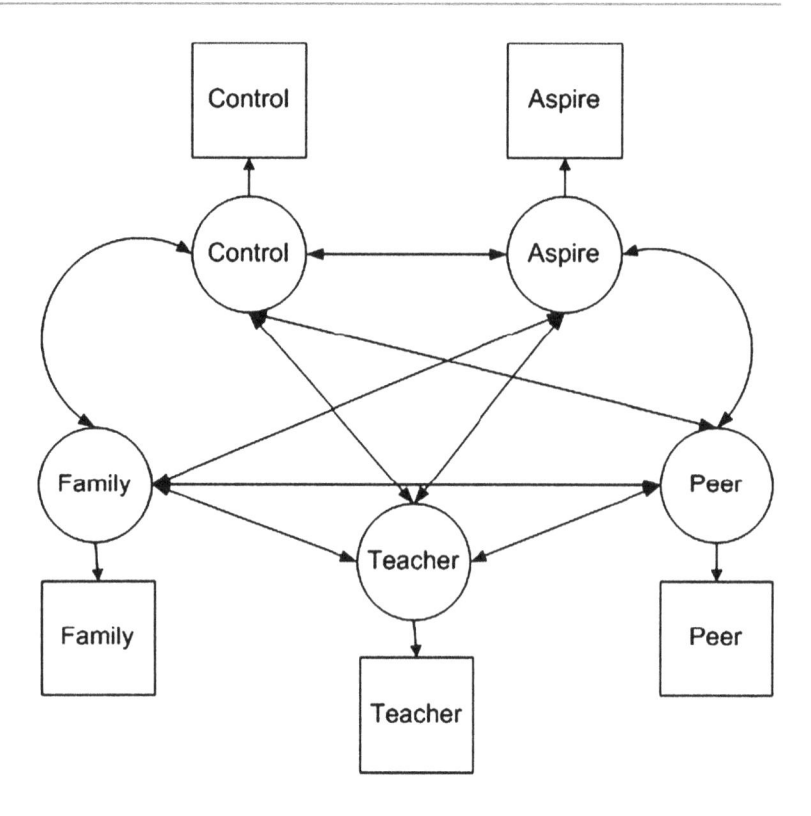

Cross-Validation of the SEI Using the Congeneric Measurement Model

Figure 38.2 is a visualization of the expected factor structure of the SEI. To evaluate the extent to which this model holds for the sample of middle and high school students, a CFA model was specified to test the correspondence between the intended measurement model based on the theoretical structure of the SEI and the observed response data. In Fig. 38.2, the boxes represent the set of items measuring the factors (shown in circles); however, rather than simply summing the items in the set to get a total score for each subtypes, the relationship was structured to be like that in Fig. 38.1 showing the congeneric measurement model. Thus, each factor in Fig. 38.2 has the measurement model structure of Fig. 38.1, and each factor was specified to be correlated (represented by the double-headed arrows) with all other factors. For this model, simple structure was enforced with all items measuring only the one intended factor with no cross-loadings. The first item on each scale had its unstandardized factor loading set to unity to set the scale for that factor, but all other factor loadings were freely estimated. Additionally, the correlations between factors were freely estimated.

Results suggested good to excellent fit of the data to the model, $\chi^2(485) = 6839.98$, CFI = .92, TLI = .92, RMSEA = .047, and SRMR = .044. The probability that the RMSEA was less than or equal to .05 was >.99 suggesting that the RMSEA was probably below the level suggesting excellent model fit. All the fit indexes suggested that the intended model fit the observed data very well and could probably not be rejected. Thus, this cross-validation sample provided evidence of the stability of the SEI in a new sample from the intended population of use. Table 38.1 provides the reliability estimates for the factors (the first entry on the diagonal) and the correlations between the factors (below the diagonal on the lower triangle). These reliability estimates and

Table 38.1 Reliabilities and correlations between factors in the 5-factor SEI model

	Teacher	Control	Peer	Aspire	Family
Teacher	**.74/.84**	.64	.47	.43	.47
Control	.70	**.70/.79**	.38	.56	.51
Peer	.49	.39	**.76/.76**	.39	.41
Aspire	.48	.71	.41	**.80/.70**	.52
Family	.54	.62	.47	.61	**.79/.67**

Note: IRT model results are above the diagonal, and CFA results are below the diagonal. Reliability estimates are given in bold on the diagonal with CFA results before the IRT results

correlation levels are similar to those found in previous research on the SEI (Appleton et al. 2006; Betts et al., 2010), providing evidence of score stability and interrelations between factors to be similar in this sample when compared to other samples.

Utilizing the Rating Scale Model for the SEI

We calibrated the items for each factor independently for the RSM in order to derive five independent scales. Table 38.2 provides the item level statistics for all 33 items. The Measure variable in Table 38.2 provides the calibrated value for each item, with the lower values suggesting somewhat easier ability for respondents to make positive responses. For instance on the Teacher-Student Relationships scale, the item "At my school, teachers care about students" has a value of −0.44 which suggested it was somewhat easier to agree with than the item asking, "The school rules are fair," which had a value of 0.74.

Figure 38.3 provides an example of the response model for the "I feel safe at school" item from the Teacher-Student Relationships scale. The vertical axis is a probability metric and the horizontal axis is the person ability score, or in this case, a linear measure of affective engagement related to teacher-student context. The figure shows the relationship between levels of engagement and the probability of answering with one of the four categorical answer choices. For instance, if one had a low level of engagement, say a value of −2.00, then the most likely category response for the student would be within the Strongly Disagree. However, a student with a higher level of engagement with a score of 1.75 would be more inclined to agree with the statement.

To evaluate the fit of the data to the intended measurement model, mean-square-based statistics called Infit and Outfit were utilized. Common interpretations of these fit statistics suggest that values between 0.5 and 1.5 are deemed productive for measurement, values less than 0.5 or between 1.5 and 2.0 are less productive but not degrading to measurement, but values over 2.0 are deemed to degrade the measurement system (Linacre, 2007). Using these heuristics as lower and upper bound magnitudes, all items appear to provide useful measurement of the intended factors. Additionally, all the items show a good level of relationship between item scores and the total score for the factor with all item-total correlations (given in the last column) except two below .60. The two items with item-total correlations of .58 also show higher levels on both Infit and Outfit statistics, but not high enough to be considered to degrade measurement.

Utilizing the Bifactor Model for the SEI

The bifactor model was originally developed as a model for exploring individual differences in the domain of intelligence assessment (Holzinger & Swineford, 1937; Thomson, 1948) and has recently been incorporated into a general psychometric model for educational and psychological measurements (Gibbons & Hedeker, 1992). Figure 38.4 provides a visualization of the model using the SEI and shows that each set of items written to measure a specific and unique subtype in the boxes is caused by two factors, a general and group level factor. The group level factors in this example are the five SEI subtype/factors that represent specific aspects of engagement. The general factor is seen as a factor underlying all the items and could be interpreted as a general engagement variable.

Table 38.2 RSM item calibration values, fit statistics, and item-total correlations by scale for the five-factor SEI model

Items	Measure	Infit	Outfit	Item-total
Teacher-student relationships (teacher)				
Overall, adults at my school treat students fairly	0.08	0.89	0.87	.74
Adults at my school listen to the students	0.13	0.91	0.89	.73
At my school, teachers care about students	−0.44	0.75	0.71	.77
My teachers are there for me when I need them	−0.22	0.85	0.83	.73
The school rules are fair	0.74	1.22	1.25	.67
Overall, my teachers are open and honest with me	−0.41	0.89	0.85	.73
I enjoy talking to the teachers here	0.08	1.00	0.99	.72
I feel safe at school	−0.46	1.36	1.32	.63
Most teachers at my school are interested in me as a person, not just as a student	0.51	1.07	1.08	.70
Control and relevance of school work (control)				
The tests in my classes do a good job of measuring what I am able to do	0.37	1.00	0.99	.64
Most of what is important to know you learn in school	0.14	0.88	0.90	.66
The grades in my classes do a good job of measuring what I am able to do	0.19	1.18	1.16	.66
What I am learning in my classes will be important in my future	−0.87	0.94	0.90	.68
After finishing my schoolwork, I check it over to see if it is correct	1.09	0.96	1.01	.63
When I do schoolwork, I check to see whether I understand what I am doing	−0.19	0.84	0.84	.65
Learning is fun because I get better at something	0.12	0.93	0.92	.67
When I do well in school, it is because I work hard	−1.31	0.98	0.96	.62
I feel like I have a say about what happens to me at school	0.46	1.29	1.31	.58
Peer support at school (peer)				
Other students at school care about me	0.64	0.79	0.75	.81
Students at my school are there for me when I need them	1.05	0.91	0.92	.73
Other students here like me the way I am	0.07	0.97	0.92	.75
I enjoy talking to the students here	−0.87	1.07	1.07	.72
Students here respect what I have to say	1.62	0.99	1.05	.73
I have some friends at school	−2.52	1.31	1.40	.58
Future aspirations and goals (aspire)				
I plan to continue my education following high school	−0.31	0.87	0.87	.79
Going to school after high school is important	0.00	0.99	0.97	.76
School is important for achieving my future goals	0.32	0.87	0.87	.79
My education will create many future opportunities for me	0.05	1.05	1.06	.74
I am hopeful about my future	−0.06	1.18	1.15	.70
Family support for learning (family)				
My family/guardian(s) are there for me when I need them	−0.57	1.06	1.01	.76
When I have problems at school, my family/guardian(s) are willing to help me	0.26	0.83	0.80	.83
When something good happens at school, my family/guardian(s) want to know about it	0.88	1.01	1.03	.79
My family/guardian(s) want me to keep trying when things are tough at school	−0.57	1.10	1.08	.72

It is also noticeable from the model that the group factors and the general factor are uncorrelated. This model assumes the general factor extracts what is common to all the items on the scale and then extracts the group factors from the residual correlations between the items measuring a specific engagement factor. The utility of this type of a model might help to parse out some of the concern about the relationship between engagement and motivation. For instance, if motivation is a necessary condition for engagement, then some sense of motivation should underlie all aspects of engagement, as the student would be motivated and goal directed to act in a manner that suggests engagement. Therefore, it might be hypothesized that a common factor underlying all specific and potentially unique aspects of engagement would be some type or level of motivation. The use of the bifactor model could potentially be used to evaluate a model

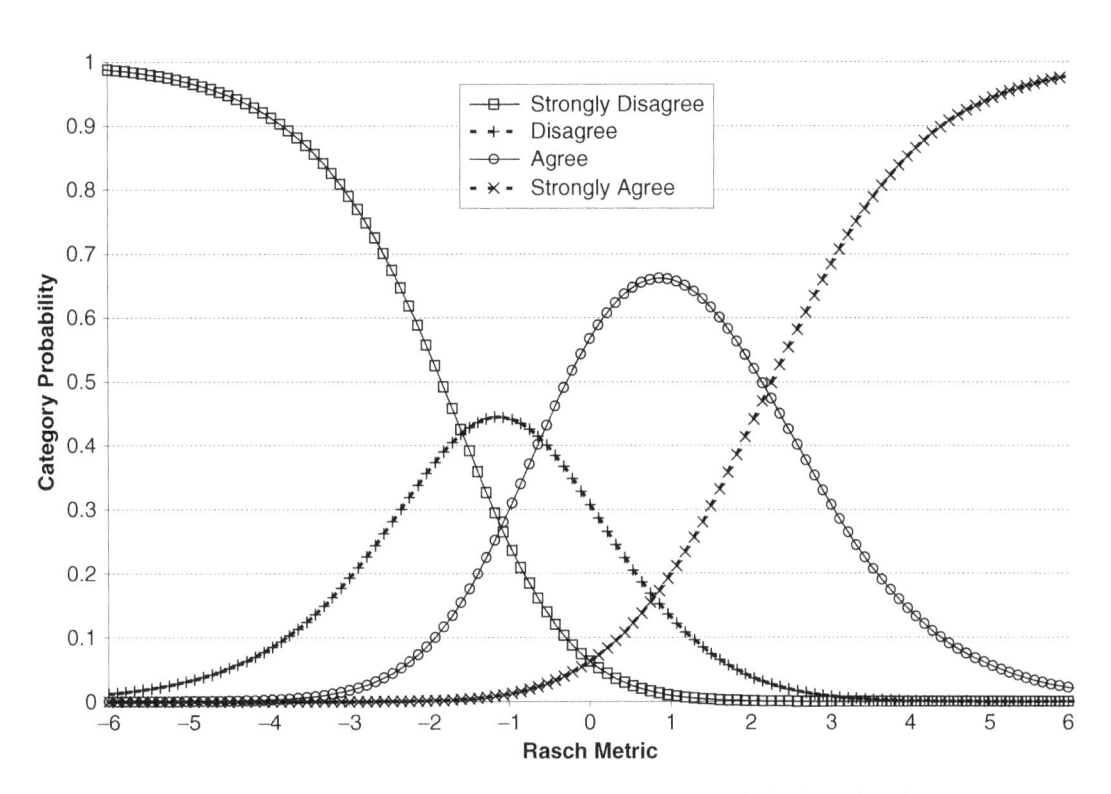

Fig. 38.3 Category probabilities and the smoothed response curves for item "I feel safe at school"

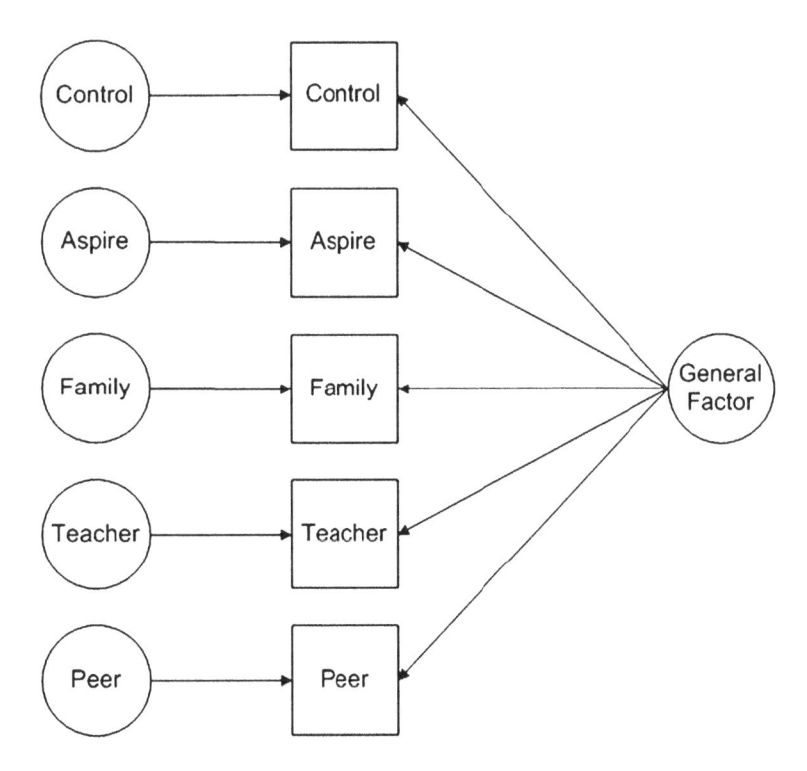

Fig. 38.4 Visualization of the bifactor model for the SEI where the general factor is a latent factor underlying responses to all the items and the group factors, control to peer, are group factors that explain the variance over and above the general factor for independent sets of items. *Note*: (1) The error terms for the latent variables have been left off the figure for clarity, and (2) there is no correlation between any of the factors, as the bifactor model assumes the factors are independent and therefore uncorrelated

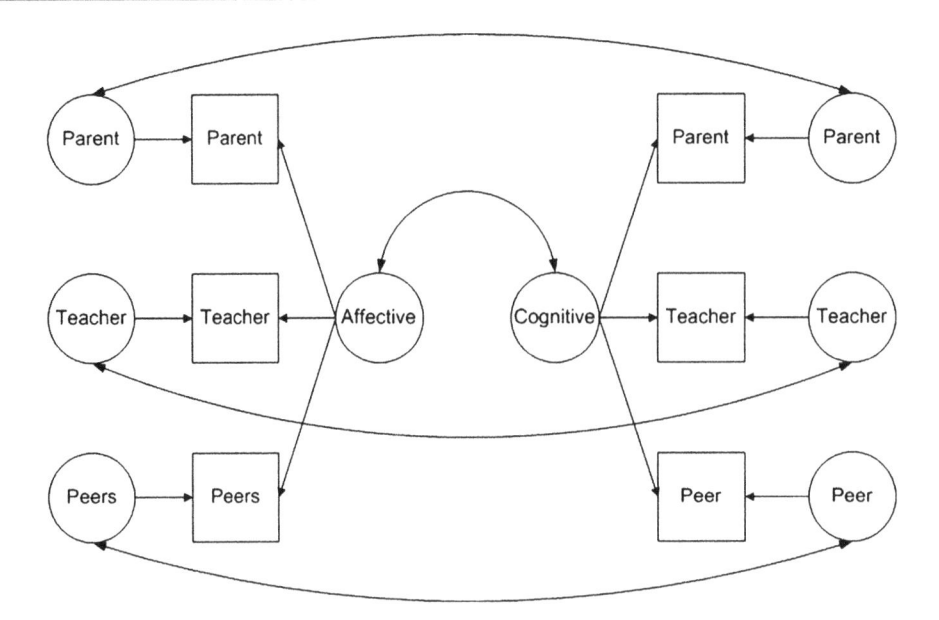

Fig. 38.5 Hypothetical use of the bifactor model to measure relationships between important types of engagement and social relations

such as this by entertaining the hypothesis that the general factor underlying all the engagement variables is a proxy for motivation and therefore would be more highly related to motivation than the group factors, which would be more specific aspects of engagement. Additionally, the model could be used to support a measurement model that had, for instance, a general factor related to one of the broad types of engagement such as cognitive engagement and group factors related to specific aspects of cognitive engagement.

Furthermore, this model could be extended beyond just measurement models to testing relationships between variables of interest. Figure 38.5 provides a possible approach to generalizing the bifactor model to measure two broad types of engagement, cognitive and affective, along with three specific contexts related to important social relationships, with parents, teachers, and peers. Here, the bifactor model could represent the relationships with the cognitive and affective engagement factors independently, and then allow for there to be a correlations between these general engagement factors. Furthermore, it could allow for correlations between the group factors of each type of engagement that were related to a similar context or subtype/component of the broad engagement type. For instance, there might be a specific factor related to parents that affect cognitive engagement and a specific factor that affects emotional engagement independently, but, as both are related to the same parental context, there might be some level of relationship between the two factors over and above that relating simply to engagement. We will explore a model similar to this with the SEI data as represented in Fig. 38.6 but without the restriction of having similar group level variables across cognitive and affective engagement.

Initial Bifactor Results

Using the bifactor structure in Fig. 38.4, the data were analyzed to evaluate the extent to which the SEI fits this intended model. To specify the model, all initial items on a factor were set to unity to set the scale, and all correlations were fixed at zero to model independent factors. Results suggested there was evidence of good fit of the data to the model, $\chi^2(462) = 6054.19$, CFI = .93, TLI = .92, RMSEA = .045, and SRMR = .047. The probability

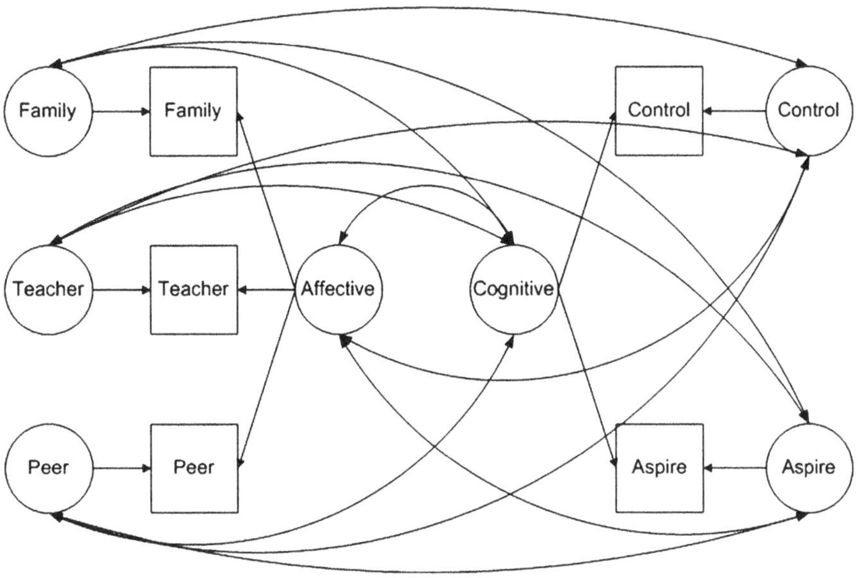

Fig. 38.6 Extended bifactor model for analyzing the SEI. The affective and cognitive factors act as general factors from the bifactor model. The group factors for affective are family, teacher, and peer, and the group factors for cognitive are control and aspire. In this model, there are correlations between the general and group factors of affective with the general and group factors of cognitive

that the RMSEA was less than or equal to .05 was >.99 suggesting that the RMSEA was probably below the level suggesting excellent model fit.

Thus, a model that posits a general engagement factor underlying item responses and unique factors related to the five group factors appeared to represent the structure in the data rather well. These results suggest that it could be possible to conceive of an engagement model with a broad general factor accounting for variation in student responses across various important areas of engagement types, but also allow for the measurement of those specific factors of interest. This could also provide initial evidence for a few hypotheses: (1) Is the general factor really a factor related to motivation that underlies all impetuses to enact in goal-oriented behavior?; or (2) Is there really a single engagement factor that broadly defines engagement and that the types of engagement, as suggested by the modifiers cognitive, behavioral, or emotional, are specific instances of that broad factor expressed in different contexts?; or (3) Is engagement really a multidimensional construct or, as the bifactor model suggests, some space between a single dimension and multidimensional?

Extended Bifactor Model

Evaluating the model for the SEI represented in Fig. 38.6 suggested good fit of the data to this model also, $\chi^2(451) = 5658.19$, CFI = .93, TLI = .92, RMSEA = .044, and SRMR = .074. The probability that the RMSEA was less than or equal to .05 was >.99 suggesting that the RMSEA was probably below the level suggesting excellent model fit. While the model fit very well, there were some interesting results from the correlations between the factors (see Table 38.3). Four of the 12 correlations were not significantly different from zero. It is important to note that the correlations here will be different, in most cases, from the correlations presented earlier in Table 38.1. The reason for this is that the correlations between the group factors in this model are computed after the variation related to the general factor has been extracted.

Table 38.3 Correlations between factors in the bifactor model

	Affective	Teacher	Peer	Family
Cognitive	.41	.12	--	.41
Control	.53	.10	--	--
Aspire	.08	--	.17	.12

Note: Correlations significant at the $p < .05$ level are given, and "--" indicates nonsignificant correlations. No adjustments were made for multiple comparisons

The general factors for affective and cognitive engagement were found to have a significant correlation ($r=.41$). Thus, whatever the general source of variation underlying the cognitive factor and the variation underlying the affective factor only have moderate levels of correlation. This might suggest that the affective and cognitive types have some moderate level of relationship but also have some distinct differences.

Looking at the group variables, the largest correlation was found between the general Affective factor and the Control and Relevance of School Work group factor of cognitive domain ($r=.53$). This might suggest that there is some correspondence between emotional sense of well-being and positive relationship to school when the student feels in control of their work and sees the relevance for the work in which they are engaged. There was also a moderately high correlation ($r=.41$) between the general Cognitive factor and the Family Support group factor of the affective domain. This might suggest that some sense of support from one's family helps to elicit a sense of focus and willingness to exert cognitive effort to tackle difficult or new skills.

The Peer Support group factor was only slightly related to Future Aspirations ($r=.17$). This suggests that after partitioning out the general Affective factor from the Peer variable and the Cognitive factor from Future Aspirations, there was some level of residual correlation between these two group variables. This might suggest that as students feel more support from their peers in school, the more they aspire to maintain a commitment to furthering their education. Thus, a sense of well-being with peers might engender an aspirational outlook for future learning and educational achievement.

The results from this extension of the bifactor model provides for various theoretical positions to be evaluated. Only a few have been outlined here briefly. Not only would the significant correlations be interesting to follow up but also so would the nonsignificant relationships as these might suggest truly orthogonal variables. Moreover, nonsignificant relationships can be used to help elucidate theory. For instance, the lack of relationship between Teacher-Student Relationships and Control and Relevance of School Work has potentially interesting implications. However, any relationships found in the present research would need further evaluation and more rigorous replication in order to move beyond conjecture and would need to be contextualized within a useful theoretical framework.

Conclusion

This chapter highlighted some of the basic issues related to measuring student engagement. While the study of student engagement is just beginning, this line of research can profit from decades of inquiry in areas of psychology that have direct bearing on three main types of engagement: emotional, cognitive, and behavioral. The chapter has also hinted at some potentially interesting avenues of future research. The study of engagement could bear great fruit as it is not only an important variable in educational and psychological research but it also has potentially interesting intersections with other areas of well-established research lines.

At present, the measurement of engagement is still inchoate and thus provides unparalleled opportunity to explore the structure of the multifarious nature of engagement. Appropriate measurement is vital to support the ongoing investigation of engagement, as poor measurement leads to poor and potentially difficult to interpret results. Some possible research-related scenarios within the context of developing useful and meaningful measures were presented. It is quite likely that the development of appropriate measures of the different types and subtypes of engagement can also foster a more coherent theory of engagement as the abstract must contend with reality, but such is the nature of science.

Two general models for constructing and evaluating measures of engagement were highlighted. The congeneric measurement model was displayed within the context of confirmatory factor analysis (CFA). This model provided an extension of the classical theory of test and is robust to violations of the stringent assumptions of the classical test theory. Using CFA has a direct benefit of numerous and historically documented approaches to evaluating model fit which can be beneficial for evaluating expected results. Modern item response theory (IRT) was used to exemplify a methodology for calibrating items on a rating scale to provide a linear measure. This chapter used only one of a number of potentially useful models for rating scale data called the rating scale model.

These statistical methods for evaluating engagement instruments can be used productively together. While the above analysis was done to show the basics of each approach, combining the CFA and IRT approaches can be complementary. For instance, the CFA model can help to provide information about the overall measurement model expected from the instrument, and the IRT model can help to identify items that appear to degrade measurement. Thus, the ongoing development of a measuring instrument can use both approaches in a reciprocal and recursive manner to evaluate the items and the scales being constructed.

This chapter also described a potentially useful CFA model called the bifactor model. Not only can this model provide an interesting approach to instrument development, it can also provide a unique method for evaluating complex relationships. Two different types of models were highlighted here: the basic bifactor model for all five subtypes of engagement on the SEI and an extension of the model thought to describe the relationships between two general types and their related subtypes of engagement. This type of modeling can also be useful in disentangling the relationship between cognitive engagement and motivation and would constitute an interesting line of research.

Overall, the study of student engagement is an important venture in educational and psychological research. Many open questions still exist, and basic definitions and relationships between important variables remain open for investigation. However, measurement of the variables of interest is a necessity before any quantitative research program can move forward, and appropriate measurement is needed to ensure that the research is based on a firm foundation. Hopefully this chapter will provide insights or inspirations to engender the development of new and important measures of student engagement to move the field forward and beyond.

Appendix

Glossary of Terms

Bifactor model a model devised in early research into individual differences in intelligence. The model posits that there is a general factor that underlies responses and that there are also uncorrelated group factors that account for substantial residual variation between the responses.

Bijective is a functional relationship that places all elements of one set into a one-to-one correspondence with all of the elements of another set.

Confirmatory factor analysis a robust and well-researched method of analyzing the relationship between observed variables and latent variables where restrictions are placed on the model to test or provide confirmatory evidence of latent structure.

Congeneric measurement an extension of the classical theory of tests that allowed for relaxation of restrictions inherent in classical test theory and elucidated the relationship between confirmatory factor analysis and test analysis.

Cross-loadings when items have significant positive factor loadings across two or more latent factors.

Factor loadings the relationship between an observed variable and the hypothetical latent variable.

Fit indexes statistical tests that evaluate the extent to which observed data conform to an intended model structure. Infit and Outfit are two examples of fit indices used to examine the Rasch models.

Item response theory a modern method of test scoring that utilizes an underlying probability model to place examinee ability and item difficulty on the same scale.

Latent variable a variable that is not directly observable. A variable hypothesized to underlie responses to sets of items or variables, often designated as a hypothetical construct.

Rating scale a method of obtaining and scoring responses to items that have response categories that represent increases in the magnitude of the variable those items define.

Score reliability stability or consistency of scores on a test.

Score validity the ongoing process of gathering evidence to support the inferences from scores and all intended interpretations.

References

Alexander, K., Entwisle, D., & Horsey, C. (1997). From first grade forwards: Early foundations of high school dropouts. *Sociology of Education, 70*, 87–107.

Andersen, E. (1997). The rating scale model. In W. van der Linden & R. Hambleton (Eds.), *Handbook of modern item response theory* (pp. 67–84). New York: Springer.

Andrich, D. (1978a). A rating formulation for ordered response categories. *Psychometrika, 43*, 561–573.

Andrich, D. (1978b). Applications of a psychometric rating model to ordered categories which are scored with successive integers. *Applied Psychological Measurement, 2*, 581–594.

Andrich, D. (1999). Rating scale analysis. In G. Masters & J. Keeves (Eds.), *Advances in measurement in educational research and assessment* (pp. 110–121). New York: Pergamon.

Appleton, J., Christenson, S., & Furlong, M. (2008). Student engagement with schools: Critical conceptual and methodological issues of the construct. *Psychology in the Schools, 54*, 369–386.

Appleton, J., Christenson, S., Kim, D., & Reschly, A. (2006). Measuring cognitive and psychological engagement: Validation of the Student Engagement Instrument. *Journal of School Psychology, 44*, 427–445.

Balfanz, R., Herzog, L., & Mac Iver, D. (2007). Preventing student disengagement and keeping students on the graduation path in urban middle-grades schools: Early identification and effective intervention. *Educational Psychologist, 42*, 223–235.

Bartholomew, D., & Knott, M. (1999). *Latent variable models and factor analysis* (2nd ed.). New York: Oxford Press.

Battistich, V., Solomon, D., Watson, M., & Schaps, E. (1997). Caring school communities. *Educational Psychologist, 32*, 137–151.

Betts, J. E., Appleton, J. J., Reschly, A. L., Christenson, S. L., & Huebner, E. S. (2010). A study of the factorial invariance of the Student Engagement Instrument (SEI): Results from middle and high school students. *School Psychology Quarterly, 25*, 84–93.

Bloom, B. (Ed.). (1985). *Developing talent in young people*. New York: Ballantine Books.

Blumenfeld, P., Kempler, T., & Krajcik, J. (2006). Motivation and cognitive engagement in learning environments. In R. K. Sawyer (Ed.), *The Cambridge handbook of learning sciences* (pp. 475–488). New York: Cambridge University Press.

Bollen, K. (1989). *Structural equations with latent variables*. New York: Wiley.

Bond, T., & Fox, C. (2001). *Applying the Rasch model: Fundamental measurement in the human sciences*. Mahwah, NJ: Lawrence Erlbaum.

Brown, T. (2006). *Confirmatory factor analysis for applied research*. New York: The Guildford Press.

Cameron, J., & Pierce, W. (1994). Reinforcement, reward, and intrinsic motivation: A meta-analysis. *Review of Educational Research, 64*, 363–423.

Catalano, R., Kosterman, R., Hawkins, J., Newcomb, M., & Abbott, R. (1996). Modeling the etiology of adolescent substance use: A test of the social development model. *Journal of Drug Issues, 26*, 429–455.

Cheung, G., & Rensvold, R. (2002). Evaluating goodness-of-fit indexes for testing measurement invariance. *Structural Equation Modeling, 9*, 233–255.

Christenson, S., Reschly, A., Appleton, J., Berman, S., Spanjers, D., & Varro, P. (2008). Best practices in fostering student engagement. In A. Thomas & J. Grimes (Eds.), *Best practices in school psychology* (5th ed., pp. 1099–1119). Bethesda, MD: National Association of School Psychologists.

Crocker, L., & Algina, J. (1986). *Introduction to classical and modern test theory*. New York: Holt, Rinehart and Winston.

Davis, H. (2003). Conceptualizing the role and influence of student-teacher relationships in children's social and cognitive development. *Educational Psychologist, 38*, 207–234.

DeVellis, R. (2003). *Scale development: Theory and applications* (2nd ed.). Thousand Oaks, CA: Sage.

Downing, S., & Haladyna, T. (Eds.). (2006). *Handbook of test development*. Mahwah, NJ: Lawrence Erlbaum.

Embretson, S. (1995). The new rules of measurement. *Psychological Assessment, 8*, 341–349.

Embretson, S., & Reise, S. (2000). *Item response theory for psychologists*. Mahwah, NJ: Lawrence Erlbaum.

Finn, J. (1989). Withdrawing from school. *Review of Educational Research, 59*(2), 117–142.

Finn, J., & Rock, D. (1997). Academic success among students at risk for school failure. *Journal of Applied Psychology, 82*, 221–234.

Fischer, G., & Molenaar, I. (Eds.). (1995). *Rasch models: Foundations, recent developments, and applications*. New York: Springer.

Franken, R. (2001). *Human motivation* (5th ed.). Pacific Grove, CA: Brooks/Cole.

Fredricks, J., Blumenfeld, P., & Paris, A. (2004). School engagement: Potential of the concept, state of the evidence. *Review of Educational Research, 74,* 59–109.

Gibbons, R., & Hedeker, D. (1992). Full-information item bi-factor analysis. *Psychometrika, 57,* 423–436.

Gulliksen, H. (1950). *Theory of mental tests.* New York: Wiley.

Guo, J., Hawkins, J., Hill, K., & Abbott, R. (2001). Childhood and adolescent predictors of alcohol abuse and dependence in young adulthood. *Journal of Studies on Alcohol, 62,* 754–762.

Hambleton, R., Swaminathan, H., & Rogers, H. (1991). *Fundamentals of item response theory.* Newbury Park, CA: Sage.

Harman, H. (1967). *Modern factor analysis* (2nd ed.). Chicago: The University of Chicago Press.

Hawkins, J., & Weis, J. (1985). The social development model: An integrated approach to delinquency prevention. *Journal of Primary Prevention, 6,* 73–97.

Holzinger, K., & Swineford, F. (1937). The bi-factor method. *Psychometrika, 2,* 41–54.

Hu, L., & Bentler, P. (1999). Cutoff criteria for fit indexes in covariance structure analysis: Conventional criteria versus new alternatives. *Structural Equation Modeling, 6,* 1–55.

Jensen, A. (1998). *The g-factor: The science of mental ability.* Westport, CT: Praeger.

Jöreskog, K. (1969). A general approach to confirmatory maximum likelihood factor analysis. *Psychometrika, 34,* 183–202.

Jöreskog, K. (1971). Statistical analysis of sets of congeneric tests. *Psychometrika, 36,* 109–133.

Kane, M. (2006). Validation. In R. Brennan (Ed.), *Educational measurement* (4th ed., pp. 17–64). Westport, CT: Praeger.

Keeves, J., & Masters, G. (1999). Introduction. In G. Masters & J. Keeves (Eds.), *Advances in measurement in educational research and assessment* (pp. 1–19). New York: Pergamon.

Kleinginna, P., & Kleinginna, A. (1981). A categorized list of motivation definitions, with suggestions for a consensual definition. *Motivation and Emotion, 5,* 263–291.

Linacre, J. (2007). *A user's guide to WINSTEPS.* Author.

Lord, F. (1980). *Applications of item response theory to practical testing problems.* Hillsdale, NJ: Lawrence Erlbaum.

Lord, F., & Novick, M. with A. Birnbaum. (1968). *Statistical theories of mental test scores.* Reading, MA: Addison-Wesley.

McDonald, R. (1985). *Factor analysis and related methods.* Hillsdale, NJ: Lawrence Erlbaum.

McDonald, R. (1999). *Test theory: A unified treatment.* Mahwah, NJ: Lawrence Erlbaum.

Muthén, L., & Muthén, B. (1998–2005). *Mplus statistical analysis with latent variables: User's guide.* Los Angeles, CA: Muthén & Muthén.

Rasch, G. (1980). *Probabilistic models for some intelligence and attainment tests.* Chicago: The University of Chicago Press.

Reschly, A., Betts, J., & Appleton, J. (2011). An examination of the validity of two measures of student engagement. Manuscript submitted for publication.

Shadish, W., Cook, T., & Campbell, D. (2002). *Experimental and quasi-experimental designs for generalized causal inference.* New York: Houghton Mifflin.

Spector, P. (1992). *Summated rating scale construction: An introduction.* Newbury Park, CA: Sage.

Thomson, G. (1948). *The factorial analysis of human ability.* New York: Houghton Mifflin.

Thorndike, R. (1982). *Applied psychometrics.* Lawrenceville, NJ: Houghton Mifflin.

van der Linden, W., & Hambleton, R. (Eds.). (1997). *Handbook of modern item response theory.* New York: Springer.

Wainer, H., & Braun, H. (Eds.). (1988). *Test validity.* Hillsdale, NJ: Lawrence Erlbaum.

Wentzel, K. (1997). Student motivation in middle school: The role of perceived pedagogical caring. *Journal of Educational Psychology, 89,* 411–419.

Wentzel, K., & Wigfield, A. (2007). Motivational interventions that work: Themes and remaining issues. *Educational Psychologist, 42,* 261–271.

Wilson, M. (2005). *Constructing measures: An item response modeling approach.* Mahwah, NJ: Lawrence Erlbaum.

Wright, B. (1999). Rasch measurement models. In G. Masters & J. Keeves (Eds.), *Advances in measurement in educational research and assessment* (pp. 85–97). New York: Pergamon.

Wright, B., & Masters, G. (1982). *Rating scale analysis: Rasch measurement.* Chicago, IL: MESA.

Yen, W., & Fitzpatrick, A. (2006). Item response theory. In R. Brennan (Ed.), *Educational measurement* (4th ed., pp. 111–153). Westport, CT: Praeger.

Part V Commentary: Possible New Directions in the Measurement of Student Engagement

Karen M. Samuelsen

Abstract

Karen Samuelsen, a respected researcher and methodologist, provided commentary on the chapters in Part V of this volume. She described the difficulty of measuring latent constructs like student engagement. She argued for greater complexity in study designs and hypotheses to account for the complex nature of proposed relationships between engagement, contexts, and outcomes. She provided examples of how various statistical methods (Structural Equation Modeling, Differential Item Functioning) may be used to address some of the current measurement issues in engagement and outlined several areas of future research to advance the study of engagement.

Physical scientists would undoubtedly be frustrated if faced with inexact measurement instruments or inaccessible subjects. As an example, let us consider NASA scientists attempting to measure a crater on a distant planet. They would rail about the inaccuracy of the measurement of the depth of that crater, but they would have little doubt that it was depth they were attempting to measure. The only thing in question would be the level of accuracy they would be able to achieve.

The measurement of a psychological construct is a much trickier business, one that is so laden with error it is a wonder we ever attempt it at all. The first step in this process should be simple; it is to fully define what we are attempting to measure. Once that is done, we can write items explicating the said construct, pilot test the instrument, run statistical tests to investigate the inferences that can be drawn from it, and so on. Of course, those items will not cover every aspect of that psychological variable, no matter how carefully they are written. So what we are left with is a measurement of something related to our original construct but not exactly identical. The correlation between what we set out to measure and what we end up measuring is limited by the quality of our definition of that construct, with ill-defined constructs being measured more poorly than those that are well defined.

It is not really simple at all to define a construct in full since that definition often includes multiple dimensions that may be related to each other or to other constructs. Unfortunately, this is a step that is often glossed over by researchers who think that the definition of their construct must be evident to all. Given that construct definition is so important, I was particularly gratified

K. Samuelsen (✉)
Department of Educational Psychology and Instructional Technology, University of Georgia, Athens, GA, USA
e-mail: ksam@uga.edu

to see the extent to which all of the authors in this section explained their conception of engagement and clarified how this construct differs from motivation. Still, further discussion of construct definition seems relevant, so part of this chapter will be devoted to possible explorations that might help provide more nuance to our definitions of engagement.

Once we have adequately defined our construct, we give the items developed to a sample from the population of interest. At that point, more error creeps into our measurement. The people in our sample may respond inaccurately due to construct-irrelevant factors such as difficulty reading or a different understanding of certain ideas. This commentary will address the issue of construct-irrelevant item-specific factors, particularly as those pertain to differential item function. More systematic issues such as social desirability, acquiescence, and central tendency may also impact our measurement precision. Social desirability (the propensity to respond in a manner that would be deemed appropriate by most people) and acquiescence (the propensity to answer positively to all questions) will not be discussed in this commentary. However, central tendency will be addressed as it pertains to the investigation of differential item function.

Further Definition of the Construct

It occurs to me that the definition of engagement embodied in the Student Engagement Instrument (SEI: Appleton, Christenson, Kim, & Reschly, 2006) and other similar instruments may be more complex than is currently being modeled. Specifically, it seems that there could be compensatory relationships that are useful to consider. I will address two of these. First, consider the potential for a compensatory relationship between affective and cognitive engagement, particularly as these relate to the behavioral manifestations of engagement (e.g., days present at school, lack of negative incidents reported). Students with high levels of cognitive engagement and a low sense of affective engagement would still evidence high levels on those behavioral outcomes due to their need to get high grades or their need for cognitive stimulation. Similarly, students who are not cognitively engaged but have high levels of affective engagement might also evidence the same high "scores" on those behavioral outcomes because they want to please their parents or teachers.

This same rationale could hold true for the different sources of affective engagement: teacher-student relationships, peer support at school, and family support for learning. Students with high levels of peer and family support might be able to make up for poor teacher-student relationships. Likewise, the three measures of cognitive engagement encompassing control and relevance of school work, future aspirations and goals, and intrinsic motivation could interact in a compensatory fashion.

Whatever the nature of the compensatory structure, if such relationships exist, then reports such as the one provided by Appleton (2012) must be considerably more complex. It might not be appropriate to say that a student is at high risk because they evidence low levels of peer support at school. If the other forms of affective engagement were high enough to compensate for low levels of peer support, then that student might not be at high risk after all. On the other hand, there may be a threshold for peer support below which the other forms of affective engagement cannot compensate, in which case very low peer support is an important indicator. The point here is not to suggest precisely what the compensatory relationship is but rather to note that the possibility of such relationships means that the model for building and refining a dynamic, engagement-based assessment-to-intervention report might need to be more nuanced to isolate students who are truly at high risk. As Appleton (2012) noted, it is crucial to ensure that students designated for an intervention actually are in need of that intervention so that resources are not incorrectly and inefficiently allocated.

These sorts of structures can be modeled using compensatory IRT (item response theory) models, wherein the contributions of the different dimensions are additive. These models are sometimes applied to achievement tests where there are multiple ways to solve problems. For example, in mathematics there could be questions that can either be solved using addition or multiplication. In that case, students who do not know how to multiply can still respond correctly by adding. Students who respond incorrectly would be those who are low in terms of both addition and multiplication proficiency. It is important to note that the inferences made about students may be incorrect if a unidimensional model is applied in a situation that is actually multidimensional (Ackerman, 1992).

Compensatory structures, should they exist, could also be modeled within a structural equation modeling (SEM) framework; however, certain assumptions would need to be made. One such assumption could be that students who were high on affective engagement but low on cognitive engagement evidenced the same overall level of engagement as those who were high on the cognitive but low on affective. If this were the case, an interaction model could be employed with the levels of affective and cognitive engagement having both direct and interactive effects on engagement outcomes (Bandalos, 2011, personal communication). In this situation, the interactive effects would, in essence, be compensatory. If this assumption cannot be made, then it would be necessary to categorize both the levels of affective and cognitive engagement. From those categories, groups representing the different combinations (e.g., low cognitive/medium affective or high cognitive/low affective) can be formed, and hypotheses can be tested regarding each combination. Though making these assumptions seems less than optimal, the ability to use SEM and model causality is a compelling reason to want to try this method.

One final consideration in terms of fully explicating the construct of engagement is in considering the stability of the different dimensions over time. Questions such as the following should be investigated. Precisely how much variation in the different dimensions is "normal"? Is there more variability in some than in the others? Is this variation consistent across groups (gender, ethnic, socioeconomic status, etc.)? An understanding of this variation is vital if one is to create and use change reports similar to the one presented by Appleton in this volume.

The results from any psychological instrument are really just blurry snapshots of what is occurring at any given time. When constructs are stable, we expect to see similar snapshots at different time points. The problem in this case is that it seems unrealistic to expect the constructs to be stable. For example, it would be natural for teacher-student relationships to vary greatly, even within the same school year. Students may become disenchanted with a teacher if their grades are not good, or they may become more attached over time. In either case, the relationship is changing, meaning student responses on the SEI would change. To create change reports that are meaningful, it is necessary to quantify the difference between normal and problematic change and not just to classify problems based on a norm-referenced interpretation of change. Appleton noted that, "The current student-focused reports of academic year changes in engagement did not account for measurement error and further development is needed to include that consideration." I would concur and add that measurement error may be more complex and come from more sources than one might think.

Differential Item Function

Two of the chapters in this section touch on cultural diversity and the issue of whether the inferences one can draw about all respondents will be correct. Fredericks and McColskey (2012, pg. 779) stated, "If measures of engagement behave differently by race, SES, gender, and grade, and these differences are not taken into account, comparisons in the level of engagement or effects across groups are invalid" (Glanville & Wildhagen, 2007). Betts (2012) also discusses the idea of validity and introduces the concepts of measurement invariance and differential item function as one source of validity evidence. Though both chapters introduce this topic, neither gives it the attention I believe it merits.

A study of the equivalence of the Rosenberg Self-Esteem Scale (RSES) across cultures, which compared responses of almost 17,000 respondents across 53 countries (Schmitt & Allik, 2005), provides a case in point. Though the authors found the factor structure of the RSES to be replicated across most countries, they cautioned that differences between cultures can make using that scale problematic under certain conditions. Specifically, they noted that there is a tendency for individuals from some cultures to report lower levels of self-esteem on the negatively worded items on the scale, meaning their overall levels of self-esteem will be underreported. The authors also uncovered a neutral response bias in which people from collectivist cultures tended to avoid the extremes of the rating scale as compared to those from more individualistic cultures. Perhaps the most important finding was that the two dimensions of self-esteem, typically self-competence and self-esteem, seemed to vary across cultures, once again in a manner that was related to the individual/collectivist nature of the culture. As an example, Portes (2011) reported that when the RSES is administered to Japanese females, a two-factor solution emerges wherein the one factor is again self-respect, but the other factor is negative in nature. That second factor is characterized by feelings like uselessness, incompetence, praise rejection, and diffidence. In this structure, those who are dissatisfied with their own accomplishments and achievements may be the ones with the highest aspirations.

An open question is whether these sorts of findings regarding the RSES would be replicated in cross-cultural studies of either the SEI or, in a similar fashion, the *Me and My School* survey. Two recent studies may help to answer that. Moreira, Vaz, Dias, and Petracchi (2009) examined the psychometric properties of the SEI for a population different from that of the original validation study (Appleton et al., 2006); specifically, their study looked at 760 Portuguese high school students. Though the 6-factor structure of the original instrument was confirmed, the authors noted that some of the items loaded on different subscales. This raises questions about the comparability of the definitions of those dimensions across the original population of interest and this new group.

Another study (Betts, Appleton, Reschly, Christenson, & Huebner, 2010) investigated the factorial invariance of the SEI and confirmed the factor structure (3 affective and 2 cognitive), latent factor relationships, and score reliability across grades 6–12 and genders. However, these authors found issues when examining the item-level results in terms of a cross loading and more complicated error structure. Betts et. al (2010) stated (pg. 91), "These results portend the need for further replication research to examine the extent to which these deviations from expectations exist in different samples or whether it was just a byproduct of the present sample." I believe they are correct but would add that their findings could be caused by cultural differences in their samples.

Backing this empirical research on noninvariance is the literature on culture and engagement (for an overview, see Bingham and Okagaki, 2012). Cultural discontinuity theory posits that children raised in a distinct, minority culture often find themselves in schools where the values of the majority culture are endorsed at the expense of their own. According to the cultural discontinuity theory, this dissonance may make the child feel the need to choose one culture over the other, thereby making it impossible to be successful in both cultures. Cultural ecological theory asserts that the type of cultural minority is key, with involuntary minorities being the ones at risk when immersed within a dominant culture. Though these theories provide rationales for why the differences between the minority (sometimes ethnic) and mainstream cultures may influence student engagement, it seems less clear precisely how these cultural mismatches impact engagement. Does choosing to act like those in the dominant culture impact one's attitude regarding the relevance of school work and one's future aspirations and goals? Or are future aspirations the driver when it comes to student engagement regardless of cultural background? Do those from the cultural minority view teacher-student and peer relationships through the same lens as those from the cultural majority? Or do they see a relationship with a teacher or peer as a choice of another culture over one's own? The research on the impact of culture on engagement is inconclusive in terms of answering the sorts of questions I just posed, but there seems to be evidence that culture is related to engagement in some way.

Given that, it seems clear that studies must be undertaken to investigate this issue. One such type of study involves investigating differential item functioning (DIF). In educational settings, we say that DIF occurs "when examinees from different groups have different probabilities or likelihoods of success on an item, after they have been matched on the ability of interest" (Clauser & Mazor, 1998, pg. 31). Put more simply within the context of an example, if DIF is not present and we look at only the most able students, we find that males and females are equally likely to get an item right. This would hold true across the ability continuum. If DIF is present, at some abilities we might find that females have a higher probability of correctly answering an item than males; meaning the item is more difficult for males.

This concept is readily transferrable to instruments measuring psychological constructs, but our notion of what constitutes DIF must be expanded. In his chapter, Betts provided an explanation of the Rating Scale Model (RSM: Andrich, 1978). That will serve as a useful springboard for my discussion of DIF, starting with the RSM and extending to the more general Partial Credit Model (PCM: Masters, 1982).

As Betts (2012) noted, the RSM includes two item parameters: one describing the scale or location value for each item and the other capturing the threshold values. Examples from the SEI may help to explain the differences between these item parameters for those not accustomed to these types of models. Based on the output provided by Betts (2012), the following items are starkly different in terms of their scale values:
- What I'm learning in my classes will be important in my future.
- After finishing my schoolwork, I check it over to see if it's correct.

Not surprisingly, students are much less likely to agree with the latter item than the former. If we placed these items on a horizontal scale, the latter would be to the right since it is "more difficult" to agree with that item, or conversely, it is easier to disagree with it. If DIF were to exist with regard to this scaling parameter, we might see that minority students are less likely to see what they are learning to be important than their majority counterparts, *even after they are matched in terms of their levels of cognitive engagement.*

In terms of the threshold values describing the items, it is useful to refer to Fig. 38.3 provided by Betts (2012, pg. 797). The thresholds are the locations where the probabilities of choosing a specific category are equal. Graphically, we see that there are curves for each of the response options: strongly disagree, disagree, agree, and strongly disagree. The first threshold is where the strongly disagree curve crosses the disagree curve; this occurs at approximately −1.7 on the Rasch metric. Another threshold occurs where the disagree curve crosses the agree curve (at approximately −0.6), and the final threshold is where the agree curve crosses the strongly agree curve (at approximately 2.3 on that same metric). This figure represents a single item, but the RSM assumes the same pattern of the first two crossing locations being relatively close together, and the final one quite distant, would be found for all items, just shifted up or down the x-axis for the different items.

This pattern indicates that people with extremely low levels of affective engagement will tend to strongly disagree with the items. A relatively small percentage of people are likely to disagree; those are the respondents whose level of affective engagement would measure between −1.7 and −0.6 on a standardized metric. We can contrast this with the relatively large percentage of respondents, between −0.6 and 2.3 on this metric, who are most likely to agree with the items. The respondents above that level would most likely strongly agree with the affective engagement items. An alternative way to express this would be to say that relatively small changes in one's level of affective engagement would result in a change from strongly disagreeing to agreeing, while a larger change is necessary for one to go from disagreeing to strongly agreeing.

Schmitt and Allik (2005), in their study of the RSES, found that people from collectivist cultures may exhibit a neutral response bias, meaning they have a tendency to not use extremes on that psychological scale. If the same were to hold true with regard to student engagement, we might see DIF with regard to these thresholds, meaning the locations of those thresholds would be different for those from collectivist versus individualist cultures. Specifically, we would expect to see the first and last thresholds pushed further to the extremes, meaning one from a collectivist culture would need to have an extremely low level of affective engagement (as an example) before he/she would be willing to strongly disagree or an extremely high level of engagement to be willing to strongly agree. Under this scenario, it would be very difficult to make appropriate inferences about respondents, especially those with average levels of affective engagement. One would have to wonder whether those average levels were due to the truth about the respondents or were aberrant findings due to the neutral response bias.

The PCM frees the constraint on the RSM that the pattern of thresholds is the same across items. Instead, these patterns are estimated freely for each item. Using the PCM, we can again have DIF at the item level, but even more specifically at the level of the threshold. As an example, let us consider the item from the SEI that states "I feel safe at school." It seems possible for minority and nonminority students who are matched in terms of their affective engagement to respond to this item differently. Only nonminority students who were extremely disengaged might strongly disagree with this statement, meaning the threshold between disagree and strongly disagree would be extremely low. Minority students, on the other hand, might think about safety quite differently, and highly engaged students might still feel unsafe, meaning that the threshold under consideration would be higher.

The presence of DIF, whether at the item or threshold level, means that scores from different groups are not comparable. Therefore, the inferences made regarding respondents are compromised. In educational assessment, differential item functioning indicates that multidimensionality exists due to the presence of some nuisance dimensions (Ackerman, 1992). For psychological measurement, where multidimensionality is often the norm, the presence of DIF could again signal the presence of a nuisance dimension or dimensions. However, it could also mean that there are differences in the manner in which respondents utilize the rating scale itself, or that the underlying factor structure differs between the groups under consideration.

In the mid-1990s, researchers began applying DIF procedures that had traditionally been used with dichotomous items to the examination of polytomous, generally ordinal, items (see Zwick & Thayer, 1996 as an example of research from that time). The problem with these traditional methods was that they yielded a single measure of DIF for each item, thereby providing no information regarding what about the item or items was problematic. The body of research on methods for examining DIF for polytomous items has grown significantly over the last several years. One of the two predominant frameworks that have emerged would be differential step function (see Penfield, Gattamorta, & Childs, 2009 for an overview) which provides the more nuanced information discussed in the prior paragraphs. Polytomous DIF can also be studied within an SEM framework using the Multiple Indicators/Multiple Causes (MIMIC) models (see Finch, 2005 for a comparison with non-SEM methods). This too provides a mechanism for examining DIF from a variety of perspectives.

Final Thoughts

This chapter has focused on potential new directions for the study of student engagement and in doing so discussed some rather complicated models. As the substantive and measurement models for engagement get more complex, it is useful to remember the assumptions that underlie these models and to test those assumptions or at least question them. Evidence regarding linearity, normality, and factor analyzability can be gathered quite easily with scatter plots, descriptive statistics, and simple statistical tests. This evidence should be provided so the reader knows the degree to which solutions might be degraded. On that same topic of providing the reader with information, standard errors should also be calculated and reported whenever possible.

Assumptions go beyond these well-known statistical ones, however. For example, consider something as simple as the fact that a 4-point

Likert-like scale is used in the SEI with strongly disagree, disagree, agree, and strongly agree being the response options. This choice is also an assumption of a sort and as such should be tested. The question should be: Is 4 scale points the appropriate number? The even number pushes respondents to choose to either agree or disagree without giving them the option of neither agreeing nor disagreeing. When a middle or neutral option is provided, it does become a catchall for respondents who are truly neutral, those who are unsure, and those who are confused; so I understand trying to avoid the neutral option. But what about 6 scale points? Since data from SEI have been factor analyzed and 5 or more ordinal levels are generally recommended to minimize bias in the parameter estimates, 4 seems an odd choice. However, it is possible that if 6 scale points were used, respondents would not use two of the options, resulting in a 4-point scale anyway.

I come back to my initial point that the measurement of latent variables is difficult. It requires patience and a commitment to continually gather evidence. I encourage researchers to continue to develop a richer model of the relationships between and within the affective and cognitive dimensions of student engagement and to more fully investigate the invariance of this model. At the same time, those researchers must be diligent about investigating all of the assumptions underlying that model and communicating information related to the reliability of their measurements to the reader. Without this foundation to rest upon, that rich model has little value.

References

Ackerman, T. A. (1992). A didactic explanation of item bias, item impact, and item validity from a multidimensional perspective. *Journal of Educational Measurement, 29*(1), 67–91.

Andrich, D. (1978). Application of a psychometric model to ordered categories which are scored with successive integers. *Applied Psychological Measurement, 2*, 581–594.

Appleton, J. J. (2012). Systems consultation: Developing the assessment-to-intervention link with the Student Engagement Instrument. In S. L. Christenson, A. L. Reschly, & C. Wylie (Eds.), *Handbook of research on student engagement* (pp. 725–741). New York: Springer.

Appleton, J. J., Christenson, S. L., Kim, D., & Reschly, A. L. (2006). Measuring cognitive and psychological engagement: Validation of the Student Engagement Instrument. *Journal of School Psychology, 44*, 427–445.

Betts, J. E. (2012). Issues and methods in the measurement of student engagement: Advancing the construct through statistical modeling. In S. L. Christenson, A. L. Reschly, & C. Wylie (Eds.), *Handbook of research on student engagement* (pp. 783–803). New York: Springer.

Betts, J. E., Appleton, J. J., Reschly, A. L., Christenson, S. L., & Huebner, E. S. (2010). A study of the factorial invariance of the Student Engagement Instrument (SEI): Results from middle and high school students. *School Psychology Quarterly, 25*(2), 84–93.

Bingham, G. E., & Okagaki, L. (2012). Ethnicity and student engagement. In S. L. Christenson, A. L. Reschly, & C. Wylie (Eds.), *Handbook of research on student engagement* (pp. 65–95). New York: Springer.

Clauser, B. E., & Mazor, K. M. (1998). Using statistical procedures to identify differentially functioning test items. *Educational Measurement: Issues and Practice, 17*(1), 31–44.

Finch, H. (2005). The MIMIC model as a method for detecting DIF: comparison with Mantel-Haenszel, SIBTEST, and the IRT likelihood ratio. *Applied Psychological Measurement, 29*, 278–295.

Glanville, L., & Wildhagen, T. (2007). The measurement of school engagement: Assessing dimensionality and measurement in variance across race and ethnicity. *Educational and Psychological Measurement, 6*, 1019–1041. doi:10.1177/0013164406299126.

Masters, G. N. (1982). A Rasch model for partial credit scoring. *Psychometrika, 47*, 149–174.

Moreira, P. A. S., Vaz, F. M., Dias, P. C., & Petracchi, P. (2009). Psychometric properties of the Portuguese version of the Student Engagement Instrument. *Canadian Journal of School Psychology, 24*(4), 303–317.

Penfield, R. D., Gattamorta, K., & Childs, R. A. (2009). An NCME instructional module on using differential step functioning to refine the analysis of DIF in polytomous items. *Educational Measurement: Issues and Practice, 28*(1), 38–49.

Portes, P. R. (2011). *Examining the problem of cultural validity in psychological measures: The case of the Rosenberg Self-Esteem Scale and implications for practice*. Paper presented at the American Educational Research Association 2011 Annual Conference, New Orleans, LA.

Schmitt, D. P., & Allik, J. (2005). Simultaneous administration of the Rosenberg self-esteem scale in 53 nations: Exploring the universal and culture-specific features of global self-esteem. *Journal of Personality and Social Psychology, 89*(4), 623–642.

Zwick, R., & Thayer, D. T. (1996). Evaluating the magnitude of differential item functioning in polytomous items. *Journal of Educational Statistics, 21*(3), 187–201.

Epilogue

The purpose of this handbook was to convene and engage international scholars on the topic of student engagement with the goal of enhancing future research and the potential for interventions to positively affect student outcomes. Authors of 34 chapters and the 5 commentaries for each of the sections of this handbook have contributed to the dialogue about research on student engagement, namely, how it is defined, the nature or degree of relationship with motivation to learn, role of contextual influences, and future research directions for the construct. As we contacted authors and read submissions, it became clear that there are a variety of perspectives and several points of agreement, as well as a number of areas that warrant clarification through future scholarly efforts. In addition, the esteemed scholars in this volume have provided excellent suggestions for future research in student engagement. We have attempted to distil what we see as primary themes in this epilogue.

Big Ideas in Engagement

Apparent in the scholarship represented by these authors is that more and more attention is being paid to the construct of student engagement by both developmental and educational psychology researchers and practitioners. Although common ground – some similarities – exists with respect to dimensions of student engagement, differences surfaced in how it is conceptualized and measured – often unique to the programmatic line of research.

It was clear that student engagement is no longer just of interest in relation to high school dropout. Rather, student engagement is associated with academic achievement, lower-risk health and sexual behaviors, social emotional well-being, and long-term outcomes, such as work success. Thus, engagement is relevant for *all* students who cross our school doors. Scholars study engagement from a variety of levels and structures – instructional methods, curricula, individuals and groups, family and peers, the person-environment fit, and so on. The authors in this volume clearly endorsed the importance of context for either enhancing or hindering student engagement at school and with learning; however, it is increasingly apparent that there is also an important role for individual student responsibility and investment, which may have been underemphasized or even absent from earlier work.

In Search of Definitional Clarity

In recent years, it is clear that there are several conceptualizations of student engagement, from those that are very narrow to those that are quite broad, subsuming other historically prominent constructs, such as motivation. A lack of definitional clarity has hindered efforts to synthesize results of studies, understand effects of interventions, and more accurately detail what is needed in future research. In this volume, we asked authors to define student engagement. The vast majority endorsed a three-part typology offered by Fredricks, Blumfeld, and Paris (2004). Thus, most engagement scholars view student engagement as multidimensional, comprised of observable behavior, internal cognition, and emotion. Many scholars also endorsed the notion that these types of engagement are interrelated. However, conceptualizations become more differentiated when these subtypes of engagement are operationalized into items and scales for measurement purposes. Or in other words, one author's conceptualization of the components of behavioral engagement is another's operationalization of cognitive engagement. In the future, it will be necessary to clearly detail how engagement is operationalized in measurement so as to facilitate understanding across authors.

A major point of contention has arisen in the conceptual and theoretical overlap between the constructs of motivation and engagement. We asked authors to offer their perspectives on this engagement-motivation issue. As with definitions, a few essentially endorsed engagement as a meta-construct, with cognitive engagement subsuming previous work on intrinsic motivation. However, most authors – motivation and engagement researchers alike – postulated that motivation is an antecedent or precursor of engagement, echoing a view offered several years ago by Russell, Ainley, and Frydenberg (2005) that motivation is intent and engagement is action. This view allows for the merging and coexistence of the rich, distinguished history of motivational research with the more nascent and intervention-focused field of engagement, thereby linking motivation to engagement and, in turn, to important outcomes of interest to scholars, parents, and educational personnel.

And yet, as with the operationalization of definitions of engagement, the overlap between engagement and motivation remains murky in measurement and, by extension, in intervention research. Consensus across scholars regarding all theoretical models, measurement, and definitions may not be possible, or even desirable, as we firmly believe the perspectives of scholars from different disciplines add to the richness and quality of scholarly inquiry around the topic of student engagement. What is, in our view, imperative is that, hereafter, all scholars provide detailed information about the models they espouse, their definitions of engagement, and their measurement tools.

Future Directions

Several common themes are apparent in the authors' thoughts of where and how student engagement research could most fruitfully develop. Longitudinal studies were recommended by quite a few authors. Studies of engagement over time were recommended by those wanting to go beyond descriptive, correlational studies to establish causality (both for the role of student engagement in learning and in the factors that predict or determine student engagement). Others were interested in seeing how different aspects of student engagement develop over time, how they influence each other, and how they may react to changing school contexts, particularly through developmental transitions, for example, from elementary to middle school, middle school to secondary school. Authors suggested that a worthy focus of investigation would address the question, "how and which students change (i.e., become more or less engaged)?"

Another question around student engagement lies in gaining further evidence over time about the interaction of different influential factors (e.g., out-of-school and school experiences, family and teacher expectations and support). Student engagement data were recommended as an important accompaniment to the collection of student achievement data, particularly to understand differential levels of student performance; the impact of policy, including high-stakes assessment; and the impact of school-level interventions designed to improve student performance.

Another set of themes for the next stage of development of research on student engagement as noted by most authors addresses the desirability of more clarity and consistency in its conceptualization as well as the relation among subtypes of engagement. Authors desired a better sense of *how student engagement works and when it works* to have an impact on student learning and developmental outcomes. There was recognition that definitional clarity is needed to advance research on student engagement and to build a research-oriented community. There was, however, no recommendation that a specific definition of student engagement be shared among the research community.

Consensus about the universality of the engagement construct for all students offers hope to see how engagement affects student groups (e.g., ethnicity, culture, general or special education) similarly or differently. At the same time, authors recognize that the need to know more about student engagement for specific student groups and cultures is a void in the research. Hence, there is an awareness that the field needs to check the universality of measures of student engagement, and that it is important to undertake studies with a range of students from different backgrounds, at different achievement levels, as well as cross-culturally. There is also an interest in mixed methods studies and an awareness of the value of both qualitative and quantitative research and of the importance of being able to link a close-grained focus (e.g., of self-regulation and goals during the completion of a particular task) with the layers of context. For example, contextual influences that have a bearing on student capability for self-regulation and goal-setting, include class learning opportunities; assessments; relations with teacher, peers, and parents; and out-of-school interests and experiences.

Finally, there is a strong interest and support for having the results of current research put to practical, evaluated use. Many authors noted that more student engagement interventions must be developed, evaluated, and refined, striving to establish the efficacy of these interventions. Some authors referred to the void of interventions as "the practice gap." Both the implementation of interventions already in practice with success (as described in some of the chapters) as well as research-derived implications for teaching and parental practices would advance the impact of student engagement research. Additionally, authors called for new approaches that tackle the intersections between individual students, school and class programs and approaches, and school-family interactions in particular. There should be an eye toward examining the effect of student engagement on the student-teacher interaction (or parent-adolescent or family-school) as well as the impact of these interactions on student performance data; bidirectional effects are an area for future research.

Our Position: A Call for Action

Working with the authors of the chapters and the commentaries has been a wonderful professional and learning experience. Each of the coeditors believes that her understanding and knowledge of student engagement has been embellished as a result of coediting this handbook. For these reasons, we extend our appreciation to the authors.

We have reflected on the contents of the chapters, in particular, the responses of the authors to the questions that framed the purpose of the handbook. It is our hope that this will be a call for action to advance the quantity and quality of research on student engagement to improve learning outcomes. We offer the following recommendations to advance the quality and utility of research on the construct of student engagement:

1. Researchers must provide their definition and conceptualization of student engagement in each investigation conducted. Given the level of consensus across researchers about the multidimensional nature of student engagement, the engagement subtype should be specified; basically, the adjective (e.g., cognitive, behavioral, affective, academic) and operationalization of this adjective are important to clarify in research. Hence, reporting of scientific findings should avoid the vague use of engagement (e.g., 'increases in engagement'), substituting rather the subtype of engagement.
2. Researchers must not only define student engagement but use measures that align with their specific definition of engagement.
3. Student engagement is best understood when contextualized; therefore, researchers must specify information about the learning, school, or family context under study.

4. Of the various subtypes noted by authors, it is clear that more information on the effect of cognitive engagement on academic learning and how affective engagement develops are needed areas of study. Cognitive and affective engagement require understanding the student perspective and voice.
5. Adopting an engagement orientation, due to the multidimensional nature, integrates students' thoughts (cognitions), feelings, and behaviors toward achieving positive learning outcomes and/or improving one's academic competencies. It is not sufficient to focus only on completion of learning activities (e.g., behavior) to foster a student's identity as a learner. Student feelings, interests, and attitudes as well as self-perceived competence on the task or use of strategy for doing one's best are part of this identity.
6. Many aspects of student engagement, irrespective of subtype, need to be better understood. For example, is student engagement separate from disengagement? Is it linear? Is more really better? Is there a tipping point with disengagement where it is very hard to recover? Is there a fairly wide band of useful engagement levels?
7. Interventions to enhance engagement subtypes must be developed and evaluated. Student engagement is not immutable – it can change – but for whom and under what conditions is still unclear. Establishing a person-environment fit whether for individual students or student groups (e.g., Maori, Native American) is inherent to fostering varied engagement outcomes. The interaction of both student and environment are critical targets for change to achieve increased student engagement.
8. Whether student engagement is conceptualized as an input, mediator, or desired outcome needs to be specified in the research design. Engagement may be any of these. There is no need to delineate engagement only as a process or outcome.
9. Engagement seems to be embedded in thinking about what one wants to achieve, whether in the classroom or as the link between present performance and later goals. The role of goals – whether student or teacher goals – is evident, plays a seminal part in much student engagement research, and warrants increased attention in theoretical models and interventions.
10. As we move forward, focus must be on the complex systems – learners, classrooms, schools, and communities that characterize development and human interaction. We identify disengaged learners, but we also need to identify disengaged learning environments. What makes learning engaging for students? What is an engaging context? How do engaging contexts differ across age and student differences?
11. Because context matters, it is important to examine for whom schools exist. Martin Maehr and Carol Midgley (1996) suggested that too often they are designed for creating positive conditions for teachers and the staff versus positive conditions for the student. School policies and practices will have to change if schools are to increase their holding power – and research must document the impact of such contextual influences.
12. The effect of discontinuity across environments for students (e.g., classroom, home) should be documented with an eye toward understanding how students resolve incongruent messages about the role of schooling and learning.
13. Although no recommendation that a specific definition of student engagement be shared among the research community surfaced from authors, we contend that to define student engagement solely as multidimensional with specified indicators for each subtype dances around, unfortunately, a definition. Additionally, enhancing clarity to what student engagement refers was embedded in the purpose of the handbook and reinforced by the commentary from Eccles and Wang (2012). Therefore, we offer this definition:

Student engagement refers to the student's active participation in academic and co-curricular or school-related activities, and commitment to educational goals and learning. Engaged students find learning meaningful, and are invested in their learning and future. It is a multidimensional construct that consists of behavioral (including academic), cognitive, and affective subtypes. Student engagement drives learning; requires energy and effort; is affected by multiple contextual influences; and can be achieved for all learners.

As coeditors, from different countries and professional backgrounds, we share a common interest in engagement as being the most promising means for understanding students' school experiences and outcomes and, most importantly, that by understanding engagement, we can improve educational and life outcomes for youth. It is our hope that this handbook advances the field so that we may someday accomplish this goal.

Respectfully submitted,
Sandra L. Christenson
Amy L. Reschly
Cathy Wylie

References

Eccles, J., & Wang, M. -T. (2012). Part I commentary: so what is student engagement anyway? In S. L. Christenson, A. L. Reschly, & C. Wylie (Eds.), *Handbook of research on student engagement* (pp. 133–145). New York: Springer.

Fredricks, J. A., Blumenfeld, P. C., & Paris, A. H. (2004). School engagement: Potential of the concept, state of the evidence. *Review of Educational Research, 74*, 59–109.

Maehr, M. L., & Midgley, C. (1996). *Transforming school cultures*. Boulder, CO: Westview Press.

Russell, V. J., Ainley, M., & Frydenberg, E. (2005). Schooling issues digest: Student motivation and engagement. Retrieved November 9, 2005, from http://www.dest.gov.au/sectors/school education/publications resources/schooling issues digest/schooling issues digest motivation engagement.htm.

Index

A

Academic achievement, 177, 332–333
   emotional engagement, 211
   GPA, 211–212
   graduation/dropping out, 212
   long-term effects, 568–569
   researchers, 568
Academic Case Management (ACM) system, 332
Academic coping, 32
Academic emotions
   achievement, 262
   appraisals as proximal antecedents, 271–272
   description, 259
   emotion, mood and affect, 260–261
   epistemic, 262–263
   functions, SE and achievement
      behavioral, 266–267
      cognitive-behavioral engagement, 267
      engagement, cognitive, 264–265
      motivational, 265–266
      negative activating emotions, 269–270
      negative deactivating emotions, 270–271
      neuroscientific and cognitive research, 263
      positive emotions, 269
      social-behavioral engagement, 268–269
   orientations and achievement-related goals
      controllability and value, 274
      motivation, 274
      performance approach and avoidance, 274–275
      reciprocal causation, 272–273
   psychological functions, 262
   reciprocal causation, regulation and therapy, 277–278
   social, 263
   and specific mood, 262
   task and environments
      autonomy support, 276
      cognitive quality, 275
      feedback and consequences, achievement, 276–277
      motivational quality, 276
      structures and social expectations, 276
   topic emotions, 263
   valence and activation, 261–262

Academic engaged time (AET), 3
   components and determinants continuum, 661–662
   description, 654
   enhancement
      description, 663–664
      instructional design, 667–668
      instructional strategies, 666
      interactive teaching, 666–667
      managerial strategies, 664–666
      student-mediated strategies, 668–670
   NECTL analysis, 662
   task, 663
   theoretical foundations, 655
Academic engagement, 102, 116, 117, 120, 269, 389–391, 424–425, 548, 564, 568–569, 697, 726, 750, 767
   engagement-achievement connections, 108
   extracurricular activities, 108–109
   homework, 108
   studies, inattentiveness, 107
   and teacher-reported, 107
Academic mediation theory, 495–496
Academic motivation, 105, 138, 173, 220, 496
Academic work, 28–29, 35, 496
Achievement/attainment, SE, 69, 99, 123, 211–212, 461, 528, 606, 786
   attendance, 114
   high school, 114–115
   longitudinal studies, 114
   research categories, 106–107
Achievement goal theory, 134, 141, 644
   academic motivation, 173
   academic tasks, 187
   classroom climate (*see* Classroom climate)
   collaborative efforts, 187
   description, 173–174
   educational psychology, 1980s and 1990s, 173
   Four-Factor Model, 175–176
   goal orientations, 174–175, 177–180
   historical developments, 174
   learning types, 187
   original development, 174
   relationships, goal orientation and engagement, 187

Achievement motivation theory, 134, 458
Adolescent student engagement
　academic achievement, 568–569
　behavioral engagement
　　definition, 55
　　extracurricular and school activities, 55–56
　　individual interactions and characteristics, 56
　　platonic and romantic peer relationships, 55
　CDC document, 579
　and childhood
　　early childhood, 47
　　middle childhood, 47–48
　　positive child development, 48
　　societal expectations, 47
　cognitive engagement, 56
　conduct problems/violence, 570
　definitions, 564
　emotional engagement
　　decrease, GPA, 56
　　description, 56
　　family factors, 57
　　participating, after-school programs, 57
　　research, 57
　　schools and disciplinary policies, 56
　emotional/psychological aspects, 563
　engaged and disengaged, 565–567
　high-risk behaviors, 563, 578–579
　and motivation, 564–565
　prevention and intervention
　　mechanisms, 574–575
　　school context, 578
　　school-wide and targeted, 575–577
　　student-teacher relationships, 577–578
　　utilizing system level, 575
　process, 565
　risk and factors, 570–573
　school dropout, 55, 569–570
　substance use and physical and mental health, 569
　troubling and high-risk behaviors, 567–568
AET *See* Academic engaged time
Affective engagement, 102, 103, 116–122, 415
　identification, school, 113
　multilevel logistic regression analysis, 121–122
　self-report measures, student, 112
　valuing, 113
Appraisals as proximal antecedents
　attributional theory, 271–272
　control-value theory, 272
　emotions causes and modulation, 271
　nonreflective induction, 272
　test anxiety research, 271
Assessment, 366, 677, 681
　CB tests and testing, 461–467
　classroom-based practices, 471
　cognitive engagement, 103
　description, 457–458
　environment, 276
　instruments, 278
　needed research, practice and policy, 472
　package, 125
　popularization, high-stakes standardized tests
　　dropout crisis, 469–471
　　exaggerated emphasis, 468–469
　　NCLB, 467
　　and student motivation, 467–468
　reform and curriculum
　　local curriculum planning, 443–444
　　origins, NZC key competencies, 443
　　vision and principles, 443
　standardized testing
　　low-stakes, 460–461
　　norm and criterion-referenced, 460
　　psychologists, 459
　　use, 459–460
　strategies, 483
　"structured" and "spontaneous", 459
　struggling and talented students, 472
　use, 111–112
Assessment-to-intervention *See* Student engagement instrument (SEI)
Attributional theory, 134, 271–272
Authentic enquiry
　application, 689
　learning, 690
Authority systems/classroom management techniques, 465
Autonomy, 27, 153–154, 359–360, 370
　adolescents, 144
　charting, NCEA, 451
　vs. control, 350–352
　educational practices and supporting students
　　competence, 422–423
　　components, 421–422, 437
　　contributions, 437
　　emotional experience, 422
　　formation, inner compass, 423
　　freedom, coercion and optional choice, 423
　　motivation, 422
　　SDT and motivation, 421
　environments, 346
　feelings, 642
　formative assessment practices, 467
　individual, 206, 271
　learner, 453
　psychological needs, 345
　self-system model, 100
　student, 103, 205, 453, 465
　support, 276, 603
　teachers, 206

B

Bandura's theory, 232, 241
Basic needs theory, 158
　affecting students' perceptions, 154
　autonomy, 153–154
　competence, 154
　description, 153
　relatedness, 154
　satisfaction, 154
　student active engagement, learning activities, 154

Behavioral engagement, 47, 51, 53–56, 119–122, 180, 182–184, 208–209, 266–268, 405, 564, 618–624, 626–627, 726 *See also* Engagement and achievement, reading
Behavioral learning theory, 518
Behavior management
  description, 374
  positive student, 374–375
  self-regulations, 375
Bifactor model, SEI, 793
  correlations, 799–800
  factors, 796
  hypothetical use, 798
  initial items, 798–799
  RMSEA, 799
  SEI data, 798, 799
  visualization, 795, 797
Biopsychosocial development
  definition and conceptual boundaries, 699
  disengagement, 700
  motivation, 700
  school dropout, 700
Bloom's theory, 656–658
Bronfenbrenner's ecological systems theory, 334

C

Cardiovascular disease (CVD), 98
Carroll's model, 660, 661, 668
  Cooley-Leinhardt model, 657
  school learning
    appeal, 656
    description, 655
    factors, 655
    time, 655–656
  Wiley-Harnischfeger model, 657
Catholic schools, 72, 332–333, 507
  academic achievement, low-income students, 333
  higher achievement and parent participation, 333
  NAEP data, 333
  in 1980s, 332–333
  warmth and care, teachers, 333
Causality orientations theory, 153, 157, 158
CDP *See* Child Development Project
Centers for disease control (CDC), 98, 579
Check & Connect (C&C), 7–8, 548, 576–577
Child Development Project (CDP), 207
Choice
  and autonomy, 467
  and behavior, 113
  behavioral engagement, 615
  career and course plans, 198
  curriculum, 533
  educational and occupational, 142
  family, 586
  feelings, individual subjects, 454
  friends, 485
  learning options and pathways, 455
  learning resources, 442
  NCEA, 451, 453
  neutral, 451
  parental, 516
  personal, 200, 202
  and preparatory activities, 533
  reforms, voluntary, 99
  regulatory process, 466
  students' perceptions, 449
  and task engagement, 142
Circumplex models, 261
Classic psychological theory, 195, 197
Classroom activities, 86, 157, 391, 464
  analysis, engagement, 285
  distinctions, motivation and engagement, 285–286
  dynamic systems perspective, 299–300
  educational levels and activities, 299
  and high school courses, 528
  indicators, engagement, 284
  interconnections and exploration, 284
  motivation, educators, 283–284
  SE, 630
  talent development sites, 530
  tests and tasks, 464
  theoretical orientation
    achievement behavior, 288
    achievement goals, 294–296
    complexity, 288
    context and relations, 296
    contribution, interest, 291–292
    developmental phases and stages, 290–291
    dynamic systems perspective, 287, 288
    educational domain, 288
    emotions, 294
    individual interest and trajectories, 292–294
    learning situation and motivation schemas, 288
    PISA 2006, 297–299
    process schemas and task engagement, 288–289
    proposals, 287–288
    role, interest, 289–290
    task perceptions, 288
Classroom-based (CB) tests, 458–459
  formative tests and SE, 465–467
  student and classroom goals structures, 462–465
  value, 461–462
Classroom climate, 35, 373, 378
  cooperative, 275
  engagement theory
    description, experiences, 368
    enthusiasm and passion, 368
    impressions, 368
    instructional exchanges, 368–369
    NRC report, 368
    perspective and motivation, 369
    relational setting and capacity, 369
  goal structures, 181–184
  teacher practices
    mastery goal structure, 185
    performance goal structure, 186
Classroom community, teachers' impact on, 206–207

Classroom practices, 167, 207, 372, 481, 604
   achievement, 627
   autonomy-supportive communication, 630
   behavioral engagement, 626–627
   CORI, 627–628
   effects, 617–624
   global quality, 630
   motivation, 629, 631
   perceived emotional support, 628–629
   perceived relevance, 617, 625
   SDT, 627
   students
      achievement, 631
      behaviorally engaged/disengaged, 629
      devaluing, 625
      minority, 631
      self-efficacy, 625
   teacher
      caring, 629
      teacher-student relationships, 625
   teaching, 617
Classroom setting and youth development
   achievement outcomes, 367
   engagement and intrinsic motivation, 367
   fifth grade, nature and quality, 367
   high school, 367
   improvement and enhancement, 367
   school reform, 368
   supportive relationships, 368
Classroom strategies
   AET, 654, 661–663
   Bloom's theory, 656–657
   Carroll's model, 655–656
   classroom setting and youth development, 367–368
   Cooley and Leinhardt's classroom-process model, 657–658
   description, 653
   enhancement AET, 663–670
   Huitt model, 658
   language and instructional discourse
      children's ability, 377
      classrooms offering, 377
      positive language development, 377
      social medium, 378
      verbal interactions, 377–378
   NECTL, 654
   process-product paradigm, 658–661
   theoretical foundations, 658
   time and learning, 654–655
   Wiley and Harnischfeger's model, 657
Coaching conversation, 683, 685
   identity and authorship, 686–687
   profile, 686
Cognitive dissonance theory, 199
Cognitive engagement, 10–11, 15, 47, 52, 54, 56, 102–103, 179–180, 182, 184, 238–240, 408, 564, 602, 747, 764, 772, 793
   and achievement, 111
   attention and flow, 264
   measures, 112
   mood-congruent memory recall, 265
   observable indicators, 111
   retrieval-induced forgetting and facilitation, 265
   studies, self-regulation and use, 111
   "think alouds", 111
Cognitive evaluation theory, 153, 158
   autonomy-supportive *vs.* controlling way, 156
   classroom conditions and student motivational processes, 156
   external events and functions, 156
   student and classroom conditions, 156
Cognitive/motivational model, 263, 266, 269
Comer's SDP and HCZ project
   Academic Case Management (ACM) system, 332
   community investment services, 331
   impacts, HCZ project, 332
   mesosystemic approach, 331
   negative effects, poverty, 331
Competency development
   affordances, 442
   curriculum and assessment reform, New zealand, 442–444
   description, 441
   engagement determination
      classroom component, 446
      teachers *vs.* students perception, 446–448
   expectations and engagement
      classes, students association, 450
      least enjoyed classes, 451
      NCEA, 450, 451
      student and teacher items, 450
   pedagogy changes
      learning-to-learn connections, 444–445
      NZC framework, 444
      sociocultural framing, 445
   self-managing behaviours, 452
   students engagement, 448–450, 453–455
   teaching, traditional, 451–452
Competency levels
   attitudinal and cognitive, 593, 594
   average scores, trajectory groups, 592, 593
   competent learners study, 591–592
   track engagement levels, 586
Competent learners, 445, 446, 596
   childhood education, 587
   data collection, 586–587
   motivation, 588
   SE patterns, school
      behavioral and cognitive, 588
      changes, education experience, 589
      changes, engagement levels, 589
      enjoyment, learning, 590
      mean score, items, 589
      measure, items, 588–589
      New Zealand data, 590
      students, school experiences, 587
Concept-Oriented Reading Instruction (CORI)

classroom practices, 627–628
defined, 603
goal, 628
reading comprehension outcomes, 630
Conceptualizing engagement, 308
controlling grades, 319
experience types, 319
flow theory and experiences, 318–319
observer ratings, 318
procedural and substantive, 318
Conceptualizing motivation, 308
beliefs, 319–320
goal theory, 320
learning and achievement, 319
mastery-avoidance goals, 320
Confirmatory factor analysis (CFA), 793, 801
application, 791–792
congeneric measurement model, 791
description, 790–791
Constructivist theories, 375, 445
Continuum/continua, 12–13, 567, 661, 662
Control-value theory, 272, 274
Cooley and Leinhardt's classroom-process model, 657–658
Coping
 behaviors types, 135
 description, 31
 educational implications
  developmental aspects, 34
  engagement and disaffection, 33
  intrinsic motivation and engagement, 33
  larger school, 37
  motivation and engagement, teachers, 36–37
  nature, academic work, 35
  SDT, 33
  social learning environment, 35–36
  student disaffection and failure, 34–35
  teachers enthusiasm and excitement, 36
  teacher-student interactions, 36
  tracking, 33
 motivational model, 31
 response, 135
 skills, 520, 524
 students' ability, school life, 31
CORI See Concept-Oriented Reading Instruction
Cultural discontinuity, 67, 68, 83, 808
Curriculum and assessment reform, 442–444
CVD See Cardiovascular disease
Cyclical feedback loop, 239–243
 academic applications, 247
 empirical advantages
  achievement differences, 246–247
  effects, self-regulatory training, 246
  goal setting, 246
  SRL phase processes, 246
 SCL, 247–248
 self-regulated strategy development (SRSD), 247
 SREP, 248–250

D

Deep engagement, 317, 686–687, 689, 692
 consensus, 679
 description, 675–676
 engagement and motivation, learning, 679–680
 identity, 681–682
 learning power and engagement (see Learning power and engagement)
 participation, 678–679
 perezhivanie, 680–681
 personal
  and community stories, 682–683
  qualities, 683
 worldview challenges
  ELLI, 677–678
  epistemology and anthropology, 676
  ideology, 676
  understanding engagement, 677
Developmental context
 early childhood
  education and intervention programs, 50–51
  participation, education programs, 51
  school context, 51
 middle childhood
  behavioral engagement, 53–54
  cognitive engagement, 54
  description, 53
  emotional engagement, 54
  individual student characteristics, 53
  research, 54–55
  role, parents and teachers, 53
  schooling and learning environments, 53
Developmental dynamics
 academic development, 24
 children and youth involvement, 22
 classroom, 22–23
 construction, academic engagement, 21–22
 coping (see Coping)engagement and disaffection, motivation
  cycles, 30–31
  parents and peers, 30
  teachers, 29–30
  trajectories, 31
 everyday school experiences, students, 24
 meaning, engagement, 22
 motivational dynamics model (see Motivational dynamics model)motivation and psychological processes, 22
 proximal processes, 23–24
 youth development and children protection, 22
Developmental periods
 adolescence (see Adolescent student engagement)application and policy implications
  growth and development, SE, 59
  manifestation, 58–59
  recognition, educators and policymakers, 58
 behavioral engagement, 51
 "chain of events", 46

Developmental periods (*cont.*)
  childhood and adolescence, 47–48
  cognitive engagement, 52
  contribution and human development, 57–58
  definition, student engagement, 47
  description, 45–46
  vs. developmental tasks
    codevelopment, 48–49
    emotional engagement and deficits, 48
    friendship, middle childhood, 48
    group cooperation, 48
    motivation, 49
    relationship, school-related activities, 48
    restrictions, 48
    schoolwork and extracurricular activities, student, 49
    social skills, 48
  early childhood, 50–51
  emotional engagement, 52
  individual's own capacities, 58
  middle childhood, 53–54
  participation-identification model, 57
  person-environment fit perspective, 58
  prominent developmental tasks, 46
  social and structural resources, 58
  social skills, children, 46
  theoretical considerations
    activity participation, 50
    bioecological theory, 49
    characteristics, child/adolescent, 50
    congruence/synchrony, 50
    encourage engagement, 50
    manifestation, 50
    person-environment fit, 49–50
    proximal processes, 49
  understanding growth, 46–47
Developmental task, childhood and adolescence, 48–49, 51, 327
  description, 47
  early childhood, 47
  middle childhood, 47–48
  positive child development, 48
  societal expectations, 47
Deviance model, 495–496
Deviant affiliation theory, 496
DIF *See* Differential item function
Differential item function (DIF), 806
  collectivist *vs.* individualist cultures, 809–810
  cultural discontinuity theory, 808
  PCM, 810
  polytomous, 810
  RSES, 807–808
  RSM, 809
  threshold values, 809
Disengagement, 71, 86, 88, 99, 106, 107, 219, 310, 315–316, 395
  areas, research and development, 124–125
  empirical research, 123
Dropout prevention
  difference, theory and direct intervention, 5

Finn's seminal theory, 7
high schools, 5
participation-identification model, 7
predictive variables, 6–7
publicity and interest, 5
Dropout prevention theory, 99–100
Drugs and relaxation techniques, 277

E
Eccles et al.expectancy-value theoretical (EEVT) model
  See Engagement theory (ET)
Educational practices, 34, 555, 565, 656, 676, 699
  components and contributions, 423
  cross-cultural research, 231–232
  FIV processes, 436–437
  high-stakes testing, 471
  IVD, 427–429
  minimizing controls
    colleagues and expected behaviors, 425
    external control, behaviors, 424
    impact, teachers external controls, 424–425
    internal compulsion, 425
    psychological control, 425
  negative feelings, 425–426
  rationale, 426–427
  self-efficacy
    benefits, instructional and social practices, 228
    competence beliefs, 228
    description, 228
    effect, children's achievement and persistence, 228
    lower-ability students, 228–229
    role models, 228
    sociodemographics, 229
    teacher bias and obstacles, 228
    transition periods, schools, 229
  supporting choice and initiation, 427
  SVE, 430–435
Educators' beliefs and practices, 81–87, 181, 185–186, 356–358, 376, 416, 425, 443, 458, 461, 464–466, 484, 486, 541, 544, 547, 549, 625
  fear, 557–559
  learning and teaching, 556–557
  mindset, 550
  opportunities, help, 557
  themes and exercises, 550–555
Effective lifelong learning inventory (ELLI) programme, 677, 678, 683, 684, 691
Emotional engagement, 10–12, 14, 46–49, 52, 54–58, 66, 72, 74, 76, 78–80, 82–87, 142, 150, 161, 162, 167, 179–184, 211, 238, 260, 268, 285, 304–306, 309, 497, 588, 602, 605, 621, 642, 644, 645, 696–698, 709, 726, 750, 764, 766, 769–772, 776, 778, 784, 785, 787, 789, 798
Engaged time, 3, 86, 101, 187, 618, 653–671, 699
Engagement and achievement, reading, 108, 120, 262, 423, 548
  behavioral, emotional and cognitive, 601–602
  behavioral engagement

effects, 605–608
GPA, 609–610
motivations impact, 610–615
reading comprehension, 609
reading, motivational processes, 605
students' aversion, 609
variety, studies, 609
classroom practices, 626–631
conceptual knowledge and social interactions, 603
conditions and classroom practices, 604, 605
instructional practices, 603–604
model, classroom contexts, 604
and motivation, 602–603
motivations impact, competence, 615–617
real-world interactions, 603
Engagement models, 12, 105, 238, 247, 493–496, 604, 648
Engagement outcomes, 625, 814
biopsychosocial development, 699–700
description, 695–696
learning activities and school
academic, 697
definition and measurement, 697
description, 696
determinants, intervention and contexts, 698–699
emotional, cognitive and behavioral, 698
Finn's model, 698
outcomes and contexts, 696–697
person-centered approach, 701
Engagement theory (ET), 10, 53, 133–136, 725
and EEVT
achievement behaviors, 142, 143
description, 141
goal, 142
personal and social identification role, 144
person-environment fit, 142
research and policy/practice communities, 145
SDT, 144
and SDT, 135, 142
Epstein theory, 323, 335, 355, 357, 358, 360
ESM *See* Experience sampling method (ESM)
ET *See* Engagement theory (ET)
Ethnicity, 5, 6, 98, 108–110, 117–119, 203, 327, 329, 330, 336, 470, 485, 496, 568, 590, 718, 719, 744, 751, 770, 813 *See also* Ethnicity and student engagement
Ethnicity and student engagement, 136, 327, 329, 330, 336, 485, 590, 719, 744, 813
children's educational experiences, 88
cultural discontinuity, 67, 88–89
discontinuity framework and ecological model, 68
discrimination, 88
ethnic groups, 66
motivation processes, 66
parents role, 74–79
poor school achievement, 68
public education, 89
researchers and ethnic groups, 66
schools role, 79–87
secondary discontinuity model, 67–68
socioeconomic differences, 67
student attitudes and emotional engagement, 66
students role, 68–74
variation, ethnic group, 67
Every-day resilience
academic coping as mechanism, 32
academic resources
educators and parents responsibility, 32
mindsets and ages, 32
positive motivational dynamics, 33
qualitative changes, early adolescence, 32–33
Expectancy-value theory, 134, 136, 141–145, 198, 610
Expectancy X value theory, 415, 416, 458, 461
Experience sampling forms (ESFs), 321
Experience sampling method (ESM), 321, 327, 766
Extant theory, 133
Extracurricular activities, 81, 108–109, 333, 387–398, 405, 530, 698, 726, 750
academic, 100, 102, 116
effectiveness, 140
engagement, 139
high school reforms, 530
involvement, 647
ISAO, 108–109
participation, 115, 500, 643
policy makers, 139
talent development high school model, 530

F
Family, 5–8, 10, 15, 32, 48–50, 57–59, 75, 76, 82, 88, 124, 226, 232, 297, 317, 321–324, 327–334, 343–361, 407, 479, 483, 494, 497, 502, 557, 565, 569, 574, 578, 586, 595–597, 646, 676, 698, 730, 751–753, 771, 772, 784, 785, 790, 793, 796, 800, 806, 811, 813
care, 101
and communities, 486
EEVT, 144
environments, 110
factors, 505
and friends, 596
history, 98
income and material qualification levels, 596
interdependence and closeness, 485
members, 485
practices, 505–506
problems, 520
relations, 113
resources, 505, 590
school
connectedness, 197
contextual features, 141
environments, 586
levels, 500
practices, 507–508
resources, 507
structure, 506–507
student composition, 506
socialization theory, 496
structure, 98, 110, 505

Family influences, 317
    children motivation, 225
    cultural capital, 225
    mastery experiences, 226
    resources and assets, capital, 225
    responsibility and support, 226
    vicarious influence, 226
Family socialization theory, 496
Fear, 56, 73, 223, 262, 264, 272, 320, 463, 516, 550
    challenge, 559
    commitment, 558–559
    control, 559
    description, 557
    middle school English teacher, 558
Feedback, 8, 9, 24, 29–31, 34, 36, 85, 153, 156, 158, 159, 163, 221–223, 228–248, 252, 271, 275–277, 296, 305, 309, 320, 346, 352, 353, 357, 407, 409, 426, 428, 447, 453, 461, 463–465, 467, 471, 472, 534, 535, 547, 552, 555, 603, 625, 637, 639, 656, 658–660, 664, 666, 667, 686, 699, 770
    behavior, 376–377
    forms, 377
    high-quality and quantity, 377
    learning, 376
Finn's seminal theory, 3, 4, 7, 139, 493, 698
Flow theory, 136, 319, 322
Fostering inner-directed valuing (FIV) processes, 422
    additive influence, reflective value and goal examination, 436
    authentic decision making, 436
    components, 436
    correlates and potential benefits, 436
    educator's behaviors and student attention, 436
    implications, 436–437
    joint contribution, 437
Four-factor model, 306
    approach/avoid orientations, 176
    distinctions, mastery and performance goals, 175–176
    mastery-avoid goals, 176
    measures, 176
    mid-1990s, 175
    PALS, 176

G
GCPS *See* Gwinnett County Public Schools (GCPS)
General deviance theory, 496
Goal contents theory, 150, 153, 158
    explanation, 155
    extrinsic goals, 155–156
    personal growth and interpersonal relationships, 155
Goal theory, 134, 141, 150, (173–187), 304, 306, 320, 610, 765
GPA *See* Grade point average (GPA)
Grade point average (GPA), 26, 56, 108, 110, 115, 116, 139, 198, 228, 322, 326, 329, 330, 333, 606, 608–610, 738, 739
    engagement measures, 211
    and school environment, 212

Gwinnett County Public Schools (GCPS), 726, 729, 733, 734
    IMD, 727
    SEI, 728
    student population, 727

H
High-performing schools and self-efficacy, 232
High school, 4, 5, 7, 9, 11, 12, 17, 22, 30, 31, 54, 69, 70 *See also* High school dropout; High school reform
    analysis, 596
    assessment, 590
    Baltimore and Philadelphia, 519
    Chinese and German, 277
    criterion-referenced, 592
    curriculum design opportunities, 444
    diploma, 470, 491
    dropout rate, 199
    final years, 442, 444, 586
    graduation exams, 139, 470
    graduation rate, 491–492
    Houston school district, 201
    low-SES, 212
    mathematics and science, 203
    mathematics instruction, 523
    and middle students perception, 626
    multiteacher format, 589
    postsecondary program, 115
    predictors sets, 114–115
    program tracking, 518
    qualifications and post-school learning experiences, 586
    reading instruction, 522
    school belonging, 389
    student motivation and engagement
        comprehensive reforms, 534–535
        preparation, 532–533
        reform priorities and sequences, 533–534
    student performance, 498–499
    teachers, 204, 451
High school completion, 119
    demographic risk, 5
    participation processes, 4
    postsecondary outcomes, 5
    skills and behaviour, 4–5
High school dropout, 5, 6, 17, 119, 316, 502, 811
    attitudes, 502
    behaviors
        attendance, 500
        participation, extracurricular activities, 500
        school misbehavior, 501
        sophomores, 501
        student mobility, 501
    deviance model, 495–496
    engagement-related predictors, 500
    factors, 492
    families, 505–508
    Finn's models, 493

goals, 502–503
institutional factors, 505
life course models, 493–494
median annual earnings, 492
models, factors types identification, 493
national crisis and "silent epidemic", 491
preschool and early elementary school, 509
research literature, factors, 508
risk factors, 503–504
role
    adolescent development and school performance, 498
    behavioral, emotional and cognitive, 497
    educational context impact, 497
    factors and students' experiences, 497
    SE, 496
    Wehlage and NRC models, 497
scholars, 499
self-perceptions, 503
structural models, 504
student performance, 498–499
student's behavior and performance, 508
student's decision, 508
Tinto model, 494–495
typologies, 504
Wehlage and colleagues' model, 495

High school reform, 4, 10, 17, 515–535
academic/personal needs, 520
behavioral and cognitive engagement, 10–11
behavioral learning theory, 518
communal engagement, 530
comprehensive reforms, 534–535
continuum/continua, 12–13
criteria, grades and recognition, 520–521
diplomas, 520
engagement and motivation, 14–15
external and internal conditions
    dimensions, student engagement, 517
    motivation and engagement, 516–517
    policy levers, 516
functional relevance, learning
    career academies, 524–525
    career applications, blending, 525–526
    school work, 524
group interventions, small, 520
indicators and facilitators, 13–14
personal expression and nonacademic interests, 528–530
process/outcome, 11–12
prominent engagement models, 12
reform priorities and sequences, 533–534
rules and disciplinary practices, 531
school-wide interventions, 520
school work, 521–524
student engagement, 11
student involvement, decision-making, 532
student motivation and engagement, 532–533
teacher-student relations, 526–528
theory and intervention, 10
transitional preparation courses

    "double math", 519
    high-standards curriculum, 518, 519
    students grouping, 519
    talent development high school reform model, 519
types and definitions, 11

High School Survey of Student Engagement (HSSSE), 744, 747, 760, 768–770, 773–775
boredom, 752
cognitive/intellectual/academic, 750
data analysis, 751
data sample, 750–751
description, 749–750
emotional, 750
NSSE, 750
pedagogy, 753–754
potential, dropping out, 753
reasons, going to school, 751–752
social/behavioral/participatory, 750
students' words
    instructional methods, 755
    multiple-option questions, 754
    open-response question, 755–756
    schools, 755
    teachers power, 755

High-stakes standardized tests
dropout crisis, 469–471
exaggerated emphasis, 468–469
NCLB, 467
role, 467
and student motivation, 467–468

HLM model, 117, 118, 198

Home-school partnership, 335, 360
Catholic schools, 332–333
Comer's SDP and HCZ project, 331–332
out-of-school time programs, 333–334
perceptions and development, 331
school-based family centers, 332

Home-school partnership model
autonomy support *vs.* control, 350–352
description, 343–344
engagement
    academic resilience, 345
    definitions, 344–345
    motivational perspective, 345
innovative approaches, 360–361
interventions
    NNPS, 358
    TIPS design, 358–359
involvement, challenges
    individual, contextual and institutional factors, 356
    low-income and less educated parents, 355
    social networks, 355–356
motivational perspective, engagement
    children's motivational resources, 346
    context effects, 346–347
    SDT, 345
    self-system processes, 345–346
parental structure, 352–354
parent autonomy support, 359–360

Home-school partnership model (cont.)
  parent involvement, 347–350
  schools, 356
  supports, student engagement
    characterization, 354
    parent involvement, 354–355
    role, 354
  teacher beliefs and practices
    attitudes and practices, 357–358
    "leaders", 356–357
    teaching-learning process, 358
HSSSE See High School Survey of Student Engagement (HSSSE)
Huitt model, 658
Human development theories, 597
Humanity, data
  challenges
    policy, 759
    practice, 759–760
    research, 759
  characteristics, 758
  description, 743–744
  input–output model, 758
  listening, students, 757–758
  schools, 760
  student engagement (see Student engagement)
  student perception data, 758
  "Tech High School", 744–745

I
ICLE See International Center for Leadership in Education (ICLE)
IMD See Information management division (IMD)
Indicators and facilitators, 13–14, 25–26
Information management division (IMD), 727–729
Inschool academic extracurricular activities (ISAO), 108, 109
Instructional interaction domain
  cognitive and language development, 375
  distinctions, 375–376
  student learning outcomes, 376
Intelligences, 76, 173–187, 417, 463, 554, 556, 608, 609, 795, 801
  bodily-kinesthetic and musical, 528
  "National Intelligence Test", 459
  spiritual and existential, 528
  test items, 270
Interactive teaching, enhancement AET, 664
  academic focus, 666
  feedback, 667
  question, 666–667
Interest
  behavioral engagement, 609
  creative leisure, 595
  disciplinary thinking, 523
  and enjoyment, 108
  and enthusiasm, 496
  extracurricular, 643
  individual, 198

intrinsic motivation, 521–522
mastery performance goals, 522
and motivation, 263
personal expression and nonacademic
  course planning and selection, 529–530
  exploration, 529
  extracurricular activities, 530
  high school reforms, 528, 529
  multiple intelligences, 528
  vocational psychologists, 528
and personal lives, 481
project-based learning, 523–524
reading, 616, 617
and relationships, 597
research, emotions, 259–260
and self-regulation, 585
students, 101, 106, 144, 442, 449, 454, 596, 626
teaching
  curriculum specialists, 522
  high school mathematics instruction, 523
  reading instruction, high school, 522
  reading/math wars, 522
texts, 603, 615
valuing, 198, 626
Interest and students' engagement, 144, 266, 269
  achievement behavior, 288
  achievement goals
    classroom engagement and disaffection, 296
    classroom peers, 296
    description, 294
    mastery and performance goals, 295
    personal orientations and characteristics, 296
  complexity, 288
  definitions, 286
  developmental phases and stages
    definition, 290
    emerging and well-developed individual interest, 290
    identification and features, 291
    personal interest, 290
    progression, 290–291
    selection and profiles, 291
    triggered and maintained situational interest, 290
  dynamics, 296
  dynamic systems perspective, 287
  educational domain, 288
  emotions, 294
  individual interest, 287
  learning situation and motivation schemas, 288
  macrocontext and relations, 297
  metaphor and ranges, 286
  microsystem, 296
  on-task interest, 292–294
  PISA 2006, 297–298
  and processes, 291–292
  process schemas and task engagement
    achievement goal orientations, 289
    assessment, 289
    mood, 288–289
    post-task reflections, 289

proposals, 287–288
relationship, person and task, 286
role
    classroom learning, 296
    component processes, 289
    experiences, 289
    interest schema, 289–290
    significance, positive emotions, 289
schema and form, 287
self-regulatory function, 287
situational interest, 286–287
task perceptions, 288
Interference models, 264
International Center for Leadership in Education (ICLE), 549
Intrinsic value demonstration (IVD), 422, 435, 437
    adolescents' perceptions, 428
    Conditional Positive Regard (CPR), 428
    development, 428
    general attitudes and skills, students, 428
    identification, 427
    individual interests, 429
    lack of IVD, 427–428
    parents behaviors, 429
    people behavior, 427
    prosocial acts and empirical research, 428
    role and accumulating experience, 429
    SDT perspective, 428
IRT *See* Item response theory (IRT)
Item response theory (IRT), 784, 788, 792, 795, 801, 806

J
Jingle, Jangle, 3–17

K
Knowledge construction process, 682, 684
    application, 689
    choose, 687
    connection, 688–689
    mapping, 688
    observing/describing, 687–688
    pedagogy, 687
    questioning, 688
    reconciling, 689
    schooling, 690
    stages sequence, 687, 688
    storying, 688
    validating, 689

L
Learning power, 247–248, 687, 690
Learning power and engagement, 677–678
    coaching conversation, 686–687
    Indigenous Australian communities, 684, 685
    knowledge construction process, 687–690
    language and place, 685–686
    pedagogical moments, 685
    practice, 690–691
    research, 685
    work
        cyberspace, 684
        description, 683
        ELLI tool, 684
Life course models
    Euro-American families, 493–494
    long-term longitudinal studies, USA, 493
    preschool participation, 494
Low-stakes standardized tests, 460–461

M
MacArthur measures, 775
Managerial strategies, enhancement AET, 664–665
Mastery goal structure, 185, 186
    behavioral engagement, 182–183
    emotional and cognitive engagement, 182
    perceptions and student influences, 182
    students, learning and understanding, 181–182
Me and My School survey, 709, 714, 722
Measurement, 15, 404–405
    approaches, SEI (*see* Student engagement instrument (SEI))
    cognitive engagement, 641
    components, engagement and indicators, 103, 104
    instruments, 196
    and interpretation issues, 137
    uses, engagement models, 105
Measuring student engagement, 9–10, 793
    assessment tools, 707–708
    definition, 709–710
    Me and My School scale, 714
    middle response categories, 714
    national trial data, analysis
        final threshold calibrations, 713
        fit indicators, 713
        infit statistic, 714
        item calibration, scale, 714, 715
    New Zealand, 708
    NZCER, 708
    perceived engagement, national patterns, 718–722
    piloting, 712
    Rasch measurement and *Me and My School*, 710–711
    scale
        description, 716–717
        descriptors, 715–716
Mentors, 8
MES *See* Motivation and Engagement Survey (MES)
Mindsets, 32, 34
    commonalities, 549–550
    description, 541
    educators, 542
    educators' beliefs and practices (*see* Educators' beliefs and practices)engaged, motivated students, 543–544
    motivation, 544–547
    questions, consideration, 543
    resilience, 542–543

Mindsets (cont.)
  resilient children and adolescents, 544
  student engagement
    Check & Connect, 548
    components, 548
    description, 547–548
    ICLE, 549
    subtypes, 548
  teacher, 542
Models, SE, 134, 136
  dropout prevention theory, 99–100
  participation-identification, 100–105
  school reform, 99
  self-system process, 100
Motivation, 150–151, 220
  academic, 134, 138, 496
  achievement, 138, 139, 142, 194, 198, 462, 503, 645
  autonomy
    people's perception and experience, 422
    quality and differentiation, 422
    SDT, 421
  and behavioral engagement, characterization, 610, 615
  beliefs
    attribution types, 416–417
    goal orientations, 416
    self-efficacy, 416
  classroom goal structures, 464–465
  classroom practices
    devaluing, student, 625
    effects, 617–624
    perceived relevance, 617, 625
    students' self-efficacy, 625
    teacher-student relationships, 625
    teaching, 617
  cluster analysis, 588
  cognitive and metacognitive processing, 644
  competition and cooperation, 464
  comprehensive reforms
    individual school-level reforms, 535
    research and development, 535
    SE, 534
  defined, 639
  development, 136
  effects, behavioral engagement and reading competence, 610–614
  and effort, 113
  energy and direction, 441
  and engagement, 265–266, 445, 785–786
  extrinsic and intrinsic, 746
  flow concept, 547
  formative tests and SE
    assessment links and processes, 466–467
    SDT, 466
    self-regulation, 465–466
  high school students, 497
  instructional contexts, 408–409
  intrinsic, 135, 195, 199, 200, 610, 615
  levels, 594–595, 796
  and membership, 212
  performance and mastery goals, 533

performance-approach/avoidant goals, 463
performance orientation, 463
preparatory activities, 533
preschool class, 545–546
purpose and commitment, 547
reading competence
  behavioral engagement, 616
  comprehension, 617
  devaluing, 617
  self-efficacy, 616–617
  students' interests, 616
reform priorities and sequences
  classroom learning activities, 533
  learning environment, 533–534
  student attendance, 533, 534
school program, 531–532
and school success, 139
SDT, 546–547
shaping student, 201
strategies, 646
student and high-stakes tests, 467–468
student engagement, 544–545
students' achievement goals, 463
summative feedback and goals, 463–464
task and ego orientation, 175
tenets, 546
tests, students
  cue seekers and conscious, 462
  curriculum content and evaluation practices, 462
  expectancy X value theory, 461
theorists, 141
Motivational dynamics model, 33, 37
  action and behavioral dimension, 24–25
  emotional reactions, 25
  engagement and disaffection
    cycles, 30–31
    parents and peers, 30
    reciprocal feedback effects, 29
    school contexts, 29
    self-system processes, 29
    teachers, 29–30
    trajectories, 31
  indicators vs. facilitators, 25–26
  nature, academic work, 28–29
  parents shape engagement, 28
  peers shape engagement, 28
  SDT, 26–27
  social contexts, 27
  teachers shape engagement, 27–28
Motivation and engagement, 27, 139, 152, 265–266
  cognition and behavior, 307
  components, 303
  contributions, 303
  description, 303
  disengagement and engagement, 310
  frameworks, 304–305
  measurement tools, 307
  role, 305–306
  theories, 304
  time and space

analysis, sequence × space learning, 309–310
sequence × space learning map, 308–309
Motivation and Engagement Survey (MES), 773, 775
Motivation and Engagement Wheel, 306, 307
Motivation engagement, 14–16
Multilevel logistic regression analysis, 120, 121

N

National Certificate in Educational Achievement (NCEA), 592, 594
  assessment, 450, 451, 453
  NQF, 444
  qualification, 450
National Education Commission on Time and Learning (NECTL), 654
National qualifications framework (NQF), 444
National Student Clearinghouse (NSC), 737, 739
NCLB See No Child Left Behind Act (NCLB)
NECTL See National Education Commission on Time and Learning (NECTL)
Negative activating emotions, 269–270
Negative deactivating emotions, 270–271
Negative feelings
  children and adolescents, 426
  disagree, teachers/parents, 426
  feelings and opinions, 426
  opposite views and beliefs, 426
Negative social experiences, 388
  direct and mediated effects, 395
  emotion, 395–396
  engagement and academic performance, 396
  kindergartners, 395
  literature, 394
  peer rejection and nominations, 394–395
  teachers academic engagement, 395
Network of partnership schools (NNPS), 358
New Zealand Council for Educational Research (NZCER), 708
New Zealand Curriculum (NZC), 452
  achievement objectives set, 443
  defined, 442, 444
  local design and review, 444
NNPS See Network of partnership schools (NNPS)
No Child Left Behind Act (NCLB), 460, 467, 469
NSC See National Student Clearinghouse (NSC)
NZCER See New Zealand Council for Educational Research (NZCER)

O

Office of Research and Evaluation (ORE), 728
On-task interest
  achievement and classroom behaviors, 293
  changing reactions, 292
  inspection, trajectories, 293
  learning program, 292–293
  measures, 292
  medium and low interest groups, 293–294
  relationship, student and text, 292
  self-report ratings, 292
  trajectories, 293
Optimal support for Value Examination (OSVE), 435
ORE See Office of Research and Evaluation (ORE)
Organismic integration theory, 158
  description, 154
  external and integrated regulation, 155
  extrinsic motivation and types, 154
  identified and integrated regulations, 155
  societal norms, rules and behaviors, students, 154
Out-of-school misbehavior, 208
  adolescent substance use, 210–211
  connectedness, 210
  "normlessness" and "school isolation", 210
  school bonding, 209–210
Out-of-school time programs
  BEST program, 334
  develop youth talents, 334
  effectiveness, 334
  extracurricular activities, 333
  social networking, 334

P

Parental influences
  administrative support, 335
  Bronfenbrenner's ecological systems theory, 334
  conceptualizing engagement, 318–319
  contextual influences
    child development, 321–322
    development, belief systems, 322
    micro and mesosystem, 322
    proximal processes, 322
  difficulties, public school, 335
  educational practices, 430
  engaging students, families, and communities, 336
  interactions, deep engagement and motivation, 317
  low-income ethnic minority groups, 320–321
  measurements, 318
  motivation, 319–320
  parental involvement, 328–330
  perspectives, 317–318
  pragmatic assistance, teachers, 334–335
  programs modeling and home-school partnerships, 331–334
  relational support, 335
  research and future directions
    achievement motivation, 336
    complex nature, classroom learning, 335
    deductive approach, 335–336
    educational socialization practices, 336
    limitations, 335
  school reform, 335
  theoretical approaches
    benefits, 322–323
    Epstein theory, 323
    positive academic and motivational outcomes, 322
    psychosocial development, 323
    relationships, homes and schools, 323
    school conditions, 323

Parental influences (*cont.*)
  underachievement and school disengagement, 315–317
  well-being and engagement, 324–328
Parental involvement, 74, 116, 407
  Asian American families, 348–349
  children's schooling, 347
  communication, 348–349
  culture and student learning, 330
  "deficit model" approaches, 330
  description, 328–329
  direct effects and motivational model, 347–348
  effects, 349
  knowledge framework, 330
  low-income and middle-class parents', 329
  meta-analysis, 347
  middle-class peers and working class parents, 329
  motivational model, 349–350
  Ogbu's contribution, 329–330
  perspectives, 330
  social networks use, 329
  tangible and intangible resources, 329
Parental structure
  components, 353
  maladaptive control beliefs, 353–354
  rules and expectations, 354
  SDT, 352
Parent autonomy support, 351, 352
  mother-child dyads, 359
  pressure, 359–360
Parents role, 317, 334, 356
  adolescent's "job", 77
  and child relationship, 75–76
  cultural model education, 78
  cultural socialization, 77–78
  diversity, 79
  encourage child's learning, Asian American, 77
  ethnic identities, girls, 78–79
  expectation and school achievement, 75
  family support and cohesion, 76
  hierarchical regression analyses, 76
  identify relationship, teacher and student, 75
  immigrant, 76–77
  involvement, 74–75
  low-income students, 75
  measure, racial socialization, 78
  national data analysis, 77
  students' engagement and support, 75
Parents shape engagement, 28
Partial credit model (PCM), 712, 713, 809
Participation-identification model, 7, 194
  academic engagement, 102
  affective engagement, 102–103
  behavioral component, 100
  cognitive engagement, 102–103
  components, engagement and indicators, 103, 104
  developmental cycle, 101
  measurement issues
    affective and cognitive engagement, 103
    antecedents consequences, engagement, 103
  uses, engagement models, 105
  motivation and engagement, 105
  normlessness measures and school isolation, 102
  social and academic engagement, 102
  types, 100
Participation-identification theory, 133, 134
Patterns of Adaptive Learning Survey (PALS), 176
PCM *See* Partial credit model
Peers selection and socialization
  effects, 390
  extracurricular engagement
    helping students, 391–392
    mechanisms, 392
    motivation, 391
  friends and relations characteristics, academic engagement
    academic orientation, 390–391
    adjusted friends improve grade point, 391
    behaviors and attribution, 391
    classroom activities, 391
    opposite effect, 390
  maintain school engagement, 397–398
  positive and negative effects, 397
  support and quality friendships
    develop positive attitudes, 392
    effects, 392
    encourage student engagement, 392
    and extracurricular involvement, 393
    social and academic support, 392–393
Peers shape engagement, 28
Perceived engagement, national patterns
  class, 719, 720, 722
  description, 718
  ethnic group, 719–720
  listening, 722
  Me and My School survey, 722
  school, 719, 721
  year level and gender
    median scale scores, 718, 719
    scale descriptors comparison, 719
Perezhivanie, 680–681, 684
Performance goal structure, 186
  beliefs and behaviors, 183
  characteristics, 183
  cognitive and behavioral engagement, 184
  distinctions, 183
  emotional engagement, 183–184
  grades, 183
  student learning, 183
Person-centered approach, 136, 616, 696, 701
Positive behavior interventions support (PBIS), 575–576
Process-product paradigm
  AET, 658, 659
  BTES, 659–660
  learning time research, 660–661
  low engagement, 661
  outcome research, 658–659
  teachers' use, 659
Programme for International Student Assessment (PISA) 2006

accepted variable structures, 298
achievement measure, 297
administered science, 297
behavior and individual interest, 298
coefficients and personal value, 298
future oriented motivation, 298
historical and cultural traditions, 299
modeling techniques, 299
out-of-school science activities, 298
Provided student ID (PSID), 728
PSSM See Psychological Sense of School Membership
Psychological motivation theory, 134
Psychological Sense of School Membership (PSSM), 211
Psychological well-being, 323–324
Psychometric information, 768
    HSSSE, 775
    reliability, 775
    validity, 775–777
Psychometric techniques, 467

Q

Quality of friendships
    extracurricular activities, 394
    lack of close friendships, 394
    school-based friendships, 393
    school transitions, 393–394
    social skills, 393

R

Race theory, 136
Rasch measurement and *Me and My School*
    assumption, 710
    fit model, 710–711
    survey item, scale, 711
Rating scale model (RSM), 809
    infit and outfit, 795
    item calibration values, 795, 796
    response model, 795, 797
Reading, 603–631
    achievement, 107, 109, 111
    and analysis, 593
    comprehension instruction, 522
    eighth-grade, 117, 119
    enjoyment, 595
    levels, 519
    and mathematics, 469
    and mathematics achievement, 212
    and math lessons, 111
    mystery novels, 521
    strategies inventory, 111
Reciprocal feedback effects, 29
Regression analysis, SE, 122, 123
Resilience *See also* Every-day resilience
    adolescents, 643
    defined, 115
    and engagement, 116
    student, 116
Resilience theory, 7–8
Resource allocation model, 264
Responsiveness, school and classroom, 105–106
Root mean square error of approximation (RMSEA), 298, 299, 791, 794, 799
Rosenberg self-esteem scale (RSES)
    factors, 808
    structure, 807–808
RSES *See* Rosenberg self-esteem scale
RSM *See* Rating scale model (RSM)
Ryan and Deci's motivation, 321

S

School belonging, 568, 596–597
    high school students, 389
    increase academic engagement, 389
    relationships, 388
    research, 388
    strengthen, 389–390
    stronger associations, 389
    techniques, hierarchical linear modeling, 389
School identification, 100
    and academic achievement/attainment, 211–212
    attitudes and behavior, 199
    and behavioral engagement
        belongingness, 208
        classroom participation, 208
        "school delinquency", 208
        types, misbehavior, 209
    children, 201
    classroom community, teachers' impact, 206–207
    components
        belonging and valuing, 195
        education researchers, 197
        motivation and behavior, 196
        personal and practical value, 198–199
        psychological theories, human needs, 195
        school community, 196, 197
        sense of belonging, 195–196
        student success, 196
    development
        behaviors, 200–201
        and consequences, 200
        student, 201
    educators and administrators, 213
    engagement form, 194–195
    feeling safe, 202–203
    mechanisms, 207
    and out-of-school misbehavior, 209–211
    positive attitudes, 193
    teachers' relationships, students, 205–206
    treatment
        African-American students, 203, 204
        defined, 203
        discipline policies, 204
        multilevel modeling, 204

Schools culture, 76, 79, 89, 559
  adults, 749
  conceptualization, 748
  experience, 748
  leaders, 749
  learning and achievement, 748–749
Schools role
  academic orientations, 80
  children's friendships, 79
  extracurricular activities, 80
  identification, children, 81
  individual engagement, 79
  Latino and White students, 80
  Mexican American youth, 80–81
  nature, schools, 81
  racial and ethnic minority youth, 79
  same-race/ethnic group peers, 79–80
  school friendship, 80
  social networks and possible friendship systems, 81
School success profile (SSP), 773
  engagement scales, 776
  MacArthur measure, 775
School-wide and targeted interventions
  Check & Connect, 576–577
  PBIS, 575–576
SDT *See* Self-determination theory (SDT)
SE *See* Student engagement (SE)
SEI *See* Student engagement instrument (SEI)
Self-determination theory (SDT), 345
  autonomy support, 603
  basic needs theory, 153–154
  causality orientations theory, 157
  cognitive evaluation theory, 156
  differences, conceptualization, 169
  distinction, motivation and engagement, 151
  empirical effort, 169
  and ET, 135, 142
  features, 546
  functional claim, 169
  functions, student engagement
    concept and functions, 162
    engagement changes and motivation, 165–166
    learning and prediction, 162
    learning environment and engagement changes, 165
    motivation and achievement relation, 163–165
    positive student outcomes, 162–163
    student-teacher dialectical framework, 162, 163
    teachers efforts, 162
  goal contents theory, 155–156
  human and social activities, 26–27
  implications, teachers, 167–169
  intrinsic motivation, 26
  motivation, 150–153
  organismic integration theory, 154–155
  overarching theoretical framework, 151–152
  positive motivational development, 26
  precursors, behavioral and positive engagement, 135
  produce changes, student motivation, 170
  relatedness and competence and autonomy, 27
  reliability, validity, and potential contribution, 169
  SE, 466
  and self-reflection, 466–467
  and self-regulation, 471
  self-system processes, 27
  student engagement
    autonomous motivation, 161
    components, 161
    description, 150
    learning activities, 161
    during learning activity, 150, 151
  student-teacher dialectical framework, 157–161
  student-teacher relationships, 152
  teacher role, 152
Self-efficacy, 244, 410
  Bandura's theory, 232
  consequences of, 223–224
  contextual influences
    description, 230
    effects, learning environments, 231
    political factors, 231
    school transitions and learning, 231
  cross-cultural research
    difference, cultures and countries, 231
    ethnic students' experiences, 231
    individualism and collectivism, 231–232
    social policies and programs, 231
  description, 222
  disadvantaged adolescents, 220
  dropout rate, 219–220
  engagement, 220
  high-performing schools, 232
  identification, 220
  information sources
    anxiety and stress, 223
    description, 222
    interpretations, 222–223
    observations, 223
    outcome expectations and values, 223
  learning and performing, 220
  motivation, 220
  perceived confidence, 222
  predictors, 220
  processes
    self-regulatory, 222
    symbolic, 222
    vicarious, 221–222
  reciprocal interactions, 221
  research, 220
  school dropouts, 219
  school success, 221
  and self-evaluations, 224–225
  social cognitive theory, 220–221, 232
  and student engagement
    educational influences, 228–229
    familial influences, 225–226
    learning, 225
    sociocultural factor, 226–228

students' skills, 232
student success, 232
underachievement, 229–230
Self-efficacy theory, 134
Self-evaluations, 245, 249–250, 667
   behavior, 224
   learning and performance, 224–225
   positive, 224
   students, 225
Self-perception theory, 199
Self-regulated learning (SRL), 465
   academic behaviors, 647
   areas
      cognitive and metacognitive strategies, 639
      motivation, 639–640
      time management strategies, 640
   behaviors, 244
   categorization, students, 646–647
   control and monitoring, 245
   description, 635
   evaluation, 647
   integration and opportunities, research, 647
   microanalysis
      aptitude measures, 250
      attribution and adaptive inference, 251
      components, 251
      cyclical event assessment method, 250–251
      definition, 250
      differences, metric and categorical, 252
      "event" conceptualization, 250
      forethought, self-monitoring and evaluation, 251
      hierarchical regression analysis, 252
      single-item scales, 251–252
   performance and impacts, 245–246
   phases
      learners, 639
      monitoring, 637
      planning, 637
      reaction/reflection, 639
      use and management, 637
   reflection processes, 245
   and SE
      academic functioning, 645–646
      behavioral engagement, 642–643
      cognitive engagement, 641, 644
      emotional and affective processes, 641–642
      motivation, 644
      positive and negative emotions, 642
      researchers, 641
      students agency, 645
      students indicators, academic involvement, 643
      treatment, constructs, 643
   self-efficacy, 244, 644
   self-evaluative standards, 245
   strategic attributions, 246
   students, metalevel knowledge, 646, 647
   success, research, 648
Self-regulated strategy development (SRSD), 247
Self-regulation, 51, 222, 238–240
   and achievement, 112
   cognitive functioning, 646
   and cognitive strategies, 103, 111, 112
   computerized task, 111
   defined, 616
   and engagement, 647
   environment, 648
   learning, 267, 269, 644
   metastrategies, 267
   SDT theories, 471
   and social and emotional skills, 479
   strategies, 211, 636
Self-regulation and student engagement
   academic behaviors and functioning, 237
   cognitive engagement and motivation
      academic tasks, 239
      assessment methodology, 240
      cyclical feedback loop, 239
      future research, 240
      impact, social environment, 239
      learning engagement, 240
      motivation and behaviors, 239–240
      school-based academic interventions, 240
      SRL, 239
   cyclical feedback loops, 240–243
   definition, student, 238
   description, 237–238
   importance and applications, dynamic feedback cycle, 243–244
   learning activities
      and academic tasks, 240
      classroom environments, 238
   research directions
      changes, students' regulatory processes, 252
      educators' knowledge, 253
      environmental factors, 252–253
      professional development training, 253
      psychology programs and report, 253
      self-efficacy perceptions, 253
   school-based professionals, 238
   SRL engagement and motivation, 244–246
   SRL microanalysis, 250–252
   theoretical framework, 238
Self-Regulation Empowerment Program (SREP)
   components, 248–249
   development, 248
   evidence-based learning, 248
   primary instructional mechanism, 249
   self-evaluation, 249–250
   self regulation graph, 249
   tutors guide, 250
Self-system model, 136
Self-system process model, 100
Sequence × space learning map, 308–310
Social-behavioral engagement, 268–269
Social cognitive theory, 610, 645
Social-competence, 197, 324–325
Social control theory, 197, 209

Social emotions, 3, 260, 263, 278, 324, 414, 415, 480, 542, 550, 551
Social engagement, 102, 119, 268
   attendance, 110
   behavior rules, 109
   classroom (and antisocial) behavior, 110–111
Socio-cultural contexts, 679, 681
   cognitive and social functioning, 479
   goals and objectives, education
      behavioral engagement, 482
      peers role, 481
      research, engagement, 481
   and interactions, 479
   interpersonal relationships, 482–483
   models, influence, 483–485
   NICHD child care study, 485
   schools, 486
   self-efficacy
      habits, 227
      intrinsic and extrinsic benefits, 226–227
      longer-term goals and self-schemas, 226
      peers groups, 227
      personal development, 227
      stress and anxiety, 228
      students, lower-income families, 226
      teachers perspective, 227
      youth and children, future-oriented conceptions, 226
   social competence, school, 480–481
Sociocultural theories, 445
SRL *See* Self-regulated learning (SRL)
SSP *See* School success profile (SSP)
Stage-environment fit theory, 141
Statistical model, 333
   contemplating and defining engagement
      behavioral, 784–785
      cognitive, 785
      theoretical framework, 784
      types, 784
   description, 783–784
   measurement issues, 786–787
   measures construction, 787–789
   motivation and engagement, 785–786
   rating scale and intended measurement model
      congeneric measurement model, 790–792
      description, 790
      item response theory, 792
   SEI, 793
   student engagement, 783
Statistical modeling, 500
Status and academic risk factors, 123–124
   conditions, participating schools, 115
   nationwide American study, 116
   resilient, 115
   "role strains", 116
Strategic content learning (SCL)
   description, 247–248
   instruction principle, 248
   performance phase, 248
   self-reflection, 248
   skills, 248
Structural equation models, 211
Structural strains theory, 496
Student' academic and extracurricular participation, 108–109
   conceptual framework, 388
   definition, student engagement, 388
   high-quality friendships and peer support, 392–393
   implications, research and school policies, 398
   maintaining school engagement, 397–398
   negative social experiences, 394–396
   peer selection and socialization, 390–392
   peers relationship, 387–388
   positive and negative peer effects, 397
   quality of friendships, 393–394
   school belonging, 388–390
   social alienation and dropping out, 396–397
Student engagement (SE), 47, 50–57, 68–74, 161–163, 183–184, 263–271, 453–455, 699–700 *See also* Academic emotions
   academic motivation, 107–108, 138
   achievement and attainment, 106–107, 114–115
   achievement and competencies, 598
   affective, 112–113, 121–122
   analysis
      odds ratios, 118
      variables used, HLM, 117, 118
   behavioral and graduation/dropout, 119, 121
   categorisation and analysis, 586
   cognitive, 111–112
   competency levels, 591–593
   competent learners study, 586–590
   complexity, 745
   context importance, 756–757
   correlations, variables, 119, 120
   definition, 3
   description, 133–134, 745
   discrepancy, 745
   and disengagement, 123–125
   dropout prevention, 5–7
   effects, status and academic risk factors, 115–116
   enhancement, educational performance, 97
   enjoyment, school, 591
   ET and EEVT, 141–145
   and ethnicity, 136
   extracurricular activities, 139
   future directions, 15–16
   graduation rates, sample, 119
   high school completion (*see* High school completion)
   HSSSE (*see* High school survey of student engagement (HSSSE))
   human development model, 140
   intervention, components, 7
   learning and belonging, school, 596–597
   learning opportunities, 597
   levels and time frames, 137
   measurement, 9–10, 117
   motivational theorists, 141

motivation levels, 594–595
multilevel logistic regression analysis, 120, 121
neuroscience, brain growth and development, 135
participants, 117
participation-identification model, 139
person-centered approaches, 136
policy makers and lay educational pundits, 138
post-school study, 595
primary research questions, 116–117
regression analysis, 122, 123
research
    definitions and models, 747
    schooling, K-12 level, 747
    student achievement, 748
    three-component model, 748
research, school success, 134
resilience theory, 7–9
responsiveness, school and classroom, 105–106
school achievement, 134
school and experience, 595–596
school leaving age and highest qualification, 593–594
school reform (see High school reform)
schools culture, 748–749
SDT theory, 135
SE and learning, 136–137
self-reports, 597
social characteristics, 590–591
student learning, 3
student participation, 125–126
teacher conversations
    competent learners research, 454–455
    learning opportunities, 453
    most and least enjoyed subjects, 454
    subject identification, 454
trajectories, five, 590, 591
whole-class settings, 448–449
Student engagement instrument (SEI), 773
    administration standardization procedures, 728–729
    bifactor model, 796–800
    cross-validation
        congeneric measurement model, 791, 794
        factor structure, 794
        reliabilities and correlations, 794–795
    evaluation, 793
    factors, 730–731, 793, 794
    introductory text, 727–728
    likert-like scale, 811
    ORE, 728
    properties, 808
    reliability and validity, 793
    RSM, 795–797
Student engagement measurement, 404–405
    behavioral, 771
    cognitive, 772
    compensatory relationships, 806
    construct definition
        affective, sources, 806
        cognitive engagement, 807
        IRT models, 806–807
        psychological instrument, 807
    description, 764–765, 805–806
    developmental difference, 778
    DIF, 807–810
    emotional, 771–772
    ESM, 766
    interview, 766–767
    malleability assessment, 778
    motivation, 765
    observations, 767–768
    operationalization, 777–778
    psychological construct, 805
    psychometric information, 775–777
    scholars, 763–764
    SEI, 810–811
    self-report measures comparison
        description, 768
        instrument names, 768, 769
    self-report methods
        survey measurement, 765
        usage, 765–766
    subscales, sample items, 768, 770, 771
    teacher ratings, 766
    variation, groups, 778–779
    varieties, 769
Student-mediated strategies, 664
    cognitive engagement, 668–669
    "countoons", 669
    description, 668
    goal-setting, 670
    self-management skills, 670
    self-monitoring methods, 669–670
    structure and routines, 670
Student participation questionnaire, 125–126
Student performance, 105, 812
    attitudes, 499
    background characteristics, 499
    behaviors range, 498–499
    educational, 498
Students' perspectives, 751, 757
    classrooms and interactions, 373–374
    formative role, 374
    positive feelings, 374
    responsibility, 374
    teacher control, 374
Students role, 181, 586
    academic efficacy, 72
    adolescents' daily lives, 74
    African Americans students, 70
    Asian American students', 73
    assimilation, 70
    awareness, racism, 72
    beliefs, 73
    bicultural efficacy, 73–74
    black students, 69
    color perceive/experience discrimination, 71
    components, racial identity, 69
    discrimination scale, 73
    disengagement, schools, 71–72
    diversity, ethnic group, 69
    education and behavioral engagement, 72

Students role (cont.)
  education value, 72–73
  elementary school students, 72
  engagement and achievement, 73
  gender, 71
  identity and discrimination, 68–69
  individuals identities, 74
  instruments, school and student, 74
  measurement, 69
  middle school students, 74
  minority students, 70
  pragmatic benefits, 73
  values, 71
Student-teacher dialectical framework, 169–170
  autonomous engagement and synthesis, 157–158
  autonomy support, student motivation, 159
  high-quality student engagement, 158
  learning environment and inner motivational resources, 157
  learning environment, opportunities and hindrances, 158–159
  longitudinal research design, 160
  organismic integration, 158
  quality, student's motivation, 158
  survey, 159
  teacher's motivating style and reports, 159
Student-teacher relationships, 205–206, 526
  classroom environment, 578
  classroom interventions, 577
  engagement, 578
  opportunities, 578
  teaching techniques, 577
Support for value examination (SVE), 436, 437
  adolescents' perceptions, 430
  authentic value, 432
  direction, values and goals, 430
  effects, SVE and modern orthodox Jewish youth, 434
  examination and reflection process, 430
  inspection model, 430–432
  integration, religious values, 434
  intrinsic/extrinsic values importance, 432
  limitation, 432
  OSVE, 435
  parents' support, 430
  promote autonomy and positive effects, 432–433
  qualitative analysis, 433
  quantitative study and valid questionnaires, 433
  religious education, 435
  revisionist and orthodox, 434–435
  structural equation modeling and mediation analyses, 432
  women's role, 433–434
  youth movement activities, 432
Systems consultation
  Ad Hoc results, 736
  aggregated results
    description, 735
    school and district report, 735–736
  context
    data privacy issues and limitations, 727
    GCPS, 726–727
  data integration
    administration standardization procedures, 728, 729
    aggregated results, 729–730
    cognitive and affective engagement, 729
    IMD and ORE staff, 728
    introductory text, 728
    PSID and CLC, 728
  description, 725
  limitations, 739–740
  progress, 739
  student engagement
    definition, 726
    vs. motivation, 726
  student-focused results
    advisor-advisee change report, 730, 732
    advisor-advisee level report, 730, 731
    data interpretive guide, 734–735
    datasets, 732–733
    SPSS, 734
    standardization, 732
    TSR and SEI factors, 731–732
  vision
    GPA, 739
    graphical representation, 737–738
    iterative process, 739
    NSC data, 737
    student engagement, 736–737

T
Teacher and peer support, 409
Teacher-made (TM) tests *See* Classroom-based (CB) tests
Teacher practices, classroom goal structures, 181–183
  mastery
    instructional approaches, 185
    learning environment, 185
    'set of practices', 185
    social relationship, 185
    support student learning, 185
    TARGET, 185
    teaching principles and strategies, 185
  performance
    description, 186
    high and low performance, 186
    instructional practices, 186
    paucity information, 186
    societal messages, 186
Teachers' beliefs, 356–358
  adult relationships, school, 85
  advantages, same-race teachers, 83
  behavioral engagement, minority college students, 82
  child and cultural norms, 83
  cultural discontinuity perspective, 83
  description, 81–82
  diversity, 82

effect, same-race teachers and student achievement, 82–83
  ethnic match, teachers and students, 82
  expectations and minority students' engagement, 84
  family support, 85
  hypothesis, 83
  interactions, 84
  limitation, teacher-student racial match, 82
  minority teachers, 82
  students' perceptions, 85
  students' positive feelings, 85
  student-teacher relationship, 82
  supporting, 84–85
  teacher perceptions and expectations, 83–84
  white teachers and emotional engagement, 82
Teachers implication, 444, 455
  accuracy scores and teachers' ratings, 168
  autonomy-supportive motivating style, 167
  capacity increases, 167
  classroom engagement, 168
  high-quality student engagement, 169
  instructional effort, 168
  monitoring and enhancing students' motivation, 167
  motivation aspects, 167–168
Teachers involve parents in schoolwork (TIPS), 358–359
Teachers shape engagement, 27–28
Teachers-students relationship, 806, 807
  adolescents efforts, 371
  adult mentors and advisors, 527–528
  appreciation, 206
  autonomy/competence supports, 370
  behavior management, 374–375
  bias, adolescents' experience evaluation, 371
  caring, 205
  changing interactions, 379
  classroom assessment scoring system, 366
  classroom organization, 374
  classroom setting and youth development (*see* Classroom strategies)
  concept development, 376
  conceptualization and measuring, 372
  consistent expectations, 206
  disengagement, 371
  effects, student outcomes, 371
  emotion
    climate, 373
    interactions, 372
  encouragement modes, 205
  engagement theory (*see* Classroom Climate)
  failures, 381
  feedback, 376–377
  high school reforms, 526
  improving interactions, 379–380
  instructional interaction domain, 375–376
  interactions and development, 366
  interdisciplinary teams, 527
  language and instructional discourse, 377–378
  learning communities, 526–527
  measuring interactions, 378–379
  NRC report, 366
  productivity, 375
  programs, 205
  quality, 105, 625
  real-world connections, 371
  relational supports, 369–370
  research, teacher involvement and caring, 526
  standardized observation method, 380–381
  students' perspectives, 373–374
  teacher sensitivity, 373
  theory, classroom, 381
  understanding engagement and behavioral expression, 366–367
Themes and exercises
  description, 550
  empathy, 554
  feedback and input, 555
  observation, 553
  ownership, 555–556
  personal control, 553–554
  student's social/emotional development, 551
  teachers and school administrators, 551
  teachers position, 552
  workshops, 554–555
Tinto model, 494–495, 498
TIPS *See* Teachers involve parents in schoolwork (TIPS)
TLI *See* Tucker-Lewis Index (TLI)
Topic emotions, 263
Tracking engagement, 34
Transactional stress model, 271, 272
Tucker-Lewis Index (TLI), 791
Two-component model, 194

U
Underachievement, 220
  beliefs and behaviors, 316
  Bronfenbrenner's ecological systems theory, 316–317
  description, 315–316
  discriminatory forces, 230
  education and socialization, 316
  effectiveness, 230
  exit examination, 316
  family support, 229
  high-risk dropout populations, 230
  interventions, 230
  poor academic performance, students, 230
  positive educational outcomes, 317
  poverty, 316
  role and contributing factors, 229
  socialization and caste systems, 229–230
Understanding student engagement, 380–381
  abundant evidence, 404
  antecedent factors and outcomes
    factors, social environment, 412–413
    intraclass correlations, 411
    motivational beliefs, 413

Understanding student engagement (cont.)
    subscale and full-scale scores, engagements, 411–412
    variables, outcomes student, 413–414
    conceptualization and measurement
        behavioral and cognitive engagement, 405
        feelings and learning activities, 405
        indicators *vs.* facilitators, 404
        indicators *vs.* outcomes grades, 404
        metaconstruct and multiple dimensions, 404
        typology and consequences, 405
        uniqueness and redundancy, 404–405
    contextual factors
        dynamics and relationships, 406
        ecological system theory, 405–406
        family and parent support, 407
        social-relatedness factors, 406–407
        validation, contextual model, 406
    description, 403–404
    instructional and social context
        affective, behavioral and cognitive engagement, 415
        peers and negative association, 415
        real-life significances, 415
        subscales and engagement, 414–415
        teacher support, 415
    limitations and directions, 417
    methods and measures
        academic performances and conduct, 411
        affective engagement subscale, 408
        aggression from peers, 409–410
        aggressive behaviors, 409
        attribution, beliefs, 410
        emotional functioning, 411
        learning and performance goals, 410
        motivating instructional contexts, 408–409
        participants, 408
        performance avoidance goals, 410
        procedures, 408
        self-efficacy, 410
        teacher and peer support, 409
    motivational beliefs
        attribution types, 416–417
        goal orientations, 416
        self-efficacy, 416
    personal factors, 407
    student outcomes, 407

V

Validity, 775
    confirmatory factor analyses, 776
    engagement measurement, 776
    engagement scales and constructs, 775–776
    psychometric information, 777
    SEM-MacArthur, 777

W

Wehlage and colleagues' model, 495
Well-being and engagement, 437
    caring and supportive relationships, 324–325
    foster adaptive achievement beliefs, 325
    homework, 325–326
    parenting styles, 326–327
    psychological well-being, 323–324
    relations and psychological, 323–324
    transmission, educational values, 327–328
Wentzel's model, 483, 484
Whole-class settings, 464
    frequencies, student recognition, 449
    'hands-on' learning, 449
    learning conditions, 448
Wiley and Harnischfeger's model, 657

Z

Zimmerman's model, 640

Lightning Source UK Ltd.
Milton Keynes UK
UKOW04f0002140916

282946UK00011B/229/P

9 781461 467915